Brief Contents

FOURTH EDITION

DAVIS ADVANTAGE for

FUNDAMENTALS OF NURSING

Thinking, Doing, and Caring

VOLUME 2

Judith M. Wilkinson, PhD, ARNP

Leslie S. Treas, PhD, RN, CPNP-PC, NNP-BC

Karen L. Barnett, DNP, RN

Mable H. Smith, PhD, JD, MN, NEA-BC

F.A. DAVIS

Philadelphia

F. A. Davis Company
1915 Arch Street
Philadelphia, PA 19103
www.fadavis.com

Printed in the United States of America

Last digit indicates print number: 10 9 8 7 6 5 4 3 2 1

Publisher, Nursing: Lisa B. Houck
Senior Content Project Manager: Adrienne D. Simon
Electronic Project Manager: Eric Van Osten
Design and Illustrations Manager: Carolyn O'Brien

Library of Congress Control Number: 2019946356

Preface

We chose our book title carefully. We have used the words *theory, concepts, application, thinking, doing,* and *caring* because we believe that excellent nursing requires an equal mix of knowledge, thought, and action. Nurses use all of these to express caring. It is knowledge and its application—not just the tasks nurses do—that delineate the various levels of nursing. Even so, skillful performance of tasks is essential to full attainment of the nursing role.

We present our material in two volumes to enable students to focus on material suitable for use in specific venues. Volume 2 was designed to be a compact, easy-to-carry reference to use in the skills lab and in clinical experiences. This volume contains practical, step-by-step, "how to" information for safely performing nursing actions and interacting with real patients. Rationales for each action explain the "why behind the what" to help you practice nursing based on concepts rather than cookbook-style action. Volume 2 offers practice-based forms, assessment questionnaires, and other clinical tips, but it is not limited to skills and procedures. It includes both thinking and doing, the same as does Volume 1; however, the emphasis is different in each volume. Volume 2 works seamlessly with Volume 1, the Skills Videos, and Davis Advantage to provide a user-friendly learning experience that will surely stimulate new enthusiasm for learning. For example, throughout Volume 2, students are offered a family case study, known as Caring for the Nguyens, through which they apply our full-spectrum model of nursing to learn about the nursing role, the healthcare system, and the real-world application of the content in Volume 1.

Other features in each chapter of this volume include critical-thinking activities (Critical Thinking and Clinical Judgment), step-by-step procedures and clinical insights (with rationales); Thinking About the Procedures exercises to tie the procedures to the skills videos are available on the Davis's Nursing Skills Videos Web site on FADavis.com; assessment guidelines and tools; a summary of the main points that were covered in Volume 1; and a knowledge map of the concepts discussed in the chapter. All of these features will be useful during a student's clinical day.

Volume 2 (as does Volume 1) will appeal to nontraditional students of the technological generation, encourage independent learning, promote critical thinking, support a variety of learning styles, and assure students that it is possible to achieve excellent nursing despite today's challenges.

We hope you will read the Preface and other introductory material in the front of Volume 1. It explains the philosophical underpinnings for this text and describes in more detail how to use the various pieces of this highly integrated learning package, which is flexible enough to accommodate a variety of teaching styles and curriculums.

Contents

CHAPTER 21

CHAPTER 22

CHAPTER 23

Meet the Nguyens

Throughout this text, you will be applying what you learn as you care for the Nguyen family. In Chapter 1, you will meet Nam Nguyen, a supervisor of construction workers, who arrives at the Family Medicine Center for his first physical exam in more than 10 years. His knee pain has caused him to seek help because it affects his work. But as you will see, Nam will discover that he has other serious health problems that require him to be more vigilant about his health. As you read and work through the exercises in Caring for the Nguyens, you will also come to know Nam's wife, Yen Nguyen, his grandchild, Kim Phan, other members of his extended family, and his friends as they all deal with health issues and life changes.

Your experience in caring for the Nguyens will show you that every client comes to you with symptoms, but each person brings unique values, lifestyles, problems, and relationships to the encounter. From the Nguyens, you will learn what it means to care for the whole person and how to be a full-spectrum nurse.

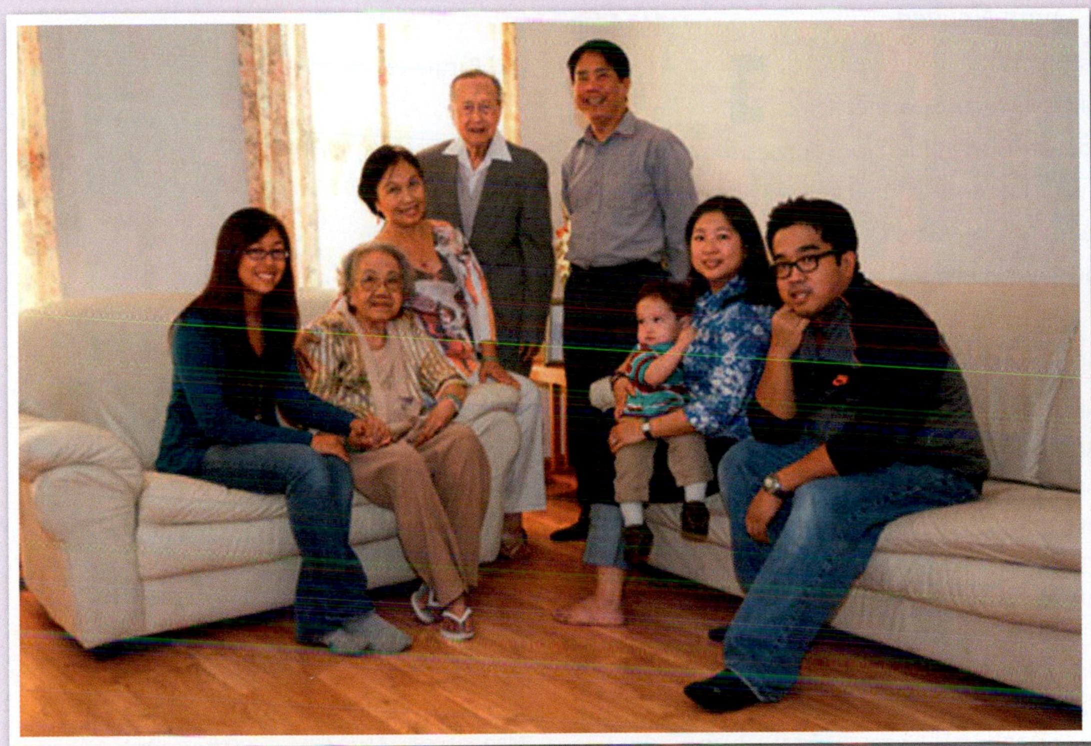

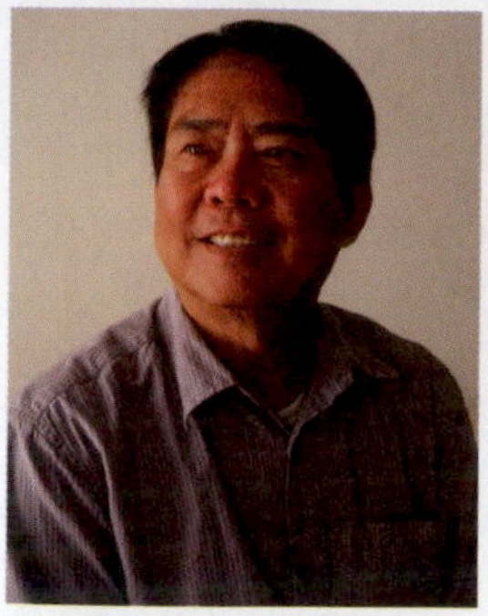

Mr. Nam Nguyen is a new client at the Family Medicine Center. He arrives at the center for a scheduled physical exam and completes the following admission questionnaire:

Name: *Nam Nguyen* Age: *56*

Marital Status S (M) W D Partnered

If applicable, spouse/partner name: *Yen*

Occupation: *Construction supervisor* Spouse/partner occupation: *Day-care teacher*

Does your spouse or partner have any healthcare problems? If so, please list:

High blood pressure

Do you have children? *Yes* Ages? *30, 27, 22*

Please circle yes if you have had the following or no if you have not.

AIDS/HIV +	YES	(NO)	Headaches	YES	(NO)
Allergies	(YES)	NO	Heart Disease	YES	(NO)
Anemia	YES	(NO)	Hernia	(YES)	NO
Anorexia	YES	(NO)	Herpes	YES	(NO)
Anxiety	YES	(NO)	High Cholesterol	YES	(NO)
Arthritis	YES	(NO)	High Blood Pressure	YES	(NO)
Bleeding Disorder	YES	(NO)	Kidney Problems	YES	(NO)
Breast Problems	YES	(NO)	Liver Problems	YES	(NO)
Cancer	YES	(NO)	Abnormal Mammogram (N/A)	YES	NO
Chicken Pox	(YES)	NO	Menopause (N/A)	YES	NO
Colon Disorder	YES	(NO)	Mononucleosis	YES	(NO)
COPD/Emphysema	YES	(NO)	Multiple Sclerosis	YES	(NO)
Depression	YES	(NO)	Osteoporosis	YES	(NO)
Diabetes	YES	(NO)	Pneumonia	YES	(NO)
Epilepsy/Seizures	YES	(NO)	Polio	YES	(NO)
Eye Problems	(YES)	NO	Prostate Problems	YES	(NO)
Gallbladder Disorder	YES	(NO)	Skin Problems	YES	(NO)
Stomach Problems/Ulcer	YES	(NO)	Stroke	YES	(NO)
Gout	YES	(NO)	Suicide Attempt	YES	(NO)
Gynecological Problems	YES	(NO)	Thyroid Problems	YES	(NO)
Sexually Transmitted Disease	YES	(NO)	Other	YES	(NO)

Please list your current medications and dosages. Also list over-the-counter and herbal products you use regularly.

Ibuprofen

Multivitamin 1 per day

Acetaminophen

Ben-Gay Balm on knees

The Diagnosis

During the visit, the clinic nurse records the following information in Mr. Nguyen's medical record:

Height	5 ft 4 in.
Weight	165 lb (75 kg)
Blood pressure	162/94 mm Hg
Pulse	84 beats/min
Respiratory rate	20 breaths/min
Temperature	98.2°F oral

Presenting Complaint: Client states he is here to become established as a client at the center and that he has not had a physical exam in more than 10 years. Wife accompanies. He is currently experiencing bilateral knee pain that is affecting his work performance. "I supervise construction workers. To check on things, I have to climb up and down ladders, lift things, and crawl around a lot." Has not missed any work but has been using increasing amounts of acetaminophen and ibuprofen "to get through the day." The medications provide only limited relief. States pain occurs daily even if not at work and is achy and dull. Feels best when he is off his feet. Desires pain relief and checkup. Explains that both parents have heart disease, his father had cancer, and his mother has diabetes. Wife expresses worry that he may be developing heart problems "because he's so tired after work and gets short of breath easily."

The nurse explains to Nam that he will be seen by the nurse practitioner shortly. She asks him whether he would like his wife to be present for the exam. He answers yes.

Zach Miller, DNP, MSN, FNP-BC, is on duty at the center today. Zach has 10 years of experience as a registered nurse (RN) in the emergency department and urgent care clinic. He has been a family nurse practitioner (FNP-BC) for 5 years and completed his Doctor of Nursing Practice (DNP) 2 years ago. Zach enters the room and introduces himself to Mr. and Mrs. Nguyen. To begin the exam, Zach reviews the information Mr. Nguyen supplied on the admission form and then asks Nam about his family history.

Zach: Are your parents still living?

Nam: Yes, they're both alive. My father is 80 years old and my mother is 76.

Zach: I'd like to hear a little more about your family history. Tell me about your father's cancer. How old was he when he was first diagnosed? Has he had treatment?

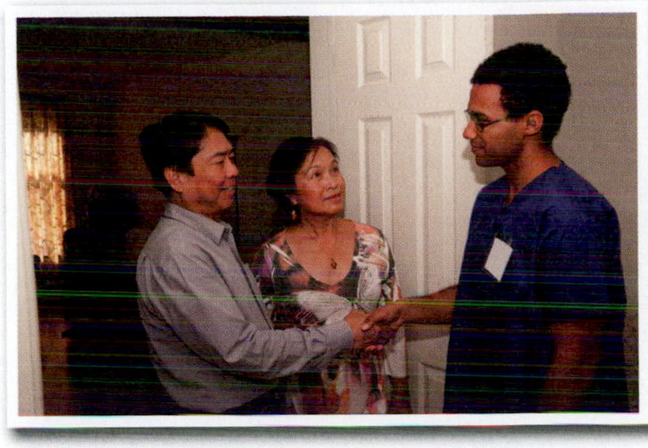

Nam: He was probably about 60 when he first found out about it. I know he had some kind of surgery and takes medicines, but I don't know the details. He seems all right though.

Zach: Your father also has high blood pressure and heart disease. Please tell me a little more about that.

Nam: My father and mother both have high blood pressure and heart disease. They both take medicines for their blood pressure. My father had a minor heart attack about 10 years ago. My mother has never had a heart attack that I know of, but she sometimes has chest pain.

Zach: Your mother also has diabetes?

Nam: She's had that for a long time. A lot of people in my family have diabetes, especially on my father's side—but nobody in my mother's family. Yet my mother is the one with diabetes!

Yen: A lot of people in my family have diabetes, too. But so far I'm okay, I think.

Zach: Have you had a health exam lately, Mrs. Nguyen?

Yen: Not in about a year, but I'm going to schedule an appointment here.

The Nguyens and Zach continue to review the health information. After reviewing the history and discussing current complaints, Zach performs a complete physical exam on Nam.

UNIT 1

How Nurses Think

CHAPTER 1

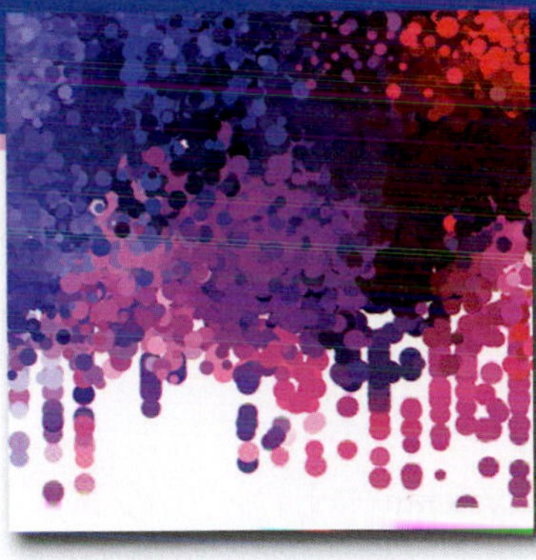

Evolution of Nursing Thought & Action

STUDENT RESOURCES

The questions and exercises in this book allow you to practice the kind of thinking you will use as a full-spectrum nurse. Critical-thinking questions usually have more than one right answer, so we do not provide "correct answers" for these features. Try to answer these questions yourself. It is more important to develop your nursing judgment than to just cover content. You will learn more by discussing the questions with your peers. If you are still unsure, see the Davis Advantage chapter resources for suggested responses.

To explore learning resources for this chapter,

Go to Davis Advantage and find:

- **Answers and Suggested Responses for all questions in this chapter**
- **Concept Map**
- **Knowledge Map**
- **References and Bibliography**
- **Lists of NOC Outcomes and NIC Interventions**

Key Concepts

Contemporary nursing education
Contemporary nursing practice
Healthcare delivery system
Nursing
Nursing history

Related Concepts

See the Concept Map on Davis Advantage.

Caring for the Nguyens

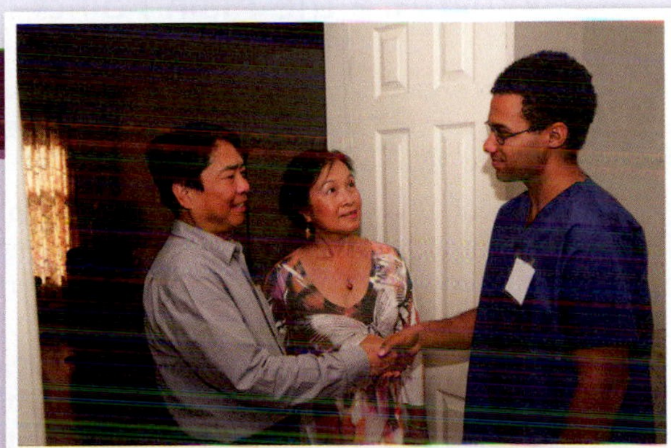

Review the opening scenario in the front of the book. In Nam Nguyen's preliminary visit to the Family Medicine Center, he is examined by Zach Miller, DNP, MSN, FNP-BC.

A. How would you respond to Mr. Nguyen's concerns that he was examined by someone who is "just a nurse"? How do you think Zach's introduction of himself as a Doctor of Nursing Practice will impact those concerns?

B. What factors might cause Mr. Nguyen to question care provided by "a male nurse"?

CLINICALJUDGMENT
Critical Thinking and Clinical Judgment

1. At a holiday family gathering, you are at the dinner table with your 60-year-old aunt, your 85-year-old grandmother, and your 15-year-old sister-in-law. Your aunt and grandmother are retired registered nurses (RNs). Your sister-in-law aspires to be a nurse, and you are in school studying to be a nurse.
   a. What factors will influence how each of you views nursing?
   b. Your sister-in-law asks you to define nursing. What would you say?
   c. How would you explain to her how a nurse is different from a nurse's aide or a physician?
2. Review the information on educational pathways into nursing.
   a. What do you believe is the minimum level of education that should be required to practice nursing?
   b. What reasons can you give to support your opinion?
3. Review the description of the National Student Nurses Association (NSNA). If your program has a local chapter of the NSNA, consider attending a meeting or consulting the association's Web site for more information. Identify at least three potential benefits of joining this organization.
4. For each of the following concepts, use critical thinking to describe how or why it is important to nursing, client care, or the evolution of nursing thought and action. Note that these are *not* to be merely definitions.

   The Nightingale era

   International Council of Nurses (ICN) and American Nurses Association (ANA) definitions of nursing

   Regulation of nursing practice

   Benner's stages of nursing skill

   Nursing organizations

   The national economy

   Better-informed healthcare consumers

   Use of nursing assistive personnel

   Use of life-extending, high-technology equipment

What Are the Main Points in This Chapter?

- Religious organizations and the military have played a major role in the development of nursing and healthcare organizations.
- Initially the role of the nurse was limited to bathing, feeding, and supporting the patient; keeping the patient environment clean and orderly; and providing support for the physician.
- Contemporary nursing care includes activities that are performed in collaboration with other members of the healthcare team and also independently.
- Licensed practical nurses (LPNs or LVNs) are nurses who have successfully completed an LPN/LVP program of study and have passed a licensure exam (NCLEX-PN). They are prepared to give direct client care.
- RNs are nurses who have successfully completed an RN program of study and have passed a licensure exam (NCLEX-RN). There are several types of RN education programs.
- Graduate nursing education is designed to prepare the RN for advanced practice, expanded roles, nursing education, or research.
- Benner has identified a five-step progression of skill acquisition in nurses: novice, advanced beginner, competence, proficiency, and expert.
- Nurse practice acts are laws that regulate the practice of nursing at the state level.
- Nurses engage in health promotion, illness prevention, health restoration, and care of the dying.
- Nurses work in a variety of inpatient and outpatient settings, including hospitals, extended care facilities, ambulatory care, and community or home health settings.
- Nurses provide care by using either the case method or the functional, team, primary, or differentiated model.

- The economy, technology, an aging population, increased consumer involvement in healthcare, the women's movement, and the change in nursing role are all forces that have strongly affected nursing.
- The healthcare delivery system is complex and involves a multitude of players.
- Managed care models of insurances (HMOs, PPOs, POS, IDNs) reimburse providers at discounted, predetermined rates and limit the consumer's choice of providers.
- Government funded programs, such as Medicare, Medicaid, and CHIP, provide health insurance for persons with disabilities, are 65 years of age or older, or have a low income.
- Nurses care for sicker inpatients because of changes in rates of reimbursement to hospitals.
- Nurses are essential members of the interprofessional healthcare team.
- Nurses must engage in lifelong learning activities to remain knowledgeable of and competent in professional practice.

Knowledge Map

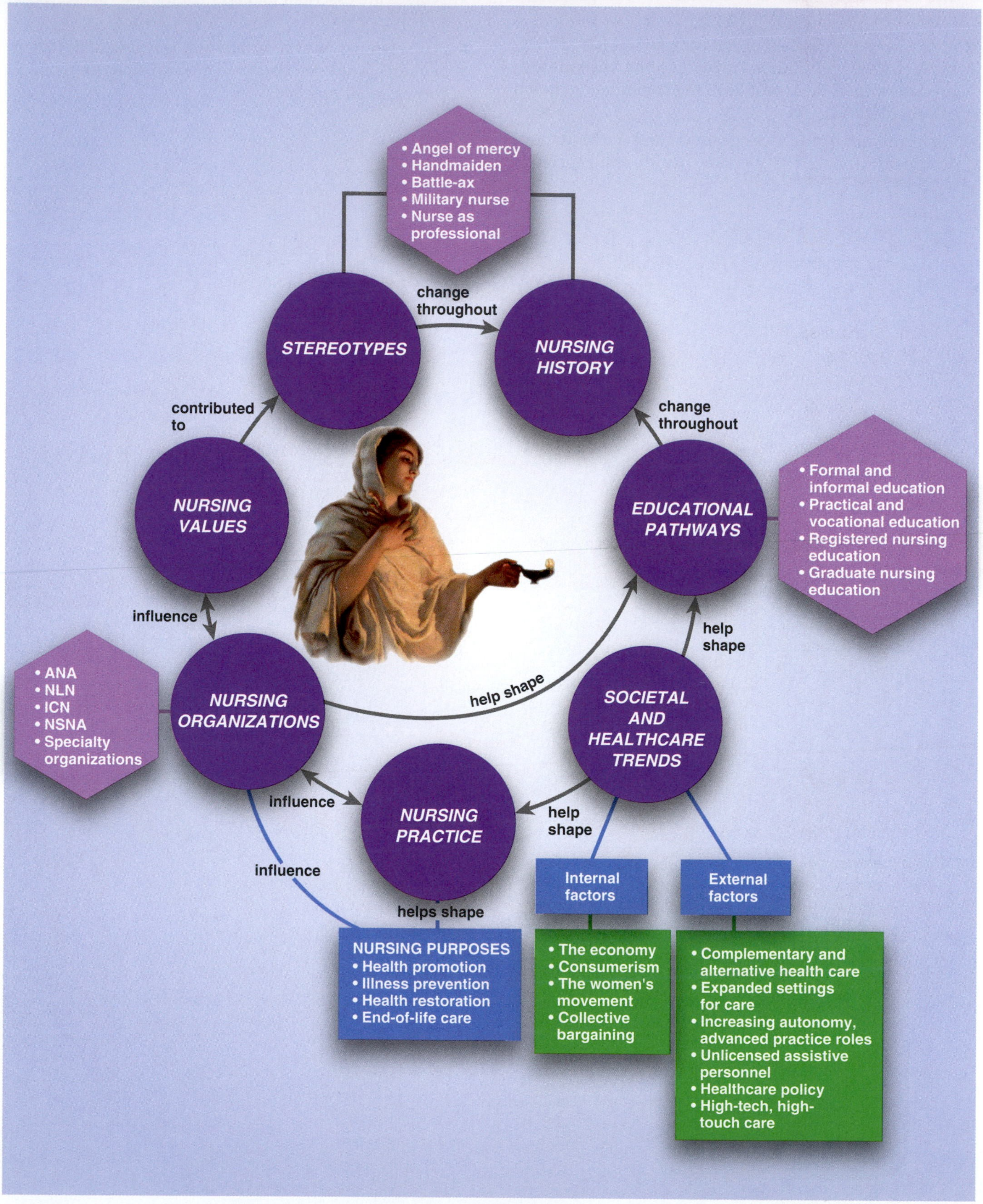

CHAPTER 2

Critical Thinking & Nursing Process

STUDENT RESOURCES

The questions and exercises in this book allow you to practice the kind of thinking you will use as a full-spectrum nurse. Critical-thinking questions usually have more than one right answer, so we do not provide "correct answers" for these features. Try to answer these questions yourself. It is more important to develop your nursing judgment than to just cover content. You will learn more by discussing the questions with your peers. If you are still unsure, see the Davis Advantage chapter resources for suggested responses.

To explore learning resources for this chapter,

Go to Davis Advantage and find:

Answers and Suggested Responses for all questions in this chapter
Concept Map
Knowledge Map
References and Bibliography
Lists of NOC Outcomes and NIC Interventions

Key Concepts

Critical thinking
Full-spectrum nursing
Nursing knowledge
Nursing process

Related Concepts

See the Concept Map on Davis Advantage.

Caring for the Nguyens

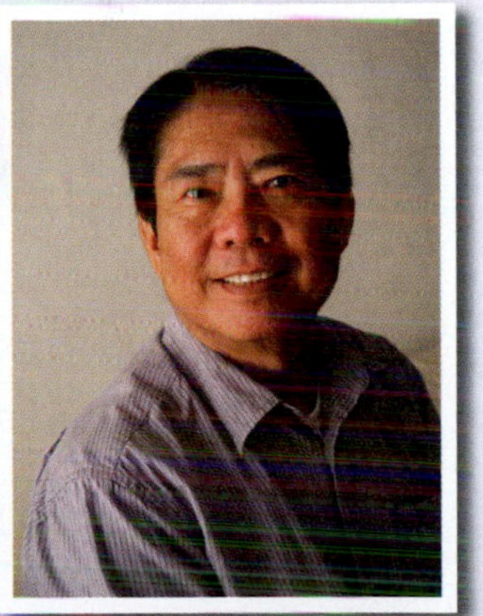

Review the opening scenario of Nam Nguyen in the front of this book. Imagine that you are the clinic nurse at the Family Medicine Center. On the basis of the information presented in the scenario, work through the following questions:

(Continued)

Caring for the Nguyens (continued)

A. **Patient Situation**
- Why is Mr. Nguyen at the clinic?
- What are his wife's concerns?
- Are his wife's concerns similar to or different from his?

B. **Critical Thinking**
- How do I go about getting the data I need? What sources should I use?
- Are my data congruent?
- What is one possible explanation for what is happening in this situation? What is an alternative explanation for what is happening in this situation?

C. **Nursing Knowledge**
- What type of nursing knowledge (theoretical, practical, ethical, or self-knowledge) is needed to answer the following questions?
  - What health concerns does Mr. Nguyen have that should be addressed by the healthcare team?
- What is the role of Zach Miller on the healthcare team?
- What role will you play in the care of Mr. Nguyen?

D. **Nursing Process**
- When you are asking Mr. Nguyen about the reason for his visit, what phase of the nursing process are you using?
- What activities are involved in the diagnosis phase? In planning outcomes? In planning interventions?
- Why would you not, at this point, be using the evaluation phase?

CLINICALJUDGMENT
Applying the Full-Spectrum Nursing Model

PATIENT SITUATION

Mrs. Castillo has late-stage cancer and is not expected to live more than a few months. With chemotherapy, she could live perhaps 1 or 2 more years. She cannot decide what to do. She knows that the chemotherapy will have unpleasant side effects and will be very expensive, and she wants to protect her family from the emotional and financial hardships of a lingering illness. She is showing physical signs of anxiety and distress (e.g., increased heart rate, restlessness, tearfulness). You want to provide support for her decision, whatever it may be.

THINKING

1. *Theoretical Knowledge*: What theoretical knowledge do you need to help Mrs. Castillo?

2. *Critical Thinking (Contextual Awareness)*: What details in the scenario represent *patient situation* or *context*?

DOING

3. *Practical Knowledge*:

   a. What practical knowledge do you need to help Mrs. Castillo?

   b. Which skills can you already perform? Which skills would you need to learn or review before caring for this patient?

CARING

4. *Ethical Knowledge*: Depending on Mrs. Castillo's decision, can you think of one ethical issue that might arise for you or for her family members later on?

Critical Thinking and Clinical Judgment

1. At the end of your first nursing class, your instructor gives an overview of a long-term assignment. She informs you that each semester of the program the class is required to complete a project that provides some type of service to the college community or the local community and that demonstrates the role or importance of nursing. The instructor asks you to begin discussing potential projects and come to class next week prepared to discuss several proposals for your community and the potential benefits of each option. You and several friends gather to talk about the assignment. "What an odd assignment!" you tell your classmates. "How can we possibly do this now? We aren't nurses. We don't have any skills. What could we possibly do?" Your classmates echo similar views.

This exercise is designed to help you actually work through the imaginary assignment you have just read. Use the *critical-thinking model* shown in Figure 2-1 in Volume 1 and the sample questions in Box 2-2 of Volume 1 to complete the assignment.

Go to Volume 1, **Chapter 2: Critical Thinking and Nursing Process.**

a. *Contextual awareness* is one concept in the critical-thinking model. Consider the context in which the assignment was given.
   - What exactly is this assignment?
   - Your instructor is perfectly aware of your knowledge and skill levels. Why do you think she would ask students to complete such an assignment so early in their nursing studies?

   To complete this assignment, you would need to gather information to find ways to answer the following questions. You would also need to use credible sources (another task of critical thinking) to address these questions.

b. What sources might you use to answer the following two questions?
   - What will I learn this semester?
   - What skills will I have by the time this assignment is due?

c. What are some ways in which you could answer the following two questions?
   - What do nurses do?
   - How do nurses interact with the community?

d. List some ways in which you could obtain information to answer this question: What does my community need?

e. If you had gathered the preceding information, you would then need to consider possible solutions. One way would be to develop a list of community needs, a list of activities that nurses engage in, and a list of skills and knowledge that you will have at the end of the term. Then, look at the overlap between the lists. This should help you to get some ideas for projects. Imagine that you have a list of possible projects similar to the following:
   - Take blood pressure measurements at a neighborhood grocery store for a day.
   - Hold a health fair at a neighborhood shopping center.
   - Create some materials for teaching about a healthy diet, and distribute them at a community event.

Now, think critically about this list of projects (this involves *reflective skepticism* and *exploring and imagining alternatives*). What questions could you ask about each project to help you decide which project to actually do?

2. Review the following scenarios. Is critical thinking occurring? If so, which part of the critical-thinking model is the student using, or which critical-thinking skill or attitude from Chapter 2 in Volume 1? If there is no evidence of critical thinking, revise the scenario to include it.

   a. Juan is a first-year nursing student. His clinical rotation is at a skilled nursing facility (SNF). He arrives at the unit at 0700 for the start of the day shift. After hearing the shift change report, he prepares to give his client a bedbath per the unit policy.

b. Lily is teaching her patient, Mr. Johannsen, about the medications he will be taking when he is discharged from the hospital. When Lily reviews the list with him, he says, "That's too many medicines. It's too confusing." Lily prepares a schedule and information sheet about the medicines and gives them to her client. She reviews the medications and their schedules with Mr. Johannsen and his wife before discharge.

c. Erin is caring for a young man who has had orthopedic surgery after a skiing accident. She is unable to hear his blood pressure when she attempts to take his vital signs. He is alert and able to converse with her. Because she is unable to hear the blood pressure, she records "0" in the client record.

d. As you are walking down the hall on the hospital unit, you hear a patient call out, "Nurse!" When you enter the room, you notice that the bedside is crowded with equipment. The patient is receiving several fluids intravenously, and a unit of blood is hanging from the intravenous (IV) pole. Because you have limited clinical experience, you say to the patient, "I'll get you some help."

3. For each of the following concepts, use critical thinking to describe how or why it is important to nursing, patient care, or critical thinking in the nursing process. Note that these are *not* to be merely definitions.

Caring

Critical-thinking skills

Critical-thinking attitudes

Exploring alternatives

The nursing process

Assessment phase

Planning outcomes phase

Planning interventions phase

Implementation phase

Evaluation phase

Theoretical knowledge

What Are the Main Points in This Chapter?

- Nursing involves thinking, doing, and caring, and all are equally important.
- Critical thinking is a combination of reasoned thinking, openness to alternatives, an ability to reflect, and a desire to seek the truth.
- Critical thinking involves both attitudes and cognitive skills.
- Critical thinking attitudes include intellectual autonomy, intellectual curiosity, intellectual humility, intellectual empathy, intellectual courage, intellectual perseverance, fair-mindedness, intellectual integrity, and confidence in reasoning.
- Nurses use critical thinking in all aspects of their practice.
- Practical knowledge (knowing what to do and how to do it) and theoretical knowledge (knowing why) are equally important in nursing.
- The nursing process is a systematic problem-solving process that guides all nursing actions.
- The nursing process consists of six overlapping and interdependent phases: assessment, diagnosis, planning outcomes, planning interventions, implementation, and evaluation.
- Critical thinking is used in each phase of the nursing process; it is related to, but not the same as, the nursing process.
- Your ability to think critically depends on your theoretical knowledge about critical thinking, your motivation to practice it, and your amount of nursing knowledge.
- In full-spectrum nursing, the nurse applies thinking, doing, and caring to the patient situation to help achieve positive patient outcomes.

Knowledge Map

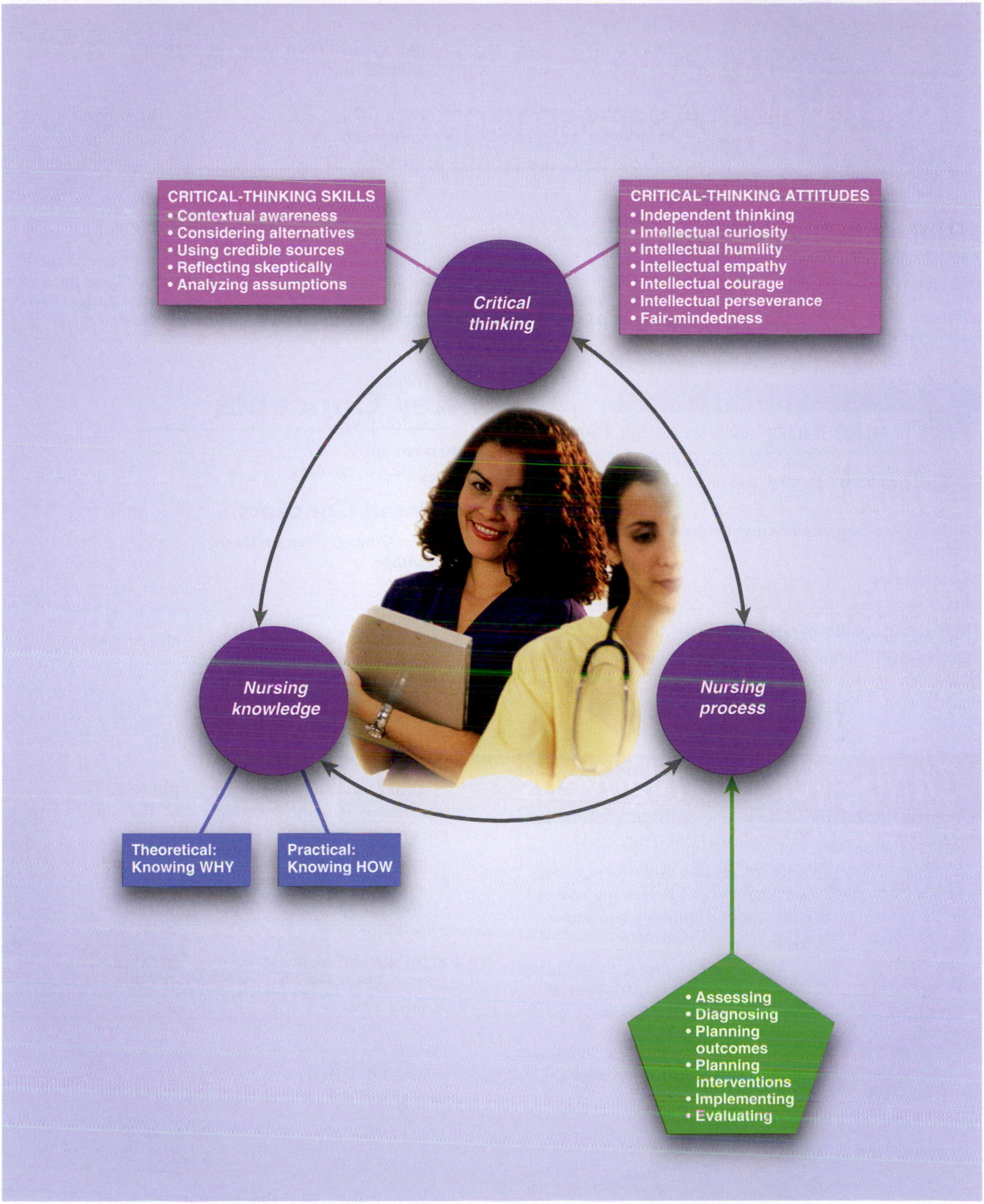
CRITICAL-THINKING SKILLS
• Contextual awareness
• Considering alternatives
• Using credible sources
• Reflecting skeptically
• Analyzing assumptions
CRITICAL-THINKING ATTITUDES
• Independent thinking
• Intellectual curiosity
• Intellectual humility
• Intellectual empathy
• Intellectual courage
• Intellectual perseverance
• Fair-mindedness
Critical thinking
Nursing knowledge
Nursing process
Theoretical: Knowing WHY
Practical: Knowing HOW
• Assessing
• Diagnosing
• Planning outcomes
• Planning interventions
• Implementing
• Evaluating

CHAPTER 3

Assessment

STUDENT RESOURCES

The questions and exercises in this book allow you to practice the kind of thinking you will use as a full-spectrum nurse. Critical-thinking questions usually have more than one right answer, so we do not provide "correct answers" for these features. Try to answer these questions yourself. It is more important to develop your nursing judgment than to just cover content. You will learn more by discussing the questions with your peers. If you are still unsure, see the Davis Advantage chapter resources for suggested responses.

To explore learning resources for this chapter,

Go to Davis Advantage and find:

Answers and Suggested Responses for all questions in this chapter

Concept Map

Knowledge Map

References and Bibliography

Lists of NOC Outcomes and NIC Interventions

Key Concepts

Assessment

Data

Related Concepts

See the Concept Map on Davis Advantage.

Caring for the Nguyens

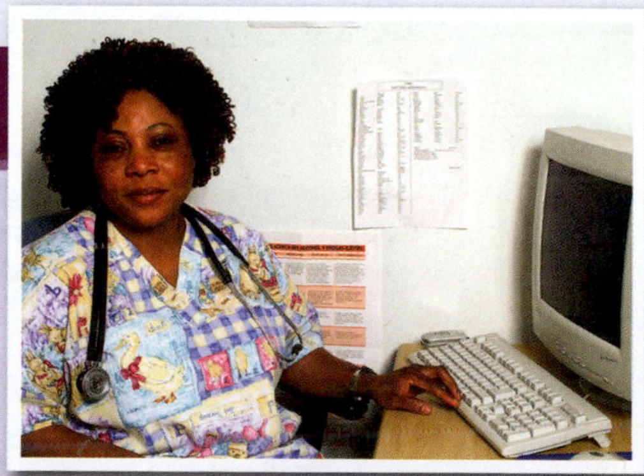

Review the opening scenario of Nam Nguyen in the front of Volume 2. Imagine that you are the clinic nurse at the Family Medicine Center. Using the information presented in the scenario, work through the following questions:

A. What type of assessment, comprehensive or focused, is being performed at this clinic visit? Explain your thinking.

B. Identify the types of data (e.g., subjective/objective, primary/secondary) that have been gathered so far. Give an example of each type.

Caring for the Nguyens (continued)

C. How might you verify data that Mr. Nguyen provided on the intake sheet?

D. Based on what you know about Mr. Nguyen, what follow-up assessments would provide useful data to help with the care of Mr. Nguyen? Why would you make these assessments?

PracticalKnowledge Clinical**Application**

In this chapter, practical knowledge pertains to your skill in applying the concepts of assessment and data, for example, by using structured and unstructured methods of data collection.

Clinical Insight 3-1 ➤ Preparing for a Patient Interview

Prepare Yourself

- **Know your purpose.** Be sure you know why you are conducting the interview and how the data will be used. As a student, this process may simply mean preparing thoroughly for your clinical assignment.
- **Read the patient's chart.** These data will give you an idea of where to start with the interview and keep you from covering topics already assessed by other caregivers. Be careful to keep an open mind, though. If you approach an interview with preconceived ideas, you may overlook important data.
- **Form some goals** for the interview.
- **Think of some opening questions.**
- **Schedule some uninterrupted time** for the interview. Giving the patient your undivided attention builds rapport and helps her feel freer to share information with you.
- **Gather the necessary assessment forms and equipment.** You will need a stethoscope, pen, pencil, blood pressure cuff, and thermometer.
- **Take a deep breath, and compose yourself** just before entering the room.

Prepare the Space

- **Provide privacy** (e.g., ask visitors to wait outside, shut the door). Unless you need information from the visitor (e.g., when the client cannot communicate clearly), you may wish to postpone the interview until it can be done in private. The presence of even a close family member may inhibit the client in some situations. For example, a wife may not want her husband to know that she had a miscarriage before they were married.
- **Keep the focus on the client** as much as possible. If others must be present, sometimes the client's spouse, family, or partner will offer information that may or may not be pertinent. Focus on the client, but do not ignore the information provided by others.
- **Remove distractions** (e.g., turn off the television, arrange for someone to watch the children for a while, if they are present).
- **Sit down. Do not hover over the bed.** Position yourself at the same level as your client, even if the client is in bed.

Prepare the Patient

- **Introduce yourself** to the patient and others in the room.
- **Call the patient by name.** First, ask what name the patient prefers. Don't use terms of endearment, such as "grandma," "dear," and "sweetie." You may think you are being friendly or expressing caring, but many people feel belittled by these terms.
- **Tell the patient what you will be doing and why.** Explain that you will be taking notes and that you will keep all information confidential.
- **Assess and provide comfort** (e.g., assess and medicate for pain, offer the bedpan, offer a drink of water).
- **Assess for anxiety.** Be sure the patient is comfortable emotionally as well as physically. A very anxious person cannot provide good information, so you may need to provide intervention to relieve anxiety before proceeding.
- **Assess readiness to discuss health issues.** If the patient indicates that now is not a good time, reschedule (e.g., if the patient has just received some bad news about his condition or in his personal life, he may need some time to process that information before he can concentrate on interview questions).
- **Interviews** are recorded only when done during research projects. The researcher must be sure to obtain institutional review board approval and written permission from the patient by using an approved consent form.

Clinical Insight 3-2 ➤ Conducting a Patient Interview

- **Individualize your approach.** Ask yourself, for example, "What approach is best considering the client's age and developmental level?" Respect the generational differences of a person older or younger than you are.
- **Be sensitive to cultural differences** (e.g., comfort with eye contact, the need for space).
- **Begin with neutral topics**, such as the biographical data (e.g., address, contact person, occupation). Ask more personal or sensitive questions after you and the client are more comfortable with each other.
- **Key Point:** *Use active listening. This is the most important interviewing technique. Focus intently on trying to understand what the client is saying, rather than thinking ahead to what your response to a statement will be.*
- **Use the mnemonic FOLK** to remember other active listening behaviors:
  Face the patient (either sitting or standing).
  Open, relaxed posture (arms and legs uncrossed).
  Lean toward the patient.
  Keep eye contact.
- **Do not get caught up in note taking.** Excessive writing interferes with eye contact and may inhibit the client's responses, especially when you are discussing personal issues, such as sexuality or drug and alcohol use.
- **Pay attention to nonverbal communication.** Body language may signal that the person is tired or in pain but is too polite to say so. If the person is fatigued, you may need to end the interview and finish it at another time.
- **Use open-ended questions** as much as possible to encourage the client to talk.
- **Avoid asking too many questions.** This may make you seem merely curious instead of genuinely interested in the client.
- **Use neutral statements instead of questions** (e.g., instead of asking, "How many children do you have?" say, "Tell me about your family").
- **Avoid asking "why"** (e.g., "Why have you stopped taking your pills?"). For some people, "why" suggests disapproval and causes them to become defensive.
- **Do not use healthcare jargon** (e.g., say, "I want to take your temperature and blood pressure" instead of "I want to take your vital signs").
- **Do not "talk down" to the client** (e.g., Don't say, "How often do you go potty?" when interviewing an adult).
- **Be sure your client understands what he says.** Confirm that clients actually understand the terminology they use. If a client says, "It's the inflammation that causes me the trouble, you know," you might say, "Tell me where the inflammation is and what happens when you have it." People may repeat words they hear from care providers without really knowing what those words mean.
- **Refocus and redirect the client as needed** (e.g., when a response becomes scattered or does not produce useful information). Encourage the client to talk about the topics of importance to her, but direct her to topics that need to be covered (e.g., "We haven't talked about your surgery. What do you expect to happen?").
- **Curb your curiosity.** Do not get caught up in the details of the client's story. Focus on the information you need to plan care.
- **Do not give advice or voice approval or disapproval.** Even if the advice is good (e.g., "It is good that you take your pills on time"), it may cause the client to be less open because he may feel that you are judging him. This can interfere with gathering of data.

Clinical Insight 3-3 ➤ Closing a Patient Interview

- Prepare the patient for closure. Begin by informing her that the interview is nearly finished.
- Summarize the key points of the interview.
- Be sure you have recorded all the important data. Ask the patient, "Is there anything else you would like to tell me?" or "Is there anything else we should talk about?"
- Thank the patient for answering the questions.
- Encourage the patient to keep you informed. For example, you might say, "Please let us know if you think of anything else we should know."
- Tell the patient what to expect next. Let the patient know when you will be leaving, when you will see him again, and what he can expect for the rest of the day (e.g., tests, treatments).
- And, finally, ask, "Is there anything I can do for you before I leave?"

ASSESSMENT GUIDELINES AND TOOLS

You can use the guidelines and forms in this section to perform a focused assessment of activities of daily living and to perform a comprehensive patient assessment.

Comprehensive Admission Assessment

Nursing Admission Data Form

Name: Ben J. Ivanos Age: 24 Phone #: 618-445-2300 Date: mm/dd/yyyy Time: 10:30

Primary Physician: Charles Katz Phone #: 618-446-8160

Chief Complaints/Procedure: ORIF fx (L) leg, Fx (R) femur + (R) ulna Height: 5' 10" Weight (lbs.): 155

Historian: Patient Temp: 100 Pulse: 90 Resp: 16 BP: 140/82

Religious Affiliation: Catholic Hospitalized within 30 days: Yes ☒ No ☐

UNABLE TO OBTAIN HISTORY ☐
Reason:

NEUROLOGICAL/SENSORY PERCEPTION
- Glaucoma ☐
- Hearing Loss/Deaf ... Right ☐ Left ☐
- Motion Sickness ☐
- Paresthesia ... Right ☐ Left ☐
- Fibromyalgia/Migraine ☐
- Spina Bifida ☐
- Stroke/CVA/TIA ☐
- Altered Mental Status ☐
- Other:

CARDIOVASCULAR/HEMATOLOGY
- Bleeding Problems ☐
- Blood transfusion in the past 3 months ☐
- Chest Pain/Angina ☐
- Heart Attack/Date: ☐
- Heart Disease ☐
- High Blood Pressure ☐
- Irregular Beats/Pacemaker/AICD ☐
- Mitral Valve Prolapse ☐
- Murmur ☐
- Peripheral Vascular Disease ☐
- Sickle Cell Disease ☐
- Venous Access Device/Type ☐
- Other:

RESPIRATORY
- Asthma ☐
- Bronchitis ... 6 months ago ☒
- COPD/Emphysema ☐
- Post Nasal Drip/Rhinitis/Sinusitis ☒
- Pneumonia ☐
- Tracheostomy ☐
- Other:

GASTROINTESTINAL
- Dysphagia ☐
- Hiatal Hernia ☐
- Liver Disease/Jaundice ☐
- Pancreatitis ☐
- Gall Stones ☐
- Ostomy ☐
- Last Bowel Movement: 5/19/2020
- Other:

GENITOURINARY/RENAL
- Kidney Disease/Urogenital ☐
- Prostate Problems ☐
- Voiding Problems ☐
- Other:

MUSCULOSKELETAL
- Arthritis ☐
- Back/Disc Problem ☐
- Fractures ... present admission ☒
- Other:

ENDOCRINE
- Diabetes/type: ☐
- Thyroid Disease ☐
- Other:

INFECTIOUS DISEASE
- Fevers ☐
- Hepatitis/type/active ☐
- HIV/AIDS ☐
- Recent Cold ☐
- Sexually Transmitted Disease/type ☐
- Tuberculosis/Active: ☐
- Other:

- Pregnant ☐
- Lactating ☐
- LMP/Date:

VACCINATION/DATE
Flu: Hepatitis B:
Pneumonia:

BEHAVIORAL HEALTH
- Anxiety Disorder ☐
- Depression ☐
- Suicide (thoughts/attempts) ☐
- Patient is a Baker Act ☐
- Other:

CANCER
- Type ☐
- Radioactive Seeds/Implant ☐
- Date:
- Other:

SOCIAL HISTORY
- Tobacco ☒
  - Number of years: 3
  - # of packs per day: 1/2
  - Year Quit: 2017
- Would you like smoking cessation info? ☒ No ☐ Yes ☐ information provided
- Alcohol ☒
  - Drinks per day: 1
  - Amount:
  - Type:
- Recreational Drug ☐
  - Amount:
  - Type:
  - Year Quit:
- Detoxification Protocol Initiated ☐

ALLERGIES & REACTION None Known ☒ Allergy Bracelet on ☐

Medications: none	Symptoms:
	Blood Reaction: ☐
Food/Shellfish/other allergies: No	Latex: ☐
Contrast/Dye: No	Latex Allergy Protocol Initiated: ☐

PAST HOSPITAL/PROCEDURE (Surgical/Medical/Behavioral Health)
None

CURRENT MEDICATIONS (include ASA/Anticoagulant, over the counter medications, ointments, patches, eye drops, herbal, vitamins and nutritional supplements)

Medication	Dose	Frequency	Last Dose
ASA	"2"	occasionally for HA	

Food/Drug Interaction information provided ☐

Initiate Social Service Consult

(Note: Additional medication can be listed on last page)

ADDRESSOGRAPH

Nursing Admission Data Form *(continued)*

PAIN HISTORY

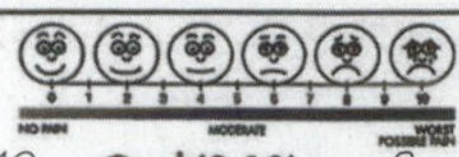

Have you been experiencing pain? ☒ Yes
If yes, when *Now* Intensity (0-10): *10* Goal (0-10): *2*
Location: *Legs and arm, muscles in back*
Radiation: *No*
Duration: *Constant*
Quality: *Sharp, aching*
Aggravating factors *Movement*

What medications/interventions are effective in relieving your pain?
Taking PCA Demerol

Acute Pain Management - It is Your Right brochure provided ☒

PSYCHOSOCIAL ASSESSMENT

☒ Lives alone ☐ Lives with spouse/SO ☐ Nursing Home/ALF
☐ Homeless ☐ Rehab Facility ☐ Other:
Marital Status ☒ Single ☐ Married ☐ Divorced ☐ Widowed ☐ Separated
Next of Kin: *Mother, Clara Ivanos* **Phone #:** *618-446-3816*
Supportive Adult: - **Phone #:** -
Has anybody threatened/hit/abused you within the last year?
☐ Yes **(refer to policy RA 004015 mauve manual)** ☒ No

EDUCATIONAL LEARNING ASSESSMENT

Learner ☒ Patient ☐ Family ☐ Significant Other
Readiness to learn ☐ Eager to learn ☒ Asks questions
☐ Extremely anxious ☐ Denies need for Education
Knowledge of current health status ☐ No knowledge
☒ Partial understanding ☐ Full understanding
Barriers to learning ☒ Physical ☐ Emotional
☐ Language ☐ Religious ☐ Cultural
☐ Reading Ability ☐ Changes in Short Memory
☐ None
Preferred Learning Method ☒ Reading ☐ Lecture
☒ Video ☒ Demo/Practice
Communication ☒ English ☐ Spanish ☐ Creole
☐ Sign Language ☐ Other:
Do you have any religious/cultural practices that are important to you or may alter your care or education? ☒ No ☐ Yes

☒ **Patient Handbook provided** ☒ **Patient safety information provided**
☒ **Patient's Bill of Rights and Responsibilities information provided**
Other Educational Materials:

PERSONAL EFFECTS: Do you use the following:

	YES	WITH PT.	FAMILY/SO
Wheelchair	☐	☐	☐
Braces	☐	☐	☐
Cane/Crutches	☐	☐	☐
Walker	☐	☐	☐
Prothesis	☐	☐	☐
Medications	☐	☐	☐
Dentures: (Full)	☐	☐	☐
Upper	☐	☐	☐
Lower	☐	☐	☐
Glasses	☐	☐	☐
Contacts	☒	☒	☐
Hearing Aids	☐	☐	☐
Other:			

Initiate Social Service Consult

ADVANCE DIRECTIVES

Do you have an Advance Directive?
(must check one)
☒ **No** Information provided to patient
☐ **No** Patient elects not to receive information
☐ **Yes** (check advance directive patient states he/she has)
☐ **Living Will** ☐ **Health Care Surrogate** ☐ **State DNAR form**
☐ **Durable Power of Attorney** ☐ **Organ Donation**
(If patient has an Advance Directive, inform patient to provide copy within 24 hours or they may complete a new advance directive or verbalize their wishes)
Do you have a guardian? ☐ **Yes name**
(Inform patient to provide guardianship form within 24 hours)
☐ **Patient unable to respond/family not available**

FALL SCREEN: ***If any of the following are checked, initiate Safety/Protective Intervention Protocol***

Inability to understand or follow instructions	☐
Impaired mobility, visual impairment, drug therapy, surgical procedure, unsteady gait, incontinence *Casts, Traction*	☒
Unable to use call light	☐
Altered mental status *Taking Demerol PCA*	☒
Nocturnal/urgency/frequency in elimination	☐
Dizziness	☐
History of falls	☐
No Criteria Met	☐

NUTRITIONAL SCREEN: ***If any of the following are checked, enter in the computer request for Nutritional Consult***

Nausea/vomiting > 5 days	☐
No food/drink for 3 days	☐
Recent unexplained weight loss > 10 lbs.	☐
Difficulty swallowing/dysphagia	☐
Evidence of Stage III - IV pressure ulcer	☐
Feeding tube	☐
New onset diabetes	☐
TPN	☐
Pregnant/lactating	☐
Surgical patients > 70 years of age	☐
Ethnic diet/special needs **(include in diet order and order for Preference consult)**	☐
Difficulty chewing **(include in diet order and order for Preference consult)**	☐
No Criteria Met	☒

FUNCTIONAL SCREEN: ***If any of the following are checked, please request physician order for physical therapy consult.***

New onset of paralysis	☐
New onset stroke/CVA	☐
New amputation	☐
Unsteady gait	☐
Decreased mobility *Casts, Tx for Fx*	☒
Dysphagia	☐
No Criteria Met	☐

Page 2 of 4

Nursing Admission Data Form *(continued)*

MARK LOCATION

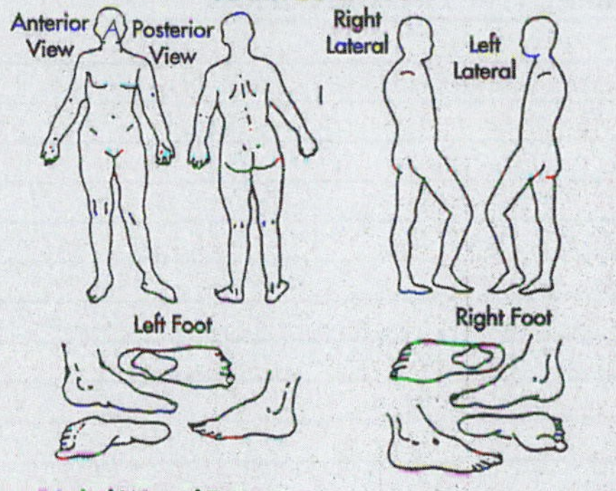

* Label Wound Type

WOUND TYPE

P = Pressure ulcer	A = Abrasions
ST = Skin tear	LU = Leg/Foot ulcers
S = Surgical	BR = Bruising
L = Laceration	M = Maceration
B = Burns	O = Other

STAGE

Pressure ulcer only

I: Reddened area, does not resolve with pressure relief.
II: Blister or superficial break in skin.
III: Full thickness wound into subcutaneous tissue.
IV: Full thickness with muscle, bone or tendon tissue exposed.
U = Unable to stage: Necrotic

COLOR WOUND BED

R = Red (new tissue)	Y = Yellow (slough)
P = Pink	B = Black (eschar)

EXUDATE

O = None	SS = Serosanguinous
S = Serous	P = Purulent

ODOR

N = None S = Slight F = Foul

SURROUNDING SKIN

OK = Clean & Intact Ra = Rash
C = Cellulitis (red & tender)
R = Raw & denuded
M = Maceration
I = Induration

Skin Breakdown Present ☐ Consent Obtained ☐ Photograph Taken ☐ Acute/Chronic Wound Flow Sheet Initiated ☐ Swat Consult Initiated ☐

BRADEN SCALE - PRESSURE ULCER RISK ASSESSMENT

SENSORY PERCEPTION Ability to respond meaningfully to pressure-related discomfort	**1. Completely Limited:**	**2. Very Limited:**	**3. Slightly Limited:**	**4. No Impairment:**	4
MOISTURE Degree to which skin is exposed to moisture	**1. Constantly Moist:**	**2. Very Moist:**	**3. Occasionally Moist:**	**4. Rarely Moist:**	4
ACTIVITY degree of physical activity	**1. Bedfast:**	**2. Chairfast:**	**3. Walks Occasionally:**	**4. Walks Frequently:**	1
MOBILITY ability to change and control body position	**1. Completely Immobile:**	**2. Very Limited:**	**3. Slightly Limited:**	**4. No Limitations:**	3
NUTRITION usual food intake pattern	**1. Very Poor:**	**2. Probably Inadequate:**	**3. Adequate:**	**4. Excellent:**	4
FRICTION AND SHEAR	**1. Problem:**	**2. Potential Problem:**	**3. No Apparent Problem:**		2

RN Signature: [signature] Date: mm/dd/yyyy **TOTAL SCORE:** 18

NOTE: Patients with a total score of 16 or less are considered to be at risk of developing pressure ulcers. Implement Skin Care Protocol. Refer to Surface Bed Decision Tree. (12 or less = high risk)

ANTICIPATED DISHARGE NEEDS

☒ Transportation ☐ Placement needed

Medical Equipment: ☐ Oxygen ☐ CPAP ☐ Nebulizer ☐ Blood Glucose Meter Other: Crutches, Wheelchair

Community Services: (Home Health, Reach to Recovery, Meals On Wheels, etc.): Home Health for f/u on cast care and pain medication. Transportation to physicians office for return visit.

Nurse Signature: [signature] Unit: 3E Date: mm/dd/yyyy Time: 10:45

Nurse Signature: ____ Unit: ____ Date: ____ Time: ____

Page 3 of 4

Nursing Admission Data Form *(continued)*

DATE & TIME	INTERDISCIPLINARY NOTES/ADVANCE DIRECTIVES INFORMATION
mm/dd/yyyy, 11:00	Healthy young adult, on no meds, admitted via E.D. p̄ motorcycle accident, and reduction and casting of multiple fx ((L) tibia + fibula, (R) femur, and (R) elbow and ulna). Experiencing severe pain r/t fx, bruises and muscle spasms. Plan:
	(1) Traction per Rx; check weights q̄ 4th
	(2) Control pain w/PCA Demerol. Assess + instruct prn
	(3) Neurovascular + circulatory checks, all extremities, q̄ 2h
	(4) Monitor edema of extremities; re-cast after 3 days if edema has subsided.

Nurse Signature: [signature] Unit: 3E Date: mm/dd/yyyy Time: 11:00

Nurse Signature: ______ Unit: ______ Date: ______ Time: ______

Current Medications: (Continued)

Medication	Dose	Frequency	Last Dose

Page 4 of 4 WHITE - INPATIENT/OUTPATIENT LITE GREEN - OUTPATIENT ONLY DARK GREEN - ANESTHESIA LITE BLUE - INPATIENT ONLY

Functional Ability Assessment

Functional ability is especially important in discharge planning and home care. Future rehabilitation needs are derived from initial and ongoing functional ability assessments. The Joint Commission (2018) requires an initial functional ability assessment "based on the patient's condition." These three functional assessment tools are commonly used:

- **The Karnofsky Performance scale (Karnofsky & Burchenal, 1949).** This tool is used primarily in palliative care settings to assess functional abilities at the end of life. To see the scale,

  Go to **http://www.hospicepatients.org/karnofsky.html**

- **The Katz Index of ADL scale (1963).** This instrument is one of the best for assessing independent performance in very basic areas. It assigns one point for independence in each of the following areas: bathing, dressing, toileting, transfer, continence, and feeding (Shelkey & Wallace, revised 2012). Nurses often use the data to plan staffing and appropriate placement of clients. The following Focused Assessment box addresses functions similar to those assessed by the Katz scale. However, to see the Katz scale,

  Go to the ConsultGeri Web site at **https://consultgeri.org/try-this/general-assessment/issue-2.pdf**

Focused Assessment

Special Needs Assessment: Questions for Assessing Independence in Activities of Daily Living

Mobility

Does the client require devices (e.g., cane, crutches, walker, wheelchair) for support?

Transfer

Can the client get in and out of bed and in and out of a chair without assistance?

If not, how much help does the client need?

Is the client completely confined to bed?

Bathing

Can the client perform a sponge bath, tub bath, or shower bath with no help?

If not, specifically what assistance does the client need?

Dressing

Can the client get all necessary clothing from drawers and closets and get completely dressed without help?

If not, specifically what assistance does the client need?

Feeding

Can the client feed self without assistance?

If not, specifically what assistance does the client need (e.g., help with cutting meat, tube feeding)?

Toileting

Can the client go to the bathroom, use the toilet, clean self, and rearrange clothing without help?

If a bedpan or commode is used during the night, can the client empty it and clean it independently?

If the client needs help with these activities, specifically what does it include?

Continence

Can the client independently control urination and bowel movements?

If not, how often is the client incontinent of bladder or bowel?

Does the client require an indwelling urinary catheter?

- **Lawton Instrumental Activities of Daily Living (IADL) scale (1969).** This easy-to-use tool is particularly helpful in assessing a person's ability to independently perform the more complex tasks of everyday life, such as shopping. Identifying early functional decline is important for discharge planning. The Lawton scale is especially useful for use in older adults, who may begin to experience functional decline within 48 hours of hospital admission (Graf, 2008; Lawton & Brody, 1969).

Patient Assessment Tool—Lawton Instrumental Activities of Daily Living (IADL).

Date:__________ Name:____________________

Please check the box that most applies for each activity:

Activity	**Needs no help (2 pts. each)**	**Needs some help (1 pt. each)**	**Unable to do at all (0 pts. each)**
1. Using the telephone	___	___	___
2. Getting to places beyond walking distance	___	___	___
3. Grocery shopping	___	___	___
4. Preparing meals	___	___	___
5. Doing housework or handyman work	___	___	___
6. Doing laundry	___	___	___
7. Taking medications	___	___	___
8. Managing money	___	___	___
Total score: ___ =	(___ × 2 =) ___ +	(___ × 1 =) ___ +	0

A patient is awarded 2 points for each area in which he/she can function totally without help, 1 point in those areas that they need some help, and 0 points for those activities that somebody else must do completely for them. The maximum score is 16, minimum score is 0.

Like other evaluations, the IADL scale provides a baseline of data that can be compared with the results of future evaluations. (Note that some activities may be gender specific. Omit these items if the patient does not usually perform those tasks.)

Permission obtained from M. Powell Lawton, Ph.D., Philadelphia Geriatric Center, Philadelphia, PA. May be used freely for patient assessment. Formatted and posted May 25, 1996, to www.acsu.buffalo.edu/~drstall/assessmenttools.html by Robert S. Stall, M.D.

CLINICALJUDGMENT

Applying the Full-Spectrum Nursing Model

PATIENT SITUATION

As the intake nurse in a community-based clinic, your role is to complete a comprehensive nursing assessment and initiate a plan of care for the clients. Your first client is a 24-year-old single woman, Sami, who is requesting clinic services for her general healthcare needs. Sami is Cuban-American and lives alone in a one-bedroom apartment. She works as a fitness trainer at the local fitness club while attending college part time. Her family lives in another town across the state. Sami's earnings place her at the poverty level. She realizes that she must have healthcare to prevent health problems and to detect them and receive treatment if they arise.

THINKING

1. *Theoretical Knowledge:* To care for Sami, what knowledge would you need that you do not already have? Can you list the URL for at least one online reputable source for this information?

2. *Critical Thinking:* You ask Sami, "If you can't afford healthcare, couldn't you get a roommate to save some money on rent?" What are some critical-thinking questions you should ask yourself when reflecting on this question later?

DOING

3. *Practical Knowledge:* What practical knowledge will you, as the nurse, use in this scenario?

4. *Nursing Process:* What kind of assessment will you perform for Sami (e.g., comprehensive, focused, special needs, discharge, etc.)?

CARING

5. *Self-Knowledge:* In what ways are you like Sami? In what ways are you different?

Critical Thinking and Clinical Judgment

1. Recall the definition of subjective data. Make a list of the kinds of patients from whom you might not be able to get subjective data and those who might give unreliable data. One example of the former is a baby who cannot talk yet. How many other types of patients can you think of?

2. What are some factors that might make it difficult, but not impossible, for a patient to provide you with subjective data? One example is when the person is severely anxious.

3. For each of the factors in question 2, state what you could do to facilitate collection of reliable subjective data from that person.

4. List your present assessment skills, and indicate your comfort level in using each skill. Include observation, physical assessment, and interviewing skills. Use a scale of 1 to 5 (1 = slightly comfortable; 2 = somewhat comfortable; 3 = moderately comfortable; 4 = fairly comfortable; and 5 = very comfortable).

5. For any skill that you score as 3 or lower, write a plan describing what you need to do to move to the higher comfort level.

6. The following are some of the criteria in the American Nurses Association (ANA) (2015) professional practice Standard 1. For each of the criteria, write an example of what would constitute evidence (proof) that the standard is being followed in a healthcare agency. The first one is done for you.

   a. "Collects data … in a systematic and ongoing process."
   I would look in the care plan for nursing orders that call for some kind of assessment on a scheduled basis. For example, an order might read, "Temperature q4hr" or "Check dressing for drainage once per shift." I would also look at the nursing notes, especially flow sheets (e.g., vital sign flow sheets, input and output records, neurological checks) to see whether assessment findings were recorded at regular intervals. I would look for nursing diagnoses or other conclusions that have been charted in the nurses' notes (e.g., stating that the medication has effectively relieved pain). Other evidence would be to observe the nurses doing systematic and ongoing data collection. I would also perform my physical assessment in a systematic way, using the same order (unless otherwise indicated).

   b. "Engages the healthcare consumer and other interprofessional team members in holistic, culturally sensitive data collection."

   c. "Prioritizes data collection based on the healthcare consumer's immediate condition, or the anticipated needs … ."

   d. "Uses evidence-based assessment techniques, instruments, tools, available data, information, and knowledge relevant to the situation to identify patterns and variances."

   e. "Documents relevant data accurately and in a manner accessible to the interprofessional team."

7. Your client, Sami (Meet Your Patient, in Volume 1), was born in Cuba. Having worked with many clients of Cuban heritage and being familiar with the nursing literature regarding various cultural patterns, you are aware of the following:

   - Many Hispanic people who live in Sami's city are bilingual.
   - When communicating, especially with strangers, it is not unusual for Hispanic women not to maintain eye contact. (During the interview, Sami speaks rapidly and does not maintain eye contact with you.)
   - Many people of Cuban descent are Catholic and may consider birth control taboo.
   - Many Cuban American women do not seek annual physical examinations (Purnell & Paulanka, 2013).

   a. Looking at the four points from the literature, how is Sami's cultural background similar to or different from your own? Remember that you are looking at cultural patterns, not Sami's individual and personal values and behaviors.

   b. On the basis of your understanding of your own culture and Sami's culture, what questions might you want to ask Sami to support her reproductive health?

8. What physical examination techniques would you use to:

   a. Assess for a distended bladder?

   b. Get information about a patient's headache?

   c. Obtain data about a patient's ankle edema?

   d. Obtain subjective data?

9. For each of the following concepts, use critical thinking to describe how or why it is important to nursing, patient care, or assessment. Note that these are *not* to be merely definitions.

Active listening

Agency policies

ANA standards of practice

Assessment

Comprehensive assessments

Focused assessments

Nursing frameworks/models

Pain assessment

Recording data

Reflecting critically about your assessment

Special needs assessments

Spiritual health assessment

The Joint Commission

The nursing health history

Validating data

Wellness assessment

What Are the Main Points in This Chapter?

- Assessment is a systematic, ongoing process of collecting, categorizing, and recording holistic data about client health status.
- Accurate, complete data are essential to effective nursing diagnosis and care planning.
- Nursing assessments focus on client responses to illness and stressors rather than on identifying disease processes.
- ANA standards of practice state that professional nurses are responsible for assessing clients.
- A comprehensive assessment provides information about the client's overall health, whereas a focused assessment provides data about a particular topic, body part, or functional ability.
- Special needs assessments provide in-depth information about a particular area of client functioning (e.g., nutrition, pain, lifestyle).
- Subjective data can be perceived only by the client; objective data are measurable or observable by the nurse or other healthcare providers.
- Nurses obtain data through observation, interviewing, and physical assessment.
- The formats and frameworks for the nursing health history vary among agencies; however, all have essentially the same components (e.g., chief complaint, family history, review of body systems).
- Effective interviews require nurse's preparation and the use of both closed-ended and open-ended questions.
- Active listening is one of the most important interviewing techniques.
- Validating data helps ensure that they are accurate, complete, and factual.
- Documentation of assessment findings is of critical importance and has professional and legal implications.
- When documenting assessments, the nurse should record cues (observations), not inferences (conclusions).

Knowledge Map

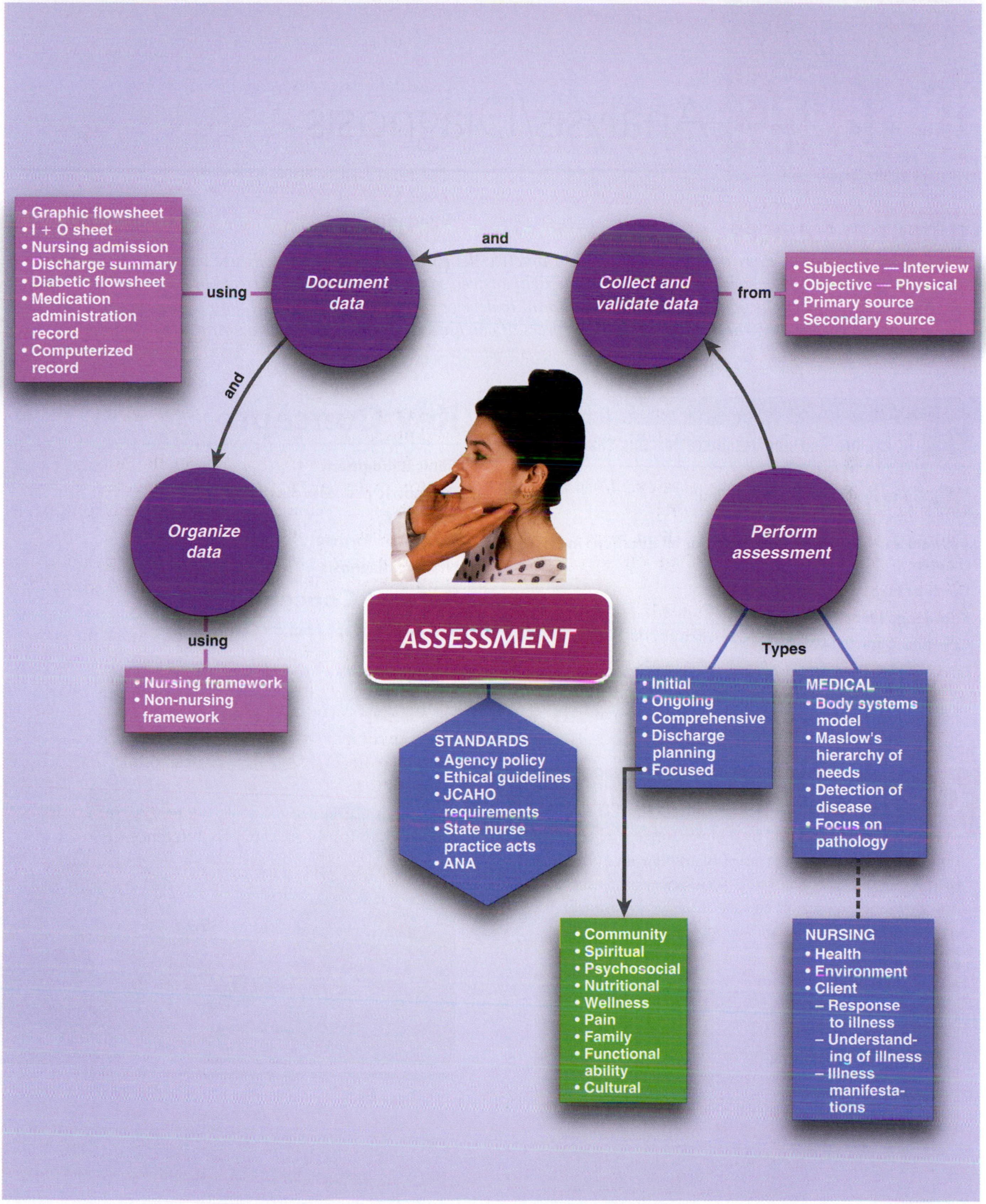

CHAPTER 4

Analysis/Diagnosis

STUDENT RESOURCES

The questions and exercises in this book allow you to practice the kind of thinking you will use as a full-spectrum nurse. Critical-thinking questions usually have more than one right answer, so we do not provide "correct answers" for these features. Try to answer these questions yourself. It is more important to develop your nursing judgment than to just cover content. You will learn more by discussing the questions with your peers. If you are still unsure, see the Davis Advantage chapter resources for suggested responses.

To explore learning resources for this chapter,

Go to Davis Advantage and find:

Answers and Suggested Responses for all questions in this chapter
Concept Map
Knowledge Map
References and Bibliography
Lists of NOC Outcomes and NIC Interventions

Key Concepts

Clinical judgment
Diagnostic process (diagnostic reasoning)
Diagnostic format
Nursing diagnosis

Related Concepts

See the Concept Map on Davis Advantage.

Caring for the Nguyens

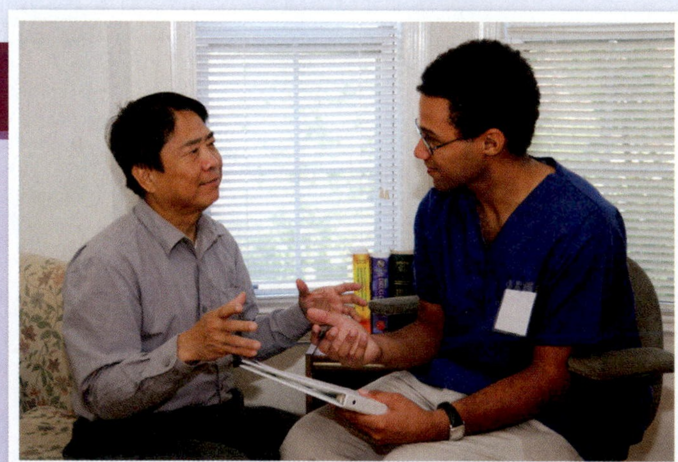

Review the opening scenario of Nam Nguyen in the front of Volume 1. After the nurse practitioner completed the interview and physical examination of Mr. Nguyen, he listed the following diagnoses on the problems list:

- Hypertension
- Obesity
- Musculoskeletal pain
- Tobacco abuse
- Family history of prostate cancer
- Family history of cardiovascular disease
- Family history of diabetes mellitus (DM)

(Continued)

Caring for the Nguyens (continued)

A. What type of problems list does this represent? How is it similar to or different from a problems list that you might generate?

B. On the basis of the data in the scenario, identify at least one actual diagnosis, one potential diagnosis, and one wellness diagnosis for Mr. Nguyen. Identify the NANDA-I labels and describe the cues that support your choices.

C. The nurse has identified the problem Overweight for Mr. Nguyen.
- What information do you need to determine the etiology of this problem?
- Because you do not have that information, write a two-part diagnostic statement describing Mr. Nguyen's nutritional status.

D. Now, rewrite the nutrition statement as a three-part statement, including the phrase "*as evidenced by.*"

E. The nurse has identified the problem Acute Pain (knees) for Mr. Nguyen. If the pain were caused by a medical condition, such as osteoarthritis, how would you write a two-part diagnostic statement to describe this health status?

CLINICALJUDGMENT

Recall from Chapter 2, that **clinical reasoning** is:

- Reflective, concurrent, creative thinking about patients and patient care.
- Logical thinking that links thoughts together to create meaning.

Analysis, problem-solving, and diagnostic process are all aspects of clinical reasoning, all of which require critical thinking (see Table 2-1).

Applying the Full-Spectrum Nursing Model

PATIENT SITUATION

You have now admitted Todd from the emergency department (ED). His admitting medical diagnosis is chronic renal failure. Refer to the Meet Your Patient scenario in Volume 1 for the data you need to answer the following questions.

THINKING

1. *Theoretical Knowledge:* What theoretical knowledge will you need to identify the collaborative problems and nursing diagnoses for Todd?

2. *Critical Thinking (Inquiry Based on Credible Sources):*

   a. What resources would you use to find out more about the pathophysiology of renal failure? How do you know the source is credible?

   b. When you are making your assessments of Todd, who is your best source of data? Why?

DOING

3. *Nursing Process (Diagnosis):*

   a. Write one collaborative problem for Todd. If you do not know the potential complications of chronic renal failure, look them up in a medical–surgical or pathophysiology textbook. Explain why you would not use nursing diagnosis terminology to describe the problem.

b. After further assessment, you observe that Todd's skin is intact and without redness or lesions. Write a nursing diagnosis (problem and etiology) to describe your concerns regarding his skin.

c. According to Maslow's Hierarchy of Needs, which problem has the highest priority?

CARING

4. *Ethical Knowledge:* The scenario does not provide enough information for you to identify the ethical dimensions of Todd's care. However, on the basis of what you already know about him, speculate about some things that might create ethical issues for you.

PATIENT SITUATION

5. *Patient Preferences:* Think critically about the patient's preferences and concerns. Suppose that Todd's main concern is not the same as the high-priority problem you identified. Speculate about some other concerns he might have. What other things might he want to have resolved that could—for him—be more important than his chronic renal failure? Besides his physical condition, what life concerns do you think Todd might have right now?

Critical Thinking and Clinical Judgment

1. Sally Jones, a 45-year-old woman, was admitted to your surgical unit directly from the surgical suite. She had been in a motorcycle accident this evening. In the emergency department, her blood pressure was falling, and she was bleeding profusely from many sites. She was sent directly to the operating room for a splenectomy, internal fixation of a compound fracture of bilateral femurs, and traumatic amputation of the right hand. During surgery, she lost 2,000 mL of blood and received three units of packed red blood cells (volume = 750 mL) along with 1,000 mL of fluid administered intravenously.

   You receive the report on the client at 1900. Sally is receiving IV fluid through several peripheral lines and through a central line (a catheter inserted into a major vein leading to the heart). She has a Foley catheter, which is draining 30 mL of concentrated urine each hour. Sally's vital signs are as follows: temperature, 102.8°F (39.3°C) (rectal); heart rate, 120 beats/min; respirations, 28 breaths/min; and blood pressure, 160/86 mm Hg. Her skin is flushed, dry, and warm to the touch. On assessment, you find the following: skin turgor > 3 seconds, dry mucous membranes, and bloodstained dressing on right upper extremity.

   She is complaining of thirst, weakness, and pain at a level of 10 on a scale of 1 to 10 (10 highest). Sally is receiving a continuous infusion of morphine. She refuses to deep-breathe, cough, or attempt to turn. She is lying very still, and her body is rigid. Sally drifts in and out of sleep but remains asleep for less than 30 minutes each time. She is irritable and restless. She communicates with one-word answers only. Frequently, she displays facial grimaces, and her body becomes increasingly stiff. Her eyes appear dull. She complains of severe pain with any passive or active movements. In answering the following questions, use a nursing diagnosis handbook to look up the NANDA-I defining characteristics, definitions, and so forth, as needed.

   a. On the basis of the data provided, which of the following NANDA-I labels would you use for Sally? Explain your reasoning.
   Deficient Fluid Volume or Risk for Deficient Fluid Volume

   b. For Sally, what cues are present for a diagnosis of Deficient Fluid Volume? What related factors are present?

   c. Using your responses to (a) and (b), write a diagnostic statement that includes problem, etiology, defining characteristics (cues), and the medical condition that the problem is "secondary to."

   d. Think of other explanations for these cues: temperature, 102.8°F (39.3°C); heart rate, 120 beats/min; respirations, 28 breaths/min; blood pressure, 160/86 mm Hg.

   e. Sally certainly has the defining characteristics for the nursing diagnosis Impaired Physical Mobility. If you use this problem label, what would the etiological factors be?

f. Which of those etiological factors could you treat with independent nursing interventions?

g. Sally has the nursing diagnoses (problem labels only are listed) and collaborative problems listed below. Answer the two following questions about that list:
- From Sally's perspective, which problem is probably of the highest priority?
- Using an urgency (or threat to life) criterion, name Sally's three most important problems and why you consider them most important.

Problems:
Deficient Fluid Volume
Acute Pain (abdominal incision, amputation site, fractures)
Risk for Disturbed Body Image
Potential Complication of trauma, surgery, and IV lines: infection
Risk for Ineffective Airway Clearance

h. Examine your theoretical knowledge. To care for Sally, what additional theoretical knowledge do you need?

i. What practical knowledge will you need to use in her care?

2. You have a homebound client with diabetes mellitus (DM) who is exhibiting the beginnings of a pressure injury. You have been treating the client for Impaired Skin Integrity related to decreased circulation and mobility. However, the client's skin continues to break down.

a. Your client has DM type 2. What type of problem is that (medical, nursing, or collaborative)?

b. What is the nursing diagnosis for this client?

c. The client has Impaired Skin Integrity. The break in the body's first line of defense (intact skin) increases the risk for infection. Write a problem statement reflecting the nursing diagnosis of that risk.

3. For each of the following concepts, use critical thinking to describe how or why it is important to nursing, patient care, or nursing diagnosis. Note that these are *not* to be merely definitions.

The diagnosis step of the nursing process

NANDA International

Patient strengths

Maslow's hierarchy

Documenting priorities

Nursing diagnoses

Possible nursing diagnoses

Collaborative problems

Wellness nursing diagnosis

Cues

Diagnostic label definition

Defining characteristics

Risk factors

Etiological factors

Theoretical knowledge

Standardized nursing languages

What Are the Main Points in This Chapter?

- Nursing diagnosis is the unique obligation of the professional nurse; it cannot be delegated.
- An accurate nursing diagnosis is the foundation for the plan of care because it directs the choice of client-centered goals and nursing interventions.
- A nursing diagnosis is a statement of health status that nurses can identify, prevent, or treat independently.
- A medical diagnosis describes a disease, illness, or injury. A nursing diagnosis, in contrast, more holistically describes human responses to disease, illness, or injury.
- Collaborative problems are potential physiological complications of diseases, treatments, or diagnostic studies that nurses monitor and help to prevent but that cannot be treated primarily by independent nursing interventions.
- You must determine the "status" of each nursing diagnosis—that is, actual, potential, or possible problem; wellness diagnosis; or syndrome—because each status requires (1) different wording and (2) different nursing interventions.
- Diagnostic reasoning involves analyzing and interpreting data, verifying problems with the patient, and prioritizing the problems.
- You can never be certain that an inference is accurate, but you can have more confidence in an inference that is well supported by data.
- A problem's etiology consists of the factors causing or contributing to the problem.
- You should involve patients in verifying and prioritizing their problems.
- Sound diagnostic reasoning is based on critical thinking and good theoretical knowledge and self-knowledge.
- A diagnostic statement consists basically of "problem + etiology"; however, a variety of formats is needed to describe client health status.
- A NANDA-I nursing diagnosis consists of a diagnostic label, a definition, defining characteristics, and related or risk factors.
- To choose the correct NANDA-I problem label, match the patient's cue clusters to the NANDA-I definition and defining characteristics.
- In general, the problem side of the diagnostic statement directs the choice of goals; the etiology directs the choice of nursing interventions.
- Diagnostic statements should be descriptive, accurate, clear, concise, and nonjudgmental.

Knowledge Map

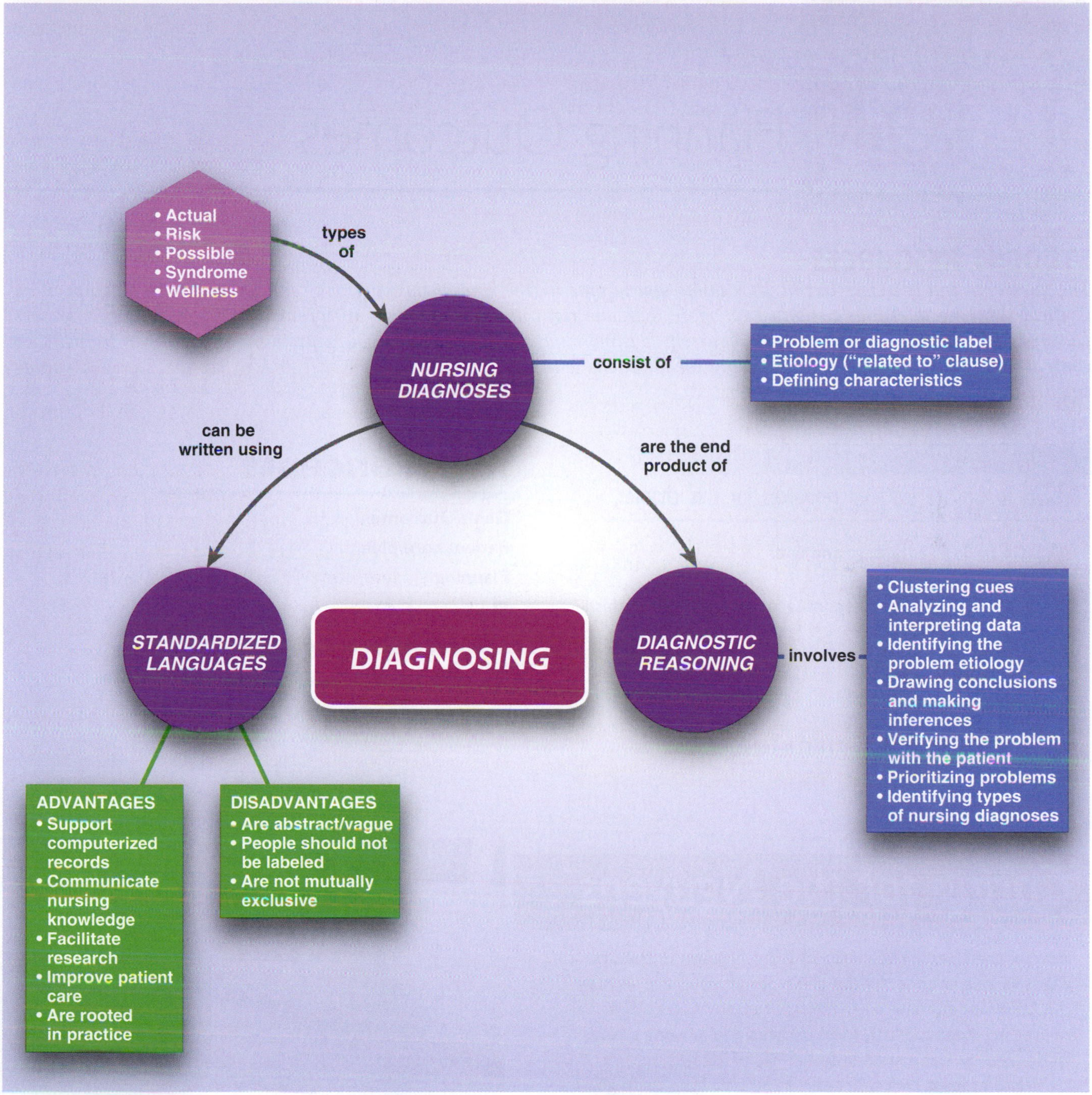

CHAPTER 5

Planning Outcomes

STUDENT RESOURCES

The questions and exercises in this book allow you to practice the kind of thinking you will use as a full-spectrum nurse. Critical-thinking questions usually have more than one right answer, so we do not provide "correct answers" for these features. Try to answer these questions yourself. It is more important to develop your nursing judgment than to just cover content. You will learn more by discussing the questions with your peers. If you are still unsure, see the Davis Advantage chapter resources for suggested responses.

To explore learning resources for this chapter,

Go to Davis Advantage and find:

Answers and Suggested Responses for all questions in this chapter
Concept Map
Knowledge Map
References and Bibliography
Lists of NOC Outcomes and NIC Interventions

Key Concepts

Goals/Outcomes
Patient care plan
Planning

Related Concepts

See the Concept Map on Davis Advantage.

Caring for the Nguyens

Review the opening scenario of Nam Nguyen in the first pages of this volume. As the clinic nurse, you have written the following nursing diagnostic statement: Overweight related to inappropriate food choices and serving size, as evidenced by body mass index (BMI) of 28.5.

Write at least two short-term and two long-term goals for Mr. Nguyen on the basis of this diagnostic statement. Remember that your goals must be realistic and consider Mr. Nguyen's other health problems.

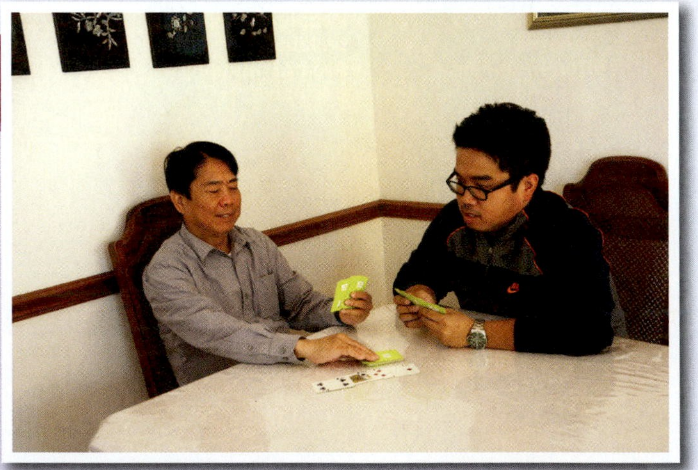

Practical Knowledge Clinical Application

Practical knowledge in the planning phase of the nursing process requires you to use a variety of care planning forms and, in some organizations, standardized language. This section includes a discharge planning form, as well as a table of Nursing Outcomes Classification (NOC) measurement scales. The remainder of the chapter consists of activities to help you apply critical thinking and clinical reasoning to the concepts you learned in Volume 1.

ASSESSMENT GUIDELINES & TOOLS

Discharge Planning Form

FOLLOW -UP CARE

When to call the doctor; symptom management (pain, nausea); plan for meeting outcomes not met during hospitalization:

Call your primary physician to find out if an insurance referral form is needed for follow-up appointments.
After discharge, you need to call for an appointment to see physician.

Clinic/Physician	Phone #	Date	Time				
______	______	______	______	or	____days	____weeks	____months
______	______	______	______	or	____days	____weeks	____months
______	______	______	______	or	____days	____weeks	____months

Plans for follow-up Labs/Tests/Treatments

Date	Time	Test/Treatment	Location	Ordered by

PERSONAL CARE

Bathing: ❑ No restrictions ❑ Other:

Treatment/Therapy/Wound or Skin Care/ Supplies Needed 2-Day Supply Sent Home ? ❑ Yes

ACTIVITY/ REHAB

❑ No restrictions ❑ Do not climb stairs ❑ Drive________ ❑ Return to Work ________
❑ Do not lift ❑ May lift up to ______lbs ❑ Weight Bearing ______# ❑ Other

DIET

❑ No restrictions ❑ Other:

Food/Drug Interactions: ❑ Coumadin ❑ MAO Inhibitors ❑ Other:

MEDICAL EQUIPMENT

❑ 2nd pair of TED hose given

COMMUNITY RESOURCES

Referral Resource	Agency	Phone #
Home IV Therapy	______	______
Home Health	______	______
Home Oxygen	______	______
Home PT/OT/Speech	______	______
Ask-A-Nurse	______	816-932-0000

Transportation Arrangements for discharge: ____

Education/Community Resources:________

Preprinted Discharge Instruction Sheet given to patient ❑ NA ❑ Yes
List Instruction Sheets:

I understand these instructions and agree with this plan of care ______________
Patient/SO Signature

MULTIDISCIPLINARY DISCHARGE INSTRUCTIONS
Shawnee Mission Medical Center
9100 W. 74th Street
Shawnee Mission, Kansas 66204

Form # 60869 Revised: 4/01 PILOT Page 1 of 2

Source: Courtesy of Shawnee Mission Health System, Shawnee Mission, KS

STANDARDIZED LANGUAGE

By combining the following scale with NOC labels and indicators, you can write observable, concrete patient goals to use in evaluating a patient's responses to care.

NOC Measurement Scales

SCALE NUMBER & DEFINITION	1*	2*	3*	4*	5*
01 Extent of Impairment of Health or Well-Being	Severely compromised	Substantially compromised	Moderately compromised	Mildly compromised	Not compromised
02 Extent of departure from an established norm or standard	Severe deviation from normal range	Substantial deviation from normal range	Moderate deviation from normal range	Mild deviation from normal range	No deviation from normal range
06	Not adequate	Slightly adequate	Moderately adequate	Substantially adequate	Totally adequate
07 Number of occurrences	10 and over	7–9	4–6	1–3	None
09 Range over which an entity extends	None	Limited	Moderate	Substantial	Extensive
11 Frequency of an affirmative and accepting perception of characteristics	Never positive	Rarely positive	Sometimes positive	Often positive	Consistently positive
12 Extent of intensity	Very weak	Weak	Moderate	Strong	Very strong
13 Frequency of making clear by report or behavior	Never demonstrated	Rarely demonstrated	Sometimes demonstrated	Often demonstrated	Consistently demonstrated
14 Extent of a negative or adverse state or response	Severe	Substantial	Moderate	Mild	None
17 Extent of proximity to a desired state	Poor	Fair	Good	Very good	Excellent
18 Extent of perception of positive expectations	Not at all satisfied	Somewhat satisfied	Moderately satisfied	Very satisfied	Completely satisfied
19 Frequency of making clear by report or behavior	Consistently demonstrated	Often demonstrated	Sometimes demonstrated	Rarely demonstrated	Never demonstrated
20 Extent of cognitive information that is understood	No knowledge	Limited knowledge	Moderate knowledge	Substantial knowledge	Extensive knowledge

Source: Moorhead, S., Swanson, E. Johnson, M., & Maas, M.: *Nursing Outcomes Classification (NOC)*, ed. 6. St. Louis, MO, C.V. Mosby, 2018. p. 12. Used with permission.
*The scores (1 through 5) are constructed so that 5 is usually the most desirable, and 1 is the least desirable condition relative to the outcome.

CLINICALJUDGMENT

Applying the Full-Spectrum Nursing Model

PATIENT SITUATION

Ivan Benjamin has just been admitted to an orthopedic unit after an automobile accident. He was the driver of the vehicle. Mr. Benjamin is 80 years old and has been living at home. His pre-existing comorbidities are type 2 diabetes and osteoarthritis. He has casts and traction on both legs and a cast on one arm. He is receiving morphine sulfate intravenously via a PCA (patient-controlled analgesia) pump. Imagine that you are an orthopedic nurse and must plan care for Mr. Benjamin. The admitting nurse wrote the following nursing diagnoses and goals on the plan of care:

NURSING DIAGNOSES	GOALS/EXPECTED OUTCOMES
1. Acute Pain secondary to musculoskeletal trauma (arms, legs, body) and muscle spasm	▪ Demonstrates correct use of PCA pump ▪ Rates pain not higher than 4 on a scale of 1 to 10 at all times
2. Risk for Impaired Peripheral Neurovascular Function secondary to casts/traction	▪ Peripheral pulses palpable ▪ Fingers and toes warm ▪ Fingers and toes without pallor or cyanosis ▪ No edema of fingers and toes ▪ Capillary refill less than 3 seconds

THINKING

1. *Theoretical Knowledge:* What general *theoretical knowledge* will you need to care for this patient? Identify just the topics in about 150 words.

2. *Critical Thinking (Considering Alternatives):* Older adults are especially sensitive to certain medications, including morphine sulfate. What is one thing you could do to ensure Mr. Benjamin's safety while managing his acute pain?

3. *Critical Thinking (Inquiry):* List at least two more things you need to know about Mr. Benjamin to begin his discharge planning.

DOING

4. *Practical Knowledge:* What general practical knowledge will you need? What would you do to obtain this knowledge?

5. *Nursing Process:*

   a. *Diagnosis:* What is another nursing diagnosis you might want to assess for Mr. Benjamin?

   b. *Planning Goals:* On the care plan, rewrite the goals/expected outcomes for Acute Pain so that they will have all the required components. Assume that today's date is January 4.

CARING

6. *Self-Knowledge:* What beliefs, values, biases, or emotional responses might interfere with your ability to provide the best care to Mr. Benjamin?

CONTEXT

7. Think critically about the context. Is there anything in this situation that you have seen before? Identify any familiar elements. For example, you may have an older male relative, even if you have never cared for an 80-year-old patient before.

Critical Thinking and Clinical Judgment

1. Merle Quinn is visiting a family planning clinic, where she has just been informed that she is 6 weeks pregnant. She looks worried and makes the following statements: "This is a shock. I've just started a new business, and I need to work 7 days a week to make it go. . . . I don't know if I am ready to be a mother. . . ." Her husband agrees: "I just don't see how we can afford this. We don't even have any insurance now."

   "Still," Mrs. Quinn says, "I don't see how I could deal with having an abortion. My parents would be devastated. I'm sure they'd never speak to me again." Her husband says, "Not to speak of the fact that the Church forbids it. It would be a sin."

   A week later, Mrs. Quinn calls the clinic in tears. She says she has not been able to eat or sleep and that she does not know what to do about her pregnancy. "I don't want this baby, but I can't bring myself to have an abortion." You diagnose her with Decisional Conflict related to unexpected/unwanted pregnancy, possibly assuming that she believes that abortion is her only alternative, as evidenced by statements of indecision, tearfulness, and inability to sleep. You make an appointment to see Mr. and Mrs. Quinn that same day. Imagine that you are writing the care plan for the Quinns.

   a. Analyze your assumptions. What values and beliefs do you have that may influence the goals you write for the Quinns? Specifically, how could your values affect the goals you write?

   b. Develop a short-term goal to address the problem clause of this nursing diagnosis. The goal should be one you expect the Quinns to be able to achieve during their appointment that same day.

   c. You also write a goal stating: "By the end of this visit, clients will verbalize and demonstrate decreased anxiety and stress." Which part of the nursing diagnosis does this goal address?

   d. The NOC standardized outcomes linked to the diagnosis of Decisional Conflict are as follows (definitions are given):
      Decision Making: Ability to choose between two or more alternatives
      Information Processing: Ability to acquire, organize, and use information
      Participation: Health Care Decisions: Personal involvement in selecting and evaluating health care options
      Which of those outcomes is most important for the Quinns to achieve *today*? Why?

   e. Now imagine that you have written the following individualized goals/outcomes for today's visit with the Quinns:
      By the end of this visit, clients will:
      1. Verbalize and demonstrate decreased anxiety and stress.
      2. Verbalize awareness that they have options for coping with whatever decision they make about the pregnancy.
      3. Discuss with the nurse options for continuing or terminating the pregnancy.
      4. Verbalize intent to discuss their feelings with family (i.e., their parents).
      5. Verbalize intent to discuss feelings with a member of the clergy.
      6. Decide whether to continue the pregnancy.
         - Why is outcome 2 so important?
         - What would you have had to assume to write outcome 4?
         - What would you have had to assume to write outcome 5?
         - Which of the outcomes is/are probably *not* appropriate for today's visit? Why?

2. For each of the following concepts, use critical thinking to describe how or why it is important to nursing, patient care, or the process of planning care. Note that these are *not* to be merely definitions.

Discharge planning

A written, individualized nursing care plan

Standardized care-planning documents (e.g., protocols)

Critical pathways

Computerized care planning

Goals (expected outcomes)

Short-term goals

Long-term goals

Action verbs (in goals)

Essential patient goals

The Nursing Outcomes Classification (NOC)

Aggregate goals

Wellness goals

Concrete, specific goal/outcome statements (as opposed to vague statements)

What Are the Main Points in This Chapter?

- During the planning outcomes phase, you will derive goals/expected outcomes from identified nursing diagnoses.
- Goals/expected outcomes (1) suggest nursing interventions, (2) serve as criteria for use in the evaluation step of the nursing process, and (3) provide motivation for patients and nurses.
- To ensure continuity of care, you should begin discharge planning with the initial patient assessment.
    - Discharge planning is especially important for older adults and patients with complex needs.
- A holistic, individualized patient care plan contains information needed to address (1) basic needs and activities of daily living (ADLs), (2) medical and collaborative therapies, (3) nursing diagnoses and collaborative problems, and (4) special teaching and/or discharge needs.
- Ideally, a care plan consists of a combination of standardized and individualized goals and interventions.
- Standardized approaches to care planning include institutional policies and procedures, protocols, unit standards of care, standardized care plans, critical pathways, and integrated plans of care (IPOCs).
- Computer-assisted care planning helps ensure that the nurse considers a variety of interventions and does not overlook common and important interventions; it reduces the time spent on paperwork.
- Nursing-sensitive goals (expected outcomes, predicted outcomes, desired outcomes) describe the changes in patient health status that are intended to result from and can be influenced by nursing interventions.
- Goals for collaborative problems are usually not nursing sensitive and should not be included on a nursing care plan.
- A goal statement should include a subject, an action verb, a performance criterion, a target time, and special conditions, if needed.
- For every nursing diagnosis, you must state one "essential" goal—one that, if achieved, would demonstrate problem resolution or improvement.
- Among the American Nurses Association (ANA)–recognized standardized vocabularies/taxonomies for describing patient outcomes are NOC, the Omaha System, and the Clinical Care Classification System.
- Goals should be concrete, specific, and observable; they should be valued by the patient/family; and they should not conflict with the medical treatment plan.

Knowledge Map

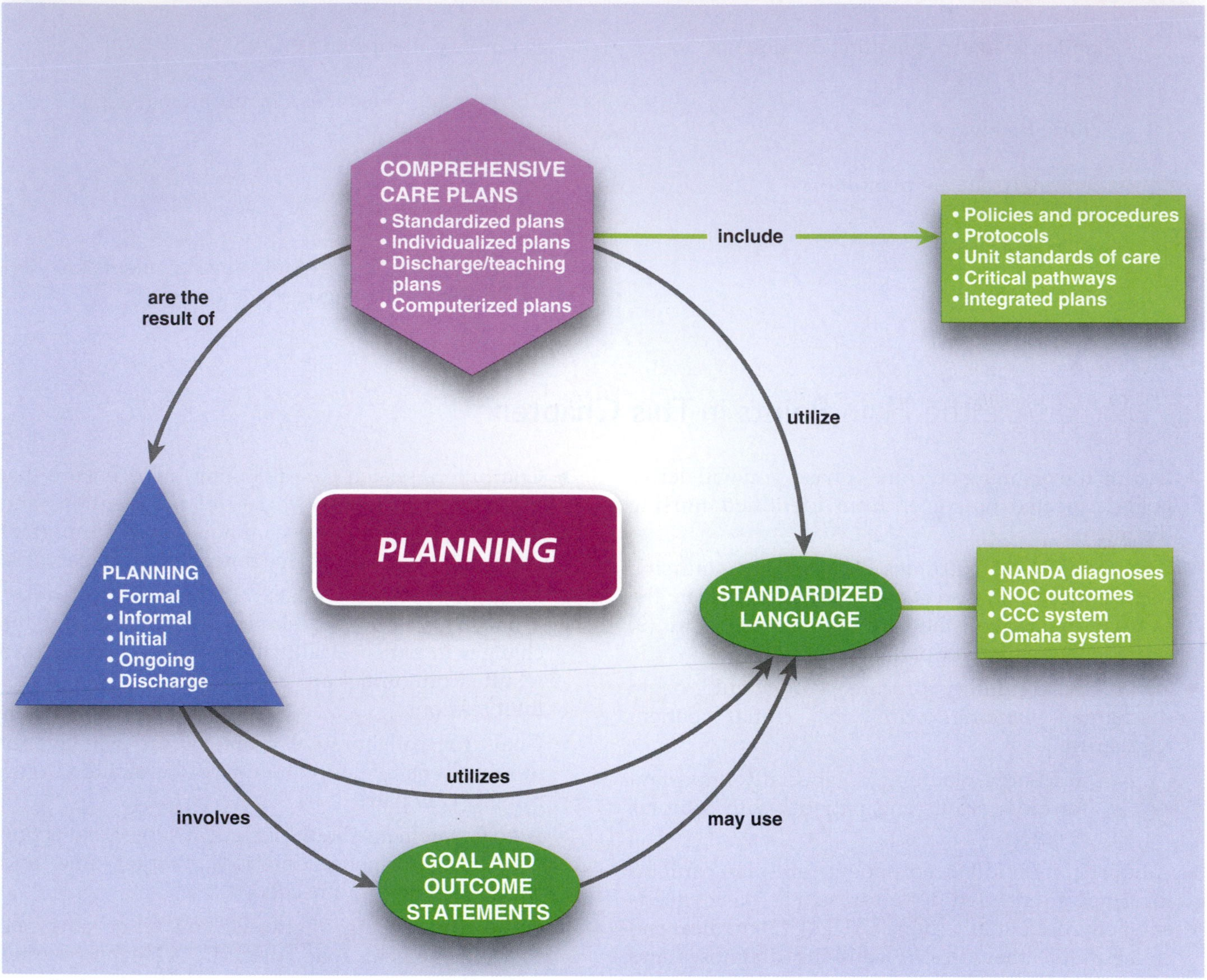

CHAPTER 6

Planning Interventions

STUDENT RESOURCES

The questions and exercises in this book allow you to practice the kind of thinking you will use as a full-spectrum nurse. Critical-thinking questions usually have more than one right answer, so we do not provide "correct answers" for these features. Try to answer these questions yourself. It is more important to develop your nursing judgment than to just cover content. You will learn by discussing the questions with your peers. If you are still unsure, see the Davis Advantage chapter resources for suggested responses.

To explore learning resources for this chapter,

Go to Davis Advantage and find:

Answers and Suggested Responses for all questions in this chapter
Concept Map
Knowledge Map
References and Bibliography
List of NOC Outcomes and NIC Interventions

Key Concepts

Evidence-based practice
Nursing interventions

Related Concepts

See the Concept Map on Davis Advantage.

Caring for the Nguyens

Recall that you have written the following nursing diagnosis for Mr. Nguyen:

Overweight related to inappropriate food choices and serving size, as evidenced by body mass index (BMI) of 28.5.

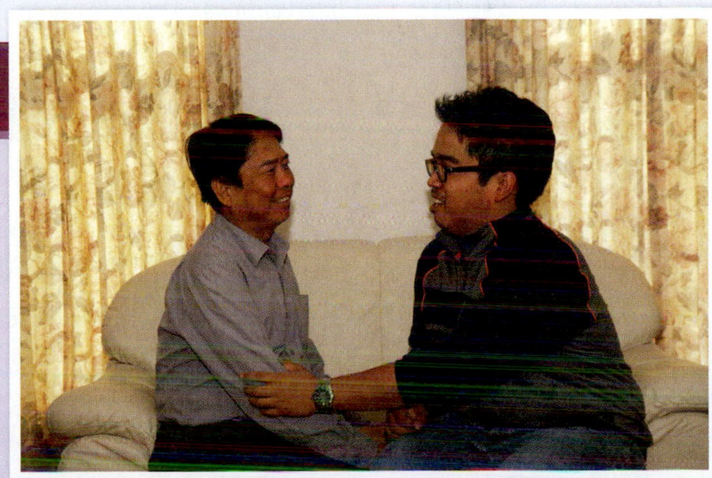

(Continued)

Caring for the Nguyens (continued)

A. On the basis of the outcomes you wrote in Chapter 5, Planning Outcomes, identify four possible interventions to address the diagnosis and outcomes.

B. Review the interventions, and identify two that would be most appropriate for Mr. Nguyen given all of the information you have about his health status.

C. Write a nursing prescription for each of the two interventions you identified above.

CLINICALJUDGMENT

Applying the Full-Spectrum Nursing Model

PATIENT SITUATION

Mr. Sanborn is a 65-year-old man who has come to the clinic for a complete physical checkup. He has no health complaints, and his physical examination results are negative for any problems except for a few minor changes associated with aging. During the interview, he tells you that he has had a same-sex partner for 5 years. On further questioning, he reveals that he has had numerous sex partners during his lifetime. He says, "I was wondering if I should be tested for HIV" and "Mike, that's my partner, says I ought to get a flu shot and maybe a hepatitis shot. What do you think?"

THINKING

1. *Theoretical Knowledge:* What principles and concepts do you need to know to help Mr. Sanborn today?

2. *Inquiry:* Which of those do you already know enough about, and which ones will you have to study further?

DOING

3. *Practical Knowledge:* What psychomotor and communication skills will you need to help Mr. Sanborn?

4. *Nursing Process (Assessment):* What further data do you need about Mr. Sanborn's sexual activity?

5. *Nursing Process (Planning Interventions):* What is one important nursing intervention for today?

CARING

6. *Self-Knowledge:* How do you feel about same-sex relationships? Would you be able to care for Mr. Sanborn effectively?

7. *Ethical Knowledge:* What does the American Nurses Association (ANA, 2015b) *Code of Ethics for Nurses* say about relationships to patients and the nature of patient health problems? For access to the *Code of Ethics for Nurses,*

Go to http://www.nursingworld.org/MainMenuCategories/EthicsStandards/CodeofEthicsforNurses/Code-of-Ethics-For-Nurses.html

Critical Thinking and Clinical Judgment

1. Recall the Quinns from Chapter 5. Merle Quinn is visiting a family planning clinic, where she has just been informed that she is 6 weeks pregnant. She looks worried and makes the following statements: "This is a shock. I've just started a new business and I need to work 7 days a week to make it go. . . . I don't know if I am ready to be a mother. . . ." Her husband agrees: "I just don't see how we can afford this. We don't have any insurance now."

"Still," Mrs. Quinn says, "I don't see how I could deal with having an abortion. My parents would be devastated. I'm sure they'd never speak to me again." Her husband says, "Not to speak of the fact that the Church forbids it. It would be a sin."

A week later, Mrs. Quinn calls the clinic in tears. She says she has not been able to eat or sleep and that she does not know what to do about her pregnancy. "I don't want this baby, but I can't bring myself to have an abortion." The nurse diagnoses Decisional Conflict related to this unexpected/unwanted pregnancy and inability to accept the only perceived alternative (abortion), as evidenced by statements of indecision, tearfulness, and inability to sleep. You make an appointment to see Mr. and Mrs. Quinn that same day. Imagine that you are writing the care plan for the Quinns.

a. *Critical Thinking and Self-Knowledge (Analyzing Assumptions):* To set aside your assumptions and care for the Quinns, you will need to focus on the Quinns' immediate problem, Decisional Conflict, rather than thinking about what they "ought" to do. Remember, the nurse's role is not to make decisions for clients but to provide information, clarification, and support.

- What questions must you ask in this case to analyze your assumptions?
- What are the answers to those questions?

b. *Critical Thinking (Contextual Awareness) and Knowledge of Patient Situation (Context):*

- What is going on in the Quinns' lives that may affect your choice of interventions?
- What is going on with Mrs. Quinn's health status that may affect your choice of interventions?

Now, imagine that you have written the following care plan for today's visit with the Quinns:

OUTCOMES	INTERVENTIONS
Nursing Outcomes Classification (NOC) Decision Making Participation: Health Care Decisions	**Nursing Interventions Classification (NIC)** Decision Making Support Family Planning: Contraception Family Planning: Unplanned Pregnancy
Individualized Goals By the end of this visit, patients will: 1. Verbalize and demonstrate decreased anxiety and stress. 2. Verbalize awareness that they have options for coping with whatever decision they make about the pregnancy. 3. Discuss with the nurse options for continuing or terminating the pregnancy. 4. Verbalize intent to discuss their feelings with family (i.e., their parents). 5. Verbalize intent to discuss feelings with a member of the clergy.	**Computer-Generated Nursing Activities** 1. Offer emotional support. 2. Inform patient(s) of alternative views or solutions. 3. Help to identify advantages and disadvantages of each alternative. 4. Encourage patient(s) to explore options, including termination, keeping the infant, or adoption. 5. Provide information as requested by patient(s). 6. Serve as liaison between patient and family. 7. Assist in identifying support system. 8. Refer to community agency for counseling, if needed (e.g., family-planning clinic). 9. Discuss factors related to unplanned pregnancy (e.g., no use or misuse of contraceptives). 10. Teach and clarify misinformation about contraceptive use. 11. Teach regarding preparation and procedures. 12. Monitor for complications of procedure.

c. *Nursing Process:* Which NIC intervention, on the basis of its label alone, does *not* appear to be relevant to producing the stated goals. (Note that it also does not appear that it would relieve the problem, reduce the etiology, or relieve Mrs. Quinn's symptoms of anxiety and distress.)

d. *Nursing Process:* Which of the computer-generated nursing activities is/are *not* appropriate for today's visit with the Quinns?

e. *Nursing Process:* For which individualized outcome is there apparently *not* a computer-generated nursing activity?

f. *Critical Thinking:* Look at nursing activity 6 ("Serve as liaison between patient and family"). What critical-thinking questions should you ask about that intervention/activity with regard to:
- Contextual awareness?
- Credible sources?
- Reflecting skeptically?

g. *Critical Thinking (Prioritizing):* Which of the computer-generated nursing activities will you probably need to do first today?

h. *Critical Thinking (Prioritizing):* Look at computer-generated nursing activities 2, 3, and 4. Which of these is most important to do today? Which one could you encourage the Quinns to do during the next week or so? Why?

i. *Nursing Process (Planning Interventions):* What would you need to do to nursing activity 1 to turn it into a nursing order that another nurse could use to care for the Quinns?

j. *Nursing Process (Assessment):* What questions would you need to ask to individualize nursing activity 1 for the Quinns' care plan?

2. For each of the following concepts, use critical thinking to describe how or why it is important to nursing, patient care, or the process of planning interventions. Note that these are *not* to be merely definitions.

Nursing interventions/strategies/activities/actions

Individualized interventions

Independent interventions

Collaborative interventions

Dependent interventions

Theories

Research

Evidence-based practice

The patient's problem status

The nursing diagnosis etiology

Client outcomes

Critical thinking (e.g., contextual awareness, reflecting skeptically)

Computerized care planning program

Standardized intervention vocabularies

Nursing Interventions Classification (NIC)

Wellness interventions

Spiritual care interventions

Nursing orders

What Are the Main Points in This Chapter?

- Nursing interventions are treatments that nurses perform (1) in response to nursing diagnoses and (2) for the purpose of achieving client outcomes.
- Nursing interventions include such activities as teaching, counseling and emotional support, referral, physical care, and environmental management.
- Independent interventions are nurse-initiated treatments—those that nurses perform or delegate on the basis of their knowledge and skills.
- Nursing interventions are performed for the purpose of assessing health status, preventing and treating disease/illness, and promoting health.
- The registered nurse (RN) is responsible for choosing interventions and writing nursing orders; however, the RN can delegate actual performance of some interventions to unlicensed assistive personnel (UAP) and licensed practical nurses or licensed vocational nurses (LPNs/LVNs).
- Theories influence your perspective: What you notice and identify as a problem, as well as how you define a problem, more or less determines your choice of interventions.
- Ideally, a nursing intervention should have a sound basis in research.
- When generating interventions, nurses use critical-thinking skills, such as making interdisciplinary connections, predicting, generalizing, explaining, and making therapeutic judgments.
- The ANA has approved the following three standardized vocabularies for nursing interventions: (1) the Nursing Interventions Classification (NIC), (2) the Omaha System (developed for community health nursing), and (3) the Clinical Care Classification (CCC).
- Standardized vocabularies are especially useful in agencies that have computerized care planning systems.
- Some standardized vocabularies include terminology for describing wellness interventions and spiritual interventions.
- Nursing orders, written on the nursing care plan, consist of the detailed instructions for performing nursing interventions.

Knowledge Map

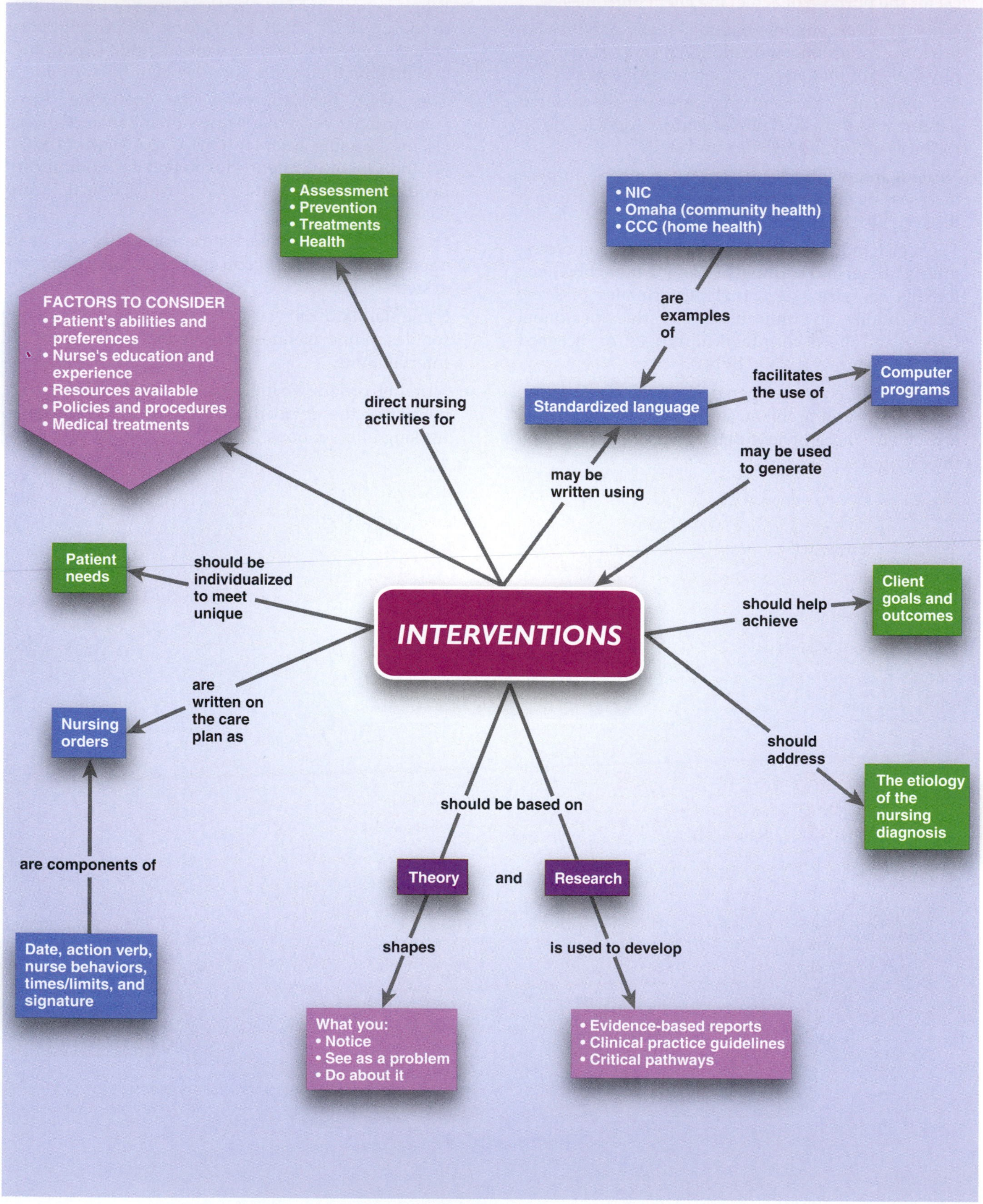

CHAPTER 7

Implementation & Evaluation

STUDENT RESOURCES

The questions and exercises in this book allow you to practice the kind of thinking you will use as a full-spectrum nurse. Critical-thinking questions usually have more than one correct answer, so we do not provide "correct answers" for these features. Try to answer these questions yourself. It is more important to develop your nursing judgment than to just cover content. You will learn by discussing the questions with your peers. If you are still unsure, see the Davis Advantage chapter resources for suggested responses.

To explore learning resources for this chapter,

Go to Davis Advantage and find:

Answers and Suggested Responses for all questions in this chapter
Concept Map
Knowledge Map
References and Bibliography
Lists of NOC Outcomes and NIC Interventions

Key Concepts

Evaluation
Implementation
Quality improvement

Related Concepts

See the Concept Map on Davis Advantage.

Caring for the Nguyens

The following information is recorded on Mr. Nguyen's clinic health record:

9/1/2020 Imbalanced Nutrition: More Than Body Requirements related to inappropriate food choices and serving size, as evidenced by BMI of 28.5
Outcome: Will lose 5 lb by 10/15/2020
Interventions:

- Collect 3-day nutrition history 9/2/2020 through 9/4/2020.

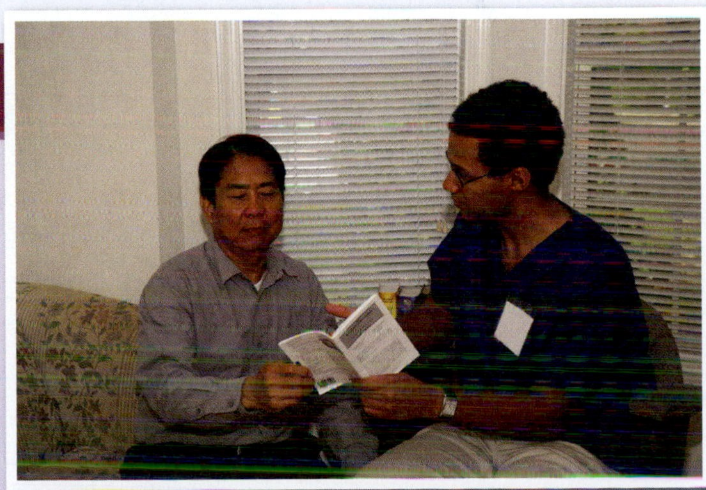

(Continued)

Caring for the Nguyens (continued)

- Have patient meet with clinic nurse for diet review and nutrition instruction 9/8/2020.
- Provide sample meal plans at 9/8/2020 instruction.
- Phone patient 9/22/2020 to discuss nutrition questions and review progress.
- Have patient return to clinic 10/15/2020 for follow-up visit.

A. What must you do before implementing each nursing intervention?

B. Identify at least two strategies that will help promote Mr. Nguyen's participation in and adherence to the plan.

C. How will you determine whether Mr. Nguyen has met his goal?

Practical Knowledge: Clinical Application

When implementing and evaluating care, you will need to make good decisions about administering and delegating care. In this section, you will find forms to help you delegate, implement, and evaluate patient care.

Delegation Decision-Making Grid

Elements for review		**Client A**	**Client B**	**Client C**	**Client D**
Activity/Task Level of client stability	Describe activity/task: Score the client's level of stability: **Client condition:** 0 – Is chronic/stable/predictable 1 – Has minimal potential for change 2 – Has moderate potential for change 3 – Has unstable/acute/strong potential for change				
Level of NAP competence	Score the NAP competence in completing delegated nursing care activities in the defined client population: **NAP is:** 0 – Expert in activities to be delegated, in defined population 1 – Experienced in activities to be delegated, in defined population 2 – Experienced in activities but not in defined population 3 – Novice in performing activities and in defined population				
Level of licensed nurse competence	Score the licensed nurse's competence in relation to both knowledge of providing nursing care to a defined population and competence in implementation of the delegation process: 0 – Expert in the knowledge of nursing needs/activities of defined client population *and* expert in the delegation process 1 – Either expert in knowledge of needs/activities of defined client population and competent in delegation *or* experienced in the needs/activities of defined client population and expert in the delegation process 2 – Experienced in knowledge of needs/activities of defined client population *and* competent in the delegation process 3 – Either experienced in knowledge of needs/activities of defined client population *or* competent in the delegation process 4 – Novice in knowledge of defined population *and* novice in delegation				
Potential for harm	Score the potential level of risk the nursing care activity has for the client *(risk is probability of [the client] suffering harm):* 0 – None 1 – Low 2 – Medium 3 – High				
Frequency	Score based on how often the NAP has performed the specific nursing care activity: 0 – Performed at least daily 1 – Performed at least weekly 2 – Performed at least monthly 3 – Performed less than monthly 4 – Never performed				
Level of decision making	Score the decision-making needed, related to the specific nursing care activity, client (both cognitive and physical status) and client situation: 0 – Does not require decision making 1 – Minimal level of decision making 2 – Moderate level of decision making 3 – High level of decision making				
Ability for self care	Score the client's level of assistance needed for self-care activities: 0 – No assistance 1 – Limited assistance 2 – Extensive assistance 3 – Total care or constant attendance				
Total Score					
Scoring: A low score on the grid suggests that an activity can be safely delegated. For example if a client's stability is ranked 3 (unstable) and the level of NAP competence is also 3 (novice in the activity), then you probably should *not* delegate to that NAP. Each agency should establish a policy regarding the individual and/or total scores to be considered acceptable for delegating.					
Source: Used by permission from the National Council of State Boards of Nursing (NCSBN), Chicago, IL (1997). Retrieved February 1, 2008, from the NCSBN web site (www.ncsbn.org)					

Evaluation Checklist

Evaluation Checklist

Instructions: Check the appropriate response and follow the associated instructions

Assessment Review

1. Were the assessment data complete and accurate?
   __ YES. No action.
   __ NO. Reassess client. Record the new data. Change care plan as indicated
2. Have all data been validated, as needed?
   __ YES. No action.
   __ NO. Validate with client (by interview and physical examination), significant others, or other professionals. Record validation (or failure to validate). Change care plan as indicated.
3. Have new data become available that require changes in the plan (e.g., a different problem etiology, new goals/ outcomes, new medical orders)?
   __ NO. No action.
   __ YES. Record the new data in the progress notes; redefine problem, goals, nursing orders, as needed.
4. Has the patient's condition changed?
   __ NO. No action.
   __ YES. Record data about present health status. Change care plan as indicated.

→ ***Move to a review of the diagnosis step.*** ←

Diagnosis Review

1. Is the diagnosis relevant and related to the data?
   __ YES. No action.
   __ NO. Revise the diagnosis.
2. Is the diagnosis well supported by the data?
   __ YES. No action.
   __ NO. Collect more data. Support or revise diagnosis.
3. Has the problem status changed (actual, potential, possible)?
   __ NO. No action.
   __ YES. Restate the problem.
4. Is the diagnosis stated clearly?
   __ YES. No action.
   __ NO. Revise the diagnostic statement.
5. Does the etiology correctly reflect the factors contributing to the problem?
   __ YES. No action.
   __ NO. Revise the etiology.
6. Is the problem one that can be treated primarily by nursing actions?
   __ YES. No action.
   __ NO. Label as collaborative and consult appropriate health professional.
7. Is the diagnosis specific and individualized to the patient?
   __ YES. No action.
   __ NO. Revise diagnosis. Revise outcomes and nursing orders as suggested by the new nursing diagnosis.
8. Does the problem (diagnosis) still exist?
   __ YES. No action.
   __ NO. Delete diagnosis and related outcomes and nursing orders.

→ ***Proceed to a review of client goals.*** ←

Planning Review: Outcomes

1. Have nursing diagnoses been added or revised?
   __ NO. No action.
   __ YES. Write new outcomes.
2. Are the outcomes realistic in terms of patient abilities and agency resources?
   __ YES. No action.
   __ NO. Revise outcomes.
3. Was sufficient time allowed for outcome achievement?
   __ YES. No action.
   __ NO. Revise time frame.
4. Do the outcomes address all aspects of the client's problem?
   __ YES. No action.
   __ NO. Write additional outcomes.

Evaluation Checklist *(continued)*

5. Do the expected outcomes, as written, demonstrate resolution of the problem specified in the nursing diagnosis?
   __ YES. No action. __ NO. Revise outcomes.
6. Have client priorities changed, or has the focus of care changed?
   __ NO. No action. __ YES. Revise outcomes.
7. Is the client in agreement with the goals?
   __ YES. No action. __ NO. Get client input. Write outcomes valued by the client.

→ ***Proceed to a review of nursing orders.*** ←

Planning Review: Nursing Orders

1. Have nursing diagnoses or outcomes been added or revised in previous review steps?
   __ NO. No action. __ YES. Write new nursing orders.
2. Are the nursing orders clearly related to the stated patient outcomes?
   __ YES. No action. __ NO. Revise or develop new nursing orders.
3. Is the rationale sufficient to justify the use of the nursing order?
   __ YES. No action. __ NO. Revise or develop new nursing orders.
4. Are the nursing orders unclear or vague, so that other staff may have had questions about how to implement them?
   __ NO. No action. __ YES. Revise nursing orders. Add details to make more specific or individualized to the patient.
5. Do the nursing orders include instructions for timing of the activities?
   __ YES. No action. __ NO. Revise nursing orders: add times, schedules.
6. Was an order clearly and obviously ineffective?
   __ NO. No action. __ YES. Delete it.
7. Are the orders realistic in terms of staff and other resources?
   __ YES. No action. __ NO. Revise orders or obtain resources.
8. Have new resources become available that might enable you to change the goals or nursing orders?
   __ NO. No action. __ YES. Write new goals or nursing orders reflecting the new capabilities.
9. Do the nursing orders address all aspects of the client's health goals?
   __ YES. No action. __ NO. Add new nursing orders.

→ ***Proceed to a review of implementation step*** ←

Implementation Review

1. Did the nurse [or NAP] get client input at each step in developing and implementing the plan?
   __ YES. No action. __ NO. Obtain client input, revise plan and implementation as needed. [Coach NAP or role model, as needed.]
2. Were the nursing interventions acceptable to the patient?
   __ YES. No action. __ NO. Consult patient; change nursing orders or implementation approach.
3. Did the nurse [NAP] prepare the patient for implementation of the nursing order (e.g., explain what the patient should expect or do)?
   __ YES. No action. __ NO. Continue same plan, but prepare patient before implementing. Reevaluate.
4. Did the nurse [NAP] have adequate knowledge and skills to perform techniques and procedures correctly?
   __ YES. No action. __ NO. Continue same plan. Have someone else implement or help the nurse [or NAP] to acquire the needed knowledge or skills. If neither of these is possible, delete nursing order.

(continued)

5. Did client or family comply with the therapeutic regimen? Were self-care activities performed correctly?
   — YES. No action.
   — NO. Reassess motivation, knowledge, and resources. Add outcomes and nursing orders aimed at teaching, motivating, and supporting, patient in carrying out the regimen. Set time for reevaluation.
6. Did other staff members follow the nursing orders?
   — YES. No action.
   — NO. Implement the omitted nursing orders or ensure that others will do so. Set time for reevaluation. Find out why order was not carried out.
7. Was the plan of care implemented in a manner that communicated caring?
   — YES. No action.
   — NO. This is a problem that must be addressed by personal and staff development.

After making the necessary revisions to the care plan, implement the new plan and begin the nursing cycle again.

Source: Wilkinson, J. (2011). *Nursing process and critical thinking* (5th ed.). Upper Saddle River, NJ: Prentice Hall, pp. 325–327.

CLINICALJUDGMENT
Applying the Full-Spectrum Nursing Model

PATIENT SITUATION

Recall Jeannette Wu from Meet Your Patient in Volume 1. She is a very thin, 80-year-old woman who is in the hospital after fracturing her hip. Her hip was repaired 4 days ago, but because of her overall fragile health and some postsurgery confusion, her recovery is slower than expected. One of her nursing diagnoses is bathing/hygiene deficit related to weakness, pain, confusion, and decreased mobility. Her nursing orders (Nursing Intervention Classification [NIC]) include self-care assistance: bathing/hygiene/toileting.

As the nurse is helping an unlicensed assistive personnel (UAP) with Mrs. Wu's bath, she notices a reddened area on Mrs. Wu's sacrum. Realizing that this may be the beginning of a pressure injury, the nurse observes closely and notes a small skin excoriation (abrasion) in the area. She repositions Mrs. Wu to prevent further pressure on her sacrum. After finishing the bath, the nurse records her findings and enters on Mrs. Wu's care plan the nursing diagnosis "skin integrity alteration related to mechanical forces (e.g., shearing forces, pressure, physical mobility), alteration in skin turgor, and pressure over bony prominences." She writes appropriate nursing orders, including an order to observe skin over bony prominences every 4 hours, and then delegates to the UAP the task of turning and repositioning Mrs. Wu every 2 hours. The nurse also places Mrs. Wu on a pressure-relief mattress and obtains a foam cushion for her wheelchair.

THINKING

1. *Theoretical Knowledge:*
   a. What facts and principles do you already know about the causes of pressure injuries?
   b. Do you have enough information to provide interventions for Mrs. Wu's actual skin integrity alteration? If not, what do you still need to find out?
2. *Critical Thinking (Inquiry):* What resource would be best to use to find out exactly what is meant by Mrs. Wu's diagnosis of bathing/hygiene deficit? Why?

DOING

3. *Practical Knowledge:* What do you know about positioning patients? How would you explain to the UAP about how to position Mrs. Wu "to prevent further pressure on her sacrum"?

4. *Nursing Process (Evaluation):*

   a. To evaluate Mrs. Wu's skin integrity problem, what reassessments would you make?

   b. To evaluate Mrs. Wu's bathing/hygiene problem, what reassessments would you make? Who can or should make them? How often, or when, would you reassess?

CARING

5. *Self-Knowledge:* How comfortable would you be in caring for Mrs. Wu, who is a frail older adult? What is one problem that might arise that is not described in the scenario?

Critical Thinking and Clinical Judgment

1. You are working a 12-hour shift (1900 to 0700) on a medical unit at a local hospital. You will be caring for six adult patients. Make a list of the theoretical and practical knowledge you need about the patients to begin organizing your work for the shift. You may not yet have enough experience to make a complete list, but speculate about the kinds of information you think you might need. For example, to organize your work, you will need to know whether you have a UAP or a licensed vocational nurse/licensed practical nurse (LVN/LPN) to assist you or whether you are providing total care for the patients.

2. Create a form for organizing your work. You will need to use a separate sheet of paper for this. Be sure it has space for at least six patients. You might begin by making a column for each patient's name and age, for example. Be sure to leave enough room to write the necessary information. For example, you will need more room to write the patients' tests and treatments than for writing in age and gender.

3. Alma Newport, who is 80 years old, has diabetes, severe arthritis, and mild dementia secondary to Alzheimer's disease. She lives alone. She refuses to consider an assisted living facility or nursing home, although her primary provider and her children, who live out of town, believe it would be safer for her to do so. On more than one occasion, she has forgotten to turn off a stove burner while cooking, burning the contents of the pan and smoking up the house.

   A home health nurse visits Mrs. Newport once a week. The physician wants Mrs. Newport to check and record her blood sugar levels before each meal. When the nurse asks her about it, Mrs. Newport says her blood sugar level is "OK" and shows the nurse the record she has kept, on which she has recorded many extremely low readings (e.g., 17, 20, 80, 24, 17 mg/dL). When the nurse checks Mrs. Newport's blood sugar, she obtains a reading of 210 mg/dL. After calibrating the glucose meter, the nurse writes the following care plan:

   Nursing Diagnosis:
   Deficient Knowledge related to cognitive deficits secondary to dementia
   Desired Outcomes:
   Mrs. Newport will demonstrate correct method for checking her blood sugar by next visit.
   Mrs. Newport will obtain correct readings.
   Nursing Orders:
   Teach correct method of fingerstick and checking blood glucose.
   Evaluate patient's technique at each visit.

   Over the next few weeks, the home health nurse checks Mrs. Newport's log and fingerstick method at each visit. The logs continue to show low readings, and Mrs. Newport remains unable to perform a fingerstick blood glucose test correctly in spite of repeated demonstrations.

   a. Evaluate Mrs. Newport's progress. Has she met, partially met, or not met the desired outcome?

   b. What possible reasons may account for your evaluation (of Mrs. Newport's outcome status)?
   Hints:
   (1) Use your theoretical knowledge and personal experience with regard to physical changes that occur with aging.
   (2) Use the data you have about Mrs. Newport.
   (3) Use your practical knowledge about nursing diagnoses.

4. A UAP is helping a patient with a shower when her pager goes off. After ensuring the patient's safety, the UAP goes into the hallway and answers her page. You observe that the UAP is still wearing her gloves. How would you handle this situation?

5. For each of the following concepts, use critical thinking to describe how or why it is important to nursing, patient care, or the processes of implementing and evaluating. Note that these are *not* to be merely definitions.

Overlapping (of implementation and other nursing process steps)

Preparing for implementation

Client participation and adherence

Coordination of care

Delegation of care

The "five rights" of delegation

Supervision

Reflecting critically about implementation

Evaluation

Outcomes evaluation

Evaluative statements

Quality assurance programs

What Are the Main Points in This Chapter?

- Implementation is the nursing process phase in which you perform or delegate the nursing activities that were planned in preceding steps.
- Before performing interventions, you should organize supplies and equipment and ensure the client's readiness.
- While implementing care, you will continue to make assessments and evaluate client responses.
- Collaboration and coordination of care are important nursing functions.
- Delegation is the transfer of responsibility for an action while retaining the accountability for the outcome—this implies that you must supervise those to whom you delegate care.
- The "five rights" of delegation are right task, right circumstance, right person, right direction/communication, and right supervision.
- The final activity in the implementation step is documentation of the care provided. Documenting client responses is actually a part of the evaluation phase; however, you will document both at the same time, often in the same note.
- Evaluation is the final step of the nursing process; it is a planned, ongoing, systematic activity in which you use predetermined standards and criteria to make judgments about (1) patient progress toward health goals; (2) the effectiveness of the nursing care plan; and (3) the overall quality of care on a unit, in an organization, or in a geographical area.
- When evaluating client health status, you will compare the client's present data/responses to the desired outcomes (goals) set in the planning outcomes phase.
- When evaluating the effectiveness of the nursing care plan, remember that you cannot control all of the variables that influence the success of a nursing activity.
- Quality improvement programs are specially designed to promote excellence in nursing; they include structure, process, and outcomes evaluation.

Knowledge Map

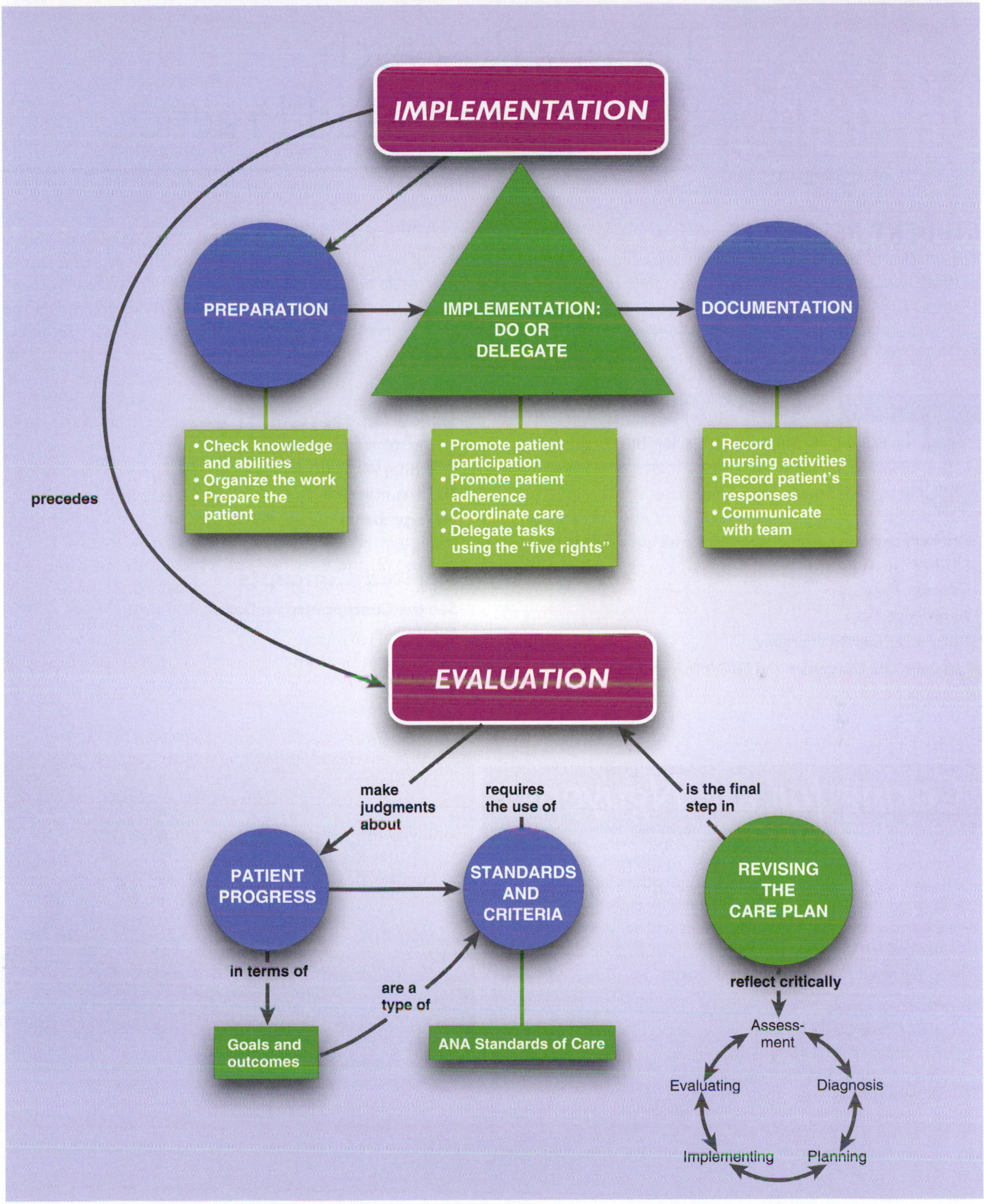

CHAPTER 8

Theory, Research, & Evidence-Based Practice

STUDENT RESOURCES

The questions and exercises in this book allow you to practice the kind of thinking you will use as a full-spectrum nurse. Critical-thinking questions usually have more than one right answer, so we do not provide "correct answers" for these features. Try to answer these questions yourself. It is more important to develop your nursing judgment than to just cover content. You will learn more by discussing the questions with your peers. If you are still unsure, see the Davis Advantage chapter resources for suggested responses.

To explore learning resources for this chapter,

Go to Davis Advantage and find:

- **Answers and Suggested Responses for all questions in this chapter**
- **Concept Map**
- **Knowledge Map**
- **References and Bibliography**
- **Lists of NOC Outcomes and NIC Interventions**

Key Concepts

Evidence-based practice
Nursing research
Nursing theory
Theory

Related Concepts

See the Concept Map on Davis Advantage.

Caring for the Nguyens

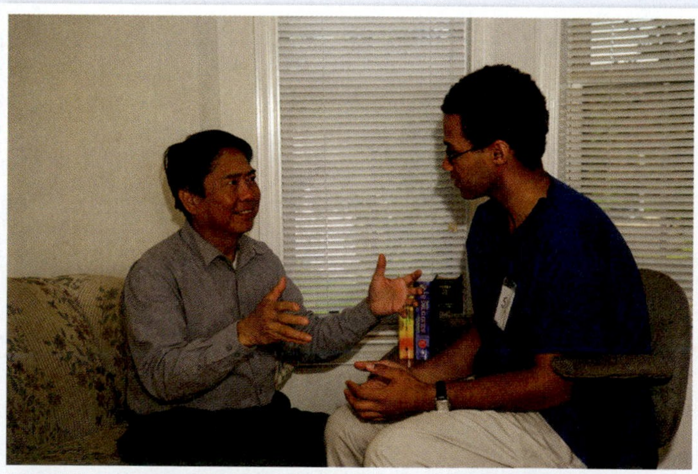

Nam Nguyen arrives at the clinic for a follow-up visit. As you may recall, he has been diagnosed with hypertension. At a previous visit, you wrote the nursing diagnosis Obesity related to inappropriate food choices and serving size, as evidenced by a body mass index (BMI) of 28.5. Today you have gathered the following intake data:

Blood pressure: 174/96 mm Hg
Heart rate: 88 beats/min
Respiratory rate: 18 breaths/min
Temperature: 98.5°F
Weight: 175 lb

Caring for the Nguyens (continued)

A. What observations can you make about today's data in comparison with those of his initial visit?

B. As part of the treatment plan for Mr. Nguyen, you have been asked to educate him about a diet to assist with weight loss and hypertension management. How would you determine the most appropriate diet to include in your treatment plan?

C. A number of sources recommend the DASH (Dietary Approaches to Stop Hypertension) eating plan. Go online and search for "Dietary Approaches to Stop Hypertension." Is there sufficient research to support incorporating this information into Mr. Nguyen's treatment plan? If so, describe the research, and summarize the DASH eating plan.

CLINICALJUDGMENT

Applying the Full-Spectrum Nursing Model

PATIENT SITUATION

You are caring for a 90-year-old patient in a long-term care facility. He is completely dependent for performing activities of daily living (ADLs). In addition, he has been unresponsive, cannot swallow safely, and has been receiving fluids and nutrition for many months through a feeding tube. His adult grandson has recently discovered a living will in which the patient had stated that he does not wish to be kept alive by "artificial means, including being tube fed." The grandson, John, insists that the patient's wishes be honored, but the patient's son (Mr. Lee) threatens a lawsuit if the caregivers discontinue the feedings. They argue loudly, and Mr. Lee yells to his son, "You just want him gone because you're in a hurry to get his money! You know you're getting the major part of it."

THINKING

1. *Theoretical Knowledge:* What facts are important to know to decide whether or not to stop the feedings?

2. *Critical Thinking (Analyzing Assumptions):* Without thinking too much, what is your first thought about what is causing the disagreement between Mr. Lee and his son John? Examine your assumption. How certain are you that it is valid? What else might be going on in their lives to cause father and son to disagree on this issue?

DOING

3. *Nursing Process (Assessment):* To provide some information about the patient that might be helpful in restoring peace between Mr. Lee and John, what patient assessments should you make?

CARING

4. *Ethical Knowledge:* State one ethical issue involved in this case—or one moral problem that the case would present for you if you were involved in it.

Critical Thinking and Clinical Judgment

1. Recall the scenario about Mr. Khatri (Meet Your Patient) in Volume 1. Imagine you are the home health nurse providing care to a frail older man in his home. Mr. Khatri is visibly upset and is grabbing at the belt around his waist as he sits in the chair. He is crying out to his deceased mother to come and take him to her. Use any nursing theory you wish, or your own idea, and describe each of the four concepts of a theory as they apply in this scenario:

   a. Patient (Who is the patient? How do you know?)

   b. Nurse (Who is the nurse? What is she doing that is "nursing"?)

   c. Health (Is the patient healthy? What is the patient's state of health?)

   d. Environment (Where is the nurse–patient encounter occurring?)

2. Recall Maslow's Hierarchy of Needs. Give one example of a specific nursing intervention a nurse could do to meet each of those needs. If you think the nurse cannot address a need, explain why.

   a. Physiological

   b. Safety and security (mental and physical protection)

   c. Love and belonging

   d. Self-esteem (achievement, reputation)

   e. Cognitive needs (knowledge, self-awareness)

   f. Aesthetic needs (beauty, balance, form)

   g. Self-actualization (personal growth, fulfillment)

   h. Transcendence (helping others to self-actualize)

3. You are an emergency department nurse taking care of a 4-year-old child who has had a bike accident. The child has an open abrasion and a few cuts that will require some minor care. However, he is frightened and crying.

   a. Using Nightingale's theory, what interventions might you use?

   b. Using Watson's theory, what might you do?

   c. Using Henderson's theory, what would be the focus of your interventions?

   d. Choose one of the following theories: Neuman, Orem, or Rogers. Describe how that theory would direct you in this case.

4. You are working the night shift, and while making your 0200 rounds, you are surprised as you look into the room of 22-year-old Angela Kindred and see her mother sitting at her bedside and sobbing. Visits are not encouraged at that time of night, and you did not know Mrs. Kindred was on the unit. Even though Angela's leukemia is terminal, you understood from the day nurse that the family, as well as Angela, had accepted the inevitable outcome.

   a. Explain how you can demonstrate caring to this mother who will soon lose her beloved daughter.

   b. Look at Watson's (1988) 10 caring processes, repeated below from the textbook. How can you use them to demonstrate caring to this mother and daughter? Be specific in your answers.

   Watson's 10 Caring Processes:

   1. Forming a humanistic–altruistic system of values
   2. Instilling faith and hope
   3. Cultivating sensitivity to self and others
   4. Forming helping and trusting relationships
   5. Conveying and accepting the expression of positive and negative feelings
   6. Systematic use of the scientific problem-solving method that involves caring process
   7. Promoting transpersonal teaching–learning
   8. Providing for supportive, protective, and corrective mental, physical, sociocultural, and spiritual environment
   9. Assisting with gratification of human needs
   10. Sensitivity to existential–phenomenological forces

5. You are a nurse in an urgent care clinic taking care of a 3-year-old with wounds from a dog bite. The child is frightened, even though his mother is sitting in the treatment room with him. You ask the mother to hold the child while he is being treated and restrain him, if necessary.

In reflecting on this intervention afterward, you decide to find the best evidence for your intervention to be certain that you will want to use it in similar situations in the future. Write a PICOT question to guide your literature search. Write each part, then write the full statement.

P—

I—

C—

O—

T—

Full statement of the question:

6. Read analytically an article in a research journal. Answer the following questions about the article:
   a. What is the article about as a whole? Answer using one sentence.
   b. What are the author's main conclusions?
   c. Do you think these conclusions are true? If not, why not?
   d. Is this article of any significance in nursing? That is, how could it be used to improve patient care or nursing education?

7. For each of the following concepts, use critical thinking to describe how or why it is important to nursing, patient care, or nursing theory and research. Note that these are *not* to be merely definitions.

Nursing theory

The science of human caring

From novice to expert

Culturally competent care

Evidence-based practice

Nursing research

Institutional review board

Informed consent

Research utilization

Analytical reading

What Are the Main Points in This Chapter?

- According to Florence Nightingale, nursing theories describe "what is" and "what is not" nursing.
- The four basic components of a nursing theory are person, nurse, environment, and health.
- A theory is developed by recognizing a need in nursing or by having an idea, using research to determine whether the idea is effective, and then using the research results to define a theory.
- Theories help nurses (1) find meaning in their experiences of nursing; (2) organize their thinking around pertinent ideas; and (3) develop new, evidence-based ideas and insights into the work they do.
- Nurses use theories as an evidence-based framework for their nursing practice.
- Three leaders in nursing caring theories are Dr. Jean Watson, Dr. Patricia Benner, and Dr. Madeleine Leininger.
- Nursing research is a systematic, objective process of analyzing phenomena of importance in nursing.
- Quantitative research may be generalized to populations similar to the one studied. It has tight controls and large numbers of participants, and the data are statistically analyzed.
- Qualitative research analyzes the lived experience of a person or group of people by examining the words and actions of a small number of participants.
- The research process is a systematic way of organizing, preparing, and presenting research.
- Research participants (people in a research study) are protected from harm by specific laws and regulations.
- Research reports are critiqued by reading analytically and using preselected criteria.
- Nursing research evolved slowly. The advanced education currently available to nurses is speeding up the evolution of research.
- Evidence-based nursing requires evaluating research to find the best evidence and then applying it in practice.
- The process of finding best evidence consists of identifying a clinical nursing problem, formulating a searchable question, searching the literature, evaluating the quality of the research, and integrating the research into practice.
- The parts of a PICOT question are: **P**atient problem, **I**ntervention, **C**omparison intervention, **O**utcome, and **T**ime.

Knowledge Map

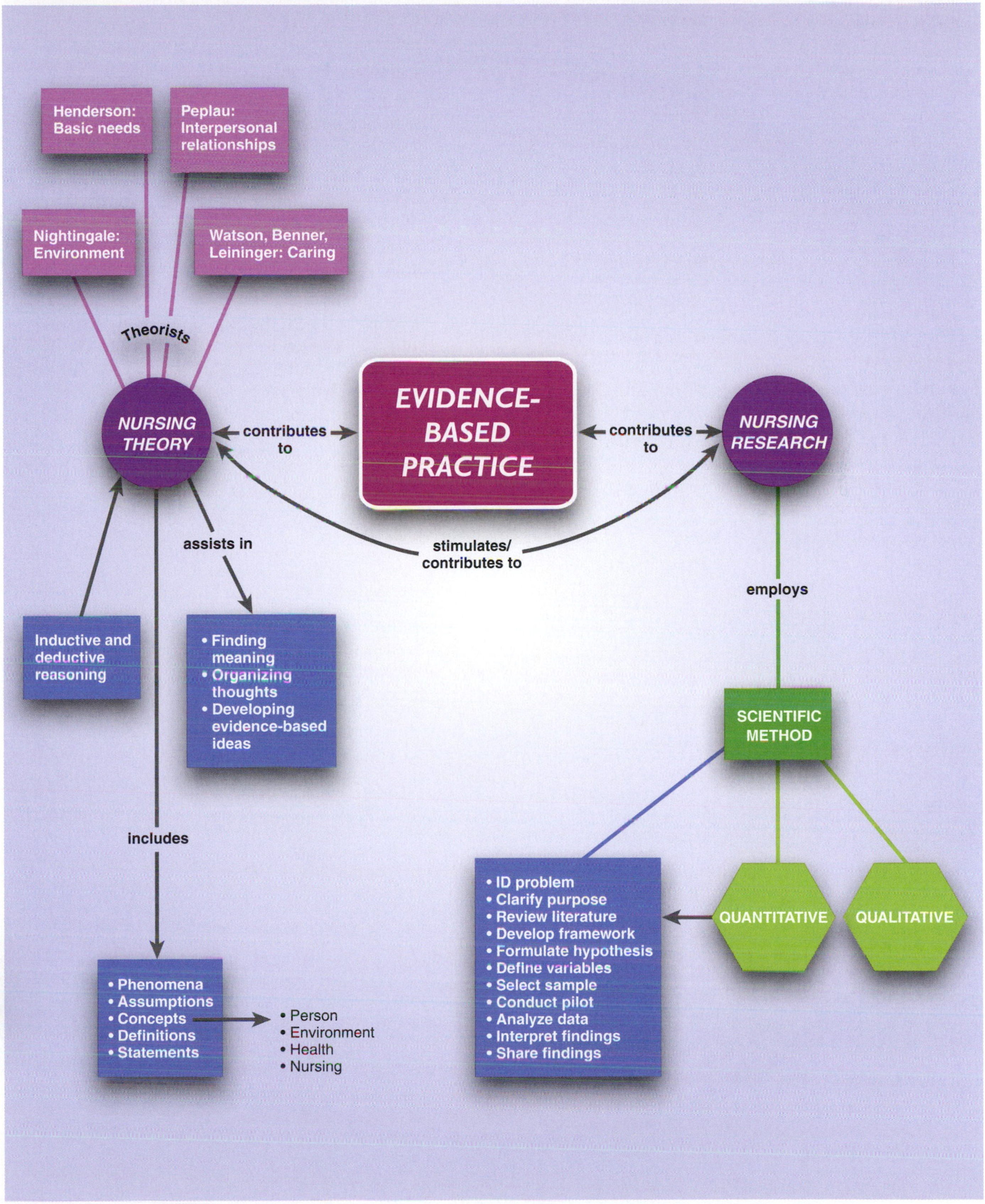

UNIT 2

Factors Affecting Health

CHAPTER 9

Life Span: Infancy Through Middle Adulthood

STUDENT RESOURCES

The questions and exercises in this book allow you to practice the kind of thinking you will use as a full-spectrum nurse. Critical-thinking questions usually have more than one right answer, so we do not provide "correct answers" for these features. Try to answer these questions yourself. It is more important to develop your nursing judgment than to just cover content. You will learn more by discussing the questions with your peers. If you are still unsure, see the Davis Advantage chapter resources for suggested responses.

To explore learning resources for this chapter,

Go to Davis Advantage and find:

Answers and Suggested Responses for all questions in this chapter
Concept Map
Knowledge Map
References and Bibliography
Lists of NOC Outcomes and NIC Interventions

Key Concepts

Growth
Development
Stages

Related Concepts

See the Concept Map on Davis Advantage.

Example Problems

Abuse, Neglect, and Violence
Substance Abuse

Caring for the Nguyens

Review the scenario of Nam Nguyen, in the Meet the Nguyens section before Chapter 1 in the front of this book. Answer the following questions based on that scenario:

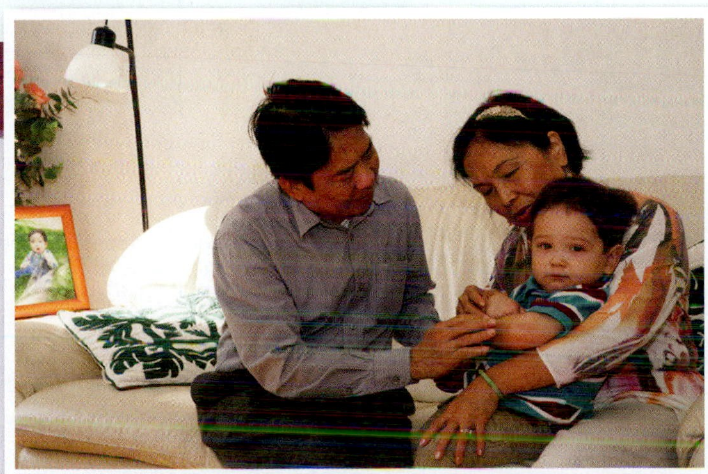

(Continued)

Caring for the Nguyens (continued)

A. Evaluate Mr. Nguyen's physical health status in comparison with what is expected for someone in his age group.

B. Mr. Nguyen and his wife are raising their 3-year-old grandson. What effect might this have on Mr. Nguyen's ability to accomplish his developmental tasks?

Practical Knowledge clinical application

One important aspect of developmental care across the life span is to identify abuse and intervene for patients who are being abused.

Keep in mind that if there is an injury, there is the possibility that it was inflicted. The following flow chart and Procedure 9-1 will aid you in identifying cases of abuse.

Possible Abuse Flow Chart

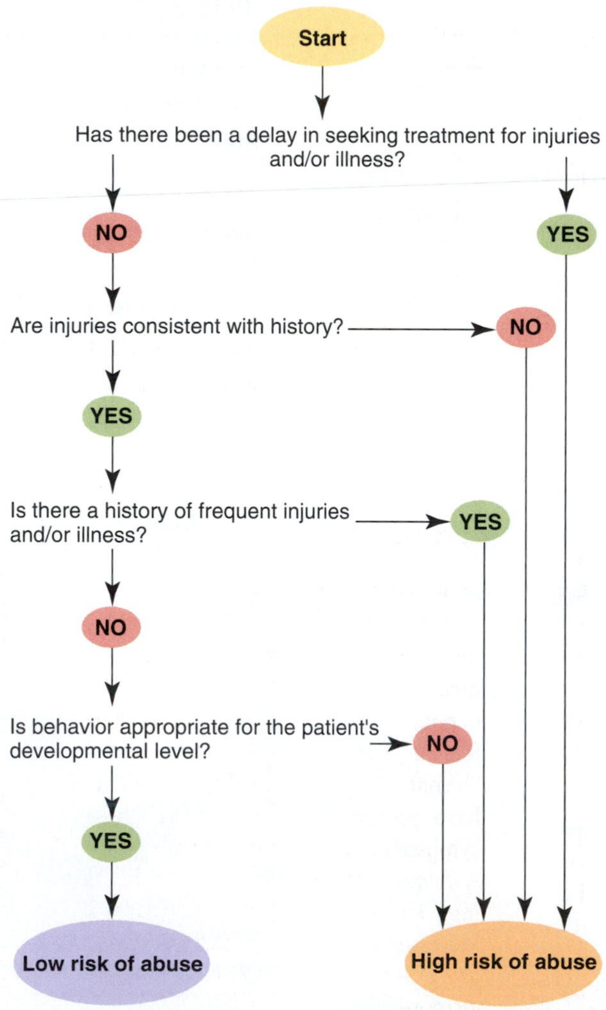

PROCEDURES

You will find information on elder abuse in Chapter 10; however, the following procedure can be used for patients of all ages.

Procedure 9-1 ■ Assessing for Abuse

➤ For steps to follow in *all* procedures, refer to the Universal Steps for All Procedures found on the inside back cover of this text.

Pre-Procedure Assessments

- If you suspect sexual abuse, request a forensic nurse or sexual assault nurse examiner (SANE) be present.
  A forensic nurse and an SANE are specially trained to identify findings that indicate abuse, to support the patient, and to handle the evidence to ensure validity in a court of law.
- Assess for abuse routinely in older or vulnerable adults and women of childbearing age, and any time a child, dependent person, or spouse has an injury.
  Even in the absence of a strong base of evidence to support screening, The Joint Commission requires that all patients be screened for abuse and domestic violence.

Delegation

Key Point: ***Assessment is a nursing responsibility and cannot be delegated.***

➤ When performing the procedure, always identify your patient, according to agency policy, by using two identifiers, and be attentive to standard precautions, hand hygiene, patient safety and privacy, body mechanics, and documentation.

➤ Privacy and confidentiality are extremely important for this procedure.

Procedure Steps

Obtain a Focused Health History.

1. **Interview the patient and family members or caregivers separately.** In case of more than one caregiver, separate them for the interview.
   An abused person may be afraid to talk in the presence of the abuser. Victims have often been intimidated and will usually support the abuser's version of events. If two adults accompany a child, it may be that one of them is abusing both the partner and the child. To help rule that out, separate the caregivers to be certain that they tell the same story.
2. **Approach the subject in a nonthreatening and caring manner.** For example, you might say: "The law requires us to ask about certain injuries. We are not accusing you of anything. I know you care about your child/parent/spouse and want to do everything possible for her health."
3. **Consider the patient's developmental and cognitive level** in assessing whether the story of how the injury occurred is consistent with the injuries.
   The patient must be developmentally capable of performing an activity in the situation where the injury occurred. For example, an infant is not likely to have opened a medication bottle and taken the pills; if a child cannot yet walk, it is not likely that he reached up to pull a hot pan off the stove.
4. **Observe the patient's behavior.** Is it inconsistent with his developmental level?
   In the presence of the abuser, it is common for the abuse victim to appear passive and withdrawn and avoid eye contact. The victim may exhibit anxiety or fear; may look to the parent or caregiver before answering questions; may be overly compliant; or may let the abuser answer the questions for him.
5. **Ask about the injury or incident.** Ask detailed questions about how and when the injury occurred or the illness began: "When did this injury happen?" "When did you first begin to feel ill?" "How did you get this injury?" "What happened to you?" "What have you been doing to treat your symptoms since you first became ill?"
   A delay in treatment of 12 to 18 hours may indicate abuse. If the details of the history of an injury change during the interview, the likelihood of abuse increases.
6. **Ask about past injuries or incidents:** "Have you ever had similar injuries?" "Have you ever required emergency care in the past?"
   Abusive behavior typically occurs over and over. If an injury is caused by abuse, the patient is most likely to have experienced abuse in the past and will have evidence of old injuries.
7. **Ask about the patient's usual diet:** "What do you usually eat for breakfast? Lunch? Dinner? What kind of snacks do you have during the day?"
   Neglect and/or abuse may be in the form of an inadequate or inappropriate diet.

Assess for Sexual Abuse.

8. **Ask directly whether the patient has been touched** inappropriately or forced to have sexual relations.
   Whenever possible, question the patient directly so that your question will not be misunderstood.
9. **Ask whether the patient has genitourinary symptoms:** "Have you had any burning or itching when you urinate? How about any vaginal discharge?"
   In a child, genitourinary symptoms may indicate sexual abuse or neglect.

(continued on next page)

Procedure 9-1 ■ Assessing for Abuse (continued)

10. Does the child display knowledge or interest in sexual acts inappropriate to his or her age or even seductive behavior?

11. Does the child appear to avoid another person, or display unusual behavior—either very aggressive or very passive?

12. Does the victim display destructive behaviors, such as alcohol or drug abuse, self-mutilation, or suicide attempts?

13. Is the victim pregnant, particularly if no intimate relationship is known or the victim is very young?

Assess for Psychological Abuse.

14. Ask parents or caregivers, "Are there family members or friends who help you with problems?"
Isolation is a risk factor for abuse. Parents or caregivers may not have the support they need.

15. Ask the patient, "Whom do you talk to when you are having problems?"
An abuser will try to isolate the victim from family and friends over time. Ask questions to determine what the relationship is between the victim and family and friends.

16. Ask, "Tell me how you feel about yourself."
An abuser demeans and degrades the victim so that the victim has low self-worth and feels that the "punishment" is deserved; conversely, the victim may desire the attention of the abuser, even if it is in the form of abuse.

17. Observe if the child acts fearful, shies away from touch, or appears to be afraid to go home.

18. Ask, "Who manages the family finances, and how are decisions made regarding spending?" (for adults)
An abuser frequently controls all the finances and restricts the resources of the victim. Abusers typically seek control of victims by fostering dependency and powerlessness.

Perform a Focused Physical Assessment.

19. If sexual abuse is suspected from the interview, have a forensic nurse or SANE present, if possible.
For any sexual examination, always have a witness in the room to protect the patient and the examiner.

20. Assess the current injury, and look for evidence of previous injuries. Look for the following cues:

a. Bruises that form an outline of a hand, cord loop, buckle, or belt
Injuries of different ages and multiple injuries may show a pattern of abuse. Be careful to assess the bruise accurately. Some home treatments may cause what looks like bruising. For example, ***moxibustion*** *(includes such actions as firmly rubbing a warm spoon down the affected area) is used in some Asian cultures.*

b. Injuries that are inconsistent with the history of the injuries or are of varying ages (e.g., bruises of different colors, cuts in varying stages of healing)

c. Obvious nonaccidental burns, such as burns to both feet and lower legs from immersion in hot water
One method of abuse is to immerse the victim's hands or feet into scalding water. The resulting injury has a well-defined border and usually seen on both extremities.

d. Circular burns, possibly from cigarettes
Burns at several locations on the body are signs of abuse.

e. Bite marks

f. Oral ecchymosis or injury from forced oral sex
Forced oral sex will cause injuries to the mouth.

g. Bruising at the crease above the eyelids, tense fontanel if the victim is an infant, hyphema, subconjunctival hemorrhage or retinal bleeding, detached retina, ruptured tympanic membrane
Key Point: ***Injuries to the head are common in abuse. Abusive head trauma (AHT, previously referred to as shaken-baby syndrome) is one of the most common and most serious injuries in a young child.***

h. Bleeding or bruising of genitalia, poor sphincter tone, encopresis (poor bowel control), and bruises on inner thighs

i. Positive culture result for sexually transmitted infection (STI) or positive pregnancy test result
STI, particularly in a child, can indicate sexual abuse.

j. Bruises on wrists and ankles from being restrained
Abused individuals may be tied or locked in a closet or other small space.

k. Refer to the figure for typical features of injuries that may be nonaccidental:

Injuries to both sides of the body

Injuries to soft tissues

Injuries in the "triangle of safety": ears, side of face, neck, and top of the shoulders
Accidental injuries in the triangle of safety are unusual. Accidental injuries are usually over bony prominences. One suspicious pattern is the "swimsuit zone" on the trunk, breast, abdomen, genitalia, and buttocks. ➤

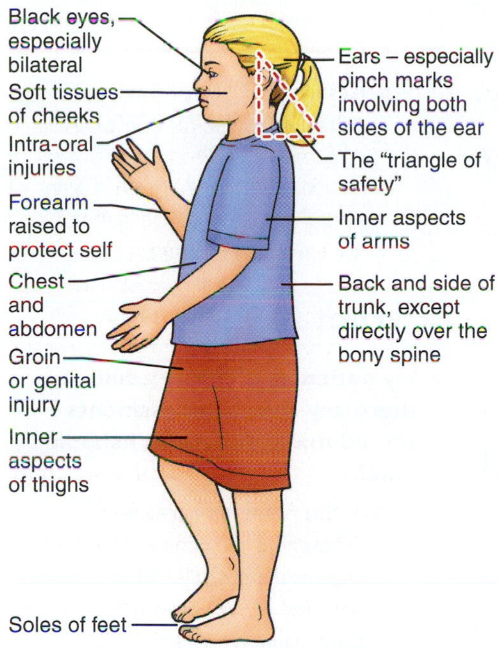

21. Assess whether the injuries are consistent with the history.
If the injuries are not consistent with the history, you must assume abuse.

22. Observe for signs of neglect:
- Malnutrition, such as a distended abdomen, or weight markedly below ideal body weight
- Excess body weight for height and age
- Poor hygiene, including oral hygiene
- Ingrown nails
- Untreated sores or pressure sores or other medical conditions
- Matted hair
- Dehydration
- Confusion
- Clothing that is inappropriate for the weather, such as heavy, full-length pants and long-sleeved shirts on hot days
- Long periods a young child or a frail older adult is left alone without care or supervision

Signs of neglect occur because of long-term starvation or underfeeding, poor personal care, untreated sores or injuries, and inadequate fluid intake. Neglect can also result in childhood obesity as a result of food of poor quality, erratic eating patterns, and poor supervision of the diet.

After the Examination.

23. If the forensic nurse or primary care provider determines that abuse has occurred, follow legal procedures to ensure that all evidence is secured. If possible, have a forensic nurse and social worker work with the patient.
In situations where a violation of the law has occurred, strict procedures are essential to ensure that your findings can be used in a court of law and to protect yourself against legal liability.

24. Provide referrals, if appropriate, for the abused person, partner, family member, or caregiver to obtain assistance in escaping the abusive situation and/or stopping the abuse.
Resources are available to assist the abused individual and to assist the parent or caregiver to stop the abuse. Be aware of local and national resources.

25. Report concerns regarding abuse, according to agency and state guidelines.

Key Point: ***Suspected child and elder abuse must be reported to the appropriate agency, according to federal and state laws. Spousal abuse may be mandatory to report, depending on state law. The Joint Commission has mandated that all cases of possible abuse or neglect be immediately reported in the hospital.***

26. Treat physical injuries, or refer to the primary care provider for medical care, as needed.
Detection and prevention of abuse require the collaborative efforts of the healthcare team.

? What if . . .

- **My patient is a child? Are there any special assessments I should make or actions I should take?**

Follow steps 1 through 6 above, with these modifications:

NOTE: The interview is important in ruling out sexual abuse in children. Physical findings are often absent, even when the perpetrator admits to penetration of the child's genitalia. Most expert interviewers do not interview children younger than age 3 years.

a. To assess for sexual abuse, ask whether the patient has been touched inappropriately:
   - *Child older than age 2 years:* Ask about being touched in the "private parts."
   - *Older child:* Ask, "Sometimes people you know may touch or kiss you in a way that you feel is strange or wrong. Has this ever happened to you?"
   - *Adolescent:* Ask, "Sometimes people touch you in ways you feel are wrong. This can be frightening, and it is wrong for people to do that to you. Has this ever happened to you?"

b. Ask the parent or caregiver:
   - "Has the child started wetting the bed or soiling himself?"

(continued on next page)

Procedure 9-1 ■ Assessing for Abuse (continued)

- **"Does the child have fears that seem unreasonable?"**
  Abuse may result in regression to former behaviors. Symptoms of sexual abuse in children may be general and nonspecific, such as sleep disturbances, bed-wetting, or excessive fears.
- **"Has the child been masturbating or sexually acting out with other children?"**
  A child who is sexually abused may exhibit inappropriate sexual behavior.
- **"Has the child ever run away? If she leaves, does she go somewhere safe?" "Is the child/adolescent sexually active?"**
  An abused child may have feelings of low self-worth and may demonstrate risk-taking behaviors, such as running away to places that are unsafe.

c. To assess for psychological abuse, ask the parent or caregiver:

- **"Was the child a result of a planned pregnancy? What were the pregnancy, birth, and postpartum period like?"**
  Risk factors for abuse include an unplanned pregnancy, complications during pregnancy, stressors (e.g., moving, illness, loss of job, divorce), a difficult pregnancy or birth, and lengthy stay in the neonatal intensive care unit.
- **"How would you describe the child now?"**
  An abusive parent may describe the child as a "problem child" who is always doing something wrong. The opposite is sometimes seen, when the child is described as "perfect."
- **"How does the child's behavior compare with that of others in the family?"**
  Determine whether the parent sees the child differently from his siblings. This is a risk factor for abuse.
- **"Has the child experienced physical or emotional problems in the past?"**
  A history of physical or emotional problems may indicate abuse.
- **"What are your expectations of the child's behavior [e.g., school performance, following instructions]?"**
  The expectations of parents or caregivers who are more likely to abuse a child may be that the child will "always be a problem" or will be a "perfect" son or daughter.
- **"What form of discipline works best with the child?"**
  Determine whether the parents or caregivers use physical or emotional punishment that may be abusive or disproportionate for the act or situation.
- **"Do you have any history of depression, anxiety, difficulty coping with situations or everyday life, or other history of mental health problems?"**
  Mental health disorders interfere with a person's ability to perceive others and situations in a realistic and appropriate way. When coping is compromised, the risk for abuse escalates.

d. Perform a physical assessment. Signs of physical abuse and neglect in children include the following:

- **Bruises on head, face, ears, buttocks, and lower back that are inconsistent with the history of the injury and are at varying stages of healing (different colors)**
- **Hemorrhage of the eye, detached retina, ruptured ear drum**
  Bruising may occur in different patterns. One pattern is the "swimsuit zone" on the trunk, breast, abdomen, genitalia, and buttocks. Children often have accidental bruises over bony areas, but usually not on the abdomen. Injuries to the head are common in abuse. AHT syndrome may cause detached retina(s), hemorrhages, and subdural hematomas.
- **Assess for abdominal pain and other nonspecific complaints.**
  Abdominal pain may be a symptom of sexual abuse in children. Signs of sexual abuse may be general and nonspecific in children.

? What if . . .

- **My patient is an older adult? Are there any special assessments I should make or actions I should take?**

a. Ask the patient's caregiver:

- **"Describe the patient's personal support network. Who visits the patient? How often does the patient have visitors?"**
  As in spousal abuse, people who victimize older people often isolate the person from any support network.
- **"Who is the patient's primary healthcare provider?"**
  Multiple healthcare providers, or lack of a provider, can be an indication of abuse. The caregiver may bring the patient to a different physician with each injury or illness to avoid discovery.
- **"Has the patient ever received the wrong dose of medication?"**
  Getting the wrong medication or dosage of medication (especially oversedation) may indicate abuse or inability to provide safe care.
- **"Who manages the patient's finances?"**
  Financial abuse is a fairly common form of abuse in this population. Determine who has control of the older person's finances and makes the decisions regarding spending.

b. Ask the patient:

- **"Do you feel safe in your home?"**
  The patient who is being abused does not feel safe. Keep in mind that abandonment is a form of abuse.

- "Tell me about your usual day." "Are you able to take care of yourself?" "Who helps you shower and dress?" or "Do you require help with showering or dressing?" "Who is responsible for grocery shopping and cooking in your home?" "How do you get to your appointments or other places you want or need to go?"
  To determine the patient's usual level of self-care

c. Observe for signs of self-neglect.

? *What if . . .*

- **You feel that you are or the patient is in immediate danger?**

  If the patient's safety or your safety is at risk, immediate intervention is required. You may need to secure the area (e.g., by closing the door), notify the in-house security officer, and then call the police.

Evaluation

- Determine whether abuse may have occurred.
- Ensure that appropriate agencies have been notified of the possible abuse.
- Evaluate whether it is safe to let the patient leave the facility.

Patient Teaching

- Inform the patient, parent, partner, and/or caregiver of local resources for prevention or intervention in situations of child, spousal, or elder abuse.
- Inform the patient that abuse is suspected. Ask for her perceptions of the situation.
- Emphasize to the patient that her safety is the primary concern.

Home Care

- If potential abuse is identified in the home, follow agency and state legal guidelines.
- If the patient's safety is at risk, immediate intervention is required. You may need to notify the police or call an ambulance. Be sure to carry a fully charged cell phone with you.
- If you believe that you are at risk for harm (common in abusive situations), leave the setting before notifying the police.

Documentation

- Follow legal requirements for documenting possible abuse, including disposition of potential evidence.
- If possible, take pictures of the injuries by using a digital camera, and include them in the charting. Place a ruler or other common object next to the injury for reference by a third party viewer.
  Photos must be saved and stored in-house because of the requirement to protect confidentiality.

  Chart all findings factually—do not add any interpretations. For example:

Do Chart:

4-year-old boy admitted with second-degree burns to both feet, extending to midpoint of shins. Father says, "I put him in the bathtub and didn't realize how hot the water was."

Do Not Chart:

4-year-old boy admitted with immersion burns to both feet, extending to midpoint of shins, as found in abuse.

Practice Resources

Louwers, Korfage, Affourtit, et al., 2014; Tiyyagura, Gawel, Koziel, et al., 2015; U.S. Preventive Services Task Force, March, 2013, June 2013.

ASSESSMENT GUIDELINES & TOOLS

Fetal Development

STAGE	DESCRIPTION
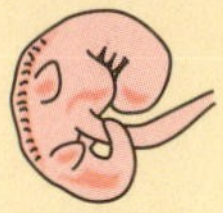 **Week 4** End of first lunar month	Length: ¼ in. (0.6 cm) Appearance: Curled upon itself with head touching tail. Signs of formation of arm and leg buds. Liver formed. Heart present. Begins to pulsate about the 14th to 24th day. Primitive blood cells present. Beginnings of brain present.
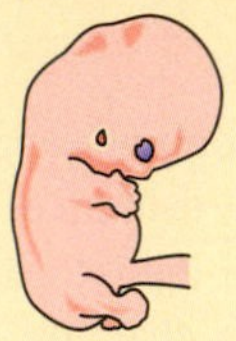 **Weeks 6–8** Second lunar month	Length: 1 in. (2.5 cm) Weight: 1/30 oz (1 g) Chambers of heart develop. Rapid brain development occurring. Primitive limbs present. Fingers and toes begin to form. Face develops. Eyes, ears, nose appear. Palate and upper lip forming. Gastrointestinal tract developing. Part of intestine still in umbilical cord. Urogenital systems forming. Head disproportionately large due to rapid brain development. Organogenesis completed.
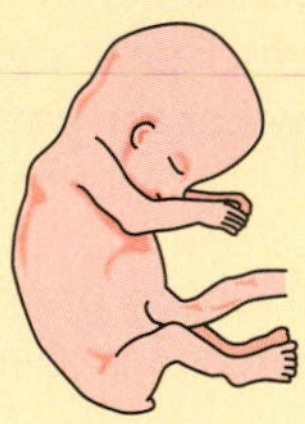 **Weeks 9–12** Third lunar month	Length: 3 in. (7.5 cm) Weight: 1 oz (28 g) Growth and maturation of structures continues. Head disproportionately large. Brain shows structural features. Eyelids fused. Nail beds form on fingers and toes. Bile present in intestines. Spontaneous movements present. Ossification centers in bones begin to appear. Enamel-forming cells and dentin forming. Kidney secretion by 10th week. Bone marrow begins to form blood cells. Distinguishing sexual traits evident. Respiratory-like movements (reflex activity) present. Intestines retracted from umbilical cord into abdomen. Palate completed fused. Neck well defined.
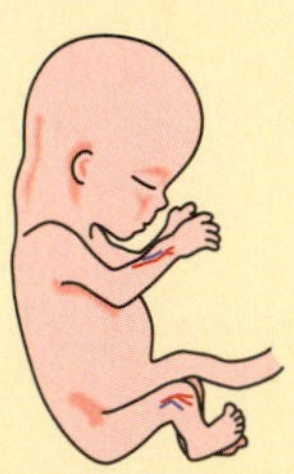 **Weeks 13–16** Fourth lunar month	Length: 6 to 7 in. (15.2 to 17.7 cm) Weight: 4 oz (112 g) Fetus active. Mother may experience quickening. Skeleton calcified and visible on x-ray film. Downy lanugo on head. Placenta distinct. Blood vessels visible beneath transparent skin. Heart actually circulating blood through fetal body. Increasing amount of respiratory movements can be detected by sonogram. Enzymes ptyalin and pepsin being secreted. Fetal thyroid gland begins functioning by the 14th week. Total body blood volume: Less than 100 mL. Amount of amniotic fluid present: 150 to 280 mL.

Fetal Development—cont'd

STAGE	DESCRIPTION
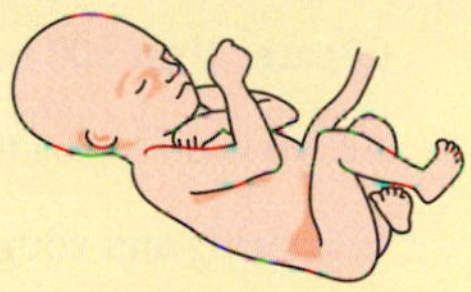 **Weeks 17–20** Fifth lunar month	Length: 10 in. (.5 cm) Weight: 8 to 10 oz (224 to 280 g) Fetal heart sounds evident with stethoscope. Scalp hair visible. Lanugo present, especially on shoulders. Skin less transparent. Eyebrows present. Vernix caseosa present. Fingernails and toenails apparent. Some fat deposits present.
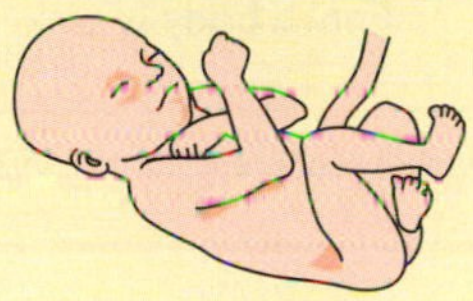 **Weeks 21–24** Sixth lunar month	Length: 12 in. (30.5 cm) Weight: 1½ lb (672 g) Skin wrinkled, pink, translucent. Increasing amounts of vernix caseosa present. Eyebrows and eyelashes well defined. External ear soft, flat, shapeless. Lanugo covering entire body. Some breathing effort evident.
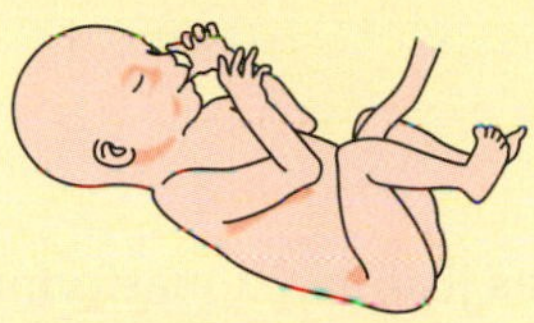 **Weeks 25–28** Seventh lunar month	Length: 15 in. (37.5 cm) Weight: 2½ lb (1120 g) Skin red, wrinkled, covered with vernix caseosa. Looks like a "little old man." Membranes disappear from eyes. Eyelids open. Scalp hair well developed. Fingernails and toenails present. Subcutaneous fat present. Testes at internal inguinal ring or below.
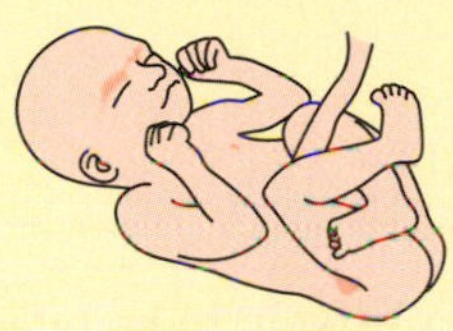 **Weeks 29–32** Eighth lunar month	Length: 15 to 17 in. (37.5 to 42.5 cm) Weight: 3½ to 4 lb (1568 to 1792 g) Skin pink and smooth. Areola of breast visible but flat. Testicles begin descent down inguinal canal (may be in scrotal sac), or Labia majora small and separated, clitoris prominent. Hair fine and wooly. One or two creases evident on anterior portion of soles. Deposits of subcutaneous fat present. Can be conditioned to respond to sounds outside of mother's body.
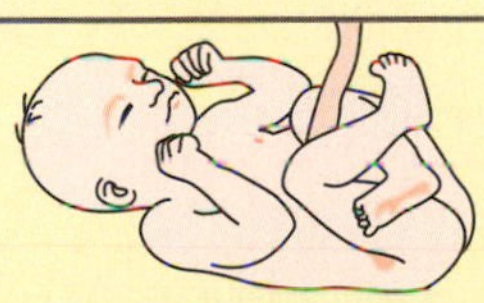 **Weeks 33–36** Ninth lunar month	Length: 19 in. (47.5 cm) Weight: 5 to 6 lb (2240 to 2688 g) Increased fat deposits give body and limbs a more rounded appearance. Skin thicker, whiter. Lanugo disappearing. Sole creases involve anterior two thirds of foot. Breast tissue develops beneath nipples.
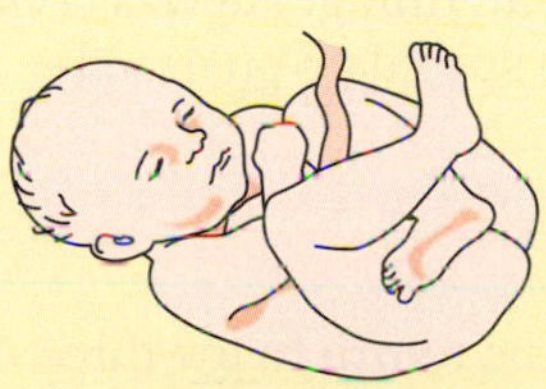 **Weeks 37–40** Tenth lunar month	Length: 20 in. (50 cm) Weight: 7 to 7½ lb (3136 to 3360 g) After 38 weeks, considered full term. Body plump. Lanugo gone from face. Vernix caseosa disappearing, present in varying amounts. Testes in scrotum (male). Labia majora meet in midline and cover labia minora and clitoris (female). Ear well defined. Erect from head. Uniform color to eyes (a slate hue). Acquires antibodies from mother.

Source: Polan, E. & Taylor, D.: *Journey Across the Life Span: Human Development and Health Promotion*, ed 5. Philadelphia: F.A. Davis, 2015.

Apgar Scoring

CATEGORY	0	1	2
Breathing effort	Not breathing	Respirations slow (less than 30 breaths/min) or irregular	Infant cries well
Heart rate (by stethoscope)	None	Less than 100 beats/min	Greater than 100 beats/min
Muscle tone	Loose and floppy	Some muscle tone, weak flexion	Active motion, full flexion
Grimace response or Reflex irritability (response to stimulation such as mild pinch)	No reaction	Grimacing	Grimacing and cough, sneeze, or vigorous cry
Skin color	Pale blue	Pink with blue extremities	Entire body is pink

Source: Medline Plus, U. S. National Library of Medicine, National Institutes of Health. Retrieved from http://www.nlm.nih.gov/medlineplus/ency/article/003402.htm

CLINICALJUDGMENT

Applying the Full-Spectrum Nursing Model

PATIENT SITUATION

Lani Ettinger is a 30-year-old woman, married, with three school-age children. She has just had a mastectomy (removal of a breast) after a positive biopsy result for cancer. There were no complications during surgery; the cancer was removed at an early stage, and she is expected to recover completely. As you are helping her prepare to leave the hospital, she begins crying.

THINKING

1. *Theoretical Knowledge:* What are Havighurst's developmental tasks of young adulthood?

2. *Critical Thinking (Contextual Awareness):* Which of those developmental tasks is/are most likely to be affected by Lani's mastectomy and her emotional reaction to it?

DOING

3. *Nursing Process (Assessment):* When you see Lani crying, what do you need to do?

CARING

4. *Self-Knowledge:* Suppose Lani tells you, "My husband has gone to get the car, but when he was here, he didn't want to hug me or kiss me. I asked him if he still loves me, and he didn't say anything. He was crying when he left." What would your feelings be about the husband? You do not need to speculate on exactly what his actions meant; just imagine what your initial feelings would be.

Critical Thinking and Clinical Judgment

1. Now that you have an understanding of the stages of growth and development, let us return to the three pediatric patients you met in Meet Your Patients, in Volume 1. All three children have been diagnosed with pneumonia. You have introduced yourself to Tamika's grandmother and Miguel's mother and have spoken by phone to Carrie's mother. Each is asking you how this hospitalization will affect their child or grandchild.
   - Tamika, a 3-year-old, lives with her grandparents. Her grandmother is present only during the afternoon visiting hours because she has to care for her husband, who suffers from numerous health problems.

- Miguel, a 2-month-old, lives with his mother. Since his admission yesterday, his mother has stayed at his bedside and provided most of her son's care. Miguel's mother is 17 years old and is very concerned about her son's condition.
- Carrie, a 13-year-old, lives with her parents. Both parents are able to visit only during the evening visiting hours after they leave work.

a. Based on Erikson's stages of development, compare the developmental stages of Tamika, Miguel, and Carrie.

b. How will nursing care differ for each child?

c. Analyze each caregiver's developmental stage, and discuss the impact it may have on health teaching.

d. Would it be a good idea to have the children's caregivers meet for a group teaching session to provide information about pneumonia? Explain.

2. For each of the following concepts, use critical thinking to describe how or why it is important to nursing, patient care, or growth and development. Note these are *not* to be merely definitions.

Ego defense mechanisms

Cognitive development

Psychosocial development

Fetal development

Infant development

Reflexes

Toddler development

Preschooler development

School-age development

Puberty

Adolescent development

Young adult development

Middle adult development

What Are the Main Points in This Chapter?

- Growth and development occur across the life span in a predictable pattern.
- Developmental theories help nurses identify what to expect behaviorally, cognitively, socially, and morally from patients at various ages.
- Fetal growth begins at the time of conception and continues for 10 lunar months until birth.
- Critical adaptations at birth include the establishment of respirations and independent circulation, thermoregulation, and the production of urine.
- Between birth and 1 year, infants develop a sense of trust when the caregiver provides the child with love, warmth, and food.
- The toddler period (1 to 3 years) is the time when the child explores the environment and attempts to become autonomous.
- In the preschool period (4 to 5 years) children are able to separate from their parents, communicate needs through language, and control bodily functions.
- The school-age child (6 to 12 years) begins to develop relationships outside the home. This leads to increasing confidence and independence.
- In the adolescent period (12 to 18 years) children establish their own identities and begin to make decisions that will affect their future.
- The young adult (20 to 40 years) leaves home and begins to function as an independent person.
- Middle adulthood (40 to 65 years) is a time when people balance aspirations with reality. It is often a time when the needs of their children diminish, whereas the needs of their aging parents increase.
- Growth and developmental differences result in each age group's having specific health problems requiring specific assessment techniques. Data from these assessments are used to plan and provide care and anticipatory guidance that are developmentally appropriate.
- Abuse of both children and adults is common. Assess all patients for signs of abuse.

Knowledge Map

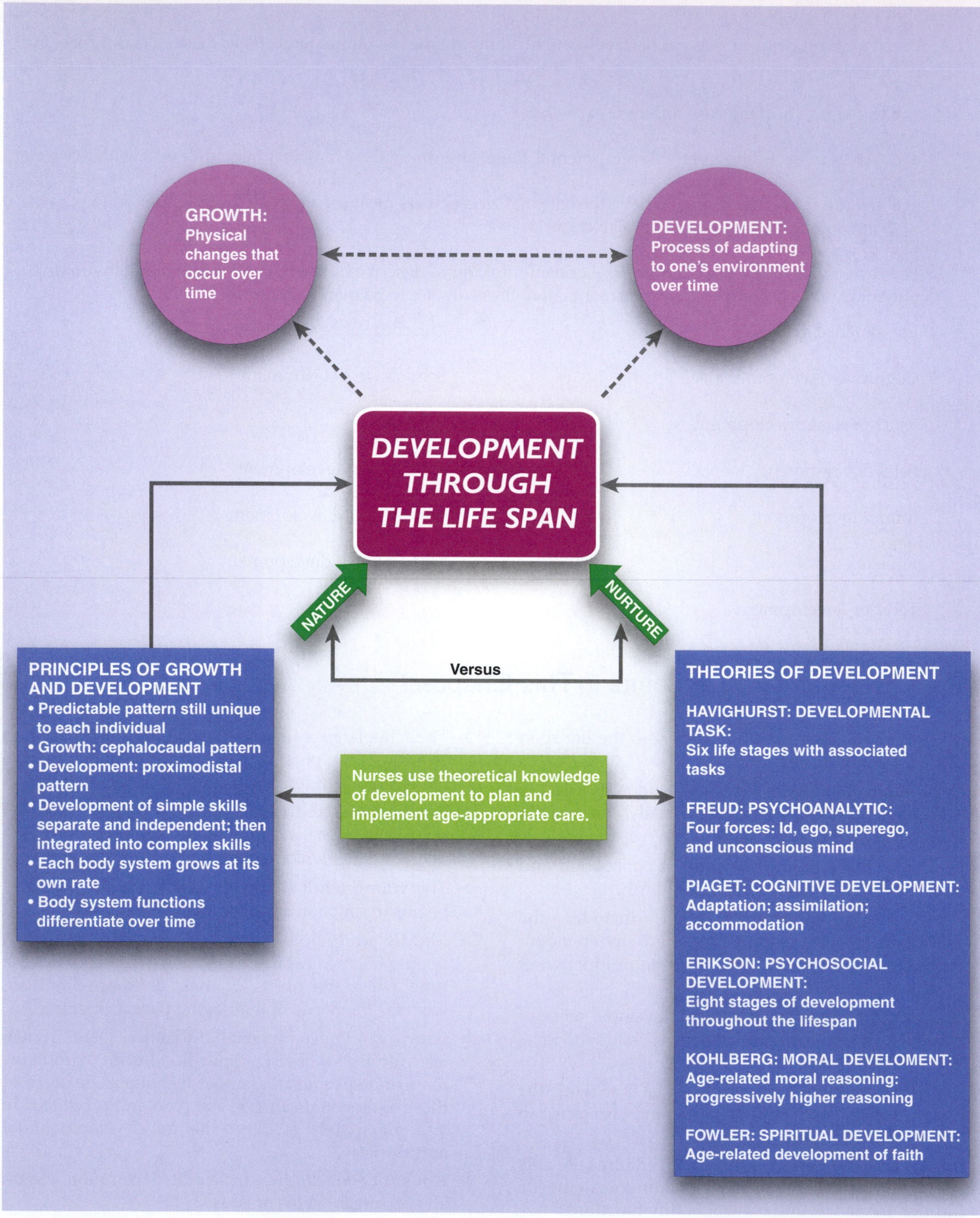

CHAPTER 10

Life Span: Older Adults

STUDENT RESOURCES

The questions and exercises in this book allow you to practice the kind of thinking you will use as a full-spectrum nurse. Critical-thinking questions usually have more than one right answer, so we do not provide "correct answers" for these features. Try to answer these questions yourself. It is more important to develop your nursing judgment than to just cover content. You will learn more by discussing the questions with your peers. If you are still unsure, see the Davis Advantage chapter resources for suggested responses.

To explore learning resources for this chapter,

Go to Davis Advantage and find:

Answers and Suggested Responses for all questions in this chapter
Concept Map
Knowledge Map
References and Bibliography
Lists of NOC Outcomes and NIC Interventions

Key Concepts

Developmental changes
Functional status
Older adulthood

Related Concepts

See the Concept Map on Davis Advantage.

Example Problems

Dementia
Elder Abuse
Frail Elderly

Caring for the Nguyens

Nam Nguyen's father, Binh, is 80 years old and has multiple health problems, including hypertension and heart disease. Although he had surgery for prostate cancer many years ago, the cancer has now metastasized. Because Binh's health was declining rapidly, Nam and Yen moved him and his wife, Mai, into their home last year. Both Nam and his wife work outside the home, so the elderly Mai cares for her husband as much as she can during the day. Binh is too weak to get out of bed without help, and his wife is not strong enough to support him. She cooks for him, but he eats only a few bites and then pushes the plate away. Nam telephones today to say, "We can't take care of him safely at home any longer. Can you tell me how to get him admitted to a hospital or a nursing home?"

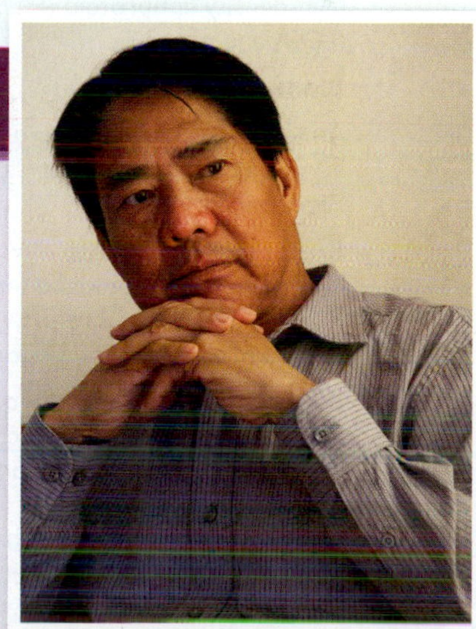

(Continued)

Caring for the Nguyens (continued)

A. What other ideas do you have for helping the Nguyens to care for or to find care for Binh other than by placing him in a hospital or nursing home?

B. Nam's first concern seems to be about getting help for his father. What do you think his next concern will be?

C. What actual data do you have about Binh Nguyen's nutritional status?

D. What else do you need to know to fully assess Binh's nutritional status? If you do not know the answer to this, you will find some information in the Assessment sections of this chapter in Volume 1. For more complete information, refer to Screening for Nutritional Problems and Focused Nutritional Assessment, in Chapter 27 of this volume.

Go to **Assessment,** in Chapter 27 of Volume 1.

E. Would you consider Binh Nguyen to be a frail elderly person? Why, or why not?

PracticalKnowledge clinical **application**

ASSESSMENT GUIDELINES AND TOOLS

Focused Assessment

Assessments for All Older Adults

- ***Vital signs***—Be aware that the normal ranges for vital signs are slightly different for older adults (see Chapter 20). For example, average body temperature in older adults is lower.
- ***Height measurement***—Compare with previous height (as a screen for osteoporosis). Especially important past age 65 years.
- ***Weight and body mass index (BMI),*** *calculated.*
- ***Lipid panel screening***—total cholesterol, triglycerides, high-density lipoprotein (HDL), low-density lipoprotein (LDL), and ratios.
- ***Blood glucose screening.***
- ***Annual clinical breast examination***—for women 40 years of age and older (U.S. Preventive Services Task Force, January 2016).
- ***Breast self-awareness***—Women should know how their breasts normally look and feel and report any breast changes to a healthcare provider right away. Breast self-examination is a lifelong option for women.
- ***Biannual mammography or thermography***—for women 55 years of age and older. Screening should continue as long as the woman is in good health and is expected to live 10 more years or longer.

  The ACS recommends that women with average risk for breast cancer should undergo regular screening mammography starting at age 45 years. Women ages 45 to 54 years should be screened, whereas women 55 years of age and older should transition to biennial screening or have the opportunity to continue screening annually (Oeffinger, Fontham, Etzioni, et al., 2015).
- ***Cervical cancer screening (Pap test)***—Women over age 65 years who have had regular cervical cancer testing in the past 10 years with normal results should not be tested for cervical cancer. Once testing is stopped, it should not be started again. Women with a history of serious cervical precancer should continue to be tested for at least 20 years after that diagnosis, even if testing goes beyond age 65 years.
  - A woman who has had her uterus and cervix removed (total hysterectomy) for reasons not related to cervical cancer and who has no history of cervical cancer or serious precancer should not be tested (American Cancer Society, n.d., last revised 2015).
- ***Colon cancer screening***—The USPSTF (June 2016) recommends screening for colorectal cancer with fecal occult blood testing, sigmoidoscopy, or colonoscopy in adults, beginning at age 50 years and continuing to age 75 years. Intervals for recommended screening strategies include the following:
  - ***Annual screening with high-sensitivity fecal occult blood testing.***
  - ***Sigmoidoscopy—every 5 years, with high-sensitivity fecal occult blood testing every 3 years.***

Focused Assessment

Assessments for All Older Adults—cont'd

- ***Screening colonoscopy*—every 10 years.**
- ***Screening computed tomography (CT) colonography***, or "virtual colonoscopy" is particularly safe in older adults as a noninvasive test that requires no sedation or anesthesia. The American Cancer Society considers CT colonography a first-line colon-cancer screening test that is as effective as traditional colonoscopy. The USPSTF (June 2016) recommends that the decision to screen older adults ages 76 to 85 years be individualized, taking into account the patient's overall health and prior screening history.

- ***Digital rectal exam (for males)*** may be done to detect an enlarged prostate. Enlargement can indicate either benign prostatic hypertrophy or prostate cancer. It is no longer recommended for routine screening in men.
- ***Serum prostate-***specific antigen (PSA) level (for men) is a more sensitive indicator than is the digital rectal exam. Some guidelines encourage yearly screening for men over age 50 years, some caution against routine screening, and some recommend making decisions on an individual basis. The USPSTF recommends that men ages 55 to 69 years discuss the potential benefits and harms of PSA screening for prostate cancer with their healthcare provider but recommends against PSA screening for men 70 years of age and older (USPSTF, 2018).
- ***Eye exam***—every 2 years if there are no problems; otherwise annually, particularly if the older adult has chronic conditions, such as hypertension, cardiovascular disease, or diabetes.
- ***Bone-density scan***—recommended for all women 65 years of age and older for routine screening for osteoporosis. For women at increased risk for osteoporotic fractures (postmenopausal, tobacco smoking, history of fragility fractures, low body weight), screening should begin at age 60 years (National Guideline Clearinghouse, 2011, updated 2013). The test is also recommended for men older than age 70 years.

CLINICALJUDGMENT

Applying the Full-Spectrum Nursing Model

PATIENT SITUATION

Alvin Bell, 82 years old, was just discharged from the hospital after treatment for a myocardial infarction (heart attack). On your first home visit to supervise his medication regimen, you notice that the house appears not to have been cleaned in weeks. Piled on every flat surface, including the floor, are what appears to be months' accumulations of newspapers, magazines, and other clutter. Dishes are piled in the sink, apparently from the time before his hospitalization. There is hardly any food in the cupboards. When you weigh Mr. Bell, you see that he has lost 3 lb in the 3 days he has been home. He admits he has not been eating: "I'm not hungry, and it's too much trouble." As you talk with him, you learn that his wife had died of cancer 7 months ago. He says, "I don't know what to do without her. I hate living alone. I don't have much reason for going on." Mr. Bell is alert and oriented but talks and moves very slowly.

THINKING

1. *Theoretical Knowledge:*
   a. What do you know about depression in older adults? Do you have enough knowledge of that topic to be able to assess whether Mr. Bell is depressed? If not, what resources would you use to make the assessment? (List specific resources; that is, give the URL, don't just say "the Internet"; give the name or author of the book, not just "my psych-nursing book").

   b. You will also need to know whether it is normal for appetite to decrease in older adults and what their caloric needs are compared with those of other age groups. Where can you find this information?

2. *Critical Thinking (Considering Alternatives):*
   a. As you survey Mr. Bell's overall situation, what is your first impulse with regard to improving his situation? What questions come to your mind?

   b. What community services might be helpful to Mr. Bell?

   c. How would you handle referrals? Would you leave a list of telephone numbers? Would you call the agencies yourself? Explain your thinking.

DOING

3. *Practical Knowledge:* In your physical examination of Mr. Bell, you find no old or recent bruises or other injuries. However, because he is depressed and losing weight, you wonder if he is suffering neglect or financial abuse. What questions could you ask to find out if that is true?

CARING

4. *Self-Knowledge:* Think of one other patient you have cared for who has something in common with Mr. Bell. Describe the way(s) in which they are alike.

Critical Thinking and Clinical Judgment

1. Margaret O'Malley, age 67 years, tells you that even though she has new reading glasses, she still cannot see as well as she would like to for reading or sewing. She says, "My eyes often feel dry and scratchy. I wonder if something is wrong."
   a. What would you advise her to do to improve her reading ability?
   b. What age-related change do you think may be causing Mrs. O'Malley's eyes to feel dry and scratchy?
2. Tony King, age 78 years, is having difficulty controlling his diabetes. Because he leads a sedentary life, his physician has advised him to take daily walks to help regulate his blood sugar. Mr. King says, "Doc, I can't do that. With arthritis in my back and hips, every step is agony. I walk just enough to take care of myself, get to the store, come here, and do whatever I have to. I'm already taking a lot of drugs for the pain; I can't take more when I walk." What kind of program could the physician recommend to Mr. King?
3. For each of the following concepts, use critical thinking to describe how or why it is important to nursing, patient care, or growth and development. Note that these are *not* to be merely definitions.
   a. Gender disparities in life expectancy
   b. Age distribution in the population (population pyramid)
   c. Aging in place

What Are the Main Points in This Chapter?

- The number of older adults (65 years of age and older) in the United States has risen significantly because of increasing life expectancy.
- Older adulthood is a time of transition. Most health problems experienced by older adults are chronic in nature and often affect the person's ability to live independently.
- Most older adults live independently.
- Aging can be examined from a life expectancy, percentage of total population, or life-span perspective.
- *Aging in place* means that as people age, they continue to live in their own elder-friendly residences and receive supportive services for their changing needs, rather than moving to another location or alternative type of housing.
- Retirement communities are planned and built specifically to provide elder-friendly dwellings and environments for independent living and allow older adults to "downsize" their dwelling.
- Continuing care retirement communities (CCRC) offer a wide range of living accommodations, including residential living, assisted living, skilled nursing care, rehabilitation, and dementia care on a large campus-like setting.
- Assisted-living facilities (ALFs) are congregate residential settings that provide or coordinate personal services, 24-hour supervision and assistance, activities, and health-related services for older adults.
- Nursing care facilities, or nursing homes, provide skilled and unskilled nursing care for older adults and adults with disabilities.
- The stages of older adulthood are referred to as the ***young-old*** (ages 65 to 74 years), ***middle-old*** (ages 75 to 84 years), and ***oldest-old*** (age 85+ years).
- The fastest growing segment of older adults is the oldest-old, some of whom are the frail elderly and ***centenarians*** (people over 100 years of age).
- Older adults learn new material more slowly. However, there is no loss of intelligence as a person ages.
- Disengagement theory and activity theory attempt to explain the psychosocial development of older adults.
- **Dementia**, or loss of cognitive ability, is not a normal result of aging. It is important to differentiate dementia from depression, acute confusion, or delirium that may be precipitated by dehydration, infection, or a medication side effect or overdose. Alzheimer's disease is the primary form of dementia.
- Developmental differences result in each age group's having specific health problems requiring specific assessment techniques. Data from these assessments are used to plan and provide care and anticipatory guidance that are developmentally appropriate.
- Older adults should have an annual physical examination, including a focused assessment of functional status.
- Frailty is set of characteristics that describe a heightened state of vulnerability for developing adverse health outcomes.
- Abuse of adults is common. All patients should be assessed for signs of abuse.
- Suspicion of elder abuse must be reported to adult protection services and/or the authority designated by law in each state.

Knowledge Map

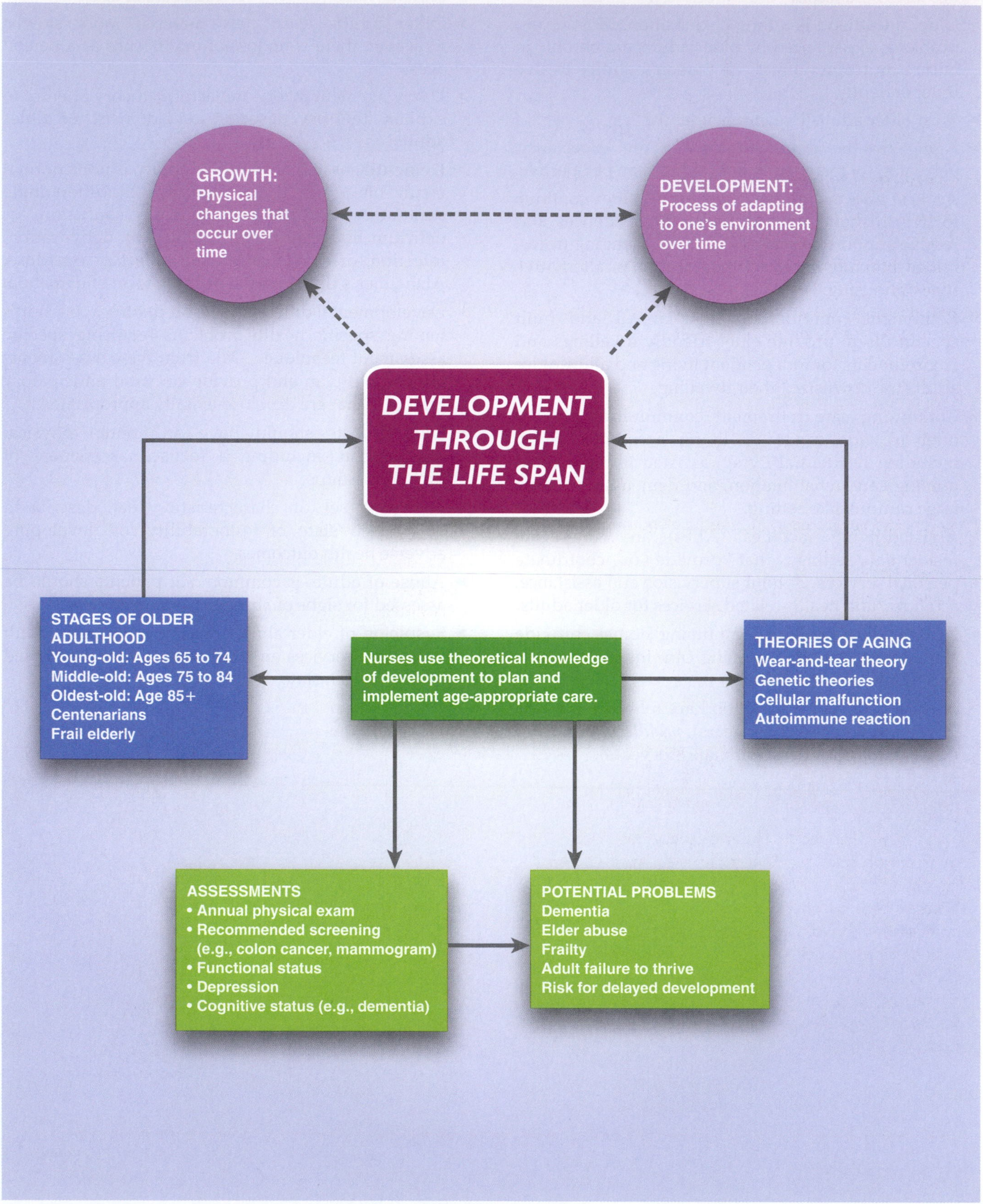

CHAPTER 11

Experiencing Health & Illness

STUDENT RESOURCES

The questions and exercises in this book allow you to practice the kind of thinking you will use as a full-spectrum nurse. Critical-thinking questions usually have more than one right answer, so we do not provide "correct answers" for these features. Try to answer these questions yourself. It is more important to develop your nursing judgment than to just cover content. You will learn more by discussing the questions with your peers. If you are still unsure, see the Davis Advantage chapter resources for suggested responses.

To explore learning resources for this chapter,

Go to Davis Advantage and find:

Answers and Suggested Responses for all questions in this chapter
Concept Map
Knowledge Map
References and Bibliography
Lists of NOC Outcomes and NIC Interventions

Key Concepts

Health
Health experience
Illness
Illness experience

Related Concepts

See the Concept Map on Davis Advantage.

Caring for the Nguyens

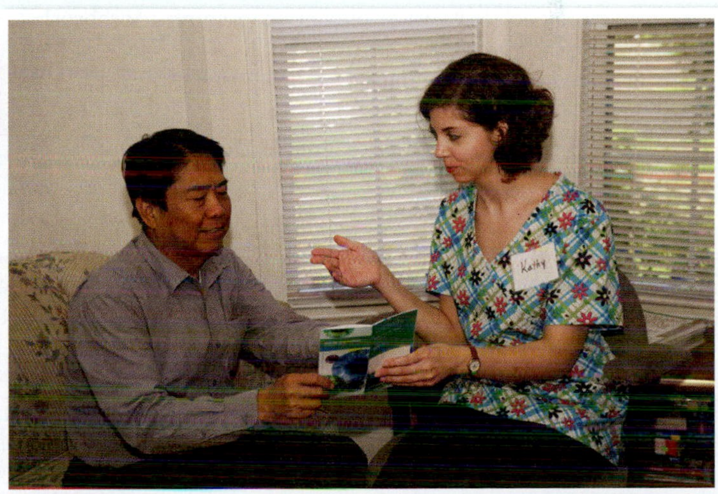

Nam Nguyen has recently been diagnosed with hypertension, obesity, and degenerative joint disease (DJD). He is struggling with these diagnoses. He tells his wife, Yen, "I feel so old now. These are the kind of things my parents are dealing with." At a clinic visit Nam tells you, "It's hard to think of myself as sick. I've been depressed ever since Zach told me about his findings. Now he's asked me to get some laboratory work. I'm afraid he may find even more problems." If you need help answering the following questions,

Go to Chapter 11, Figures 11-1 and 11-2, The Health-Illness Continuum and **Dunn's Health Grid** in Volume 1.

(Continued)

Caring for the Nguyens (continued)

A. Identify the disruptions that Mr. Nguyen must deal with on the basis of these diagnoses. Explain your reasons for choosing these disruptions.

B. How would you evaluate Mr. Nguyen's health status?

C. What kinds of activities could you suggest to Mr. Nguyen to improve his health status?

D. What stage of illness behavior is Mr. Nguyen exhibiting with regard to his recent medical diagnoses?

PracticalKnowledge clinical **application**

Practical knowledge in this chapter means using the nursing process to apply what you have learned about how people experience health, wellness, and illness.

PROCEDURES

The procedures in this chapter are designed to help you admit, transfer, and discharge patients in such a way that you can begin to establish trust at the first patient contact.

Procedure 11-1 ■ Admitting a Patient to a Nursing Unit

➤ For steps to follow in *all* procedures, refer to the Universal Steps for All Procedures found on the inside back cover.

Equipment

- Identifying armband (if this has not been supplied by the admissions department)
- Patient's chart, including physician's orders and nursing admission record
- Thermometer, blood pressure cuff, and stethoscope
- Scales for height and weight
- Gown
- Admission pack (e.g., water pitcher, soap, comb, toothbrush, mouthwash, and facial tissues)
- Nursing care plan or clinical pathway, if one has already been made
- Hospital brochures, Patient Care Partnership, and other forms
- Admission assessment form

Delegation

A registered nurse is responsible for managing medical orders and assessing the patient's need for nursing care in all settings, although this may vary in some specifics according to hospital policy, the law, and regulations. Most other admission activities can be delegated to unlicensed assistive personnel (UAP) if the patient is stable.

Pre-Procedure Assessments

- Assess for signs of emotional distress and/or physical distress.
- Assess ability to ambulate and/or move.
- Assess ability to communicate and understand what is occurring.

➤ When performing the procedure, always identify your patient according to agency policy, using two identifiers, and be attentive to standard precautions, hand hygiene, patient safety and privacy, body mechanics, and documentation.

Procedure Steps

1. **Ensure placement of patient labels** (e.g., on the chart, at the bedside, outside the door).

2. **Introduce yourself to the patient and the family.** Explain who you are. Do not be afraid to tell a client that you are a nursing student.
Many clients are aware that students have more time to spend with them. Talking to the patient and family reassures them and provides information about the patient's level of consciousness and awareness, social relationships, and so on.

3. **Assist the patient into a hospital gown.**
If the patient is able to stand, assist him or her into a gown before weighing the patient to obtain the most accurate weight.

4. **Measure height and weight** while the patient stands on a floor scale, if possible. If the patient is unable to stand, transfer him or her into the bed and measure weight by using a bed scale.
Weigh in the same manner each time to ensure accuracy.

5. **Assist the patient into bed.**
Get the patient comfortable before continuing the admission to prevent overtiring him or her.

6. Check the patient's identification band to ensure that the information, including allergies, is correct. Verify this information with the patient or the family.
Questioning the patient about allergies and verifying with the family will ensure that the information is accurate and documented on the wristband and the chart.

7. **Measure vital signs.**
Measuring the vital signs before completing the rest of the admission ensures that you will be aware of the patient's status. If the vital signs are abnormal, further assess the patient's condition before continuing. Report your findings to the admitting care provider.

8. **Complete the nursing admission assessment**, including health history and physical assessment. Be sure to include the patient's expectations and concerns. For inpatients, this must be completed within 24 hours after admission. All patients should be screened on admission for risk for pressure injuries. (Chapter 22 provides a step-by-step approach to physical assessment.)
An admission assessment is needed to identify problems and establish a baseline. The Joint Commission requires that each patient have an admission assessment performed by a registered nurse.

9. **Check that the list of the patient's current medications** (created in the admissions department) is complete and accurate. Usually the patient's own medications are sent home with the family, or they may be sent to pharmacy for storage.
It is important to know what medications the patient has been taking. The pharmacy will identify medicines brought from home, when necessary. When medications are ordered and given during the patient's stay, they are compared with those on the list so that any discrepancies can be resolved.

10. **Orient the patient to the room.**
These actions ensure that the patient and family will be able to call for assistance if needed and increase the patient's and family's level of comfort and ability to function in the hospital setting. Remember that one of the disruptions associated with illness is anxiety about the unknown. If you tell your client what to expect, you help minimize anxiety.
    a. Make sure the client knows how to use the bed, the call light, and any equipment that you expect him or her to use.
    b. Point out the location of personal care items.
    c. Show the client the location of the restroom.
    d. If you will be measuring the client's intake and output, tell him or her so during your orientation.
    If the client is alert, he or she may be able to assist you with these measures.

11. **Explain hospital routines**, including the use of siderails, meal times, and so on. Answer the patient's and family's questions.
Hospitalization takes away control of basic decisions. Knowing the routines and available choices increases patient and family comfort.

12. **Verify with the patient all other admission data** on the chart for completeness and accuracy.
Basic data, such as name, address, marital status, name of admitting physician, admitting diagnosis, consent to treatment, and so on, will usually be obtained in the admissions office. However, you will need to be sure all the admitting information is complete, and complete it if it is not.

13. **Ask if the patient has an advance directive** (e.g., power of attorney or living will). If so, place a copy in the hospital record. If not, explain the purpose of the document, and give the patient a form to fill out if he wishes to do so. (See Chapters 17 and 45, Volume 1, if you need more information about advance directives.)
Advance directives enable patients to indicate their preferences about treatments and prolonging life.

14. **Advise the patient of his privacy rights under the Health Insurance Portability and Accountability Act (HIPAA, 1996).** See that he has a written explanation of his privacy rights (see Chapter 45 as needed).

15. **Inventory the patient's belongings.** Encourage the family to take home valuable items and money. If that is not possible, arrange to have valuables placed in the hospital safe. Most agencies require money in excess of $5 to be sent home or to the cashier's office.
Patient belongings, including valuables, are frequently lost during hospitalization. Documenting the disposition of everything ensures ability to return the belongings to the patient upon discharge.

16. **Complete or ensure that all admission orders** have been completed (e.g., laboratory tests, medications, diet and fluid orders).
Unless it is an unscheduled admission, diagnostic tests are usually completed on an outpatient basis before admission to the hospital. However, there may still be some orders that need to be implemented immediately, whereas others can be delayed. Make sure the orders are completed in the most appropriate time frame.

17. **Ensure patient comfort** (e.g., positioning, pain, water at bedside).

18. Make one last safety check (i.e., call light within reach, bed in low position, siderails up as appropriate, equipment functioning properly).

19. **Before leaving, ask if you can do anything else** for the patient and the family.

20. **Initiate the care plan or clinical pathway.**
Identifying the patient's priority problems enables the nurse to develop the most appropriate nursing orders.

(continued on next page)

Procedure 11-1 ■ Admitting a Patient to a Nursing Unit (continued)

? What if ....

- **The patient is at risk for falls?**
  Perform a fall risk assessment, as appropriate to the patient and according to agency policy.
  Falls are common in inpatient facilities, especially among older adults. If a patient has fall risk factors, risk reduction measures can be instituted.

- **The patient has special care needs?**
  When the patient has special needs, such as allergies, a nothing by mouth (NPO) order, or an "intake and output" order, post patient care reminders at the head of the bed or at the door to remind other care providers of such needs.

- **The patient needs a more in-depth assessment in some areas?**
  Perform special needs assessments as relevant to the care and condition of the patient (social situation, nutrition and hydration status, functional abilities, spiritual and cultural variables). If these are warranted, they must be completed within 24 hours after admission or prior to surgery.
  In-depth assessment of these topics is not a part of all admission assessments but should be done if the patient's condition warrants.

- **The patient has a learning disability?**
  If possible, preadmissions should be arranged for the patient and main caregiver. This allows more time to discuss issues of consent, alleviate anxiety, and set up links with a learning disability specialist or social worker.
  Allow more time for the admission process, or the preadmission process if that has been arranged.
  Use short sentences, presenting one idea at a time.
  Include the caregiver in the admission process, but encourage the patient to participate as much as possible.
  Document the main caregiver's name and contact numbers.
  Expect the patient to be anxious.
  Include special communication and personal needs in the plan of care.
  Give the patient hospital information with pictures, such as those given to children, if appropriate for her developmental level.

- **The patient is an older adult?**
  Ask all older adults if they have had any falls in the past year. If they report a fall, observe them as they stand up from a chair without using their arms, walk several paces, and return ("get up and go"). If they are steady, no further assessment is required. If there is unsteadiness or if the person reports more than one fall, further assessment is required.
  The incidence and severity of fall-related complications rise steadily after age 60 years. Fall rates in nursing homes and hospitals are almost three times the rate for those living at home.

- **The patient is a child?**
  Use a friendly approach.
  The first priority is to establish a trusting relationship with the child and the parents to help relieve fears and anxiety. Children younger than 3 years of age may fear being separated from parents. Older children usually worry more about what is going to happen to them.
  Explain the visiting and rooming-in policies to the parents.
  Ask about the child's usual routine (e.g., toileting, bedtime rituals, favorite foods).
  Speak to the child directly if he or she is old enough to understand.
  Direct the family to the bathroom, playroom, television, and snack room, if those are available.
  Encourage the parents to bring toys and other favorite items from home.
  It helps the child feel more comfortable in the unfamiliar surroundings.

Documentation

- Document all assessment findings on the admission database provided by the institution.
- Document an admission note and any teaching or other interventions in the nursing notes or flowsheet (according to agency policy).
- Recall that a discharge plan is created on admission. You will find forms for discharge assessment and teaching in the Forms section, after the Procedures section, in this chapter.

Practice Resources

The American Geriatrics Society (n.d.); The Joint Commission (2008, 2018a); McKenzie, Lasater, Delander, et al., 2017).

Procedure 11-2 ■ Transferring a Patient to Another Unit in the Agency

➤ For steps to follow in all procedures, refer to the Universal Steps for All Procedures found on the inside back cover.

Equipment

- Medical record or chart
- Care plan
- Patient's medications
- Supplies for any ongoing treatments
- Patient's belongings, clothes, and personal care articles
- Standardized handoff form, if available
- A utility cart, if belongings are numerous
- Wheelchair or transfer cart
- If patient must be transferred with equipment running (e.g., portable oxygen), obtain it ahead of time and set it up for the transfer.

Delegation

If the patient's condition allows, you can delegate the physical transfer of the patient and have the UAP move the patient's belongings to the other room. However, as the nurse, you are responsible for obtaining and completing the necessary records, making the final assessment, and gathering and checking the medications. You must also give the handoff report to another nurse.

Pre-Procedure Assessments

- Make a final, brief focused physical assessment.
- Assess the patient's mobility and ability to assist.
- Assess for emotional and/or physical distress (administer medications, as needed).
- Assess the patient's ability to communicate and understand what is occurring.

➤ When performing the procedure, always identify your patient according to agency policy, using two identifiers, and be attentive to standard precautions, hand hygiene, patient safety and privacy, body mechanics, and documentation.

Procedure Steps

1. **Obtain the number of personnel needed** to make a safe transfer.
   For efficiency and patient and staff safety.
2. **Gather the patient's medications and label them** correctly for the new room.
   Ensures availability of medications when the patient arrives at the new unit; helps prevent medication administration errors.
3. **Notify the receiving unit** of the time to expect the transfer. Also notify other departments (e.g., dietary, pharmacy, admitting), primary care provider, and the family of the transfer.
   You need to schedule the transfer with the receiving nurse so that he or she can plan the work and you can arrange the transfer at a time that will limit the number of interruptions during the handoff. Limiting interruptions minimizes the risk of communication errors (e.g., forgetting information). Other departments must have the transfer data so that such services as meals and physical therapy treatments will not be interrupted. The primary care provider and the family, of course, need to know where to find the patient.
4. **Gather the patient's personal belongings and supplies,** including treatment-related supplies and equipment (e.g., isolation supplies, clean dressings), and patient records. Place them on a utility cart, if necessary.
   Having the supplies and equipment "ready to go" makes the transfer more efficient for you and less stressful for the patient.
5. **Bring the wheelchair or transfer cart** to the bedside, and assist the patient to the chair or cart. If using a wheelchair, the patient can hold the pan of supplies; if using a bed or cart, place the supplies on the bed.
6. **Take the patient to the new room,** and give the handoff report. Follow agency procedure for handoff reports. However, the method chosen should allow both the giver and the receiver of patient information the opportunity for any clarifications needed.
   a. If you need to review the contents of an oral handoff report, see Chapter 18. In general, the report should include name, age, and gender of the patient, physicians involved, surgical procedures, medical diagnoses, medications, allergies, laboratory data, special equipment (e.g., oxygen, suction), the patient's current health status, and whether there are advance directives and resuscitation orders. Identify the nursing diagnoses and priorities for nursing care.
   b. Consistently use a structured framework or memory aid to guide the handoff process and the oral report.
   The objective of a handoff is to provide accurate information about the patient. The information communicated must be accurate to ensure patient safety.
   c. Be sure to point out to the receiving nurse if the patient is taking corticosteroids, anticoagulants, antidiabetes medications, antibiotics, or narcotic analgesics.
   These medications can have serious side effects and need careful monitoring.

(continued on next page)

Procedure 11-2 ■ Transferring a Patient to Another Unit in the Agency (continued)

? What if...

- **The patient has intravenous (IV) lines and other equipment that cannot be turned off?**

It is common to transfer patients with IV lines. Some wheelchairs are equipped with an IV pole; for others, you may need to obtain a rolling pole from the unit supply room. The patient may be able to maneuver the rolling pole. Most beds and transfer carts also have portable IV poles, sometimes stored in the underside of beds and transfer carts. Portable oxygen and suction are also available for patients who must have them even during transfer. Be sure to obtain these, set them up, and check their functioning prior to moving the patient from his bed.

- **The patient has too many personal belongings for one person to carry?**

If the patient's condition requires two staff members for the transfer, one person can manage the utility cart while the other manages the patient. If only one person can make the actual move, load a utility cart, and move all the supplies and belongings to the new room before transferring the patient.

- **The patient is being transferred to the intensive care unit (ICU)?**

If this is an urgent transfer, you may need to notify the receiving nurse and move the patient with his or her records and medications. Later, you can make the other notifications, finish the charting, and move patient belongings and other supplies. Some ICUs may require the family to take the patient's personal belongings home.

Evaluation

With the receiving nurse, evaluate the patient's response to the move. The receiving nurse will take vital signs and make a preliminary admission assessment.

Documentation

- Just before moving, document as much information as you can, including the patient's status at that time.
- After the handoff, document the information reported in the handoff, the name and title of the person who received the patient, and your report.
- Sign the note. Some agencies have a standardized form for the transfer note.

Example documentation

3/13/21 1615 Client transferred to room 501 by stretcher, with both siderails up, with assistance of one. Temperature 104.8°F, pulse 100 beats/min, and BP 138/88, respirations 20 breaths/min and shallow. Drowsy upon arrival. Responds to verbal stimuli with moaning. Last pain medication given at 1515. Denies pain when asked. No urine noted since 12:00 p.m.; will encourage voiding by offering urinal every 2 hr. #22 IV in RAC and #18 IV in R hand flushed with 3 mL of normal saline; flushes without redness, edema, or induration. Receiving 3 L/min of oxygen during transfer. Placed on 3 L/min in room; will wean oxygen as tolerated. Handoff report given to Linda Hamm, RN.——————————Sarah Fields, RN

Practice Resources

Ernst, McComb, & Ley (2018); The Joint Commission (2018a, 2018b); Patton, Tidwell, Falder-Saeed, et al. (2017)

Procedure 11-3 ■ Transferring a Patient to a Long-Term Care Facility

➤ For steps to follow in *all* procedures, refer to the Universal Steps for All Procedures found on the inside back cover.

Equipment

- Health record or chart
- Care plan
- Patient's medications
- Supplies for any ongoing treatments
- Patient's belongings, clothes, and personal care articles
- Standardized transfer form, if available
- A utility cart, if belongings are numerous
- Wheelchair or transfer cart

Delegation

If the patient's condition allows, you can delegate the physical transfer of the patient and have the UAP move the patient's supplies and belongings. However, as the nurse, you are responsible for obtaining and completing the necessary records, making the final assessment, and gathering and checking the medications. You must also give the handoff report to another nurse.

Pre-Procedure Assessments

- Make a final, brief focused physical assessment.
- Assess the patient's mobility and ability to assist.
- Assess for emotional and/or physical distress (administer medications, as needed).
- Assess the patient's ability to communicate and understand what is occurring.

➤ When performing the procedure, always identify your patient according to agency policy, using two identifiers, and be attentive to standard precautions, hand hygiene, patient safety and privacy, body mechanics, and documentation.

Procedure Steps

1. **Notify the patient and the family well in advance** of the upcoming transfer to another facility. Include information about the reasons the patient is being transferred, as well as any alternatives to transfer. You will also need to determine which agency is to arrange transportation of the patient.
Allows the patient and the family time to adjust emotionally and to make any necessary plans.

2. **Prepare the patient's records.** You may need to send a copy of the patient's chart to the receiving facility. The original remains with the hospital. You will usually also send a copy of the comprehensive nursing assessment and a detailed nursing care plan, as well as prescriptions and cards for future appointments (e.g., with physicians or social workers).
Ensures continuity of care, thus minimizing patient stress.

3. **Gather and pack the patient's personal items** and treatment supplies to send to the long-term care facility with the patient.
Having the supplies and equipment "ready to go" makes the transfer more efficient for you.

4. **Be certain the medications are labeled correctly.**
Ensures availability and correct administration of medications when the patient arrives at the new facility.

5. **Coordinate the transfer.** Notify the receiving facility of the time to expect the transfer and of any special equipment the patient will need (e.g., IV pole, portable oxygen); notify other hospital departments (e.g., dietary, pharmacy, admitting), primary care provider, and the family of the transfer.
You need to schedule the transfer with the receiving agency so that they can plan their work and you can arrange the transfer at a time that will limit the number of interruptions during the transfer. Other in-house departments must have the transfer data so that such services as meals and physical therapy treatments will be discontinued. The primary care provider and the family, of course, need to know where to find the patient.

6. **Just before transfer, make your final quick assessment, and sign off your charting** (usually there is a preprinted, standardized discharge form for this purpose).
It is important to complete documentation in a timely manner, but it is also important to provide the most recent assessment data to the long-term care facility.

7. **Take the patient off the unit** and out of the hospital after you are notified that transportation has arrived (or delegate this task). Alternatively, a transporter may come to your unit to get the patient. (Note: Some agencies ask you to remove the patient's identification band at the time of transfer.)
Keeping the patient on the unit as long as practical helps minimize his or her anxiety and fatigue that may occur as a result of a long wait in the hospital lobby.

8. **Give an oral report** to the nurse at the long-term care facility. You will usually give a telephone report unless a nurse comes to your hospital to accompany the patient. The report should include, as appropriate for the care, treatment, and services provided, the following:
   a. The reason the patient is being transferred
   b. The patient's physical and psychosocial status
   c. A summary of care, treatment, and services provided and progress toward outcomes
   d. Referrals and community resources provided to the patient
   A report helps ensure continuity of care and provides a baseline for assessing later changes in the patient's health status.

- **It is best to consistently use a structured framework or memory aid to guide the handoff process and the oral report.**
The objective of a handoff report is to provide accurate information about the patient. The information communicated must be accurate to ensure patient safety.

- **Notify the long-term care agency** if the patient is colonized or infected by methicillin-resistant *Staphylococcus aureus* (MRSA) or other contagious microorganisms.
The facility can arrange for and communicate any special isolation or care activities to its staff. MRSA is a serious problem for long-term care residents.

- **Be sure to point out to the nurse** if the patient is taking these medications: corticosteroids, anticoagulants, antidiabetes medications, antibiotics, or narcotic analgesics.
These medications confer a particularly high risk of adverse postdischarge drug events, and the long-term-care nurses will need to continue careful monitoring.

? What if…

- **The patient has IV lines and other equipment that cannot be turned off?**
It is common to transfer patients with IV lines. Some wheelchairs are equipped with an IV pole, or you may need to hold the IV bag while taking the patient to the transporting vehicle. If so, always hold the bag well above the patient's chest and arm so that blood does not back up in the tubing. Also, you should notify the long-term care facility so that its staff will have the necessary equipment in the transport vehicle. Portable oxygen and suction are also available for patients who must have them. Usually, the receiving facility will bring these, but you need to coordinate that in advance.

- **When you are ready to transfer the patient, the patient's condition worsens and he or she becomes unstable?**
Perform interventions to stabilize the patient; call for help, if needed; and notify the medical provider. Notify the transporter and the long-term care center of the change in patient status, and postpone the transfer until further medical assessment is done.

(continued on next page)

Procedure 11-3 ■ Transferring a Patient to a Long-Term Care Facility (continued)

Evaluation

The receiving nurse at the long-term care facility will evaluate the patient's response to the move.

Documentation

- Just before the transfer, document your final assessment, and complete the agency's discharge summary.
- You will probably put your final nursing note on a transfer or discharge summary, similar to the ones shown in the Forms section later in this chapter.

Practice Resources

Ernst, McComb, & Ley (2018); The Joint Commission (2018a); Patton, Tidwell, Falder-Saeed, et al. (2017)

Procedure 11-4 ■ Discharging a Patient From the Healthcare Facility

➤ For steps to follow in *all* procedures, refer to the Universal Steps for All Procedures found on the inside back cover.

Equipment

- Health record or chart
- Patient's medications
- Supplies for any ongoing treatments
- Patient's belongings, clothes, and personal care articles
- Standardized discharge form, if available, with instructions for patient
- A utility cart, if belongings are numerous
- Wheelchair

Delegation

If the patient's condition allows, you can delegate to the UAP such tasks as packing belongings, helping the patient dress, and taking the patient out of the facility. However, as the nurse, you are responsible for obtaining and completing the necessary records, making the final assessment, gathering and checking the medications, and coordinating care.

Pre-Procedure Assessments

- Make a final, brief focused physical assessment.
- Assess the patient's mobility.
- Assess for emotional and/or physical distress.
- Assess the patient's ability to communicate and understand what is occurring.

➤ When performing the procedure, always identify your patient according to agency policy, using two identifiers, and be attentive to standard precautions, hand hygiene, patient safety and privacy, body mechanics, and documentation.

Procedure Steps

1. **Notify the patient and the family** as much in advance of the discharge as possible. This is often done early in the hospital stay.
   Allows them time to adjust emotionally and to make any necessary plans.

A Day or Two Before Discharge (Steps 2 and 3)

2. **Make or confirm necessary arrangements.**
   a. Arrange for or help the family arrange for services (e.g., home healthcare, physical therapy, IV therapy, social worker) that will be needed at home.

   NOTE: To reimburse for home care, insurers require a physician's order for all services, and the patient must meet certain eligibility criteria.

   b. Confirm or arrange for equipment needed in the home (e.g., portable oxygen).
   c. Confirm or arrange for transportation.
   d. Make necessary referrals (e.g., medical specialists, physical therapists); book appointments, if necessary and if in line with agency policy.
   Hospital stays are short, and many patients are still ill enough to require continuing complex treatments as well as care by family members when they go home.

3. **Communicate and provide teaching** to the patient and caregivers.
   Patients who have a clear understanding of their after-hospital care (e.g., medications, follow-up visits) are 30% less likely to visit the emergency department or be readmitted compared with patients who lack this information (Agency for Healthcare Research and Quality [AHRQ], 2014b).
   a. Discuss the patient's diagnosis, care needs, and functional abilities with the family/caregiver.
   b. Train the patient and the caregiver in the use of equipment. Arrange for follow-up evaluation at home to check that the equipment is working and being used correctly and that further training is given, if needed.
   With the stress caused by illness and the disruption of transition home, patients may not retain what they have been taught in the hospital. Therapies will be ineffective if equipment is used incorrectly, so follow-up is essential to help avoid further illness and hospital readmission.
   c. Provide education about medication use and side effects.
   Medication errors at home are a frequent cause of adverse events and readmissions to the hospital.

d. Ask relatives or the caregiver to bring clothing for the patient to wear during transport to the home, if needed.
If this was an unplanned admission, the patient may have come to the hospital in nightwear and a robe.

Day of Discharge (Steps 4 Through 16)

4. **Make and document final assessments.**
   a. Assess to ensure that the patient's condition remains as expected.
   b. Confirm that the patient has house keys, that heating has been turned on, and that food is available.
   c. Follow up on diagnostic and laboratory test results.

5. **Bring a wheelchair or other transport** device to the bedside.

6. **Make final notifications.**
   a. Contact the family or the guardian; confirm transportation.
   b. Notify community service agencies and home health nursing of the discharge, as needed.

7. **Gather prescriptions and instruction sheets**, including a list of current medications and appointment cards; give the list to the patient along with the discharge instructions at discharge. **Key Point:** Be certain that either the patient or the caregiver can read the instructions. Inadequate literacy has been shown to be a risk factor for readmission.

8. **Gather and pack the patient's personal items** and treatment supplies.
Having the supplies and equipment ready to go makes the transfer more efficient for you and less stressful for the patient and the family.

9. Prepare the patient's medications. Be certain the medications are labeled correctly; pack them; and record which medications the patient is taking home.
This ensures availability and correct administration of medications when the patient arrives home. It also provides a legal record that the patient left the facility with the medications.

10. **Review discharge instructions** with the patient and the caregiver (and provide a written copy to take home):
    a. Medication instructions
    b. Symptom management and treatments
    c. Information about provider and location for the follow-up appointment(s)
    d. How to obtain further care, treatment, and services, as needed
    e. How and when to call the physician or primary care provider, including instructions on how to recognize signs of a change in condition
    f. Emergency contact
    g. Diet restrictions
    h. Maintenance of hydration
    i. Activities of daily living, focusing on safety and mobility
Teaching should occur throughout the hospital stay. However, it is important to reinforce with a last-minute summary and written instructions to take home. With the stress caused by their illness and the anticipation of discharge, patients may not retain what they have been taught.

11. **Address any questions or concerns** of the patient and the caregiver.
Ensures the patient's ability to safely transition to home.

12. **Give new prescriptions to the patient**, as well as reminder cards for outpatient appointments (e.g., with physicians, social services) to the patient.
Ensures continuity of care, thus minimizing patient stress.

13. **Document your final nursing note, and complete the discharge summary** (the patient often receives a copy of the summary). The patient needs a copy of (1) instructions for care at home, which may be called a *discharge plan*, and (2) a discharge summary, which is a summary of the progress of his illness as well as the treatment received from admission through discharge. Some agencies combine these into one form.
It is important to document the patient's condition at the time he or she leaves the unit. This provides a baseline for comparison if the patient's condition should deteriorate after discharge.

14. **Accompany the patient off the unit** and out of the hospital (or delegate this task) when you are notified that transportation has arrived.
Keeping the patient on the unit as long as practical helps minimize the anxiety and fatigue that may occur as a result of a long wait in the hospital lobby while a family member or other caregiver brings the car to the door.

15. **Notify the admissions department** of the discharge. Depending on agency policy, notify the primary care provider or the admitting physician.
This will discontinue all scheduled services, such as meals, and notify the housekeeping department that the room needs to be cleaned.

16. **Ensure the patient's records are sent** to the medical records department.
Whether paper or electronic, the chart is a legal document and remains permanently in storage in the medical records department.

? What if...

- **Near the time of discharge, the patient's condition worsens and he or she becomes unstable?**
  Perform interventions to stabilize the patient; call for help, if needed; and notify the provider.
  Notify the family that discharge will be delayed.
  Communicate with other hospital departments and community agencies, as necessary.

- **The patient is an older adult?**
  Allow for more time for the patient to dress and leave the hospital.
  Allow for more time to communicate, teach, and answer questions.
  Obtain feedback to ensure that the caregivers have heard and understood the instructions.

(continued on next page)

Procedure 11-4 ■ Discharging a Patient From the Healthcare Facility (continued)

Consider having a geriatric nurse specialist make follow-up home visits.
Hearing, visual, and mobility deficits become more common with advanced age.

■ **The patient is taking "high-risk" drugs after discharge?**

Medications with a high risk of postdischarge adverse events include corticosteroids, anticoagulants, antidiabetes medications, antibiotics, antianxiety agents, sedatives, and narcotic analgesics. Provide teaching for patient, family, and other caregivers throughout the hospital stay. A day or two before discharge, review teaching with patient and family; evaluate their understanding. On discharge, summarize medication precautions, and provide clear written instructions. Be sure that the patient and the family can read them.

Evaluation

A few weeks after discharge, the facility will contact the patient to evaluate the quality and appropriateness of the discharge process. This may be done through a home visit, a telephone interview, or a questionnaire sent to the patient. As a nurse, you may or may not be involved in this evaluation. The best way to evaluate the multidisciplinary care will be based on the need for the patient to be readmitted to the acute care facility.

Documentation

- **For the health record, the primary provider will write a discharge progress note that contains the following information:**
  Reason for hospitalization
  Significant findings during the stay, including significant changes in status since admission
  Procedures performed; care, treatment, and services provided during the stay
  Status of goals for the stay
  Condition at discharge
- **Agency policy determines the format and content of nursing documentation.** This is often a combination of a structured discharge form or checklist and a narrative progress note. Regardless of format, you should document the following information:
  - Your final assessment of the patient's health status
  - Information and teaching provided to the patient and the caregivers
  - Referrals, medications
  - How the patient left the unit (e.g., in wheelchair) and who accompanied him (e.g., wife, staff member)

  The Joint Commission recommends standardized formats for documentation (2008, p. 367).

To see examples of discharge summaries, see the Forms section, later in this chapter.

Practice Resources

Agency for Healthcare Research and Quality (2014a, 2014b); Alper, E., O'Malley, T.A., & Greenwald, J., 2017; The Joint Commission (2018a); Kronick, Arnold, & Brady (2016); Lim, F., Foust, J., & VanCleave, J. (2016).

CLINICAL INSIGHTS

Clinical Insight 11-1 ➤ Preparing the Room for an Admission

Delegation

As a general rule, these tasks can be delegated to unlicensed assistive personnel (UAPs). The nurse is responsible for evaluating and supervising as well as for setting up special equipment (although the UAP may obtain it from storage).

Clean the Room

Although there are differences among agencies, it is common for the housekeeping department to clean the room and change the bed linens when a patient is discharged, so you should find the room ready for your preparations. The rest of these guidelines assume that fact.

Prepare the Bed

- Position the bed according to patient status. If the patient is ambulatory, put the bed in the lowest position, and lock the wheels. If the patient will arrive on a stretcher, place the bed at stretcher height.
- If necessary, rearrange the furniture to allow easy access to the bed.
- Fold back the top linens to "open" the bed (see figure).
- The patient may need to be placed in the bed immediately, so it should be ready when he or she arrives.

Prepare Routine Supplies

- Most agencies have an admission pack containing a lotion, tissues, water pitcher, and a drinking cup. Open the pack, and place its contents in the room.
- Place a hospital gown on the bed and nonslip footwear by the bedside. Some patients may choose to wear their own sleep clothing.

Prepare Equipment

You will need:

- A stethoscope, a thermometer, and a blood pressure cuff in the room for taking vital signs
- A scale for measuring and weighing the patient
- If the patient is not ambulatory, a bedpan, a urinal, and perhaps a bedside commode
- A clean-catch urine specimen container if laboratory work has not already been done
- Set up and check special equipment (e.g., oxygen, suction, cardiac monitor, pulse oximeter, IV pump).

Prepare the Environment

Turn on the lights, and adjust the room temperature. Open or close curtains, as needed.

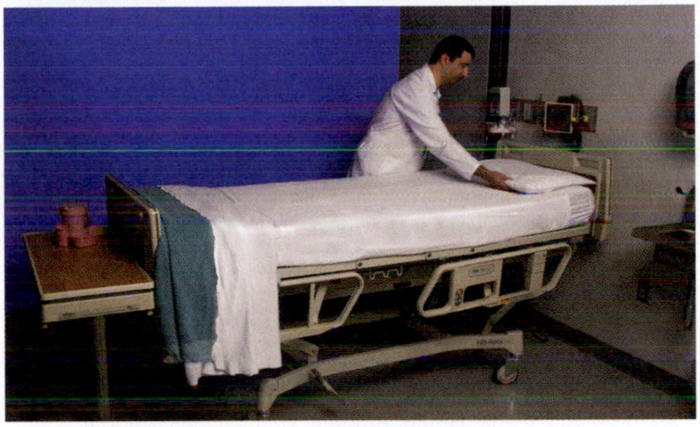

FORMS

The forms in this section are copies that are put into the patient's permanent record in paper form. Many agencies, however, have computer-based discharge processes.

Fishermen's HOSPITAL

Discharge Assessment/Instructions

Date of Discharge	Time of Discharge	Mode of Discharge ☐ Ambulatory ☐ Wheelchair ☐ Stretcher ☐ Ambulance	Accompanied by:
Belongings sent with patient/family ☐ Yes ☐ No		Personal Medications sent with patient family ☐ Yes ☐ No	
Temp	P	Discharge Destination ☐ Home ☐ AMA ☐ Facility______ ☐ Home Health	Transfer Information Sent ☐ Yes ☐ No
R	BP		
Special Instructions			

Patient Assessment and Health Status

	Yes	No		Yes	No		Yes	No
Afebrile	☐	☐	Skin Intact	☐	☐	Hygiene	☐	☐
Able to live independently	☐	☐	Eating Well	☐	☐	Self-Care	☐	☐
Pain Controlled	☐	☐	Adequate Hydration	☐	☐	Assist	☐	☐
Oriented	☐	☐				Total Care	☐	☐
Appropriate Behavior	☐	☐				Adequate Elimination	☐	☐
Functions Independently	☐	☐						

Additional Comments:

Weight monitoring daily **Avoid all tobacco products**

Instructions

Diet ☐ No Restrictions	
Activity ☐ No Restrictions	
Special Equipment/Treatment ☐ No Restrictions	
Discharge Medications (Name, Amount, Special Instructions) ☐ No Meds See Patient Education	
Special Instructions/Discharge Summary **Call MD or go to the ER if symptoms worsen**	
☐ Pt or Caregiver given instructions about and counseled on potential for drug-food interactions	
Physician Follow-up Appointment	Outpatient Visit
Referral ☐ None Required	

I have received all personal belongings.
I have received a copy and understand the above Instructions.
I have received a copy of the Patient Education form.

Patient Identification

____
Signature/Responsible Party

____
Physician/Nurse Signature **Date**

0916065

Fishermen's HOSPITAL

3301 Overseas Highway, Marathon, FL 33050 • Ph 305-743-5533 • Fax 305-743-3962

Allergies/Reactions	No known drug allergies ☐			**IN-PATIENT** Circle Y to continue or N to not continue and sign below to authenticate order.			**AT DISCHARGE** Circle Y to continue at same dose or N to not continue or document any changes in dose.		
MEDICATION NAME (Include Herbal, OTC, Vitamins)	Dose / Route / Freq	Reason Taken	LAST DOSE DATE/TIME	Continue on Admission		Continue at home on same dose		Continue with the following changes:	
Patient takes no medication ☐									
				Y	N	Y	N		
				Y	N	Y	N		
				Y	N	Y	N		
				Y	N	Y	N		
				Y	N	Y	N		
				Y	N	Y	N		
				Y	N	Y	N		
				Y	N	Y	N		
				Y	N	Y	N		
				Y	N	Y	N		
				Y	N	Y	N		
				Y	N	Y	N		
				Y	N	Y	N		
				Y	N	Y	N		

Source-of-Medication list *(check all used)*:

___ Bottles/List
___ Patient/Family
___ Retail pharmacy ______________________
______
___ MD office records
___ Previous discharge medical record
___ Medication Administration Record from ____________
______
___ Med Reconciliation Form

Meds:

___ Sent home with ______________________
___ Removed
Sent to Pharmacy for approval

New medications prescribed for patient discharge:

Meds	Dose / Route / Freq	Reason

ADMITTING NURSE SIGNATURE	DATE	DISCHARGE NURSE SIGNATURE	DATE

Patient Education Form

Page _____ of _____

FORM N-100, Rev. 12-07 White: Chart Yellow: Patient

CLINICALJUDGMENT

Applying the Full-Spectrum Nursing Model

PATIENT SITUATION

Recall Evelyn's case (Meet Your Patient in Volume 1). She is 87 years old and has lived in a nursing home for the past 5 years. She suffers from congestive heart failure (CHF), hypertension, diabetes, macular degeneration resulting in near blindness, a severe hearing deficit, urinary incontinence, and immobility resulting from a hip fracture. Despite these limitations, she keeps current with regard to the lives of all of her family members and friends. At the nursing home, staff members confide in Evelyn, and she knows about their children, their romances, and the gossip around the nursing home. Whenever there is an election, she makes sure that she gets to vote. She "reads" every audio book she can get her hands on.

Recently, Evelyn was admitted to the hospital for severe CHF. When leaving the nursing home, she told her pastor, "I don't want to die yet. I'm having too much fun!" You notice that the papers from the nursing home do not contain an advance directive, and it was not mentioned in the nursing home's report to you.

THINKING

1. *Critical Thinking (Considering Alternatives):*
   a. What are some possible reasons that there is no advance directive?
   b. Which of those seems most likely to you?
   c. How might you find out about the status of Evelyn's advance directive?

DOING

2. *Nursing Process (Nursing Diagnosis):* On the care plan from the nursing home, there were two nursing diagnoses:
   - Urge Urinary Incontinence, related to difficulty ambulating to the bathroom
   - Impaired Skin Integrity, related to immobility and incontinence

   Which of these can you remove from the care plan for now? Explain your decision.

CARING

3. *Self-Knowledge:* The next day, despite aggressive treatment, Evelyn's condition worsens. She is not responding to verbal stimuli, and her oxygen level is decreasing. There is discussion about putting her on a ventilator.
   a. What would be your feelings?
   b. If Evelyn has an advance directive that says "no ventilator," how would that change your feelings?
   c. If there is an advance directive that says, "Do everything possible to keep me alive," how would that change your feelings?

   Note: We are not asking you what you would do; rather, you should consider how you would feel.

Critical Thinking and Clinical Judgment

1. Describe your personal view of health.
2. Identify an individual in your life, personally or professionally, who personifies health. What characteristics do you identify in this individual that represent health? What factors do you think contribute to this individual's health status?

3. Use the nursing process to develop a plan to improve your personal health.

4. What attributes, resources, or life experiences do you have as an individual to offer in your role as a nurse?

5. For each of the following concepts, use critical thinking to describe how or why it is important to nursing, patient care, or experiencing health and illness. Note that these are *not* to be merely definitions.

   Health

   Wellness

   Illness

   Disruptions

   Hardiness

   Responses to illness

   Health–illness continuum

What Are the Main Points in This Chapter?

- Health is a complex phenomenon that involves physical, mental, and spiritual aspects. Having good health is an almost universal desire.
- Wellness is a way of life oriented toward optimal health and well-being.
- Life and wellness require nourishment. Nourishment comes in the form of food, exercise, sleep, relationships, meaningful work, the environment, and memories.
- The person with an illness rarely perceives the experience as a medical diagnosis. Instead, illness is usually described in terms of how it makes the person feel, such as pain, sadness, loss, fatigue, or being overwhelmed.
- People dealing with life-threatening illnesses have to figure out how to live even while dying. Dealing with death is one of the most difficult experiences you will face as a nurse.
- One aspect of persevering through illness and life disruption is maintaining as much normalcy as possible. Normalcy helps clients cope with illness.
- Nurses deal with people who have been thrust into new life situations—situations they did not ask for and for which they were not prepared.
- People who are suffering illnesses experience loneliness, part of which can be related to the actual physical separation, part to a sense of the world going on without them, and part to a sense of no one really being in their world.
- Several factors influence a person's responses to disruptions. These factors include age; family patterns; culture; hardiness; support; access to healthcare resources; the stage and nature of the illness; and the intensity, duration, and multiplicity of the disruption.
- Chronic illnesses are a large and growing healthcare concern, especially among older adults.
- You can ease the disruptions experienced by the patient during admission, transfers, and discharge from a healthcare setting through effective discharge planning, communication, coordination, and teaching.
- As a nurse, you will need to cultivate a healing presence. Listening, being attentive, being willing to learn from those in your care, and recognizing and respecting others' ways of coping are behaviors associated with a healing presence.
- Most people experience health, illness, and wellness as an ever-changing continuum through which they move.
- Communicating genuine care, concern, and sensitivity comes from who you are as a person, not from assuming a professional persona that you "put on" to fulfill a role.
- Patients and families may not recognize the strengths and creative abilities that they bring to a situation. Part of the art of nursing is to envision the strengths and potential in patients and families who may be too overwhelmed to identify them on their own.
- Your healing presence may be the most memorable aspect of nursing care that you have to offer.

Knowledge Map

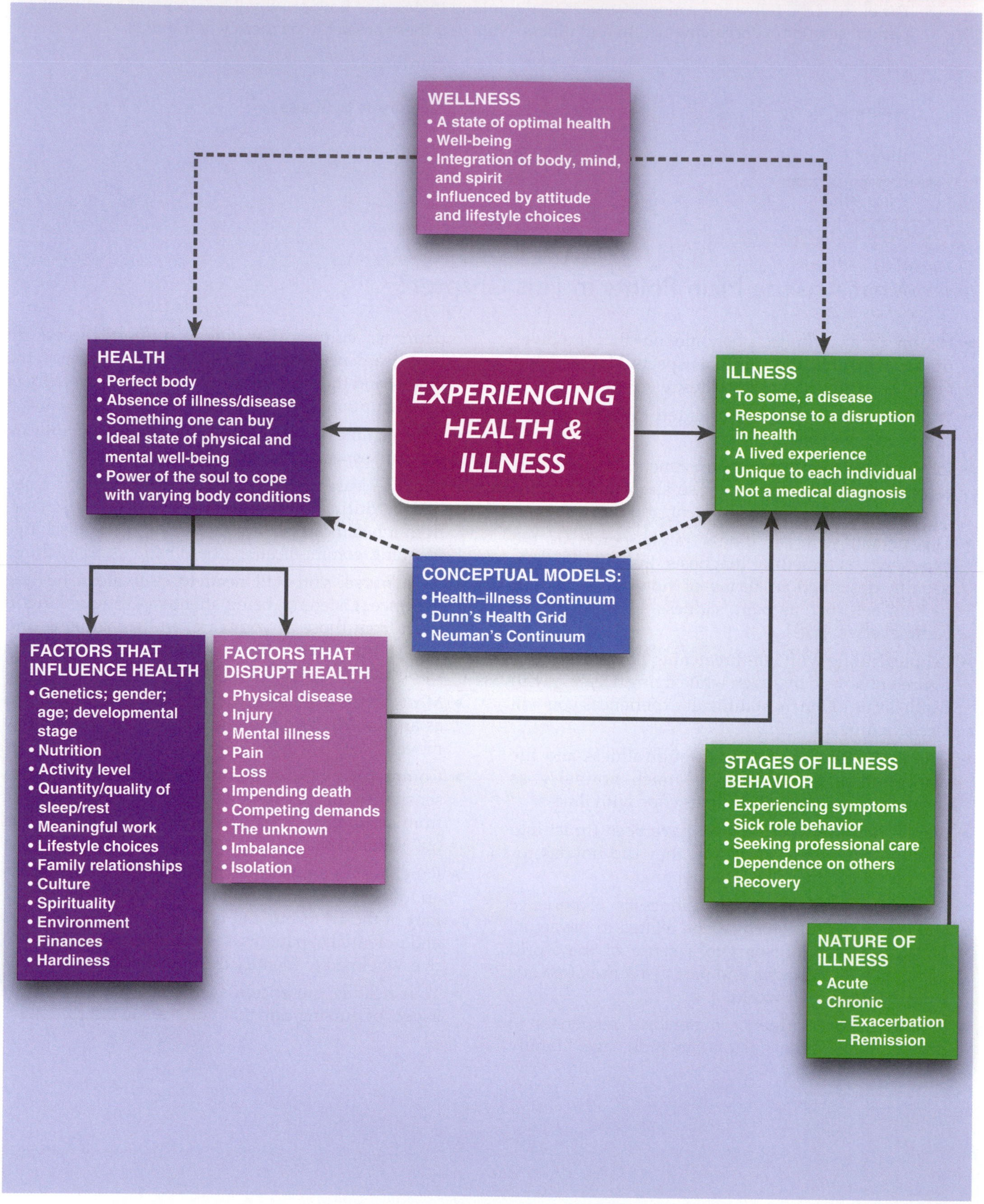

CHAPTER 12

Stress & Adaptation

STUDENT RESOURCES

The questions and exercises in this book allow you to practice the kind of thinking you will use as a full-spectrum nurse. Critical-thinking questions usually have more than one right answer, so we do not provide "correct answers" for these features. Try to answer these questions yourself. It is more important to develop your nursing judgment than to just cover content. You will learn more by discussing the questions with your peers. If you are still unsure, see the Davis Advantage chapter resources for suggested responses.

To explore learning resources for this chapter,

Go to Davis Advantage and find:

Answers and Suggested Responses for all questions in this chapter
Concept Map
Knowledge Map
References and Bibliography
Lists of NOC Outcomes and NIC Interventions

Key Concepts

Adaptation
Anxiety
Coping
Fear
Stress

Related Concepts

See the Concept Map on Davis Advantage.

Example Problem

Post-Traumatic Stress Disorder (PTSD)

Caring for the Nguyens

After having a comprehensive physical examination at the family health center, Yen Nguyen has been scheduled to have a mammogram and screening laboratory work. When she arrives at the clinic for her mammogram, she tells you she is very nervous. "I have a good friend who just found out she has breast cancer. She's very depressed now. Do I really have to do this test?"

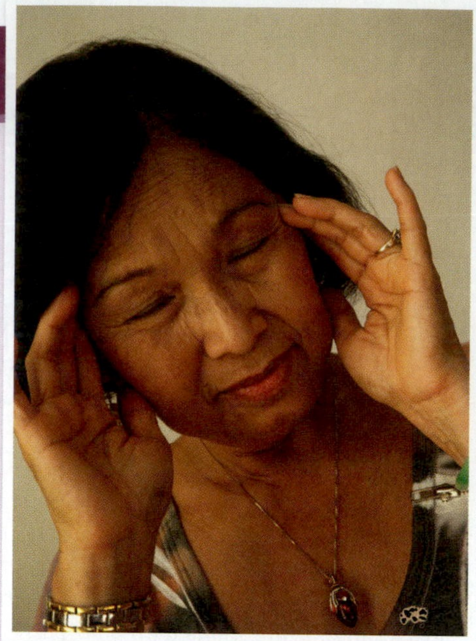

A. What kind of stress is Yen experiencing?

B. Three days later, the radiologist contacts Yen requesting that she return to the family health center for additional films of the upper outer quadrant of the right breast. "There are some calcifications I want to check out," explains the radiologist.
- What factors might affect Yen's adaptation to this stress?
- Evaluate what you know about Yen's perception of her stress, her overall health status, her support system, and her coping methods. What more do you need to know about these topics to fully answer this question?

C. Later, Yen calls the office frantically explaining that she is very upset about this recent event. She says, "Not knowing is killing me. I'm so nervous I can't stand it. I can't sleep. I can't eat." She asks how she can handle the stress until she comes in for the additional tests next week. What strategies would you recommend to help Yen deal with the stress?

PracticalKnowledge clinical **application**

CLINICAL INSIGHTS

Clinical Insight 12-1 ➤ Dealing with Angry Patients

- **Be aware of how you are responding to angry patients.** Are you relieving your own stress, or are you relieving the client's stress? If you respond angrily to relieve your own stress, you may provoke further anger in the patient and even escalate the situation to the point of aggression.
- **Remind yourself not to take anger personally;** remind family members and colleagues of this as well.
- **Recognize that anger and anxiety are normal feelings when facing adversity,** such as a life-threatening or debilitating illness. Do not discount feelings by saying something like, "Please, don't be so angry," or "You shouldn't talk like that." Or, "Everything will be OK. Don't worry."
- **Encourage the client and family to express feelings** verbally and appropriately.
- **Listen instead of defending.** If the patient says, "Everything about this place stinks," *don't defend.* Don't respond with a comment such as, "We really are all trying to do the best we can for you."

Clinical Insight 12-1 ➤ Dealing with Angry Patients *(continued)*

Do encourage the person to express his feelings or give you more information: "You seem really angry; what's going on?" or "Maybe I can help. Tell me a little more about what stinks."

- **Do not take responsibility for the patient's anger.** It is not your fault, so don't apologize—unless you really *do* have something to apologize for.
- **Remain calm;** this reassures the patient and also keeps the emotion from escalating.
- **Help the patient identify what is causing the anger,** and try to meet those needs.
- **Be alert to your own and the patient's safety needs.**

Do not allow a patient to get between you and the door if the person seems to be violent.

Do not wear a stethoscope around your neck, dangling jewelry, or anything a patient might use to hurt you.

Do not go into a room alone with a patient who seems to have the potential for violence.

Do not turn your back on an angry patient.

Remain at least an arm's length away from an angry and potentially violent patient.

Key Point: ***Be sure you know how to call for help from staff or security personnel if you think you or someone else is in danger.***

Key Point: ***If you believe the patient's anger may escalate to violence, your priority is your own safety and the safety of others in the area.***

Also refer to the NIC intervention, Anger Control Assistance (Butcher, Bulechek, Dochterman, et al., 2018, pp. 69-70).

Clinical Insight 12-2 ➤ Crisis Intervention Guidelines

For nurses who are at an entry level of practice, the goals of crisis intervention include the following (Brammer & MacDonald, 2003; Gorman & Anwar, 2014):

Assess the Situation.

What is the nature of the patient's condition and the severity of the crisis?

Ensure Safety.

- Call for help if you or the patient is in physical danger.
- Do not leave the patient unless you think you are in imminent danger.
- First ensure your own safety; then provide for the patient's safety.

Defuse the Situation.

- Keep in mind that a person in crisis may not be in control of his or her actions.
- Try to calm the person verbally.
- Attempt physical restraint only as a last resort and only when there is enough help to do it safely for both the staff and the patient.

Decrease the Person's Anxiety.

- Reassure the person that he or she is in a safe place and that you are concerned and want to help.
- Explain gently but firmly that you need the person's help and cooperation.
- Help the person to vent feelings of fear, guilt, and anger.
- Use physical contact very cautiously. The person in turmoil may interpret touch as aggression or a sexual approach.

Determine the Problem.

- Find out what the patient believes to be the cause of the crisis.
- Remain calm, and do not pressure the patient to give reasons. Any tension on your part will create further panic in the patient.

Decide on the Type of Help Needed.

- You may be able to calm the person enough for him to understand what just happened, or you may not. Evaluate your ability to calm the patient on the basis of your assessment of his or her coping skills and resources.
- Put in place the help needed to restore the person to a minimal level of functioning. This may require long-term treatment. In that case, make the necessary referrals.

Return the Person to his or her Precrisis Level of Functioning. This May Involve Crisis Counseling and/or Home Crisis Visits.

- *Crisis counseling.* The goal is to provide immediate relief, solve the most urgent problems, and give long-term counseling, if needed. Crisis centers often rely on telephone counseling ("hotlines").
- *Home visits.* If telephone counseling is not adequate or if observations of the home environment are needed, home visits may be necessary.

ASSESSMENT GUIDELINES AND TOOLS

Focused Assessment

The Holmes-Rahe Social Readjustment Scale

This is a way to check your stress level, measured in "life change units." Of course, it is not possible to score the exact "amount" of stress. However, this will give you a general idea of your stress level and should provide some insight into the sources of your stress. The following are based on the number of life change units over a 1- to 2-year period:

- Over 300 points (Major amount of change): 80% chance of major illness
- 200–299 (Moderate amount of change): 50% chance of major illness
- 150–199 (Mild amount of change): 33% chance of major illness
- 0–149 (Insignificant amount of change): Minimal chance of major illness

Of course, your personality and your ability to cope also determine the likelihood of your becoming ill.

Life Event	Life Change Units	Life Event	Life Change Units
Death of spouse	100	Son or daughter leaving home	29
Divorce	73	Trouble with in-laws	29
Marital separation	65	Outstanding personal achievement	28
Imprisonment	63	Spouse begins or stops work	26
Death of a close family member	63	Beginning or ending school	26
Personal injury or illness	53	Change in living conditions	25
Marriage	50	Revision of personal habits	24
Dismissal from work	47	Trouble with boss	23
Marital reconciliation	45	Change in work hours or conditions	20
Retirement	45	Change in residence	20
Change in health of family member	44	Change in schools	20
Pregnancy	40	Change in recreation	19
Sexual difficulties	39	Change in church activities	19
Gain of new family member	39	Change in social activities	18
Business readjustment	39	Minor mortgage or loan	17
Change in financial state	38	Change in sleeping habits	16
Change in number of arguments with spouse	35	Change in number of family reunions	15
Major mortgage	32	Change in eating habits	15
Foreclosure of mortgage or loan	30	Vacation	13
Change in responsibilities at work	29		

Source: Reprinted from Holmes, T., & Rahe, R. (1967). Social readjustment rating scale. *Journal of Psychosomatic Research, 11*(2), 213–218. Reprinted with permission from Elsevier.

Focused Assessment

Assessing for Stress: Questions to Ask

1. **Assess stressors and risk factors.** Ask the client to complete a stress inventory, such as the preceding Holmes-Rahe Social Readjustment Scale. Then ask the client the following questions:
   - What is causing the most stress in your life?
   - On a scale of 1 to 10 (where 1 is "not much" and 10 is "extreme"), rate the stress you are experiencing in each of these areas: work or school, finances, community responsibilities, your health, health of a family member, family relationships, family responsibilities, relationships with friends.
   - How long have you been dealing with the stressful situation(s)?
   - Can you track the accumulation of stress in your life?
   - How long have you been under this stress?
   - Note the client's developmental stage, and determine whether he is functioning as expected for this stage. Review Chapter 9 if you need help to identify developmental milestones. To help you assess for stressors that can be predicted to occur in each stage, you might ask questions such as:

     What challenges do you face as a result of your life and your age?

     Have you had recent life changes?

     Do you anticipate any life changes?

To review developmental stage milestones and changes,

Go to **Chapters 9 and 10,** in Volume 1. Also see Chapter 12, **Box 12-1: Stressors Throughout the Life Span,** in Volume 1.

2. **Assess coping methods and adaptation.**
   - What coping strategies have you used previously? What was successful, and what was not successful?
   - Tell me about previous experiences you have had with stressful situations in your life.
   - What do you usually do to handle stressful situations? (If the client needs prompting, you can ask, "Do you cry, get angry, avoid people, talk to family or friends, do physical exercise, pray? Some people laugh or joke, others meditate, others try to control everything, and others just work hard, or look for a solution. What is your usual response?")
   - How well do these methods usually work for you?
   - What have you been doing to cope with the present situation?
   - How well is that working?
   - During the interview, you should also observe for the use of psychological defense mechanisms.

To review psychological defense mechanisms,

Go to Chapter 12, **Table 12-1: Psychological Defense Mechanisms,** in Volume 1.

   - If the patient has not exhibited any defense mechanisms, you could ask about the common ones. For example, "Do you ever cope with a situation by denying it exists or just by trying to put it out of your mind?"
   - Also ask the client about physiological changes and diseases caused by ongoing stress. Check the client's records for a history of somatoform disorders. Ask the client:

     What physical illnesses do you have? How long have you had them?

     What, if any, physical changes have you noticed?

     Do you have other physical conditions, for example, hypertension, cardiac disease, diabetes, arthritis, joint pains, or cancer?

To review findings that might indicate maladaptation to stress,

Go to Chapter 12, **Table 12-2: Organic Disorders Brought About by Failure of Adaptive Mechanisms,** in Volume 1.

3. **Assess physiological responses to stress.**

The following are examples of questions you should ask:

- What do you do to stay healthy?
- Tell me about your health habits.
- How often do you have a checkup?
- What are your health concerns?

4. **Assess emotional and behavioral responses to stress.**

Emotional Responses

Observe for:

- Anger
- Anxiety
- Depression
- Fear
- Feelings of inadequacy
- Low self-esteem
- Irritability
- Lack of motivation
- Lethargy

Behavioral Responses

Observe for:

- Crying, emotional outbursts
- Dependence
- Poor job performance
- Substance use and abuse
- Sleeplessness (or sleeping too much)
- Change in eating habits (e.g., loss of appetite, overeating)
- Decrease in quality of job performance
- Preoccupation (i.e., daydreaming)
- Illnesses
- Increased absenteeism from work or school
- Increased number of accidents
- Avoiding social situations or relationships
- Rebellion, acting out

(Continued)

Focused Assessment

Assessing for Stress: Questions to Ask—cont'd

Examples of Assessment Questions

- Do you smoke tobacco products?
- How much alcohol do you drink per week?
- What do you eat? What is your typical eating pattern?
- How much fluid do you drink daily?
- How many hours do you sleep at night? Do you feel rested when you wake up? Do you take naps?
- Do you often wake up very early in the morning and have difficulty getting back to sleep?
- What prescribed medications, vitamins, over-the-counter medications, or herbs do you take?
- What regular physical activity or exercise do you engage in?
- How much time do you spend at work versus at leisure and play?
- Do you constantly take work home with you? Or think about work almost all the time?
- How do you relax?
- Have you given up activities and relationships you previously enjoyed because you "don't have enough time" or are too tired?
- How do you express anger? What typically causes you frustration?
- Do you try to be perfect?
- Would you describe yourself as having the stress-filled lifestyle of a type A personality?
- How often do you find yourself feeling hopeless? Sad?

5. **Assess cognitive responses to stress.**

   Observe for the following responses when you assess other functional areas:

   - Difficulty concentrating
   - Poor judgment
   - Decrease in accuracy (e.g., in counting money)
   - Forgetfulness
   - Decreased problem-solving ability
   - Decreased attention to detail
   - Difficulty learning
   - Narrowing of focus
   - Preoccupation, daydreaming

6. **Assess support systems.**

   Ask the following questions:

   - Tell me about your home. Describe your living environment. (Make a home visit, if possible, or contact the case manager or social worker to arrange a home evaluation.)
   - Who are the persons who provide the most support for you? In what ways do they support you?
   - What support is available from family, friends, significant others, community agencies, and clergy that you may not have required until now?
   - Do you have or do you seek spiritual support?
   - How has your stress affected the family?
   - What are your financial resources? What are your financial obligations?

CLINICALJUDGMENT

Applying the Full-Spectrum Nursing Model

PATIENT SITUATION

Mrs. Williams, a 76-year-old woman, was admitted yesterday after suffering a stroke that paralyzed her right side. She has had diabetes and high blood pressure for many years. Since the stroke, she has been unable to speak clearly and becomes frustrated as she attempts to communicate her needs. Her daughter says Mrs. Williams is a proud, independent, and tidy woman, who has been living alone since her husband's death last year. Until her stroke, she had been driving her car, cleaning the house, doing her grocery shopping, and maintaining the yard and garden. She wears eyeglasses for reading and driving and has a hearing aid, although she rarely uses it.

THINKING

1. *Theoretical Knowledge:*

   a. What stroke risk factors probably functioned as stressors for Mrs. Williams? (*Hint:* Look up stroke risk factors in a medical-surgical nursing or pathophysiology text, or online.)

   b. What are common stressors for patients who must be hospitalized?

2. *Critical Thinking (Contextual Awareness):*

   c. Now that Mrs. Williams is in the hospital, what new stressors might she have?

DOING

3. *Practical Knowledge:* What might you advise Mrs. Williams's daughter to do to help her mother adapt more comfortably to the stressors in the hospital?

4. *Nursing Process (Diagnosis):* Based on only the data in the scenario, write one actual nursing diagnosis for Mrs. Williams. Do not use potential diagnoses. Remember, the defining characteristics must be present in the scenario. State the data you would need in order to make the diagnosis more descriptive.

CARING

5. *Self-Knowledge:* Imagine yourself in Mrs. Williams's situation.

   a. What is the one thing that would cause you the most stress? Why would that be the most stressful thing?

   b. What is the single most important thing you would want your nurse to do for you?

Critical Thinking and Clinical Judgment

1. Gloria and her husband John (Meet Your Patient, in Volume 1) live in a residential community, and John commutes from there to work in a nearby city. Gloria runs an accounting business from their home. They have two teenage boys, who are active in sports, church activities, Boy Scouts, and the school band. The boys need transportation to their various activities. Gloria and John teach Sunday school and are Boy Scout leaders. Gloria's mother needs knee replacement surgery and so cannot take care of Gloria's father, who is in the early stage of Alzheimer's disease. In addition to her own home responsibilities, Gloria must go to her parents' house to prepare meals and to provide care for her parents during the day. Gloria's sister comes at 8:00 p.m. to sleep in the parents' home during the night.

   a. What resources may be available to help Gloria?

   b. What stress-reducing techniques can you suggest to help Gloria?

   c. What may reduce John's stress?

   d. On a scale of 1 to 10 (1 being low and 10 being high), what number will you give to Gloria's stress level?

2. Look again at Gloria and John's situation. Using the following list of defense mechanisms, create a possible scenario for each. That is, what might Gloria (or John) say and/or do if using one of the defense mechanisms in this situation? If you need to review psychological defense mechanisms,

Go to **Table 12-1,** in Volume 1.

   a. **Avoidance**—unconsciously staying away from events or situations that might open feelings of aggression or anxiety.

   b. **Conversion**—changing emotional conflict into physical symptoms that have no physical basis.

   c. **Denial**—transforming reality by refusing to acknowledge thoughts, feelings, desires, or impulses. This is an unconscious response; the person is *not* consciously lying.

   d. **Displacement**— "Kicking the dog." Transferring emotions, ideas, or wishes from one original object or situation to a substitute inappropriate person or object that is perceived to be less powerful or less threatening.

e. **Reaction formation**—similar to compensation, except the person develops the exact opposite trait. The person is aware of his or her feelings but acts in ways opposite to what he or she is really feeling.

3. Mary is a nursing student. She works part time to maintain health insurance coverage for herself and her children and to earn tuition money for school. She has to do her studying after the children are in bed, so she gets little sleep herself. Her grades are low and do not reflect Mary's true knowledge level. The Nursing faculty suggest that Mary seek counseling for dealing with examination anxiety and learn about test-taking strategies. Mary realizes she may fail out of nursing school without this counseling, but she does not know how she will fit weekly sessions into her already full schedule.

   a. List Mary's stressors.

   b. *Self-Knowledge*:

   - What life experiences do you have that may help you to understand Mary's situation?
   - How could these same life experiences interfere with your empathy for and understanding of Mary?
   - How much of Mary's story can you identify with as being part of your own experience now?

   c. Which type of intervention do you think would be most helpful to Mary: (1) helping her to change her perception of her stressors, or (2) the health promotion activities discussed in Volume 1? Explain your reasoning.

   d. Before deciding specifically how to help Mary, what data do you still need?

   e. Based on the information you have, what do you think Mary's two most important goals are?

   f. If you discover that Mary's most important goals actually are to (1) provide for her children and (2) succeed in nursing school, how might you use this information to help her?

4. *Self-Knowledge:* In Volume 1, you listed your stressors. Let's assess further.

   a. What are your two (or three) *most* important goals? List them in order of importance.

   b. What support do you have that can help you to achieve each of these goals?

5. *Self-Knowledge and Theoretical Knowledge:* Lead a partner through a visualization exercise; then reverse roles, and have your partner lead you through it.

   a. Before beginning, what were your thoughts and feelings about the exercise?

   b. After doing the visualization exercise, how did you feel? Did you feel more relaxed?

   c. How do you think your attitudes and perceptions prior to the exercise affected how you felt *after* the exercise?

6. For each of the following concepts, use critical thinking to describe how or why it is important to nursing, patient care, or stress and adaptation. Note that these are *not* to be merely definitions.

Stress

Developmental stressors

Coping strategies

Psychological defense mechanisms

Inflammatory response

Somatoform disorders

Relaxation techniques for stress reduction

What Are the Main Points in This Chapter?

- Stress is a disturbance in normal homeostasis caused by internal or external stimuli called *stressors*.
- Adaptive coping techniques are those that offer healthy choices to the person and reduce the negative effects of stress.
- Approaches to coping include altering the stressor, adapting to the stressor, and avoiding the stressor.
- Whether the outcome of stress is positive (adaptation) or negative (disease) depends on the balance between the strength and duration of the stressors and the effectiveness of the person's coping methods.
- The three stages of Selye's general adaptation syndrome (GAS) are alarm, resistance, and exhaustion. Each stage in GAS produces different physical or psychological responses.
- In the alarm stage of GAS, responses are produced primarily by adrenal hormones, epinephrine, mineral-ocorticoids, and the sympathetic nervous system.
- The exhaustion stage can lead to stress-induced illness, burnout, or death.
- The two most common responses of local adaptation syndrome (LAS) are the reflex pain response and the inflammatory response.
- Examples of psychological responses are anxiety, fear, anger, and ego defense mechanisms.
- Psychological defense mechanisms are unconscious mental mechanisms that help decrease the inner tension associated with stressors; when overused, they are maladaptive.
- Unsuccessful adaptation can lead to crisis, organic disease (e.g., stomach ulcers), somatoform disorders (e.g., hypochondriasis), and psychological disorders (e.g., mental illness).
- Crisis exists when (1) an event in a person's life drastically changes his or her routine and is perceived as a threat to self, and (2) the person's usual coping methods are ineffective, resulting in high anxiety and reduced ability to function.
- Burnout occurs when nurses or other professionals cannot cope effectively with the demands of the workplace.
- You should assess for data about the patient's stressors, risk factors, coping and adaptation, support systems, and psychosocial and physiological responses to stress.
- Interventions for stress must be individualized to the patient. They include (1) health promotion activities for preventing and improving the ability to cope with stressors; (2) managing anxiety, fear, and anger; (3) stress management techniques that focus on discharging tension or producing relaxation; (4) techniques to alter perception (i.e., cognitive restructuring and positive self-talk); (5) identifying and using support systems; (6) reducing the stress of hospitalization; (7) providing spiritual support; (8) crisis intervention; (9) stress management in the workplace; and (10) making referrals.

Knowledge Map

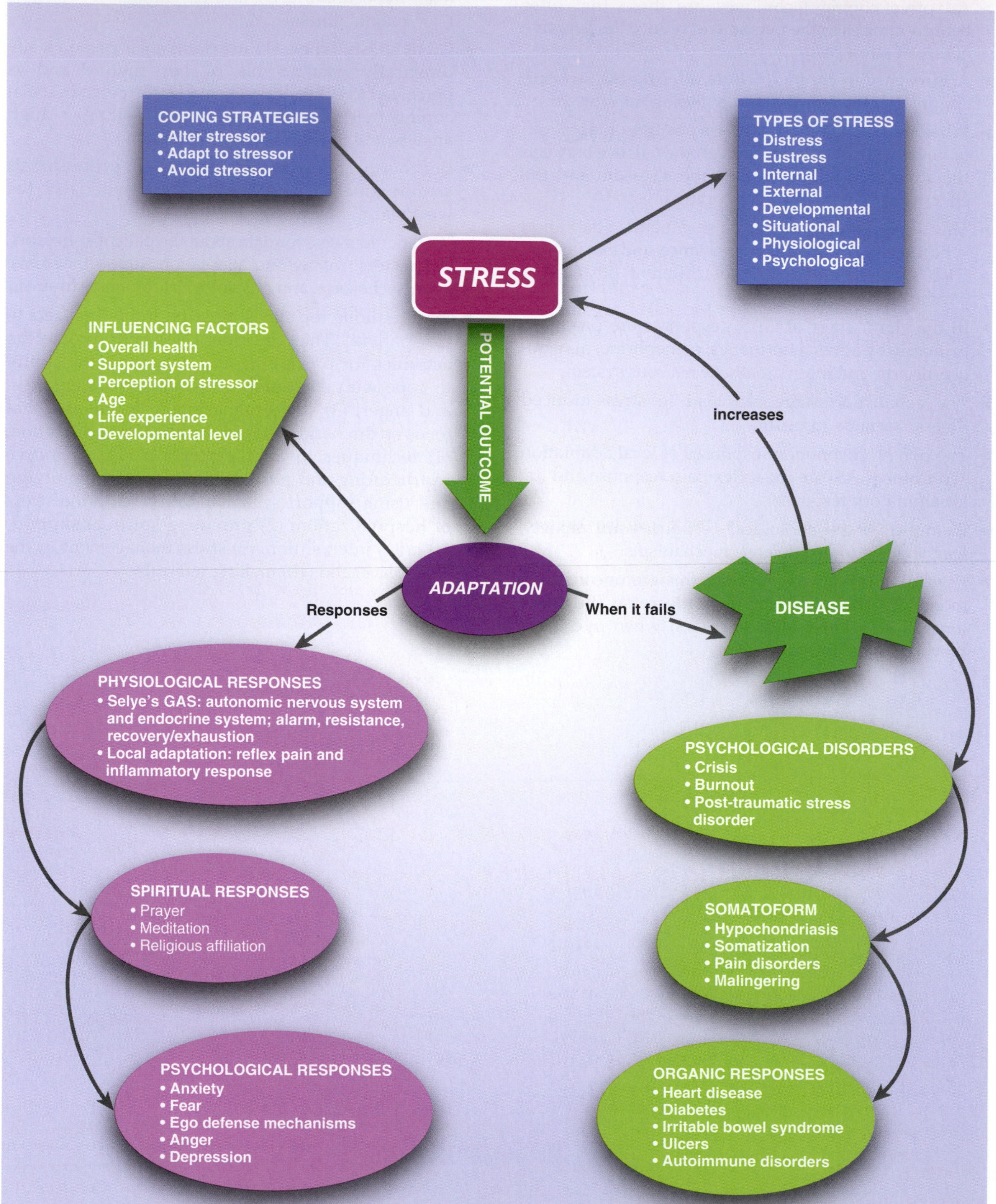

CHAPTER 13

Psychosocial Health & Illness

STUDENT RESOURCES

The questions and exercises in this book allow you to practice the kind of thinking you will use as a full-spectrum nurse. Critical-thinking questions usually have more than one right answer, so we do not provide "correct answers" for these features. Try to answer these questions yourself. It is more important to develop your nursing judgment than to just cover content. You will learn more by discussing the questions with your peers. If you are still unsure, see the Davis Advantage chapter resources for suggested responses.

To explore learning resources for this chapter,

Go to Davis Advantage and find:

Answers and Suggested Responses for all questions in this chapter

Concept Map

Knowledge Map

References and Bibliography

Lists of NOC Outcomes and NIC Interventions

Key Concepts

Anxiety

Depression

Psychosocial health

Self-concept

Related Concepts

See the Concept Map on Davis Advantage.

Example Problems

Anxiety

Depression

Self-Concept Disturbance and Low Self-Esteem

Caring for the Nguyens

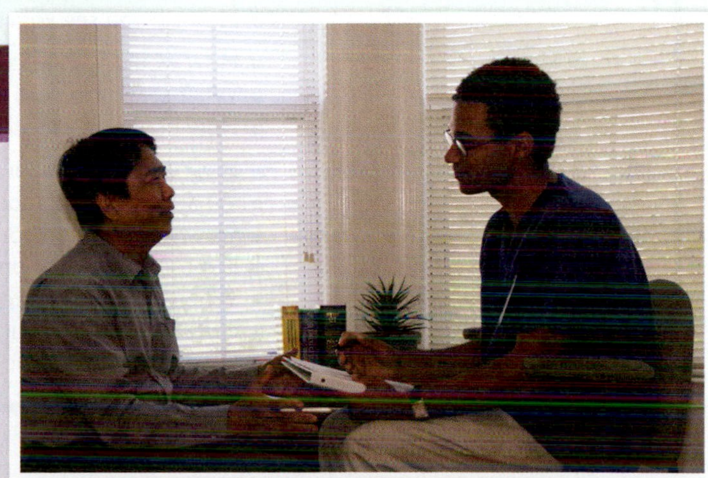

Recall the case of Nam Nguyen. Mr. Nguyen has been diagnosed with hypertension, obesity, and degenerative joint disease. At clinic visits he has made the following comments: "Every time I come in here, I get some new diagnosis. I guess it's amazing I'm not dead yet. I thought I had a lot more time left, but I'm not so sure anymore." When you ask him what his main concerns are, he tells you, "Just take a look at me! I'm a mess. Nothing is turning out the way I planned. I might as well just die now. It would save my family a lot of grief."

(Continued)

Caring for the Nguyens (continued)

A. What information do you need in order to respond to Mr. Nguyen?

B. How should you respond to Mr. Nguyen?

C. What actions should you take?

D. What conclusions can you make about Mr. Nguyen's self-concept (body image, role performance, personal identity, and self-esteem)? What additional information do you need about his self-concept?

PracticalKnowledge clinical application

This section provides guidelines and forms for assessing self-concept, self-esteem, anxiety, and depression, which are basic to psychosocial health and illness. In addition, you will find tables of selected standardized outcomes and interventions to consider when planning care for patients with problems related to anxiety and depression.

CLINICAL INSIGHTS

Clinical Insight 13-1 ➤ Assessing Self-Concept

Assessment Category	Examples of Assessment Questions
Body image	■ When you look in the mirror, what do you see? ■ How do you think others see you? ■ How does your current ability to engage in work and leisure activities compare with how you would like to be?
Role performance	■ What are your three or four major roles (e.g., daughter, student)? ■ How successful are you in each of these roles? ■ How important is it to you to be successful in each of these roles? ■ What is interfering with your ability to perform any of these roles? What can you do about it? ■ How did you see yourself before your illness/injury/loss? ■ How do you see yourself now?
Personal identity	■ How would you describe yourself to others? ■ What special abilities do you have? ■ How do you think others see you?
Self-esteem (also refer to the Assessment Box, Performing a Self-Esteem Inventory)	■ How do you feel about yourself? ■ What do you like about yourself? ■ To what extent do you feel you are in control of your life? ■ If you could change one thing about yourself, what would it be? ■ Where would you like to be 5 years from now? ■ How realistic are your expectations of yourself? ■ How do you see your illness/injury/loss in relation to yourself?

Clinical Insight 13-2 ➤ Performing a Self-Esteem Inventory

Place a check mark in the column that most closely describes the client's answer to each statement. Each check is worth the number of points listed.

	3 Often or a great deal	2 Sometimes	1 Seldom or occasionally	0 Never or not at all
1. I become angry or hurt when criticized.				
2. I am afraid to try new things.				
3. I feel stupid when I make a mistake.				
4. I have difficulty looking people in the eye.				
5. I have difficulty making small talk.				
6. I feel uncomfortable in the presence of strangers.				
7. I am embarrassed when people compliment me.				
8. I am dissatisfied with the way I look.				
9. I am afraid to express my opinions in a group.				
10. I prefer staying home alone rather than participating in group social situations.				
11. I have trouble accepting teasing.				
12. I feel guilty when I say no to people.				
13. I am afraid to make a commitment to a relationship for fear of rejection.				
14. I believe that most people are more competent than I am.				
15. I feel resentment toward people who are attractive and successful.				
16. I have trouble thinking of any positive aspects about my life.				
17. I feel inadequate in the presence of authority figures.				
18. I have trouble making decisions.				
19. I fear the disapproval of others.				
20. I feel tense, stressed out, or "uptight."				

Problems with low self-esteem are indicated by items scored with a 3 or by a total score higher than 46.

Source: Townsend, M. C. (2015). *Psychiatric mental health nursing: Concepts of care in evidence-based practice* (8th ed., p. 250). Philadelphia: F.A. Davis.

Clinical Insight 13-3 ➤ Identifying Depressed Patients Who Should Be Referred for Evaluation

Two Yes/No Questions

One way to identify depression that is more than simple, situational depression is to ask the following two questions. A yes answer merits a referral.

1. "Over the past 2 weeks, have you felt down, depressed, or hopeless?"
2. "Over the past 2 weeks, have you felt little interest or pleasure in doing things?"

SIGECAPS

Another method is to use the mnemonic SIGECAPS, a concise version of the *DSM-IV-TR* diagnostic criteria. Ask the patient whether he has experienced, for 2 or more weeks:

Sleep increase/decrease
Interest in formerly compelling or pleasurable activities diminished
Guilt, low self-esteem
Energy poor
Concentration poor
Appetite increase/decrease
Psychomotor agitation or retardation
Suicidal ideation

Both of the following require referral for evaluation and treatment:

Major depression = depressed mood or interest *plus* 4 SIGECAPS for 2 or more weeks

Mild depression (mood disorder) = depressed mood or interest *plus* 3 SIGECAPS most days for 2 or more years

Source: U.S. Preventive Services Task Force. (2016). Depression in adults: Screening. Retrieved from https://www.uspreventiveservicestaskforce.org/Page/Document/UpdateSummaryFinal/depression-in-adults-screening1

IN SAD CAGES

Some people prefer a mnemonic from an older source, IN SAD CAGES, which you would use in essentially the same way. Ask the patient whether he has experienced, for 2 or more weeks:

Interest reduced
Negative thoughts
Sleep disturbance
Appetite change
Decreased confidence or self-esteem
Concentration reduced
Affect blunt or flat
Guilt
Energy reduced
Suicidal ideas

The original reference does not include a suggested total that requires referral. However you can assume that the more symptoms, the more severe the depression. We suggest the following:

IN (reduced interest and negative thoughts or depressed mood) plus 4 of the other **SAD CAGES** requires referral.

Do not try to differentiate mild and major depression with this method.

Adapted from: Leng, L. B. (2011). Overview of major depressive disorder. *The Singapore Family Physician, 37*(4), 18–21.

ASSESSMENT GUIDELINES AND TOOLS

Focused Assessment

Anxiety Assessment Guide

Rating Scale: None = 0, Mild = 1, Moderate = 2, Severe = 3, Disabling (Panic) = 4

PHYSIOLOGICAL EFFECTS	Rating	PSYCHOLOGICAL EFFECTS	Rating
Shortness of breath (dyspnea)	____	Depersonalization (unreal)	____
Choking sensation	____	Feeling "on edge"	____
Dry mouth	____	Poor concentration	____
Pounding heart, increased heart rate	____	Poor memory	____
Chest pain	____	Depressed mood	____
Increased sweating and clamminess	____	Loss of interest	____
Feeling faint, dizzy, unsteady	____	Restlessness	____
Nausea and abdominal upsets	____	Sense of panic	____
Numbness (pins and needles)	____	Worry, anticipation of the worst	____
Hot/cold flashes	____	Irritability	____
Trembling, shaking	____	Nightmares	____
Muscle tension and aches	____	Feeling of fear and foreboding	____
Exaggerated startle response	____	Excessive apprehension	____
Difficulties in falling asleep and staying asleep	____	Feeling lack of control	____

Assessing Overall Scores

0–28	Mild anxiety
29–56	Moderate anxiety
57–84	Severe anxiety
85–112	Disabling anxiety

Creating a total score from this table can help you assess whether overall anxiety is mild, moderate, severe, or disabling. However, individual physiological or psychological symptoms that are rated as severe (3) or disabling (4) may be more important and relevant to your nursing assessment. For example, your patient's overall or total assessment may be 26 (in the mild range, 0–27) but she has rated "Excessive apprehension" as 4 (disabling).

Focused Assessment

Depression Assessment Guide: Patient Health Questionnaire (PHQ-9)

This is a valid and reliable measure of depression developed in 1999 by Pfizer, Inc. It can be self-administered (Kroenke, Spitzer, & Williams, 2001). It may be useful across cultures (Chen, Huang, Chang, et al., 2006).

Over the past 2 weeks, how often have you been bothered by any of the following problems? (Check or circle your answers.)

	Not At All	Several Days	More Than Half the Days	Nearly Every Day
1. Little interest or pleasure in doing things	0	1	2	3
2. Feeling down, depressed, or hopeless	0	1	2	3
3. Trouble falling or staying asleep, or sleeping too much	0	1	2	3
4. Feeling tired or having little energy	0	1	2	3
5. Poor appetite or overeating	0	1	2	3
6. Feeling bad about yourself—or that you are a failure or have let yourself or your family down	0	1	2	3
7. Trouble concentrating on things, such as reading the newspaper or watching television	0	1	2	3
8. Moving or speaking so slowly that other people could have noticed. Or the opposite—being so fidgety or restless that you have been moving around a lot more than usual	0	1	2	3
9. Thoughts that you would be better off dead or of hurting yourself in some way	0	1	2	3
ADD COLUMNS		☐	+ ☐	+ ☐
TOTAL:	☐			

10. If you checked off any problems, how difficult have these problems made it for you to do your work, take care of things at home, or get along with other people?

    Not difficult at all _____

    Somewhat difficult _____

    Very difficult _____

    Extremely difficult _____

(Healthcare professional: For interpretation of TOTAL, please refer to the accompanying score card. [Note to students: Interpretation requires training. You should report the patient's score to your instructor or your immediate supervising nurse.])

Source: Pfizer, Inc. Retrieved from http://www.phqscreeners.com/.

Focused Assessment

Differentiating Depression from Dementia

Use this tool to help identify older adults who should be referred for further evaluation to determine whether symptoms are related to depression or dementia.

- To determine whether the patient should be referred to a mental health professional, refer to the Clinical Insight 13-3: Identifying Depressed Patients Who Should Be Referred for Evaluation.
- To determine whether the patient should be referred to a mental health professional, refer to Clinical Insight 13-3.

Key Point: ***Confusion may be present in patients with depression as well as those who have dementia or delirium.***

Characteristic	Depression	Dementia
Cause/triggers	Loss (e.g., of spouse, of independence); stress	Physiological causes (e.g., Alzheimer's disease, brain infarcts)
Onset	Acute or chronic; can be related to specific events	Chronic, gradual, and insidious
Course	Varies, depending on cause	Progressive, over a long period of time
Alertness	Usually reduced	Usually normal
Memory	Memory loss and forgetfulness	Recent and remote memory impaired; loss of recent memory is first sign; some loss of common knowledge
Thinking	Inability to concentrate	Difficulty with abstraction and word finding, especially nouns; difficulty with calculations; decreased judgment
Response to questions	Often says, "I don't know."	Answers inappropriately or with "near misses"
Language	Speaks slowly; slow to respond to verbal stimuli	Disoriented, rambling, incoherent; difficulty using nouns
Sleep	Difficulty falling asleep, early morning awakening, much day sleeping	Sleep fragmented; awakens often during night
Reversibility	Potential	Irreversible, progressive

Source: Adapted from Edwards, N. (2003). Differentiating the three D's: Delirium, dementia, and depression. *MedSurg Nursing: Official Journal of the Academy of Medical-Surgical Nurses, 12*(6), 347–357.

STANDARDIZED LANGUAGE

You can use the tables in this section when planning care for patients with problems of self-concept, anxiety, and depression. The tables provide standardized wording for nursing outcomes and interventions. You can use the Nursing Outcomes Classification (NOC) indicators with the outcomes to write goals. Non-NOC outcomes are also suggested. In addition to the broad Nursing Interventions Classification (NIC) interventions, the tables provide specific nursing activities suggested by the NIC.

Self-Concept Diagnoses: Selected NIC Interventions and Nursing Activities

NIC INTERVENTION	SELECTED NURSING ACTIVITIES (NIC)
Anticipatory Guidance	Assist the patient to adapt to anticipated role changes. Suggest printed literature and electronic sources for the patient to read, as appropriate. Schedule visits at strategic developmental or situational points.
Behavior Modification	Develop a change behavior program. Reinforce constructive decisions. Offer positive reinforcement for independent decisions.
Body Image Enhancement	Use anticipatory guidance to prepare patient for predictable changes in body image. Monitor frequency of statements of self-criticism. Assist patient to separate physical appearance from feelings of personal worth, as appropriate.
Coping Enhancement	Use a calm, reassuring approach. Assist the patient in developing an objective appraisal of the event. Encourage the acceptance of the limitations of others.
Decision-Making Support	Inform patient of alternative views or solutions in a clear and supportive manner. Help patient identify the advantages and disadvantages of each alternative. Obtain informed consent, when appropriate.
Delusion Management	Establish a trusting, interpersonal relationship with patient. Avoid arguing about false beliefs. State doubt matter-of-factly. Avoid reinforcing delusional ideas.
Developmental Enhancement **Child**	(Depends on developmental stage) Assist each child to become aware that he or she is important as an individual. Provide activities that encourage interaction among children.
Grief Work Facilitation	Identify the loss. Encourage expression of feelings about the loss. Instruct in phases of the grieving process, as appropriate.
Hallucination Management	Maintain a safe environment. Provide patient with opportunities to discuss hallucinations. Provide antipsychotic and antianxiety medications on a routine and PRN (as-needed) basis.
Hope Inspiration	Assist patient or family to identify areas of hope in life. Inform the patient about whether the current situation is a temporary state.
Mood Management	Evaluate mood initially (e.g., signs, symptoms, personal history), and on a regular basis, as treatment progresses. Determine whether patient presents a safety risk to self or others. Provide opportunity for physical activity (e.g., walking or riding the exercise bike).
Parent Education: Childrearing Family	Facilitate parents' discussion of methods of discipline available, selection, and results obtained. Instruct parent on normal physiological, emotional, and behavioral characteristics of child.

Self-Concept Diagnoses: Selected NIC Interventions and Nursing Activities—cont'd

NIC INTERVENTION	SELECTED NURSING ACTIVITIES (NIC)
Reality Orientation	Inform patient of person, place, and time, as needed. Provide a consistent physical environment and daily routine. Recommend patient wear personal clothing and assist, as needed.
Role Enhancement	Assist patient to identify usual role in family. Assist patient to identify role insufficiency. Assist patient to identify positive strategies for managing role changes.
Risk Identification	Review data derived from routine risk assessment measures. Determine availability and quality of resources (e.g., psychological, financial, education level, family and other social, and community). Identify typical coping strategies.
Self-Esteem Enhancement	Monitor patient's statements of self-worth. Convey confidence in patient's ability to handle situation. Refrain from negative criticism.
Values Clarification	Pose reflective, clarifying questions that give the patient something to think about. Encourage patient to make a list of what is important and not important in life and the time spent on each. Avoid use of cross-examining questions.

Source: Butcher, H. K., Bulechek, G. M., Dochterman, J. M., & Wagner, C. M. (Eds.). (2018). *Nursing interventions classification (NIC)* (7th ed.). St. Louis, MO: Elsevier. Used with permission.

Anxiety-Related Diagnoses: Selected NOC Outcomes and NIC Interventions

CUE CLUSTER	NOC OUTCOMES*	SELECTED INDICATORS	NIC INTERVENTIONS AND SPECIFIC ACTIVITIES†
Susan is pacing the floor and does not make eye contact when she speaks to you. Her hands are shaking. Her blood pressure is 140/88 mm Hg ***Diagnosis:* Anxiety**	Anxiety Self-Control ***Other Outcomes*** Anxiety Level Concentration Coping	(Often demonstrated) ▪ Monitors intensity of anxiety ▪ Maintains concentration	Anxiety Reduction ▪ Use a calm, reassuring approach. ▪ Explain all procedures, including sensations the patient is likely to experience during the procedure. ▪ Help the patient identify situations that precipitate anxiety. ***Other Interventions*** Anger Control Assistance Anticipatory Guidance Calming Technique Coping Enhancement Emotional Support
Martin has a terminal illness. He looks very sad. He states that he is worried that his dying will be prolonged and difficult for his family and that he is afraid of dying. ***Diagnosis:*** **Death Anxiety**	Acceptance: Health Status ***Other Outcomes*** Anxiety Self-Control Comfortable Death Depression Level Dignified Life Closure Fear Self-Control Hope Spiritual Health	(Often demonstrated) ▪ Appears peaceful ▪ Reports positive self-regard ▪ Clarifies personal values	Emotional Support ▪ Listen to/encourage expressions of feelings and beliefs. ▪ Provide support during denial, anger, bargaining, and acceptance phases of grieving. ***Other Interventions*** Anxiety Reduction Coping Enhancement Decision-Making Support Dying Care Hope Inspiration Pain Management: Acute Pain Management: Chronic Presence Religious Ritual Enhancement Spiritual Support
Ms. Eng says, "I just don't know whether to have this chemotherapy or not. I know I could live a little longer, but the side effects …." She has decided twice to do it and each time has changed her mind. She says, "I just can't focus on anything else." ***Diagnosis:*** **Decisional Conflict**	Decision-Making ***Other Outcomes*** Information Processing Participation in Health Care Decisions Personal Autonomy	(Not compromised) ▪ Identifies alternatives. ▪ Identifies needed resources to support each alternative.	Decision-Making Support ▪ Determine whether there are differences between the patient's view of his or her own condition and the views of the healthcare providers. ▪ Serve as a liaison between patient and family. ▪ Serve as a liaison between patient and other healthcare providers. ***Other Interventions*** Assertiveness Training Health System Guidance Learning Facilitation Mutual Goal Setting

Anxiety-Related Diagnoses: Selected NOC Outcomes and NIC Interventions—cont'd

CUE CLUSTER	NOC OUTCOMES*	SELECTED INDICATORS	NIC INTERVENTIONS AND SPECIFIC ACTIVITIES†
Bryan is to have his burns debrided today. He is crying. He says, "I wish my mom was here. It hurts so bad when they do that. I'm so scared." ***Diagnosis:*** **Fear**	Fear Self-Control ***Other Outcomes*** Fear Level Fear Level: Child	(Often demonstrated) ■ Uses relaxation techniques to reduce fear ■ Maintains concentration ■ Controls fear response	Coping Enhancement ■ Use calm reassuring approach. ■ Encourage family involvement. ■ Hold a young child or infant, as appropriate. ***Other Interventions*** Anxiety Reduction Calming Technique Presence
Mr. Paul's blood pressure remains dangerously high, yet he does not make the changes in diet and exercise that are needed, and he often fails to take his pills. "I feel OK. This is a bunch of mumbo jumbo. My folks ate fried foods, and they lived to be over 80." ***Diagnosis:*** **Ineffective Denial**	Health Beliefs: Perceived Threat ***Other Outcomes*** Acceptance: Health Status Anxiety Self-Control Fear Self-Control Symptom Control	(Strong) ■ Perceived threat to health ■ Perceived vulnerability to progressive health problems ■ Perceived impact on functional status	Self-Awareness Enhancement ■ Assist the patient to identify the values that contribute to self-concept. ■ Assist the patient to identify the effect of illness on self-concept. ■ Verbalize the patient's denial of reality, as appropriate. ***Other Interventions*** Anxiety Reduction Calming Technique Coping Enhancement Counseling Emotional Support Health Education Self-Modification Assistance Self-Responsibility Facilitation Teaching: Disease Process

*Johnson, M., Bulechek, G., Butcher, H., et al. (2011). *NANDA, NOC, and NIC linkages: Nursing diagnoses, outcomes, and interventions* (3rd ed.). St. Louis, MO: Elsevier; and Moorhead, S., Swanson, E., Johnson, M., & Maas, M. L. (Eds.). (2018). *Nursing outcomes classification (NOC)* (6th ed.). St. Louis, MO: Elsevier. Used with permission.
†Johnson, M., Bulechek, G., Butcher, H., et al. (2011). *NANDA, NOC, and NIC linkages: Nursing diagnoses, outcomes, and interventions* (3rd ed.). St. Louis, MO: Elsevier; and Butcher, H. K, Bulechek, G. M., Dochterman, J. M., & Wagner, C. M. (Eds.). (2018). *Nursing interventions classification (NIC)* (7th ed.). St. Louis, MO: Elsevier. Used with permission.

Depression-Related Nursing Diagnoses: Selected NOC Outcomes and NIC Interventions

CUE CLUSTER	NOC OUTCOMES*	SELECTED INDICATORS	NIC INTERVENTIONS AND SPECIFIC ACTIVITIES†
John has AIDS and is dying. He sleeps most of the time. During care activities (e.g., bath), he closes his eyes and remains passive. When asked to move or participate, he sighs and says, "I can't." When friends visit, he turns away from them; when they talk to him, he just shrugs. He has stopped eating. He says, "It doesn't matter what I do. Nothing can change the way this is going to turn out."	Hope ***Other Outcomes*** ▪ Depression Level ▪ Depression Self-Control ▪ Mood Equilibrium ▪ Psychomotor Energy ▪ Quality of Life ▪ Will to Live	(Often demonstrated) ▪ Expresses meaning in life ▪ Expresses inner peace ▪ Expresses belief in self ▪ Expresses belief in others ▪ Expresses sense of self-control	Hope Inspiration ▪ Demonstrate hope by recognizing the patient's intrinsic worth and viewing the patient's illness as only one facet of the individual. ▪ Help the patient expand spiritual self. ▪ Create an environment that facilitates patient practicing religion, as appropriate. ▪ Facilitate the patient's/family's reliving and savoring past achievements and experiences. ▪ Teach the family about the positive aspects of hope (e.g., develop meaningful conversational themes that reflect love and need for the patient). ▪ Avoid masking the truth. ***Other Interventions*** Coping Enhancement Counseling Mood Management Resiliency Promotion Self-Modification Assistance Spiritual Growth Facilitation Values Clarification
Jennifer is 16 and pregnant. She does not follow good health practices. She angrily says, "It's my body, and I don't want this baby. But my parents say abortion is a sin. I should honor my parents, but I hate them. I hate having to depend on them, and I hate being pregnant."	Health Beliefs: Perceived Control ***Other Outcomes*** ▪ Depression Self-Control ▪ Family Participation in Professional Care ▪ Health Beliefs ▪ Health Beliefs: Perceived Ability to Perform ▪ Health Beliefs: Perceived Resources ▪ Hope	(Strong) ▪ Requested involvement in health decisions ▪ Efforts at gathering information ▪ Belief that own actions control health outcomes ▪ Willingness to designate surrogate decision maker	Self-Responsibility Facilitation ▪ Discuss with the patient the extent of responsibility for present health status. ▪ Determine whether patient has adequate knowledge about healthcare condition. ▪ Encourage verbalizations of feelings, perceptions, and fears about assuming responsibility. ▪ Discuss consequences of not dealing with own responsibilities. ▪ Encourage patient to take as much responsibility as possible for own self-care. ▪ Provide positive constructive feedback for accepting additional responsibility for behavior change. ***Other Interventions*** ▪ Cognitive Restructuring ▪ Emotional Support ▪ Family Involvement Promotion ▪ Financial Resource Assistance

Depression-Related Nursing Diagnoses: Selected NOC Outcomes and NIC Interventions—cont'd

CUE CLUSTER	NOC OUTCOMES*	SELECTED INDICATORS	NIC INTERVENTIONS AND SPECIFIC ACTIVITIES†
	■ Participation in Health Care Decisions ■ Personal Autonomy		■ Health Education ■ Health System Guidance ■ Hope Inspiration ■ Mood Management ■ Mutual Goal Setting ■ Patient Rights Protection ■ Self-Esteem Enhancement ■ Values Clarification
Tim has attempted suicide twice. He now says, "I will get it right this time. I know where I can get a gun."	Suicide Self-Restraint ***Other Outcomes*** ■ Mood Equilibrium ■ Will to Live	(Often demonstrated) ■ Obtains assistance as needed ■ Exhibits impulse control ■ Expression of determination to live ■ Expression of sense of control ■ Interest in one's own treatment ■ Expression of hope	Suicide Prevention ■ Refer patient to mental healthcare provider … for evaluation and treatment. ■ Administer medications to decrease anxiety, agitation, or psychosis and to stabilize mood, as appropriate. ■ Conduct mouth checks after medication administration to ensure that patient is not "cheeking" medications to use later for an overdose attempt. ■ Initiate suicide precautions (e.g., ongoing observation and monitoring of the patient, provision of a protective environment) … ■ Limit access to windows, unless locked and shatterproof, as appropriate. ■ Monitor patient during use of potential weapons (e.g., razor). ■ Assist patient to identify network of supportive persons and resources (e.g., clergy, family, providers). ***Other Interventions*** ■ Behavior Management: Self-Harm ■ Hope Inspiration ■ Mood Management ■ Spiritual Support

*Johnson, M., Bulechek, G., Butcher, H., et al. (2011). *NANDA, NOC, and NIC linkages: Nursing diagnoses, outcomes, and interventions* (3rd ed.). St. Louis, MO: Elsevier; and Moorhead, S., Swanson, E., Johnson, M., & Maas, M. (Eds.). (2018). *Nursing outcomes classification (NOC)* (6th ed.). St. Louis, MO: Elsevier. Used with permission.

†Johnson, M., Bulechek, G., Butcher, H., et al. (2011). *NANDA, NOC, and NIC linkages: Nursing diagnoses, outcomes, and interventions* (3rd ed.). St. Louis, MO: Elsevier; and Butcher, H. K, Bulechek, G. M., Dochterman, J. M., & Wagner, C. M. (Eds.). (2018). *Nursing interventions classification (NIC)* (7th ed.). St. Louis, MO: Elsevier. Used with permission.

CLINICALJUDGMENT
Applying the Full-Spectrum Nursing Model

PATIENT SITUATION

Matthew has been admitted to the emergency department with extensive wounds to both forearms, including tendon and vascular damage, as a result of a suicide attempt. Matthew seems very quiet, almost withdrawn, and answers most of your questions in monosyllables.

Matthew reports the following: He is the third child in a family of five. Matthew's middle-class parents are now retired, and his brothers and sisters are scattered across the country in various large cities. Although Matthew claims his schooling years were unremarkable, he reminisces about several occasions when he was bullied and physically beaten by gangs of older adolescents.

Matthew further states that he graduated from Harvard Law School and became vice president of an influential law firm. Despite his apparent success in life, he has continued to question his self-worth since childhood. Plagued by worries and depression that have increased over the past few years, he says he wrote a note indicating that he now realizes what a failure he is and proceeded to slash both of his forearms with a sharp razor. Matthew reports that he has not been eating much, feels tired all the time, and has no interest in going outside the house. He says, "I just don't feel like doing anything; I just want to sleep all the time."

THINKING

1. *Theoretical Knowledge:* Using just the information you have in the Patient Situation, use the SIGECAPS method outlined in Clinical Insight 13-3 to assess Matthew's level of depression. You will need to assume that he is reporting what he has experienced in the past 2 weeks (unless he is obviously referring to the past).

2. *Critical Thinking (Inquiry):* What items of the SIGECAPS cannot be completed with the information in the Patient Situation? What do you need to ask Matthew to complete them?

DOING

3. *Nursing Process (Interventions):* Based on your SIGECAPS data, what do you need to do right away (or be certain it was done in the emergency department)?

CARING

4. *Self-Knowledge:* What do you have in common with Matthew that might help you to empathize with him?

5. *Ethical Knowledge:* Try to put aside your own beliefs now, and answer the following questions from the perspective of (a) Matthew and (b) one of your nursing colleagues on the unit:

   a. Give one reason to support Matthew's claim that he has a right to commit suicide if his despair is too deep to bear.

   b. Give one reason to support a colleague's claim that Matthew does not have a right to commit suicide, no matter how he feels.

Critical Thinking and Clinical Judgment

1. Review the scenario about Karli (Meet Your Patient from Volume 1):

   You are caring for a 16-year-old patient named Karli, who is suffering from fractures to both arms and several ribs, as well as extensive first- and second-degree burns to 30% of her body following a motor vehicle accident. Karli was driving her parents' car home from her part-time job when she lost control of the car and crashed into a wall. The car exploded in flames. A passerby quickly reported the accident, and fast action by the emergency response team saved Karli's life.

   Karli is suffering from a moderate amount of shock and pain. Her mood alternates between outbursts of anger or self-directed sarcasm and despondence. She tells you that she cannot understand how the accident happened, that one moment she was adjusting the car radio, and the next moment she awoke in the hospital. Then suddenly she explodes. "It's not fair! I just took my eyes off the road for a second; that's all!" She bursts into tears. Picking at her bandages, she sobs, "No one will ever love me the way I'm going to look. My life is over. I hate myself!" You take her hand. "I used to be pretty," she says, "but now I'll look like a freak! What did I do to deserve this? I know plenty of kids who drive drunk or high all the time. I wasn't doing anything wrong! Why did this happen to me?"

a. Now that you have completed Chapter 13 in Volume 1, make a list of the multiple physical, psychological, and social issues that you would need to consider in developing a comprehensive care plan for Karli.

b. Compare your list with the one you made when you first began reading the chapter. Is the latest one different from the earlier one, or is it the same?

2. In the Meet Your Patient scenario, Karli perceives herself as unlovable "looking this way." Which of the following nursing activities do you think might be helpful in *exploring and changing her perception*? For those you *do not* choose, explain why.

Role Enhancement

- Help the patient distinguish ideal and actual self. Help her describe realistic roles and expectations tailored to specific health changes.
- Compare realistic roles with previous and less functional roles.

Conflict Mediation

- Provide a quiet, private, neutral setting for mediation to take place.
- Maintain your own neutrality in the process; do not "take sides."

Promoting Family Integrity

- Encourage and facilitate communication among family members.
- Encourage family members to care for the patient as much as possible.

Family Mobilization

- Help the family to identify strengths they can use to support the patient.
- Teach family members how to provide home care for the patient.
- Help the family identify community resources and/or support groups.
- With the patient's permission, keep the family informed about the patient's progress.

Enhancing Socialization

- Explore and reinforce the individual's established relationships.
- Provide opportunities to rehearse relationship-building skills.
- Investigate, assist, and promote any developing relationships with persons of similar interests and goals.
- Provide information and links to community activities that relate to the person's past, current, and future interests.
- Promote access to education in social skills development.
- Encourage the patient to communicate and engage in interpersonal relationship activities by providing ongoing positive feedback.

- Organize small, cohesive group activities.
- Provide or act as a role model, where appropriate.

3. Mrs. King is being admitted into the orthopedics unit for a scheduled total knee replacement. Even though she appears to be in good health for a 72-year-old woman, you are concerned about her excessive weight, which can be described as moderate to severe obesity. You are troubled by how the obesity may negatively affect postsurgical recovery, wound healing, and mobility.
   a. What theoretical knowledge will you draw on to plan care to meet her biopsychosocial needs?
   b. What assumptions are you making? What stereotypes do you have that might affect your understanding of Mrs. King's situation?
   c. What do you think might be contributing to Mrs. King's obesity?
   d. What facts do you have to support those ideas?
   e. How could you find out for sure what is contributing to Mrs. King's obesity?
4. You notice that day by day your patient is eating less and complaining about constipation and tiredness. You carefully review her nutritional requirements against the food menu, as well as check nursing records for bowel movements. You have exhausted your initial search for obvious reasons your patient's appetite has changed. While sitting next to your patient, you cannot help noticing how tired she looks.
   a. What psychosocial problem do you suspect (low self-esteem, depression, anxiety, or disturbed personal identity)?
   b. What data do you have to support your inference in (a)?
   c. Objective data in her chart indicate that the patient has been eating very little and that she has been having bowel movements only every 3 or 4 days—and even then only with a laxative or enema. What other symptom do you need to investigate further?
   d. How could you obtain more information about that symptom?
   e. Think of depressed people you have known or depressed patients you have cared for. What have you found to be difficult about dealing with them?
5. Edna Jackson is 42 years old. She has had a hysterectomy (removal of her uterus). Her surgery was uncomplicated, her overall health is good, and she is expected to make a full and rapid physical recovery. Her husband was not present when she was admitted and has not been to see her since the surgery. He did not want her to have the surgery. He had told Edna that he didn't know whether he would want to have sex with her when she is no longer "a whole woman." During their marriage, he has had numerous casual affairs, which Edna has tolerated because she feels that her difficulty is balanced by the many positive benefits of their relationship, including a "good sex life."

   Edna has seven brothers and sisters, and she has five children of her own, ages 23, 21, 18, 6, and 4. She comes from a culture and a religion that value children and motherhood. She believes she is a good mother, although she must work full time outside the home. Edna is an office manager—respected by her boss and by those who work for her. She has an internal locus of control and evaluates her job performance as "better than most people would do."
   a. Look at the context. What aspects of this situation may negatively impact Mrs. Jackson's recovery?
   b. Based on your answers in (a), what nursing diagnoses might be useful in describing the psychosocial aspects of Mrs. Jackson's health? (State both the problem and the etiology.)
   c. What strengths does Mrs. Jackson have that may help her to avoid and/or overcome those problems?

6. Matthew has been admitted to the emergency department with extensive wounds to both forearms, including tendon and vascular damage, as a result of a suicide attempt. Matthew seems very quiet, almost withdrawn, and answers most of your questions in monosyllables.

Matthew reports that he is the third child in a family of five. Matthew's middle-class parents are now retired, and his brothers and sisters are scattered across the country in various large cities. Although Matthew claims his schooling years were unremarkable, he reminisces about several occasions when he was bullied and physically beaten by gangs of older adolescents.

Matthew graduated from Harvard Law School and became vice president of an influential law firm. Despite his apparent success in life, he has continued to question his self-worth from early childhood. Plagued by worries and depression that have increased over the past few years Matthew wrote a note indicating that he now realized what a failure he is and proceeded to slash both his forearms with a sharp razor.

During the nursing assessment, Matthew reports that he has not been eating much, feels tired all the time, and has no interest in getting outside the house. He says, "I just don't feel like doing anything; I just want to sleep all the time."

a. After Matthew's tendon and vascular repair, he is admitted to your medical-surgical unit. What, broadly speaking, are your first two priorities for Matthew's care?

b. Which of these nursing diagnoses—Suicide Risk or Risk for Self-Harm—would you use, and why?

c. Prioritize the following interventions for Matthew. Rank them (1 = highest rank, 4 = lowest rank). Explain your thinking.

____ Refer to a mental health professional for help with his depression.

____ Examine Matthew's belongings and the room for anything he might use to harm himself.

____ Encourage Matthew to tell you if he begins having thoughts of suicide.

____ Begin establishing a therapeutic relationship and gaining his trust.

d. Evaluate your self-knowledge. To plan comprehensive care for Matthew, in what areas do you need to increase your theoretical and practical knowledge? How will you do that?

7. For each of the following concepts, use critical thinking to describe how or why it is important to nursing, patient care, or psychosocial health and illness. Note that these are *not* to be merely definitions.

Self-concept

Self-esteem

Body image

Biopsychosocial well-being

Anxiety

Defense mechanisms

Depression

Therapeutic relationships

Hopelessness

What Are the Main Points in This Chapter?

- Health and well-being are influenced by psychological, social, and spiritual development.
- Psychosocial theory provides a way to understand people as interactions of psychological and social events.
- Self-concept is one's overall view of oneself; it answers the question, "Who do you think you are?"
- Self-concept is developed throughout the life span and is influenced by multiple factors. Four dimensions contribute to self-concept: body image, role performance, personal identity, and self-esteem.
- Body image is a person's mental image of his physical self.
- Role performance consists of the actions a person takes and the behaviors he or she demonstrates in fulfilling a role, such as the role of a student.
- Personal identity is a person's view of himself as a unique human being, different, and separate from all others.
- Self-esteem evaluations arise from the differences between the ideal self and the actual self.
- Communication skills are important because psychosocial information is personal and sometimes sensitive.
- When you formulate psychosocial diagnoses it is difficult, but important, to determine what the cause is and what the effect is.
- Many of the NOC standardized psychosocial outcomes are found in the domains of Psychosocial Health and Family Health.
- Many of the NIC standardized psychosocial interventions are found in the Behavioral and Family domains.
- Anxiety is a common emotional response to a (usually unknown) stressor; it results from psychological conflicts, and it is accompanied by physical symptoms (e.g., trembling).
- Assessment should identify the presence, level, and cause of anxiety.
- Interventions for anxiety should help the patient become aware that he is anxious, identify the source of anxiety, and deal with the symptoms it produces.
- Depression is characterized by diminished interest or pleasure in previously enjoyed activities, sadness, emptiness, a flat or hollow feeling (absence of feeling), tearfulness, difficulty concentrating, feelings of worthlessness, and some physical symptoms (e.g., constipation).
- Assessment of depression includes a comprehensive history of mood, thoughts, behavior, and physical status.
- If you suspect severe depression, you should refer the patient to a mental health specialist; if there is a risk of suicide, referral should be immediate.
- In communicating with depressed persons, it is important to not to be overly cheerful and to avoid phrases such as "Cheer up."

Knowledge Map

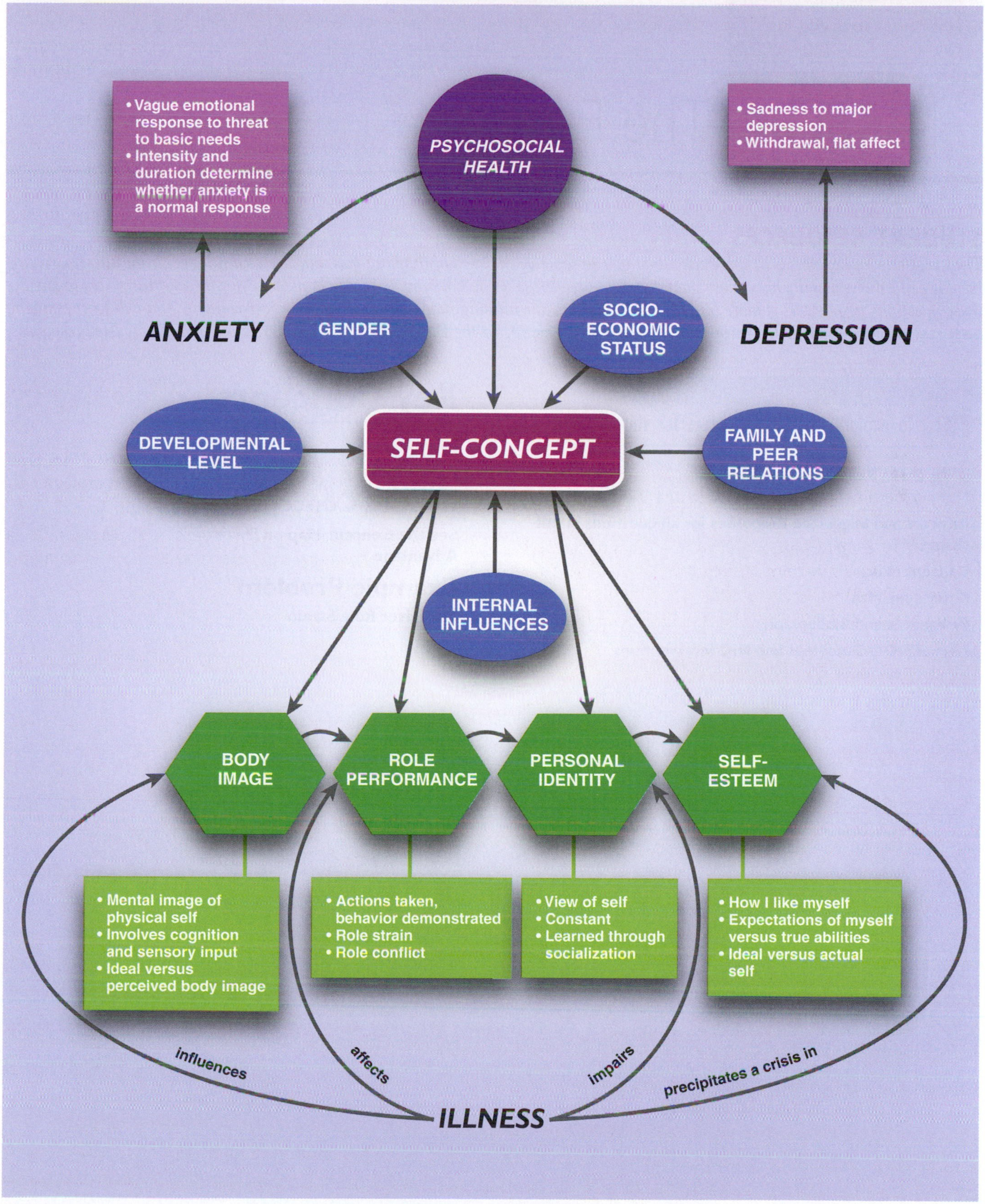

CHAPTER 14

The Family

STUDENT RESOURCES

The questions and exercises in this book allow you to practice the kind of thinking you will use as a full-spectrum nurse. Critical-thinking questions usually have more than one right answer, so we do not provide "correct answers" for these features. Try to answer these questions yourself. It is more important to develop your nursing judgment than to just cover content. You will learn more by discussing the questions with your peers. If you are still unsure, see the Davis Advantage chapter resources for suggested responses.

To explore learning resources for this chapter,

Go to Davis Advantage and find:

Answers and Suggested Responses for all questions in this chapter
Concept Map
Knowledge Map
References and Bibliography
Lists of NOC Outcomes and NIC Interventions

Key Concepts

Family
Family nursing

Related Concepts

See the Concept Map on Davis Advantage.

Example Problem

Caregiver Role Strain

Caring for the Nguyens

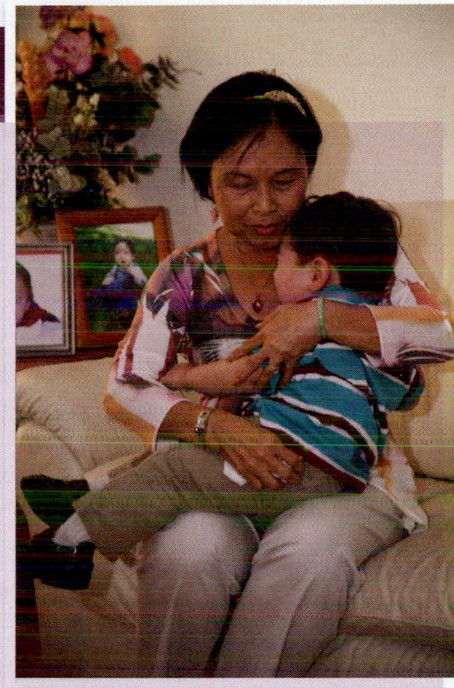

Kim Phan, 3 years old, is the first grandchild for Nam and Yen Nguyen. Until recently, Kim lived with his mother, Trinh Phan, the Nguyen's daughter. Trinh had been diagnosed with schizophrenia at age 18 years. Initially she was functioning adequately on her medications; however, she has not been taking her medications, and her condition has been worsening for the past year. When Trinh became unable to care for Kim, Nam and Yen assumed the child's care. Trinh rarely visits Kim. Nam and Yen convinced Trinh to obtain residential care at a mental health facility. Nam tells you at a clinic visit that he wishes his family were "normal."

A. What do you need to clarify about Nam's statement about his family?

B. What do *you* think Nam means by a "normal" family?

C. How would you respond to Nam's comments?

D. What effect might this new family structure have on Nam's and Yen's health?

E. How might you promote family functioning for the Nguyens? What assessments should you make? What interventions should you consider?

F. What personal values or biases do you have that may affect your ability to care for the Nguyens?

PracticalKnowledge clinical **application**

Material in this section will help you to assess and plan care for families.

CLINICAL INSIGHTS

Clinical Insight 14-1 ➤ Conducting a Family Assessment

In general, a family assessment should include the following:

Identifying Data Include such information as name, address, phone number, cultural/ethnic background, religious identification, social affiliation.

Family Composition For each member of the family, include gender, age, relationship, date and place of birth, occupation, and education.

(Continued)

Clinical Insight 14-1 ➤ Conducting a Family Assessment *(continued)*

Family History and Developmental Stage	This refers to the stages and developmental tasks in the Focused Assessment: Assessing Family Development Tasks.
Environmental Data	Include a description of the home, neighborhood, larger community, family's social supports, and their transactions with the community.
Family Structure	■ *Identify the structural type* (e.g., traditional nuclear, single-parent, etc.). Also assess: ■ *Communication patterns*: Functional and dysfunctional patterns; the manner in which emotions are expressed, and contextual variables that affect communication ■ *Power and role structures* (e.g., How are family decisions made? What are the roles of each member? Have there been changes in these?) ■ *Family values* (e.g., What are their values? What are their priorities? How do they compare with the values of their cultural group? Are there value conflicts in the family?)
Family Functions	Assess the effectiveness of the family's: ■ *Nurturing* (e.g., Are the members close? Are they separate or connected?) ■ *Socialization and child rearing* (e.g., Who is [are] the socializing agent[s] for the children? What are their child-rearing practices? Are needs for play being met?)
Health Beliefs, Values, and Behaviors	■ How do they define health and illness? ■ What are their dietary, sleep, physical, and drug habits? ■ What are their dental and medical health practices, including physicals, eye exams, immunizations, and exercise patterns? ■ Do they have access to health services?
Family Stressors and Coping	■ What are their stressors (e.g., financial, family communication or relationships, neighbors, holidays, children's behavior)? ■ What successful coping strategies have they used? ■ What dysfunctional strategies?
Abuse and Violence within the Family	Because of the prevalence of abuse and because families are likely to be ashamed to discuss it, you should assess every family member to see whether any abuse or neglect is occurring. For detailed guidelines, go to Procedure 9-1, Assessing for Abuse.

ASSESSMENT GUIDELINES AND TOOLS

Focused Assessment

Assessing Family Developmental Tasks

Stages and Children's Ages	Tasks
Beginning family No children	➤ Relinquishing the family of origin as the major emotional and economic resource ➤ Gaining a sense of autonomy and independence ➤ Making the relationship/marriage work; investment in spouse as the major emotional resource ➤ Finding a place in the kin network of each partner ➤ Exploring options for career development ➤ Deciding whether to have children
Childbearing family Age: Newborn to 2 years	➤ Achieving pregnancy and birth ➤ Adjusting to life changes after birth and to the infant's needs ➤ Determining ways to meet all members' needs ➤ Renegotiating marriage ➤ Increasing contact with extended family

Focused Assessment

Assessing Family Developmental Tasks—cont'd

Stages and Children's Ages	Tasks	
"No longer newlyweds" (with no children) No children; ages not applicable	➤ Establishing a sense of the permanence of the relationship ➤ Establishing long-term residency ➤ Being involved in the community/promoting the well-being of the community ➤ Focusing on or establishing professional careers	
Family with preschool children Age 3–5 years	➤ Adjusting to increased costs associated with family life ➤ Socializing the preschoolers ➤ Coping with loss of parental energy and privacy 3–5 years	
Mature family (with no children) Ages not applicable	➤ Renegotiating relationship on basis of more maturity ➤ Adjusting to changing levels of responsibility in work and community ➤ If not done already, achieving financial security	
Family with school-age children 6–12 years	➤ Adjusting to the needs and demands of growing children ➤ Promoting joint decision making among parents and children ➤ Encouraging and supporting educational and school-related activities	
Family with teenagers and young adults Ages: 13–20 years	➤ Maintaining open communication among family members ➤ Reinforcing ethical and moral values ➤ For teens, balancing independence with parental rules	
Family launching young adults Ages: 18–30 years	➤ Maintaining support to young adults as they leave the security of family ➤ Rediscovering marriage	
Postparental family Ages: Adults	➤ Preparing for retirement ➤ Adjusting to children's moving into new phases of adulthood, marriage or other relationship, and childbearing and to becoming a grandparent	
Middle-aged couple (with no children)	➤ Accepting that it may be too late to reconsider childbearing or child rearing ➤ Reaching the peak of a career or realizing that the peak may not occur ➤ Planning for retirement	*None*
Aging family (also applies to family with no children)	➤ Adjusting to retirement and changes associated with aging ➤ Adjusting to the loss of a spouse and friendships	Adult *(or none)*

Source: Adapted from Friedman, M. M., Bowden, V. R., & Jones, E. G. (2003). *Family Nursing: Research, Theory, and Practice* (5th ed.). Upper Saddle River, NJ: Prentice Hall; Kaakinen, J., Coehlo, D. & Steele, R., et al (Eds.). (2018). *Family Health Care Nursing: Theory, Practice and Research* (6th ed.). Philadelphia, PA: F.A. Davis; McGoldrick, M. & Carter, E. (1985). The family life cycle: Its Stages and Dislocations. In J. Henslin (Ed.), *Marriage and Family in a Changing Society* (4th ed.). New York: Free Press, pp. 372–389.

CLINICALJUDGMENT

Applying the Full-Spectrum Nursing Model

PATIENT SITUATION

Sandra Jackson, a 22-year-old single mother of an 18-month-old child, has type 1 diabetes mellitus. Her blood glucose levels have been unstable, primarily during times of stress and illness. Sandra lives with her mother, two younger sisters, and a brother. At times her boyfriend stays in the home, depending on the status of their relationship. Sandra works part time at a retail chain, struggling to meet the financial responsibilities of rearing a child. She is showing physical signs of depression and distress (e.g., apathy, anorexia, excessive sleeping, and episodes of crying). During your home visit, Sandra says, "Something is really wrong with me. I can't snap out of this feeling of darkness. Life is too hard for me and is nothing but pain. I can't take it anymore and want it to be over." You believe she needs immediate mental health support.

THINKING

1. *Theoretical Knowledge:*
   a. What facts and principles do you already know about stress and depression?
   b. How does the emotional illness of one family member affect others living in the home and the family as a whole?
2. *Critical Thinking (Inquiry):*
   a. What factors in Sandra's life are possibly contributing to her feelings of hopelessness and thoughts of self-harm?
   b. Name at least three nursing diagnoses that would best suit Sandra's health needs.

DOING

3. *Practical Knowledge:* Based on the knowledge you have about stress and depression, (see #1 above), how would you explain to the family about how best to support Sandra?
4. *Nursing Process (Evaluation):* What measures would you identify to determine whether your nursing plan of care was effective?

CARING

5. *Self-Knowledge:*
   a. How comfortable would you be caring for a patient who is at risk for self-injury?
   b. What is one problem with Sandra and her family, not described in the scenario, that could possibly arise?
6. *Ethical Knowledge:* What ethical concerns might you have for a woman with a young child who is at risk for self-injury, but has no financial resources to cover the expenses of mental health care?

Critical Thinking and Clinical Judgment

1. You are caring for a 58-year-old woman who was admitted for surgery of the foot. Today is the second day you have cared for the client. You notice that the family seems quiet and subdued. You ask the client whether something is wrong. She says that her 29-year-old niece just lost her job as a TV programming assistant because her employer found out she is HIV positive. Apparently the diagnosis was revealed on her health insurance claim forms when they were processed.
   a. Name two things in this scenario that you, as a nurse, *cannot* change.
   b. Do the client and her family have a problem that you *can* help them with? How can you find out?

c. Imagine you were your client (the aunt). What concerns would you have?

d. Try to depict this situation by using systems theory. Draw circles for each system involved, and show where the systems interact.

e. Use your self-knowledge. What biases or values do you have that might affect your thinking in this case, either positively or negatively?

2. You are caring for a 45-year-old man who was involved in a serious car accident. He suffered severe head trauma and, if he lives, probably will have serious deficits. He was admitted 24 hours ago and has not made significant improvements. The family is aware of his status and likely outcome.

   a. What are some concerns this family might have?

   b. Using structural–functional theory, describe how this family might be affected.

   c. How can you help this family?

3. You are caring for a 3-year-old child who had had a fall. The child will be fine and is being discharged. As you are reviewing the discharge instructions, the mother reveals that she and the child spent last night in a hotel because of violence in the home. She tells you that her husband (the child's stepfather) drinks excessively and at times has become violent, hitting her but not the child. She did not call him when they went to the emergency room and is afraid to go home.

   a. What do you think this woman's main concerns might be?

   b. Do you think this is a common problem or an unusual problem?

   c. What is the developmental stage of this family?

   d. What theoretical knowledge do you need to help this family?

   e. What kinds of help do you think this woman might need if she decides to escape from her husband?

   f. How could you help her at this moment?

4. For each of the following concepts, use critical thinking to describe how or why it is important to nursing, client care, or the family. Note that these are *not* to be merely definitions.

Family relationships

Blended families

Communication

Systems theory

Structural–functional theories

Developmental theory

Family interactional theory

Family as the unit of care

Family health risk factors

The national economy

Health beliefs

Family coping mechanisms

Unexpected illness

What Are the Main Points in This Chapter?

- *Family* is not limited to the traditional definition of a husband, a wife, and their children; defined more broadly, it is a group of individuals who provide physical, emotional, economic, and/or spiritual support while maintaining involvement in each other's lives.
- Families are structured in a variety of ways. Three examples are the traditional nuclear family, dual-earner families, and single-parent families.
- Family nursing views the family from three perspectives: as the context for care of an individual, as the unit of care, and as a system.
- Wellness of each member is critical to the health of the family unit.
- Under general systems theory, the family is viewed as a system in interaction with other systems (e.g., other families, groups, communities, and individuals).
- Under structural–functional theories, families are viewed as social systems with a focus on outcomes.
- Developmental theories focus on family stages: beginning family, childbearing family, family with preschool children, family with school-age children, family with teenagers and young adults, family launching young adults, postparental family, and aging family.
- Family interactional theory views the family as a unit of interacting personalities with a major emphasis on family roles.
- The family teaches health beliefs, values, and behaviors to its individual members.
- Assessment of family communication patterns consists of interviewing the family and the individual seeking care, as well as astute observation by the nurse.
- How families cope with everyday life situations and hospitalization can influence the effectiveness of care rendered.
- Nurses can promote family wellness by addressing both individual and family concerns.
- The family can be a source of support or a source of difficulties for the ill person.

Knowledge Map

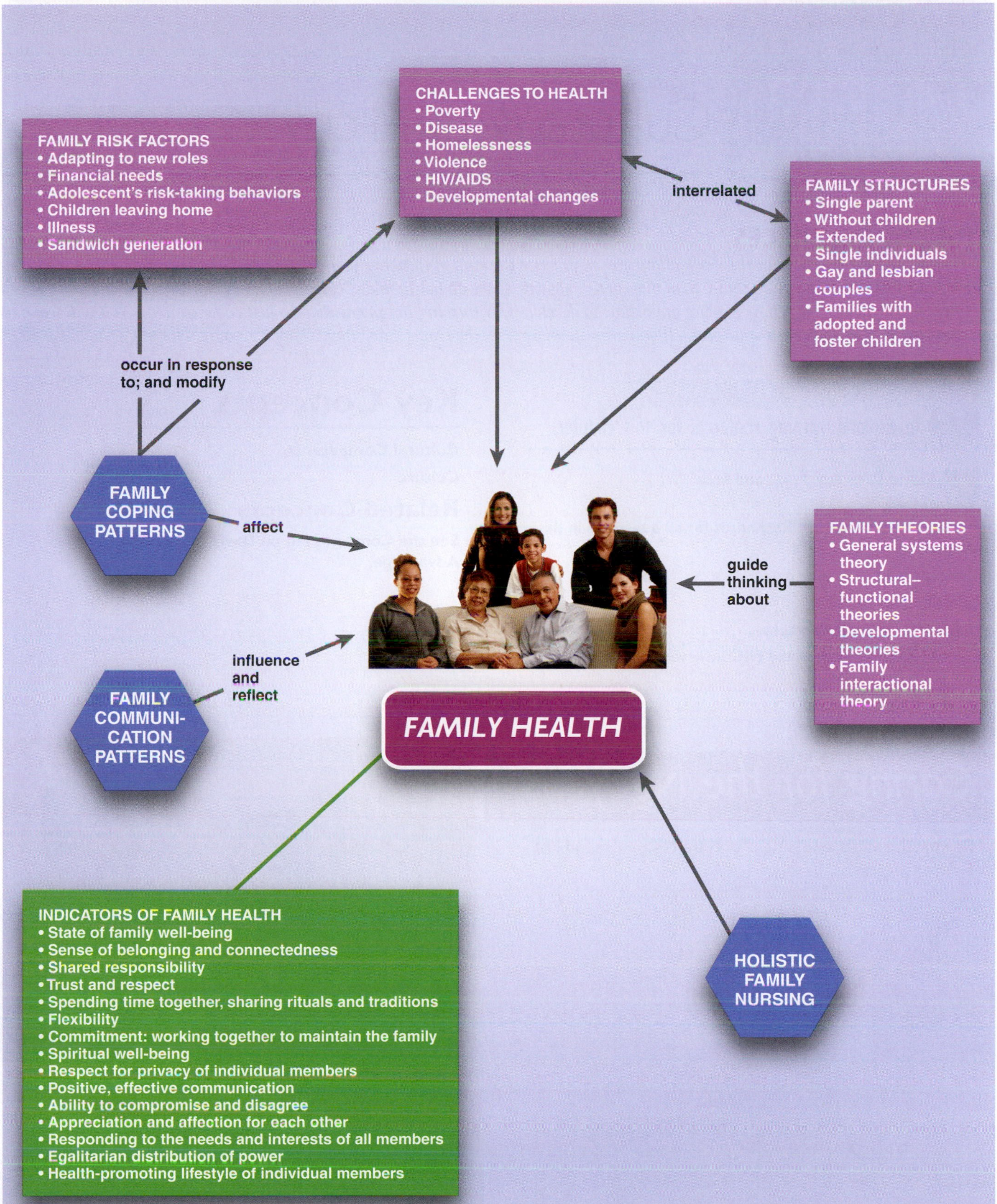

CHAPTER 15

Culture & Ethnicity

STUDENT RESOURCES

The questions and exercises in this book allow you to practice the kind of thinking you will use as a full-spectrum nurse. Critical-thinking questions usually have more than one correct answer, so we do not provide "correct answers" for these features. Try to answer these questions yourself. It is more important to develop your nursing judgment than to just cover content. You will learn by discussing the questions with your peers. If you are still unsure, see the Davis Advantage chapter resources for suggested responses.

To explore learning resources for this chapter,

Go to Davis Advantage and find:

Answers and Suggested Responses for all questions in this chapter
Concept Map
Knowledge Map
References and Bibliography
List of NOC Outcomes and NIC Interventions

Key Concepts

Cultural Competence
Culture

Related Concepts

See the Concept Map on Davis Advantage.

Caring for the Nguyens

Review the initial assessment of Nam Nguyen, found just before Chapter 1.

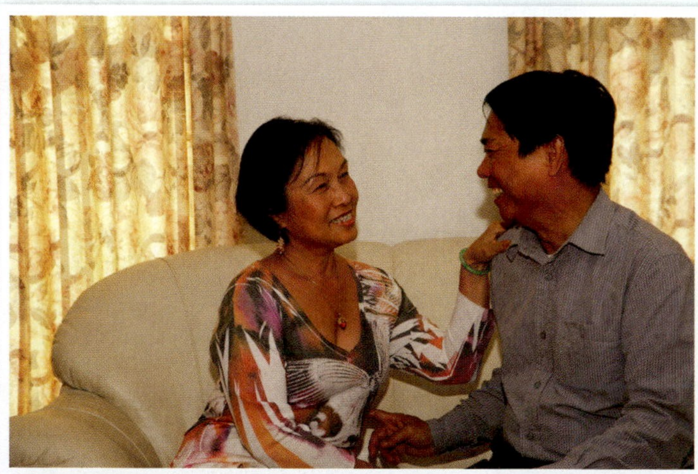

A. How might the Nguyens' cultural heritage affect their health beliefs?

B. What factors would you want to consider when performing a cultural assessment of the Nguyen family?

Practical Knowledge clinical application

Information in this section may be useful for assessing and communicating with clients of cultures different from your own.

CLINICAL INSIGHTS

Clinical Insight 15-1 ➤ Assessing for Biological Variations

People differ genetically and physiologically. Some biological variations create susceptibility to certain diseases and injuries. The following are examples:

Body Build and Structure

- 12% of Native Americans have 25 vertebrae instead of 24, which relates to an increased number of back problems.
- Lower socioeconomic status increases the likelihood of obesity.
- Black and white men are, on average, about 3.5 inches taller than Asian American men and 2 inches taller than Mexican American men.

Skin Color

- Darker skin challenges the nurse to be more observant when assessing skin color changes (e.g., when assessing oxygenation or skin rashes). Obtain a baseline skin color by asking a family member or someone who knows the patient well.
- To assess for oxygenation and cyanosis in dark-skinned people, examine the sclera, buccal mucosa, tongue, lips, nailbeds, palms of the hands, and soles of the feet.
- To assess for jaundice in Asians, examine the sclera.

Vital Signs

- The average systolic blood pressure of black men between 35 and 65 years of age is 5 mm Hg higher than that of European American men of the same age.

Laboratory Tests

- Native Americans, Hispanic Americans, and Japanese Americans, on average, have higher blood glucose levels compared with whites.
- Bone density is greater in whites than in Chinese, Japanese, and Alaska Native populations.

Susceptibility to Disease

- Blacks have a higher incidence of hypertension and sickle cell anemia compared with other groups.
- Asian Americans have a higher incidence of tuberculosis compared with the white population.
- Blacks, Native Americans, and Mexican Americans are more likely to have diabetes mellitus than their white counterparts.

Nutritional Variations

- All groups have their own food preferences.
- Soy sauce, used in many Asian foods, is high in sodium.
- There is a high incidence of diabetes mellitus in areas where sugar cane is a major crop.

Enzymatic and Genetic Variations and Body Secretions

- Lactose intolerance, caused by a deficiency of the enzyme lactase, is more commonly seen in blacks, Native Americans, and Asian Americans.

Drug Metabolism

- Native Americans and Asians are more likely to experience facial flushing and palpitations after ingesting alcohol.
- African Americans metabolize alcohol, nicotine, antihypertensives, and beta blockers differently from European Americans; they are more susceptible to side effects of haloperidol and tricyclic antidepressants; and they respond better to diuretic therapy compared with whites.
- Asian Americans tend to experience more gastrointestinal side effects from opiates, even though the analgesic effect is less.
- Chinese Americans are more sensitive to the cardiovascular effects of propranolol; they have increased absorption of antipsychotics, antihypertensives, and some narcotics.
- Recall that most drug studies in the past were normed on European Americans, so "variations" refer to differences from those norms.

Practice Resources

Andrews, M. & Boyle, J. (2015); Giger, J. (2016); Purnell, L. (2013); Purnell, L. & Paulanka, B. (2008); Spector, R. (2017); Suzuki, L. & Ponterotto, J. G. (2007).

Clinical Insight 15-2 ➤ Communicating With Clients Who Speak a Different Language

When Possible, Use a Qualified Interpreter or a Translator.

- A **translator** merely restates what has been said into the targeted language.
- An **interpreter** is specially trained to provide the meaning behind spoken words from one language to another. An interpreter can serve as a cultural broker by conveying the client's responses to questions and by providing general information about the client's culture (Centers for Disease Control and Prevention [CDC], 2018).

When Using any Type of Interpreter, it is Important to do the Following:

- Because of confidentiality issues, avoid asking a family member, especially a child or the spouse, to act as the interpreter.
- Avoid using an interpreter who is socially or politically incompatible with the client (e.g., you would not ask an Israeli to interpret for a Palestinian).
- Be aware of gender and age differences. (It usually is preferable to have an interpreter of the same gender as the client.)
- Have the interpreter spend some time alone with the patient.
- Ask the interpreter to interpret the words used by the healthcare provider as closely as possible, except where literal translation might be offensive or misunderstood. In such cases, an interpreter (as compared with a translator) would provide the meaning of your words in terms acceptable to the client.
- Do not use metaphors ("happy as a clam") or medical jargon.
- Observe nonverbal communication (e.g., body language) when the client is listening and talking to the interpreter.
- Address your questions to the client, not to the interpreter.
- Maintain eye contact with both the client and the interpreter.
- Speak slowly and distinctly, facing the client; do not speak loudly.
- Ask one question at a time; allow time for interpretation and for response from the client before asking another question.
- Use active rather than passive voice (e.g., say, "The doctor will see you tomorrow." rather than "You will be seen by the doctor tomorrow.")
- Be aware that many clients can understand more English words than they can express.
- Have health education materials translated into the client's language, or have an interpreter audiotape or videotape instructions.

If There is no One Available to Interpret for You:

In addition to the preceding strategies, you should do the following (Munoz and Luckmann, 2005; Purnell, 2014):

- Greet the client with respect. Greet the person formally, using Mr., Ms., and so forth, until given permission to do otherwise. People in some groups consider it disrespectful to use a person's first name.
- Identify the client's primary language, and use any words that you are familiar with in her language to show that you are trying to communicate.
- Use the Internet or computer software to translate words into the client's native language.
- If appropriate, use a third language that both of you speak. For example, some Vietnamese and some Cambodians speak French.
- Speak slowly and clearly, using simple sentences to discuss one question or need at a time.
- Use gestures to help convey meaning.
- Restate in different words, if needed.
- Use pictures or diagrams.
- Be aware that some clients may answer yes, even if they do not understand what you have said.

Practice Resources

Munoz, C., & Luckmann, J. (2005); Purnell, L. (2014); Centers for Disease Control and Prevention (2018).

ASSESSMENT GUIDELINES AND TOOLS

Focused Assessment

Obtaining Minimum Cultural Information

You should obtain at least this much cultural information from every client. For some, you may need a more in-depth assessment.

- Begin the interview with open-ended questions, such as the following:

  I would like to know more about your family.

  Who will be able to help you when you go home?

  What do you do to help keep yourself well?

- When you and the client are comfortable, be sure to ask a question such as, "What concerns you the most about your illness and treatment?" This allows you to focus on the individual, rather than just on his or her culture.
- You will not need to perform an in-depth cultural assessment on every patient, but you will need to recognize situations in which this is needed.

Language(s) spoken; proficiency in the language of the host country	➤ What language(s) do you speak? ➤ Are you comfortable speaking [English], or would you like to have an interpreter?
Length of time client has been here; where client was raised	➤ Where were you raised? ➤ How long have you lived here?
Ethnic affiliation and identity	➤ What racial and ethnic group(s) do you identify with? ➤ How closely do you identify with the values of those groups?
Usual religious practices	➤ What religion do you practice, if any? ➤ Are there any special beliefs, rituals, or practices you want us to be aware of?
Nonverbal communication style	➤ You will need to observe the patient and draw on your theoretical knowledge of the patient's cultural group for this information.
Family roles, primary decision maker	➤ Who is in your family? ➤ What is your role in your family? ➤ Who makes most of the decisions? ➤ How are decisions made in your family? ➤ Who should I talk to for decisions about your healthcare?
Social support in the new country	➤ Do you have family and friends here? ➤ Who can you go to when you need help? ➤ Where do you work? ➤ Will you need any help with your healthcare expenses?

Sources: Giger, J: Transcultural Nursing: Assessment and Intervention, ed. 7. St. Louis, MO: Elsevier, 2016; Spector, R: Cultural Diversity in Health and Illness, ed. 9. Upper Saddle River, NJ: Pearson Education, 2017; Suzuki, L. A., & Ponterotto, J. G.: Handbook of Multicultural Assessment: Clinical, Psychological, and Educational Applications, ed. 3. San Francisco, CA: Jossey-Bass, 2007.

Focused Assessment

Cultural Assessment Using the Transcultural Assessment Model

Assess information listed in the following categories:

Cultural Uniqueness

- Cultural and ethnic identification
- Place of birth
- Time in country

Communication

- Voice quality
- Pronunciation and enunciation
- Use of silence
- Use of nonverbal communication
- Touch
- Spoken language

Space

- Degree of comfort
- Distance in conversations
- Definition of space
- Body movement

Social Organization

- Normal state of health
- Marital status
- Number of children
- Parents living or deceased
- Friends
- Work
- Leisure

Time

- Orientation to time
- View of time
- Physiochemical reaction to time

Environmental Control

- Locus of control
- Value orientation
- Health and illness beliefs

Biological Variations

- Physical assessment (including body structure, skin color, skin discoloration, hair color and distribution, other visible physical characteristics, weight, height, laboratory variances)
- Susceptibility to illness
- Nutritional preferences
- Psychological characteristics

Other

In addition to the Giger categories, obtain information about the following:

- Educational experiences (formal and informal)
- Family patterns of healthcare
- Family role and function
- Healthcare beliefs and practices (folk and professional)
- Religious practices and beliefs
- Social networks
- Values orientation

Source: Adapted from Giger, J: Transcultural Nursing: Assessment and Intervention, ed. 7. St. Louis, MO: Elsevier, 2016.

CLINICALJUDGMENT

Applying the Full-Spectrum Nursing Model

PATIENT SITUATION

Mrs. Vasquez, a 70-year-old Mexican American woman, has diabetes mellitus and has come to the hospital because of a sore on her lower leg that will not heal. Mrs. Vasquez, a widow, cares for herself at home. She speaks only a little English and has some difficulty understanding your questions. After great effort on your part, you determine that she has missed her last appointment with her diabetes specialist because she has no transportation, so she has just been putting a dressing on the sore. Mrs. Vasquez tells you that she loves to see her grandchildren, who visit often, and that she enjoys cooking and eating Mexican food. She also says that she believes she is sick because she has displeased God. However, God is a source of comfort and assurance to her. She prays a lot and has rosary beads in her hand.

THINKING

1. *Theoretical Knowledge (Recall of Facts and Principles):* List six important culture specifics.

2. *Critical Thinking (Application of Knowledge):* Based on your theoretical knowledge, what are your expectations about communicating with Mrs. Vasquez?

3. *Critical Thinking (Compare and Contrast):* Compare your expectations to the actual data you have about her ability to communicate.

DOING

4. *Nursing Process (Assessment):* What are some pertinent cultural data that you should assess for Mrs. Vasquez?

5. *Nursing Process (Analysis/Diagnosis):* Which nursing diagnosis do you think would be best for planning Mrs. Vasquez's care? (Recall that the etiology should suggest your nursing interventions, and the diagnostic label should suggest the expected patient outcomes.) Explain your reasoning.
   - Noncompliance (with clinic appointments), related to lack of transportation
   - Skin Integrity Impairment, related to self-treatment of ulcer
   - Noncompliance (with clinic appointments), related to beliefs about God and illness

CARING

6. *Self-Knowledge:* What areas of commonality do you have with Mrs. Vasquez, around which you might form a caring relationship?

7. *Self-Knowledge:* Do you agree with Mrs. Vasquez that illness may be caused by displeasing God?

8. *Ethical Knowledge:* Suppose you do not agree with Mrs. Vasquez that she is ill because she has displeased God. Discuss whether you would explain to her that this is most likely not true and then teach her about the cause of diabetic ulcers.

Critical Thinking and Clinical Judgment

1. Mrs. Vasquez, a 70-year-old Mexican American woman, has diabetes mellitus and has come to the hospital because of a sore on her lower leg that will not heal. Review the details of Mrs. Vasquez's case in the preceding Full Spectrum Nursing Model Situation.
   a. Identify Mrs. Vasquez's cultural data, and group it under the following culture specifics:

      Communication

      Space

Time orientation

Social organization

Environmental control

Biological variations

b. You have learned that cultural data can have implications for nursing care. Answer each of the following:
   - What additional information should you assess for in this situation?
   - What biases do you have that affect your thinking in this situation?

2. An Asian woman comes to your clinic for assessment of her blood pressure. In casual conversation, she tells you that her oldest daughter is about to be married. She reveals that her daughter has some type of anemia for which she needs medication. She tells you that she has recently heard terrible stories about sickle cell anemia and is afraid that this is what her daughter has.
   a. What additional data do you need to collect to answer this client's questions?
   b. What assurances, if any, can you give this client about her daughter?

3. At times, nurses must care for clients who do not speak their language. This poses a challenge to those who strive to provide culturally competent care to all clients. Even with the assistance of interpreters, this can be difficult because of barriers such as differing dialects, street talk, and jargon. Keeping these facts in mind, answer the following questions:
   a. What options do you have when you encounter a person who cannot speak English?
   b. How do you communicate with such a client if no interpreter is available?
   c. What biases do you have about such a situation? Why?

4. Alma is of European descent; she is Caucasian. She is a Roman Catholic and believes abortion is wrong. She believes that it should be illegal to own a gun. She is a nursing student.

   Violetta's parents came to the United States from Europe. They were born in France. Before that, her great-grandparents lived in Africa. Violetta is an African American. She is Roman Catholic, and she believes that abortion is wrong. She believes that it should be illegal to own a gun. She is a nursing student.

   Darcy is of European descent; she is Caucasian. She laughs at the idea of religion, saying, "Nobody's 'up there' looking out for me; and when you're dead, you're dead." Darcy is a gang member and carries a gun in her purse or her pocket at all times. She did not finish high school, and by the age of 19, she had had two abortions.

   All of the women live in the United States. Which two women do you think share the most cultural commonalities? Explain your thinking.

5. Helen is a 52-year-old divorced African American woman. Her only child, Tamika, is incarcerated for prostitution and possession of narcotics. Helen is now raising her two grandchildren, Calvin, age 13 years, and Jevetta, age 2 years. Helen is a nursing assistant at the local hospital. It is hard for her to make ends meet because she has hypertension and diabetes, for which she takes a number of medications, including insulin—that is, when she can afford them. Helen has not applied for medical assistance because she believes she should be able to take care of herself, but she does receive assistance for Jevetta's day-care costs. In addition to her grandchildren, Helen has a large group of friends, many of whom attend her church. She has little time to spend with her friends since she took custody of the children. Jevetta has been admitted to the hospital for asthma. You are Jevetta's student nurse.
   a. Using your data collection skills, think of diagnostic labels that you could apply to Jevetta and to Helen as Jevetta's caregiver.
   b. What resources may be helpful to Helen?

6. Examine the following nursing diagnosis labels. For this set of labels, write an etiology that might be caused by cultural differences. The first one is completed for you as an example.

   - Body Nutrition (Excess), *related to patient's lack of knowledge about how to adapt his preferred ethnic foods to her prescribed low-fat diet.*
   - Health Maintenance Alterations
   - Role Performance Alteration
   - Anxiety
   - Powerlessness
   - Knowledge Deficit

7. For the following set of labels, explain or give an example of how the nurse might misdiagnose or misperceive the data because of cultural differences. The first one is done for you.

   - Decisional Conflict

The nurse might ask a woman to make some decision about her care. The woman may seem indecisive and unable to reach a conclusion. The reason might be that the husband is the decision maker in the family. When the husband arrives, the Decisional Conflict ("problem") may no longer exist.

   - Confusion
   - Socialization Alteration
   - Nonadherence
   - Pain (Acute or Chronic)

8. For each of the following concepts, use critical thinking to describe how or why it is important to nursing, patient care, or cultural competence. Note that these are *not* to be merely definitions.

Culture

Subculture

Ethnicity

Race

Religion

Acculturation

Health and illness belief

Health and illness practice

Phenomena of culture

Ethnocentric

Folk medicine

Cultural competence

Transcultural nursing

Giger and Davidhizar assessment model

Biological variations among cultures

Prejudice and racism

Professional (e.g., nursing) subculture

Cultural sensitivity

Cultural awareness

Culture universals

Culture specifics

What Are the Main Points in This Chapter?

- The cultural and ethnic composition of North America has changed dramatically over the past several decades, making it essential that nurses understand the healthcare beliefs and practices of diverse populations.
- Culture includes shared values, beliefs, norms, and practices that guide a particular group's thinking, decision making, and actions in a patterned way.
- Through acculturation, most ethnic and cultural groups modify some of their traditional cultural characteristics, values, beliefs, and practices.
- You should be familiar with the common characteristics of different cultural groups in your community.
- The U.S. Census Bureau (2018) has identified and divided the population into the following racial categories:
  White
  Black or African American
  American Indian or Alaska Native
  Asian
  Native Hawaiian or Other Pacific Islander
- The Census Bureau (2018) categories for ethnicity (or "origin") are (1) Hispanic, Latino, or Spanish and (2) Not Hispanic, Latino, or Spanish.
- **Culture universals** (commonalities) are the values, beliefs, and practices that people from *all* cultures share. **Culture specifics** (diversities) are those values, beliefs, and practices that are unique to a culture.
- A **cultural archetype**, similar to a model, is an example of something that is recurrent and has its basis in facts. A **cultural stereotype** is a widely held but oversimplified and unsubstantiated belief that all people of a certain racial or ethnic group are alike in certain respects.
- Six organizing phenomena of culture that influence health include communication patterns, space, social organization, time, environmental control, and biological variations.
- Healthcare providers cannot understand the health beliefs and practices of diverse populations if they view them through the lens of the conventional (Western, American) culture of healthcare.
- A variety of "alternative" healing systems exists. Remedies have been passed down from generation to generation and include the use of herbs, customs, and rituals.
- An understanding of cultural concepts, theories, and models can help develop cultural competence.
- Ethnocentrism, stereotyping, prejudice, and racism are barriers to culturally competent care.
- When assessing a client and making nursing diagnoses, you must consider the client's cultural values, beliefs, and practices related to health and healthcare.
- Culturally competent care requires a nonjudgmental attitude, self-awareness, sensitivity, respect for differences, theoretical knowledge, and the desire to be culturally competent.

Knowledge Map

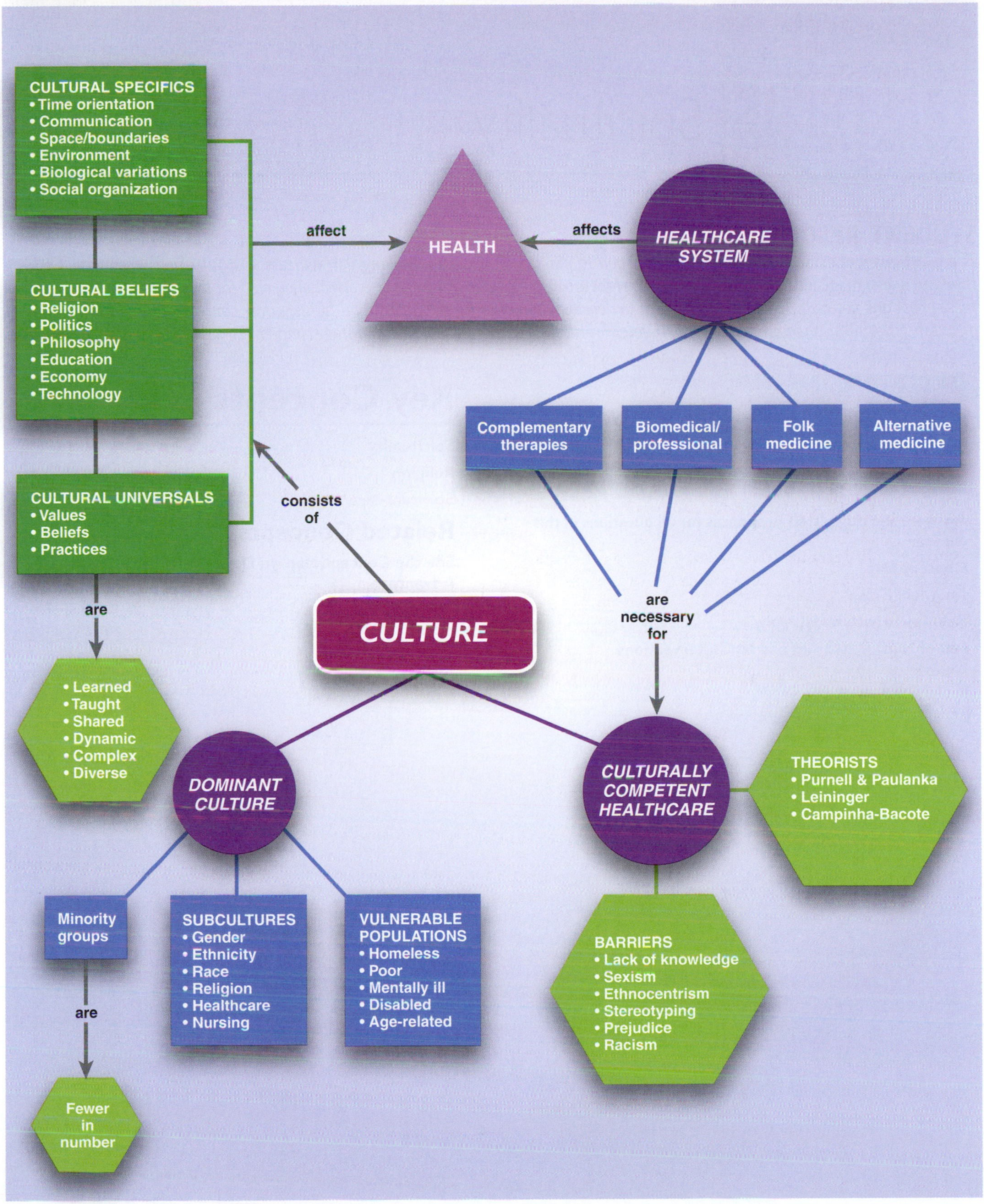

CHAPTER 16

Spirituality

STUDENT RESOURCES

The questions and exercises in this book allow you to practice the kind of thinking you will use as a full-spectrum nurse. Critical-thinking questions usually have more than one right answer, so we do not provide "correct answers" for these features. Try to answer these questions yourself. It is more important to develop your nursing judgment than to just cover content. You will learn more by discussing the questions with your peers. If you are still unsure, see the Davis Advantage chapter resources for suggested responses.

To explore learning resources for this chapter,

Go to Davis Advantage and find:

Answers and Suggested Responses for all questions in this chapter

Concept Map

Knowledge Map

References and Bibliography

List of NOC Outcomes and NIC Interventions

Key Concepts

Spirituality

Religion

Spiritual care

Related Concepts

See the Concept Map on Davis Advantage.

Caring for the Nguyens

Kim Phan is the 3-year-old grandson of Nam and Yen Nguyen. The Nguyens are both practicing Catholics. Kim's mother, Trinh, is the Nguyen's daughter. Trinh feels that Catholicism is "a waste of time" and does not attend church. Kim has had no formal religious experiences or training.

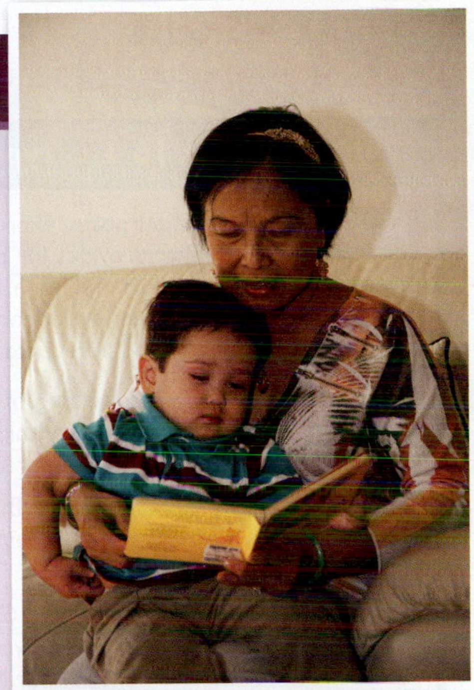

A. At a clinic visit, Nam asks you what you think about keeping religion away from a child. How would you respond?

B. Mr. Nguyen explains his views on the situation: "If anything were to happen to him, he would go to hell. I think we should take him to church and get him baptized right away. I don't know how anyone can live like that. He has no connection to God." Do you agree with this statement? Explain your views.

C. Nam asks you to pray for Kim and his mother. How would you feel about this situation? What would you say to Nam?

PracticalKnowledge clinical application

In this section, you will find guidelines for performing spiritual interventions and for performing focused spiritual assessments.

CLINICAL INSIGHTS

Clinical Insight 16-1 ➤ Types of Prayers

Prayer has a variety of purposes, expressions, and meanings to patients and their families, as well as to nurses themselves. For many people, prayer provides for periods of intimacy with God, reveals the presence and love of God, and serves as a powerful source of comfort and hope. For those who embrace the power and influence of prayer, it supports their spiritual journeys and may help them experience forgiveness, love, hope, trust, and meaning. Symbolically, a nurse engaged in prayer manifests the reality of God's presence with that patient.

Adoration	Directing of our focus and our thoughts to God, asking nothing but to enjoy the presence of God in our lives; might take the form of meditation	*I Chronicles 29: 11-12*
Praise	Belief that the love of God draws forth our praises, not to obtain anything, but simply to offer words of praise	*Luke 2:20, 11:2, 18:43*
Thanksgiving	Offered to God for all the blessings of life and living and whatever draws our attention to God's presence in our lives	*Psalm 100:4; Philippians 4:6*
Penitence	Desire to confess one's sins, with an intention to change	*Psalm 51*
Offering	Offering of all that we have (our life, our work, our hopes and dreams) to God for the purposes that God envisions for us	*Psalm 141:2*
Intercession	Praying for the needs of others	*Luke 11:5-8; Luke 18:1-5*
Petition	Presents our own needs to God	*Mark 11:24; Hebrews 5:5; 11:1*
Agreement	Need for the prayer of another believer to achieve an outcome or answer	*Matthews 18:19; Acts 1:14*
Faith	Belief that a problem will be resolved by God	*Mark 11:22-23; I Timothy 2:1;*
Fellowship	Need for companionship with God	*Corinthians 13:14*
Consecration and dedication	Seeking direction from God on an issue or to make a decision	*Luke 22: 41-42; Romans 12: 1-2; Matthew 26:39*
Forgiveness	To overcome negative emotions from being hurt or wronged by another person	*Mark 11:25*
Committal	To relieve oneself of burden (worry, fear) associated with trying to handle a problem	*Psalm 55:22; I Peter 5:6*
Imprecation	Offered to pray for our enemies, to overcome the wickedness of others	*Matthew 5: 44-48*

Adapted from *Book of common prayer*, 1979; Cheatham, D. (2008). *Kinds of prayer—a brief review*. retrieved from http://devotionalnet.faithsite.com/uploads/147/95698.pdf; Stanley, C. (2011). *Handle with prayer: unwrap the source of God's strength for living*. Colorado Springs, Co.: David Cook.

Clinical Insight 16-2 ➤ Praying With Patients

Because there is a rich diversity in religious expression, keep the following guidelines in mind when you pray for or with patients:

Ask how the patient prefers to address the divine. Some people prefer the use of parental language in their prayers, for example, *Father God* or *Divine Mother*. Some use the word *Jehovah*, *Yahweh*, or *Allah*. Hindus may address one or more of multiple Gods, each of whom has several names. So do not be afraid to seek direction from the patient in these matters: Most people are honored to be able to explain their beliefs and practices to someone who is open to the experience.

Before the prayer begins, ask the patient whether any rituals or religious items are necessary. Muslims may want water to wash the mouth, nostrils, and hands before beginning prayer. Roman Catholics may want to hold their rosary beads while praying, and some Buddhists and Hindus meditate with a set of beads called a *mala*. Others may have a prayer cloth or other item that needs to be accessible.

Always feel free to pray or not to pray. Never feel that you are being forced to do or say something that makes you uncomfortable.

Do not be a compulsive "prayer" or a compulsive avoider of prayer. Always make sure that the patient (and/or family) is comfortable with prayer if he has not yet requested it.

Know that there are appropriate times and places for the offering of prayer. Prayer at the bedside may be most appropriate, although it may make people uncomfortable in a crowded waiting room. Perhaps the statement "I will be praying for you and your family" might be more appropriate for some patients than actually praying aloud at that moment.

When a patient asks for prayer, consider using this reply: "I would be honored to offer prayer. What would you like me to *especially* address in the prayer?" Knowing what the patient hopes for in prayer gives you an idea of the type of prayer the person is requesting.

When the patient tells you what she wants you to pray for, be sure to focus your prayer around the request.

- It is always good to summarize the results of previous conversations with the patient and her needs in the course of your prayer. For example, imagine that a patient with cancer who has been treated with chemotherapy now finds that the blood counts are coming back to normal levels. The chemotherapy treatment seems to be successful at this point, but the patient is afraid of a relapse and asks you to pray for the cancer to be cured.
- Analyze the situation in terms of what has happened in the past, what is happening now, and what the patient is requesting. This will help you organize your thoughts and then put them into the form of a prayer.

Perhaps you would want to take the patient's hand in yours (if appropriate, based on your intuition and the nature of your nurse–patient relationship) and compose a prayer, for example, as follows: Dear [Lord], I give you thanks that [John] has done so well with his treatments. Please continue to help him be strong and open to your healing presence. We pray for his family, doctors, and nurses that all may be a part of [John's] continued healing and sense of comfort. I pray that the treatments that he is receiving, together with the prayers that we are offering, may all be effective in his care and in the treatment of his cancer. Watch over [John], and visit us all at this time with your healing presence. [Amen.]

When a terminally ill patient requests a prayer for a cure, total healing, or a miracle, you may feel challenged. Knowing how to offer prayers that are "realistic" allows for the occurrence of miracles and healings of all types while also keeping in perspective the physical realities of the nature of disease and the reality of death.

If composing a prayer is difficult for you, you may want to explore, for example, the use of the Psalms in the Hebrew Bible (Old Testament) or some New Testament scriptures, if appropriate for the patient. Also see, Clinical Insight 16-1, Types of Prayers. If the patient's religion is different from your own, ask whether he or she has examples of sacred writings from which you might be allowed to read. Perhaps the patient has a favorite prayer or a text from an authoritative source that brings comfort and hope.

It is always good to include in the course of your prayer a request for God's help and direction with the patient's health-care team. This expresses the reality that we are all working together for a common good and purpose and that we depend on God and others for our welfare and place in life.

Once the prayer is over, thank the patient for asking you to participate. In that way you can ask whether you can be of any further assistance.

ASSESSMENT GUIDELINES AND TOOLS

Focused Assessment

The HOPE Approach to Spiritual Assessment: Examples of Questions

Mnemonic	Examples of Questions
H—Sources of **Hope**, meaning, comfort, strength, peace, love and connection	What are your sources of internal support? What do you hold onto to get you through difficult times? For some people, religious or spiritual beliefs are a source of comfort in dealing with life's ups and downs. Is this true for you?
O—Organized religion	Do you belong to a religious or spiritual community? Does it help you? How important is this to you? What aspects of your religion are helpful to you?
P—Personal spirituality/**Practices**	Do you believe in God? What is your relationship with God? Do you have personal spiritual beliefs that are not a part of organized religion? If so, what are they? What aspects of your spirituality are most helpful to you (e.g., meditation, prayer, reading scripture, listening to music, nature)?
E—Effects on medical care and end-of-life issues	Has your illness affected your relationship with God? Or to do the things that usually help you spiritually? Are you concerned about conflicts between your beliefs and your healthcare treatment plan? Do you have any dietary restrictions or other practices I should know about in planning your care? Would you like to speak to a clinical chaplain (or community spiritual leader)?

Source: Based on Gowri, A., & Hight, E. (2001). Spirituality and medical practice: Using the HOPE questions as a practical tool for spiritual assessment. *American Family Physician, 63*, 36–41.

Focused Assessment

S-P-I-R-I-T Assessment

- Obtain information from the patient, when possible.
- For an emergency admission or if the patient cannot give information, consult the next of kin or a designated power of attorney (DPOA) as soon as possible for information.

S—Spiritual/religious belief system

Religion, tradition, sect, or denominational affiliation

Text/writing(s) providing source of authority and codes for behavior

Name and phone number of supporting or affiliated church, synagogue, temple, or other place of worship

Past experience with a belief system (positive or negative)

Beliefs related to health, illness, healthcare, healthcare providers, Western medicine, adjuvant therapies, herbal or natural healing methods or techniques

Beliefs about suffering, terminal or chronic illness, advance directives, autopsy, organ donation

Stigmas related to illness, if applicable

P—Personal spirituality

Individual beliefs and practices of affiliation that the patient or family accepts and attempts to follow (may be directly or indirectly related to above assessment areas)

Individual beliefs that may differ or even be contrary to affiliation beliefs

Whether spirituality is a part of personal experience of religion or is a separate entity

Level of comfort discussing spirituality

Whether personal spirituality is viewed positively or negatively at the present time

I—Integration within a spiritual community

Name and title of religious or spiritual leader or authority figure(s)

Names and titles of religious groups that may need to be contacted: for example, Stephen Ministry, prayer group leader, prayer chain support person, shaman, medicine man or woman, men's or women's group within denomination

Role of patient or individual in any of above named groups

R—Ritualized practices and restrictions

Activities that patient's or family's faith encourages or forbids

Needs for modesty and covering of body parts or appendages

Any special beliefs or needs in relation to drawing blood or to laboratory tests or procedures

Dietary needs and restrictions: food preferences, preparation of foods, and location of food preparation areas

Gender-specific roles and responsibilities of care providers

Prayer needs and restrictions: Who offers and delivers such practices?

Articles or other materials needed for worship, devotion, or prayer (rosaries, prayer beads, prayer books, religious tracts, Bibles, crosses, prayer shawls or cloths)

I—Implications for medical care

Beliefs and practices that healthcare providers should remember while providing care

Specific medications that may not be administered and withheld; implications for pain control

Specific medical procedures or products that may not be administered (abortion, administration of blood products)

Communication patterns and needs for effective care delivery: Who makes decisions? What is the role of parents or guardians when children or other vulnerable populations are the recipients of care? Does the guardian reflect the beliefs of patient, if these are known?

T—Terminal events planning

Wishes for advance directives (cardiopulmonary resuscitation, intubation, ventilator assistance, feeding tubes)

Wishes for transplantation or organ donation

Need for religious services (last rites, ministries of healing, baptism, initiation, confession, communion)

Clergy or ministry groups to be contacted and when

Ideas of an afterlife

Treatment of the body at the time of death

Funeral planning

Source: Adapted from Maugans, T. (1996). The SPIRITual history. *Archives of Family Medicine, 5*(1), 11–16; and Highfield, M. E. F. (2000). Providing spiritual care to patients with cancer. *Clinical Journal of Oncology Nursing, 4*(3), 115–120.

STANDARDIZED LANGUAGE

Selected NIC Interventions and Activities to Support Spirituality

NURSING DIAGNOSES

Moral Distress	Impaired Religiosity (NANDA-I)*
Spiritual Distress	Risk for Impaired Religiosity*
Risk for Spiritual Distress	Readiness for Enhanced Religiosity
Spiritual Pain	

NURSING INTERVENTIONS	NURSING ACTIVITIES
Dying Care	Facilitate obtaining spiritual support for patient and family. Support the patient and family through stages of grief (see Chapter 17). Facilitate discussion of funeral arrangements.
Emotional Support	Explore with the patient what has triggered emotions. Embrace or touch the patient supportively. Make supportive or empathetic statements. Encourage the patient to express feelings of anxiety, anger, or sadness.
Forgiveness Facilitation	Listen empathetically without moralizing or offering platitudes. Explore forgiveness as a process. Assist client to seek out an arbitrator (objective party) to facilitate the process of individual or group concern. Explore possibilities of making amends and reconciliation with self, others, and/or higher power.
Hope Inspiration	Assist patient and family to identify areas of hope in life. Help the patient expand his spiritual self. Facilitate the patient/family's reliving and savoring past achievements and experiences. Create an environment that facilitates the patient's practicing religion, as appropriate.
Presence	Be physically available as a helper. Remain physically present without expecting interactional responses. Offer to remain with the patient during the initial interaction with others in the unit. Listen to the patient's concerns. Stay with the patient to promote safety and reduce fear.
Religious Ritual Enhancement	Coordinate or provide healing services, communion, meditation, or prayer in the place of residence or other setting. Encourage the use of and participation in usual religious rituals or practices that are not detrimental to health. Assist with modifications of the ritual to meet the needs of the disabled or ill. Treat the individual with dignity and respect.
Self-Awareness Enhancement	Assist patient to realize that everyone is unique. Assist patient to identify life priorities. Assist patient to identify guilty feelings. Assist patient to identify source of motivation.

Selected NIC Interventions and Activities to Support Spirituality—cont'd

NURSING INTERVENTIONS	NURSING ACTIVITIES
Self-Esteem Enhancement	Encourage the patient to identify strengths. Provide experiences that increase the patient's autonomy, as appropriate. Explore previous achievements of success. Assist patient to identify the significance of culture, religion, race, gender, and age on self-esteem. Monitor frequency of self-negating verbalizations. Reinforce the personal strengths that patient identifies.
Spiritual Growth Facilitation	Encourage conversation that assists the patient in sorting out spiritual concerns. Assist patient with identifying barriers and attitudes that hinder growth or self-discovery. Offer individual and group prayer support, as appropriate. Encourage participation in devotional services, retreats, and special prayer/study programs. Assist the patient to explore beliefs as related to healing of body, mind, and spirit. Refer for pastoral care or primary spiritual caregiver as issues warrant.
Spiritual Support	Be open to the patient's expressions of loneliness and powerlessness. Encourage chapel service attendance, if desired. Provide desired spiritual articles, according to individual preferences. Be available to listen to the individual's feelings. Listen carefully to the individual's communication, and develop a sense of timing for prayer or spiritual rituals. Be open to individual's feelings about illness and death.
Values Clarification	Consider the ethical and legal aspects of free choice, given the particular situation, before beginning the intervention. Pose reflective, clarifying questions that give the patient something to think about. Encourage patient to make a list of what is important and not important in life and the time spent on each. Encourage patient to list values that guide behavior in various settings and types of situations. Avoid use of the intervention with persons with serious emotional problems.

OTHER NIC SPIRITUAL CARE INTERVENTIONS

Active Listening	Crisis Intervention	Meditation Facilitation	Resiliency Promotion
Anticipatory Guidance	Decision-Making Support	Mood Management	Self-Esteem Enhancement
Anxiety Reduction	Emotional Support	Music Therapy	Self-Modification Assistance
Bibliotherapy	Grief Work Facilitation	Referral	Self-Responsibility Facilitation
Coping Enhancement	Guilt Work Facilitation	Role Enhancement	Support Group
Counseling	Humor	Religious Ritual Enhancement	Touch

Sources: Butcher, H., Bulechek, G., Wagner, C. M. (Eds.). (2018). *Nursing interventions classification (NIC)* (7th ed.). St. Louis, MO: Elsevier; *Herdman, H., & Kamitsuru, S. (2018). *NANDA international nursing diagnoses: Definitions & classification*, 2018–2020 (11th ed.). New York: Thieme; Jackson, D., Doyle, C., Capon, H., et al. (2016). Spirituality, spiritual need, and spiritual care in aged care: what the literature says. *Journal of Religion, Spirituality & Aging*, DOI: 10.1080/15528030.2016.1193097. Retrieved from https://pdfs.semanticscholar.org/9990/d4bb705f50d362d2d9322e2a266977af9cf6.pdf; Martin & Scheet. (1992). *The Omaha system*. Philadelphia, W. B. Saunders Co., p. 69; Saba, V. K. (2017). *Clinical care classification (CCC) system*, version 2.5: User's guide. Retrieved from https://sabacare.com/Custom/Tables/Diagnoses.php?SF=DiagCode&SO=Asc; Millspaugh, C. (2005). Assessment and response to spiritual pain: Part II. *Journal of Palliative Medicine, 8*(5): 1110–1117; and Toivonen, K., Stolt, M. & Suhonen, R. (2015). Nursing support of the spiritual needs of older adults living with dementia. *Holistic Nursing Practice, 29*(5), 303–312.
*To make safe and effective judgments using NANDA-I nursing diagnoses, it is essential that nurses refer to the definitions and defining characteristics of the diagnoses listed in this work.

CLINICAL JUDGMENT

Applying the Full-Spectrum Nursing Model

PATIENT SITUATION

Review the Meet Your Patient scenario to answer the questions below about Charles Johnson, a 75-year-old black man with newly diagnosed cancer of the lung. He is unsure whether he wants to have the chemotherapy his physician has recommended to increase his life span.

Go to Chapter 16, **Meet Your Patient,** in Volume 1.

THINKING

1. *Theoretical Knowledge (Recall of Facts and Principles):* Define *forgiveness,* and explain the benefits of forgiving self and others.

2. *Critical Thinking (Application of Knowledge*): Based on your theoretical knowledge about forgiveness, with whom might Mr. Johnson need to reconcile? Why do you think so?

DOING

3. *Practical Knowledge (HOPE Assessment):* Use the Focused Assessment: The HOPE Approach to Spiritual Assessment: Examples of Questions, and enter Mr. Johnson's data. Identify sections for which you need additional data.

CARING

4. *Self-Knowledge:* How is your religious background similar to or different from Mr. Johnson's?

5. *Self-Knowledge:* (a) How would you feel if Mr. Johnson said to you, "Church folk are all a bunch of hypocrites, if you ask me. I choose not to be a part of any of that."? (b) How would you respond?

6. *Ethical Knowledge:* Imagine that Mr. Johnson's sister comes to visit and leaves some religious pamphlets on a chair, where he will not see them before she leaves. What would you do?

Critical Thinking and Clinical Judgment

1. A 5-year-old boy was admitted to the hospital last night with a fever of 103°F (39.4°C). He was diagnosed with a serious infection that is easily treated with intravenous (IV) antibiotics. However, his parents are Christian Scientists, and they do not want antibiotics administered to their son. They have called their Christian Science practitioner to visit as soon as possible.
   a. What practical knowledge do you have that will give you some insight into this situation?
   b. What essential piece of knowledge do you need that is *not* given in this scenario?
   c. If the parents do not agree to accept IV antibiotics for their son, what can you do to (1) ensure that he receives treatment *and* (2) support their spiritual needs?
2. A woman is admitted to the emergency department and gives birth to a premature male infant who is in severe respiratory distress. The woman is a devout Roman Catholic. What interventions could you use to ensure holistic spiritual care in this emergency situation?

3. Interview nurses in the area where you have your clinical experiences. Discuss the interviews with classmates.
   a. Ask them to describe spiritual problems their patients have had.
   b. Ask them to tell you of any spiritual interventions they have used with patients, and how effective they believe them to be.
   c. Ask them how comfortable they are in using spiritual interventions, especially prayer.
4. For each of the following concepts, use critical thinking to describe how or why it is important to nursing, patient care, or spirituality. Note that these are *not* to be merely definitions.

   Spirituality and religion

   Nursing research in religion and healthcare

   Major religions and healthcare

   The nurse and spirituality

   Assessment of the spiritual domain of care

   Spiritual care nursing interventions

   Spiritual well-being

What Are the Main Points in This Chapter?

- Spirituality is a powerful force in the lives of many patients.
- Nursing has historical roots in religion and spirituality.
- Nurses work with other disciplines to provide spiritual care.
- Religion is a sort of "map" that outlines and integrates essential beliefs, values, and codes of conduct into a manner of living.
- Spirituality, like a journey, takes place over time and involves the accumulation of life experiences and understandings. It is the attempt to find meaning, value, and purpose in life.
- Religion and spirituality affect health and well-being; in turn, health and well-being affect a person's religion and spirituality.
- Research suggests that patients' beliefs in religion and spirituality are important to healthcare outcomes; however, it does not explain *how* or *why* this is so.
- The more you know about similarities in and differences among the world's major religions, the more you will be able to offer comprehensive, compassionate care to patients.
- People, even within the same religion, vary greatly in the degree to which they follow the rituals and practices of their own religion.
- Self-knowledge helps you to avoid abuses of spiritual care (e.g., imposing your religion on a patient).
- Barriers to spiritual care include (1) lack of awareness of spirituality in general and of your own spiritual belief system, (2) differences in spirituality between you (the nurse) and the patient, (3) fear that your spiritual knowledge is insufficient, and (4) fear of where spiritual discussions might lead.
- Nursing interventions related to spiritual care require you to be self-aware, fully present, supportive, empathetic, and nonjudgmental and to have a desire to benefit the patient.
- When a patient asks you to pray, you must determine whether he wishes you to pray *for* or *with* him, and you should ask what the person would like you to *especially* address in the prayer.
- A miracle does not necessarily involve the notion of a cure; miracles are more often events that proceed according to natural law but still have a powerful impact on the person's expectations.

Knowledge Map

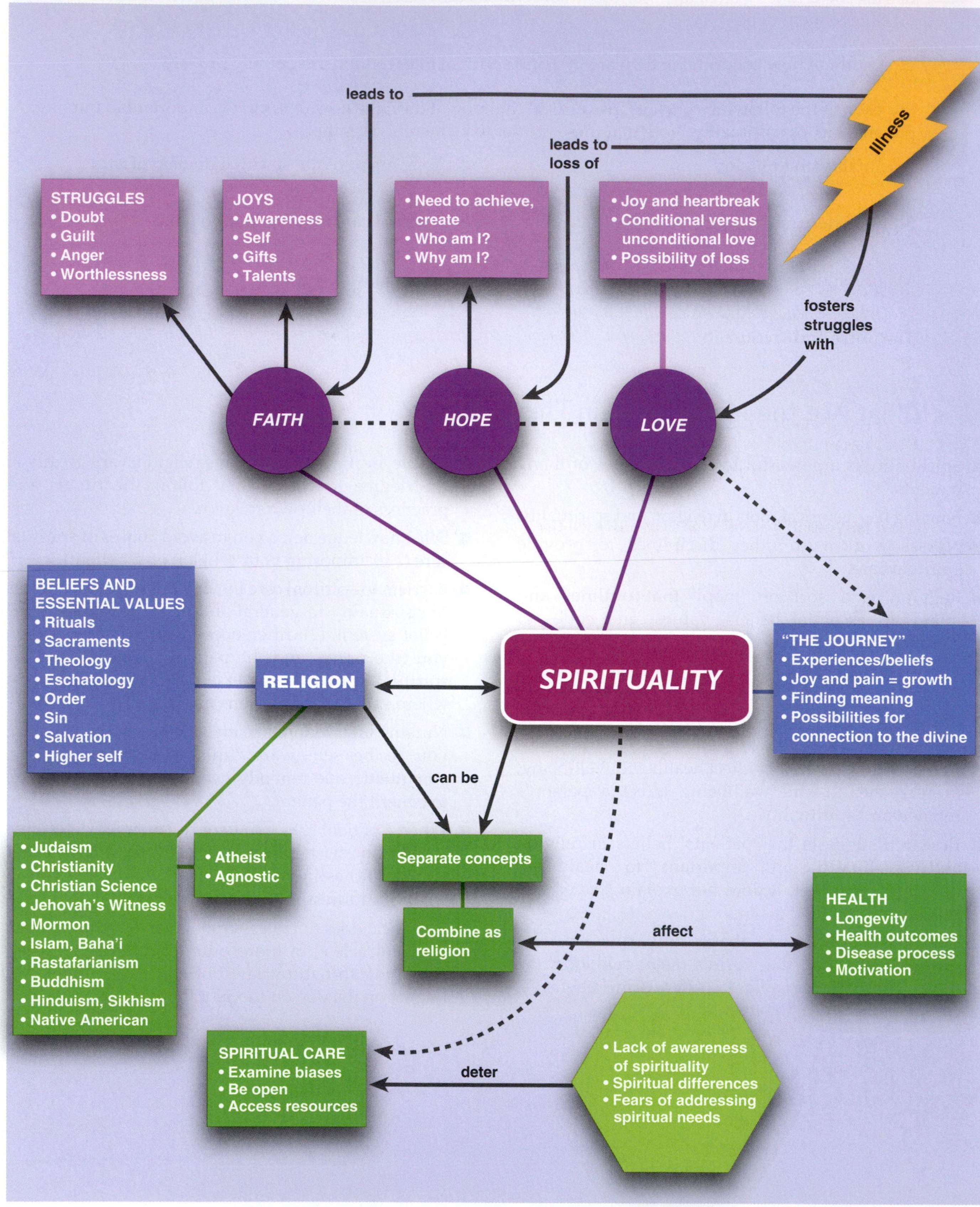

CHAPTER 17

Loss, Grief, & Dying

STUDENT RESOURCES

The questions and exercises in Volume 2 allow you to practice the kind of thinking you will use as a full-spectrum nurse. Critical-thinking questions usually have more than one correct answer, so we do not provide "correct answers" for these features. Try to answer these questions yourself. It is more important to develop your nursing judgment than to just cover content. You will learn by discussing the questions with your peers. If you are still unsure, see the Davis Advantage chapter resources for suggested responses.

To explore learning resources for this chapter,

Go to Davis Advantage and find:

Answers and Suggested Responses for all questions in this chapter
Concept Map
Knowledge Map
References and Bibliography
List of NOC Outcomes and NIC Interventions

Key Concepts

Death and dying
End-of-life care
Grief
Loss

Related Concepts

See the Concept Map on Davis Advantage.

Caring for the Nguyens

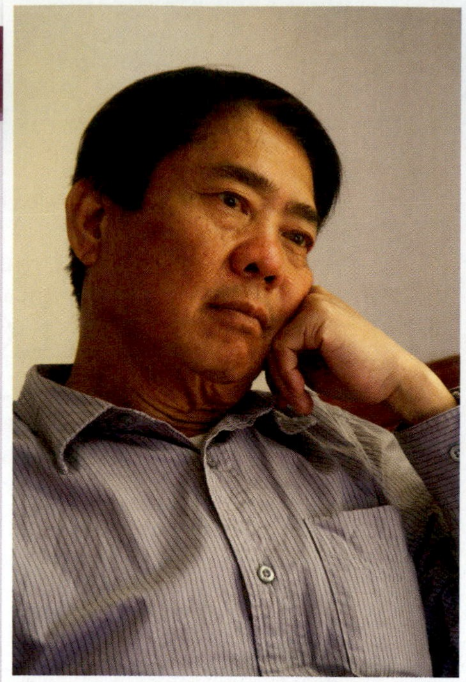

At a clinic visit, Nam Nguyen tells you that his father's health is declining rapidly. Mr. Nguyen tells you, "I thought he was doing okay. I knew he had surgery for his prostate, so I thought it was all over. Lately he's been having lots of low back and hip pain. So my mom begged him to go to the doctor, and the doctor told him he has cancer all over." Mr. Nguyen shakes his head and looks away from you. You notice tears in his eyes.

Mr. Nguyen tells you that his family has avoided discussions about serious illness and death. "It just never got discussed. The whole idea made my parents uncomfortable. When my father got sick the first time, he refused to discuss it. 'I'm going to get better. Don't even think about it,' he would say." Now Mr. Nguyen feels the need to discuss this situation with his parents but does not know how to bring up the topic. He asks for your advice.

A. What would you think and feel when you see Nam's tears and when Mr. Nguyen asks for this advice?

B. What would you advise Mr. Nguyen?

C. What type of grief is Mr. Nguyen experiencing?

D. Examine the factors that affect grief. Apply these factors to Mr. Nguyen's situation. You will need to review the family history included in the introduction to the Nguyens (in the front of this book) to fully answer this question. Indicate whether the information for any of the factors to be evaluated is insufficient.

PracticalKnowledge clinical **application**

In this section, you will find guidelines for caring for dying patients and their families, providing postmortem care, and communicating with people who are grieving.

CLINICAL INSIGHTS

Clinical Insight 17-1 ➤ Communicating With People Who Are Grieving

Perfect your listening skills. Listen for what is *not* said as well as what is said.

Be alert for and respond to nonverbal cues with appropriate touch and eye contact. A smile, a gentle touch, sitting with a patient, and eye contact all relay a message of genuine care and concern. You may not need to say very much at all.

Encourage and accept expressions of feelings.

- Receiving expressions of intense feelings (e.g., anger and guilt) may be painful for you. It may help to remember that it is therapeutic for people to express their feelings.
- You do not need to change the person's feelings or "make them better." As much as we would like to do this, it is not possible.
- You do need to validate the person's feelings (e.g., "It is normal to feel that way; it is okay").

Reassure the person that it is not "wrong" to feel anger, guilt, relief, or other feelings she may believe to be unacceptable. A dying patient might say, "I know it's awful, but I feel so angry with God for not curing this disease." Or a bereaved spouse might admit, "I shouldn't feel this way, but I'm relieved that it's finally over." Patients need to hear you say their feelings are not "wrong" or "bad" and that they are going through a normal process.

Increase your self-awareness. Become more conscious of your own attitudes and feelings regarding death and dying. *If you are comfortable with your perspective, you will be able to hear patients' expressions of anger, guilt, frustration, fear, and loneliness more comfortably.*

Continue to communicate with dying patients even if they are in a coma. Encourage family members to do so as well.

- Talk to the patient. Tell the person what is going on around him or her, what care you are providing, and when you or others enter or are about to leave the room.
- Avoid discussing the dying person as though he or she were not present. *Research indicates that patients continue to hear even though they cannot respond, sometimes up to the moment of death.*

Practice Resources

Emanuel, L., Ferris, F., von Gunten, C., et al. (2015); Gibson, A., Hyde, Y., & Kautz, D. (2016); Holms, N., Milligan, S., & Kydd, A. (2014); The Joint Commission (2015); Wittenberg-Lyles, E., Goldsmith, J., Oliver, D., et al. (2012).

Clinical Insight 17-2 ➤ Helping Families of Dying Patients

- **View the family as your unit of care.** *Family members often rate communication with clinicians as one of their most important needs.*
- **Provide information, support, and a listening ear.** Include specific facts about the patient's condition and prognosis and whom to call about changes in condition.
- **Communicate medical updates daily.** *Information can relieve anxiety and is useful to the family when making decisions.*
- **Encourage family members to help with care if they are able.** Instruct and supervise, as appropriate. If family members are not physically or emotionally able to provide care, accept that. *This helps meet their need to be useful, promotes family ties, and makes the patient more comfortable.*
- **Encourage family members to ask questions.** *They may hesitate to do so for various reasons (e.g., they may not want to interrupt busy care providers).*
- **Listen actively to the patient's and the family's concerns.** Make eye content; clarify when you do not understand. *This helps you avoid misinterpreting the family's concerns and needs.*
- **Help the family to understand the goals of care and solve problems, when needed.**
- **Follow up with other healthcare team members promptly** if the family has questions that are outside your scope of practice.
- **Arrange for a formal interprofessional meeting with the family** soon after the patient's admission, if possible. Discussions should cover personal, cultural, and religious traditions (e.g., how prayers are to be conducted, how the body is to be handled after death, and so on).
- **Encourage the family to visit the hospital chapel and to speak with a chaplain** or with their own spiritual adviser.
- **Provide anticipatory guidance regarding the stages of loss and grief,** so that they will know what to expect after their loved one dies.
- **Acknowledge the family's feelings** and the loss they are experiencing. *Many times family members begin the grieving process before the loved one dies.*
- **Help the family members explore past coping mechanisms;** reinforce successful past coping mechanisms.

(Continued)

Clinical Insight 17-2 ➤ Helping Families of Dying Patients *(continued)*

- **Refer for ethics consultation** if decision making may become a problem.
- **Remind family members and significant others to take care of themselves.** *Watching a loved one die is a very difficult experience. A sensitive, caring nurse can make it a little easier.*
  - Many times they need "permission" to go to eat or to go home and rest.
  - If the patient is near death and family and friends do not want to leave the patient's side, make them as comfortable as possible.
  - Provide comfortable chairs, coffee, and snacks (according to organizational policy), and be alert for other needs they may have.
- **Teach the family what to expect with regard to medications, treatments, and signs of approaching death.** *If family members know what is normal, they will be less likely to panic or fear the inevitable.*
- **As physical signs of death become apparent, keep the family informed.** You may say something like, "Her blood pressure is becoming difficult to hear. That is one of the signs that she is closer to death." Help the family to understand what the patient is experiencing, as this may be very different from what they are seeing.
- **Reassure families when the patient becomes withdrawn near the time of death** that this does not mean the patient is rejecting them, but only that her body is conserving energy and that the person has come to terms with dying and letting go of connections with life.
- **When the patient is very near death, ask family members directly, "Do you want to be present while he is dying?"** Tell them what to expect, if they do not know.
- **When an expected death occurs, shift the focus of your care** to the family and those who were caregivers. *Death does not end the relationship; family and caregivers need support during bereavement.*

Practice Resources

Emanuel, L., Ferris, F., von Gunten, C., et al. (2015); The Joint Commission (2014, 2015); Keely, M. (2016); Slatyer, S., Pienaar, C., Williams, A., et al. (2015); Stayer, D. (2016); Williams, B., Lewis, D., Burgio, K., et al. (2012); Yim, M., Vico, C., & Wai, C. (2013).

Clinical Insight 17-3 ➤ Caring for the Dying Person: Meeting Physiological Needs

Active dying usually occurs over a period of 10 to 14 days (although it can take as little as 24 hours). The "final hours" refer to the last 4 to 48 hours of life, when failure of body systems results in death.

- **Encourage the patient to be as independent as possible.** *This helps the patient to maintain a sense of control.*
- **Provide adequate pain control.** *This can be a major issue for patients and caregivers. In fact, dying patients are often more concerned about pain and loss of control than about dying itself. Pain is difficult to assess in semiconscious or unconscious patients. See Chapter 31 if you need more information about pain management.*
  - Dispel the myths about pain medication (e.g., addiction, overdose). Effective pain control medications exist and can be administered via various routes. Assure the patient and the family that the focus is on pain control and not addiction to analgesics.
  - Respect the patient's informed decision to refuse pain medications. For example, a patient may prefer to endure pain so that she can be awake and alert when the family is at the bedside.
  - Follow the prescribed pain protocols to ensure that pain is controlled.
  - Administer pain medication on a regular schedule instead of waiting until the patient asks (prn), to ensure pain control.
  - Teach and perform nonpharmacological pain relief measures when you judge that these may be helpful (e.g., meditation, heat/cold therapies, massage, distraction, imagery, deep breathing, and herbal-scented lotions). It may be soothing to play soft music, add "white noise," or turn off the television.
  - Patients who are near death may moan or grunt as they breathe; this does not necessarily indicate pain. Be sure that families understand this. When accompanied by agitation and restlessness, these symptoms may indicate terminal delirium, which may require medications for control.
- **Monitor the patient's energy level.** *Fatigue is a normal part of the dying process. Most dying patients sleep much of the time.*
  - Perform hygiene and other care, if the patient tires easily or lacks the energy for self-care (i.e., activities of daily living [ADLs]).
  - Remove environmental stressors that interfere with sleep (e.g., noise, too much light, a room that is too hot or too cold).
  - Identify psychosocial stressors (e.g., depression, anxiety, fear) that may keep the patient awake (see Clinical Insight 17-4).

Clinical Insight 17-3 ➤ Caring for the Dying Person: Meeting Physiological Needs *(continued)*

- **Maintain skin integrity.** *During the final hours of life, the goal changes from preserving skin integrity to providing comfort. Realize that during this time even excellent care may not prevent skin breakdown.*
  - Turn the patient frequently, unless contraindicated. Refer to the pain control interventions in the preceding list.
  - Assess for increased diaphoresis and/or incontinence.
  - Maintain adequate nutrition.
- **If the patient is comatose or unconscious, provide special care for the eyes** so that they do not become too dry. Many agencies use a form of artificial tears for this purpose.
- **If the patient is not able to take fluids, wet the lips and mouth frequently with cool water** or with a prepared product to prevent dryness and cracking of lips and mucous membranes of the nose, mouth, and eyes.

  There is some evidence that glycerin swabs dry the mucous membranes, so they should not be used.
- **Provide artificial hydration (unless the patient has an advance directive requesting no artificial hydration)** via the nasogastric (NG) or intravenous (IV) route. *IV fluids can cause edema, nausea, and even pain in a patient who is actively dying. Dehydration is thought not to cause distress during the last hours, and may even be protective* (Emanuel, Ferris, von Gunten, et al., 2015).
- **Take the vital signs often, unless contraindicated;** observe for decreased level of consciousness and pallor.
- **Assess and provide interventions for constipation, urinary retention, and incontinence.** *Constipation may be associated with decreased fluid intake, inactivity, weakness, hypercalcemia, hyperkalemia, and lack of privacy. It can contribute to pain, nausea, vomiting, and anorexia, so intervention is an important comfort measure. Incontinence may occur because of fatigue and loss of sphincter control. It can be distressing to patients and family members.*
  - Administer laxatives, stool softeners, and lubricants for constipation.
  - Catheterize the patient if she is unable to void and the bladder becomes distended.
  - Use pads for incontinence, but change them frequently to prevent skin breakdown and, near the end, to promote comfort.
  - Use a rectal tube if there is severe diarrhea.
- **Intervene for "death rattle"** if it occurs and if it is distressing to the family.
  - Turn the patient on the side, and elevate the head of the bed.
  - Administer antispasmodic and anticholinergic medications, if necessary.

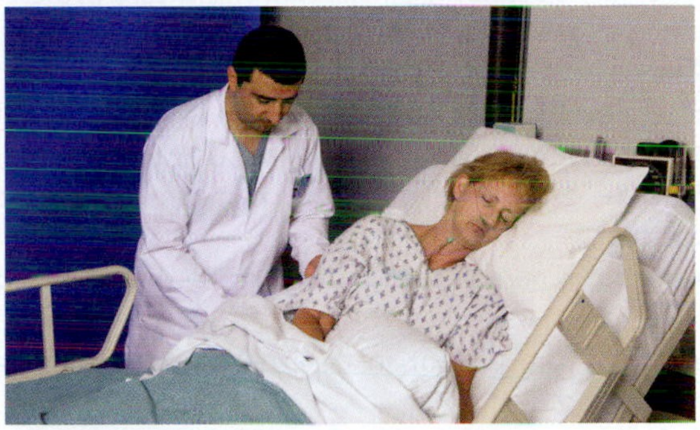

- **Provide medication for other symptoms,** such as nausea and breathlessness.
- **Continue to speak to the patient as if he can hear.**
- **Do not talk about the patient with others in her presence.** *The patient is usually able to hear even after she can no longer respond to sounds and other stimuli. Assume that the unconscious patient hears everything.*
- **Document changes in vital signs and level of consciousness.** Record intake and output, noting changes. Document the times of cardiac arrest and cessation of respirations.

Practice Resources

Brennan, C., Prince-Paul, M., & Wiencek, C. (2011); Covington, M. (2013); Emanuel, L., Ferris, F., von Gunten, C., et al. (2015); Fahlberg, B. (2015a); Higgins, I., Riet, P., Sneesby, L., et al. (2013); The Joint Commission (2014, 2015); Kisvetrová, H., _ koloudík, D., Joanovi_, E., et al. (2016); Steindal, S., Ranhoff, A., Bredal, I., et al. (2013).

Clinical Insight 17-4 ➤ Caring for the Dying Person: Meeting Psychological Needs

Patients experience many emotions at the end of life, including anger, sadness, depression, fear, relief, loneliness, and grief. At this time, communication and support are most helpful. Discussing concerns and issues is a viable means of coping.

- **If there is an advance directive or living will, locate the documents.** Review the documents to be certain you understand the patient's wishes. If you have not already done so, notify all relevant healthcare professionals of the existence of these documents.
- **Answer all questions honestly.**
- **Explain all care and treatments even if the patient is unconscious.** *He or she may still be able to hear.*
- **Realize that the patient may feel he is losing control.**
  - Help the person recognize what he does have control over.
  - Include the patient in care decisions as much as he is able.
- **Attend to social needs.** *Relationships are a priority at this time. Some patients may simply need to keep the bonds with family members and friends intact. For other patients, this may be a time to reestablish or mend relationships.*
  - Notify family members when the patient wishes to see them.
  - Allow the patient and family members to discuss death at their own pace.
  - Offer to contact a chaplain or other spiritual leader if the patient wishes.
  - Pray with the patient if he requests it and if you are comfortable doing so.
- **Encourage the patient to express feelings**. Be prepared to accept a wide range of feelings, including anger, hopelessness, loneliness, and depression.
- **Early in the dying process, assess the sources of financial support** for the patient and the family. *Finances may be a concern and may place an additional burden on the family; or the patient may feel she is a burden.*
- **Be aware of sexual needs.** Provide realistic information about these issues. For example, suggest ways a couple can be close and affectionate at this time. Be aware that expressions of sexuality may change as a person becomes closer to death. *Some people may feel it is not right to have sexual feelings when the person they love is dying. Others may be afraid of harming the patient if they are sexually intimate.*
- **When the patient is very near death, focus on relieving symptoms** (e.g., pain, nausea) and emotional distress.
- **If the person can communicate, ask about immediate concerns:**
  - "Are you in pain?" "Are you comfortable?"
  - "What are you afraid of now?"
  - "What can we do to help you go peacefully?"
  - "Who do you want in the room with you right now?"
- **If the patient asks whether she is dying, be honest and provide information that aligns with cultural beliefs and practices.**
- **If the patient cannot communicate, ask a significant other what the patient would want.** Ask the family member or person who is most likely to know.
- **When the patient is very near death, it may be helpful to say something like, "Your family will be fine**" rather than, "It is okay for you to go now." *Be aware that some people seem to wait to die until after a significant date (birthday, anniversary, and so on) has passed. Others wait for family to gather, whereas others wait until loved ones leave so they will not upset the family by dying in their presence.*

Practice Resources

Brennan, C., Prince-Paul, M., & Wiencek, C. (2011); Coolen, P. (2012); Emanuel, L., Ferris, F., von Gunten, C., et al. (2015); Finocchiaro, D. (2016); The Joint Commission (2015); Pola, A., & Nelson, R. (2014); Scogin, F., Fairchild, J., Yon, A., et al. (2014); Slatyer, S., Pienaar, C., Williams, A., et al. (2015).

Clinical Insight 17-5 ➤ Providing Postmortem Care

Supporting the Family

- **At the moment of death, do not interrupt or intrude on the family.** Wait quietly and observe, or if family members would feel more comfortable being alone with the patient, leave the room. Give them as much time as they need. When they move away from the body or have expressed their last good-byes, then it is time to assess the patient and report the lack of vital signs.
- **Immediately after death, express sympathy to the family.** This is very important. Make a simple statement, such as "I am sorry for your loss." Avoid statements that interpret the situation for the family, such as "It's God's will." Also avoid attempts to mitigate the family member's grief by saying, for example, "It will get better in time," or "You still have your son."
- **If the family wishes to be alone with the body,** straighten the bedcovers and make the patient look as natural as possible. Remove any tubes, IV lines, and so on, according to the institution's policy, and have the patient positioned in a way that appears comforting (e.g., bedcovers pulled up, hands at the side).

Clinical Insight 17-5 ➤ Providing Postmortem Care *(continued)*

- **Be accepting of family members' behavior at this time,** no matter how strange it may seem to you. A family might want to take a picture, or the spouse may lie down beside the deceased person.
- **If no family members are present, identify the next of kin,** and be sure the family is informed of the patient's death.
- **If family members arrive after the death, offer to take them to the bedside.**
- **If family members wish to be involved in postmortem care,** encourage them to do so. This can help them in their grieving process.
- **Ask whether each family member wishes to spend time alone with the deceased person,** and arrange for them to do so. Never remove the body until the family is ready. Viewing the body is helpful to many individuals.
- **Ask, "How can I help?" "What do you need?" "What would you like me to do for you?"**
- **Locate the patient's personal effects, and give them to the family/next of kin.** If you cannot remove a ring, wrap it with gauze, tape it in place, and tie the gauze to the wrist to prevent subsequent loss.

Legal Responsibilities

- **Notify the primary provider about the death.** Usually the physician must pronounce death; however, in some areas, a coroner or a nurse may also perform this task.
- **The person who pronounces death must sign the death certificate.** In some agencies, the nurse is responsible for checking to ensure that it has been signed.
- **If the patient is donating organs,** review and make any necessary arrangements.
- **If an autopsy is to be performed,** as a rule, the provider (or other person designated by the institution) is responsible for obtaining signed permission from the next of kin.

Care of the Body

- **Follow agency policies, and respect cultural and spiritual preferences.**
- **Wash the body if there has been any incontinence or drainage.** Place absorbent pads between the buttocks to absorb rectal drainage. Ask the family before washing the body. *In some cultures, the body is not washed, or family members arrange to have someone special do it.*
- **Dress the body in a clean gown, comb the hair, and straighten the bed linens.**
- **Place the body supine in a natural position.**
  - Place dentures in the mouth before rigor mortis occurs.
  - Close the eyes and mouth before rigor mortis occurs. Close the eyes by gently pressing on the lids with your fingertips. If they do not stay closed, place a moist compress on the eyelids for a few minutes, and then try to close them again.
  - Tie a strip of soft gauze (e.g., Kling) under the chin and around the head if your institution requires it (not all do). Alternatively you can place a folded towel under the chin to keep the jaws closed. *This keeps the mouth set in a natural position in case there is a viewing later.*
  - Place a pillow under the head and shoulders. *This prevents blood from settling there and causing discoloration.*
- **Be sure that dressings are clean, and unless an autopsy is to be done, remove all tubes and drains.** Be careful when removing tape or dressings. Apply small adhesive bandages to puncture sites. *After death, the skin loses its elasticity and can be torn easily.*
- **If the family asks about the coldness and color of the body, explain to them about algor mortis and livor mortis.**
- **After the family has spent time with the body, arrange to have it sent to the morgue,** where an autopsy will be performed; if not, the funeral home in charge of arrangements will arrive to transport the body.
  - Pad the wrists and ankles to prevent bruising; tie them together with gauze.
  - Wrap the body in a shroud or body wrap for transfer to the morgue.
  - If no relatives were present to receive the patient's belongings, bag them, label the bag, and send it with the body to the morgue.
  - If possible, close the doors to adjoining rooms before transport.
- **Make sure there are identification tags on the body, on the shroud or body bag, and on the patient's possessions; and that hazard labels are placed, if necessary.** Follow agency policy for number and location of tags. They will usually include the patient's name, room and bed numbers, date and time of death, and the healthcare provider's name. Misidentification can create legal problems, for example, if the body is prepared incorrectly for the funeral.
- **Follow institutional policy if the patient has died as a result of a communicable disease.** By law, there are special preparations to perform in such cases.
- **Handle the body ensuring dignity.**

Documentation

- **Documentation varies among healthcare facilities.** However you will almost always document the time that you noted the absence of heartbeat and respirations, any auxiliary equipment still present (e.g., mechanical ventilator), the disposition of the patient's possessions (especially money and jewelry), and the date and time the body is transported to the morgue or the funeral home.

Practice Resources

College of American Pathologists (2012, updated); The Joint Commission (2015); Olausson, J., & Ferrell, B. (2013); Smith-Stoner, M., & Hand, M. (2012).

ASSESSMENT GUIDELINES AND TOOLS

You can use these guidelines for assessing dying patients, as well as for assessing other types of loss.

Focused Assessment

Assessing Grief and Loss

1. Assess the patient and significant others for common grief reactions.

Physical	Emotional	Behaviors	Cognition
Loss of appetite	Anger	Forgetfulness	Decreased concentration
Weight loss/gain	Sadness	Withdrawal	Forgetfulness
Fatigue	Guilt	Insomnia or too much sleep	Impaired judgment
Decreased libido	Relief	Dreaming of deceased	Obsessive thoughts of the deceased or lost object
Decrease in immune system	Shock	Verbalizing the loss	Preoccupation
Decreased energy	Numbness	Crying	Confusion
Possibly physical symptoms, such as headache or stomach pain	Loneliness	Loss of productivity at work or school	Questioning spiritual beliefs
	Fear		Searching to understand
	Anxiety		Searching for purpose and meaning
	Powerlessness		
	Helplessness		
	Depression		

2. Assess knowledge base of patient and significant others.

a. Can they make informed decisions about healthcare choices? You might ask the following questions:
   - "Tell me what you understand about your illness."
   - "Are there any questions about your illness that you would like me to answer?"
   - "What are your options for treatment?"
   - "Do you know how to reach your provider if you have questions about your care?"

b. What and how much do the patient and the family want to know? *Some people wish to have all the details of their condition and care. For others, the details cause anxiety.*

3. Assess the history of loss. Determine whether the patient or the family has sustained recent losses or major changes (e.g., death, moving, divorce, retirement). Ask such questions as:
- "Have you had any recent changes in your life?"
- "Tell me about your family."
- "Are your parents still living?" (as appropriate)
- "What previous experiences have you had with the loss of someone you loved (or with this or a similar condition)?"

4. Assess coping abilities and support systems. Questions to assess coping include the following:
- "What do you do to reduce stress?"
- "Which family/friends can you talk with?"
- "What or who would you say is your greatest support when going through difficult times?"
- "Tell me about a previous loss, and what you did to cope with it."
- "What community resources can help you get through this? Have you contacted them?"

The way individuals have coped in the past will affect how they cope with dying or with their current loss. It may also be therapeutic for them to identify their resources and support systems.

5. Assess the meaning of the loss or illness. Be alert for statements that may indicate the patient or family is struggling to find meaning, such as:
- "I'm being punished."
- "She doesn't deserve this."
- "Why is this happening to me?"

In trying to "make sense" of their loss or their dying, people try to attach a meaning to their suffering.

6. Differentiate between grief and depressive disorder.

a. Symptoms common to both grief and depressive disorder are sadness, insomnia, poor appetite, and weight loss. Feelings of sadness and depression are a normal part of grief, provided the depression does not linger too long.

b. Symptoms that indicate grief are not constant. For example, the person may feel relatively better in certain situations, such as when he is with friends and family. However, triggers, such as the deceased person's birthday, an anniversary, or holidays, cause the feelings to resurface more strongly.

c. Symptoms that indicate depressive disorder are more intense. For example, the person is preoccupied with the loss and rarely gets any relief from the symptoms. Other symptoms include:
   - Feelings of guilt not related to the loved one's death
   - Thoughts about own death or of suicide (other than feelings the person would be better off dead now that the loved one is gone)

Focused Assessment

Assessing Grief and Loss—cont'd

- Preoccupation with own "worthlessness"
- Sluggishness
- Hesitant and confused speech
- Prolonged and marked difficulty in carrying out ADLs
- Hallucinations, other than thinking he or she hears the voice of or sees the deceased person

7. **Perform a physical assessment.** Look for signs of increased stress, such as tension, forgetfulness, distraction, increased or decreased appetite and sleep, weight gain or loss, fatigue, and decreased self-care (e.g., deficient hygiene). *A thorough physical examination provides data to help you determine how well the patient is coping with the loss or illness.*

8. **Perform a cultural and spiritual assessment.**

   a. Assess the patient's and the family's religious beliefs, any spiritual needs they may have (e.g., forgiveness, hope, meaning, love), and cultural influences that may affect the way they cope.

   b. **Key Point:** ***Do not assume that a person adheres closely to the dominant values of his religious or cultural group. Always assess.*** For example, ask: "To what religious and ethnic groups do you belong?" and "How closely do you identify with those groups?"

See Chapters 15 and 16 for details of cultural and spiritual assessment, if you need them.

9. **Perform these specific assessments for dying patients.** In addition to the other assessments in this guideline, you should also assess the following:

   a. When the patient and the family are ready, encourage them to talk about what the patient might want for burial or cremation or whether there are tasks that the person would like taken care of (e.g., giving away valuables, calling family members).

   b. Determine whether the dying person has a living will or advance directives.

   c. Discuss with the patient and the family the possibility of organ donation, if appropriate for the patient's circumstances.

   d. Observe for physical changes that indicate the approach of death:

   1 to 3 months before death: Beginning withdrawal from others, increased sleep, decreased appetite, difficulty digesting food (especially meats), and preference for liquids. *Anorexia may be protective, as the resulting ketosis can diminish pain and increase the person's sense of well-being.*

   1 to 2 weeks before death: Cardiovascular deterioration causes decreased blood pressure, pulse and respiration changes (decreased or increased), a yellowish pallor to the skin, and extreme pallor of extremities. Observe for temperature fluctuations, increased perspiration, brief periods of apnea during sleep, rattling breathing sounds caused by congestion, and nonproductive cough.

   Days to hours before death: A brief surge of energy and mental clarity, with a desire to eat and to talk with family members

   - Dehydration, difficulty swallowing, decreasing blood pressure, weak pulse
   - Mucous membranes dry and tacky; cracked lips. *Dehydration during the last hours of dying is thought to not cause distress and perhaps to stimulate endorphin release.*
   - Sagging of tongue and soft palate, diminished gag reflex, secretions accumulating in the oropharynx and/or bronchi
   - Shallow, rapid, or irregular breathing; respiratory congestion; Cheyne-Stokes respirations; apnea of 10 to 30 seconds; "death rattle." *Cheyne-Stokes breathing is a cyclic pattern consisting of a 10- to 60-second period of apnea and then a gradual increase in depth and rate of respirations. Respirations gradually become slow and shallow, and then the cycle begins again with apnea.*
   - Decreased peripheral circulation, increased perspiration, "clammy" skin; extremities cool and mottled; dependent body parts darker than the rest of the body
   - Decreased urinary output, concentrated and foul-smelling urine, secondary to decreased kidney function
   - Slack facial muscles ("drooping")
   - Retained feces; bowel and bladder incontinence *due to decreased peristalsis and relaxation of sphincters*
   - Blurred vision; eyes open but unseeing
   - Restlessness or agitation (check for impacted stool, distended bladder, pain, medications, cerebral hypoxia, unresolved emotional or spiritual issues)
   - Decreased communication, quiet, withdrawal. Some become more coherent and energized for a time.
   - Fatigue

   Moments before death: Does not respond to touch or sound; cannot be awakened. There may be a short series of long-spaced breaths before breathing stops entirely and the heart stops beating. Auscultate to determine whether apical pulse and respirations are absent.

Sources: Blinderman, C., & Billings, A. (2015). Comfort care for patients dying in the hospital. *The New England Journal of Medicine, 373*(10), 2539–2561; Carter, L. (2016). Understanding our role in bereavement. *International Journal of Childbirth Education, 31(4)*, 28–30; Emanuel, L., Ferris, F., von Gunten, C., et al. (2015). The last hours of living: Practical advice for clinicians. *Medscape*. Retrieved from http://www.medscape.com/viewarticle/716463; Finocchiaro, D. (2016). Supporting the patient's spiritual needs at the end of life. *Nursing2016, 56*(5), 46–59; Pies, R., Shear, K., & Zisook, S. (2014). Distinguishing grief, complicated grief, and depression. *Medscape*. Retrieved from http://www.medscape.com/viewarticle/836977_2; Scott, P. (2016); 10 signs death is near. Caring.Com. Retrieved from https://www.caring.com/articles/signs-of-death; and Widera, E. & Block, S. (2012). Death rattle: Prevalence, prevention and treatment. *Journal of Pain and Symptom Management, 23(4)*, 310–317.

STANDARDIZED LANGUAGE

Standardized Language

Examples of NOC Outcomes and NIC Interventions for Loss and Grieving Diagnoses

Nursing Diagnoses	Selected NOC Outcomes	Selected NIC Interventions
Grieving		
Defining Characteristics: Anger, potential loss of significant object (e.g., job status, body function), denial of potential loss, sorrow, guilt, bargaining, altered eating and sleep patterns, changes in activity level or libido, difficulty taking on new roles	Adaptation to Physical Disability Coping Family Coping Grief Resolution Psychosocial Adjustment: Life Change	Anticipatory Guidance Body Image Enhancement Coping Enhancement Emotional Support Family Integrity Promotion Family Support Grief Work Facilitation Grief Work Facilitation: Perinatal Death
➤ Does Thomas Manning (Meet Your Patient) in your textbook, have any symptoms of Grieving?		
Complicated Grieving		
Defining Characteristics: Repetitive use of ineffective coping behaviors, reliving of past experiences with little or no reduction in intensity of grief, prolonged interference with functioning, psychosomatic responses, expressions of grief (e.g., anger, sadness, crying), idealization of lost object or person, labile affect, developmental regression, denial of loss, expression of unresolved issues or guilt	Coping Family Coping Family Resiliency Grief Resolution Psychosocial Adjustment: Life Change Role Performance	Coping Enhancement Family Integrity Promotion Family Support Grief Work Facilitation Grief Work Facilitation: Perinatal Death Resiliency Promotion Role Enhancement Self-Awareness Enhancement

➤ Most of the NOC outcomes are the same for Grieving and Complicated Grieving. How do the interventions differ?

➤ Note that for both diagnoses, many of the defining characteristics include normal grief reactions. But for Grieving, the symptoms occur before the loss. For Complicated Grieving, they continue to occur for a long time after the loss, and/or they are more intense than normal.

Sources: Moorhead, S., Swanson, E., Johnson, M., & Maas, M. (Eds.). (2018). *Nursing outcomes classification (NOC)* (6th ed.). St. Louis, MO: Elsevier. Used with permission; Butcher, H. K, Bulechek, G. M., Dochterman, J. M., & Wagner, C. M. (Eds.). (2018). *Nursing interventions classification (NIC)* (7th ed.). St. Louis, MO: Elsevier. Used with permission; Herdman, H. & Kamitsuru, S. (2018). *NANDA International Nursing Diagnoses: Definitions and Classifications 2018-2020* (11th ed.). New York: Thieme Medical Publishers; and Johnson, M., Moorhead, S., Bulechek, G., et al. (2012). *NOC and NIC linkages to NANDA-I and clinical conditions* (3rd ed.). St. Louis, MO: Elsevier. Used with permission.

CLINICALJUDGMENT

Applying the Full-Spectrum Nursing Model

PATIENT SITUATION

Marie, 84 years, has had a right-sided cerebrovascular accident (CVA; also referred to as stroke or brain attack). Doctors say she is unlikely to regain much physical function, if she even awakens from the coma. She was alert and active before her stroke and was able to maintain her independence with the help of a home health aide, who assisted her with ADLs and meal preparation three times a week. Kelly and Dan, her children, have met with the provider, who has told them that Marie's chance of survival is slim. He wants to put a feeding tube into Marie and has asked whether they want Marie to be resuscitated in case of a cardiac or respiratory arrest. Kelly wants to do what is best for her mother, but she feels that Marie would not want to be kept alive in this condition. She is also concerned about putting her through uncomfortable procedures if there is no chance of recovery. Her brother, Dan, thinks Marie should have the feeding tube. Kelly asks to speak with you and wants to know the best thing to do for her mother.

THINKING

1. *Theoretical Knowledge (Recall of Facts and Principles):* If Marie and Dan agree that they do not want Marie to be resuscitated, the provider will complete a DNR (DNAR, AND) order. What do the letters *DNR, DNAR,* and *AND* represent?

2. *Critical Thinking (Problem-Solving):* At this stage of your education, you probably need more information about CVAs and tube feedings. Write a PICO (patient/population, intervention, control, and outcomes) question you could use to search the literature for information about these two topics and how they are related. See Chapter 8 if you need to review PICO questions.

DOING

3. *Practical Knowledge (Nursing Diagnosis):* Write a possible nursing diagnosis to describe Kelly's situation.

4. *Practical Knowledge (Basic Skills):* If Kelly and Dan agree to tube feedings for Marie, as her nurse, what basic nursing skills will you need to perform? How will you learn to perform these skills, if you do not already know how to do them?

CARING

5. *Ethical Knowledge:* How do you think the situation came to this? What might Kelly, Dan, and Marie have done before the stroke occurred to prevent this confusion and indecision?

6. *Self-Knowledge:* What are your responsibilities in this situation? What could you do to help Kelly and Dan?

Critical Thinking and Clinical Judgment

1. Jessie McCarthy, a 69-year-old woman, is terminally ill with multiple myeloma. She is currently hospitalized for a week of chemotherapy. Her husband of 49 years is recuperating from recent hip surgery and has difficulty getting around. Her daughter and son-in-law are very close to them, and her granddaughter, 14 years old, has a very special relationship with her "Gammie." The side effects of Mrs. McCarthy's chemotherapy include nausea and headaches. She does not like to have people around when she feels this way. Jessie's pastor comes to visit every other day, and this seems to give her comfort. Her 50th wedding anniversary will come around when she is still in the hospital. She verbalizes her fear of "not making it home this time." You are her nurse in the hospital where palliative care is being provided. Initiate a holistic plan of care for Mrs. McCarthy, addressing the main issues noted.

   a. What immediate physical problems does Mrs. McCarthy have? Do not use her medical diagnosis as an answer.

   b. What might you do to meet her physical needs?

c. What psychological needs does Mrs. McCarthy have: (1) What are her fears? (2) What social and emotional issues is she facing? (3) How might you help meet her needs?

2. You are caring for Jack Wirtz, a 37-year-old man, who was admitted to the hospital for a lumbar laminectomy (surgery of his lower spine). As you are doing Jack's preoperative assessment, he tells you that his 12-year-old son had died 6 months ago in an automobile accident and that Jack was the driver. He is a builder and has been out of work since the accident. His wife now works to help support them. Jack's affect is flat, and he talks in a monotone.
   a. What losses has Jack experienced?
   b. What further assessments need to be made for Jack, and why?

3. A patient requests your participation in a plan for assisted suicide or passive euthanasia. What are your options as a nurse? Use the Internet to get information about this.
   a. List the Web site addresses (URLs) for the pages you found to be helpful in answering the question. Beside each URL, state the name of the organization, person, or agency to which the Web site belongs.
   b. For each URL, state what you believe to be the *purpose* of the Web site.

4. Find a partner. Take 5 minutes to describe to her a personal loss you have had (e.g., a person, a pet, an object, an aspect of health). The partner must listen silently and not speak at all during this time. When you have finished, answer the following questions:
   a. What did you feel while describing your loss?
   b. Did you feel that the listener was really listening to you?
   c. How did the listener respond to you?

5. Now reverse the process; you become the listener. When you have finished, answer the following questions:
   a. What did you feel while you were listening?
   b. Did the time go quickly or seem long?
   c. What did you learn from this listening experience?

6. John, 17 years old, is a volunteer at the hospital. He has just moved from another state because of his father's work, so he is a new senior at the local high school. As you chat with him, he reveals that his mother is getting radiation and chemotherapy treatments for breast cancer and has been very ill. What are some loss issues this young man is facing?

7. Sharon, 48 years old, is in the hospital for a hysterectomy (removal of her uterus) because of fibroids and heavy bleeding. With teary eyes, she shares with you that she is feeling "down" and does not want any visitors this evening. She says, "I really thought I would feel better after having this surgery done."
   a. Why do you think Sharon is teary and feeling "down"?
   b. What should you do to begin helping Sharon cope with her loss?

8. You are having lunch with a nursing colleague, who reveals to you that her mother has Alzheimer's disease. Her mother has been placed in a nursing home because she is losing her memory and is not safe at home. Your friend describes feeling distracted, angry for no reason, and unable to shake her feelings of sadness.
   a. What might be causing your colleague to feel distracted and angry?
   b. How would you respond to her?

9. You are caring for Mr. Bishop, a 57-year-old man who is terminally ill with metastatic bone cancer. He wants to donate his organs for research after his death, but his wife is totally against this.

   a. What could you do or say to him to help resolve this issue? Go to the following Web site (http://organdonor.gov/) and download information on organ donation and transplantation to use in this situation.

   b. Now go to the top of the Web page, and look at the logo and other information. Who do you think provides and maintains the content for this Web site? What else would give you a clue about the source of the site?

   c. Look at the bottom of the Web page. What department of the U.S. government "owns" this page?

10. For each of the following concepts, use critical thinking to describe how or why it is important to nursing, patient care, or loss, grief, and dying. Note that these are *not* to be merely definitions.

Physical loss

Actual loss

Dysfunctional or Complicated grief

Disenfranchised grief

Significance of the loss

Stages of grief

Advance directives

Assisted suicide

Palliative care

What Are the Main Points in This Chapter?

- How people cope with loss directly affects their healing and well-being.
- Loss may be actual or perceived, physical or psychological, and external or internal.
- Grief comprises physical, psychological, and spiritual responses to loss.
- People do not move neatly from one stage of grief or dying to the next; there is constant movement and overlap between and among them.
- Factors that affect the grieving process include the significance and circumstance of the loss, the timeliness of the death, the bereaved support system, spiritual beliefs, cultural values, the person's developmental stage, and conflicts existing at the time of death.
- Patients experience loss of independence, body image, self-esteem, and so on, when they are ill and/or hospitalized. Recognizing these as losses, you can assist the patient with the grieving process, thus promoting physical, emotional, and spiritual healing.
- The Uniform Determination of Death Act states that death has occurred when "an individual . . . has sustained either (1) irreversible cessation of circulatory and respiratory functions, or (2) irreversible cessation of all functions of the entire brain, including the brainstem. . . ."
- Palliative care focuses on providing comfort care and symptom relief, without further efforts to stop the disease process or to prevent death.
- Hospice care is a movement and an approach that allows terminally ill persons to face death with dignity and surrounded by the comfort of their home and family.
- Healthcare providers are responsible for educating staff and patients about advance directives.
- A "do-not-resuscitate" (DNR) prescription, also called "do-not-attempt-resuscitation" (DNAR) or "allow-natural-death" (AND) prescription, is a specific prescription to *not* perform cardiopulmonary resuscitation.
- Nurses should be aware of what is involved in assisted suicide and euthanasia. You should think ahead about what your response might be if a patient wants to discuss these topics. The American Nurses Association (ANA) position statement on roles and responsibilities of nurses in end-of-life care will provide you with helpful guidance.
- An autopsy is a medical examination of the body to determine the cause of death.
- When a patient is dying or has experienced any type of loss, you should perform a thorough, holistic assessment.
- In most cases, grief is normal, not dysfunctional; you should not diagnose Dysfunctional/Complicated Grieving in every person who is grieving a loss.
- You can facilitate grief work by validating feelings ("It's normal to feel that way") and providing an opportunity and encouragement to talk about the person or object for whom the person is grieving.
- Active dying usually occurs over a 10- to 14-day period, although it can take as little as 24 hours. During the final 4 to 48 hours, failure of body systems results in death.
- When the patient is very near death, focus on relieving physical symptoms and emotional distress. If she can communicate, ask about immediate concerns, such as "Who do you want in the room right now?"
- At the moment of death, do not interrupt or intrude on the family; give them as much time as they need to say good-bye to their loved one. Express your sympathy.
- Care of the body includes making it presentable for the family, carefully placing identification tags, and arranging to have the body sent to the morgue.
- The death certificate must be signed by the person who legally pronounced the death (usually a provider).

Knowledge Map

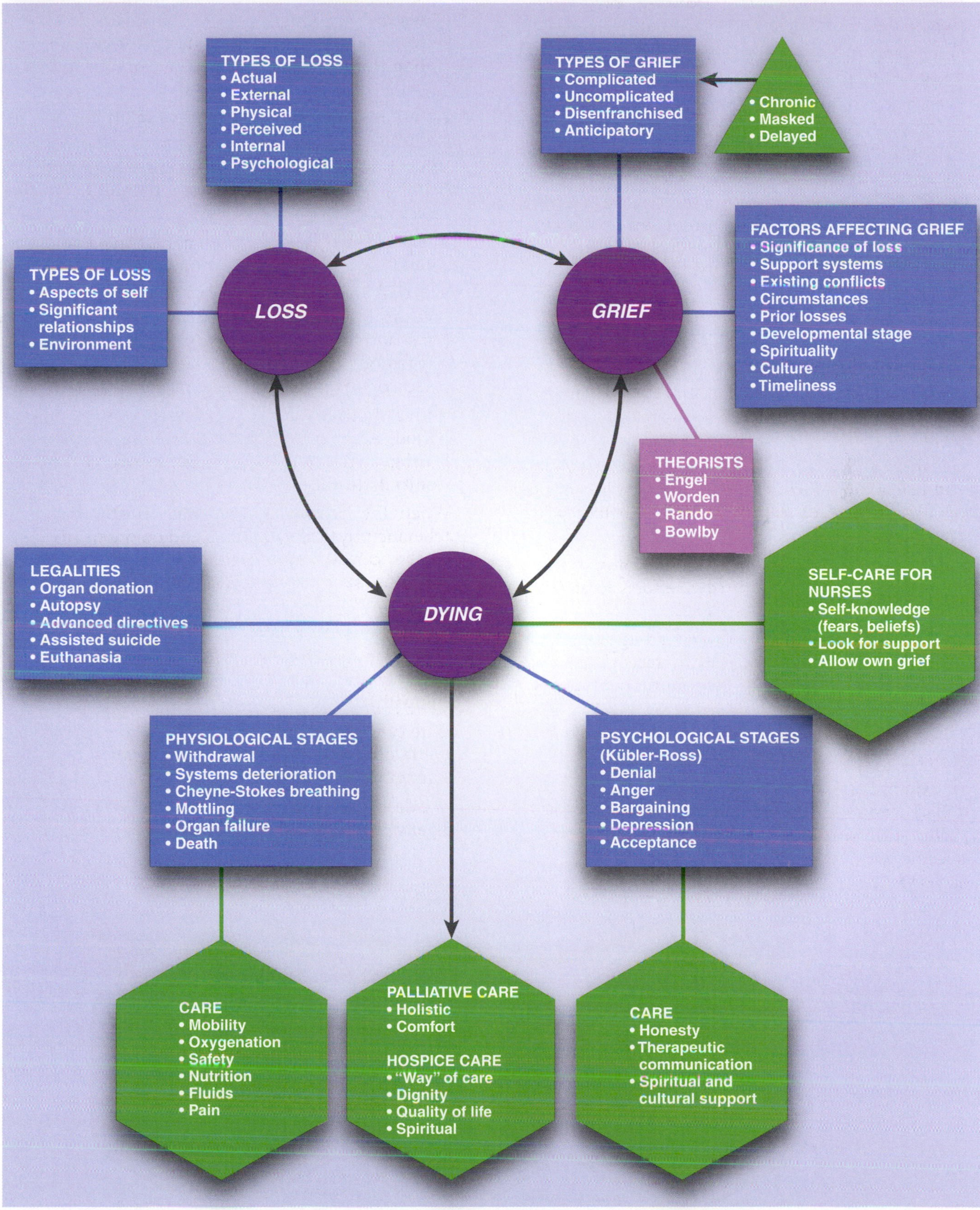

UNIT 3

Essential Nursing Interventions

CHAPTER 18

Documenting & Reporting

STUDENT RESOURCES

The questions and exercises in Volume 2 allow you to practice the kind of thinking you will use as a full-spectrum nurse. Critical-thinking questions usually have more than one correct answer, so we do not provide "answers" for these features. Try to answer these questions yourself. It is more important to develop your nursing judgment than to just cover content. You will learn by discussing the questions with your peers. If you are still unsure, see the Davis Advantage chapter resources for suggested responses.

To explore learning resources for this chapter,

Go to Davis Advantage and find:

Answers and Suggested Responses for all questions in this chapter
Concept Map
Knowledge Map
References and Bibliography
Lists of NOC Outcomes and NIC Interventions

Key Concepts

Documentation
Oral Reporting

Related Concepts

See the Concept Map on Davis Advantage.

Caring for the Nguyens

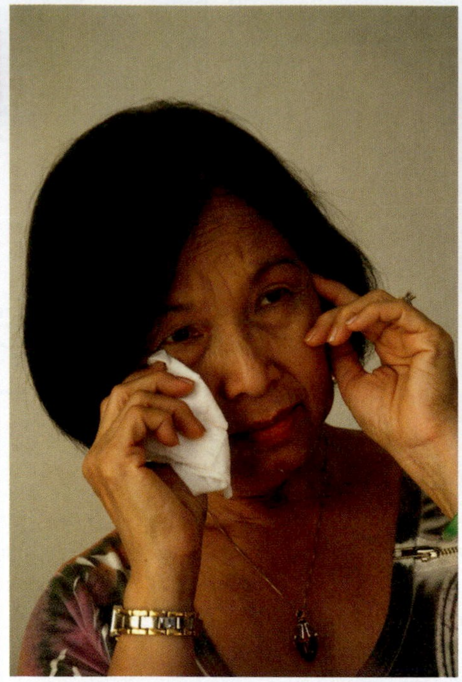

Yen Nguyen arrives at the Family Medicine Clinic complaining of pain and drainage from her right eye. She requests an appointment. As part of your clinical experience working as a triage nurse at the clinic, you must evaluate the client's status and determine whether she needs to be seen today. What follows is your conversation with Mrs. Nguyen:

Mrs. Nguyen: I don't have an appointment, but I need to see someone today. My husband is a client here. I have an appointment in 2 weeks for a physical, but I've never been here before. I just can't wait 2 weeks.

You: What seems to be the problem?

Mrs. Nguyen: My eye is killing me. My right one. It burns and stings, and there's all this nasty gunk coming out. I think I need some medicine for it.

You: Tell me a little more about this problem. When did this start?

Mrs. Nguyen: I woke up yesterday with a painful, itchy eye. I used some saline drops, but the eye seems to be worse. I work at a preschool, and they won't let me work unless I take care of this. I also think I need to be checked for other things. I haven't had an appointment in a long time. I suppose I just need some tests. My husband just found out he has high blood pressure, but I don't think I do. I guess I'm not old enough. I'm 55, but my mother got high blood pressure when she was 70.

As Mrs. Nguyen is talking, you notice a large amount of thick, yellow-green drainage in the corner of her right eye and that the eye is reddened. She is rubbing this eye vigorously and dabbing at it with a tissue. The skin is puffy around the eye as well. Her left eye is slightly red, but there is no drainage.

Mrs. Nguyen's vital signs are as follows: blood pressure, 132/76 mm Hg; heart rate, 88 beats/min; respirations, 18 breaths/min; and temperature, 98.9°F (37.2°C). On the basis of your brief assessment, you ask the receptionist to give Mrs. Nguyen an urgent appointment.

A. Make two charting entries to describe the above events. First make a brief narrative note.

B. Next construct a SOAP(IER). Be sure to follow charting guidelines when you prepare your note.

PracticalKnowledge clinical **application**

Material in this section will help you to assess and plan care for families.

CLINICAL INSIGHTS

Clinical Insight 18-1 ➤ Giving Oral Reports

For All Types of Report Formats:

Remember the acronym CUBAN (Currie, 2002):

Confidential
Uninterrupted
Brief
Accurate
Named nurse

Use a Standardized Format, Such as the Following:

PACE

Patient/Problem—Include client's name, room number, diagnosis, reason for admission, and recent procedures. State the present problem. Briefly summarize medical history relevant to the current problem.

Assessment/Actions—Nursing assessments and interventions directed to the problem.

Continuing/Changes—Continuing needs and potential changes include:

- Client care and treatments that must be monitored on other shifts (e.g., dressing changes)
- Changes in the client's condition or the care plan, recent or anticipated (e.g., new orders, changes in discharge date)

Evaluation—Evaluation of responses to nursing and medical interventions, progress toward goals, and effectiveness of the plan

SBAR/SBAR-R

Identify yourself, the client, and the agency.
S*ituation*—"Here's the situation . . ."
B*ackground*—"The supporting background information is . . ."
A*ssessment*—"My assessment of the situation is that . . ."
R*ecommendation*—"I recommend that you . . ."
[**R***ead back*—"To repeat the information and . . ."]
[**Q**uestions—Questions asked and answered]

IPASS

I llness severity—describes the patient's illness acuity level
P atient summary—a comprehensive overview of the patient (e.g., history, diagnostic test results)
A ction list—correlates with interventions (e.g., consultations, prescriptions, medications)
S ituation awareness and contingency plans—overall plan based on patient's response (condition deteriorates or improves)
S ynthesis by receiver—Confirmation of understanding; message sent is the message received (Joint Commission, 2017; Clements, 2017)

Include the Following Content:

In a Handoff Report:

- Client's name, age, and room number
- Client's admitting diagnosis—one or several may exist. Status of identified outcomes
- Client's relevant past medical history
- Treatments the client has received during this admission, such as surgery, intravenous (IV) line placements, and breathing treatments; consultations completed with other disciplines
- Upcoming consultations, diagnostic tests, surgeries, or treatments
- Client restrictions, such as diet, bedrest, isolation, activity limits
- Plan of care, such as IV therapy, pain management, current medications, wound care, client or family concerns, discharge planning
- Significant assessment findings from the previous shifts
- Teaching conducted

(Continued)

Clinical Insight 18-1 ➤ Giving Oral Reports *(continued)*

In a Transfer Report:

- Your name, facility, and phone number
- Client's name, age, gender, and admitting and current diagnoses
- Client's providers(s), if still following client
- Procedures or surgeries performed
- Current medications and last date/time each was taken/ time next dose is due
- Client status at present as well as progression since admission
- Last set of vital signs, plus any pertinent trends since admission
- Tubes in place, such as IV lines, catheters, drainage tubes, along with the intake and output of each tube or drain
- Presence of wounds or open areas of the skin plus current interventions for each
- Names and contact numbers for family and significant others
- Special directives, such as code status, presence of advance directives, preferred intensity of care, or isolation required
- Reason the client is being transferred
- Location of above information (on transfer form, in medical records, etc.)

When Your Report Is Finished:

- Ask the receiving nurse whether he has any questions.
- Get the nurse's full name, and then record it plus the transfer date and time in your transfer documentation.

Practice Resources

Cornell, P., Gervis, M., Yates, L., et al. (2014); Ernst, K., McComb, S., & Ley C. (2018); Gore, A., Leasure, A., Carithers, C., et al. (2015); The Joint Commission (2017); Schroeder, S. (2006); Shahid, S. & Thomas, S. (2018); Streeter, A. & Harrington, N. (2017).

Clinical Insight 18-2 ➤ Receiving Telephone and Verbal Prescriptions

You should accept verbal and telephone prescriptions only in specific situations when the primary care provider is not able to electronically submit, write, or enter them personally.

- **Have a second nurse listen to the prescription**, if possible, to verify its accuracy.
- **Write or enter the prescription electronically only if you heard it yourself**; no third-party involvement is acceptable.
- **Repeat the written prescription** even if you believe you have clearly understood it.
- **Spell unfamiliar names** when repeating to be sure the spelling is correct.
- **Pronounce digits of numbers separately.** For example, instead of "seventeen," say "one, seven." Mishearing a number can lead to a serious error in medication dosage.
- **Make sure the prescription makes sense,** given the client's current status.
- **Transcribe the prescription directly into the medical record as quickly as possible.** Writing it on a piece of paper and then copying it again onto a paper prescription form or into an electronic health record (EHR) can introduce an additional chance of error. If entering into an EHR, it is best to have the EHR's prescription entry area open and begin entering the prescription as the prescriber dictates it to you.
- **Write the prescription while the prescriber remains on the telephone or in the building** so that you can ask any necessary questions immediately without the need for a return call.
- **When writing on a paper prescription form, first document the date and time.** Next write the text of the prescription. Following the text of the prescription, depending on how you received the prescription, write "TO" (telephone order) or "VO" (verbal order), followed by the prescribing provider's name and then your name. The following is an example of a telephone prescription:

  12/17/20 0815 Morphine 2 mg IV push ×1 for pain now. TO Dr. Clayton Kent/Sarah Hogan, RN; prescription read back for verification and validated.

- **Sign electronically to activate the prescription.** If entering the prescription electronically, indicate during entry that it was given verbally or over the telephone, the date and time the prescription was given, and then search for and select the prescribing provider's name. Click "sign" or whatever option in your EHR indicates the prescription is signed and is now active.
- **Be sure you have the provider's phone number** so that you can reach him or her if questions arise in the future.
- **All verbal and telephone prescriptions must be countersigned** by the provider within 24 hours or according to agency policy.

Practice Resources

Buppert, C. (2012). National Coordinating Council on Medication Error Reporting and Prevention (2015); Institute for Safe Medication (2017); Kelly, S. (2017).

Clinical Insight 18-3 ➤ Guidelines for Documentation

GUIDELINE	HOW TO APPLY	RATIONALE OR EXAMPLE
	When to Document	
Documentation begins at the start of your shift.	■ *Hospital or long-term care facility*—start of shift ■ *Home visit or outpatient facility*—when you first encounter the client ■ *On first observation*—Document the condition of your client when you first observed him or her. Was the person awake? Was he or she in bed? Did the person have any complaints? What did you do?	
Document immediately.	Develop the discipline to document as soon as possible after making an observation or providing care.	The longer you wait, the more likely you will forget important details.
Never document ahead.	Never document before performing an intervention.	It is impossible to see into the future and be sure that what you expect to happen will actually happen. Doing this threatens the credibility of the medical records.
Avoid "block" documentation.	Each entry needs to be made individually; record the time each was done.	Do not document an entry time as "From 1300 to 1500."
Document chronologically.	■ *On paper:* Document times in chronological order. ■ *EHRs:* Most automatically insert the current date and time when forms are opened. Follow the documentation system's guidelines for changing those dates and times before signing.	Chronological documentation communicates the changing status of the client.
Designate late entries (paper).	■ If you forget to make an important entry while documenting, you will later need to add "late entry" to the first available line. ■ Record the time and date you are making the addition; clearly designate it is a late entry.	■ Late entry example: 5/11/20, 1400; late entry for 5/11/20, 1200
	■ If you know legal action is pending, do not place a late note in the health record without notifying the nurse manager or risk management officer first.	■ It is a criminal offense to alter a client record after the organization's approved time limit for doing so has passed.
Designate late entries (EHR).	■ Open the appropriate form and change the automatically generated current date/time to the date/time your care was actually done; then sign. ■ Follow the agency policy regarding the period for making a late entry.	
	What to Document	
Questions to aid your recall.	As your shift or visit progresses, you will perform assessments and nursing interventions. To remind yourself what to record, ask yourself these example questions.	■ What were your assessment findings? ■ Did any abnormalities exist? ■ What was the client's response to your intervention? Did any changes occur from the initial assessment?
Interventions, client responses, and evaluation of progress toward goals.	■ These are often recorded on an individualized plan of care (IPOC). ■ Clearly describe what your client is experiencing. ■ **Key Point:** *Do not document a symptom without also documenting what you did about it and how the client responded.*	(Symptom) Pt complained of pain, rated 6 on a 0–10 scale. (Intervention) Administered Tylenol 1,000 mg, by mouth, at 0900. At 1030, client rated pain as 3.

(Continued)

Clinical Insight 18-3 ➤ Guidelines for Documentation *(continued)*

GUIDELINE	HOW TO APPLY	RATIONALE OR EXAMPLE
Significant events or changes in condition.	When possible, quote the client's interpretation of the event or change.	Quoting the client directly gives all health-care providers consistent data.
Informed consent.	■ If you are asked to obtain informed consent for a procedure, document your actions. ■ In most states, your signature (paper or electronic) confirms only that the client signed the consent. ■ For further discussion of informed consent, see Chapters 44 and 45.	The primary provider conducting the procedure is legally responsible for discussing the procedure and its risks and benefits.
Client teaching.	■ Include instruction about medications and client diagnoses. ■ Include discharge teaching. ■ If the client's physical or cognitive condition prevents teaching, explain that in your documentation.	Documenting client teaching can positively affect insurance and other payments to the institution.
Spiritual or other concerns expressed by the client and/or family.	Document your interventions.	Addressing spiritual concerns ensures that the client receives holistic healthcare.
Attempts made to contact the primary care provider.	■ Contacts may, for example, be made to notify the provider of the client's condition or to clarify prescriptions. ■ If you are unable to contact the primary healthcare provider, document your contacts with your charge nurse, nurse manager, supervisor, medical director, and hospital administrator.	You must indicate that you made every effort to communicate your concerns.
Client leaving the facility against medical advice (AMA).	■ Document the client's condition, any explanations of risks and consequences given to the client, the client's destination (if known), and your notification of the client's care providers. ■ If your facility has specific forms for AMA departures, use the designated form. ■ If the form is a hard-copy one, have the client sign the form before leaving. ■ If the client refuses to sign, note this in your chart.	Your actions and responsibilities in the situation must be made clear in the record.
Client's refusal of treatment.	■ Try to determine the client's reason for refusal. ■ Quote the exact language the client used in this situation, whenever possible.	This helps ensure documentation of facts instead of inferences.
Use of restraints.	■ Most facilities have a separate form that allows you to document the reason for restraint use, the type of restraint, and frequent checks of the client. ■ You must have contacted the primary healthcare provider.	■ The primary care provider must place a signed prescription for restraints in the medical records. ■ Prescription for restraint must be re-ordered inside a specific time frame set by the organization or the restraints are discontinued (see Chapter 24).

Clinical Insight 18-3 ➤ Guidelines for Documentation *(continued)*

GUIDELINE	HOW TO APPLY	RATIONALE OR EXAMPLE
"Occurrences."	■ Document your findings accurately and objectively. ■ Fill out a separate occurrence form and send to the risk manager (paper forms). ■ Do not make reference to the occurrence form anywhere in your documentation.	■ Examples of occurrences: falls and medication errors. ■ Occurrence forms are not part of the client's health record. Go to Chapter 18, **Occurrence Reports** in Volume 1.
Complete data about medications.	■ *Paper medication administration record (MAR)*—Include the date, time, and medication given, and your initials. ■ *Electronic MAR*—Ensure your entry is accurate, then sign electronically that administration was accomplished successfully.	Accurate documentation is an essential component of the nurse's role.
prn, unscheduled, IV infusions, and STAT medications.	■ Record on the MAR. ■ Include comments regarding the medication in your narrative documentation, or insert a comment in your electronic file. ■ Document a timely evaluation of client's response to the medication.	Certain prn medications require a follow-up response be documented within a specific period set by the organization, usually 15 to 30 minutes after the medication is given.
Medications not administered.	■ Document the omission on the MAR. ■ If the client states a reason for refusing the medication: *Paper notes*—Quote the client in your narrative notes. *Electronic MAR*—Use pull-down or other menu.	■ *Examples:* "Client refuses medication; dose accidentally omitted." ■ Most electronic MARs include an explanation with a selection from a drop-down list, such as "Client refused" or "Client not available." ■ Some MARs also contain a narrative section to type a comment about why a medication was not given.
	How to Document	
Know your organization's requirements for reimbursement.	■ Requirements typically specify frequency of documentation and the type of data that must be recorded. ■ Fulfilling documentation requirements helps ensure appropriate reimbursement. ■ Home care, hospitals, clinics, office settings, and long-term care facilities have specific guidelines for documentation necessary for payment.	
Date and time all your documentation.	■ Most organizations use a 24-hour clock or military time to avoid confusion between a.m. and p.m. ■ The day begins at 0001 (1 minute past midnight) and ends at 2400 (12 midnight). ■ *Morning hours*—Most people have little difficulty with early morning hours. Example: 9:00 a.m. is 0900. ■ *Hours after 12 noon*—To convert to military time after 12 noon, simply add 12 to the clock time. Example: 7:30 p.m. + 12 = 1930 in military time.	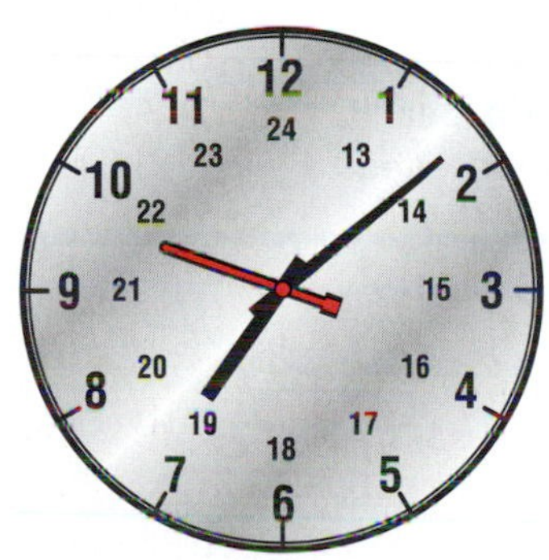 Many healthcare facilities use the 24-hour clock.

(Continued)

Clinical Insight 18-3 ➤ Guidelines for Documentation *(continued)*

GUIDELINE	HOW TO APPLY	RATIONALE OR EXAMPLE
Document accurately and objectively, using nonjudgmental language.	■ Avoid labeling clients or team members. ■ Do not document judgments about decisions made by members of the healthcare team. ■ Document objective facts, so the reader can draw an informed conclusion. ■ Quote the client in his or her own words, when possible.	■ *Document:* "I'm not taking that medicine. Take it away." ■ *Do not document:* "Client is obnoxious and refuses prescribed medication."
Avoid vague, subjective words.	■ When possible, give specific examples.	■ Such terms as *good*, *average*, or *normal* do not clearly define the status of the client. ■ Descriptive details allow caregivers to better understand your client's individual needs.
Use only the abbreviations authorized by your organization.	See below Tables, Abbreviations Commonly Used in Health Care.	
Use correct spelling and grammar.	Incorrect spelling may raise questions about what you are attempting to communicate. Incorrect grammar implies carelessness on your part and questions your competence if your documentation is reviewed.	
Document your own nursing actions.	■ Do not allow anyone to document for you. ■ Do not document the actions of others as though you had performed them.	Each nurse is responsible for documenting his or her assessments, interventions, and evaluations. A deviation from this principle can imply cover up, carelessness, or a blatant disregard of policy and standards of practice.
You may need to document the actions of someone else.	■ Try to avoid this, but if you must do it, be sure to designate clearly whose actions they are. ■ *EHRs*—You can indicate another person performed the action in an added comment or by searching for and selecting the other care provider in the appropriate field, then signing.	For example, if an NAP (nursing assistive personnel) helps the client ambulate: *Do not document:* "Client assisted to bathroom." *Do document:* "J. Scott, NAP, assisted client to bathroom."
Avoid documenting what someone else said, heard, felt, or smelled.	■ If the information is critical and you *must* document it, use quotations and attribute the remarks to the person who made them.	*Example:* "Wife stated, 'My husband told me that he is in a lot of pain, but does not want to bother the nurses.'"

TABLES

Abbreviations Commonly Used in Healthcare

ABBREVIATION	MEANING
ADLs	Activities of daily living
ad lib	As desired, if the patient desires
AKA	Above-knee amputation
Amb	Ambulation, ambulatory
Amt	Amount
ASAP	As soon as possible
bid	Twice a day
BM	Bowel movement
BR	Bedrest
BRP	Bathroom privileges
BSC	Bedside commode
$\bar{c}$	With
Cal	Calories
Cath	Catheter
CBC	Complete blood count
CCU	Critical care unit or coronary care unit
c/o	Complaint of
CO_2	Carbon dioxide
CPR	Cardiopulmonary resuscitation
CVA	Cerebrovascular accident (stroke)
D&C	Dilation and curettage
DM	Diabetes mellitus
dsg or drsg	Dressing
DX or Dx	Diagnosis
EBL	Estimated blood loss
EKG/ECG	Electrocardiogram/ electrocardiography
ED/ER	Emergency department, emergency room
EEG	Electroencephalogram/electroence-phalography
EENT	Eyes, ears, nose, throat
ETOH	Alcohol
F	Female
FBS	Fasting blood sugar
ft	Foot
Fx	Fracture
GI	Gastrointestinal
gtt(s)	Drop(s)
GU	Genitourinary
GYN	Gynecology
HA	Headache
HMO	Health maintenance organization
h/o	History of
hob or HOB	Head of bed
HOH	Hard of hearing
H&P	History and physical
hr	Hour
Ht	Height
HTN	Hypertension
Hyper	Above or high
Hypo	Below or low
ICU	Intensive care unit
I&O	Intake and output
Isol	Isolation
IV	Intravenous
IVP	Intravenous push (caution: do not use to mean "IV piggyback")
L	Liter
lb	Pound
LPN	Licensed practical nurse
LMP	Last menstrual period
LVN	Licensed vocational nurse
mcg	Microgram
MD	Medical doctor
Med	Medication

(Continued)

Abbreviations Commonly Used in Healthcare—cont'd

ABBREVIATION	MEANING
mg	Milligram
mL	Milliliter
MN	Midnight
NAS	No added salt
N/V/D	Nausea, vomiting, diarrhea
NKA or NKDA	No known allergies or no known drug allergies
NG	Nasogastric
NGT	Nasogastric tube
noc	At night
NPO	Nothing by mouth
O_2	Oxygen
OB	Obstetrics
OOB	Out of bed
OPD	Outpatient department
ortho	Orthopedics
OR	Operating room
os	Mouth, opening
OT	Occupational therapy
oz	Ounce
pc	After meals
PCA	Patient-controlled analgesia
PO	By mouth
P, $\bar{p}$	After
PPBS	Postprandial blood sugar
prn	As needed
Pt	Patient
PT	Physical therapy
q	Every
qam	Every morning
qh	Every hour
qid	Four times a day
RN	Registered nurse
R/O	Rule out
RX or Rx	Treatment or prescription
$\bar{s}$	Without
SCD	Sequential compression device
SOB	Short of breath
$\bar{ss}$	One-half
SSE	Soapsuds enema
STAT	Immediately
STI or STD	Sexually transmitted infection or sexually transmitted disease
TB	Tuberculosis
TO	Telephone order
TPR	Temperature, pulse, respirations
tid	Three times a day
VO	Verbal order
VS	Vital signs
WBC	White blood count
w/c	Wheelchair
WNL	Within normal limits
wt	Weight

Key Point: *Abbreviations vary among healthcare agencies. Furthermore, they change rather often because of regulating agency guidelines (e.g., The Joint Commission). Therefore, you will need to be familiar with the abbreviations in the agency in which you work.*

DOCUMENTATION FORMS

Adult admission history electronic screen.

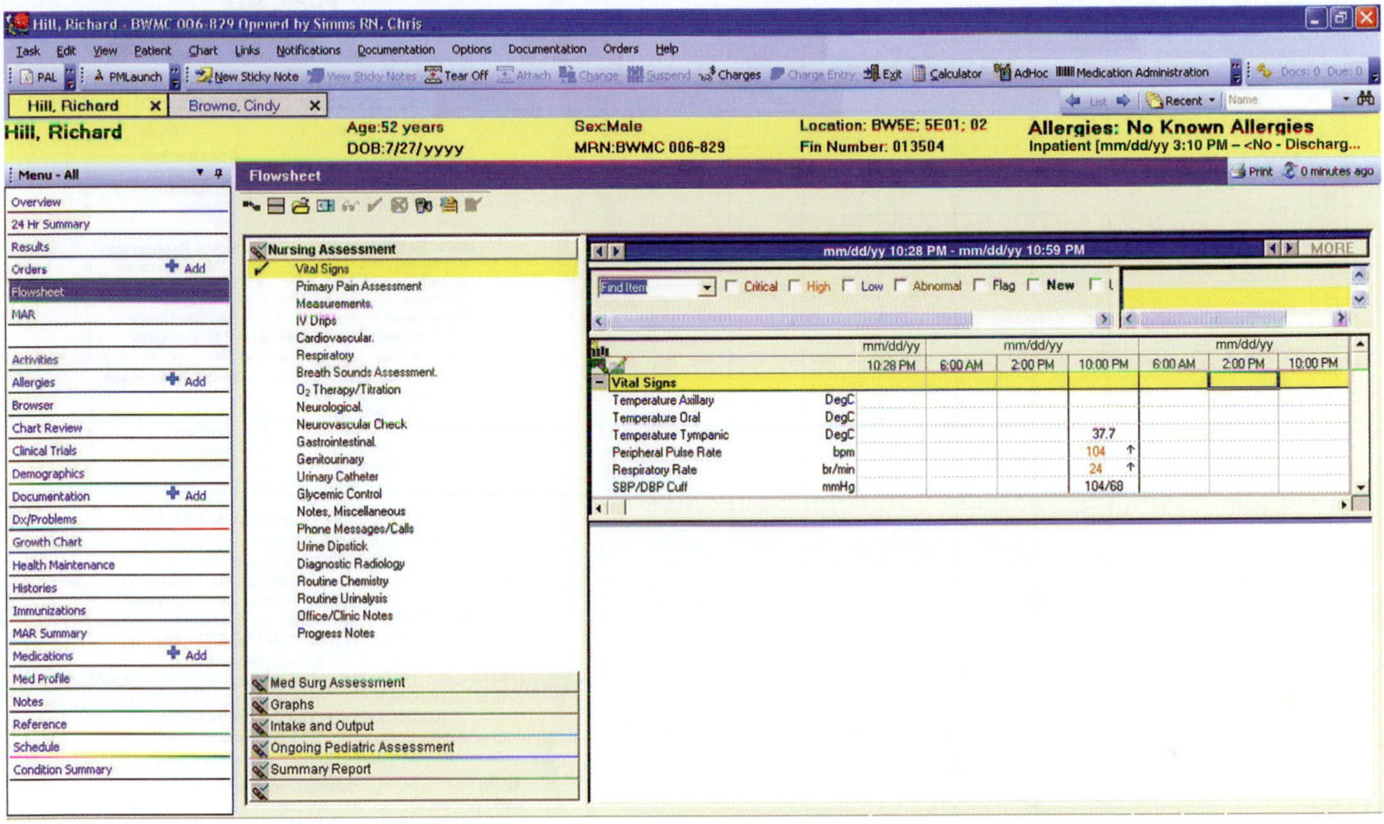

Nursing assessment flowsheets are comprehensive charting documents.

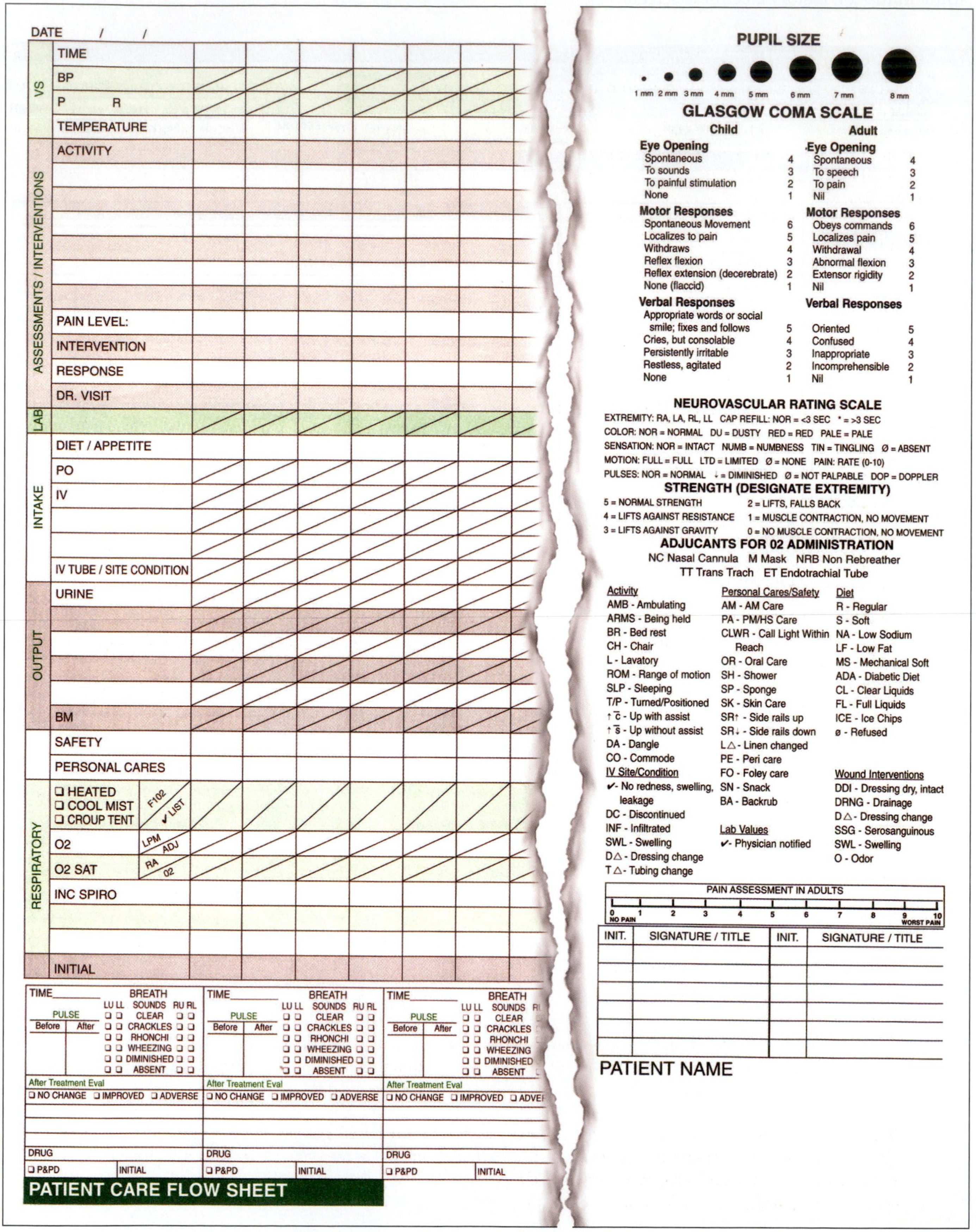

DATE / /

VS	TIME						
	BP						
	P R						
	TEMPERATURE						
ASSESSMENTS / INTERVENTIONS	ACTIVITY						
	PAIN LEVEL:						
	INTERVENTION						
	RESPONSE						
	DR. VISIT						
LAB							
INTAKE	DIET / APPETITE						
	PO						
	IV						
	IV TUBE / SITE CONDITION						
OUTPUT	URINE						
	BM						
	SAFETY						
	PERSONAL CARES						
RESPIRATORY	❑ HEATED ❑ COOL MIST ❑ CROUP TENT — FiO2 / ✔ LIST						
	O2 — LPM / ADJ						
	O2 SAT — RA / O2						
	INC SPIRO						
	INITIAL						

TIME______ PULSE Before After — BREATH SOUNDS LU LL RU RL: ❑❑ CLEAR ❑❑ / ❑❑ CRACKLES ❑❑ / ❑❑ RHONCHI ❑❑ / ❑❑ WHEEZING ❑❑ / ❑❑ DIMINISHED ❑❑ / ❑❑ ABSENT ❑❑

After Treatment Eval: ❑ NO CHANGE ❑ IMPROVED ❑ ADVERSE

DRUG

❑ P&PD INITIAL

PATIENT CARE FLOW SHEET

PUPIL SIZE

1 mm 2 mm 3 mm 4 mm 5 mm 6 mm 7 mm 8 mm

GLASGOW COMA SCALE

Child		Adult	
Eye Opening		**Eye Opening**	
Spontaneous	4	Spontaneous	4
To sounds	3	To speech	3
To painful stimulation	2	To pain	2
None	1	Nil	1
Motor Responses		**Motor Responses**	
Spontaneous Movement	6	Obeys commands	6
Localizes to pain	5	Localizes pain	5
Withdraws	4	Withdrawal	4
Reflex flexion	3	Abnormal flexion	3
Reflex extension (decerebrate)	2	Extensor rigidity	2
None (flaccid)	1	Nil	1
Verbal Responses		**Verbal Responses**	
Appropriate words or social smile; fixes and follows	5	Oriented	5
Cries, but consolable	4	Confused	4
Persistently irritable	3	Inappropriate	3
Restless, agitated	2	Incomprehensible	2
None	1	Nil	1

NEUROVASCULAR RATING SCALE

EXTREMITY: RA, LA, RL, LL CAP REFILL: NOR = <3 SEC * = >3 SEC
COLOR: NOR = NORMAL DU = DUSTY RED = RED PALE = PALE
SENSATION: NOR = INTACT NUMB = NUMBNESS TIN = TINGLING Ø = ABSENT
MOTION: FULL = FULL LTD = LIMITED Ø = NONE PAIN: RATE (0-10)
PULSES: NOR = NORMAL ↓ = DIMINISHED Ø = NOT PALPABLE DOP = DOPPLER

STRENGTH (DESIGNATE EXTREMITY)

5 = NORMAL STRENGTH 2 = LIFTS, FALLS BACK
4 = LIFTS AGAINST RESISTANCE 1 = MUSCLE CONTRACTION, NO MOVEMENT
3 = LIFTS AGAINST GRAVITY 0 = NO MUSCLE CONTRACTION, NO MOVEMENT

ADJUCANTS FOR 02 ADMINISTRATION

NC Nasal Cannula M Mask NRB Non Rebreather
TT Trans Trach ET Endotrachial Tube

Activity
AMB - Ambulating
ARMS - Being held
BR - Bed rest
CH - Chair
L - Lavatory
ROM - Range of motion
SLP - Sleeping
T/P - Turned/Positioned
↑c̄ - Up with assist
↑s̄ - Up without assist
DA - Dangle
CO - Commode

IV Site/Condition
✔- No redness, swelling, leakage
DC - Discontinued
INF - Infiltrated
SWL - Swelling
D△ - Dressing change
T△ - Tubing change

Personal Cares/Safety
AM - AM Care
PA - PM/HS Care
CLWR - Call Light Within Reach
OR - Oral Care
SH - Shower
SP - Sponge
SK - Skin Care
SR↑ - Side rails up
SR↓ - Side rails down
L△ - Linen changed
PE - Peri care
FO - Foley care
SN - Snack
BA - Backrub

Lab Values
✔- Physician notified

Diet
R - Regular
S - Soft
NA - Low Sodium
LF - Low Fat
MS - Mechanical Soft
ADA - Diabetic Diet
CL - Clear Liquids
FL - Full Liquids
ICE - Ice Chips
ø - Refused

Wound Interventions
DDI - Dressing dry, intact
DRNG - Drainage
D△ - Dressing change
SSG - Serosanguinous
SWL - Swelling
O - Odor

PAIN ASSESSMENT IN ADULTS
0 NO PAIN 1 2 3 4 5 6 7 8 9 10 WORST PAIN

INIT.	SIGNATURE / TITLE	INIT.	SIGNATURE / TITLE

PATIENT NAME

CLINICALJUDGMENT

Applying the Full-Spectrum Nursing Model

PATIENT SITUATION

Ellen, 85 years, has sustained a right-sided cerebrovascular accident (CVA; also called stroke or brain attack). Doctors say she is unlikely to regain much physical function, if she even awakens from the coma. Her children, Mary and Dale, have met with the provider, who tells them that Ellen is not likely to survive. The provider wants to insert a feeding tube and has asked whether they want Ellen to be resuscitated in case of cardiac or respiratory arrest. Mary tells you she wants to do what is best for her mother, but she feels that Ellen would not want to be kept alive in this condition. She is also concerned about putting her through uncomfortable procedures if there is no chance of recovery. Her brother, Dale, says, "Mom needs the feeding tube. I can't sit and watch her starve to death. As long as she's alive, there's hope."

THINKING

1. *Theoretical Knowledge (Recall of Facts and Principles):* You plan to use the Focus Charting® format to document this interaction.
    a. Write the focus for this note.
    b. What does the acronym DAR stand for?
2. *Critical Thinking (Contextual Awareness):*
    a. What aspects of this situation have you experienced or observed before in your role as a caregiver?
    b. How might those past experiences affect your perception in this situation?

DOING

3. *Practical Knowledge (Handoff Report):* Ellen's last name is Smith; assume her children are also named Smith. Ellen is in room 820. Using the PACE format, what would you say to the oncoming nurse during handoff report? You will be able to address only a small amount of physiological information because the scenario does not provide it.

CARING

4. *Self-Knowledge:* In what way(s) can you identify with any of the people involved in this scenario?

Critical Thinking and Clinical Judgment

1. You are caring for James Wilson, a 96-year-old patient. Mr. Wilson has been admitted to the hospital for pneumonia. Usually he is alert and oriented to place, time, and person. However, during this admission he has become confused and agitated. He frequently yells at staff and resists care by kicking and hitting. While you are providing morning care, Mr. Wilson becomes very agitated and yells and curses at you. When you attempt to provide oral hygiene, he throws his dentures at you. The dentures break when they hit the floor.
    a. Construct a nurse's note that documents this situation by using the paper format you prefer.
    b. You will need to complete an occurrence report regarding the broken dentures. The report asks you to identify actions that you might have taken to prevent this incident. Brainstorm this question with your peers. Identify one or two actions that might have prevented this incident.
2. The primary care provider has written a prescription on your client's paper medical record that you find illegible. A veteran nurse states that she can read it, and she translates it for you. What factors should you consider before determining how to proceed?

3. For each of the following concepts, use critical thinking to describe how or why it is important to nursing, client care, or documenting and reporting. Consider both paper and electronic documentation in each. Note that these are *not* to be merely definitions.

Narrative documentation	Flowsheets
SOAP(IER) documentation	Charting by exception
Nursing admission database	Signing documentation forms
Medication administration record	Handoff report
Occurrence report	Late entry

What Are the Main Points in This Chapter?

- The client record is a collection of documents that form a legal record of the client's healthcare experience.
- The client record is used by healthcare professionals to communicate information about the client's care, to legally document the care delivered to the client and the client's responses to that delivered care, to document care for reimbursement, to educate students, to determine whether care is adequate, as a data source for health research, and as the basis for determining the cost of care.
- In source-oriented records, members of each discipline record findings in a separately labeled section.
- In problem-oriented records, members of each discipline document on shared notes, and the record is organized around a problem list.
- In electronic health records (EHRs), members of each discipline all document inside the same EHR. The EHR can be organized as source oriented, problem oriented, or a combination of the two.
- The EHR can be accessed by many members of the healthcare team at the same time.
- The narrative format tells the story of what has occurred in a chronological format.
- SOAP(IER) is an acronym for Subjective data, Objective data, Assessment, Plan (and Intervention, Evaluation, and Revision). This format may be used to address a single problem or to document summative notes on a client.
- In Focus Charting®, data are entered in the Data–Action–Response (DAR) format.
- Charting by Exception (CBE) utilizes preprinted or electronic flowsheets to document most aspects of care. CBE assumes that unless a separate entry is made—an exception—all standards have been met and the client has responded as expected.
- Paper and electronic flowsheets and graphic records are used to record recurring assessments, such as vital signs, intake and output, weight, hygiene, and activities of daily living (ADLs).
- Paper progress notes are used to document the client's responses to care. They may be in the form of narrative, SOAP(IER), PIE (Problem–Intervention–Evaluation), or Focus-style notes.
- A discharge summary should be completed when the client is discharged from the organization. A transfer form should be completed when the client is transferred within the organization.
- An occurrence report, or incident report, is a formal record of an unusual occurrence or accident that is not part of the client's medical record.
- The most commonly used paper and electronic home health documentation form is OASIS (Outcome and Assessment Information Set), a federally required form that includes history, assessment, demographics, and information about the client's and caregiver's abilities.
- Federal law requires that a resident in long-term care be evaluated using the Minimum Data Set for Resident Assessment and Care Screening (MDS) within 14 days of admission. The MDS must be updated within the specified time frame and with any significant change in client condition.
- The handoff report is designed to alert the next nurse about the client's status, changes in the client condition, planned activities, tests or procedures, or concerns that require follow-up.
- To minimize miscommunication and other errors, a consistent, structured (standardized) format should be used in handoff reports that contain critical key items.
- Nurses should not take verbal and telephone prescriptions unless the prescribing provider is in a situation in which the prescription cannot be written or entered or the client is in a life-threatening situation.
- Telephone prescriptions offer more room for error because of unfamiliar terminology and differences in background noise.
- Documentation should be accurate and nonjudgmental.

- You should document as soon as possible after you make an observation or provide care.
- You should never share your electronic username or password with someone else.
- Document any significant events or changes in condition, teaching performed, use of restraints, and client refusal of treatment or medications.
- You are responsible for documenting the care you provided. Never document the actions of others as though you had performed them.
- You are legally and ethically required to question a provider's prescription that you believe is inappropriate or unsafe.

Knowledge Map

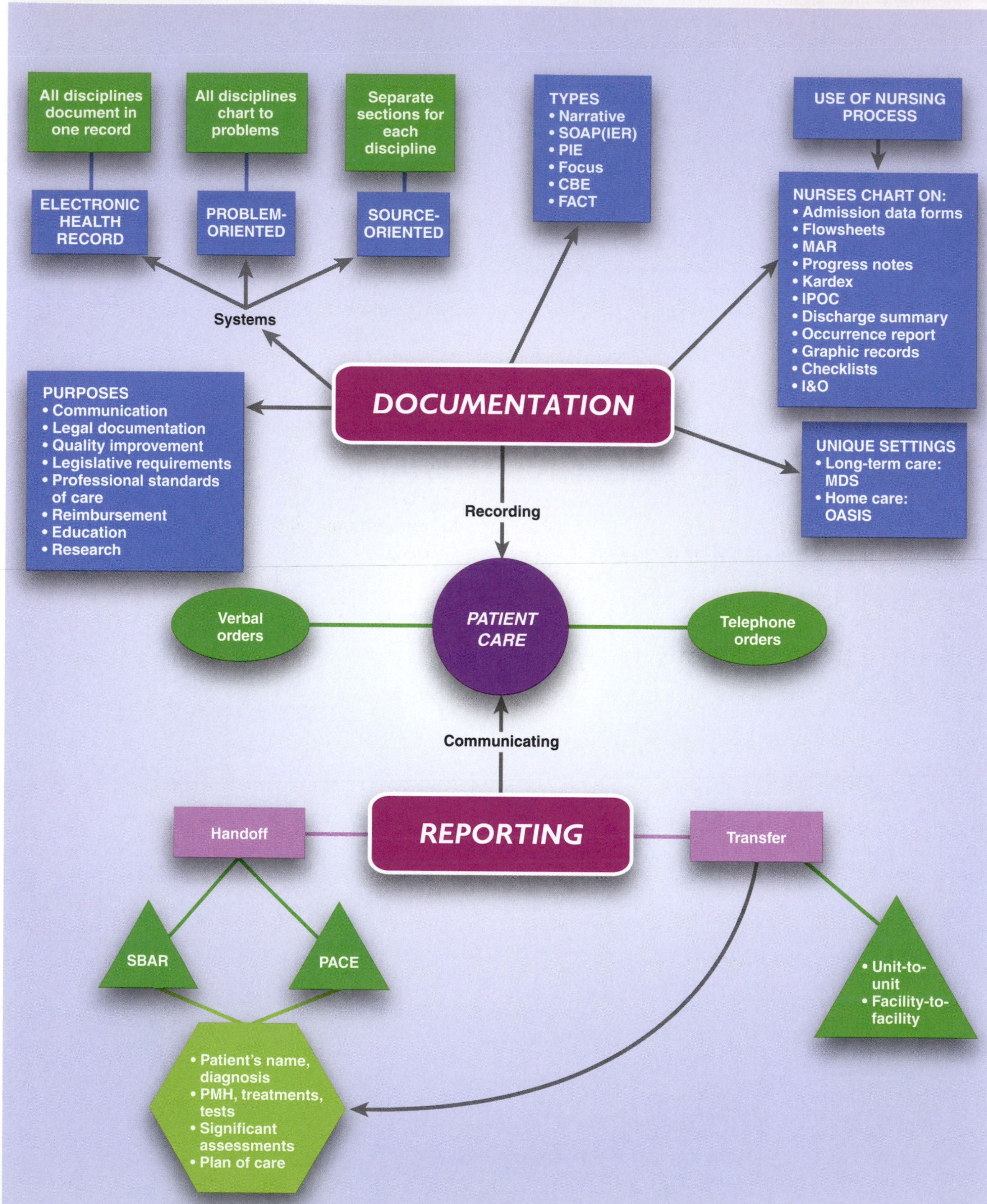

CHAPTER 19

Teaching & Learning

STUDENT RESOURCES

The questions and exercises in this book allow you to practice the kind of thinking you will use as a full-spectrum nurse. Critical-thinking questions usually have more than one right answer, so we do not provide "correct answers" for these features. Try to answer these questions yourself. It is more important to develop your nursing judgment than to just cover content. You will learn more by discussing the questions with your peers. If you are still unsure, see the Davis Advantage chapter resources for suggested responses.

To explore learning resources for this chapter,

Go to Davis Advantage and find:

Answers and Suggested Responses for all questions in this chapter
Concept Map
Knowledge Map
References and Bibliography
Lists of NOC Outcomes and NIC Interventions

Key Concepts

Health literacy
Learning
Learning environment
Teaching

Related Concepts

See the Concept Map on Davis Advantage.

Caring for the Nguyens

Nam Nguyen has medical diagnoses of hypertension, type 2 diabetes mellitus, obesity, and osteoarthritis. There is a positive history of tobacco abuse. On the basis of the information you know about Nam and his family, consider the following questions:

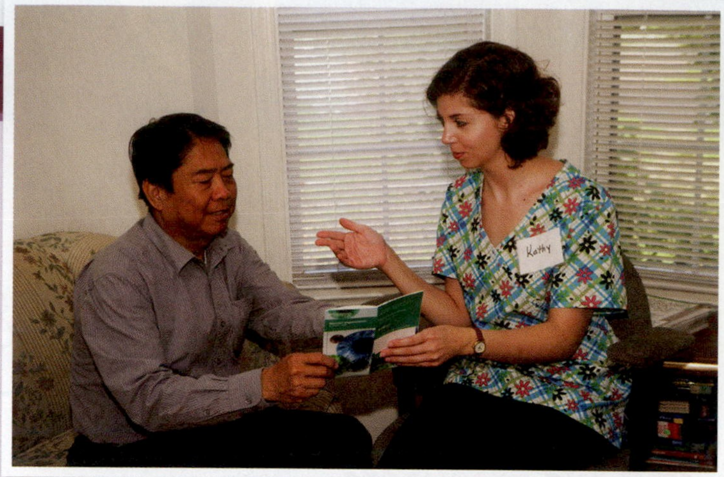

A. What kinds of information does Nam probably need?

B. What would be the best approach to teach Nam about his healthcare conditions?

C. You have been asked to teach Nam about weight loss. What theoretical knowledge must you have, and where can you obtain it?

D. What patient information do you need to know before planning your teaching?

E. Nam tells you that he feels overwhelmed with his recent diagnoses. He does not believe he can begin a weight loss program or attend any teaching sessions. How might you handle this concern?

F. Nam has been prescribed the following medicines. Devise one or more teaching sessions focused on these medications. You will need to use your pharmacology reference books to devise this plan. As you plan your teaching, keep in mind that Nam is overwhelmed by his recent diagnoses.

Lisinopril 20 mg PO daily
Hydrochlorothiazide 25 mg PO daily
Metformin 500 mg PO bid

Practical Knowledge clinical application

ASSESSMENT GUIDELINES AND TOOLS

Focused Assessment

Learning Assessment Guidelines

Pre-assessment

Before assessing the learner, think about the following:

- **Time constraints.** How much information do you need to present? How much time do you have to do it?
- **Available resources.** What equipment and supplies do you have to work with? Do you have access to the Internet? Audiovisual and projection equipment? A whiteboard? A scanner? Books? Do learners have mobile devices with downloaded applications for interactive classroom learning?

Assessing the Learner

A teaching/learning assessment should include the following:

- **Intended audience.**

  Who are you teaching?

  What are the person's age, occupation, developmental level, and cultural affiliation?

  Will you be teaching a person or a group?

- **Learning needs.**

  What is the client's health (or other) problem?

  What behavioral changes are needed?

  What self-care knowledge and skills does the client need?

- **Client's knowledge level.** Determine what the client already knows so that you can reinforce accurate information, correct misinformation, and adapt the teaching plan to the client's learning needs. Ask such questions as:

  What do you think caused or worsened your health problem?

  What are your concerns about it?

  How has the problem affected your usual activities?

  What are your concerns about treatment (tests, surgery, etc.)?

- **Health beliefs and practices.**

  Ask the client to give a general description of his or her health:

  What do you usually do to stay healthy?

  What problems do you think you are at risk for?

  What lifestyle changes would you be willing to make in order to improve your health?

- **Physical readiness.** Assess the client's concentration, manual dexterity skills, and minimal pain to be able to listen and learn.

- **Emotional readiness.**

  Find out whether the client is experiencing anxiety or emotional distress that will interfere with the learning process.

  Ask the client whether he or she would like a family member or friend to be present during the learning.

- **Ability to learn.**

  What are the learner's cognitive and psychomotor developmental level and ability? How does the client learn best (e.g., by memorization or by problem-solving or applying information)?

  How well does the client recall previously presented material?

- **Health literacy level.**

  Does the patient have the ability to understand basic health information and services needed to make appropriate healthcare decisions?

  Is the information the healthcare provider offers in the patient's primary language?

  Is the health teaching provided in a format the patient can understand?

  Is medical jargon or unnecessary technical information used?

  Can the person read and write?

- **Neurosensory factors.**

  What is the client's ability to feel, see, hear, and grasp?

  Does the client have a medical condition that causes neurosensory compromise?

- **Learning styles.**

  How do you prefer to learn new things? For example, do you prefer to read about them, talk about them, watch a video, be shown how to do it, listen to the teacher, or use a computer?

  Do you like to read?

  Where do you get information about your health—online, from books, magazines, your family, your healthcare provider?

  Do you learn best alone or with other people?

CLINICALJUDGMENT

Applying the Full-Spectrum Nursing Model

PATIENT SITUATION

Katrina Peplowsi, a 22-year-old college student from Ukraine, is transported to the emergency department of a local hospital after passing out in her dorm room. Katrina had been sick with a viral illness and had had a fever for 5 days, as well as nausea, vomiting, and diarrhea. She had been drinking large amounts of Gatorade because of her insatiable thirst, thought to be related to the fever and vomiting. Before the illness, Katrina's friends and family had been commenting about her remarkable weight loss, in spite of her increased appetite, since she started school 2 months earlier. On arrival to the emergency department, Katrina's blood sugar is found to be 585 mg/dL. She is diagnosed with diabetes mellitus, type 1. After her blood sugar is stabilized with fluid therapy and insulin infusion, Katrina regains consciousness. Although Katrina speaks some English, her proficiency is somewhat limited.

THINKING

1. *Theoretical Knowledge (Recall of Facts and Principles):* As a patient newly diagnosed with diabetes mellitus, type 1, Katrina will need healthcare education on many aspects of her condition. List at least six important topics that are relevant to her care.

2. *Critical Thinking (Application of Knowledge):* What would you consider as you are devising a teaching plan for Katrina?

3. *Critical Thinking (Synthesis of Knowledge):* What factors are important for customizing her teaching plan, considering the extent of her ability to communicate?

DOING

4. *Nursing Process (Assessment):* What are some pertinent personal factors that you should assess for Katrina when adapting a teaching plan to suit her learning needs?

5. *Nursing Process (Planning):* As you think about involving other members of the healthcare team, how would you plan to optimize Katrina's motivation to learn how to best manage her diabetes after discharge?

CARING

iCare 6. *Self-Knowledge:* What areas of commonality do you have with Katrina, around which you might form a caring relationship?

7. *Ethical Knowledge:* Suppose that Katrina refuses to receive information from you about diabetes mellitus. She states she is not interested in knowing how to give herself insulin because she does not want to give herself injections at home. How should you best respond to Katrina's needs?

Critical Thinking and Clinical Judgment

1. Recall that Heather (Meet Your Patient, in Volume 1) is a 20-year-old mother of a 4-year-old preschooler. They have come to a family practice clinic for a well-child checkup. You notice that the child speaks only in one- or two-word phrases. Heather is impatient with her and repeatedly tells her to "stop using that baby talk." Your nursing instructor tells you that you need to assess for teaching needs and provide anticipatory guidance to the mother regarding safety, nutrition, and normal preschooler growth and development.

   a. Heather says, "I don't know what I'm doing wrong. All her little friends are taller and talking more. She was small when she was born, so I suppose it's my fault." How do you assess Heather's learning needs without reinforcing her feelings of self-blame?

b. Your assessment shows that although the child is below the 5th percentile for height and weight, she has grown appropriately since her last clinic visit. What teaching could you provide that might help address her mother's learning needs related to childhood growth and development?

c. In addition to information on growth and development, your anticipatory guidance should include safety measures and nutrition for a 4-year-old. How can you evaluate whether your teaching has been effective and further promote Heather's retention of all of this new information?

2. As a student, you have learned about discharge planning. Your instructor tells you that you need to begin teaching for discharge as soon as the client is admitted. You hear the nurses complaining that they just do not have time for any teaching. So where do you begin? You will need to use the teaching process for your assigned client.

   Your client is a 9-year-old girl who is being admitted to the outpatient procedures unit for testing because of chronic recurrent urinary tract infections. She receives on a daily basis an antibiotic, lisdexamfetamine dimesylate (Vyvanse), for attention deficit disorder (ADD) and an asthma inhaler to help her participate in sports activities. She is accompanied by her mother and father, a younger sister, and her big, pink teddy bear. She is scheduled for x-ray studies and blood work. Depending on the results of her tests, she may require surgery or dilation of her ureters. The parents appear very anxious and tell you that their daughter "has a hard time understanding things and needs a lot of repetition." You have an hour to prepare her for the procedures and testing.

   a. Assessment

      (1) What information do you already have that will be significant for your teaching plan?

      (2) What other information will you need to gather?

   b. Diagnosis

      (1) What possible nursing diagnoses are involved in this situation? Consider a diagnosis for your client and another one for at least one of her family members.

   c. Planning

      (1) What information will you present first?

      (2) What teaching techniques would you use for this situation?

      (3) Who would you include in the teaching?

      (4) Where would you complete the teaching?

   d. Goals and interventions

      (1) Write an appropriate goal for your client (the child). Remember to make the goal client centered, timed, and realistic. You have only an hour to complete this teaching.

      (2) What content and methods would you include in your teaching plan?

      (3) How can you incorporate the client's stuffed teddy bear in your teaching?

   e. Evaluation

      (1) How would you determine whether your teaching was effective?

      (2) What further teaching do you need to continue to prepare your client for discharge?

3. For each of the following situations, determine which teaching techniques would be most effective.
   a. Some adolescents with diabetes are preparing for their prom. The after-prom party lasts until 6:00 a.m. and will interfere with their usual schedule for insulin administration. You need to help them decide how to manage this problem. They are all busy with after-school activities and attend three different schools.
   b. An 80-year-old man has experienced a cerebrovascular accident (CVA; also called stroke) with right-sided weakness. He will need mobility training and assessment of his home situation for safety hazards. Currently he lives alone.
   c. A new mother must learn how to feed her infant, who has a cleft palate. She is in considerable pain after an emergency cesarean section and unexpected blood loss.
4. You are assigned to a client with a diagnosis that you are unfamiliar with. You are expected to prepare a teaching session for this client and family and for your classmates. How should you prepare for this assignment?
5. Give an example of teaching content you might need to present to a 58-year-old patient who has been diagnosed with hypertension. What chapters in this text (Volume 1) might be useful if you need theoretical knowledge about hypertension to answer this question? Where would you look to find out where this information is located?
6. Do you think it is appropriate for a nurse to offer personal experiences in the teaching process? Explain your thinking.
7. A client refuses to make eye contact during a teaching session. This makes it difficult for you to determine whether she is actually paying attention to what you are saying. How can you assess whether she is focused on the teaching session?
8. For each of the following concepts, use critical thinking to describe how or why it is important to nursing, patient care, or teaching clients. Note that these are *not* to be merely definitions.

   Role of teaching in nursing practice
   Principles of teaching and learning
   Factors that affect the learning process
   Factors that affect the teaching process
   Timing
   Choice of techniques
   Relevance
   Learning styles
   Amount of information to be presented

What Are the Main Points in This Chapter?

- Teaching is an essential component of professional nursing.
- Nurses do formal and informal teaching for individuals and groups.
- To be effective, teaching requires cooperation between the learner and the teacher.
- Learning is a change in behavior, knowledge, skills, or attitudes that occurs as a result of exposure to environmental stimuli.
- Bloom and Krathwohl (1956) identified three domains of learning: cognitive, psychomotor, and affective.
- Krathwohl (2002) adapted Bloom's model describing learning using a more outcomes-based approach: remember, understand, apply, analyze, evaluate, and create.
- Teaching includes motivating the learner.
- Teaching is interactive and requires communication.
- Readiness means that the learner is both motivated and able to learn at a specific time.
- Other factors that affect learning include emotions, timing, active involvement, feedback, repetition, environment, amount and complexity of the content,

communication, developmental stage, culture, and literacy.

- Common barriers to teaching in the hospital setting include failure to see teaching as a priority and lack of time, preparation, space, privacy, poor coordination, and third-party reimbursement for teaching.
- Barriers to learning include illness, physical discomfort and fatigue, anxiety, low health literacy, environmental distraction, overwhelming amount of behavioral change needed, not enough time, lack of positive reinforcement, and feelings of discouragement.
- The teaching process is similar to the nursing process.
- The NANDA-I (2018) nursing diagnosis Deficient Knowledge may be the primary problem or the etiology of other problems; this diagnosis is often overused or used incorrectly.
- A teaching plan is similar to a nursing care plan, except that (1) interventions are actually teaching strategies and (2) the plan includes the content of the teaching, the sequencing of the content, and the materials to be used.
- Demonstration and return demonstration are the most effective strategies for teaching psychomotor skills.
- A certain amount of forgetting is normal. You can aid learner retention by using strategies that require learner participation and by providing printed materials to use at a later time.
- It is important to document specifically what teaching you did as well as your evaluation of the learning that occurred.

Knowledge Map

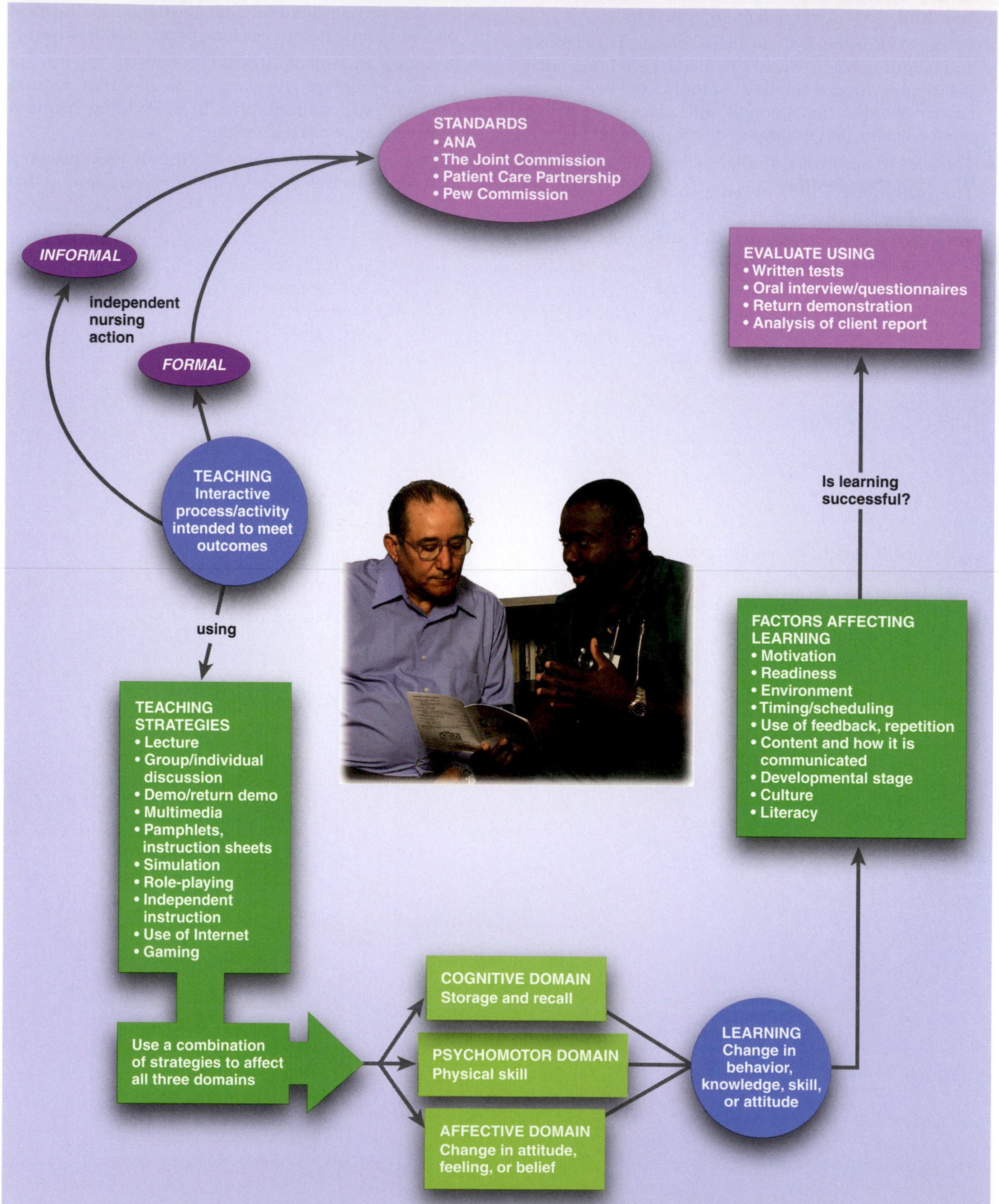

CHAPTER 20

Measuring Vital Signs

STUDENT RESOURCES

The questions and exercises in this book allow you to practice the kind of thinking you will use as a full-spectrum nurse. Critical-thinking questions usually have more than one right answer, so we do not provide "correct answers" for these features. Try to answer these questions yourself. It is more important to develop your nursing judgment than to just cover content. You will learn more by discussing the questions with your peers. If you are still unsure, see the Davis Advantage chapter resources for suggested responses.

To explore learning resources for this chapter,

Go to Davis Advantage and find:

Answers and Suggested Responses for all questions in this chapter
Concept Map
Knowledge Map
References and Bibliography
List of NOC Outcomes and NIC Interventions

Key Concepts

Oxygenation
Perfusion (pulse, blood pressure)
Thermoregulation
Vital signs

Related Concepts

See the Concept Map on Davis Advantage.

Example Problems

Hyperthermia/Heat Stroke
Hypothermia
Hypertension
Hypotension

Caring for the Nguyens

Recall that on Nam Nguyen's preliminary visit to the Family Medicine Center, his blood pressure (BP) was 162/94 mm Hg. On subsequent visits, his BP was 168/100 mm Hg and 174/96 mm Hg, and he was continuing to gain weight. Mr. Nguyen was diagnosed with hypertension and prescribed an antihypertension medication to be taken each morning. This morning Mr. Nguyen has come to the clinic for follow-up. The following information is gathered as he checks in for his visit.

VS: BP, 168/92 mmHg; pulse, 80 beats/min; respirations, 20 breaths/min; temperature, 98.4°F (36.9°C)

Weight: 180 lb (82 kg)

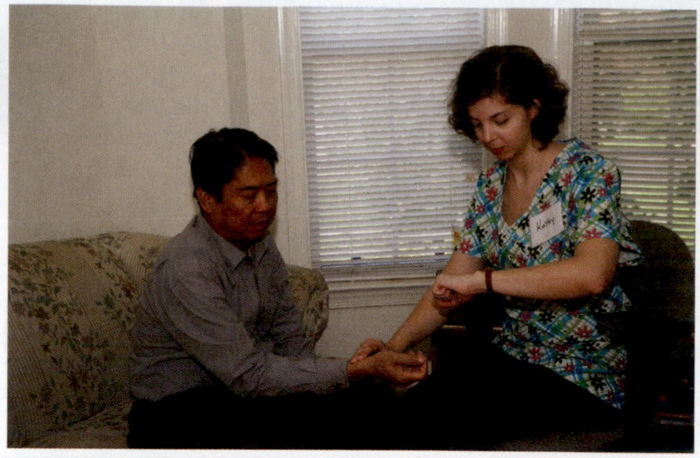

Review the preliminary data and the preceding information to answer the following questions:

A. What patterns do you see in the data?

B. Do you have enough information to draw any conclusions? If not, what other information should you gather?

C. Identify three alternatives that may explain what is happening with Mr. Nguyen's vital signs.

D. How could you determine which of these alternatives provides the best explanation of what is happening?

E. Why is it important to intervene in this situation?

Practical Knowledge Clinical Application

Use the Procedures, Clinical Insights, and tables in this section when assessing your clients' vital signs.

PROCEDURES

Procedure 20-1 ■ Assessing Body Temperature

➤ For steps to follow in *all* procedures, refer to the Universal Steps for All Procedures found on the inside back cover.

Equipment

- Thermometer (An oral thermometer generally has a blue tip. A rectal thermometer generally has a red tip.)

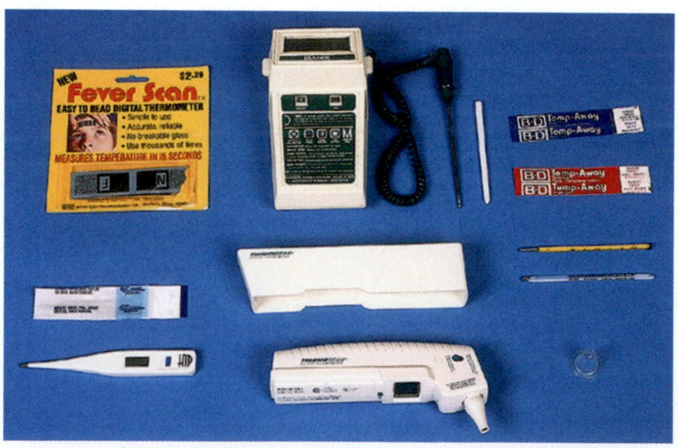

- Glass-and-mercury thermometers should not be used in any healthcare setting. However, because some people still use them at home, we include them in this procedure. They should be used with disposable covers and cleaned and sterilized regularly according to the manufacturer's instructions.
- Thermometer cover, if needed
- Procedure gloves, if taking a rectal temperature or if there is risk of contact with body fluids (e.g., saliva)
- Water-soluble lubricant, if taking a rectal temperature
- Towel, if needed (to dry the axillae), for taking an axillary temperature
- Tissues

Delegation

You can delegate temperature measurement to unlicensed assistive personnel (UAP) if you conclude that the patient's condition and the UAP's skills allow. Perform the pre-procedure assessments, and inform the UAP of the route and type of thermometer used. Explain to the UAP any special considerations (e.g., patient's oral intake in the last 20 to 30 minutes; patient is confused). Ask the UAP to document and immediately report a temperature greater than 100°F (37.8°C) or lower than 97.9°F (36.6°C).

Pre-Procedure Assessments

- Determine the most appropriate site for the patient. Consider patient comfort, safety, and accuracy of measurements. For example, do not use the oral route for a patient who is unable to hold the thermometer properly, for children or others who cannot follow instructions (e.g., unconscious patients), or for patients who use "mouth breathing."
- For taking an oral temperature—determine how long it has been since the patient smoked, had anything to eat or drink, or chewed gum. If so, wait 20 to 30 minutes before taking the temperature.
  Smoking, eating, drinking, and chewing gum can all affect an oral temperature reading.
- Assess for any contraindications to using the site you have chosen. For example:
  Tympanic: Assess for impacted earwax or hearing aid.
  Rectal: Check the patient record for diarrhea or impacted stool.
  Axillary: Check the patient record for presence of fever or hypothermia.
  Skin: Assess for the presence of conditions that require a very precise, reliable reading (e.g., fever, hypothermia).
  Some conditions increase the risk for patient injury; others contribute to inaccurate, unreliable temperature measurement.
- What were the previous recordings, if any?
  Noting changes over time is important in all patient assessments.
- Assess for clinical signs and symptoms of temperature alterations.

Procedure 20-1A ■ Taking an Axillary Temperature

➤ When performing the procedure, always identify your patient according to agency policy, using two identifiers, and be attentive to standard precautions, hand hygiene, patient safety and privacy, body mechanics, and documentation.

Procedure Steps

1. **Position the client in the supine or sitting position.**
2. **Dry the patient's axilla,** as needed.
   Moisture from perspiration alters the temperature reading.
3. **Slide the thermometer into a protective sheath** (depending on the type of thermometer).
   A protective sheath provides a barrier to prevent transmission of organisms.
4. **Place the thermometer tip** in the middle of the axilla.
5. **Position the patient's upper arm down,** with the lower arm across the chest.
   Puts the thermometer in close proximity to the axillary blood vessels, allowing it to better reflect the core temperature.

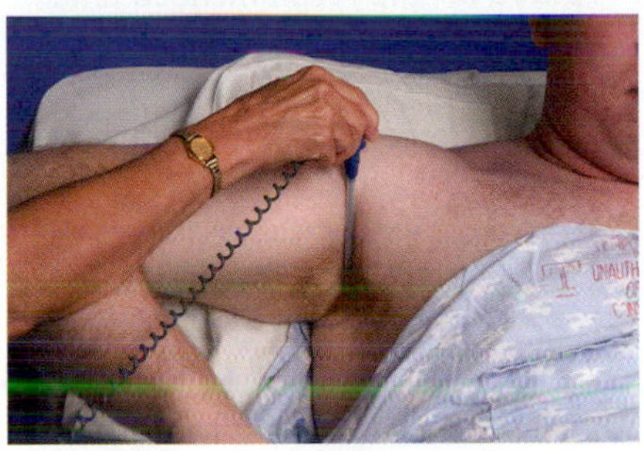

6. **Hold the thermometer in place** for the recommended time.
   a. Leave an electronic probe in place until it beeps.
   b. Leave a plastic thermometer (or a glass thermometer, if you must use it) in place for 8 minutes or according to agency policy (usually 5 minutes for children).
   Study findings differ for accuracy of temperature measurements at the axillary site. Follow agency policy.
7. **Read the temperature.**
   a. **Electronic thermometer**: Read the digital display; remove the thermometer.
   b. **Glass thermometer**: Remove the thermometer, hold it at eye level, and rotate it until the markings are clear. Avoid using a glass thermometer, if possible.
8. **After removing the thermometer,** discard the cover. If there is no cover, wipe the thermometer with a tissue.
   Removes any moisture that may have accumulated in 8 minutes' time.
9. **Clean and replace the thermometer** in the storage base, following agency policy.
   Prevents microbial growth on thermometers and recharges the battery.

(continued on next page)

Procedure 20-1 ■ Assessing Body Temperature (continued)

Procedure 20-1B ■ Taking an Oral Temperature

➤ When performing the procedure, always identify your patient according to agency policy, using two identifiers, and be attentive to standard precautions, hand hygiene, patient safety and privacy, body mechanics, and documentation.

Procedure Steps

1. **If using a glass or plastic thermometer**, shake down the liquid, if necessary.
   a. Stand in an open area away from tables and other objects.
   Prevents thermometer breakage.
   b. Hold the end opposite the bulb between your thumb and forefinger, and snap your wrist downward.
   c. Shake the thermometer until the reading is less than 96°F (36°C).
   The reading must be lower than the anticipated temperature measurement.
2. **Slide the thermometer into a protective sheath.**
   Provides a barrier to prevent transmission of microorganisms.
3. **Place the thermometer tip** under the tongue in the posterior sublingual pocket (right or left of frenulum).
   Puts the tip in close proximity to the major blood vessels under the tongue, allowing the thermometer to reflect the core temperature.

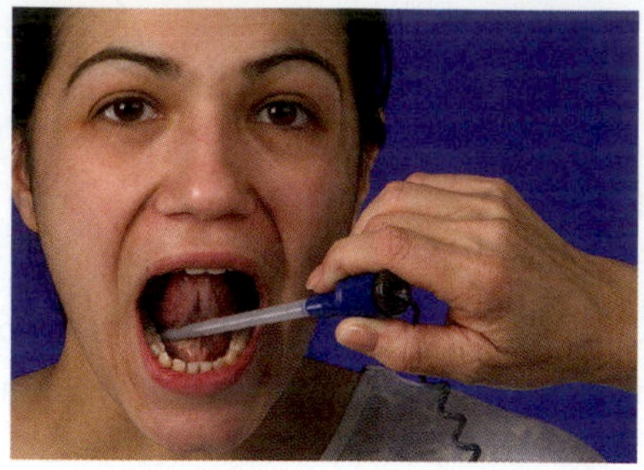

4. **Have the patient close her lips** around the thermometer, and caution the patient not to bite down on it.
   Protects the thermometer from exposure to the air, which could alter the reading. Biting may break a glass thermometer, injuring the mouth.
5. **Leave the thermometer in place** for the recommended time.
   a. Glass or plastic thermometer—5 to 8 minutes
   b. Electronic (digital) thermometer—until it beeps
   c. According to agency policy
   Research findings differ on the optimal time for measuring an oral temperature, so follow agency policy.
6. **Read the temperature.**
   a. **Glass thermometer**: Position the thermometer at eye level, and rotate it until the markings are clear. ▼

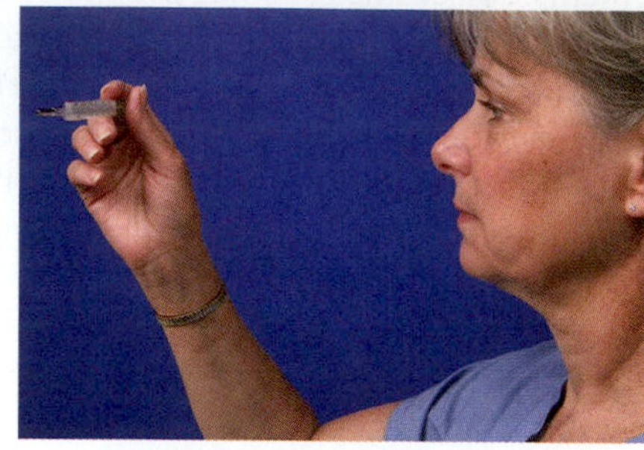

   b. **Electronic thermometer**: Read the digital display.
7. **After removing the thermometer,** discard the cover. If there is no cover, wipe the thermometer with an antimicrobial or alcohol-based wipe.
   Wiping removes mucus, which can make the markings on a glass thermometer difficult to read.
8. **Clean and replace the thermometer.** Follow agency policy.
   Prevents microbial growth on thermometers and recharges battery of electronic thermometers.

Procedure 20-1C ■ Taking a Rectal Temperature

➤ When performing the procedure, always identify your patient according to agency policy, using two identifiers, and be attentive to standard precautions, hand hygiene, patient safety and privacy, body mechanics, and documentation.

➤ *Note:* This procedure primarily describes use of an electronic (digital) thermometer.

Procedure Steps

1. **Slide the thermometer into a protective sheath.**
   A protective sheath provides a barrier to prevent transmission of microorganisms.
2. **Position an adult patient** in Sims' position (on the side with the knees flexed); Drape the patient so that only the anal area is exposed. ➤

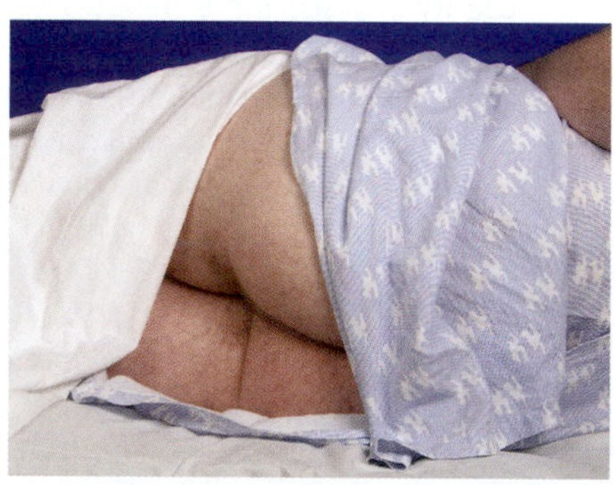

Step Variation: Taking a Rectal Temperature in a Small Child

Place a child in the prone position. You can lay the child face down across your lap or a parent's lap.
Flexing the knees helps relax the muscles to ease insertion and aid in visualization. Draping provides privacy and decreases embarrassment.

3. **Lubricate the tip** of the thermometer by squeezing water-soluble lubricant onto a tissue and then applying it to the thermometer.
Prevents injury to the rectal mucosa and eases insertion. Inserting the thermometer into the lubricant container would contaminate the contents of the container.

4. **Don a procedure glove** on your dominant hand, or on both hands, if necessary.

5. **With your nondominant hand,** separate the patient's buttocks to visualize the anus.

6. **Gently insert the thermometer,** approximately:
Adult—1 to 1.5 inches (2.5 to 3.7 cm)
Child—0.9 inches (2.5 cm)
Infant—0.5 inches (1.5 cm)
The thermometer must be placed past the rectal sphincter.
   a. Have the patient take a deep breath. Insert the thermometer as he exhales.
   Taking a deep breath helps relax the anal sphincter.
   b. If you feel resistance, do not use force.
   Inserting the thermometer too far or forcing against resistance may injure the rectal mucosa.

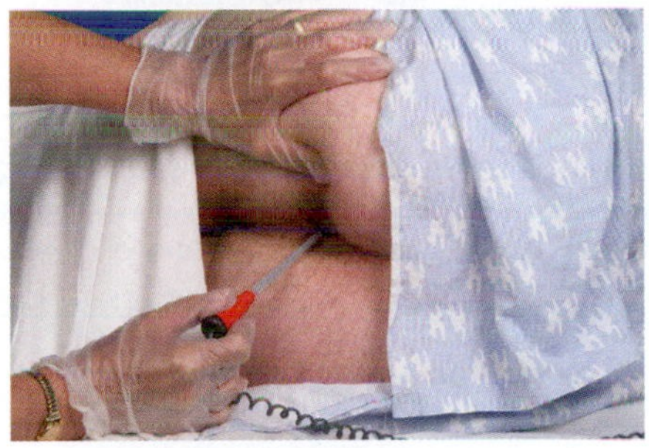

7. **Hold the thermometer in place** until it beeps. (For a plastic or glass thermometer, hold the thermometer in place for 3 to 5 minutes.
The thermometer must be held in place to prevent inadvertent injury to the patient. An electronic thermometer will beep when a constant temperature is reached. Research differs on the optimal time for measuring rectal temperature, so follow agency policy.

8. **Remove the thermometer,** discard the cover, and read the digital display.

9. **Remove the procedure gloves,** and discard them in a biohazards container.

10. **Follow agency policy** for cleaning and storing thermometers.
Prevents microbial growth on thermometers and recharges electronic thermometer battery.

Procedure 20-1D ■ Taking a Temporal Artery Temperature

➤ When performing the procedure, always identify your patient according to agency policy, using two identifiers, and be attentive to standard precautions, hand hygiene, patient safety and privacy, body mechanics, and documentation.

➤ *Note:* If the patient has been lying down, do not measure the temperature on the side that was on the pillow. Do not measure if a cap or hair has been covering the area over the temporal artery because these can prevent heat dissipation and produce a falsely high reading.

Procedure Steps

1. **Remove the protective cap** from the instrument; clean the lens/probe, according to the manufacturer's instructions.

2. **Place the probe flat** on the center of the forehead, midway between the eyebrow and the hairline.

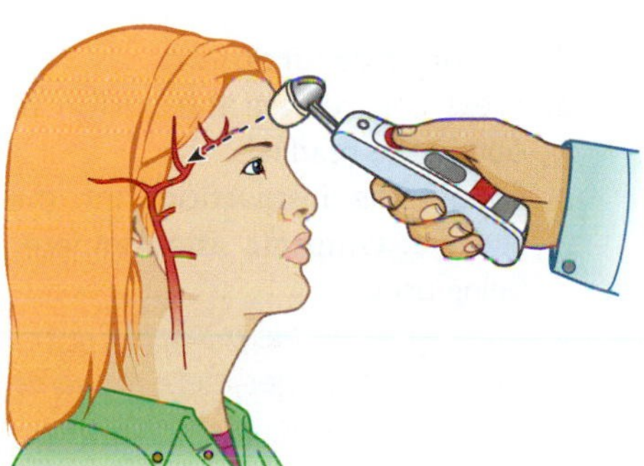

3. **Press and hold the button** while you stroke the thermometer medially to laterally across the forehead; keep the lens/probe flat and in contact with the skin, and slide in a reasonably straight line until you reach the hairline.

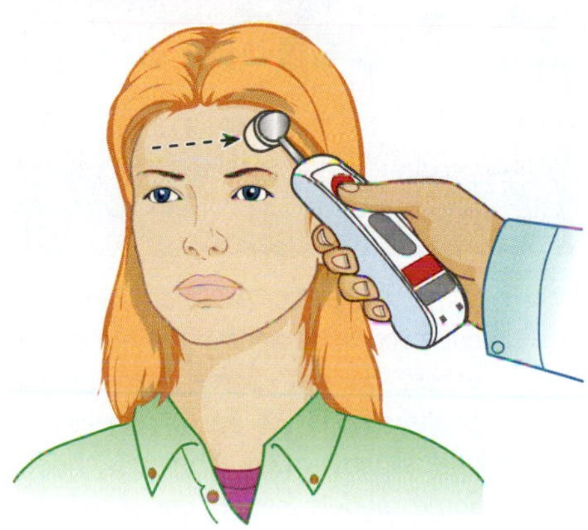

4. **Still holding the button,** touch the thermometer lens/probe behind the ear lobe, in the soft depression below the mastoid.
This step is necessary for an accurate reading if there is any moisture at all on the patient's forehead.

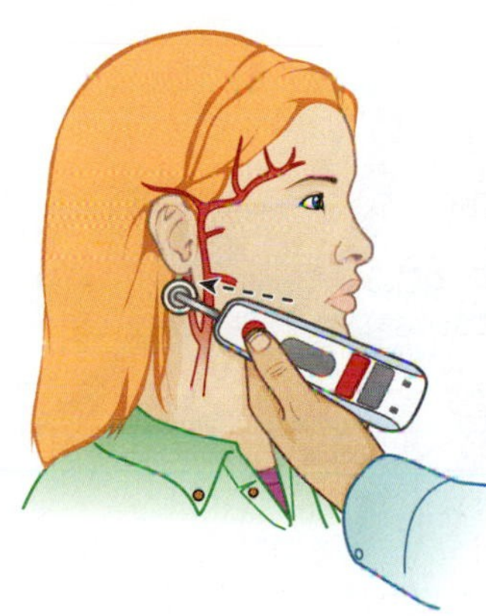

(continued on next page)

Procedure 20-1 ■ Assessing Body Temperature (continued)

5. **Release the button for** the temperature reading. ➤

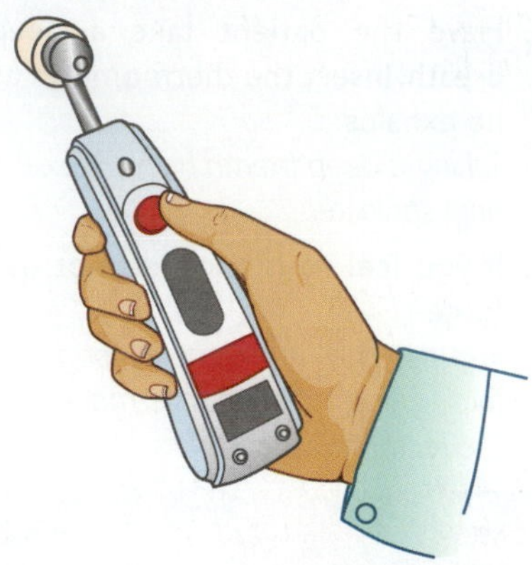

Procedure 20-1E ■ Taking a Tympanic Membrane Temperature

➤ When performing the procedure, always identify your patient according to agency policy, using two identifiers, and be attentive to standard precautions, hand hygiene, patient safety and privacy, body mechanics, and documentation.

Procedure Steps

1. **Make sure the thermometer** lens is intact and clean.
   Ensures accurate reading.

2. **Place a disposable cover tightly** over the lens, making sure the clear film is smooth across the lens.
   Ensures accurate reading and prevents cross-contamination.

3. **Position the patient's head** to one side. If you are right-handed, use the right ear; if you are left-handed, use the left ear.
   This allows you to better visualize the ear canal.

4. **Straighten the ear canal,** or follow the manufacturer's instructions. As a rule: ▼

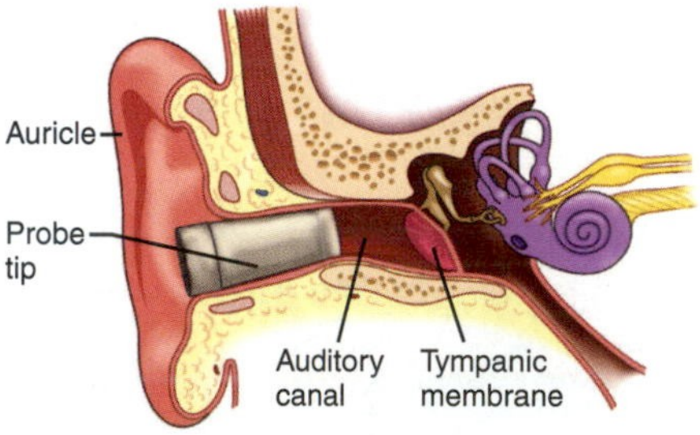

   a. **For an adult,** pull the pinna up and back. ▼

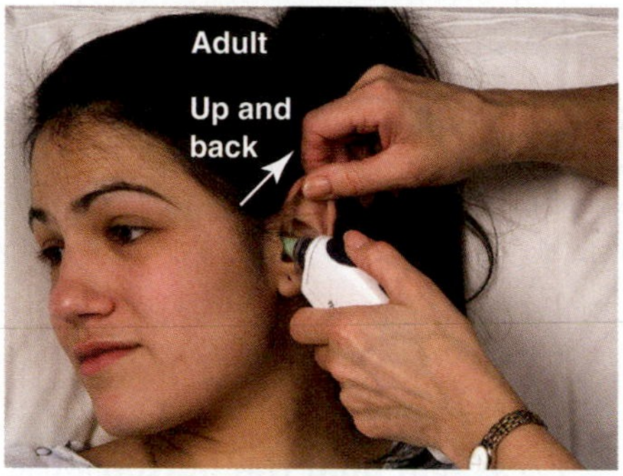

   b. **For a child,** pull the pinna down and back. ▼

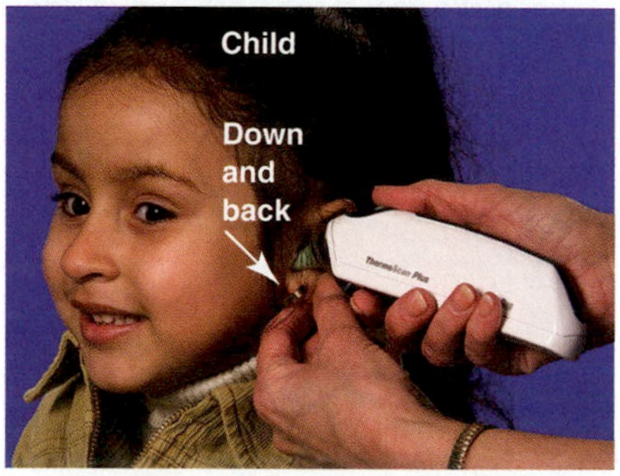

   Some tympanic thermometers require you to straighten the ear canal; others do not. Some instruct, for adults, to pull the ear up, backward, and slightly away from the head. Some models instruct, for a child, to pull the pinna straight back instead of down and back. The external auditory canal is curved upward in children younger than 3 years of age. In an adult, it is a slightly S-shaped structure.

5. **Insert the probe into the ear canal** gently and firmly, directing it toward the tympanic membrane and inserting far enough to seal the opening.
   Creates a seal to obtain an accurate reading without causing trauma to the ear canal.

6. **Rotate the probe handle** toward the jaw (for some thermometer models). Follow the manufacturer's instructions; not all models require this.
   Aims the lens toward the tympanic membrane.

7. **Take the measurement.**
   a. Press and release the button to obtain the reading.
   b. Follow the instructions for the specific tympanic thermometer being used.
   Some tympanic thermometers record the reading immediately; for some, you must wait for about 3 seconds.

8. **Remove the thermometer** when you hear a beep and the display flashes. Note the reading in the display window.
9. **Repeat the measurement** in the other ear.

Research shows a significant difference in temperature in the left ear compared with the right ear (Heusch & McCarthy, 2005; Levander & Grodzinsky, 2017).

10. **Discard the probe cover** (usually you will press an "eject" button to do this), and replace the thermometer in its charging base.
Recharges the battery to ensure its usability during the shift and protects the instrument.

Procedure 20-1F ■ Taking a Skin Temperature Using a Chemical Strip Thermometer

➤ When performing the procedure, always identify your patient according to agency policy, using two identifiers, and be attentive to standard precautions, hand hygiene, patient safety and privacy, body mechanics, and documentation.

Procedure Steps

1. **Place the thermometer strip** (paper or tape) on the patient's skin, generally on the forehead or abdomen.
The thermometer strip must be in contact with the skin to work properly. ▼

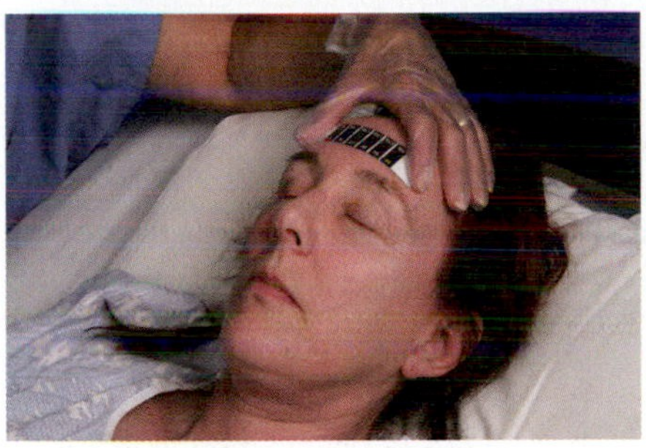

2. **Leave the thermometer strip** in place 15 to 60 seconds (or as directed by the manufacturer).
3. **Observe for color changes.**
Chemical strips have indicators that change colors to indicate temperature changes.
4. **Read the temperature before** removing the strip from the patient's skin.
Ensures the most accurate reading.
5. **Remove and discard** the thermometer strip.

? What if . . .

- **The patient's temperature is not within normal range?**

Identify whether the temperature reading indicates hypothermia, fever, or hyperthermia (e.g., heat stroke).
Perform other assessments to determine the cause or severity of the findings.
Assess for clinical signs to confirm an abnormal temperature reading.
Institute interventions to raise or lower temperature, as appropriate.
Provide comfort measures (e.g., change linens if they are wet from diaphoresis).

- **You must use a glass thermometer?**

Be sure the thermometer does not contain mercury.

Before and after use, shake down the thermometer, as needed.
Clean the thermometer before and after use with soap and water or approved solution; rinse.
Use disposable covers, if available.
When reading the thermometer, hold it at eye level and rotate it until the markings are clear and easy to read.
Handle carefully and store in an appropriate container to avoid breakage.

Evaluation

- Compare with the normal range for the developmental stage, site used, and client's baseline data.
- Look for trends to identify potential concerns.
- Notify the appropriate healthcare provider of any abnormal findings.

Patient Teaching

- Inform the patient of the temperature reading.
- Explain the significance of the temperature reading and any interventions that may be needed.

Home Care

- Clients commonly use chemical strip (disposable), glass, or tympanic membrane thermometers at home. Teach the following points:
  - Do not use an oral thermometer to take a rectal temperature. Use a specially shaped, more rounded, rectal thermometer to avoid injuring the rectum.
  - Do not use glass-and-mercury thermometers. If you find that the client has a glass-and-mercury thermometer, or any kind of glass thermometer, urge the client to replace it with a safer instrument (e.g., a plastic thermometer). Arrange for an exchange if there is a procedure for this in your agency or community.
Glass-and-mercury thermometers carry the risk of breakage, cuts, and exposure to toxic mercury.
  - If you obtain a high or low reading using a chemical strip or a tympanic thermometer, retake the temperature using a plastic or digital thermometer.
  - Teach the same procedures you have learned for measuring temperature. Observe as the client takes a temperature to ensure correct technique.
  - Clients often use the oral site. Remind them to not drink, eat, or smoke for 30 minutes before taking the temperature.

(continued on next page)

Procedure 20-1 ■ Assessing Body Temperature (continued)

- Reinforce the following points about care of reusable thermometers:
  - If you use the same thermometer for more than one person, use disposable covers, if possible. Clean the thermometer well between uses.
  - If the person has an infection or communicable illness, soak the thermometer in 70% isopropyl alcohol between uses.
  - Clean the thermometer after each use, even if it is used for only one person. Wash with soap and water, rinse with cold water, dry well, and store in a clean, dry container.
  - If you store a thermometer in alcohol, rinse it with cold water before taking the temperature.
  - Do not use the same thermometer for taking both oral and rectal temperatures.

Documentation

You will usually record temperature on a graphic flowsheet (see Flowsheets and Graphic Records in Chapter 18, Volume 1; also see Documentation Forms in Chapter 18, Volume 2). In some situations (e.g., a fever), you may need to write a nurse's note. If so, follow these suggestions:

- Document the temperature, indicating the route of measurement, according to agency policy.
- Notify the appropriate healthcare provider of abnormal findings.
- Document supporting findings, such as "Skin is hot and dry" and state whether the temperature reading is consistent with the client's condition.

Sample Documentation

mm/dd/yyyy 1230 Oral temperature 105°F: has risen steadily since the first elevation at 0630, when it was 100°F. Skin hot and dry. Voiding only small amounts, but states no burning. Urine dark but clear. No chills. I&O begun. Gave Tylenol 650 mg by mouth and notified Dr. Anderson of patient's condition and medication. ______ Mary Clinton, RN

Practice Resources

Amoore, D. (2010); Heusch, A., & McCarthy, P. (2005); Levander. M. & Grodzinsky, E. (2017); Lockwood, C., Conroy-Hiller, T. & Page, T. (2004); Medline Plus (2018); Morrow-Barnes, A. (2014); Pickering, D. (2013a); Rabinowitz, R., Cookson, S., Wasserman, S., et al. (1996)

Thinking About the Procedure

The video, **Assessing Body Temperature,** along with questions and suggested responses, is available on the ***Davis's Nursing Skills Videos*** Web site on FADavis.com.

Procedure 20-2 ■ Assessing Peripheral Pulses

➤ For steps to follow in *all* procedures, refer to the Universal Steps for All Procedures found on the inside back cover.

Equipment

- Watch with a second hand or digital readout
- Pen, pencil, and flowsheet or personal digital assistant (PDA)

Delegation

You can delegate measurement of pulses to the UAP if you conclude that the patient's condition and the UAP's skills allow. For example, if pedal circulation is critical and you suspect it may be difficult to palpate, you should not delegate assessment of the pedal pulse.

- If you do delegate, perform the pre-procedure assessments and tell the UAP which site (e.g., radial, brachial) to use. Inform the UAP of any special considerations (e.g., to note what the patient's activity has been just before taking the pulse).
- Ask the UAP to document and report the pulse to you and to report immediately if it is outside normal limits (you must specify what is "normal" for each patient).

Pre-Procedure Assessments

- Determine why assessment of pulses is indicated.
  Conditions requiring an assessment of pulses include blood loss, cardiac or respiratory disease, diabetes mellitus, and other conditions that affect oxygenation.
- Assess factors that may alter the pulse, such as activity and medications. If the client has been active recently, wait 5 to 10 minutes before measuring.
  Activity increases the pulse rate; increased intracranial pressure decreases the rate; some medications, such as digoxin, decrease the rate; other medications, such as albuterol, increase the pulse rate.

Procedure 20-2A ■ Assessing the Radial Pulse

➤ When performing the procedure, always identify your patient according to agency policy, using two identifiers, and be attentive to standard precautions, hand hygiene, patient safety and privacy, body mechanics, and documentation.

Procedure Steps

1. **With the patient sitting or supine,** flex his arm, and place the forearm across his chest.

2. **Palpate the radial artery.**
The radial site is the most frequently used to calculate the patient's heart rate because it is generally the easiest site to use.
   a. Place the pads of your index or middle fingers (or both) in the groove on the thumb side of the patient's wrist, over the radial artery.
   b. Press lightly but firmly until you are able to feel the radial pulse. Start with light pressure to prevent occluding the pulse, and gradually increase the pressure until you feel the pulse.
   The fingertips are the most sensitive parts of the hand to palpate arterial pulsations. Avoid using the thumb because it has its own pulsation and may interfere with the accuracy of your count.

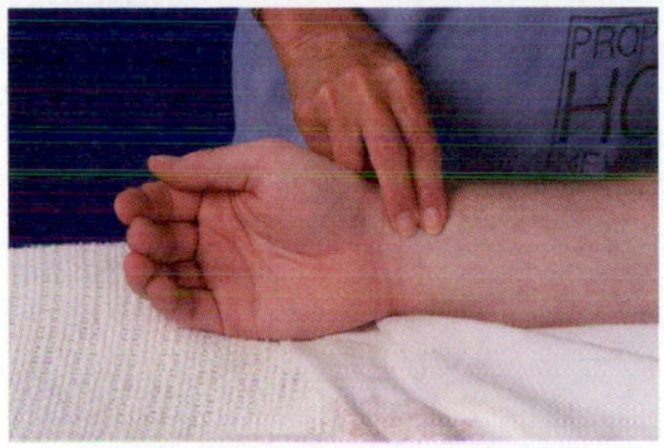

3. **Note the rhythm and quality** of the pulse. Note whether the thrust of the pulse against your fingertips is bounding, strong, weak, or thready.
The rhythm and quality of the pulse are a reflection of the patient's cardiac output. The strength of the pulse reflects the volume of the blood that is ejected against the arterial wall with each contraction of the heart. An irregular or weak pulse indicates decreased cardiac output. A bounding pulse indicates increased cardiac output.

4. **Count the pulse:**
   a. Count for 60 seconds the first time you take a patient's pulse. After that, you can count a pulse with a regular rhythm for 15 seconds and multiply by 4, or count for 30 seconds and multiply by 2 to get the beats per minute. If you do not know the patient well, count for a full minute to be certain to detect irregularities. See Step 4c rationale.
   b. Begin timing with the count of 1—starting with the first beat that you feel.
   c. Count an irregular pulse for 1 full minute (60 seconds).
   Research findings are conflicting. Some studies indicate that a 60-second count is most accurate; others suggest that accuracy is not affected by a 30-second or even a 15-second count if the pulse is regular. You must count an irregular pulse for 1 full minute to be accurate.

5. **For an admission assessment** or peripheral vascular check, palpate the radial pulses on both wrists simultaneously. Note any difference in the quality of the pulse between the two sides. Is the pulse on one side weaker than that on the other?
Palpating simultaneously enables the recognition of small differences in the peripheral circulation.

Procedure 20-2B ■ Assessing the Brachial Pulse

➤ When performing the procedure, always identify your patient according to agency policy, using two identifiers, and be attentive to standard precautions, hand hygiene, patient safety and privacy, body mechanics, and documentation.

Procedure Steps

1. **Palpate the brachial artery.**
   a. Using firm pressure, press in the inner aspect of the antecubital fossa until you palpate the brachial artery.
   b. If you have difficulty palpating the pulse, ask the patient to pronate the forearm (i.e., turn the palm of the hand downward).
   This brings the brachial artery over a bony prominence and makes the pulse easier to feel. ▼

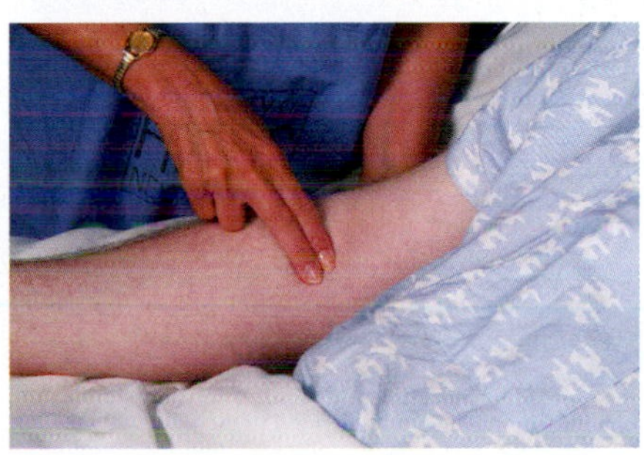

2. **Assess pulse rate, rhythm, and quality,** and assess bilaterally (see Procedure 20-2A).
The brachial pulse is used most frequently to assess BP and to identify the presence of a pulse during cardiopulmonary resuscitation (CPR) in an infant.

(continued on next page)

Procedure 20-2 ■ Assessing Peripheral Pulses (continued)

Procedure 20-2C ■ Assessing the Carotid Pulse

➤ When performing the procedure, always identify your patient according to agency policy, using two identifiers, and be attentive to standard precautions, hand hygiene, patient safety and privacy, body mechanics, and documentation.

Caution! Do not palpate the carotid pulse except during cardiopulmonary resuscitation in an adult and, in certain situations, to assess for circulation to the head. Persons not trained in CPR should not assess the carotid pulse.

Pressure on the carotid (especially in older adults) can stimulate the vagus nerve, causing the pulse and BP to drop suddenly, and perhaps fainting or circulatory arrest. It can also decrease circulation to the brain.

Procedure Steps

1. **Palpate the carotid artery lightly.** Place your fingers on the patient's trachea, and slide them to the side into the groove between the trachea and the sternocleidomastoid muscle.
   Compressing the carotid arteries can stimulate the carotid bodies and significantly decrease the patient's heart rate and BP. ▼

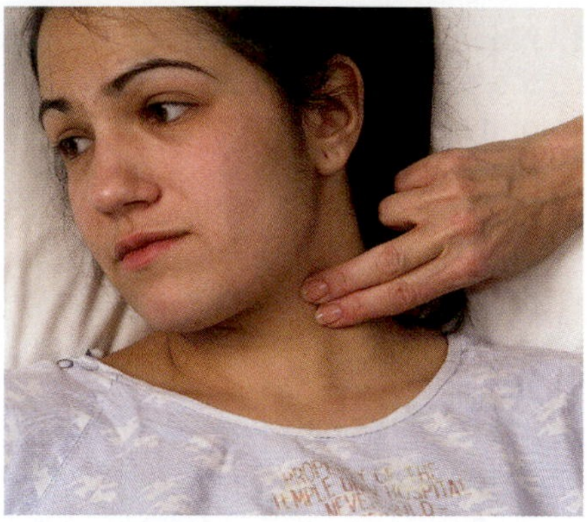

Never compress the carotid artery on both sides of the neck at the same time.

2. **Assess the rate, rhythm, and quality,** and compare bilaterally.

Procedure 20-2D ■ Assessing the Dorsalis Pedis Pulse

➤ When performing the procedure, always identify your patient according to agency policy, using two identifiers, and be attentive to standard precautions, hand hygiene, patient safety and privacy, body mechanics, and documentation.

Procedure Steps

1. **Palpate the dorsalis pedis pulse.**
   a. Run your fingers up the groove between the great and first toes to the top of the foot.
   b. Palpate very lightly.
   The dorsalis pedis pulse is easily obliterated, so use very light pressure. The dorsalis pedis pulse is used to access circulation of the foot.

As a result of atherosclerosis or hardening of the arteries, the dorsalis pedis may be difficult to palpate in older adults.

2. **Assess pulse rate, rhythm, and quality,** and assess bilaterally. ▼

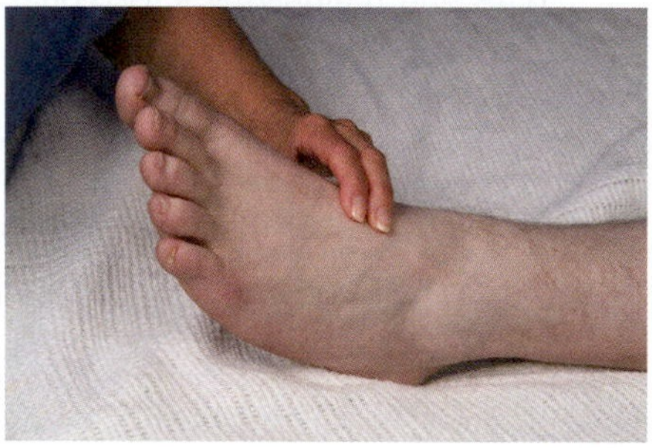

3. **If you are unable to palpate the dorsalis pedis pulse,** use a Doppler ultrasound device to assess the pulse and circulation to the lower extremity.

Procedure 20-2E ■ Assessing the Femoral Pulse

➤ When performing the procedure, always identify your patient according to agency policy, using two identifiers, and be attentive to standard precautions, hand hygiene, patient safety and privacy, body mechanics, and documentation.

Procedure Steps

1. **Palpate the femoral pulse** by pressing deeply in the groin midway between the anterosuperior iliac spine and the symphysis pubis.
The femoral artery lies very deep and requires significant pressure to palpate. You may need to use both hands to feel the pulse on an adult. ➤

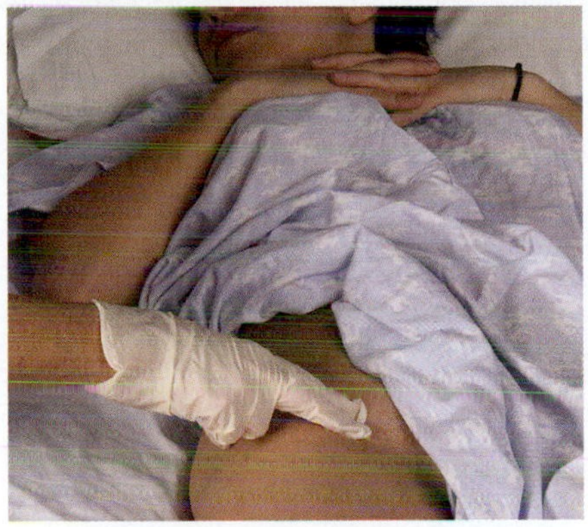

2. **Assess pulse rate, rhythm, and quality,** and assess bilaterally.
The femoral pulse is used to determine the presence of a pulse during CPR and to assess circulation to the leg.

Procedure 20-2F ■ Assessing the Posterior Tibial Pulse

➤ When performing the procedure, always identify your patient according to agency policy, using two identifiers, and be attentive to standard precautions, hand hygiene, patient safety and privacy, body mechanics, and documentation.

Procedure Steps

1. **Palpate the posterior tibial pulse** by pressing on the inner (medial) side of the ankle below the medial malleolus.
The posterior tibial pulse is usually palpated easily, but it may be deeper in some people. So, press down moderately, and then increase pressure until you feel the pulse. It is relatively easy to obliterate. ➤

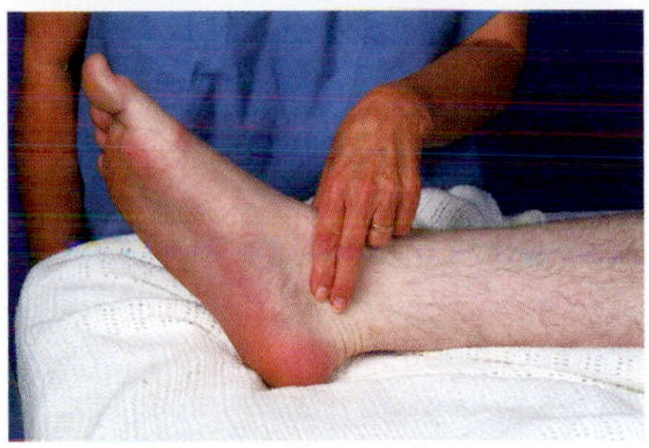

2. **Assess pulse rate, rhythm, and quality, and assess bilaterally.**
The posterior tibial pulse is used to assess circulation to the lower extremity; it is assessed along with the dorsalis pedis pulse.

Procedure 20-2G ■ Assessing the Popliteal Pulse

➤ When performing the procedure, always identify your patient according to agency policy, using two identifiers, and be attentive to standard precautions, hand hygiene, patient safety and privacy, body mechanics, and documentation.

Procedure Steps

1. **Palpate the popliteal pulse** by pressing behind the knee in the middle of the popliteal fossa.
The popliteal pulse can be difficult to feel. It is used only when specifically indicated because of absence of pedal pulses or for taking the thigh BP. ➤

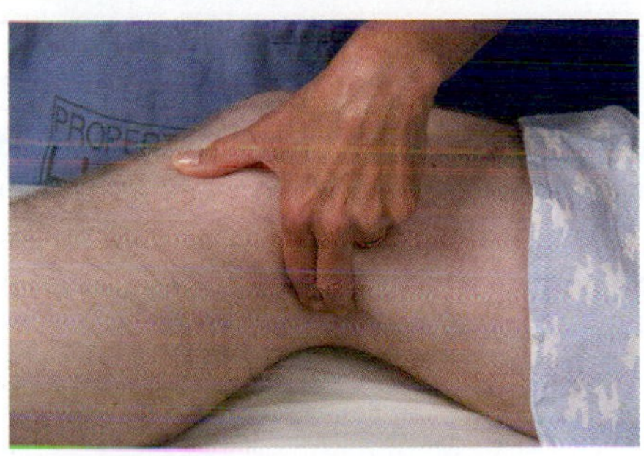

2. **Assess pulse rate, rhythm, and quality,** and assess bilaterally.
The popliteal pulse is used to assess circulation of the lower leg and auscultate the thigh BP.

(continued on next page)

Procedure 20-2 ■ Assessing Peripheral Pulses (continued)

Procedure 20-2H ■ Assessing the Temporal Pulse

➤ When performing the procedure, always identify your patient according to agency policy, using two identifiers, and be attentive to standard precautions, hand hygiene, patient safety and privacy, body mechanics, and documentation.

Procedure Steps

1. **Palpate the temporal pulse** by pressing lightly lateral (outside area) and superior to (above) the eye.

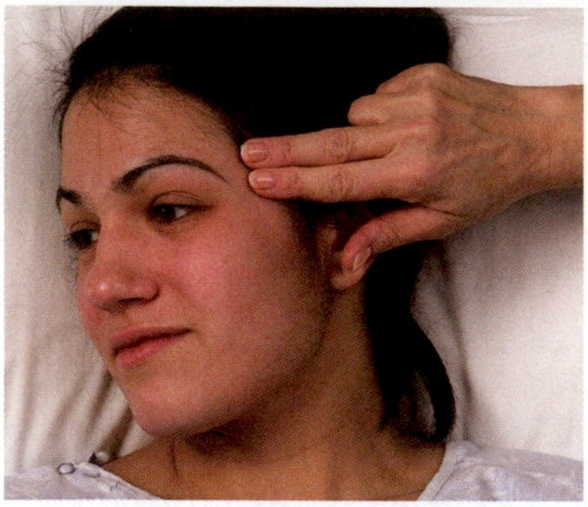

2. **Assess pulse rate, rhythm, and quality,** and assess bilaterally as for the radial pulse (see Procedure 20-2A).
   The temporal pulse is easily accessible and is used frequently in infants.

? What if . . .

- **The patient is an infant or a child younger than 3 years of age?**

  Auscultate an apical pulse rate. Rates are faster and small arteries more difficult to feel in a child or infant.

  If a parent is present, encourage the parent to hold the child to reduce anxiety.
  Fear increases the pulse rate.

- **The patient is an older adult?**

  Have the patient at rest for 15 to 20 minutes after activity and before assessing the pulse.
  The pulse tends to return to baseline more slowly in older adults.

  If the pulse is fast, take repeated measures; if a pattern of fast rate emerges, note this for the primary healthcare provider for further evaluation.
  An elevated heart rate is related to increased mortality in older women, so it is a simple index of the general health status.

- **The pulse is faint or weak?**

  Use a Doppler ultrasound device to detect blood flow.
  Lack of pulses indicates inadequate circulation to the lower extremities. If you cannot feel the pulse, you must determine whether the pulse is absent or whether you are having difficulty feeling it. To draw the conclusion that the pulse is "absent," you must use a Doppler ultrasound device.

  Apply transmission gel to the end of the probe. Do not use water-soluble lubricant as a substitute for transmission gel.

  Place the probe lightly on the skin over the artery you are using.

  Turn on the instrument, and set the volume control to the lowest setting.

  Tilting the probe to a 45-degree angle to the artery, move the probe slowly in a circular motion to locate the signal (a rhythmic hissing noise). Count for 60 seconds.
  Move the probe slowly to avoid distorting the signal.

  When you are finished, wipe the gel off the patient's skin. Clean the probe with soapy water or an antiseptic solution. Do not immerse the probe or bump it against anything hard.
  Clean the probe to prevent cross-contamination to other patients. Probes are fragile and may malfunction if bumped against a hard surface.

Evaluation

Especially if pedal pulses are decreased, observe for other indications of inadequate circulation, such as cool skin, decreased capillary refill, and bluish or ashen skin tone. You must provide supporting evidence if you document that pedal pulses are decreased or absent. The complete absence of a pulse requires immediate intervention.

Patient Teaching

- Teach the patient about the significance of any abnormalities in pulse rate or rhythm.
- Explain any interventions that may be needed.

Home Care

Assess the skill level of the person who will be assessing the client's peripheral pulses in the home, and provide instructions, if necessary.

Documentation

Usually, you will document routine vital signs, including pulse, on a flowsheet or graph. Documentation in the nurse's note must include the pulse rate, rhythm, quality, and site (e.g., "radial pulse 64 beats/min, regular, and strong bilaterally").

Practice Resources

Alexis, O. (2010); Lowry, M. & Ashelford, S. (2015); Nicholson, C. (2014); Pickering, D. (2013b)

Thinking About the Procedure

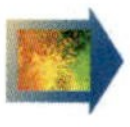

The video, **Assessing Peripheral Pulses,** along with questions and suggested responses, is available on the ***Davis's Nursing Skills Videos*** Web site on FADavis.com.

Procedure 20-3 ■ Assessing the Apical Pulse

➤ For steps to follow in *all* procedures, refer to the Universal Steps for All Procedures found on the inside back cover.

Equipment

- Watch with a second hand or second readout
- Stethoscope
- Alcohol wipes (to clean stethoscope)

Delegation

You can delegate measurement of the apical pulse to the UAP if you conclude that the patient's condition and the UAP's skills allow.

- First, perform the pre-procedure assessments.
- Then, inform the UAP of any special considerations (e.g., to note what the patient's activity has been just before taking the pulse, or to mark the time exactly so you can compare it with the patient's electrocardiography [ECG] reading).
- Ask the UAP to document and report the pulse reading to you, and to report immediately if it is outside normal limits (you must specify what is "normal" for each patient).

Pre-Procedure Assessments

- Determine why assessment of the apical pulse is indicated.
  Conditions that require assessment of the apical pulse include digitalis therapy, blood loss, cardiac or respiratory disease, or other conditions that affect oxygenation status.
- Assess factors that may alter the pulse, such as activity and medications. If the client has been recently active, wait 10 to 15 minutes before obtaining a measurement.
  Activity can increase the pulse rate. Relate above factors to baseline pulse rate to determine their effect.

➤ When performing the procedure, always identify your patient according to agency policy, using two identifiers, and be attentive to standard precautions, hand hygiene, patient safety and privacy, body mechanics, and documentation.

Procedure Steps

1. **With the client supine or sitting,** expose the left side of the chest, but only as much as necessary.
   Prevents distortion of sound from the patient's gown rubbing on the stethoscope, while also protecting the patient's privacy.

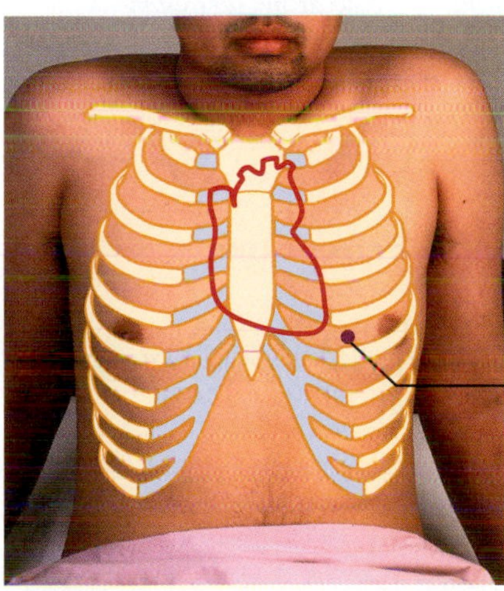

2. **Wipe the stethoscope** with a 70% alcohol or benzalkonium chloride wipe before and after examining the patient.
   Cleaning can reduce the bacterial count by up to 100%.

2. **Palpate the 5th intercostal space** at the midclavicular line for the apical pulse.
   The left ventricle of the heart and the point of maximal impulse (PMI) lie in this area. The apical pulse is generally best heard at the PMI, over the apex of the heart.
   a. To locate the 5th intercostal space, slide your finger down from the sternal notch to the angle of Louis (the bump where the manubrium and sternum meet).
   b. Slide your finger over to the left sternal border to the 2nd intercostal space.
   c. Now place your index or ring finger (depending on which hand you use) in the 2nd intercostal space, and count down to the fifth intercostal space by placing a finger in each of the spaces.
   d. Slide over to the midclavicular line, keeping your finger in the 5th intercostal space.
   The apical pulse is generally best heard at the PMI in the 5th intercostal space at the midclavicular line. The PMI is located over the apex of the heart. For an adult, this site is on the anterior chest at 3 inches (8 cm) or less to the left of the sternum, at the 4th, 5th, or 6th intercostal space at the midclavicular line.

4. **Palpate the apical pulse.**
   a. The palpated apical pulse (also called *PMI*).
   b. The pulse area should be about the size of a quarter, without lifts or heaves.
   A larger than normal pulsation may indicate ventricular hypertrophy.

5. **Warm the stethoscope** in your hand for 10 seconds. Then, place the diaphragm over the PMI, and listen to the normal S_1 and S_2 heart sounds ("lub-dub"). Count each pair of sounds ("lub-dub") as one heartbeat.
   A cold stethoscope placed on the skin may startle the patient and increase the heart rate. Heart sounds result when blood moves through the valves of the heart. The first heart sound is louder at the apical area and should be audible when the pulse is auscultated.

(continued on next page)

Procedure 20-3 ■ Assessing the Apical Pulse (continued)

6. **Count the apical heart rate** for 1 full minute.
   Ensures accuracy. Because the apical heart rate is needed as an assessment measure for the administration of some medications (e.g., digoxin), accuracy is essential. Some cardiac conditions cause either slow or irregular rates, both of which must be counted for a full minute to ensure accuracy.

7. **Clean the stethoscope** again with 70% alcohol or benzalkonium chloride wipe.

? What if . . .

- **The apical rate is less than 60 beats/min?**

  (*Note:* You may also see "bpm" as an abbreviation for "beats per minute" or for "beats/min.")

  If the patient is taking cardiac medications, withhold them and consult with a healthcare provider about any need to adjust the dosage.
  Certain cardiac medications (e.g., digoxin) are given to slow the heart rate; bradycardia may indicate that blood levels are too high.

  Assess for chest pain, dizziness, dyspnea.
  May indicate decreased cardiac output

- **The apical rate is greater than 100 beats/min?**

  Obtain a complete set of vital signs. Assess for pain, anxiety, fever, dehydration, decreased oxygenation, hypotension, and decreased exercise.
  These factors may increase pulse rate.

Evaluation

- Are the findings within normal limits?
- Are there other factors supporting the findings?
- What are the trends over time?
- Is the skin pink, warm, and dry?
- Is there any cyanosis?

Patient Teaching

- Teach the patient about the significance of any abnormalities in the pulse rate or rhythm.
- Explain any interventions that may be necessary.

Home Care

- Assess the skill level of the person who will be assessing the client's apical pulse in the home, and provide instructions, if necessary.
- Teach the home caregiver when to hold medications and/or to call primary care provider (e.g., to hold the digitalis if the rate is <60 beats/min).
- Before leaving the client's home, clean the stethoscope with detergent or disinfectant, when possible; or place it in a plastic bag for transporting to the reprocessing location.
- If the patient has an infection with a multidrug-resistant organism, reusable equipment, such as stethoscopes, should remain in the client's home. If the stethoscope cannot remain in the client's home, clean and disinfect it before leaving, using a low- to intermediate-level disinfectant. If this is not practical, place the stethoscope in a plastic bag, and transport it to another site for cleaning and disinfection.

Documentation

Document the pulse rate, rhythm, and site.

Sample documentation

mm/dd/yyyy 0800 Apical pulse regular rhythm, and strong, rate of 64. ——— Janice Jonas, RN

Practice Resources

Alexis, O. (2010); Lowry, M. & Ashelford, S. (2015).

Thinking About the Procedure

The video, **Assessing Apical Pulse,** along with questions and suggested responses, is available on the ***Davis's Nursing Skills Videos*** Web site on FADavis.com.

Procedure 20-4 ■ Assessing for an Apical–Radial Pulse Deficit

➤ For steps to follow in *all* procedures, refer to the Universal Steps for All Procedures found on the inside back cover.

Equipment

- Watch or clock with a second hand or second readout
- Procedure gloves, if indicated
- Stethoscope
- Alcohol wipes to clean the stethoscope

Delegation

Instead of delegating measurement of an apical–radial pulse to a UAP, you would most likely ask the UAP to assist you in this procedure because it is best performed by two persons working together.

Pre-Procedure Assessments

- **Determine why assessment of pulse deficit is indicated.** *Conditions that require assessment of pulse deficit include digitalis therapy, blood loss, cardiac or respiratory disease, and other conditions that affect oxygenation status.*
- **Assess factors that may alter the pulse, such as activity and medications.**

➤ When performing the procedure, always identify your patient according to agency policy, using two identifiers, and be attentive to standard precautions, hand hygiene, patient safety and privacy, body mechanics, and documentation.

Procedure Steps

1. **Wipe the stethoscope** with a 70% alcohol or benzalkonium chloride wipe before and after examining the patient.
   Cleaning can reduce the bacterial count by up to 100% and prevent the transmission of microbes.
2. **Expose the left side** of the patient's chest, minimizing patient exposure.
   Prevents distortion of sound from the patient's gown rubbing on the stethoscope and protects privacy.
3. **Place the watch such that the second hand is visible to both nurses** (if two nurses are performing the procedure).
   Using one watch increases accuracy of counts.
4. **Nurse 1 prepares to auscultate the apical pulse.** She palpates the 5th intercostal space at the midclavicular line, then holds the diaphragm of the stethoscope in place, using firm pressure until Nurse 2 says "Start."
   Aids in hearing high-pitched sounds and ensures good contact between the diaphragm of the stethoscope and the skin.

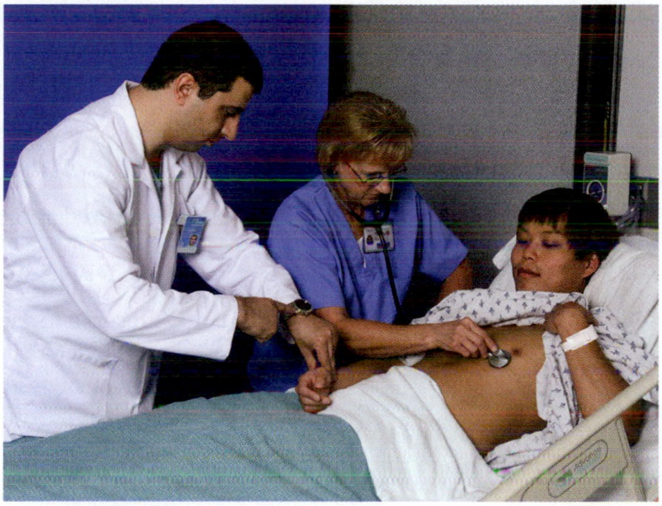

5. **Nurse 2 palpates to locate the radial pulse**, preparing to assess rate, rhythm, and quality.
6. **Nurse 2 says "Start" when ready to begin** and "Stop" when finished. Both nurses count the pulse simultaneously for 1 full minute
   Count simultaneously to ensure accuracy. Counting for 1 full minute is necessary for an accurate assessment of any discrepancies that may exist between the two sites.
7. **To obtain pulse deficit, subtract** the radial rate from the apical rate.

   Apical Rate – Radial Rate = Pulse Deficit

   Atrial and ventricular dysrhythmias may cause beats that do not perfuse, so although you hear an apical heartbeat, you do not feel a peripheral pulse. The pulse deficit is the number of heartbeats that do not perfuse.

? What if . . .

- **Another nurse is not available to assist?**
  Hold the stethoscope in place with the one hand while palpating the radial pulse with the hand wearing the watch. *Even if you cannot manage to count both rates, you should be able to feel any differences between the apical and radial pulses.*
- **There has been an increase in pulse deficit since the last measurement?**
  An increase in pulse deficit means that the patient's cardiac output has decreased.

(continued on next page)

Procedure 20-4 ■ Assessing for an Apical–Radial Pulse Deficit (continued)

Evaluation

- Identify the presence of an apical–radial pulse deficit, and compare with previous findings.
- Assess other measures of cardiopulmonary status to identify a decline in the patient's condition.
- Look for trends.
  The presence of any apical–radial pulse deficit is abnormal.

Patient Teaching

- Teach the patient about the significance of an apical–radial pulse deficit.
- Explain any necessary interventions.

Home Care

- Assess the skill level of the person(s) who will be measuring the client's apical–radial pulse deficit in the home, and provide instructions, if necessary.
- Before leaving the client's home, clean the stethoscope as described in the Home Care section of Procedure 20-3.

Documentation

Document the apical–radial pulse deficit.

Sample documentation

mm/dd/yyyy 0900 Apical–radial pulse deficit is 4 beats/min. —Jon Albertson, RN

Practice Resources

Alexis, O. (2010); Opio, M. & Kellett, J. (2017).

Thinking About the Procedure

The video, **Assessing for an Apical Radial Pulse Deficit,** along with questions and suggested responses, is available on the ***Davis's Nursing Skills Videos*** Web site on FADavis.com.

Procedure 20-5 ■ Assessing Respirations

➤ For steps to follow in *all* procedures, refer to the Universal Steps for All Procedures found on the inside back cover.

Equipment

- A watch with a second hand (or a wall clock)

Delegation

You can delegate the counting of respirations to the UAP if you conclude that the patient's condition and the UAP's skills allow.

- Perform the pre-procedure assessments, and inform the UAP of any special considerations (e.g., the need to place the patient in a certain position).
- Ask the UAP to document and report the respirations to you, and to report immediately if they are not within the normal range for this patient (specify the range).

Pre-Procedure Assessments

- Observe for signs of respiratory distress—breathing faster or slower than normal, gasping breaths, confusion, circumoral (around the month) cyanosis.
  Signs of hypoxemia may indicate that the patient is not adequately oxygenated.
- Determine the baseline respiratory rate and the character of respirations.
- Assess for factors that may affect the respiratory rate (e.g., pain, activity, fever, respiratory disorders).

➤ When performing the procedure, always identify your patient according to agency policy, using two identifiers, and be attentive to standard precautions, hand hygiene, patient safety and privacy, body mechanics, and documentation.

Procedure Steps

1. **Position the patient.** With the patient in a sitting (preferably) or in Fowler's position, flex the patient's arm, and place her forearm across her chest.
   Aids in counting the patient's pulse rate by making the rise and fall of the chest more discernible and by making the patient less aware that you are measuring the respiratory rate. The patient's awareness might alter the respiratory rate and/or pattern because respirations are partially under voluntary control.

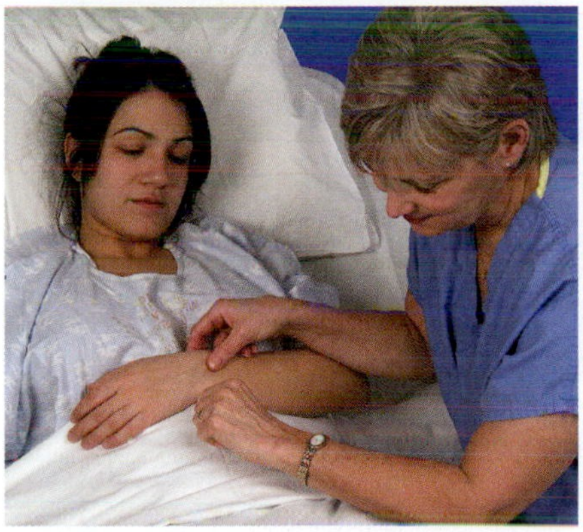

2. **Palpate and count the radial pulse;** remember that number.
3. **Then, keeping your hand** on the patient's wrist, count the respirations.
   Allows you to count the respirations unobtrusively.
4. **Observe the respiratory rate, rhythm, and depth.**
   - Rate—normal for patient's age, fast (tachypnea), or slow (bradypnea)
   - Rhythm—regular or irregular
   - Depth—normal, shallow, or deep (e.g., Kussmaul's respirations)

   All of these characteristics are necessary to evaluate respiratory status. Different pathologies affect each of these characteristics differently.
5. **Count the number of breaths** per minute. Begin timing the respirations with a count of 1, not 0 (the same as with pulse measurement).
   a. If the respiratory rhythm is regular, count the rate (one inhalation and one exhalation is one respiration) for 30 seconds, and multiply by 2.
   b. If the rhythm is irregular, count the rate for 1 full minute (60 seconds).
   Variations in rhythm may cause an inaccurate rate when counted for less than 1 minute.

? What if . . .

- **The patient is an infant?**

  Place your hand on the abdomen to assess the respiratory rate. Auscultate breath sounds with a stethoscope.
  Infants and young children breathe rapidly and are abdominal breathers, so it is difficult to see each and every rise and fall of the abdomen. Using a stethoscope increases the accuracy of the count, as well as providing information about the breath sounds.

  For infants and very young children, count for 1 full minute.
  Infants and young children have irregular respirations. Counting for a full minute provides a more accurate rate for irregular respirations.

- **The patient is receiving oxygen therapy or requires careful assessment of respiratory status?**

  Apply a pulse oximeter (see Procedure 36-2, Monitoring Pulse Oximetry).
  Evidence suggests that pulse oximetry is useful for detecting deterioration of physiological function that might otherwise be missed (e.g., during the perioperative period or in seriously ill patients).

Evaluation

- Compare the respiratory rate and rhythm with previous readings.
- Note other vital signs, especially temperature.
- Look for trends, and note whether the respiratory rate and rhythm are changing in conjunction with changes in the other vital signs.
  If the patient has an elevated temperature, the respiratory rate will increase. Corresponding elevation in pulse with respiratory rate may indicate hypoxemia. If respirations are not within normal parameters, assess oxygenation with a pulse oximeter.

Patient Teaching

Teach the patient about factors that affect respiratory status, such as smoking and activity.

Home Care

Assess the skill level of the person(s) who will be measuring the client's respiratory rate in the home, and provide instructions, as needed.

Documentation

You will document routine vital signs (including respirations) on a graph or flowsheet. When a nurse's note is needed, follow these guidelines:

- Document the respiratory rate and rhythm.
- Document that respirations are either labored or unlabored; if labored, describe in what way (e.g., intercostal retractions, use of accessory muscles, nasal flaring).

(continued on next page)

Procedure 20-5 ■ Assessing Respirations (continued)

Example of Electronic Health Record

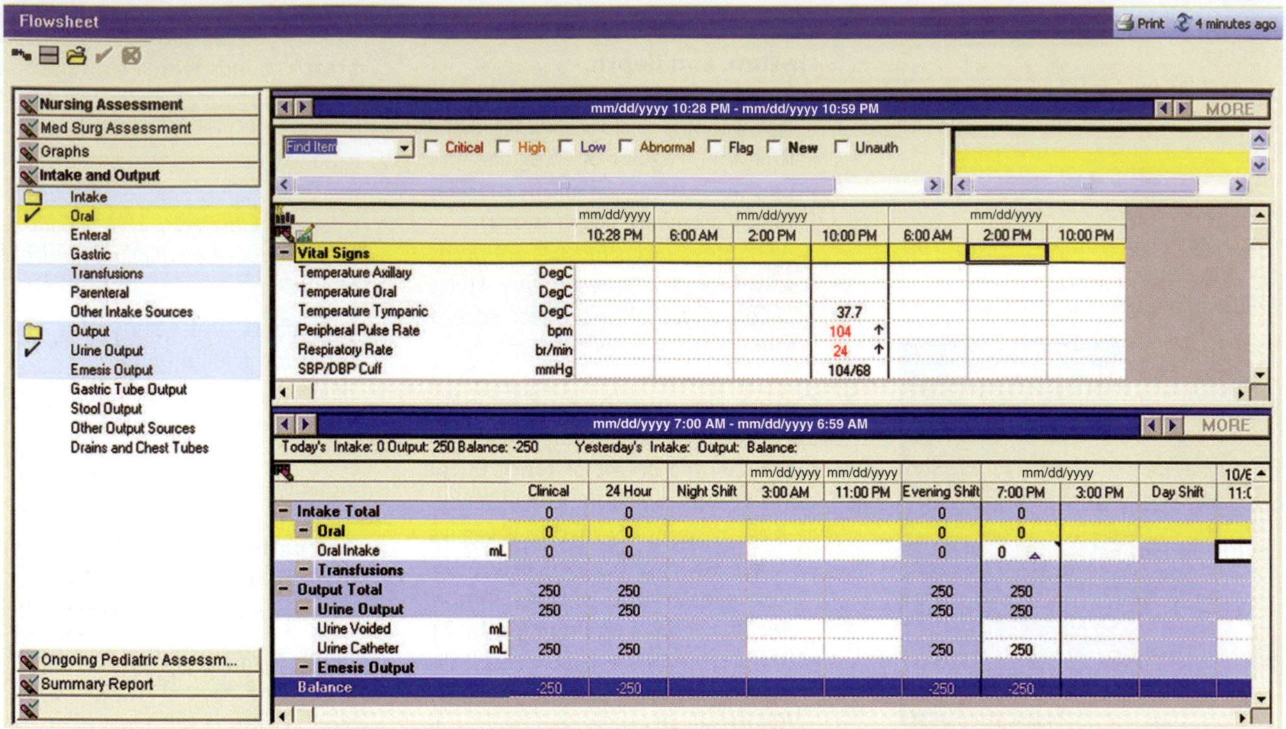

Practice Resources

Parkes, R. (2011); Royal College of Nursing (2015); Wheatley, I. (2018a)

Thinking About the Procedure

The video, **Assessing Respirations,** along with questions and suggested responses, is available on the ***Davis's Nursing Skills Videos*** Web site on FADavis.com.

Procedure 20-6 ■ Measuring Blood Pressure

➤ For steps to follow in *all* procedures, refer to the Universal Steps for All Procedures found on the inside back cover.

Equipment

- Stethoscope

Do not wear a stethoscope around your neck. *There is a slight risk that you can entangle it in intravenous and other lines. There is also a risk that a patient who is psychotic or delirious could use it to harm you. Also, wearing a stethoscope can be a source of cross-contamination.*

- 70% alcohol or benzalkonium chloride wipes.
  For cleaning stethoscope before and after use. Clean all parts.
- Sphygmomanometer with a cuff of the appropriate size. Refer to Clinical Insight 20-1.
  A cuff that is too small will result in a false-high reading; using a cuff that is too large will result in a false-low reading.
- *Note:* This procedure describes the use of an aneroid manometer or an electronic measuring device.

Delegation

You can delegate measurement of BP to the UAP if the patient's condition and the UAP's skills allow.

- Perform the pre-procedure assessments.
- Inform the UAP of the site (e.g., radial, brachial) to use.
- Inform the UAP of any special considerations (e.g., not to place a BP cuff on the same side as the site of a mastectomy).
- Ask the UAP to record and report the BP to you, and to report immediately if it is outside normal limits (you must specify what is "normal" for each patient).
- Tell the UAP that if BP is elevated, to note which arm, the patient's position during measurement, and activity immediately preceding the measurement.

Pre-Procedure Assessments

- Check for factors or activities that may alter the readings.
  Caffeine, smoking, exercise, and stress can all elevate BP. Be certain the patient has been lying or sitting for at least 5 minutes (30 minutes after strenuous exercise) and is relaxed.
- Check the previous recording, if any.
  Noting changes over time is important with all patient assessments. Because BP changes constantly and because so many factors affect it, you cannot draw conclusions from a single measurement.

➤ When performing the procedure, always identify your patient using two identifiers according to agency policy, using two identifiers, and be attentive to standard precautions, hand hygiene, patient safety and privacy, body mechanics, and documentation.

➤ *Note:* To improve the accuracy of your readings, also refer to Clinical Insights 20-1 and 20-2.

Procedure Steps

1. **Clean the stethoscope before and after** the procedure.
   Although only a small percentage of microorganisms are pathogenic, cleaning can reduce the bacterial count by 94% to 100%.

2. **Place the patient in a comfortable position**, ensuring that:
   a. The legs are uncrossed, the back is supported, and the feet are resting on the floor (if the patient is sitting in a chair); or that the patient is supine.
   This position allows for the most accurate reading. Crossing the legs may elevate the BP reading.
   b. The measurement arm is supported at heart level, slightly flexed, with the palm facing upward.
   BP will decrease if the arm is above the heart and increase if the arm is below the heart or not supported.

3. **Fully expose the arm**, being careful that clothing is not tight. Remove clothing rather than rolling up a sleeve. *Note:* There is some evidence to suggest that readings taken over sleeves do not affect BP results and that it may actually be preferable because of concerns about hygiene, privacy, and religious beliefs (Pinar, Ataalkin, & Watson, 2010). While you are learning, and until there is evidence, we advise that you will find it easier to hear the BP sounds on a bare arm.
   Clothing that is tight enough to restrict blood flow will alter the reading.

4. **Place the cuff** on the upper arm.

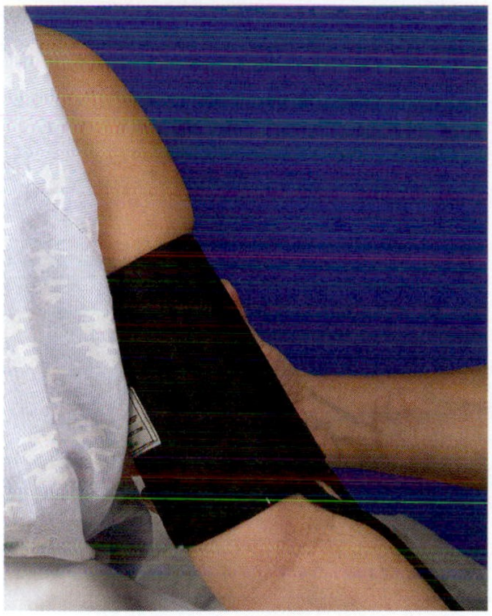

   a. Wrap the cuff snugly.
   b. Ensure that the cuff is totally deflated, and palpate the brachial artery.
   c. Place the bottom edge of the cuff approximately 1 inch (2.5 cm) above the antecubital space.
   d. Place the center of the cuff bladder directly over the brachial artery (the center is often indicated with an arrow on the BP cuff).
   The center of the cuff bladder needs to be directly over the brachial artery to obtain an accurate reading. Loose application of the cuff results in overestimation of BP.

5. **Place the stethoscope ear pieces** in your ears, pointing slightly forward.
   When the earpieces point slightly forward, they direct sound into the ear canal, making the sounds more audible.

6. **Palpate the brachial artery** on the arm with the cuff. (Use the radial artery for this step, if you so prefer.)
   For correct stethoscope placement

7. **Inflate the cuff,** as follows:
   a. Close the sphygmomanometer valve and inflate the cuff rapidly to about 80 mm Hg.
   b. Then, palpate the pulse while you continue inflating in 10 mm Hg increments until you no longer feel the pulse.
   c. As you *inflate* the cuff, the artery is occluded as the pressure of the cuff exceeds the pressure in the artery. At that point, blood flow through the artery is halted, and no sound can be heard. Note the pressure at which the pulse disappears.
   d. Go to step 8 or the variation, as you prefer.
   Palpating the artery while inflating the cuff ensures that the cuff is inflated higher than the systolic BP. If the patient has an auscultatory gap, the systolic pressure can be mistakenly identified as lower than it actually is. Palpation is particularly important if the baseline systolic BP is unknown or if the patient is hypertensive.

8. **Continue inflating the cuff** to a pressure that is 20 to 30 mm Hg above the level at which the pulse disappeared. Move to step 9.
   Helps ensure you will not miss an auscultatory gap or a faint first sound.

Variation: Cuff Inflation Technique

- Do not continue palpating after the pulse disappears; instead, deflate the cuff rapidly.
- Wait 2 minutes, and then place the stethoscope over the brachial artery and inflate the cuff to a pressure that is 20 to 30 mm Hg above the palpated level.
- Continue with steps 9 and 10.

(continued on next page)

Procedure 20-6 ■ Measuring Blood Pressure (continued)

9. **Place the stethoscope over the brachial artery,** as follows:

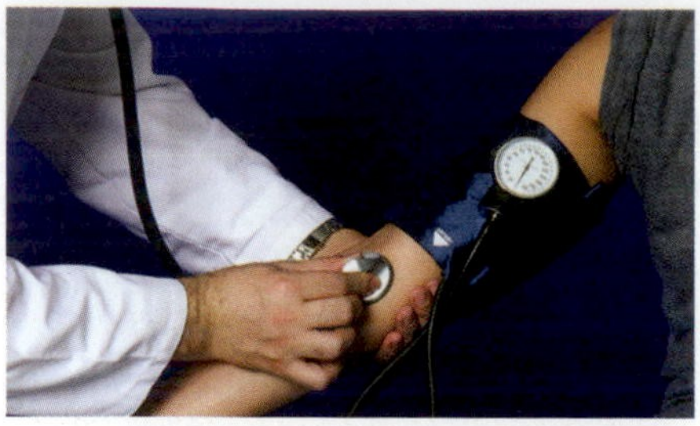

a. Be certain that the stethoscope tubing is not touching anything and that the diaphragm is not tucked under the edge of the cuff.
When the tubing rubs against clothing, for example, it produces artifact sounds that make it difficult to hear the BP sounds. Placing the bell or diaphragm under the cuff can partially occlude the brachial artery, delaying the appearance of the Korotkoff sounds.

b. Using the bell will enable you to hear BP sounds more accurately, especially at diastolic pressures. However, most healthcare providers use the diaphragm because it is easily placed and because some stethoscopes do not have a bell.

10. **Deflate the cuff slowly** (2 to 3 mm Hg per second or per beat), listening for the Korotkoff sounds as you deflate.
Deflating the cuff slowly increases patient discomfort and may alter the reading. Deflating the cuff faster may cause errors in hearing the Korotkoff sounds.

a. As you deflate the cuff, blood begins to flow rapidly through the partially open artery, producing turbulence that you will hear through the stethoscope as a tapping sound. Note the point on the manometer at which you hear the first sound. This is the *systolic BP*. (If you are using an electronic BP device, read the digital screen when the numbers appear. Follow the manufacturer's instructions.)
The 1st Korotkoff sound is the systolic pressure.

b. Continue deflating the cuff, and note the level at which the sounds become muffled and disappear. The artery is no longer compressed and sound will disappear. Record the point at which the sound disappears as the *diastolic pressure*.
The 5th Korotkoff sound (the disappearance of sound) is the diastolic BP in adults. The 4th Korotkoff sound (the muffling of sounds) is the diastolic BP in children. Note: The American Heart Association recommends recording the first sound, muffling, and the last sound in children younger than 13 years of age, pregnant women, and people with high cardiac output or peripheral vasoconstriction.

11. **If you need to repeat** the measurement, deflate the cuff completely, and wait 2 minutes before reinflating it.
Prevents venous congestion and false high readings.

? What if . . .

■ **You cannot feel the brachial pulse?**

While supporting the arm at the elbow, have the patient pronate her forearm.
This moves the brachial artery more over a bony prominence, making the pulsation easier to feel.

■ **You have difficulty hearing BP sounds in many patients?**

You may need a stethoscope with a built-in amplifier.

■ **You are not certain of the systolic reading when you begin to deflate the cuff?**

Do not stop cuff deflation to recheck the systolic reading. Deflate the cuff completely and wait 1 to 3 minutes before taking another measurement.
Stopping deflation and retaking BP too soon can lead to a muffling of the Korotkoff sounds and inaccurate results.

■ **You must use a mercury manometer?**

Because mercury is a health hazard, mercury manometers should not be found in healthcare agencies. Use an aneroid manometer or an electronic BP device, if one is available. If you must use a mercury manometer, be certain the meniscus of the mercury is at eye level when taking the reading. Take care not to bump equipment against the glass cover over the column of mercury.

■ **You are using an automatic BP device?**

Follow the same guidelines as for a manual BP device (e.g., cuff size and placement, patient position).
Turn on the machine; be sure the cuff is deflated.
Apply the cuff.
Press the button to start the measurement.
At the tone, read the digital measurement.

■ **You do not have a cuff size to fit the upper arm?**

Use the forearm, thigh, or calf. See Procedure Variations A, B, and C, respectively.

■ **The patient requires contact or isolation precautions?**

Follow agency guidelines for equipment (e.g., stethoscope, BP cuff). Generally, the equipment remains in the room with the patient; otherwise, it must be disinfected before it is taken out of the room. For information about contact precautions and protective isolation, see Chapter 23, Clinical Insights 23-2, 23-3, and 23-4.

Procedure Variation A: Measuring Blood Pressure in the Forearm

- Place a properly sized cuff on the forearm, midway between the elbow and the wrist. Auscultate over the radial artery.
- Note that a forearm reading is not interchangeable with an upper arm reading.

Procedure Variation B: Measuring Blood Pressure in the Thigh

- Use the thigh or the calf if the cuff will not fit either the upper or lower arm.
  Note: The thigh systolic measure may be 20 to 30 mm Hg higher than an arm BP reading. The diastolic reading is generally comparable.
- Place the patient in a prone position. If patient cannot be prone, place supine, with knees slightly bent.
- Choose the correct cuff size. Wrap the cuff snugly around the thigh so that the lower edge of the cuff is approximately 1 inch (2.5 cm) above the popliteal fossa and the center of the cuff bladder is positioned directly over the popliteal artery (often indicated with an arrow on the BP cuff).
- Palpate and auscultate over the popliteal artery. ➤

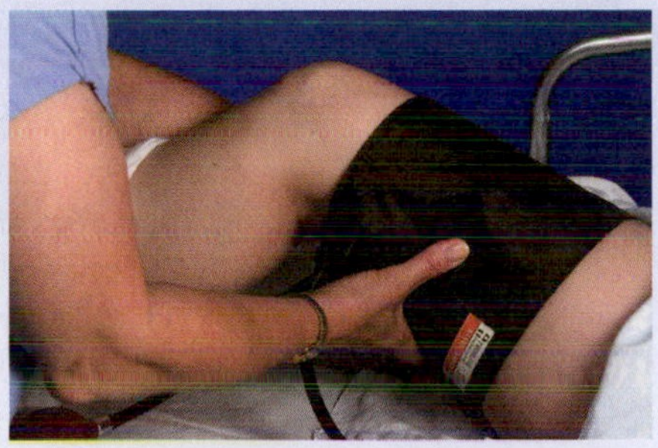

Procedure Variation C: Measuring Blood Pressure in the Calf

- Use the thigh or the calf if the cuff will not fit either the upper or lower arm.
- Place the patient supine.
- Choose the correct size cuff. Wrap the cuff snugly around the calf so that the lower edge of the cuff is approximately 2.5 cm above the malleoli or ankle.
- Place the stethoscope over either the dorsalis pedis or the posterior tibial artery.
  Note: Calf BP measurements are not equivalent to upper arm measurements in adults; they tend to produce a higher systolic BP.

Procedure Variation D: Palpating the Blood Pressure

- Apply the cuff, and palpate for the radial or brachial pulse.
- Begin to inflate the cuff. When you can no longer feel the pulse, inflate the cuff about 30 mm Hg more.
- As you release the valve and slowly deflate the cuff, note the reading on the manometer at which you once again feel the pulse.
- Document the palpated BP according to the way it was assessed (e.g., "Palpated, low Fowler's, left arm 86/——" [or "86 systolic"]).

Evaluation

- Compare the current BP reading with previous readings.
- Look for trends. Is the BP slowly decreasing (e.g., impending shock) or slowly increasing (e.g., hypervolemia)?
- Look for a corresponding change in pulse rate, indicating potential hypoxemia.
- If this is the first BP measurement for the client, check readings in both arms.
  A difference of 10 mm Hg or less is normal.
- Report any significant changes in the BP reading.

Patient Teaching

Teach the patient about:

- Normal BP values (keep in mind that prehypertension is diagnosed at a lower level when using self-monitored readings).
- Significance of the BP reading.
- Further follow-up that may be necessary.

Home Care

- The American Heart Association (AHA) and their guidelines recommend self-monitoring of BP at home. Self-measurement of BP is thought to (1) provide more reliable data compared with office BP measurement because of the ability to obtain multiple readings, and (2) to improve adherence to treatment regimens.
- If possible, use the same equipment each time to prevent false changes in measurement.
- Explain the need for frequent recalibration of the home-monitoring device.
- Assess the skill level of the person(s) who will be measuring the patient's BP in the home, and provide instructions, if necessary.
- Assess whether self-monitoring is causing the client to be anxious.
  Some clients do become overly anxious when they know they must monitor their BP, or when they obtain a high reading. Self-monitoring should not be used if it produces too much anxiety; this raises the BP even more.
- Teach clients not to change their medication dosage without consulting their primary healthcare provider when their BP goes up or down.
- Before leaving the client's home, clean the stethoscope and sphygmomanometer with detergent or disinfectant, when possible; or place them in a plastic bag for transporting to the reprocessing location.
- If the client has an infection with a multidrug-resistant organism, reusable equipment, such as stethoscopes, should remain in the home. If the stethoscope and sphygmomanometer cannot remain in the client's home, clean and disinfect them before leaving by using a low- to intermediate-level disinfectant. If this is not practical, place them in a plastic bag and transport them to another site for cleaning and disinfection.

Documentation

- You will usually document BP on a flowsheet (such as in Procedure 20-5, Documentation).
- Document the BP systolic/diastolic readings (e.g., 130/80 mm Hg).
- If you hear the 4th Korotkoff sound or muffling, document systolic/muffling/diastolic (e.g., 130/80/70 mm Hg). If you hear an auscultatory gap, document "systolic/diastolic with an auscultatory gap from . . ." For example, "170/90 with an auscultatory gap from 170 to 140."

(continued on next page)

Procedure 20-6 ■ Measuring Blood Pressure (continued)

- Follow agency policy regarding the recording of muffled sounds.
- If you chose an alternative site, document the site used and the reason for not using the upper arm.

Practice Resources

Alexis, O. (2010); Alvarez, J., Ruiz, S., Mosqueda, J., et al., (2016); American Heart Association (2016); Charbek, E. (2015); McEvoy, M. (2016)

Thinking About the Procedure

The video, **Measuring Blood Pressure,** along with questions and suggested responses, is available on the ***Davis's Nursing Skills Videos*** Web site on FADavis.com.

CLINICAL INSIGHTS

Clinical Insight 20-1 ➤ Choosing a Blood Pressure Cuff Size

- The *width* of the bladder should cover approximately two-thirds of the *length* of the upper arm (or other extremity) for an adult, and the entire upper arm for a child.
- Another method for sizing:
  1. The cuff width should be 40% of the arm circumference.
  2. The *length* of the bladder should encircle 80% of the arm.
- Perhaps the easiest sizing method is to measure *arm circumference* and follow these guidelines:

For arm circumference	Cuff should be
22–26 cm ($8\frac{1}{2} \times 10\frac{1}{4}$ in.)	"small adult" size: 12 × 22 cm ($4\frac{3}{4} \times 8\frac{3}{4}$ in.)
27–34 cm ($10\frac{1}{2} \times 13\frac{1}{2}$ in.)	"adult" size: 16 × 30 cm ($6\frac{1}{4} \times 11\frac{3}{4}$ in.)
35–44 cm ($13\frac{3}{4} \times 17\frac{1}{4}$ in.)	"large adult" size: 16 × 36 cm ($6\frac{1}{4} \times 14\frac{1}{4}$ in.)
45–52 cm ($17\frac{3}{4} \times 10\frac{1}{2}$ in.)	"adult thigh" size: 16 × 42 cm ($6\frac{1}{4} \times 16\frac{5}{8}$ in.)

Practice Resources:

Mishra, B., Sinha, N., Ur, H. (2017); Pickering, T., Hall, J., Appel, L., et al (2005); Whelton, P., Carey, R., Arownow, W., et al. (2018)

Clinical Insight 20-2 ➤ Taking an Accurate Blood Pressure

To improve your technique and accuracy of measurement, use the following tips in addition to Procedure 20-6.

- Explain the procedure, particularly on admission or when changing the routine.
  Reduces patient anxiety.
- Wait 30 minutes before assessing BP after client has ingested caffeine or has smoked.
- Have the patient empty his bladder.
- Have the patient relax and sit in a chair, with feet on the floor, back supported for at least 5 minutes
- Do not assess BP while the client is in pain.
- Apply the cuff over bare skin, if possible. Advise clients who are home monitoring to remove all clothing covering at the location of cuff placement and to apply the cuff over bare skin.
- Ensure the patient's arm is supported.
- Instruct the client to not talk during BP measurement. You should not talk either.
- Keep environmental noise and client movement to a minimum.
- Hold the stethoscope lightly but completely against the skin; do not put your thumb on top of the bell or diaphragm. Try not to allow the tubing to brush against your clothing or the bed.
- Do not be influenced by the client's previous BP measurements.
- Use the same limb for each measurement, unless you are comparing arms or averaging readings from both arms.
- For the initial reading, measure the BP in both arms and use the arm with the higher reading for subsequent measurements.
- If you obtain an elevated reading, confirm in the other arm.
- Do not draw conclusions based on one reading. Take two or more readings, at least 1 to 2 minutes apart, and average them. If the readings differ by more than 5 mm Hg, obtain and average additional readings.
- Provide the patient with his BP readings orally and in writing.

Practice Resources

Bunker, J. (2014); Tomlinson, B. (2010); Whelton, P., Carey, R., Arownow, W., et al. (2018)

Clinical Insight 20-3 ➤ Teaching Your Client About Hypertension

Teach the Client and Family About Lifestyle Changes for Preventing and Managing Hypertension

- Limit salt intake to 1 teaspoon per day (2,400 mg of sodium).
- Consume a diet high in potassium (e.g., fresh fruits and vegetables, such as bananas, potatoes, and acorn squash).
- Consume a diet high in calcium (e.g., milk and milk products [yogurt], sardines, molasses, tofu).
- Limit alcohol intake to 1 or 2 drinks per day for men; 1 for women. (One drink is a can of beer, one jigger of liquor, or one glass of wine. Wine is preferable.)
- Maintain ideal body weight; lose weight, if overweight.
- For overall cardiovascular health, reduce saturated fat and cholesterol intake.
- Eliminate smoking.
- Engage in aerobic exercise (30 to 45 minutes several days a week, or a total of 150 minutes per week).
- Try to reduce stress and stressful situations.
- Even one lifestyle change has effects similar to treatment with a single antihypertensive drug. More than one change has an even more positive effect on BP.

Teach the Client About Monitoring His Blood Pressure at Home

- Monitor blood pressure at home to determine whether lifestyle modifications and/or medications are effective.
- Keep a record of your BP readings, including date, time, systolic and diastolic measurements, and any information that you want your provider to know.
- Take your BP whenever you experience symptoms such as headaches or dizziness.
- Use an upper arm or wrist BP monitor that has been validated.
- Take your BP equipment when you visit your healthcare provider to check your BP monitor for accuracy.
- Follow the researchers' and manufacturer's guidelines for arm position and recalibration. This is especially true for wrist monitors (Dourmap, Girerd, Marquand, et al., 2010; Zheng, Huang, Sheng, et al., 2012).
- Follow-up assessments are important.

Go to **Table 20-6: Classification of Adult Blood Pressure,** in Volume 1.

Source: Whelton, P., Carey, R., Arownow, W., et al. (2017). 2017 Guideline for the Prevention, Detection, Evaluation, and Treatment of High Blood Pressure in Adults. *Journal of the American College of Cardiology, 23976*. DOI:10.1016/j.jacc.2017.07.745
Whelton, P., Carey, R., Arownow, W., et al., (2018). 2017 ACC/AHA/AAPA/ABC/ACPM/AGS/APhA/ASH/ASPC/NMA/PCNA Guideline for the Prevention, Detection, Evaluation, and Management of High Blood Pressure in Adults. *Journal of the American College of Cardiology, 71*(19), e127–e248. DOI:10.1016/j.jacc.2017.11.006. Retrieved on September 23, 2018, from: http://www.onlinejacc.org/content/71/19/e127?_ga=2.117871433.119615486.1537818239-291529677.1537536713

FORMS
Graphic Flowsheet

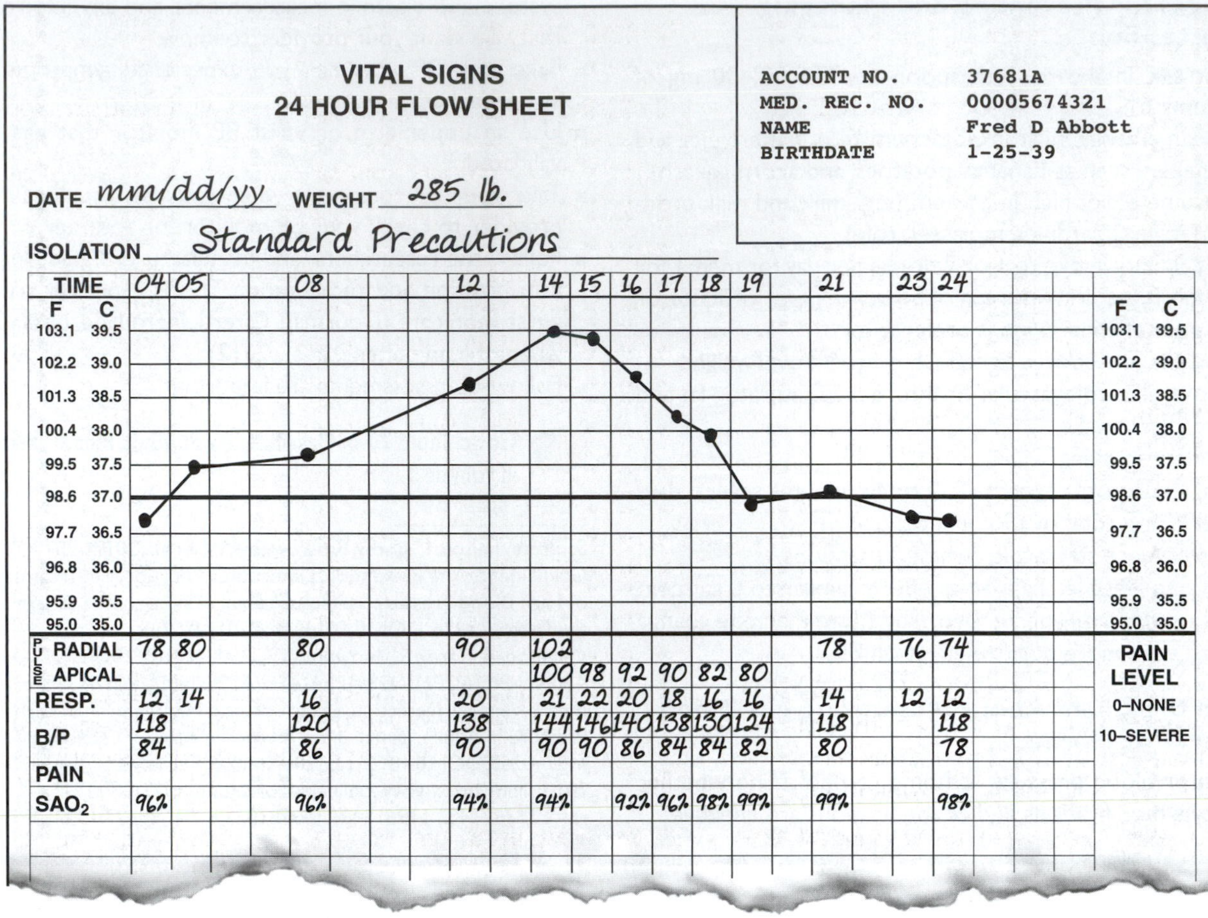

VITAL SIGNS
24 HOUR FLOW SHEET

ACCOUNT NO. 37681A
MED. REC. NO. 00005674321
NAME Fred D Abbott
BIRTHDATE 1-25-39

DATE mm/dd/yy WEIGHT 285 lb.
ISOLATION Standard Precautions

F C: 103.1 39.5; 102.2 39.0; 101.3 38.5; 100.4 38.0; 99.5 37.5; 98.6 37.0; 97.7 36.5; 96.8 36.0; 95.9 35.5; 95.0 35.0

TIME	04	05	08	12	14	15	16	17	18	19	21	23	24
PULSE RADIAL	78	80	80	90	102						78	76	74
PULSE APICAL					100	98	92	90	82	80			
RESP.	12	14	16	20	21	22	20	18	16	16	14	12	12
B/P	118/84		120/86	138/90	144/90	146/90	140/86	138/84	130/84	124/82	118/80		118/78
PAIN													
SAO_2	96%		96%	94%	94%		92%	96%	98%	99%	99%		98%

PAIN LEVEL
0–NONE
10–SEVERE

CLINICALJUDGMENT
Applying the Full-Spectrum Nursing Model

PATIENT SITUATION

A patient in the critical care unit had a stable pulse and BP for the first few days. He has become more ill, and now his pulse and BP are weak and difficult to palpate. His last BP reading was abnormally low, so it must be monitored frequently. He is receiving intravenous fluids in both arms.

THINKING

1. *Critical Thinking (Reflecting and Deciding What to Do):* Which of the patient's vital signs (TPR and BP) might you delegate to a UAP?

DOING

2. *Practical Knowledge:* How would you take the patient's blood pressure? Be specific:
   a. What site would you use?
   b. What equipment would you use?

3. *Nursing Process (Assessment):*

   a. Will you need to validate any of the vital signs you obtain? If so, why?

   b. How could you validate those vital signs?

CARING

4. Assume that you are very busy. How would you demonstrate caring to this patient while you are assessing his vital signs (the ones you did not delegate to a UAP)?

Critical Thinking and Clinical Judgment

1. Recall the clients in the Meet Your Patients scenario (in Volume 1 of your textbook). Two-year-old Jason's oral temperature was 101.8°F (38.8°C), and his skin was warm, dry, and flushed. His mother told you that he had been eating poorly and was very irritable. What cues alert you that something is wrong?

2. You have already established (in Think Like a Nurse 20-3, in Volume 1 of your textbook) what, if any, additional information you need to determine the meaning of Jason's temperature elevation.

   a. What theoretical knowledge may account for Jason's temperature?

   b. Are there any actions you should take while meeting with Jason and his mother? If so, what?

   c. What biases do you have that affect your thinking about this situation? (This requires self-knowledge.)

3. Suppose you have the following data: In a long-term care center, where most patients are older, the average normal oral temperature of the patients is 97.1°F (36.2°C). In a local well-baby nursery, the average skin temperature of the newborns ranges from 97.7°F to 98.6°F (36.5°C to 37.0°C), but it fluctuates during the first 24 hours after birth. At a walk-in surgery center, the average oral temperature of the healthy clients is 98°F (36.7°C).

   a. What conclusion might you draw about what is causing the differences in average body temperature among these three groups? (*Clue:* First list the average temperatures in order, from highest to lowest.)

   b. What theoretical knowledge did you use to answer that question?

4. Suppose you have the following data about patients' temperatures:

   Patient A, 58 years old: 0600, 97.7°F (36.5°C); 1200, 98.8°F (37.1°C); 2100, 99°F (37.2°C)

   Patient B, 14 years old: 0600, 97.5°F (36.4°C); 1200, 97.9°F (36°C); 2100, 98.4°F (36.9°C)

   Patient C, 80 years old: 0600, 96.4°F (35.8°C); 1200, 96.8°F (37.1°C); 2100, 97.2°F (36.2°C)

   What conclusion can you draw about what is probably affecting the patients' temperatures? (*Clue:* Look at the pattern for each patient. How are the patterns similar?)

5. Organize a small group of classmates. Obtain several different sizes of blood pressure cuffs for each member of the group. Practice checking blood pressure on each other. Vary the size of the cuffs used, and note the variation generated by the change in cuff size. List your findings here (for at least three different people and at least two cuff sizes).

	Cuff Size		
BP READING	**LARGE**	**MEDIUM**	**SMALL**
Person A			
Person B			
Person C			

6. Analyze the following scenario. A 46-year-old man is hospitalized for multiple trauma after a mountain bike accident.

   Vital signs on admission: BP, 138/90; P, 108 beats/min; R, 24 breaths/min; T, 98.9°F (37.2°C)

   8 hours later: BP, 162/100; P, 122 beats/min; R, 26 breaths/min; T, 37.9°C (100.2°F)

   He is restless, agitated, and in pain.

   a. What is going on in this situation that may be influencing the VS?

   b. Do you have enough patient information to determine what is happening?

   c. What nursing actions should you consider?

   d. Should you involve others in your discussion of possible actions? If so, who?

   e. What can you delegate in this situation?

   f. Should you report this change in vital signs to the primary care provider? Why, or why not?

7. Ms. Alvin is an 80-year-old patient in a long-term care facility. Her blood pressures have been in the range of 120/70 to 130/80 mm Hg for the past month. When she is newly assigned to your care, you see that according to her medical records, she has a history of hypertension. She is taking an antihypertensive medication. You observe that she is very thin, especially her extremities. She weighs only 90 lb (40.8 kg), although she is of average height.

   a. Do you think the charted BP readings are probably accurate? Why, or why not?

   b. How could you make sure that the recorded BP readings are accurate?

   c. After looking for a small BP cuff, you discover that there is only one size available in the agency: a standard adult size. What should you do?

8. For each of the following concepts, use critical thinking to describe how or why it is important to nursing, patient care, and measuring vital signs. Note that these are not to be merely definitions.

   Vital signs

   Circadian rhythm

   Metabolism

   Shivering

   Fever

   Pulse

   Stethoscope

   Radial artery

   Brachial artery

   Apical pulse

   Diaphragm

   Oxygen saturation and pulse oximetry

   Blood pressure

   Peripheral resistance

What Are the Main Points in This Chapter?

- Vital signs (temperature, pulse, respirations, and blood pressure) are indicators of a person's state of health and functioning of the body systems.
- Many factors, such as age, activity, smoking, and gender, cause normal variations in vital signs.
- Body temperature is the balance between heat production and heat loss.
- Fever is a symptom, but it is also beneficial to the immune response.
- A normal pulse rate varies widely according to age, from an average of 120 beats/min for newborns to 80 beats/min for adults.
- Assess the pulse for quality, bilateral equality, volume, and rate.
- Respiration is the process of supplying the body with oxygen and disposing of carbon dioxide.
- Assess respirations for rate, depth, rhythm, and associated clinical signs (e.g., breath sounds, chest movement, cough, pallor, and cyanosis).
- Blood pressure is the pressure of the blood as it is forced against arterial walls during cardiac contraction.
- Normal blood pressure in an adult is a systolic reading of less than 120 mm Hg and a diastolic reading of less than 80 mm Hg, based on an average of two or more readings taken on two or more occasions.
- The "elevated" classification for blood pressure has a systolic reading between 120 and 129 mm Hg systolic and diastolic reading less than 80 mm Hg, based on an average of two or more readings taken on two or more occasions.
- Hypertension, stage 1 is systolic reading between 130 and 139 mm Hg or diastolic reading between 80 and 89 mm Hg, based on an average of two or more readings taken on two or more occasions.
- Hypertension, stage 2 is systolic reading of 140 mm Hg greater or a diastolic reading of 90 mm Hg or greater, based on an average of two or more readings taken on two or more occasions.
- Clients can prevent or control hypertension through certain lifestyle changes (e.g., exercise, weight control, diet, and stress management).
- Nurses can delegate the activity of taking vital signs, but they are responsible for evaluating the meaning of the data.

Knowledge Map

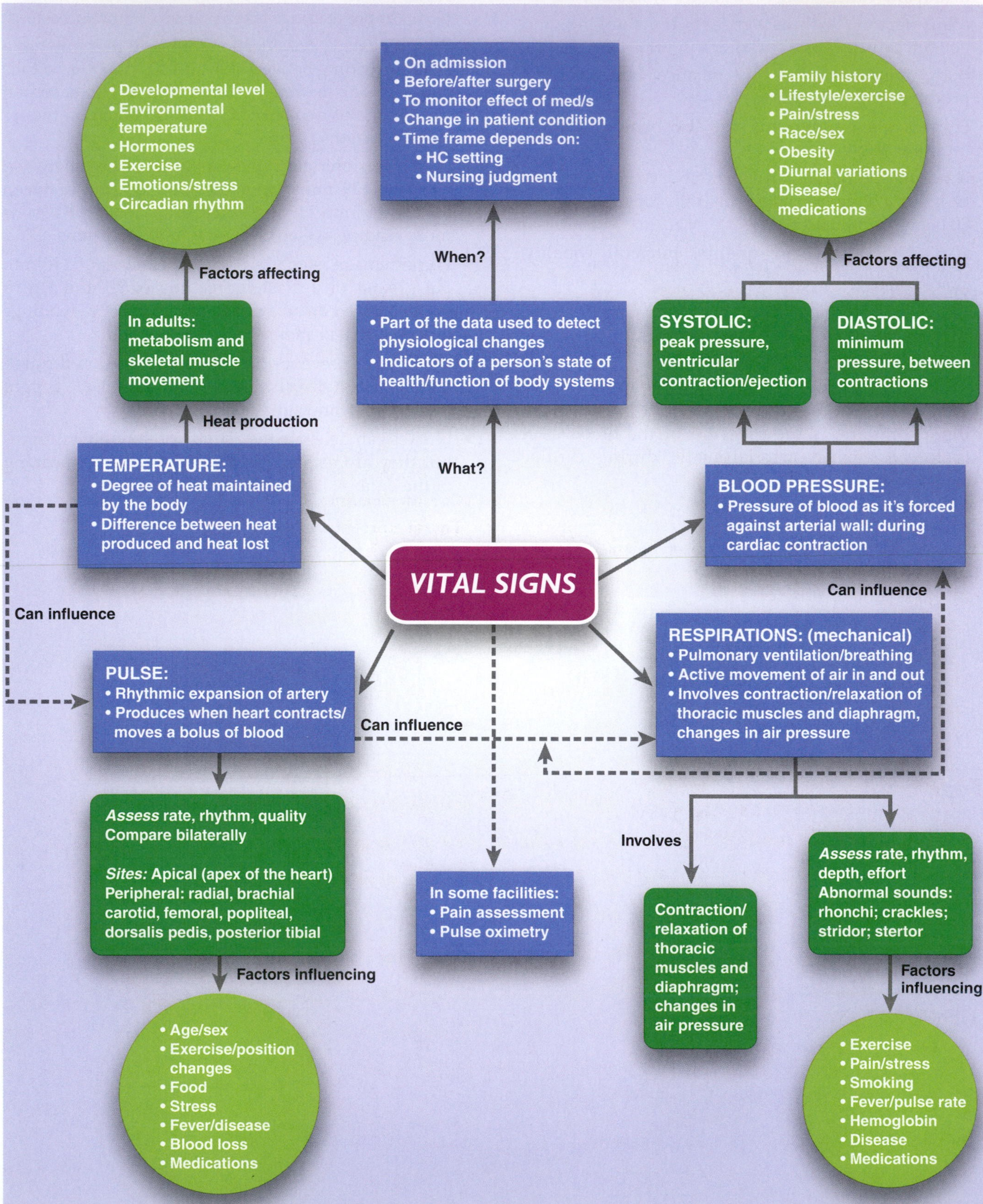

CHAPTER 21

Communication & Therapeutic Relationships

STUDENT RESOURCES

The questions and exercises in this book allow you to practice the kind of thinking you will use as a full-spectrum nurse. Critical-thinking questions usually have more than one right answer, so we do not provide "correct answers" for these features. Try to answer these questions yourself. It is more important to develop your nursing judgment than to just cover content. You will learn more by discussing the questions with your peers. If you are still unsure, see the Davis Advantage chapter resources for suggested responses.

To explore learning resources for this chapter,

Go to Davis Advantage and find:

Answers and Suggested Responses for all questions in this chapter
Concept Map
Knowledge Map
References and Bibliography
Lists of NOC Outcomes and NIC Interventions

Key Concepts

Communication
Communication techniques
Therapeutic relationships

Related Concepts

See the Concept Map on Davis Advantage.

Caring for the Nguyens

Below is a transcript of an interaction that occurred during Nam Nguyen's first visit to the family healthcare clinic. As you may recall, Zach Jackson is a family nurse practitioner who is examining Nam Nguyen. Analyze the interaction. Identify open-ended and closed-ended questions and therapeutic communication techniques. Comment on responses that Zach might have improved on.

Zach: "Are your parents still living?"
Nam: "Yes, they're both alive. My father is 80 years old, and my mother is 76."

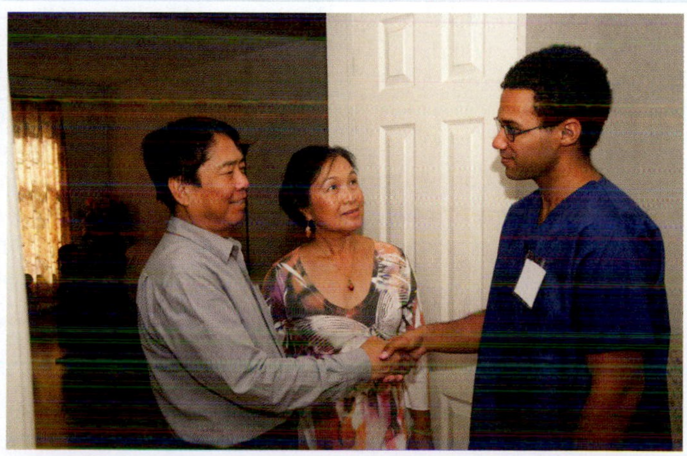

(Continued)

Caring for the Nguyens (continued)

Zach: "I'd like to hear a little more about your family's history. Tell me about your father's cancer. How old was he when he was first diagnosed? Has he had treatment?"

Nam: "He was probably about 60 when he first found out about it. I know he had some kind of surgery and takes medicines, but I don't know the details. He seems all right, though."

Zach: "Your father also has high blood pressure and heart disease. Please tell me a little more about that."

Nam: "My father and mother both have high blood pressure and heart disease. They both take medication for their blood pressure. My father had a small heart attack about 10 years ago. My mother has never had a heart attack that I know of, but she sometimes has chest pain."

Zach: "Your mother also has diabetes?"

Nam: "She's had that for a long time. A lot of people in my family, especially on my father's side, have diabetes, but nobody in my mother's family. Yet my mother is the one with diabetes!"

Yen: "A lot of people in my family have diabetes, too. But so far, I'm okay, I think.

Zach: "Have you had a health exam lately, Mrs. Nguyen?"

Yen: "Not in about a year, but I'm going to schedule an appointment here."

Practical Knowledge Clinical Application

This section provides clinical insights and assessments for communicating with patients.

CLINICAL INSIGHTS

Clinical Insight 21-1 ➤ Enhancing Communication Through Nonverbal Behaviors

Nonverbal Behaviors	Interpretation
Direct eye contact	■ Demonstrates interest and attention. Consider the client's cultural heritage when determining how much eye contact is appropriate.
Concerned facial expression	■ Lends credibility, if congruent with conversation.
Leaning forward	■ Shows interest in the conversation.
Personal space	■ Maintaining a distance of 18 inches to 4 feet allows most clients to feel comfortable during the interaction. Adjust the distance within that range, according to the client's preference.
Professional appearance	■ Gives people an impression of how you may act in your role as a healthcare provider.
Sitting down to talk	■ Communicates willingness to listen and a sense of not wanting to rush the interaction with the client.
Touch	■ Conveys caring and concern when used appropriately.

Clinical Insight 21-2 ➤ Communicating With SBARQ

Situation	In 10 seconds, identify yourself and the patient and describe the present situation that prompted you to call. State: ■ Your name ■ Your unit ■ The patient's name and room number ■ The problem
Background	Give other information pertinent to the situation—not the patient's entire history since admission, but circumstances leading up to the situation (e.g., medications, laboratory results, current symptoms).
Assessment	State the problem and what you think is causing it. This is an inference rather than traditional data collection.
Recommendation	State what you think will correct the problem, or what you need from the physician.
Question	■ Allow the patient an opportunity to ask or answer any questions. ■ Review specific concerns.

*For more information about SBARQ, see Chapter 18, Clinical Insight 18-1: Giving Oral Reports. Also,

Go to **Chapter 18,** in Volume 1.

Practice Resources

Bloom, L., Petersson, P., Hagell, P., et al., 2015; Institute for Healthcare Improvement (n. d.); Lancaster, R. J., Westphal, J., & Jambunathan, G., 2015.

Clinical Insight 21-3 ➤ Communicating With Clients From Another Culture

Cultural Sensitivity

- Most important: Be aware of your own cultural beliefs and attitudes.
- Learn about other cultures, especially those in your area.
- Convey empathy, and show respect.
- Be certain the communication strategies you usually use are culturally appropriate for the individual.
  - Is direct eye contact viewed as aggressive or impolite? Or is it perceived as being engaged and caring?
  - How much space should you maintain between yourself and the patient?
- Use touch cautiously. In some cultures, it is inappropriate to touch certain parts of the body.
- Proceed slowly. Rushing may cause the patient to be more anxious and is offensive to some.
- Smile and be polite, but not overfriendly or casual. Use the patient's title and last name when introducing yourself.
- Use short words and sentences. Do not give too much information in one sentence.
- Present one idea at a time.
- Provide written teaching materials.

If There Is a Language Barrier

- Written information provided must be appropriate to the population served and the language of the patient (The Joint Commission, 2010, p. 10).
- Use a trained medical interpreter, if possible.
- To review guidelines for communicating with clients who speak a different language, see Chapter 15, Clinical Insight 15-2: Communicating with Clients Who Speak a Different Language, in this volume.
- Some medical dictionaries or Web-based resources have a comprehensive list of English–Spanish phrases.

(Continued)

Clinical Insight 21-3 ➤ Communicating With Clients From Another Culture *(continued)*

- The following are some useful Spanish words and phrases.

English	*Spanish*	*English*	*Spanish*
How do you feel?	¿Como se siente?	Cough	Tosa
Good	Bien	Open your mouth	Abra la boca
Bad	Mal	Take a deep breath	Respire profundamente
Have you any difficulty breathing?	¿Tiene dificultad al respirar?	You may eat	Puede comer
		Tea	Té
Are you thirsty?	¿Tiene sed?	Coffee	Café
Have you any pain?	¿Tiene dolor?	I will give you something for	Le dare algo para eso
Show me where	Enséñeme dónde	A pill	Una píldora
Is it worse now?	¿Está peor ahora?		

Clinical Insight 21-4 ➤ Communicating With Clients Who Have Impaired Cognition or Consciousness

Patients Who Are Cognitively or Developmentally Impaired or With Dementia

Always try to communicate.	Make every effort to communicate, even if you think that the client cannot understand you.
Address the patient slowly (not more loudly) and from the front.	Convey nonthreatening approach with a friendly demeanor and direct eye contact. Impaired cognition does not mean the person has difficulty hearing.
Do not rush the patient.	Provide adequate time to allow the patient to communicate. Patients need time to respond to your questions or commands.
Use multiple communication modalities.	Provide verbal and written discharge instructions. Review the instructions several times with the patient before discharge, and include family members in the teaching.
Provide reminders.	Use memory aids, schedules, and reminder notices to reinforce information.
Orient the client.	Verbally orient to time, person, and place, and provide visual orientation materials, such as a calendar or schedule.
Eliminate distractions.	Background noise, such as from a TV or smartphone, can interfere with the patient's ability to concentrate and follow your communication.
Stimulate memory.	If the patient loses his or her place in the conversation, stimulate memory by repeating the last expressed thought. For instance, you might say, "We were talking about your back pain. Tell me more about your back pain." Or if the patient cannot "find" the word, encourage him to instead describe that word. This will reduce frustration.
Use short sentences.	Use short sentences containing a single thought, such as "Are you hungry?" Avoid complex statements. You could say, "You look hungry. Would you like a sandwich or a milk shake, or can you hold off until dinner?"
Ask "yes/no" questions.	Ask direct questions that require only a yes or no answer. ("Are you hungry?")
Ask one question at a time.	Likewise, when giving instructions, be sure to take a step at a time.
Limit choices.	Limit choices to avoid confusing or frustrating the patient.
Be concrete and specific.	Do not use vague comments to indicate that you are listening. The patient may be unable to interpret such comments as "I see." Instead, repeat the patient's words, and directly state your response. "You are cold. I will bring you a blanket."

Clinical Insight 21-4 ➤ Communicating With Clients Who Have Impaired Cognition or Consciousness *(continued)*

Avoid slang and jargon.	The patient may not understand these. For instance, if you say to your patient, "Are you cool?" she might think you mean body temperature when you might actually mean, "Are you feeling okay?"
Use gestures.	Model desired behaviors. You might say, "Brush your teeth now," and then enact brushing your teeth.
Do not assume.	Bear in mind that patients cannot behave differently and that they may be confused about reality. When they are talking about superficial, routine matters, they may seem more competent than they are.

Clients with Expressive Difficulties

- If you are sure of the word the person is trying to say, repeat it. Do not guess, though.
- Pay close attention to nonverbal communication.
- Assess for and anticipate unmet needs, such as hunger, thirst, and pain.
- Respond to the emotion, not the words.
- Do not reprimand the patient if he or she curses or is aggressive.

Patients Who Are Unconscious

- Touch and speak to unconscious or sedated patients; advise them of the care that you are providing. Although these patients may not be able to respond, they may be able to hear your comments.
- Consult with previous caregivers or the family to determine what the patient responds to.
- Begin each interaction by identifying yourself and addressing the patient by name.
- Speak calmly and slowly, even if the patient does not seem to be alert and oriented.
- Explain all healthcare procedures as you are performing them.
- Provide soothing music and periods of rest.

Patients Who Have Suffered a Stroke

- Remember that many stroke survivors may have trouble communicating their thoughts. They also commonly experience emotional ups and downs. Do not take these moods personally.
- With patients who have aphasia, speak more slowly, not more loudly. Be careful not to use a patronizing tone.
- Be a good listener, and allow time for the patient to express her thoughts.
- **Augmentative and alternative communication** (AAC) might be helpful to patients experiencing expressive aphasia. AAC includes all forms of communication other than speech, such as communication boards and electronic devices, to express thoughts, needs, wants, and ideas.

Practice Resources

Alzheimer's Society (2015, July); American Heart Association (2015); American Speech-Language-Hearing Association (n.d.); deVries, K. (2013, May); Zembrzuski, C. (2013, revised).

ASSESSMENT GUIDELINES AND TOOLS

Focused Assessment

Communication

A focused assessment should identify factors that alter a patient's ability to receive, understand, and transmit verbal and nonverbal messages.

Medications

- Is the patient taking medications that might interfere with speech, cognition, or level of consciousness?
- Does the patient use alcohol or other substances? Is he intoxicated?

Language Barriers

- What is the patient's primary language?
- Does the patient have sufficient command of the dominant language?
- Is an interpreter (foreign language or sign language) required?
- Can the patient read and write? At what level, and in what language?

Cognitive Function

Communication difficulties may signal cognitive impairment. Look for history of developmental delays and pathology or injury of the central nervous system.

- What is the patient's level of consciousness?
- Is there short-term memory loss or long-term memory loss, or both?
- Is intellectual function at, below, or above expectations for age?
- Can the patient read simple instructions?
- Can the patient follow simple spoken instructions?
- Can the patient understand a yes-or-no choice?
- Are there symptoms or a diagnosis of mental illness or dementia?
- If the patient is unconscious, are there nonverbal responses that indicate she can hear you (e.g., blinking, moving the head, squeezing your hand)?

Hearing

- Ask the patient, and observe, whether there are hearing problems.
- Is the patient wearing a hearing aid? If so, is it working properly? Does the patient appear to be reading your lips?
- Is the patient trying to use sign language to communicate?
- Refer to Chapter 22 for tests of hearing (e.g., ticking watch).

Vision

- Is the patient wearing glasses or contact lenses?
- Is the patient able to see adequately?
- Refer to Chapter 22 for vision tests.

Also see Chapter 22, **Procedure 22-20: Brief Bedside Assessment,** in this volume.

Aphasia

- Is there a history of stroke, or a diagnosis of aphasia?
- Is there receptive aphasia (inability to receive or interpret verbal or nonverbal messages)?
- Is there expressive aphasia (inability to express verbal or nonverbal messages)?

Physiological Barriers

Does the patient have conditions that cause difficulty speaking, such as:

- Dyspnea?
- Artificial airway?
- Oral problems, such as poorly fitted dentures?
- Cleft palate or other structural problems?

Communication Style

- Is it difficult to understand what the patient says (e.g., slurring words, stuttering, inability to pronounce certain sounds)?
- Does the patient speak readily or refuse to speak?
- Does the patient speak slowly or rapidly? Spontaneously or hesitantly?
- Is the vocabulary adequate for the purpose needed?
- Has the vocabulary changed from the person's normal vocabulary?

Other

- Are verbal communication and nonverbal communication congruent?

CLINICALJUDGMENT

Applying the Full-Spectrum Nursing Model

Choose *two* of the following communication techniques and plan to consciously use them with your next patient. Use the following thinking, doing, and caring questions to reflect on your interaction.

- Active listening
- Communicating assertively by making "I" statements
- Restating a message
- Clarifying messages
- Validating messages
- Sharing observations about body language
- Asking open-ended questions
- Using silence
- Summarizing the conversation

THINKING

1. *Critical Thinking (Contextual Awareness):* Before you have the conversation, make a note of what is going on in the situation (e.g., values, environment, culture) that might influence the effectiveness of the two techniques you will be using.

DOING

2. *Nursing Process (Assessment):* Before using the two techniques, assess for factors that might affect the patient's ability to communicate. Make a note of them.

3. *Nursing Process (Implementation):* As soon as possible after using the techniques, record the conversations. Try to remember the exact words.

4. *Nursing Process (Evaluation):* Evaluate your ability to use the two techniques you chose.
   a. Did you use them at appropriate times in the conversations—as an appropriate response to something the patient said?
   b. What effect did what you said have on the interaction? How did the patient respond to what you said?
   c. Do you think your communication was therapeutic for the patient?

CARING

5. *Self-Knowledge:*
   a. What were your thoughts and feelings before, during, and after the interaction?
   b. In what way has your comfort level with these two techniques changed?
   c. Describe the type of patient or situation in which you would be the least confident in your ability to communicate therapeutically.

Critical Thinking and Clinical Judgment

1. Mrs. Washington arrives at the clinic complaining of a painful lump in her left breast. She is 40 years old and appears very nervous. She tells you, "I was afraid to come in, but I guess I have to find out what this is."
   a. How might you acknowledge Mrs. Washington's feelings? Give examples.
   b. What might you say to clarify and validate her messages?
   c. Write a hypothetical conversation with Mrs. Washington that:
      - Acknowledges her feelings
      - Establishes trust

- Explores the issue
- Clarifies and validates her messages
- Uses silence
- Summarizes the conversation

2. Paramedics bring a 35-year-old man and his 14-year-old son to the emergency department (ED). Both have been involved in a recreational vehicle gas explosion and have suffered burns. The son is placed in one of the trauma rooms adjacent to his father. He has partial and full-thickness burns over his face, neck, chest, arms, and hands, and he is unresponsive. The father has partial-thickness burns on his right hand and forearm. He appears to be in a lot of pain and is screaming for his son in Spanish. He speaks limited English. Thirty minutes later, his wife (who is also the boy's mother) arrives at the ED. She is crying and asking whether her husband and son will be okay. Her English is fluent.
   a. Identify at least two interventions that can help you communicate with the father.
   b. What kind of body language would you expect from the father?
   c. How could you show acceptance of and establish trust with the father?
   d. Identify at least two factors that will influence communication with the son.
   e. Identify at least two communication strategies to use with the son.
   f. Explain or give an example of how to use the following techniques as you communicate with the anxious wife and mother:
      - Establishing trust
      - Using silence
      - Offering nonverbal support

3. For each of the following concepts, use critical thinking to describe how or why it is important to nursing, patient care, or communication. Note that these are *not* to be merely definitions.

Verbal communication

Nonverbal communication

Intrapersonal communication

Interpersonal communication

Group communication

Therapeutic communication

Therapeutic relationship

Barriers to therapeutic communication

Distance between sender and receiver

Communication strategies

What Are the Main Points in This Chapter?

- Communication is a dynamic, reciprocal process of sending and receiving messages.
- Communication occurs on three levels: intrapersonal, or self-talk; interpersonal (between two or more people); and group communication.
- The sender delivers a message to the receiver via verbal and/or nonverbal communication. The receiver provides feedback to the sender.
- Verbal communication is the use of spoken and written words.
- Nonverbal communication, sometimes called *body language*, communicates how someone is feeling and gives a more accurate account of an individual's true sentiment.
- Physical development, maturity, language skills, intellectual abilities, culture, gender, roles, and relationships influence the communication process.
- Collaborative professional communication is assertive without being aggressive.
- Communication is most successful in a comfortable environment. A favorable environment is quiet, private, free of unpleasant smells, and at a comfortable temperature.
- The distance between individuals engaged in communication is affected by the relationship of the individuals, the nature of the conversation, the setting, and cultural influences.
- Relationships affect the choice of vocabulary, tone of voice, use of gestures, and distance associated with the communication.
- Therapeutic communication is the use of communication skills that results in a positive effect on client care; it is the foundation of professional nursing practice.
- Therapeutic communication occurs in the context of a helping relationship. The helping relationship has four phases: preinteraction, orientation, working phase, and termination.
- Group communication occurs when you are interacting with a family, a community, or a committee. Groups may be focused on a task, self-improvement, coping skills, or work-related issues.
- To enhance communication, listen actively, establish trust, be assertive, restate messages, clarify and validate messages, interpret body language, share observations, explore issues, use silence, summarize the conversation, and make use of process recordings while you are learning.
- Barriers to communication include asking too many questions; asking why; fire-hosing information; changing the subject inappropriately; failing to listen; failing to probe; expressing approval or disapproval; offering advice; providing false reassurance; stereotyping; and using patronizing language.
- Language barriers, sensory perceptual alterations, impaired cognitive skills, and physiological barriers make therapeutic communication challenging, but nursing activities can enhance communication with these clients.

Knowledge Map

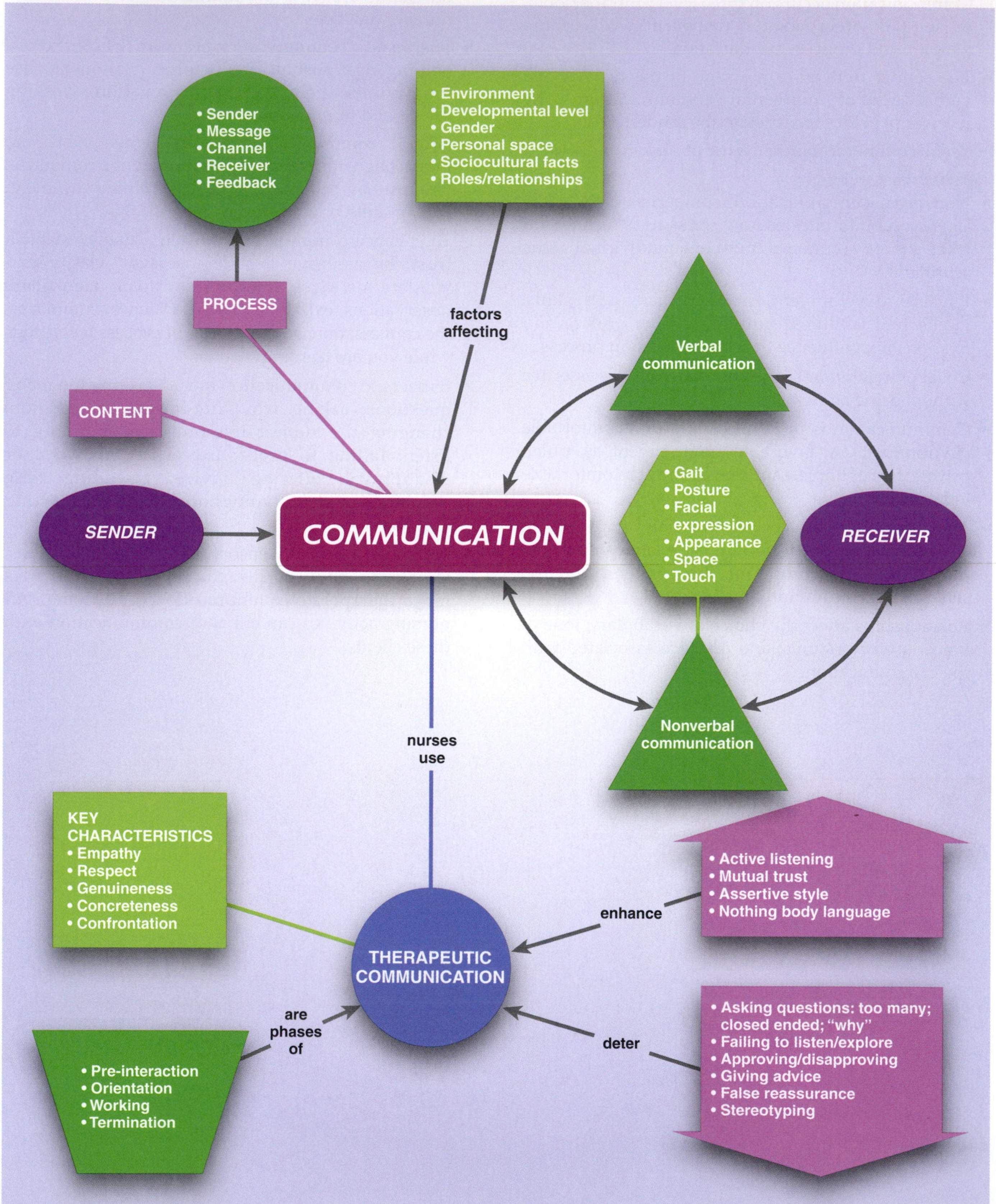

CHAPTER 22

Health Assessment

STUDENT RESOURCES

The questions and exercises in this book allow you to practice the kind of thinking you will use as a full-spectrum nurse. Critical-thinking questions usually have more than one right answer, so we do not provide "correct answers" for these features. Try to answer these questions yourself. It is more important to develop your nursing judgment than to just cover content. You will learn more by discussing the questions with your peers. If you are still unsure, see the Davis Advantage chapter resources for suggested responses.

To explore learning resources for this chapter,

Go to Davis Advantage and find:

Answers and Suggested Responses for all questions in this chapter
Concept Map
Knowledge Map
References and Bibliography
Lists of NOC Outcomes and NIC Interventions

Key Concepts

Health assessment
Nursing assessment
Physical examination

Related Concepts

See the Concept Map on Davis Advantage.

Caring for the Nguyens

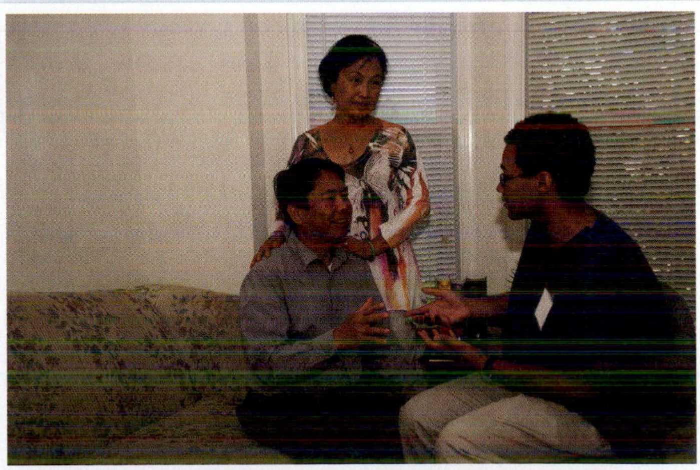

Nam Nguyen has had a comprehensive physical examination with Zach Miller, the nurse practitioner. To review the note written by Zach,

Go to Chapter 22, **Documenting Physical Examination Findings,** in Volume 1.

Also, for laboratory data for Nam Nguyen

Go to Chapter 22, **Laboratory Data for Nam Nguyen,** in Volume 1.

(Continued)

Caring for the Nguyens (continued)

A. Discuss how each of the following would differ from the examination Zach Miller conducted and what would be expected if:
- A registered nurse conducted the exam.
- A nursing student performed the exam.

B. Review Zach's documentation of the exam. Identify the abnormal findings.

C. Review the laboratory work. Identify the abnormal findings.

D. What conclusions, if any, can you draw from these findings? What actions should you consider based on these conclusions?

E. Identify at least two nursing diagnoses based on these findings.

F. Zach Miller has identified a problem of obesity for Mr. Nguyen.
- What information do you need to determine the etiology of this problem?
- Because you do not have that information, write a two-part diagnostic statement describing Mr. Nguyen's nutritional status.

G. Now rewrite the nutrition statement as a three-part statement, using "as evidenced by."

H. Zach Miller has identified the diagnosis Pain (in knees) for Mr. Nguyen. If the pain is caused by a medical condition, such as osteoarthritis, how would you write a two-part diagnostic statement to describe this health status?

I. How would the examination of Yen Nguyen differ from the exam Nam experienced?

J. How would the examination of Kim Phan, Nam's 3-year-old grandson, differ?

K. If you were responsible for examining Nam Nguyen, what aspects of the exam would you find most challenging? Explain why.

PracticalKnowledge ClinicalApplication

PROCEDURES

Key Point: ***As the RN, you are responsible for (1) performing the initial assessment to establish a baseline and (2) performing follow-up assessments for any changes.*** You can instruct unlicensed assistive personnel (UAPs) to report any changes to you. You can delegate measurement of height, weight, and vital signs to the UAP. However, you may want to obtain the first set of vital signs yourself because they will serve as a baseline.

Together, the procedures in this section represent a comprehensive physical examination you can use for initial and ongoing physical assessments. Procedure 22-20 provides a brief bedside assessment. The following procedures are described mainly for adult patients. To review ways in which to modify your examination for people of different ages,

Go to Chapter 22, **Modifications for Different Age Groups**, in Volume 1.

Also, note the following:

- **Developmental Modifications** for various age groups are given just before the procedure steps. Use these to help adapt your examination techniques to the specific patient.
- **Developmental Variations** are provided in the procedure in column 2, under Expected and Abnormal findings. Use these when you are analyzing assessment findings.

Key Point: ***Compare side to side throughout the examination.***

Procedure 22-1 ■ Performing the General Survey

➤ For steps to follow in *all* procedures, refer to the Universal Steps for All Procedures found on the inside back cover.

Equipment

See Equipment Needed for Physical Examination, below.

Equipment Needed for Physical Examination

Usual Equipment for Ongoing Assessment

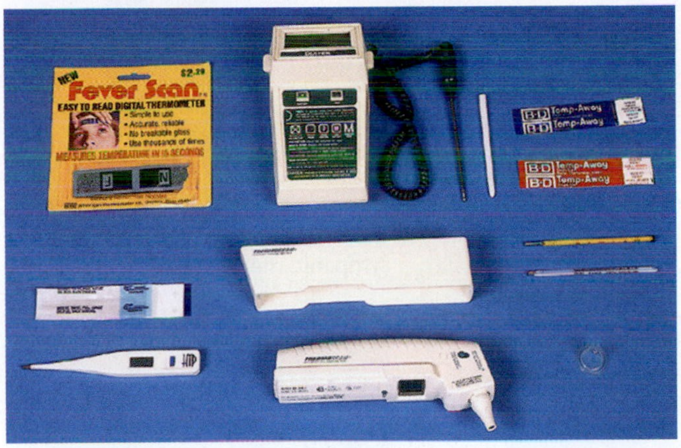

Thermometer (for measuring temperature)

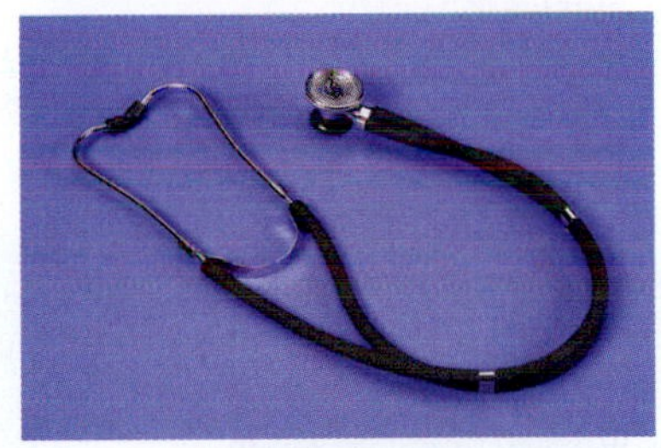

Stethoscope (for measuring blood pressure and listening to heart, lung, and bowel sounds)

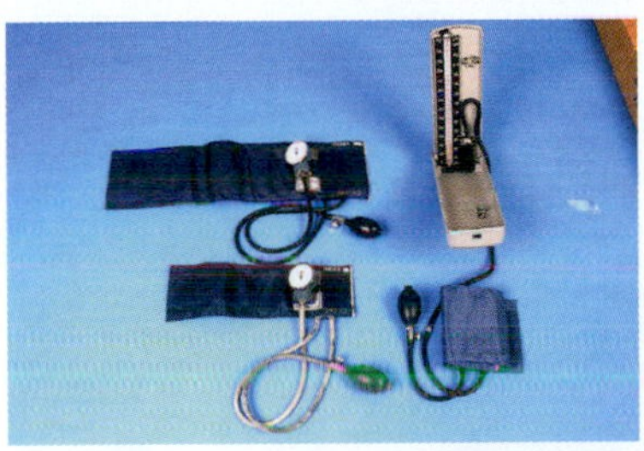

Sphygmomanometer (for measuring blood pressure)

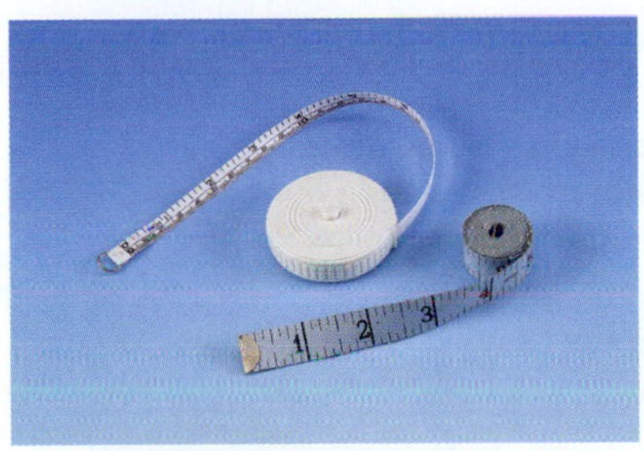

Tape measure (to measure circumference and length)

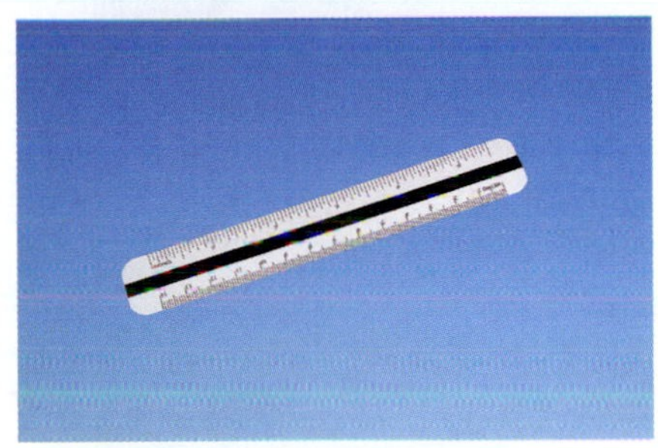

Pocket ruler (to measure size or distance)

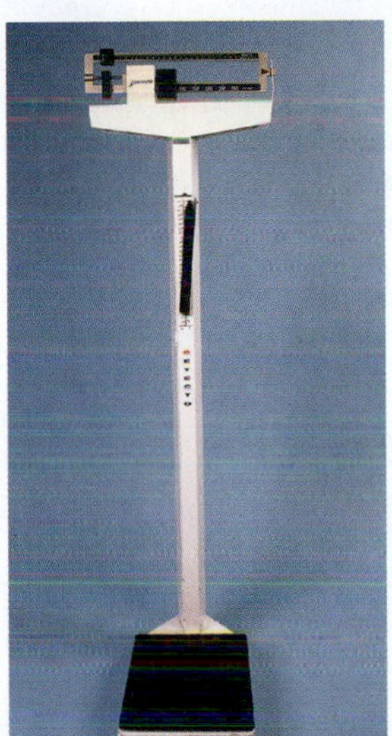

Scale (to measure weight and height)

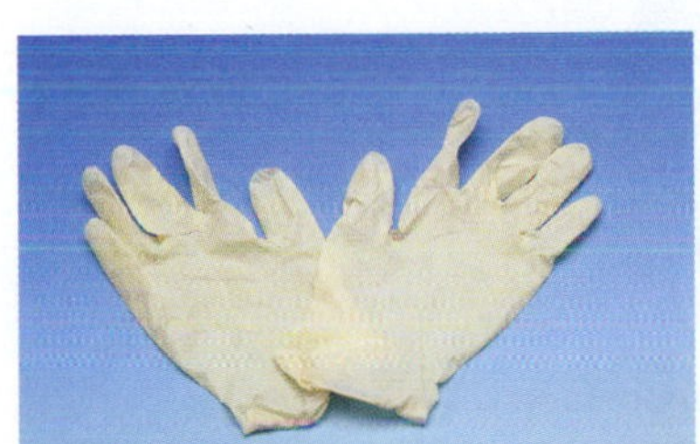

Gloves (to wear if there is any possible exposure to blood or body fluids)

(continued on next page)

Procedure 22-1 ■ Performing the General Survey (continued)

Equipment Needed for Physical Examination—cont'd

Additional Equipment for a Comprehensive Assessment

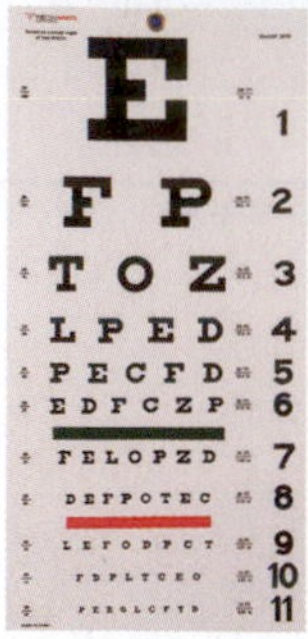

Snellen acuity chart (for screening vision)

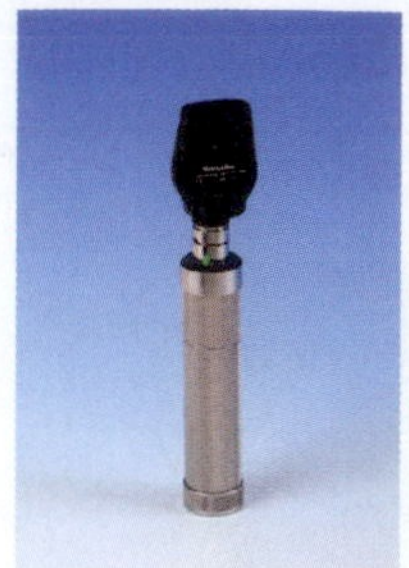
Ophthalmoscope (for inspection of the internal structures of the eye)

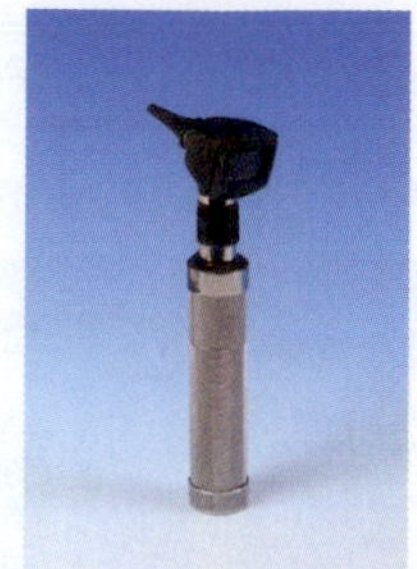
Otoscope (for examining the external auditory canal and tympanic membrane)

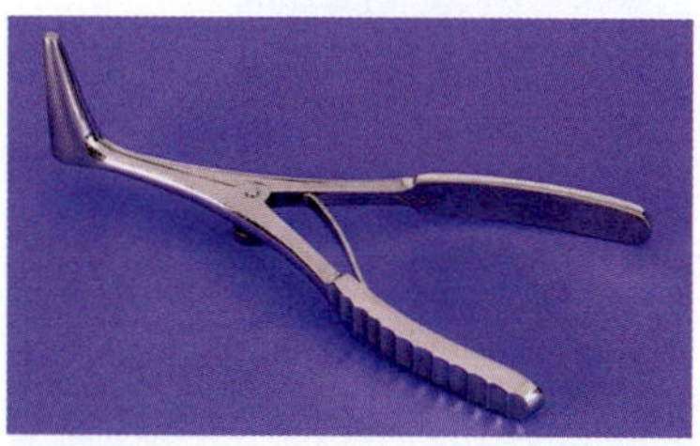
Nasal speculum (for examining the nasal turbinates)

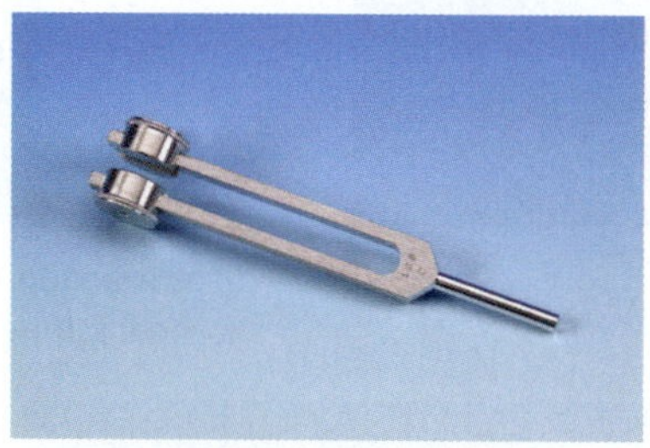
Tuning fork (for auditory screening and assessment of vibratory sensation during the neurological examination)

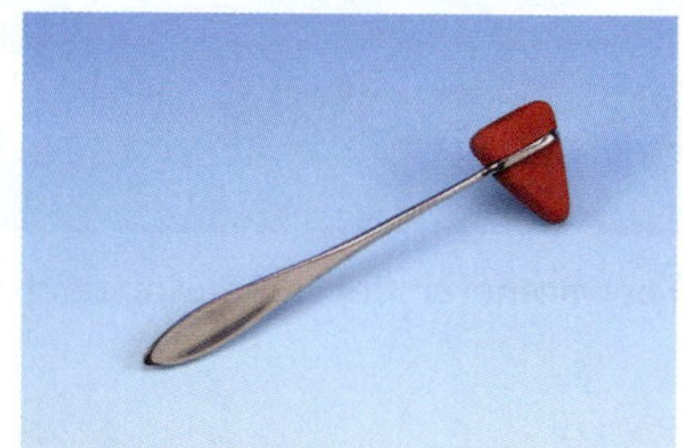
Percussion hammer (for eliciting deep tendon reflexes)

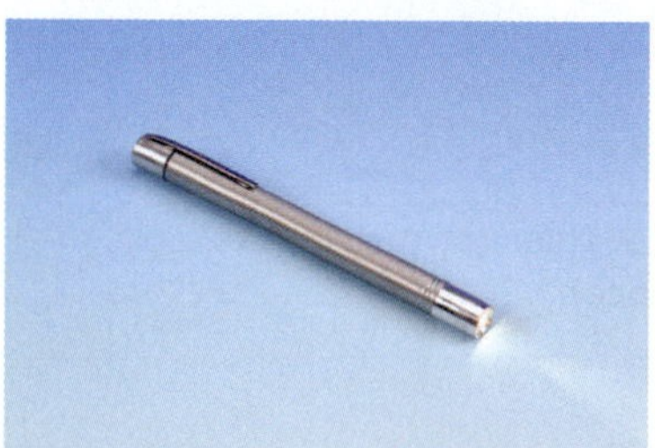
Penlight (for visualizing the eyes and inside of mouth, or highlighting a skin lesion)

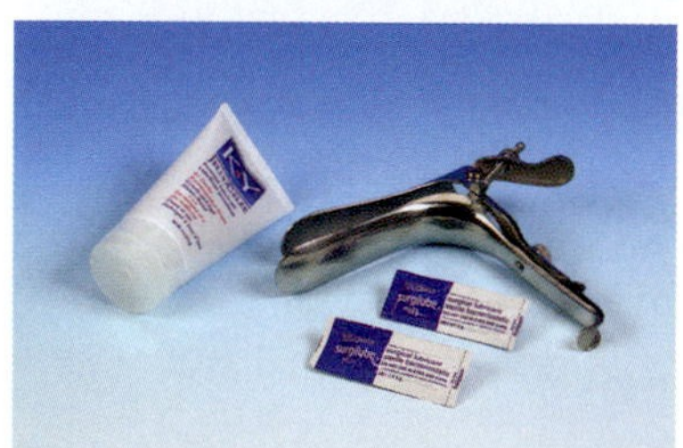
Vaginal speculum and lubricant (for examining the female pelvis; lubricant is also used for rectal examinations)

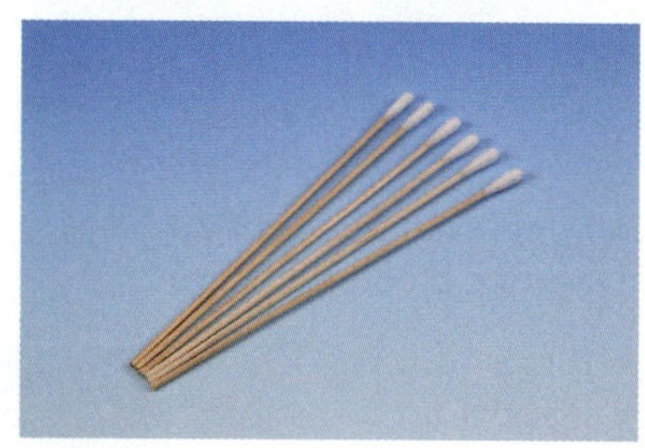
Cotton-tipped applicators (for obtaining specimens)

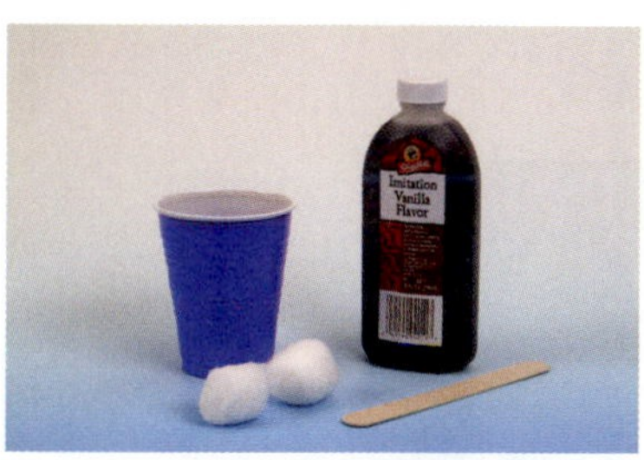
Cotton balls, tongue depressor, strong-smelling substance, a glass of water (for testing various cranial nerves)

Positioning

- Have the client seated as you begin the examination (on an examination table or on the side of the bed). Face the client, and make eye contact.
  Helps build rapport and put the client at ease.
- If the client is unable to sit, use Fowler's or semi-Fowler's position.
  An upright position allows the client to expand his lungs fully and is useful for assessing vital signs, the head and neck, the heart and lungs, the back, and the upper extremities.

Focused History Questions

- How are you feeling today?
- (If the client is an outpatient) What brings you to the clinic today?
- Are you in any discomfort or pain?
- Have you had any hospitalizations or surgeries?
- What medicines do you take? Name both prescribed and over-the-counter drugs.
- How much alcohol do you drink per day? Do you smoke cigarettes? If so, how many per day? Do you use drugs for nonmedical purposes?
- Do you use any herbal products or natural remedies?
- Do you have any difficulty falling asleep or staying asleep?

Developmental Modifications for Infants and Children

- Encourage the parents to be present during the examination.
  Infants and toddlers usually feel most secure if the parents are present.
- Adolescents should be examined without parents or siblings present, unless they request otherwise. Provide privacy.

Developmental Modifications for Older Adults

- *Older adults*—assess the older adult's functional status. You can use the Lawton Instrumental Activities of Daily Living (IADLs) found in the Assessment Guidelines and Tools in Chapter 3.
- *Older adults*—work the SPICES assessment into the examination of various body systems: **S**leep disorders, **P**roblems eating or feeding, **I**ncontinence, **C**onfusion, **E**vidence of falls, **S**kin breakdown.

➤ When performing the procedure, always identify your patient according to agency policy, using two identifiers, and be attentive to standard precautions, hand hygiene, patient safety and privacy, body mechanics, and documentation.

Procedure Steps / Findings

Observe the client's general characteristics.

1. **Identify signs of physical or emotional distress** (e.g., pain, fear, or anxiety). If signs of distress are present, perform a focused assessment, and address the immediate problem.

   Expected findings: The client is in no apparent distress. The client appears relaxed, with no evidence of pain, fear, or anxiety.

   Abnormal findings: Pain, grimacing, breathing problems, skin color changes.

2. **Observe apparent age, gender, and race.** Ask the patient, "What racial or ethnic group do you identify with?" Ask yourself,
   - Is apparent age consistent with biological age?
   - Are there cultural or gender-related factors that influence the exam or findings?

   Expected findings: Client appears his stated age. Makes eye contact consistent with his cultural norms. Is reasonably comfortable with being examined.

3. **Note facial characteristics,** including facial expression, symmetry of facial features, and the condition and color of the skin. Ask yourself,
   - What is the client's face telling me?
   - Is the facial expression appropriate to the situation?
   - Are facial features symmetrical (palpebral fissure and nasolabial folds)?
   - Are there any changes in condition or color of skin?
   - Does the client maintain eye contact?
   - Does the client appear older than his stated age?

   Expected findings: Face is symmetrical; visible skin is intact without excessive wrinkling, discoloration, or deformity.

   Abnormal findings: Excessive wrinkling may be from sun exposure, tobacco use, or illness.

(continued on next page)

Procedure 22-1 ■ Performing the General Survey (continued)

4. **Note body type and posture.** Greet the client with a handshake. Be aware that shaking hands is not acceptable in all cultures.
   Allows you to assess muscle strength and surface skin characteristics while conveying that you care.
   Ask yourself,
   - Is the body build stocky, slender, average, obese, or **cachectic** (very thin, wasted appearance)?
   - Are the body parts proportional to the client's overall size?
   - Is body fat distributed normally?
   - Does the client assume a specific position for comfort (e.g., sitting versus supine)?

Expected findings: Posture is upright, and body appears proportionate. Grip is strong.

---

5. **Observe gait, and note any abnormal movements.** If the client has Alteration in Bed Mobility, determine ability to move and amount of assistance needed. Ask yourself,
   - Does the client move in a coordinated manner?
   - Are there any obvious gait problems?
   - Does the client walk with a wide base of support or short stride length?
   - Does the client use assistive devices, such as a cane?
   - Are there any abnormal or spastic movements?

Expected findings: Movements are coordinated; gait is steady; does not use assistive devices.

Abnormal findings: Unstable or shuffling gait; spastic movements, stiff movements may be associated with joint, muscle, or neurological disorders. A slumped position may indicate fatigue, depression, osteoporosis, or pain.

---

6. **Listen to your client's speech pattern**, pace, quality, tone, vocabulary, and sentence structure while you are examining the body systems. Ask yourself,
   - Are the responses appropriate (a) to the situation, and (b) for developmental stage?
   - Is there any difficulty with speech?
   - Does the client's tone of voice match her statements?
   - Is the voice hoarse?
   - Does the client have a foreign accent; is there hesitancy and/or little verbalization?

Expected findings: Client responds appropriately to questions. Tone of voice matches responses. Speech is clear, evenly paced, and rises and falls based on content.

Abnormal findings: Rapid speech, slow speech, slurred speech, illogical responses, language barrier.

---

7. **Assess mental state and affect.**
   a. Determine level of consciousness.
   b. Determine orientation to time, place, and person.
   Ask yourself,
   - If the client is disoriented, does he reorient easily?
   - What is the client's mood? Is it appropriate for the situation?

   NOTE: If you note any abnormal findings, be sure to focus on them when you assess mental status during the sensorineurological examination.

Expected findings: Awake, alert, and oriented to time, place, person, and self. Mood is appropriate for the situation.

Abnormal findings:
- Confusion and irritability may indicate hypoxia or medication side effects.
- Inability to recall information or provide history may indicate a neurological disorder.
- Lethargy and somnolence may be caused by medications; depression; or a neurological, thyroid, liver, kidney, or cardiovascular disorder. Bizarre responses may signal a psychiatric problem.

8. **Observe dress, grooming, and hygiene.** Ask yourself,
   - Is the client appropriately and neatly dressed?
   - Is the client well groomed?
   - Are there any unusual odors?

Expected findings: Client is dressed appropriately for the climate. Skin is clean, and clothing is in good repair. No noticeable odor.

Abnormal findings: Poor hygiene, dirty skin or nails, uncombed hair, visible soiling of clothing, mismatched or wrinkled clothing, unpleasant odor; may indicate an impaired ability to care for oneself, chronic pain, fatigue, depression, or low self-esteem.

---

9. **Measure vital signs**: Blood pressure, temperature, radial pulse, respiratory rate. If your initial observations and interview indicate that the client is in pain, perform a pain assessment as well. (See Chapter 31).

Expected findings:

BP: < 120/80 mm Hg

Temperature: 97.3°F–98.6°F (36.3°C–37°C) oral

Pulse: 60–100 beats/min, regular, and easily palpated

Respiratory rate: 12–20 breaths/min, regular and even

Abnormal findings: See Chapter 20.

---

10. **Measure height and weight.**

   a. *For adults:* Calculate BMI, or use the accompanying table.

$$\frac{\text{Wt (lb)} \times 703}{\text{Ht (in.)}^2} = \text{BMI}$$

   b. *For children:* Plot height and weight on growth chart.

Developmental Modifications

Adults

- Use a platform scale with a sliding ruler, or a bed scale if the client cannot stand safely.

Infants and children

- Weigh infants without clothing; weigh older children in their underwear.
- For infants and children younger than 2 years, use a stationary measure (e.g., infant scale) if available. Position supine to measure height; ensure that the knees are extended.
- For infants and children younger than 2 years, also measure head circumference.

Expected findings: *For adults:* BMI is 18.5–24.9.

For children: Height and weight are consistent with previous trend on growth chart.

Abnormal findings:

BMI < 18.5 = underweight

BMI 25–29.9 = overweight

BMI > 30 = obese

BMI 30–34.9 = Level I, moderate obesity

BMI 35–39.9 = Level II, severe obesity

BMI > 40 = Level III, morbid obesity

NOTE: For growth charts for males and females from birth to age 20 years,

Go to the Centers for Disease Control and Prevention (CDC), National Center for Health Statistics Web site at http://www.cdc.gov/growthcharts/clinical_charts.htm

? What if . . .

- **There is an apparent language barrier?**
  Obtain an interpreter; and refer to Clinical Insight 21-4, in Chapter 21 of this volume.

(continued on next page)

Procedure 22-1 ■ Performing the General Survey (continued)

Use this table to find body mass index, based on height and weight, or use a BMI calculator, such as those found at http://www.nhlbi.nih.gov/health/educational/lose_wt/BMI/bmicalc.htm

Weight (lb)

Height (ft/in)	120	130	140	150	160	170	180	190	200	210	220	230	240	250	260	270	280	290	300	310	320	330
4'5"	30	33	35	38	40	43	45	48	50	53	55	58	60	63	65	68	70	73	75	78	80	83
4'6"	29	31	34	36	39	41	43	46	48	51	53	56	58	60	63	65	68	70	72	75	77	80
4'7"	28	30	33	35	37	40	42	44	47	49	51	54	56	58	61	63	65	68	70	72	75	77
4'8"	27	29	31	34	36	38	40	43	45	47	49	52	54	56	58	61	63	65	67	70	72	74
4'9"	26	28	30	33	35	37	39	41	43	46	48	50	52	54	56	59	61	63	65	67	69	72
4'10"	25	27	29	31	34	36	38	40	42	44	46	48	50	52	54	57	59	61	63	65	67	69
4'11"	24	26	28	30	32	34	36	38	40	43	45	47	49	51	53	55	57	59	61	63	65	67
5'0"	23	25	27	29	31	33	35	37	39	41	43	45	47	49	51	53	55	57	59	61	63	65
5'1"	23	25	27	28	30	32	34	36	38	40	42	44	45	47	49	51	53	55	57	59	61	62
5'2"	22	24	26	27	29	31	33	35	37	38	40	42	44	46	48	49	51	53	55	57	59	60
5'3"	21	23	25	27	28	30	32	34	36	37	39	41	43	44	46	48	50	51	53	55	57	59
5'4"	21	22	24	26	28	29	31	33	34	36	38	40	41	43	45	46	48	50	52	53	55	57
5'5"	20	22	23	25	27	28	30	32	33	35	38	38	40	42	43	45	47	48	50	52	53	55
5'6"	19	21	23	24	26	27	29	31	32	34	36	37	39	40	42	44	45	47	49	50	52	53
5'7"	19	20	22	24	25	27	28	30	31	33	35	36	38	39	41	42	44	46	47	49	50	52
5'8"	18	20	21	23	24	26	27	29	30	32	34	35	37	38	40	41	43	44	46	47	49	50
5'9"	18	19	21	22	24	25	27	28	30	31	33	34	36	37	38	40	41	43	44	46	47	49
5'10"	17	19	20	22	23	24	26	27	29	30	32	33	35	36	37	39	40	42	43	45	46	47
5'11"	17	18	20	21	22	24	25	27	28	29	31	32	34	35	36	38	39	41	42	43	45	46
6'	16	18	19	20	22	23	24	26	27	29	30	31	33	34	35	37	38	39	41	42	43	45
6'1"	16	17	19	20	21	22	24	25	26	28	29	30	32	33	34	36	37	38	40	41	42	44
6'2"	15	17	18	19	21	22	23	24	26	27	28	30	31	32	33	35	36	37	39	40	41	42
6'3"	15	16	18	19	20	21	23	24	25	26	28	29	30	31	33	34	35	36	38	39	40	41
6'4"	15	16	17	18	20	21	22	23	24	26	27	28	29	30	32	33	34	35	37	38	39	40
6'5"	14	15	17	18	19	20	21	23	24	25	26	27	29	30	31	32	33	34	36	37	38	39
6'6"	14	15	16	17	19	20	21	22	23	24	25	27	28	29	30	31	32	34	35	36	37	38
6'7"	14	15	16	17	18	19	20	21	23	24	25	26	27	28	29	30	32	33	34	35	36	37
6'8"	13	14	15	17	18	19	20	21	22	23	24	25	26	28	29	30	31	32	33	34	35	36
6'9"	13	14	15	16	17	18	19	20	21	23	24	25	26	27	28	29	30	31	32	33	34	35
6'10"	13	14	15	16	17	18	19	20	21	22	23	24	25	26	27	28	29	30	31	32	34	35

Less risk — More risk

Documentation

- Document BP as right or left arm, and note the patient's position: sitting, standing, or lying.
- Document temperature measurement route: oral, rectal, or tympanic membrane.
- If you need more information about documenting,

Go to **Documenting Physical Examination Findings (Nam Nguyen),** in Chapter 22, Volume 1.

- For a Graphic Flowsheet for recording vital signs,

Go to Chapter 18, **Documenting & Reporting,** in Volume 1.

Practice Resources

Centers for Disease Control and Prevention (CDC) (last updated 2015, May); CDC (last updated 2016); National Guideline Clearinghouse (NGC) (2013, May); National Heart, Lung, and Blood Institute (n.d.).

Procedure 22-2 ■ Assessing the Skin

➤ For steps to follow in *all* procedures, refer to the Universal Steps for All Procedures found on the inside back cover.

Equipment

- Nonlatex gloves (if exposure to body fluids is a possibility)
- Flexible transparent ruler
- Penlight
- Magnifier
- Pen and record form

Clean stethoscope and rulers before and after use unless they are only used for one patient.

Focused History Questions

Ask the patient about the history or presence of any:

- Rashes
- History of allergies
- Areas of skin that have changed color
- Skin lesions
- Skin with rough or unusual texture
- Skin that is always warm or cool, regardless of room temperature

Developmental Modifications for Older Adults

- Assess the level of risk for pressure injury. For assessment tools (Braden scale, Norton scale), go to Chapter 35 in this volume.

  As adults age, the subcutaneous tissue layer thins. The dermal layer loses elasticity as a result of changes in collagen fibers; and the strong bond between the epidermal and dermal layers decreases. These changes make the skin prone to breakdown.

➤ When performing the procedure, always identify your patient according to agency policy, using two identifiers, and be attentive to standard precautions, hand hygiene, patient safety and privacy, body mechanics, and documentation.

Procedure Steps

1. **Inspect skin color, including mucous membranes, tongue, and conjunctiva.**

   To assess color changes of exposed and unexposed areas. Color changes and odors may indicate underlying disease and should be fully investigated.

   a. Provide good lighting.

   b. In dark-skinned clients, look for color changes in the conjunctiva or oral mucosa, tongue, lips, nailbeds, palms of the hands, and soles of the feet.

   Skin color varies widely among individuals, depending on age and ethnicity; but in each individual, skin color is fairly uniform over her body. ▼

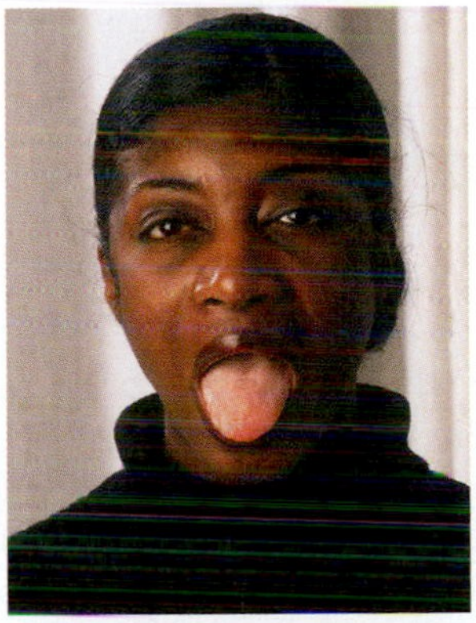

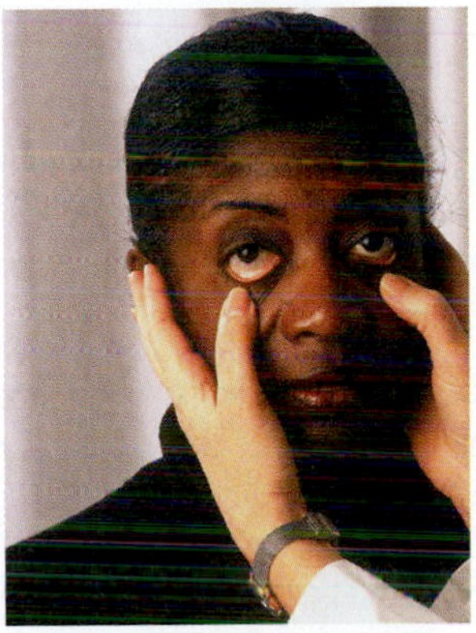

   c. Note any unusual odors.

   d. To assess for cyanosis, be sure to examine the tongue.

   Exposure to cold causes the lips to turn blue, but not the tongue. Cyanosis affects the color of the skin, mucous membranes, and tongue.

Findings

Expected findings: Skin color is uniform, with darker exposed areas. Mucous membranes and conjunctiva are pink and moist. No unusual odors.

Developmental Variations

Newborns—May be jaundiced for a few weeks. Blue-black Mongolian spots and pink-red capillary hemangiomas are common and fade with time.

Older adults—May have thin, translucent skin and wrinkles caused by loss of elasticity. Fragile skin is not uncommon among lighter-skinned, older adults.

Abnormal findings: Pallor, jaundice (may require further investigation), cyanosis, erythema, hyperpigmentation, hypopigmentation.

- Café-au-lait spots, although usually normal, may sometimes signal a genetic disorder.
- If there are abnormal findings, ask the patient (or someone who knows her well) about the baseline skin color.

For more information about skin color changes see Table 22-2 in Volume 1.

Also see the following illustrations, Skin Color Changes.

(continued on next page)

Procedure 22-2 ■ Assessing the Skin (continued)

Skin Color Changes

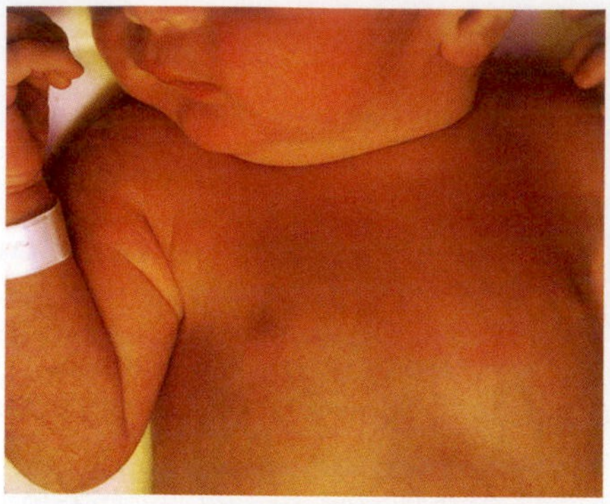
Jaundice

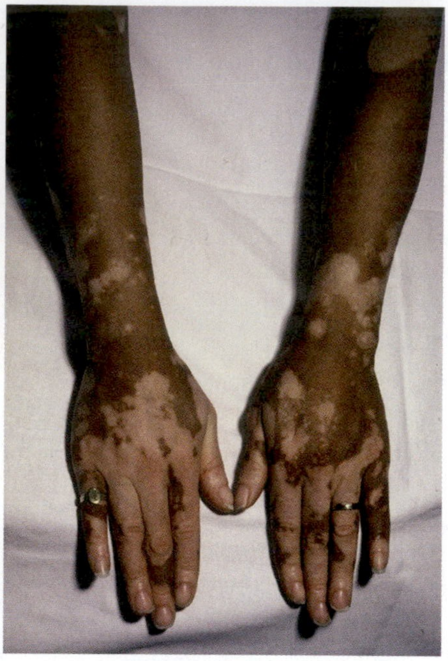
Vitiligo

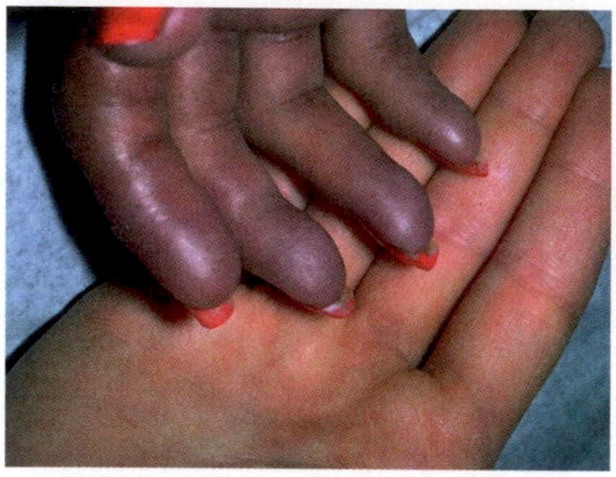
Cyanosis

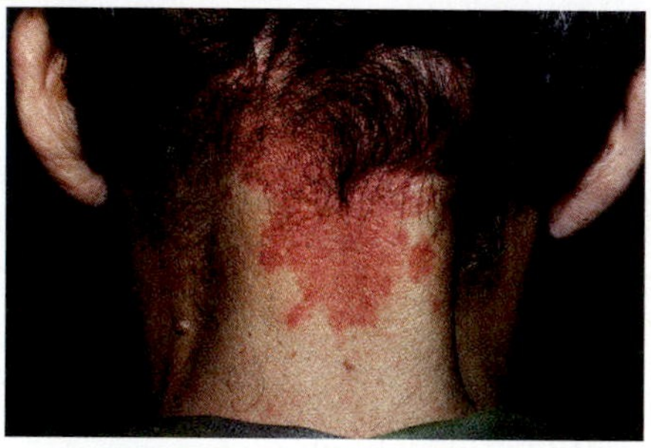
Port-wine stain (nevus flammeus)

2. Palpate skin for temperature.

a. Wear procedure gloves and discard after examining any open areas of the skin.
b. Use dorsal aspect of hand or fingers.
c. Compare bilaterally.

The dorsa of the hands and the fingers are most sensitive to temperature variations.

d. Check the skin temperature over any area of erythema.
e. If skin feels excessively warm, validate your data, and assess for fever.

Expected findings: Skin is warm; temperature is the same bilaterally.

Abnormal findings: Local area(s) that are warmer or cooler than the rest of the skin; generalized temperature increase or decrease.

- Localized warmth with erythema can indicate an infection.
- Cool skin might be a sign of compromised circulation, shock, exposure to cold, hypothyroidism, or dehydration, particularly in the older adult.

3. **Palpate skin for turgor.** Test an unexposed area, such as the area below the clavicle, inner thigh, sternum, or forehead, by gently pinching up the skin, noting its return when you release it.

Developmental Modifications

Infants—Check skin turgor on the abdomen.

Older adults—Check skin turgor over the sternum or clavicle. ▼

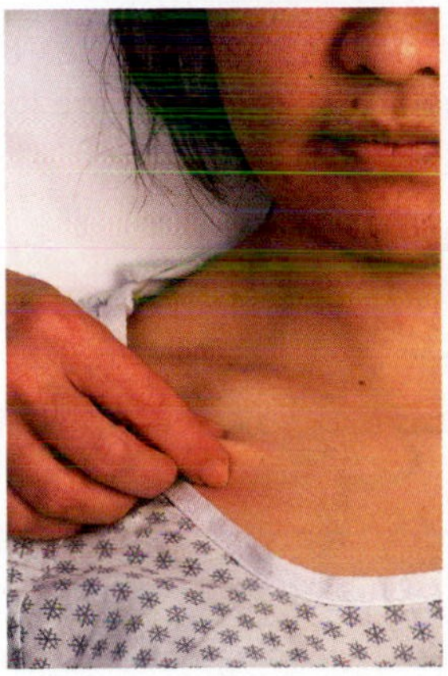

Expected findings: Skin returns immediately to its original position.

Developmental Variations

Older adults have decreased skin turgor as a result of decreased elasticity.

Abnormal findings: Decreased or increased turgor.

- *Tenting (decreased turgor):* Skin takes several seconds to return to original position.
- *Tenting:* Seen with dehydration or normal aging. It predisposes the patient to skin breakdown.
- *Increased turgor:* Skin tension does not allow the skin to be pinched up; may be caused by edema or scleroderma.

4. **Palpate the skin for texture.**
   Texture varies, depending on the area being assessed and the age of the client.

Expected findings: Skin is smooth and soft. Exposed areas and extensor surfaces (e.g., elbows and knees) are drier and coarser than other areas.

Developmental Variations

Infants and young children—have smooth skin.

Abnormal findings: Coarse, thick, rough, or dry skin; very smooth, thin, fine-textured, shiny skin.

5. **Palpate skin for moisture/hydration.** Use the dorsum of your hand.

Expected findings: Skin is warm and dry.

Developmental Variations

Older adults—Skin may be dry and flaky because of decreased activity of sebaceous and sweat glands.

Adolescents—May have skin that is oilier than normal.

Abnormal findings: Increased moisture (skin feels damp, visible diaphoresis); decreased moisture (skin feels dry).

6. **Inspect for edema.**
   a. Press firmly with your fingertip for 5 seconds over a bony area, such as the tibia.
   b. Release your finger, and observe the skin for the reaction.
   c. If edema is present, note the location, degree, and type of swelling. For example, if you observe edema in the lower leg, how far up the leg does it extend?

Expected findings: No edema. Normally there will be no evidence of the pressure once you release your finger. If pitting edema is present, you will see a depression in the skin.

Grading System

Trace: Minimal depression with pressure.

+1: 2 mm depression; rapid return of skin to position.

+2: 4 mm depression that disappears in 10–15 seconds.

(continued on next page)

Procedure 22-2 ■ Assessing the Skin (continued)

+3: 6 mm depression that lasts 1–2 minutes. Area appears swollen.

+4: 8 mm depression that persists for 2–3 minutes. Area is grossly edematous.

Abnormal findings: Edema is an abnormal finding.

7. Identify any skin lesions.

a. Inspect and palpate lesions.

b. When you notice bruises, be alert for signs of abuse (see Chapter 9).

c. Ask the client: "Do you have any new moles or other lesions? Has there been any change in existing moles/lesions?"

d. Assess for malignant lesions using ABCDE:

A) (asymmetry)
B) (irregular borders)
C) (color variations)
D) (diameter: > 0.5 cm)
E) (elevation) ▼

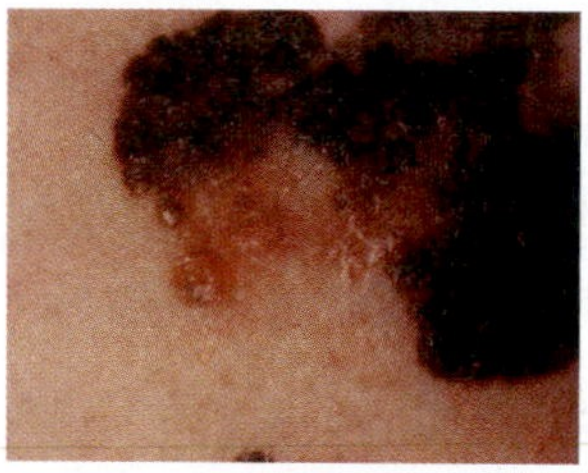

Malignant melanoma

Expected findings: No lesions are present.

Normal variations include moles, freckles, birthmarks, striae (in pregnant women or clients who have lost much weight), and wrinkles.

Developmental Variations

Newborns—***milia*** (tiny collections of sebum, usually on the face) are common.

Adolescents—Acne is a common abnormal finding among adolescents.

Adults—***acrochordons*** (skin tags) may be seen around the neck, axillae, skinfolds, or areas where clothing rubs.

Older adults—Flat beige or brown macules are common on exposed skin areas.

Abnormal findings: See the illustrations for Abnormal Skin Lesions following, and the table Describing Skin Lesions at the end of this procedure.

Abnormal Skin Lesions

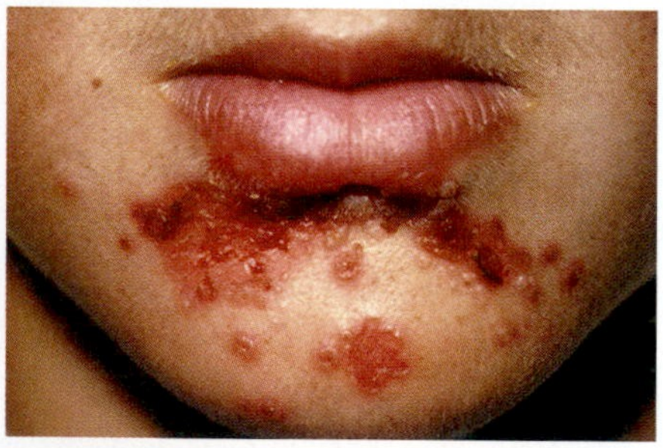

Herpes

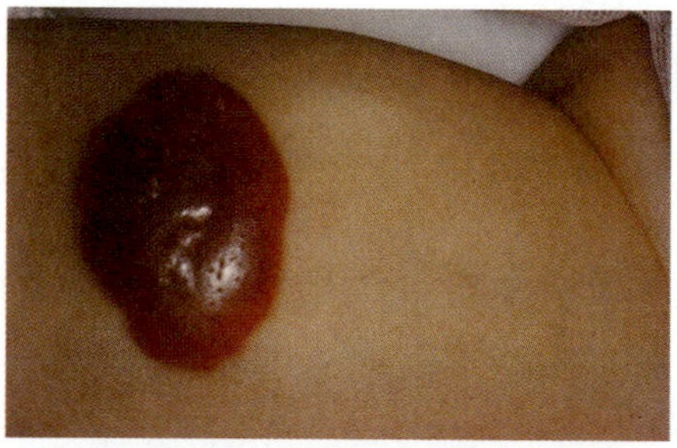

Capillary hemangioma

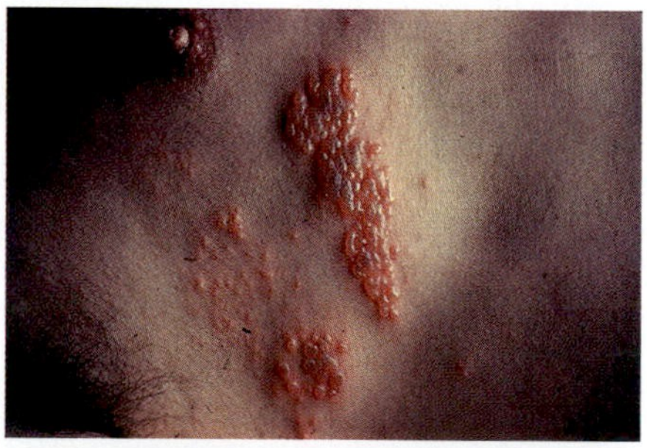

Vesicles (blisters)

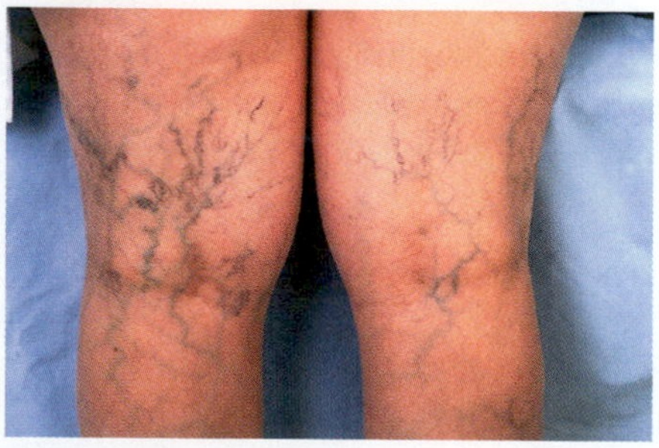

Venous star

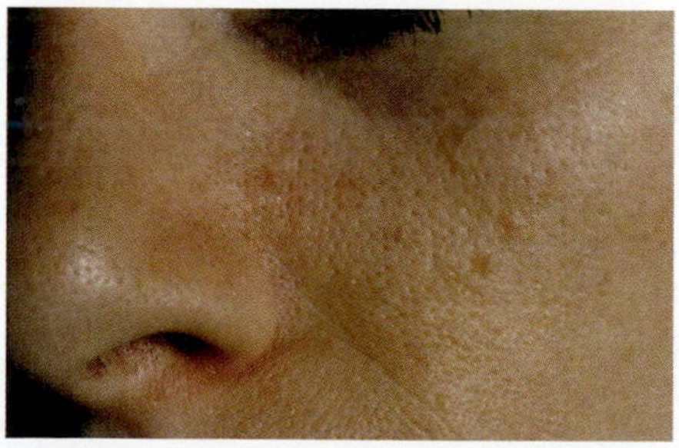

Petechiae

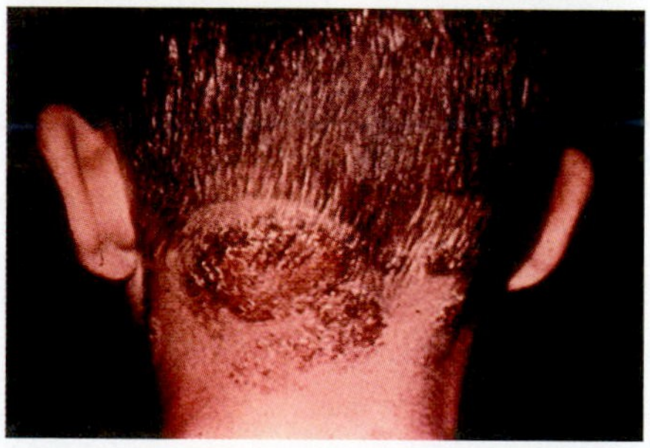

Ringworm

Describing Skin Lesions

When you observe a lesion, evaluate for and describe the following:

- ***Size.*** Measure the length, width, and depth of the lesion.
- ***Shape and pattern.*** Describe the *shape* of individual lesions. If there are clusters or groups, describe the *pattern*. Is it linear or circular? Are the *borders* distinct, or do they run together? Is the border smooth or irregular?
- ***Color.*** Describe the color of the lesion, and determine whether there is any variation of color within the lesion.
- ***Distribution.*** Are the lesions distributed over the entire body? Are they confined to a specific region? What parts of the body are affected?
- ***Texture.*** The texture (e.g., smooth, rough, scaly) of a lesion helps with classification.
- ***Surface relationship.*** To assess surface relationship, you will need to palpate the lesion. Is it flat, raised, or depressed? Is it firmly attached to the surrounding skin or mobile?
- ***Exudate.*** Examine the lesion(s) for signs of drainage. Describe the color, appearance, amount, and odor of drainage, if present.
- ***Tenderness, pain, or itching.*** Press on the lesion, and determine the patient's reaction. Does touching the lesion cause pain or discomfort?

Patient Teaching

Teach the patient the signs and symptoms of skin cancer, the importance of skin self-examination, and preventive measures.

Home Care

- Assess the skill level of the caregiver. Instruct the caregiver in the importance of skin assessment and measures to prevent skin breakdown.
- Be alert for lesions (e.g., burns, bruises) that may signal physical abuse. For more signs of abuse, refer to Procedure 9-1.

Documentation

- If lesions are present, describe the history: onset, duration, associated or aggravating factors (e.g., itching), factors that relieve symptoms, treatments that have been used, and responses to treatment.
- Sketch the location of skin lesions on body diagrams, if available (see example); or sketch a body diagram, if necessary.

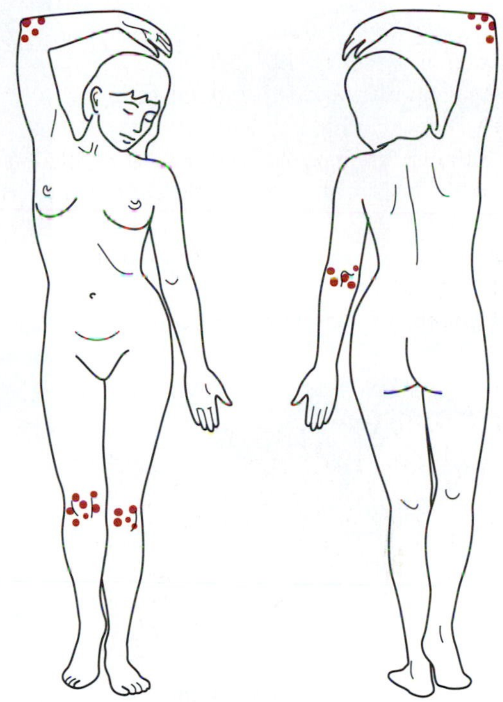

If you need more information about documenting, review Caring for the Nguyens, and

Go to Chapter 22, **Documenting Physical Examination Findings (Nam Nguyen),** in Volume 1.

(continued on next page)

Procedure 22-2 ■ Assessing the Skin (continued)

Describing Skin Lesions

PRIMARY LESIONS

Types		Description
Macule (nonpalpable, < 1 cm) 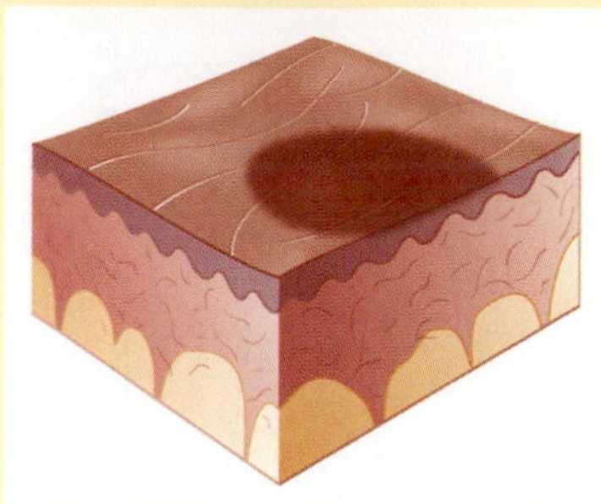	Macule (nonpalpable, < 1 cm) 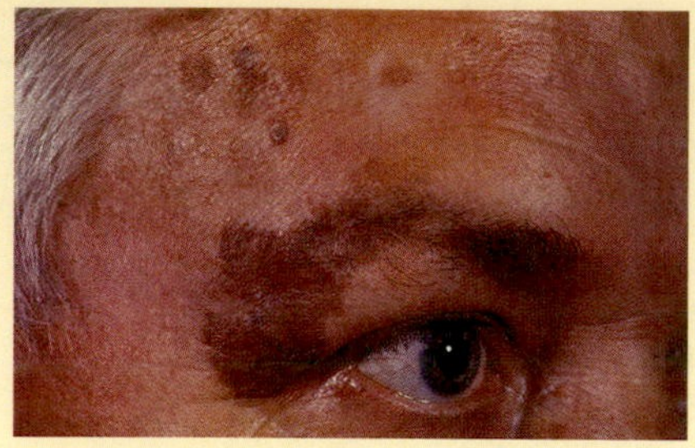	Flat and colored. Examples: freckle, petechiae, birthmark, Mongolian spot
Papule (palpable) < 1 cm; Plaque > 1 cm 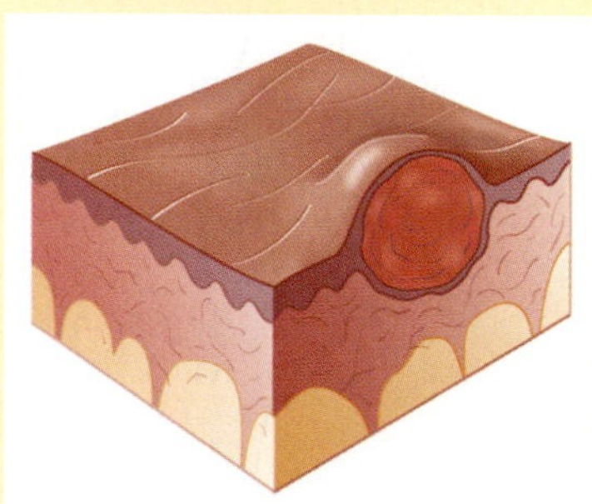	Papules (seborrheic keratosis) 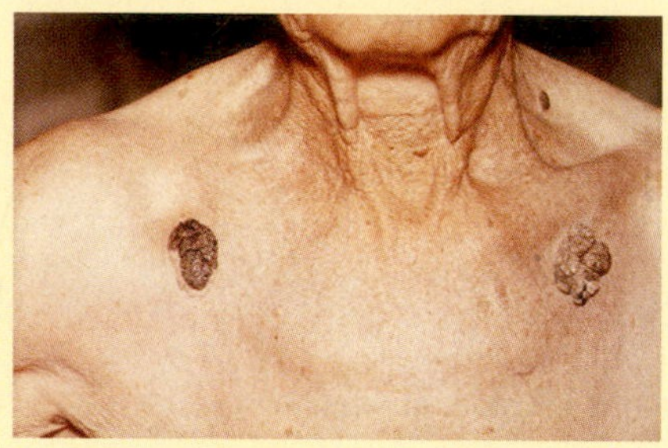	Elevated and raised, but superficial. Examples: mole, psoriasis
Vesicle (palpable), < 1 cm; Bulla, > 1 cm 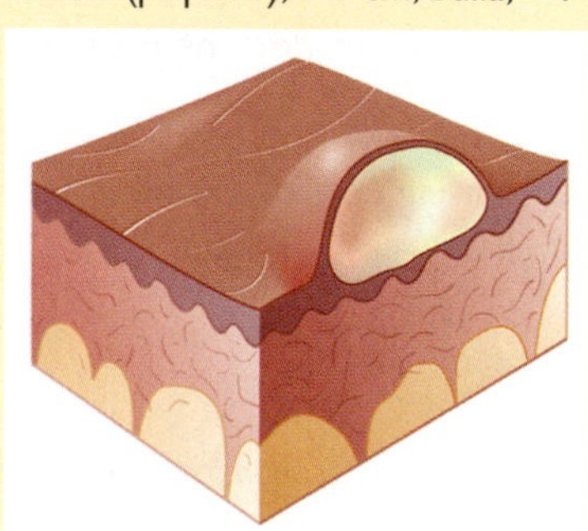	Vesicles (blisters) 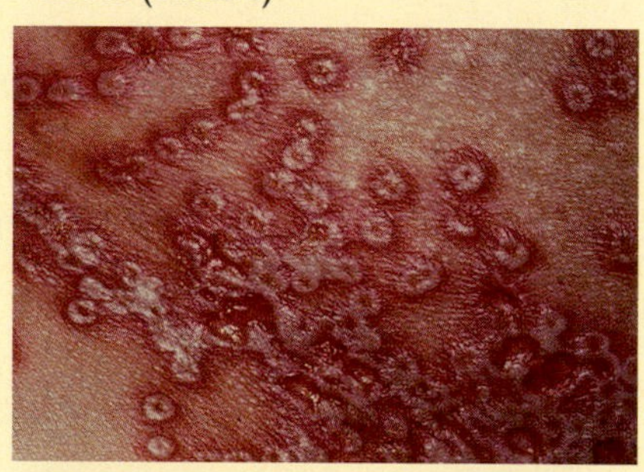 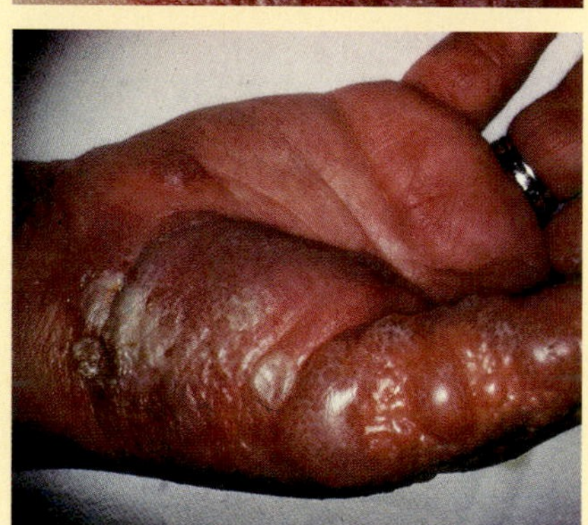	Elevated and filled with serous fluid. Examples: blister, herpes simplex

Describing Skin Lesions—cont'd

PRIMARY LESIONS

Types		Description
Cyst (palpable), < 2 cm 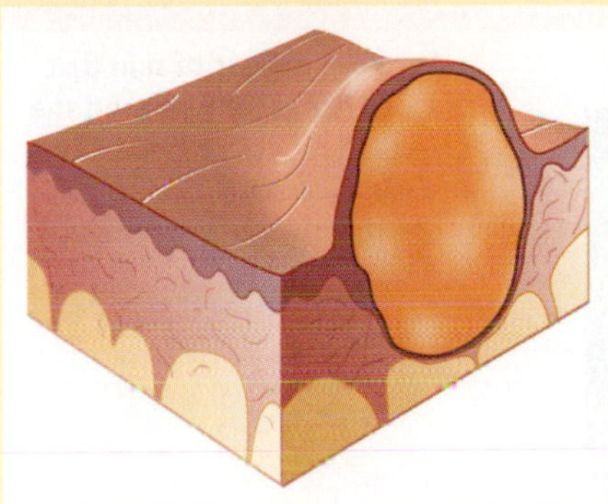	Keratogenous cyst 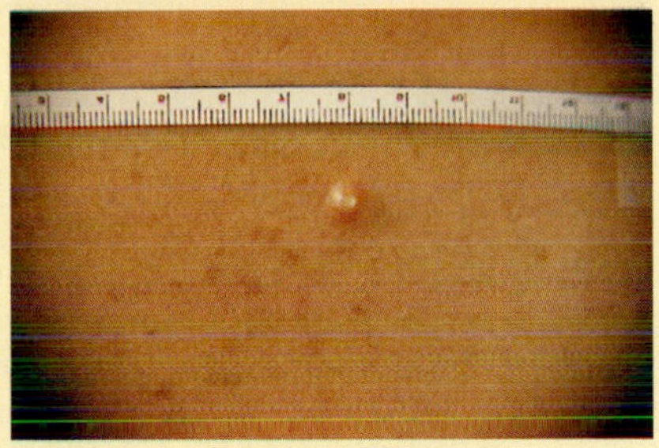	Palpable, fluid-filled, and encapsulated. If not fluid-filled, called a *nodule*
Pustule (palpable) 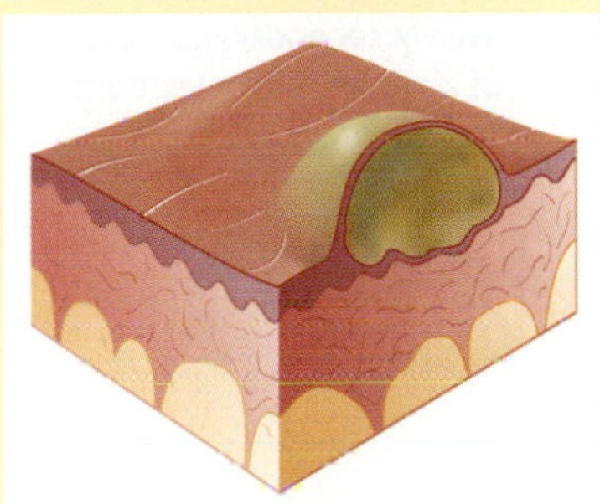	Pustules (acne) 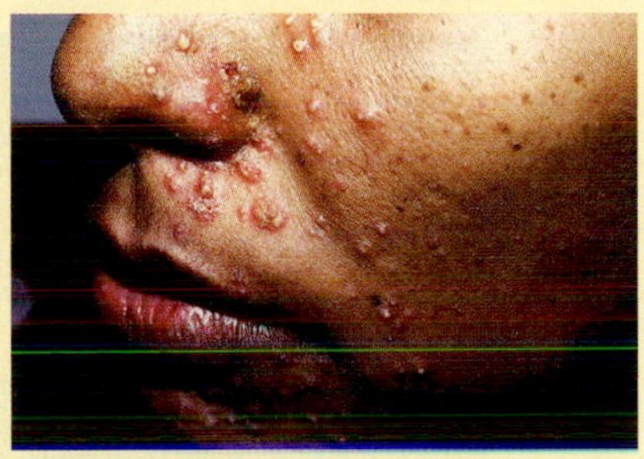	Elevated and filled with pus. Examples: acne, folliculitis, impetigo
	Nodule (palpable) 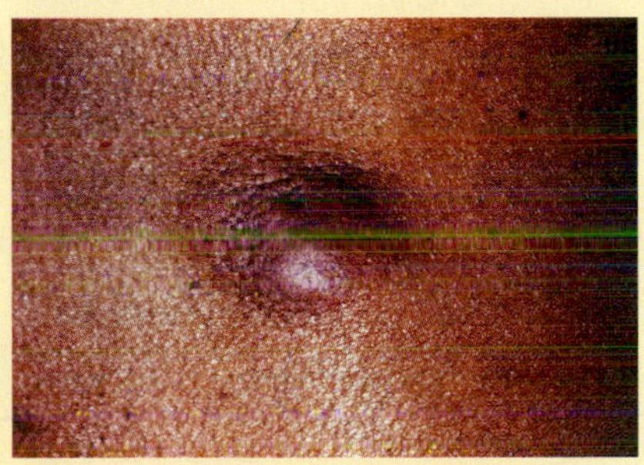	Elevated, solid, and firm, with depth into dermis. Examples: wart, lipoma (fatty cyst)
Wheal 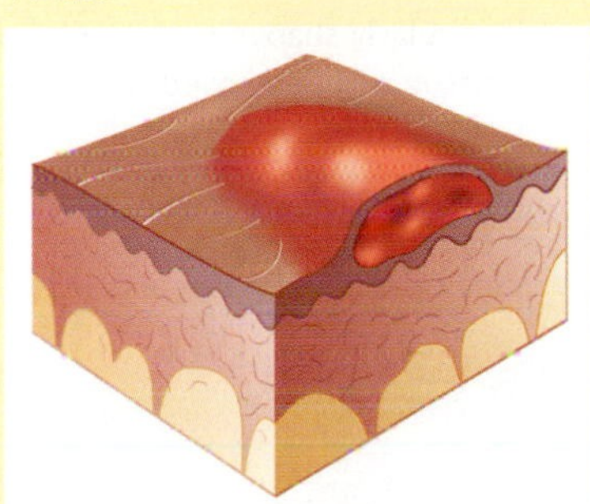	Hive 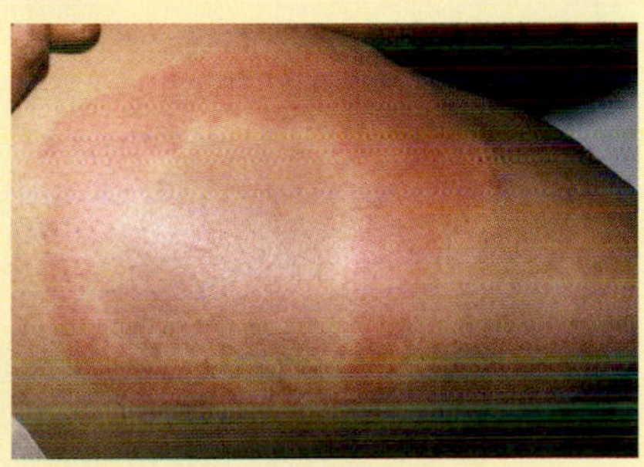	Elevated, superficial, with localized edema. Examples: insect bites, hives

(continued on next page)

Procedure 22-2 ■ Assessing the Skin (continued)

Describing Skin Lesions—cont'd

SECONDARY LESIONS

Types		Description
Excoriation 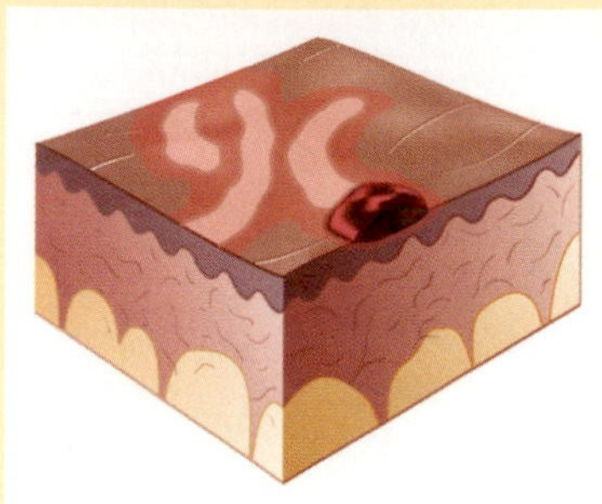	Excoriation from pruritus 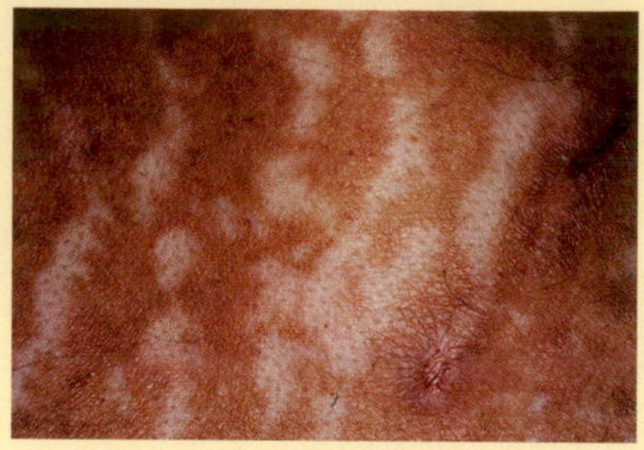	Abrasion or loss of skin that does not extend beyond the superficial epidermis. Examples: scratches, stasis dermatitis, atopic dermatitis
Erosion 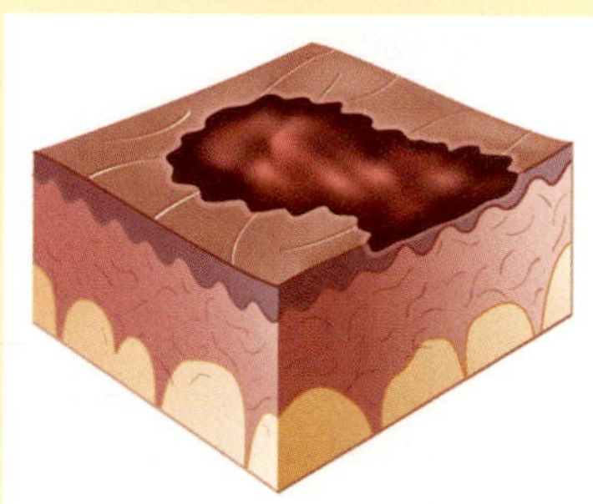	Erosions 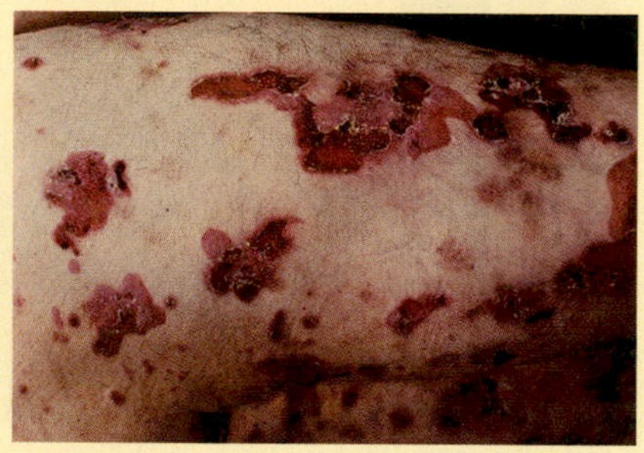	Loss of superficial epidermis, usually secondary to rupture of a blister. Examples: abrasions and impetigo
Fissure 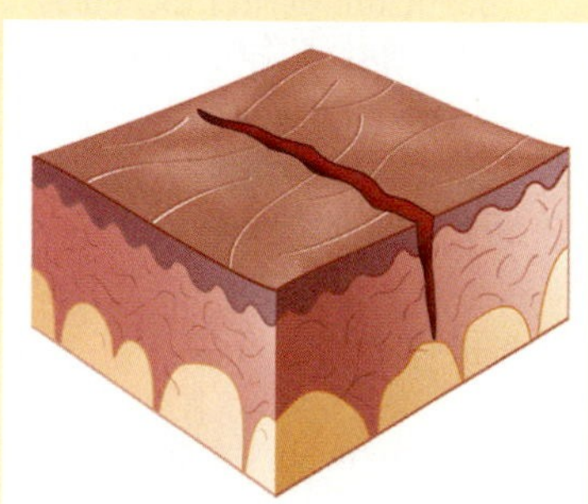	Cheilitis 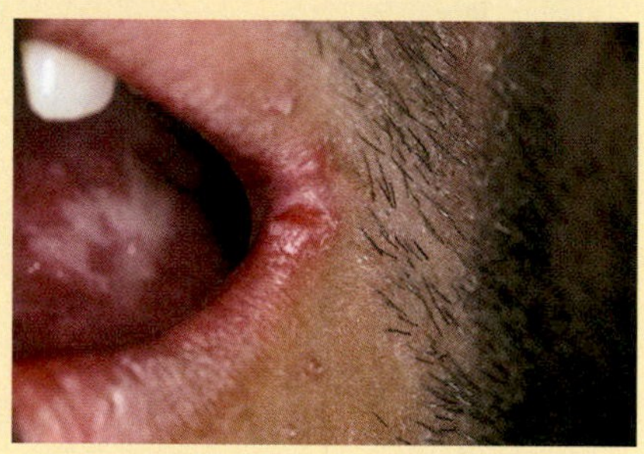	Linear break in the skin ("crack"); may extend to the dermis. Examples: athlete's foot, cheilitis
Ulcer 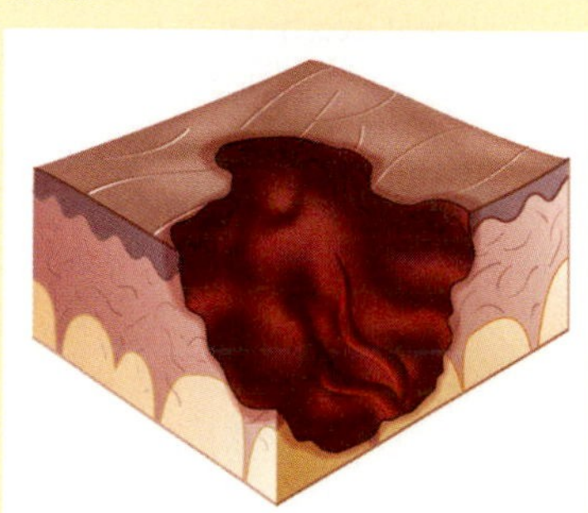	Stasis ulcer 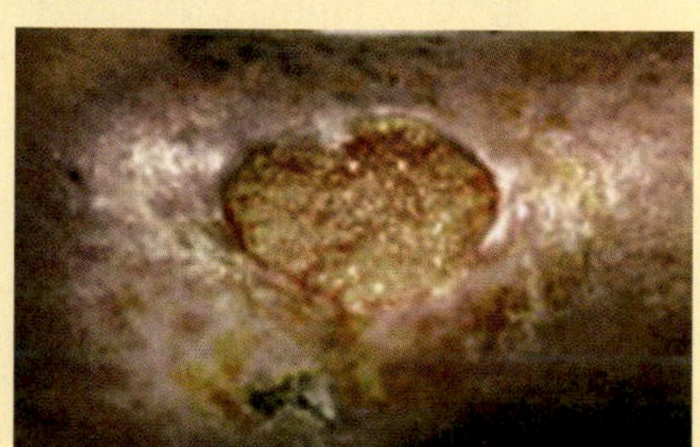	Irregularly shaped with loss of tissue. Graded based on depth and tissue involvement. Examples: pressure injury, stasis ulcers

Describing Skin Lesions—cont'd

SECONDARY LESIONS

Types		Description
Crust 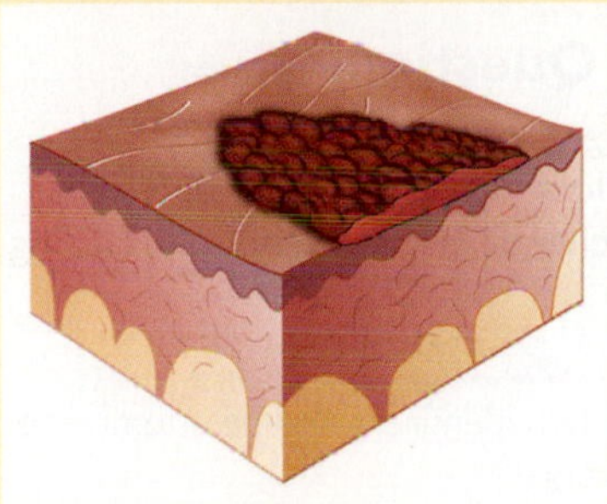	Crust 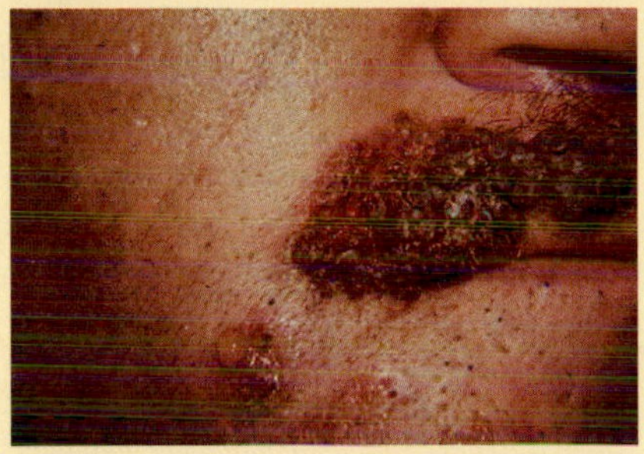	Elevated, rough texture with dried exudate. Examples: impetigo, herpes simplex
Scales 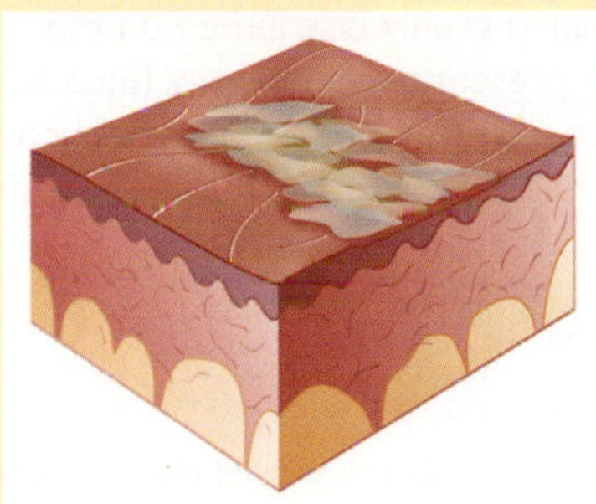	Psoriasis 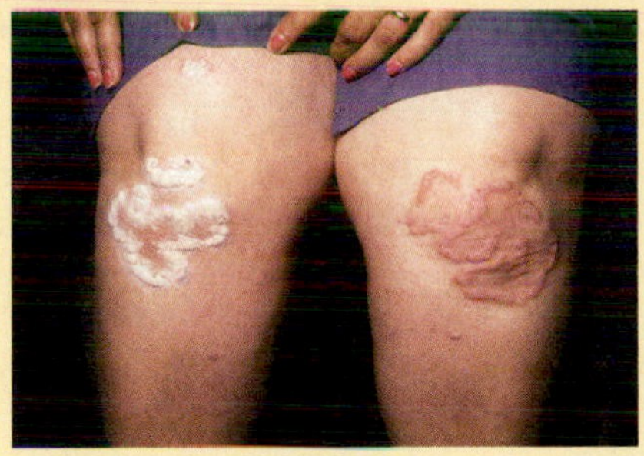	White to tan flaking, dead skin cells; may be adherent or loose. Examples: psoriasis and dandruff
Scar 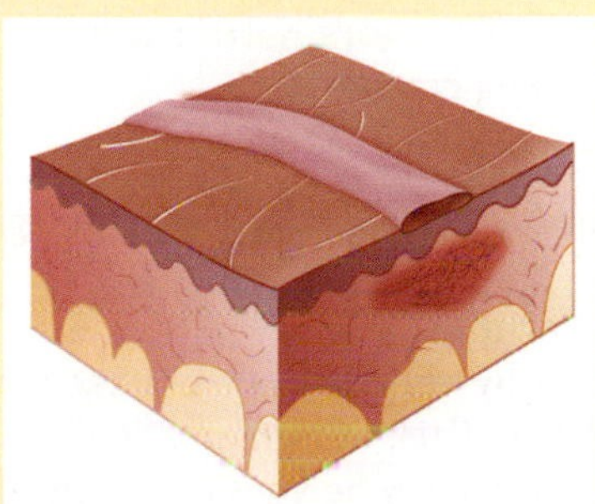		Fibrous tissue at site of injury, trauma, or surgery. Examples: surgical site, trauma site
Keloid 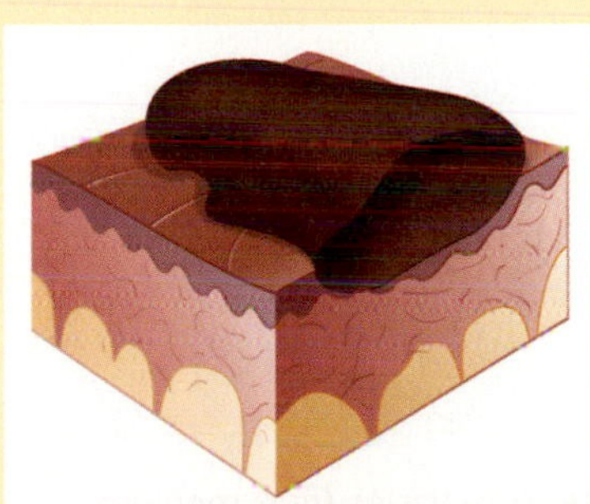	Keloids 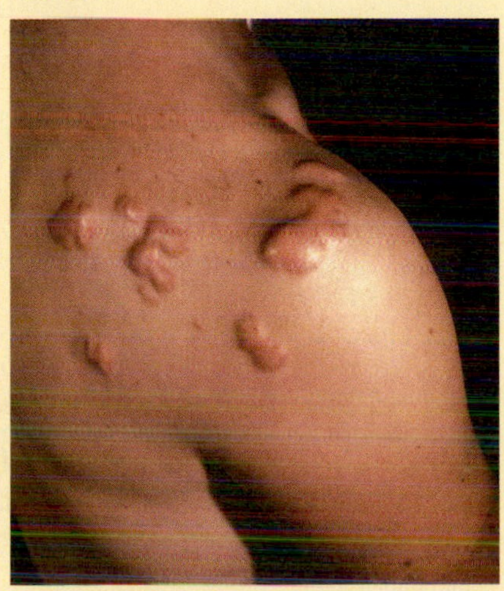	Raised and irregular scar caused by excess collagen formation. Examples: surgical scars, ear piercing

Sources: Linton, C. P. (2011). Describing the configuration of skin lesions. *Journal of the Dermatology Nurses' Association, 3*(6), 379; Reddy, M. (2008). Skin and wound care: Important considerations in the older adult. *Advances in Skin & Wound Care, 21*(9), 424–436

Practice Resources

Kottner, J., & Surber, C. (2016); Linton, C. P. (2011), Reddy, M. (2008).

Procedure 22-3 ■ Assessing the Hair

➤ For steps to follow in *all* procedures, refer to the Universal Steps for All Procedures found on the inside back cover.

Equipment

- Nonlatex procedure gloves (if exposure to body fluids is a possibility)
- Pen and record form

Focused History Questions

- Have you had any changes in hair texture?
- Have you had any hair loss?
- Do you use dyes or chemical treatments for curling or straightening?

➤ When performing the procedure, always identify your patient according to agency policy, using two identifiers, and be attentive to standard precautions, hand hygiene, patient safety and privacy, body mechanics, and documentation.

Procedure Steps

1. **Inspect the hair and scalp.** Check the color, quantity, and distribution of the hair and the condition of the scalp. Note the presence of lesions or pediculosis.
   Sex, genetics, and age affect hair distribution on the head, legs extremities, pubis, and axillae. With aging, melanocyte function declines and sebaceous gland function decreases.

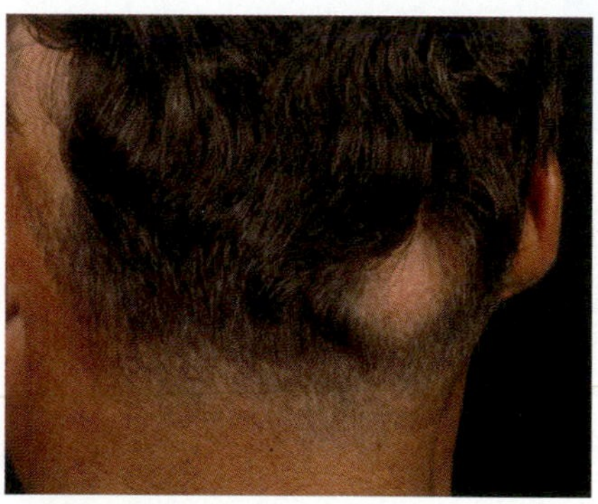

Alopecia areata

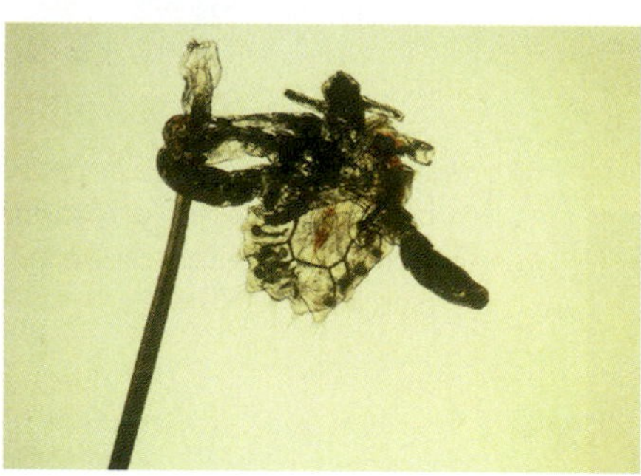

Pediculosis (lice)

Findings

Expected findings: The hair is evenly distributed on the scalp, and fine body hair is present over the body (men often have more hair on the face, chest, and back; alopecia is considered normal in men). The hair is clean and free of debris or pediculosis.

Developmental Variations

Infants—may have very little scalp hair.

Adolescents—may have oily hair. Puberty marks the onset of pubic hair growth and increased hair growth.

Older adults—Scalp, axillary, leg, and pubic hair may be dry and thin; hair of the ears, nostrils, and eyebrows may become coarse.

Abnormal findings:

- Generalized hair loss not attributed to genetics or aging; patchy hair loss.
- ***Hirsutism*** (excess facial or trunk hair).
- White hair accompanied by very pale skin is seen in a condition known as *albinism* (lack of pigmentation).
- Alterations in hair distribution may be signs of disease.

2. **Palpate the texture of the hair.**

Expected findings: Hair texture varies (fine, medium, coarse), depending on genetics and treatments.

Abnormal findings: Very dry, coarse hair may indicate hypothyroidism; thinning and very fine hair may indicate hyperthyroidism.

3. **Palpate the scalp for mobility and tenderness.**

Expected findings: Scalp is smooth, firm, symmetrical, nontender, and without lesions.

Abnormal findings: Common deviations include an asymmetrical or bumpy scalp caused by trauma or lesions, and scaly flakes or patches caused by fungal infection (e.g., dandruff), dermatitis, or psoriasis; tenderness; lesions.

Developmental Variations

Infants: In newborns, ***cradle cap***—scaly white patches over the scalp caused by secretion of sebum—is common. It can be removed with washing and gentle scrubbing.

Patient Teaching

If indicated, teach the patient to check for head lice, and provide education on preventive measures.

Documentation

If you need more information about documenting your findings, review Caring for the Nguyens, and

Go to Chapter 22, **Documenting Physical Examination Findings (Nam Nguyen),** in Volume 1.

Procedure 22-4 ■ Assessing the Nails

➤ For steps to follow in *all* procedures, refer to the Universal Steps for All Procedures found on the inside back cover.

Equipment

- Nonlatex gloves (if exposure to body fluids is a possibility)
- Pen and record form

Focused History Questions

- Have you had any recent changes in the way your nails grow or look?
- Have you had any recent trauma to your nails?
- Do you use acrylic nails?
- Do you have any medical problems, such as peripheral vascular disease or diabetes?

➤ When performing the procedure, always identify your patient according to agency policy, using two identifiers, and be attentive to standard precautions, hand hygiene, patient safety and privacy, body mechanics, and documentation.

Procedure Steps

1. **Inspect nails.**
   - Check nails for color, condition, texture, and shape.
   - Examine nails on both hands and feet. However, for efficiency you may defer examination of the toenails until the assessment of peripheral circulation. ▼

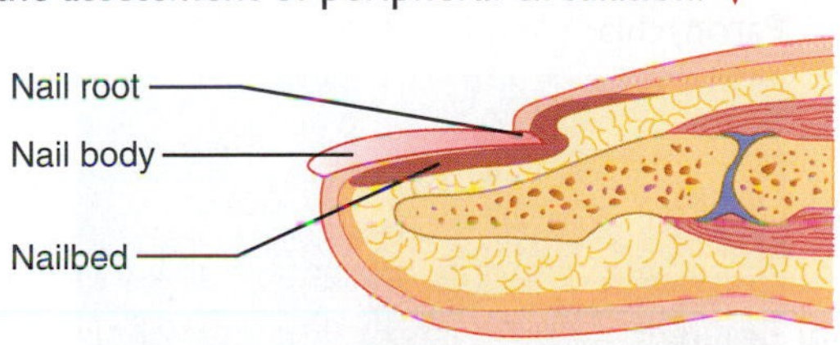

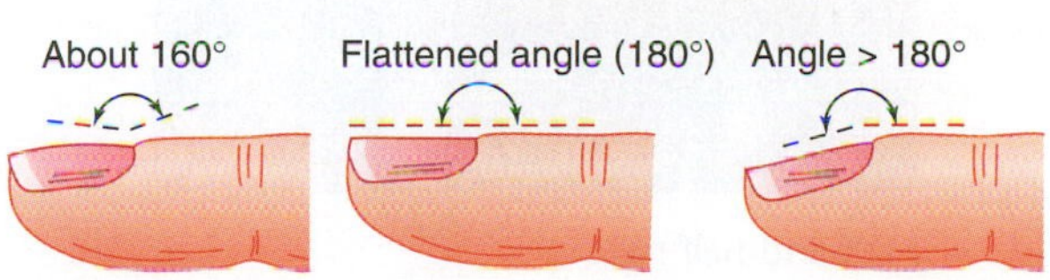

Findings

Expected findings: Healthy nailbeds are level, firm, and similar to the color of the skin. The shape is convex, with a nail plate angle of about 160°.

Developmental Variations

Newborns—have very thin nails.

Children—may bite their nails. Most children outgrow this habit.

Older adults—nails grow more slowly, become thicker, and tend to split.

Abnormal findings:
- Black discoloration resulting from blood under the nail is seen after local trauma.
- Pale or cyanotic nailbeds are seen in circulatory or respiratory disorders that result in anemia or hypoxia.
- White spots may indicate zinc deficiency.
- Spoon-shaped (concave) nails are associated with iron deficiency.

(continued on next page)

Procedure 22-4 ■ Assessing the Nails (continued)

2. Inspect and palpate for texture.
Grooves or lines in the nails provide information about nutrition and health problems.

Expected findings: Nails are smooth and uniform in texture; surrounding tissue is smooth.

Abnormal findings: Thickened nails with yellowing may indicate fungal infection, known as *onychomycosis.*
- Brittle nails are seen with hyperthyroidism, malnutrition, calcium and iron deficiencies, and repeated use of harsh nail products.
- Soft boggy nails are seen with poor oxygenation.
- Paronychia.

3. Assess capillary refill. Briefly press the tip of the nail with firm, steady pressure; then, release and observe for changes in color.
This test assesses circulatory adequacy rather than the nails themselves. However, circulatory insufficiency affects the nails and nailbeds. It is convenient to perform the assessment at this point in the exam.

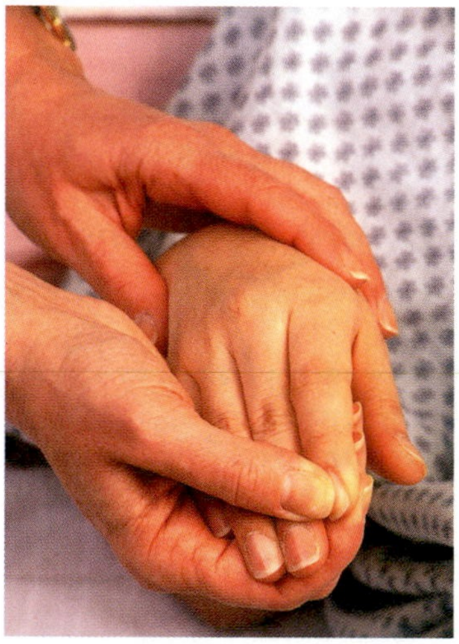

Expected findings: Normal capillary refill is < 2 to 3 seconds.

Developmental Variations

Older adults—capillary refill time (CRT) is slower.
Males—CRT faster than in women
Environment—CRT is slower in a cool environment.

Abnormal findings: Delayed capillary refill.

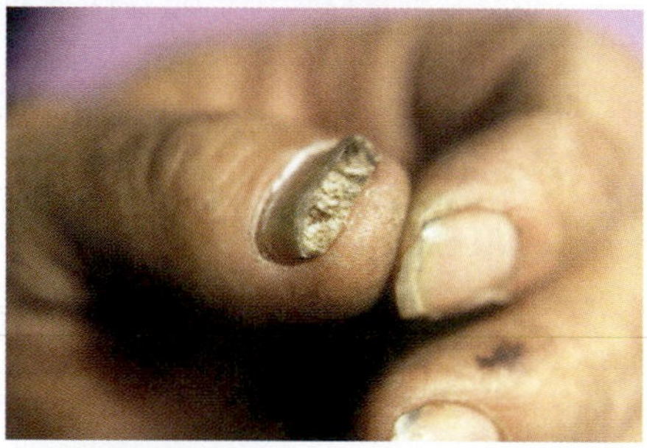

Fungal infection

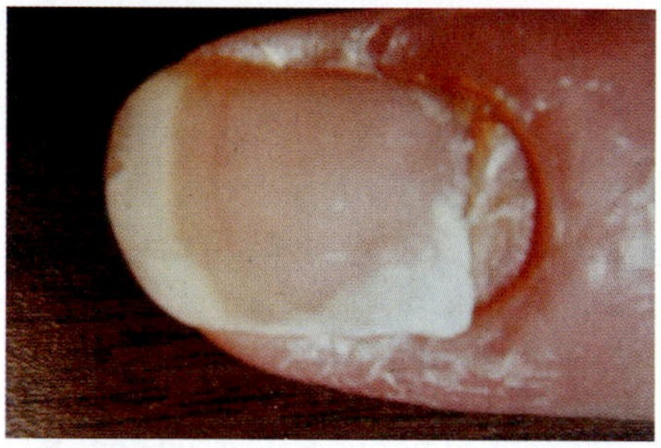

Paronychia

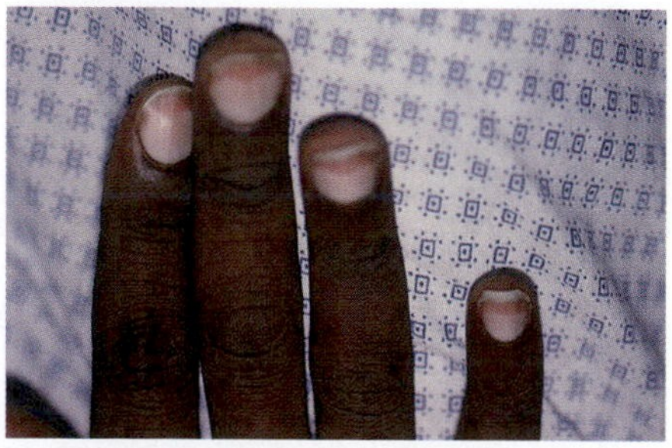

Half-and-half nails

Documentation

If you need more information about documenting your findings, review Caring for the Nguyens, and

Go to Chapter 22, **Documenting Physical Examination Findings (Nam Nguyen),** in Volume 1.

Practice Resources

Lima, A., & Bakker, J. (2015), Linton, C. P. (2012).

Procedure 22-5 ■ Assessing the Head and Face

➤ For steps to follow in *all* procedures, refer to the Universal Steps for All Procedures found on the inside back cover.

Equipment

- Nonlatex gloves (if exposure to body fluids is a possibility)
- Penlight (to transilluminate the sinuses)
- Pen and record form

Clean equipment before and after use unless used for only one patient.

Focused History Questions

- Have you had any recent headaches?
- Have you ever had a head injury or loss of consciousness?
- Have you ever had a seizure?
- Do you have jaw or facial pain?

Positioning

The client should be sitting, if possible.

➤ When performing the procedure, always identify your patient according to agency policy, using two identifiers, and be attentive to standard precautions, hand hygiene, patient safety and privacy, body mechanics, and documentation.

Procedure Steps

1. **Inspect the head. Check for size, shape, symmetry, and position.**
   If size seems unusual measure it.

Developmental Modifications

Newborns and infants—assess and transilluminate fontanels, and measure head circumference.

Findings

Expected findings: There is wide variation in head size and shape, although the shape should be symmetrical and rounded. The head should be erect, midline, and proportional to the body size based on age.

Developmental Variations

Newborns and infants—cranial bones are not fused at birth, and head shape may reflect normal pressure or trauma during vaginal birth for several weeks. The anterior fontanel ("soft spot") fuses at about 18 months; the posterior, at about 8 weeks. Infants normally cannot hold the head up until about 6 months of age.

Abnormal findings: Larger or smaller than expected size for age, asymmetry of skull.

2. **Inspect the face.** Note the client's facial expression. Ask yourself,
   - Are the facial features symmetrical?
   - Are there any abnormal facial movements?
   - Are there any visible lesions or abnormal hair distribution?

Expected findings: Facial expression is appropriate for the situation. No visible lesions. Facial features and movement are symmetrical.

(continued on next page)

Procedure 22-5 ■ Assessing the Head and Face (continued)

Helpful hint: Look for symmetry in the palpebral fissures and the nasolabial folds.

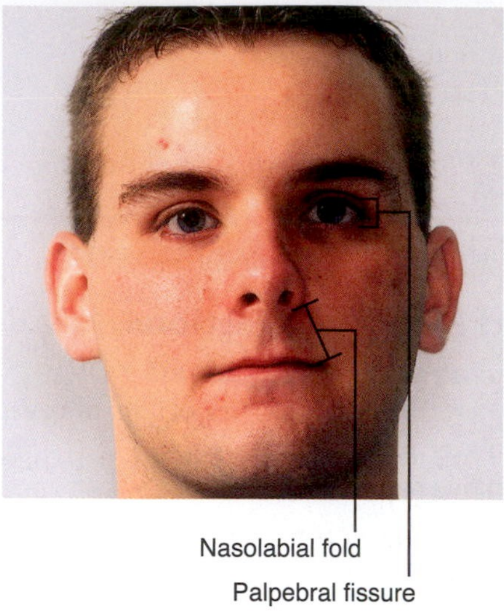

Abnormal findings: Facial appearance inconsistent with gender, age, or racial/ethnic group; asymmetry of facial features or facial movement.

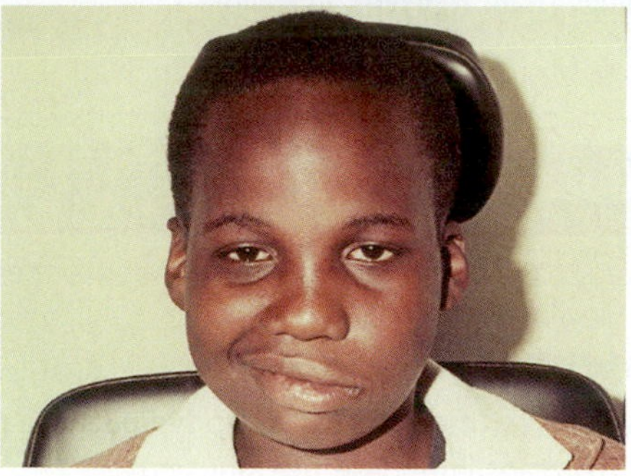

Bell's palsy

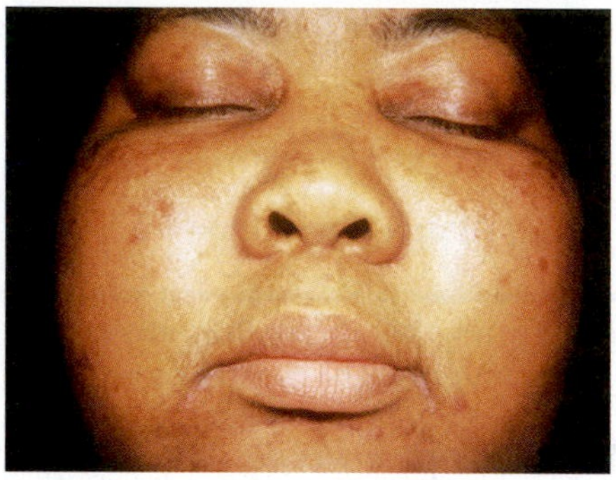

Cushing's syndrome

---

3. Palpate the head. Check for masses, tenderness, and scalp mobility.

Developmental Modifications

Newborns and infants—palpate anterior and posterior fontanels.

Expected findings: The head should be nontender, relatively smooth and symmetrical; and without unusual contours, bulges, or lesions.

Abnormal findings: Contour abnormalities (e.g., indentations, "bumps") or tenderness can result from trauma, congenital anomalies, or surgery.

---

4. Palpate the face for symmetry, tenderness, muscle tone, and temporomandibular joint (TMJ) function.

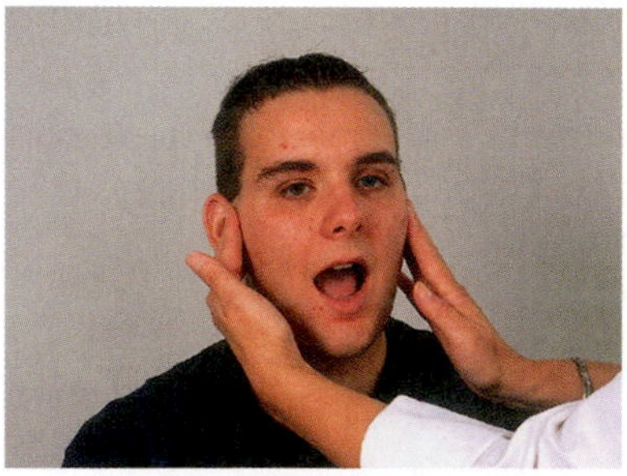

Palpating the TMJ

Expected findings: Smooth, symmetrical movement with no pain, crepitus, or clicking of the jaw

Abnormal findings: Irregular or uneven movement of the jaw; pain or popping/cracking with movement may indicate TMJ syndrome.

Documentation

- If you need more information about documenting your findings, review Caring for the Nguyens, and

Go to Chapter 22, **Documenting Physical Examination Findings (Nam Nguyen),** in Volume I.

Procedure 22-6 ■ Assessing the Eyes

➤ For steps to follow in *all* procedures, refer to the Universal Steps for All Procedures found on the inside back cover.

Equipment

- Nonlatex gloves—if exposure to body fluids is a possibility
- Visual acuity chart with color bars (Snellen)
- A card—to cover one eye during the acuity exam
- Penlight
- Cotton ball and cotton-tipped applicator
- Ophthalmoscope
- Pen and form

Clean equipment before and after use unless used for only one patient.

Positioning

The client should be sitting, if possible.

Focused History Questions

- Have you noticed any changes in your vision?
- Do you wear glasses or contact lenses?
- Have you ever had an eye injury?
- Have you ever had an eye infection or stye?
- Do you have problems with excessive tearing or dry eyes?
- Have you ever had eye surgery?
- Have you ever experienced blurred vision?
- Do you have difficulty with nighttime vision?
- Do you ever see halos of light, spots or floaters, or flashes of light?
- Do you have a history of eye problems, such as glaucoma, or medical problems, such as diabetes or hypertension?
- When was your last eye exam?
- Do you use any prescription or over-the-counter eye medications?

➤ When performing the procedure, always identify your patient according to agency policy, using two identifiers, and be attentive to standard precautions, hand hygiene, patient safety and privacy, body mechanics, and documentation.

Procedure Steps

1. Test distance vision.

- Depending on patient's age and literacy level, use the Snellen standard eye chart or Snellen E chart (for those who cannot read). Picture charts are available for preschoolers.
- If the client wears corrective lenses, they should be worn during a test.
  a. Have the patient sit or stand 6 m (20 ft) from the chart. With a card, cover the eye not being tested; ask the patient to read the smallest line of print that he can distinguish. Consider a line to be read correctly if the client makes no more than two mistakes in that line. If he hesitates when reporting the letters or symbols, document "with hesitation."
  b. Test the opposite eye.
  c. Test both eyes together.

Findings

Expected findings: 20/20 vision in the right eye, left eye, and both eyes. The top number of the fraction indicates the distance the person was standing from the chart; the bottom number is the distance from which a person with normal vision would be able to read the chart.

Developmental Variations

Children—distance vision does not reach 20/20 until around age 6 or 7 years.

Middle adults—at about middle age, the lens of the eye begins to lose some ability to accommodate to near objects.

Abnormal findings: A smaller fraction (e.g., 20/100) indicates diminished distant vision or myopia. A larger fraction (e.g., 20/15) indicates diminished near vision, called *hyperopia.*

(continued on next page)

Procedure 22-6 ■ Assessing the Eyes (continued)

d. At the end of each line of the Snellen chart is a fraction—the top line is 20/200. After each test, record the resulting fraction: the number at the end of the smallest line the patient could read with no more than two errors. If there were more than 2 errors in a line, record the number of items missed.

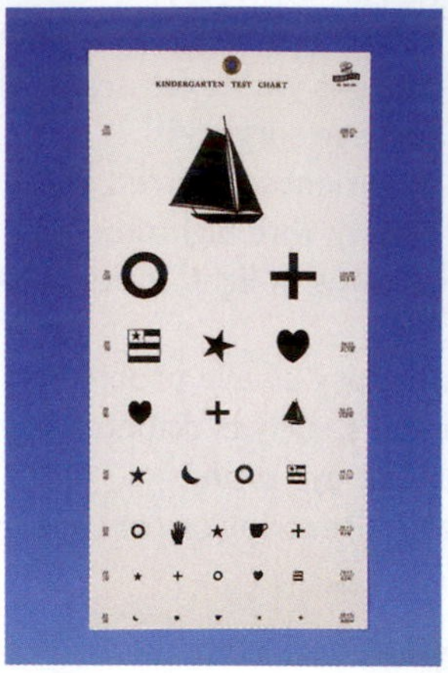

Preliterate chart

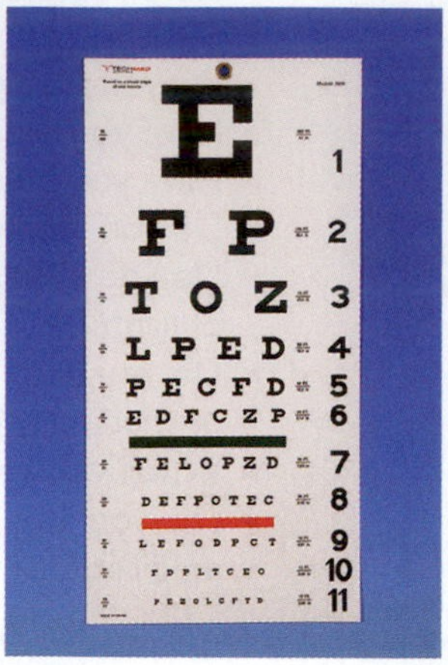

Snellen standard chart

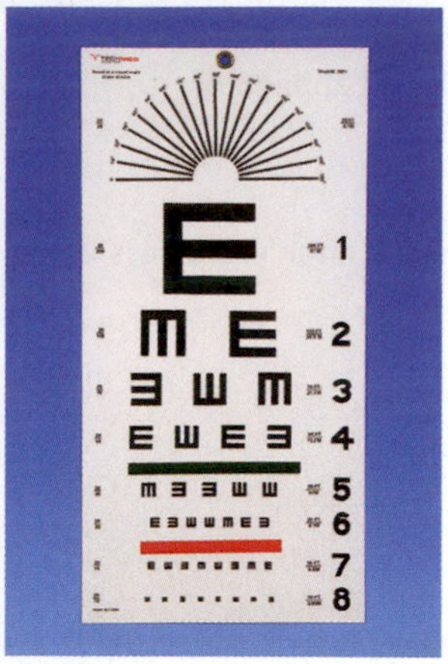

Snellen E chart

2. Test near vision. Test the client's ability to read newsprint at a distance of 35.5 cm (14 in.) from the eyes. Use print-sized pictures if the patient is unable to read.

Expected findings: The client reads newsprint at a distance of 35.5 cm (14 in.).

Developmental Variations

Adults: The lens of the eye naturally loses some ability to accommodate to near objects. In clients older than 45 years, diminished near vision is known as *presbyopia.*

3. Test color vision.

a. Have the patient differentiate patterns of colors on color cards or identify the color bars on the Snellen eye chart.

b. Inability to distinguish colors requires a thorough evaluation using the Ishihara cards to determine the scope of the color deficit.

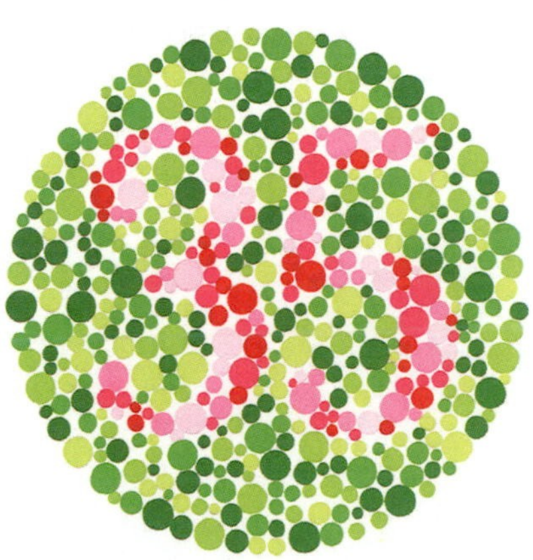

Ishihara card

Expected findings: Color vision is intact.

Developmental Variations

Older adults experience some decline in color vision, especially in the ability to see purples and pastels.

Abnormal findings: Inability to distinguish colors.

4. Test peripheral vision.

a. Seat the client 60–90 cm (2–3 ft) from you.

b. Have client cover one eye and fix the gaze straight ahead while you bring an object in from the periphery to the center of the visual fields. Be sure to begin by holding the object well outside the range of normal peripheral vision. Instruct the client to identify when the object becomes visible.

c. Repeat this in each of the four visual fields, moving clockwise.

Expected findings: Expect no deficits in the visual fields.

Abnormal findings:

- ***Strabismus*** (crossed eye) is a condition in which one or both eyes deviate from the object they are looking at. Constant strabismus of one eye may result in ***amblyopia*** ("lazy eye"), in which the brain does not fully acknowledge the images seen by the amblyopic eye. This creates reduced vision in that eye, not correctable by glasses or contact lenses.
- **Loss of peripheral vision**. Report gross deficits to an ophthalmologist for further assessment.

Developmental Variations

Infants: Strabismus is normal during the first 1 or 2 months of life. After that, it may be caused by weak intraocular muscles or a lesion on the oculomotor nerve.

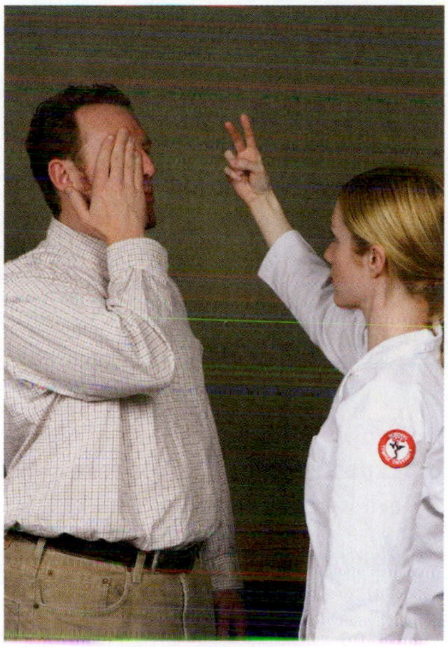

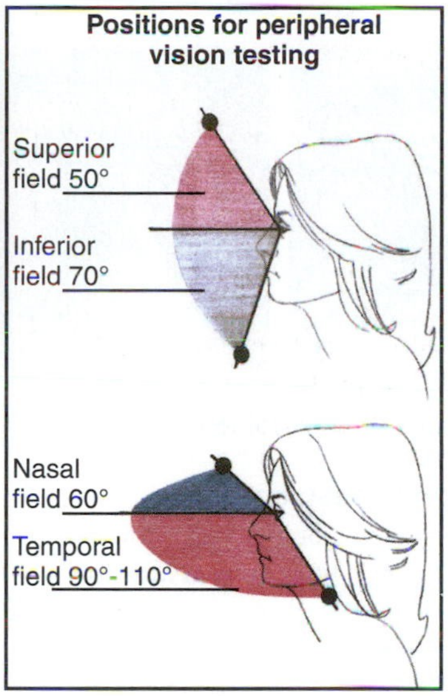

5. Assess extraocular movements (EOMs).

a. **Inspect the eyes for parallel alignment.**

a. **Expected findings:** The eyes should be in parallel alignment.

b. **Test the corneal light reflex** by shining a penlight at the bridge of the nose. Note where the light reflects on the cornea of each eye.

b. **Expected findings:** Corneal light reflex appears at the same position in each eye.

Abnormal findings: An asymmetrical corneal light reflex may indicate weak extraocular muscles or strabismus.

(continued on next page)

Procedure 22-6 ■ Assessing the Eyes (continued)

c. **Test the six cardinal fields of gaze.** Stand in front of the patient, and have the patient follow an object through the six cardinal fields without moving his head.

c. **Expected findings:** The eyes move through all six gaze positions.

Abnormal findings: Inability to move through all gaze positions.

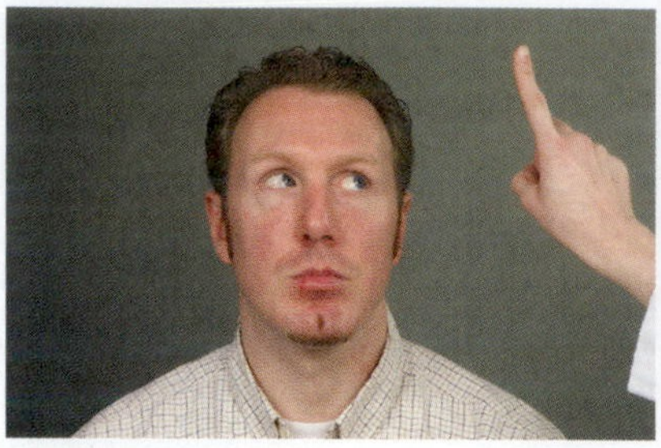
Up left

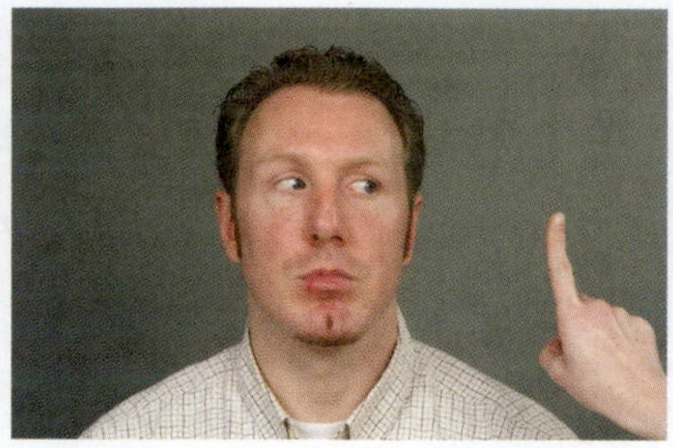
Side left

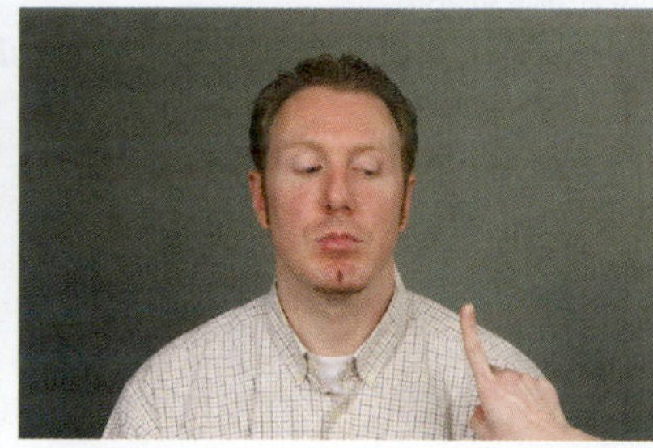
Down left

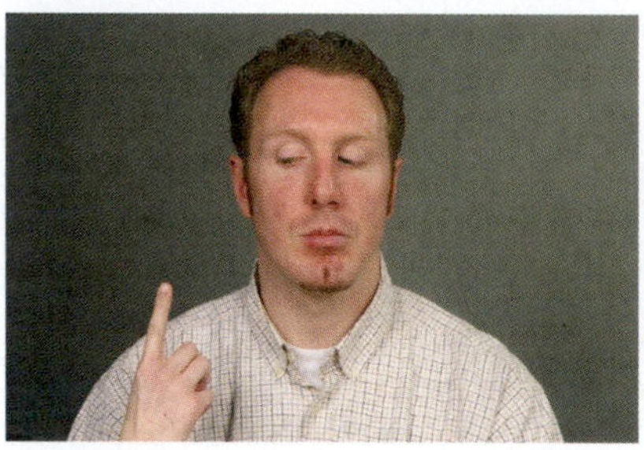
Down right

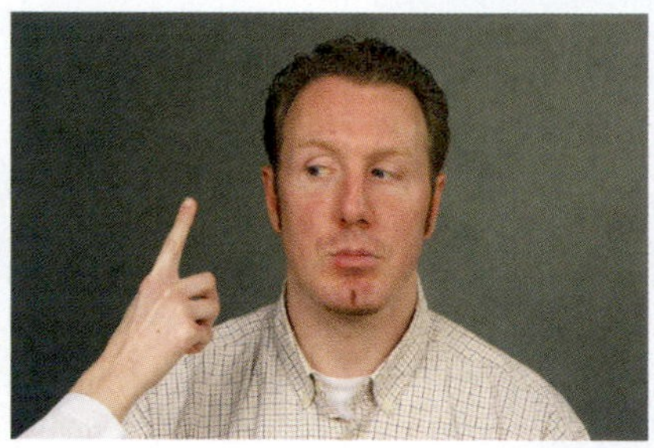
Side right

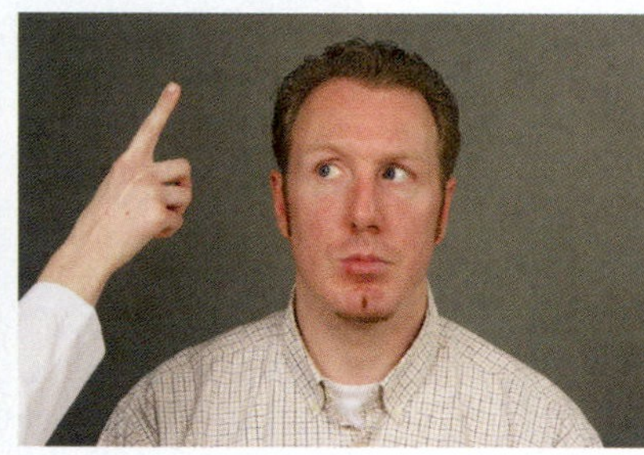
Up right

d. **Perform the cover/uncover test.** Have the patient cover one eye and gaze at a distant object. Have the patient uncover the eye and repeat on the opposite side.

d. **Expected findings:** The gaze should be steady when the eye is covered or uncovered.

Abnormal findings: A shift in gaze indicates weak eye muscles.

6. Inspect the external structures.

a. **General appearance.** Check the color and alignment of the eyes.

a. **Expected findings:** Eyes clear, bright, and in parallel alignment.

Developmental Variations

Older adults—a decrease in periorbital fat may give the eyeballs a sunken appearance.

Abnormal findings: Glazed eyes may indicate a febrile state.

b. **Inspect the eyelids.** Note the presence of any lesions, edema, or lid lag.

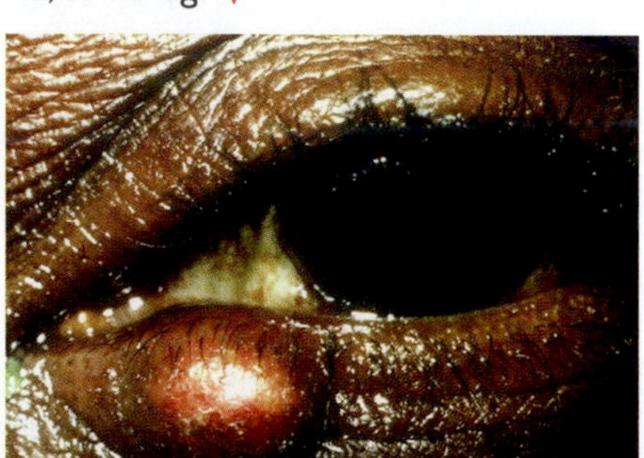
Hordeolum (stye)

b. **Expected findings:** Eyelid margins moist and pink. No crusting, scales, or lesions present; lids move freely. Upper eyelid covers half of the upper iris; lower eyelid appears at bottom edge of iris.

Developmental Variations

Older adults—the lower lids may sag; skinfolds are prominent in the upper lids.

Abnormal findings: Asymmetry of lids may result from CN III damage or from a stroke. Lesions may be benign (e.g., a stye) or pathological (e.g., basal cell carcinoma).

c. **Inspect the eyelashes.** Note symmetry and distribution.

c. **Expected findings:** Eyelashes are evenly distributed and curve outward. No crustations or infestations are present.

Abnormal findings: Inflammation of the eyelids, which may be caused by infection; inverted eyelashes (entropion); everted eyelashes (ectropion); visible sclera between the iris and upper lid.

d. **Inspect the lacrimal ducts and glands.** Note any edema, excessive tearing, or drainage.

d. **Expected findings:** No periorbital edema or lesions are present. No drainage.

Abnormal findings: Swelling, redness, drainage, or tenderness.

e. **Inspect the conjunctivae.** Note the color, moisture, and contour of the conjunctivae.

(1) The palpebral conjunctivae cover the lids. To assess, have the patient look up as you place a cotton-tipped applicator on the upper lid, gently grasp the upper lid and lashes, and evert the lid over the cotton-tipped applicator.

(2) The bulbar conjunctiva covers the eyeball. To assess, pull the lower lid down.

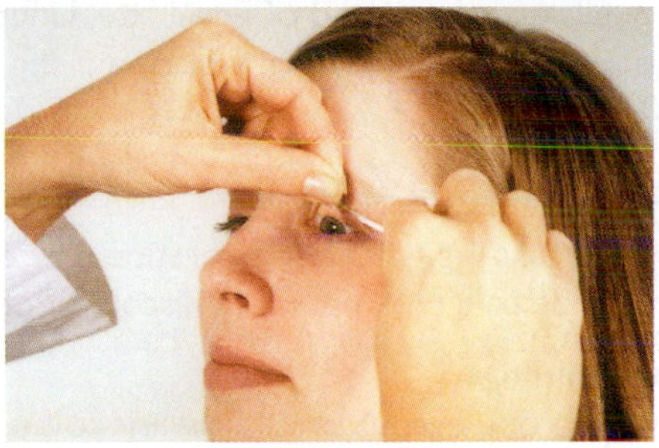

Examining the palpebral conjunctiva

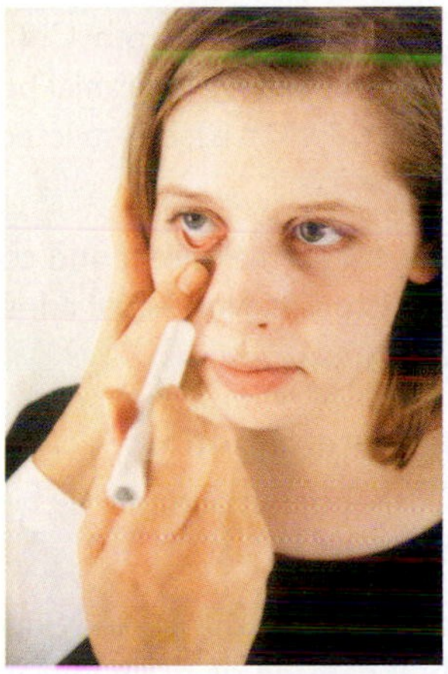

Examining the bulbar conjunctiva

e. **Expected findings:** The palpebral conjunctivae are smooth, glistening, and peach in color. Minimal blood vessels are present. The bulbar conjunctivae are clear with few underlying blood vessels and white sclera visible.

Developmental Variations

Older adults—the conjunctivae may be pale or have a slightly yellow tint as a result of fat deposits.

Abnormal findings: Pallor, dryness, edema; pterygium; subconjunctival hemorrhage.

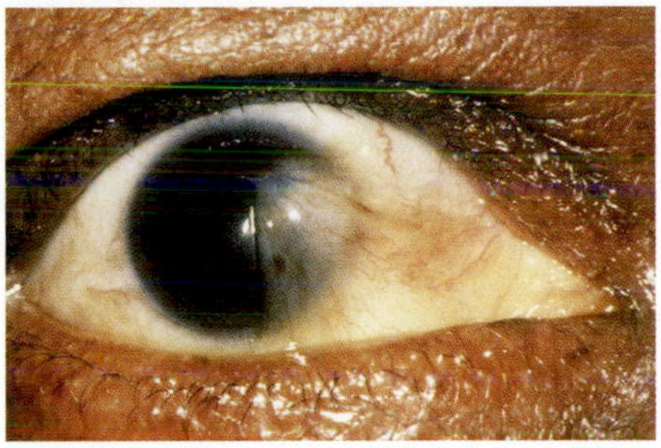

Pterygium

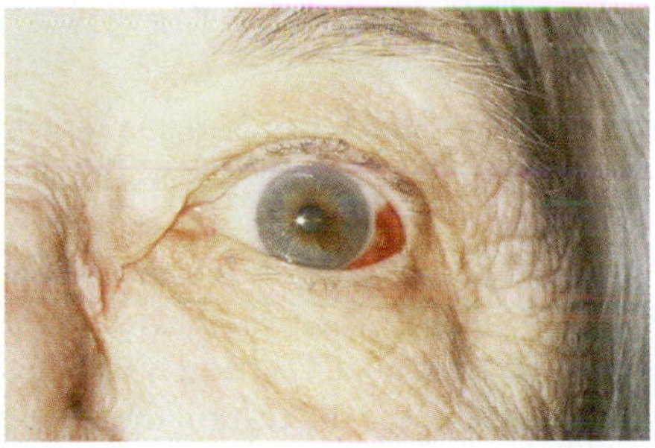

Subconjunctival hemorrhage

f. **Inspect the sclera.** Note the color of the sclera and whether any lesions are present.

f. **Expected findings:** The sclera should be smooth, white, and glistening. Dark-skinned patients may have a yellowish cast to the peripheral sclera or small brown spots more centrally.

Abnormal findings: Yellow (icteric) sclera.

(continued on next page)

Procedure 22-6 ■ Assessing the Eyes (continued)

g. **Inspect the cornea and lens.** As the client looks straight ahead, shine a penlight at an angle to the eye, and move it across the corneal surface. Note the color and whether any lesions are present.

g. **Expected findings:** The cornea and lens are clear, smooth, and glistening.

Developmental Variations

Older adults—arcus senilis (white, gray, or blue opaque ring in the corneal margin) is a normal variant.

Abnormal findings: Lens opacities (cataracts); roughness or irregularity of the cornea.

h. **Test the corneal reflex.** Touch the cornea with a wisp of sterile cotton, or use a needleless syringe to shoot a small amount of air over the cornea.

Note: This is not routinely performed on conscious patients. A conscious person can blink intentionally, so there is no need to perform this test. In addition, there is a slight risk of corneal abrasion from cotton.

h. **Expected findings:** Blink reflex is prompt.

Abnormal findings: Failure to blink may result from neurosensory deficits.

i. **Inspect the iris and pupils.** Note color, size, shape, and symmetry.

i. **Expected findings:**

- The iris is blue, green, brown, or a combination of these colors; its shape is circular.
- The pupils are round and of equal size. Unequal pupils (anisocoria) can be a normal variation if the difference is < 0.5 mm.

Developmental Variations

Older adults—pigment degeneration may cause the iris to be pale with brownish discolorations.

Abnormal findings:

- Damage to one eye may cause the iris to be a different color.
- Absence of part or all of the iris is a congenital problem.
- Unequal pupils may result from CN III damage, brain herniation, or increased intracranial pressure (ICP).
- Enlarged pupils (mydriasis); constricted pupils (myosis).
- Cloudy pupils.

j. **Test pupillary reaction.** In a dimly lighted room, have the patient look straight ahead. Bring a penlight in from the side, and shine the light onto one eye. Note the reaction, equality, and speed of response of both eyes. (For example, when you shine a light onto the right eye, the right pupil reaction is direct; the left eye is consensual). Repeat the test on the opposite eye. ▼

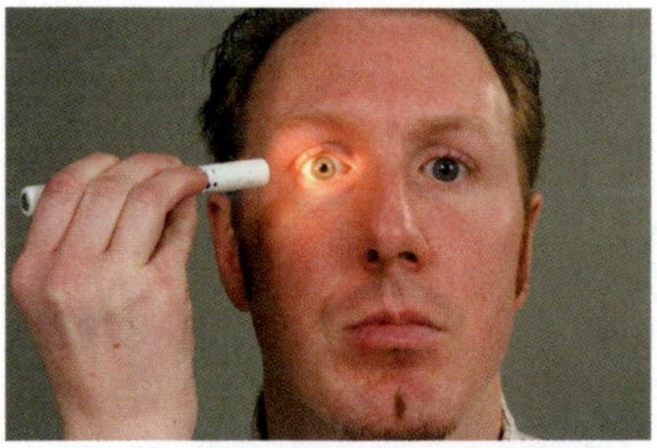

Testing pupillary reaction to light

j. **Expected findings:** Normal direct and consensual response to light is brisk, with equal constriction of both pupils.

Developmental Variations

Older adults—pupil reaction may be slower but should be symmetrical.

Abnormal findings: Sluggish or fixed pupils may result from CN II damage or brain injury. Absence of consensual response may result from nerve compression or anoxia.

k. **Test pupil accommodation.** Have the patient look straight ahead and focus on an object about 30 cm (12 in.) from his face. Slowly bring the object in toward the patient's eyes. Note pupil size and location.

k. **Expected findings:** The pupils constrict and the eyes cross as a person attempts to focus on a near object.

Developmental Variations

Older adults—accommodation may be slow.

Abnormal findings: One or both pupils fail to accommodate, or they accommodate slowly.

l. **Inspect the anterior chamber.** Shine a penlight across the eye from the side as the patient looks straight ahead. Observe color, size, shape, and symmetry.

l. **Expected findings:** The chamber should be clear and symmetrically curved.

Abnormal findings: Blood or pus in the chamber.

---

7. Palpate the external structures.

a. Gently palpate the globe (eyeball) with your fingertips on the upper lids over the sclera. Note consistency and any tenderness. ▼

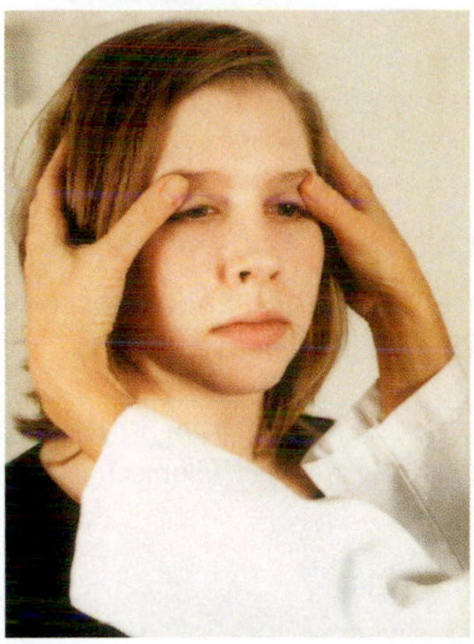

b. Palpate the lacrimal glands and ducts by palpating below the eyebrow and below the inner canthus of the eye. Note tenderness and excessive tearing or discharge.

Expected findings: The globe is firm and nontender. Lacrimal glands are nonpalpable; no tenderness is present.

Abnormal findings: Firm or tender globe; swelling and tenderness over the lacrimal glands.

---

8. Assess the internal structures via ophthalmoscopy. This is an advanced physical assessment technique.

a. Darken the room.

b. Stand about 1 foot from the patient at a 15° lateral angle.

c. Dial the lens wheel to zero with your index finger. Hold the ophthalmoscope to your brow.

d. Have the patient look straight ahead while you shine the light on one pupil and identify the red light reflex. ▼

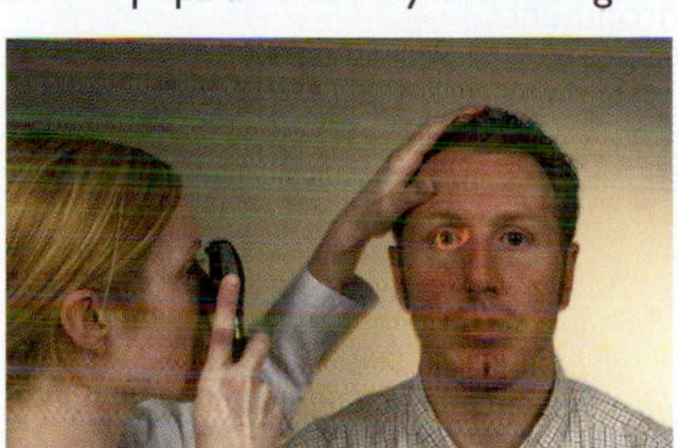

Checking red reflex

Expected findings: A positive red light reflex. On internal examination, the optic disk is round with sharp margins. There are no opacities and the cup-to-disk ratio is 1:2. The disk is yellow with a white cup.

Abnormal findings: Any findings not consistent with the above should be reported promptly.

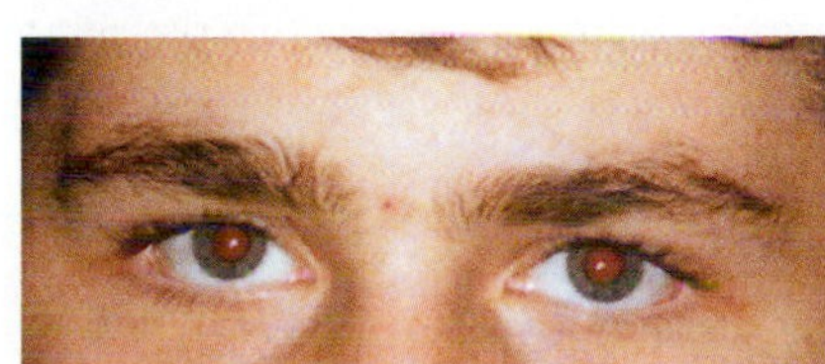

Red reflex over pupil area

(continued on next page)

Procedure 22-6 ■ Assessing the Eyes (continued)

e. Once you identify the red light reflex, move closer to within a few inches of the eye and observe the internal structures of the eye. Adjust the lens wheel to focus, as needed. Use your right eye to examine the patient's right eye, and your left eye to examine the patient's left eye. ▼

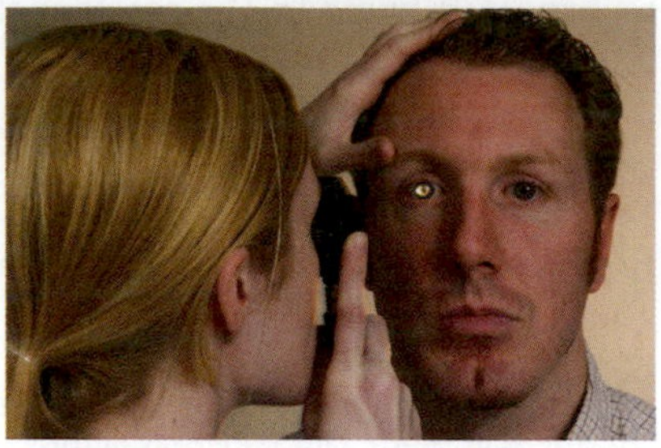

Examining internal structures of the eye

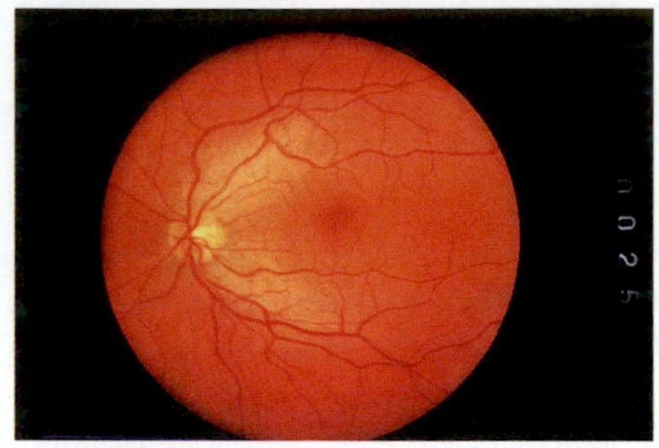

Normal fundus

f. Repeat for the opposite eye.

Patient Teaching

Teach the patient the importance of routine eye examinations.

Documentation

If you need more information about documenting your findings, review Caring for the Nguyens, and

Go to Chapter 22, **Documenting Physical Examination Findings (Nam Nguyen),** in Volume 1.

Procedure 22-7 ■ Assessing the Ears and Hearing

➤ For steps to follow in *all* procedures, refer to the Universal Steps for All Procedures found on the inside back cover.

Equipment

- Nonlatex gloves (if exposure to body fluids is a possibility)
- Tuning fork
- Watch that ticks (or a similar device)
- Otoscope with pneumatic tube
- Pen and record form

Positioning

Have the patient seated, if possible.

Focused History Questions

- Do you have any hearing problems?
- Have you ever had ringing in your ears?
- Have you had any changes in your hearing?
- Do you have any ear drainage? If yes, how much and what color?
- Do you have any ear pain?
- Do you have any balance problems, dizziness, or vertigo?
- Do you have a history of head trauma?
- Are you exposed to noise pollution at work or in your home environment?

➤ When performing the procedure, always identify your patient according to agency policy, using two identifiers, and be attentive to standard precautions, hand hygiene, patient safety and privacy, body mechanics, and documentation.

Procedure Steps / Findings

1. Inspect the external ear.

a. Check the placement and angle of attachment of the ear.

a. **Expected findings:** The normal angle of attachment is 10°.

Abnormal findings: High or low placement of the ear may be a sign of hearing deficit or genetic problems, for example, Down syndrome.

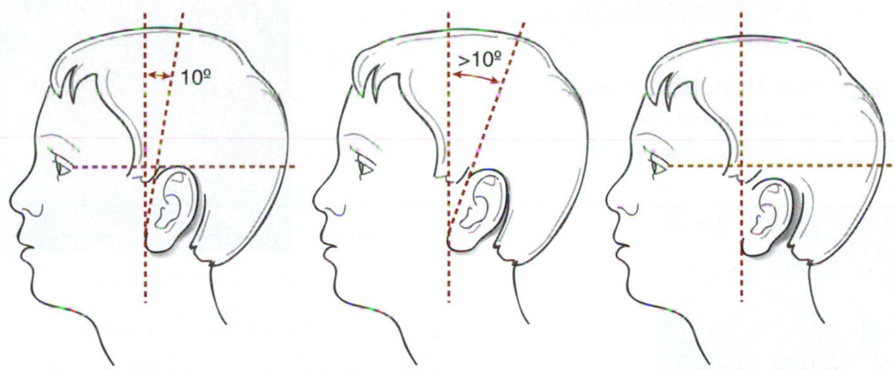

b. Note the shape, size, and symmetry of the ears.

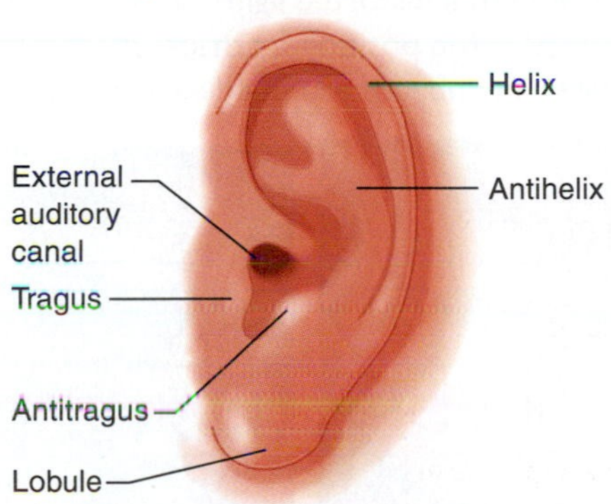

b. **Expected findings:** The helix, antihelix, antitragus, tragus, and lobule are present. The ears are 4 to 10 cm in length and symmetrical in size and shape.

Developmental Variations

Older adults—the ear changes shape as the lobe elongates.

Abnormal findings: Absence of any of the landmarks may indicate a hearing deficit. Ears that are < 4 cm long or > 10 cm long may indicate a genetic disorder.

c. Observe the color of the ear.

c. **Expected findings:** Color is consistent with skin color.

Abnormal findings: Redness may indicate inflammation or infection.

d. Observe the condition of the skin; observe for drainage and visible lesions.

d. **Expected findings:** Skin is intact with no drainage or lesions. Piercings may be present.

Developmental Variations

Older adults—may have coarse hair on the helix, antihelix, and tragus; skin may be dry.

Abnormal findings: Bloody drainage may result from trauma. Purulent drainage may be seen with infection. The ears are a common location for skin cancer.

2. Palpate the external structures of the ear. Note the consistency of the skin, the presence of lesions, and any signs of tenderness.

Expected findings: Skin is soft, pliable, and nontender. No nodules or lesions are present.

Abnormal findings: Tenderness is often associated with infection (e.g., otitis externa, otitis media).

(continued on next page)

Procedure 22-7 ■ Assessing the Ears and Hearing (continued)

3. **Perform an otoscopic exam.**
   This is an advanced physical assessment technique.
   a. Use a speculum with the largest diameter and shortest length that the ear canal can accommodate; 4 mm is a common size for adults.
   b. Have the patient tilt his head to the side not being examined.
   c. For adults, grasp the pinna and gently pull upward and back. For a child, position the pinna down and back.
   Positions the ear canal with more direct alignment, allowing for improved visualization.
   d. Insert the speculum no further than halfway into the ear canal. As you advance the speculum, examine the canal for redness, open areas, drainage, foreign objects, and so on. ▼

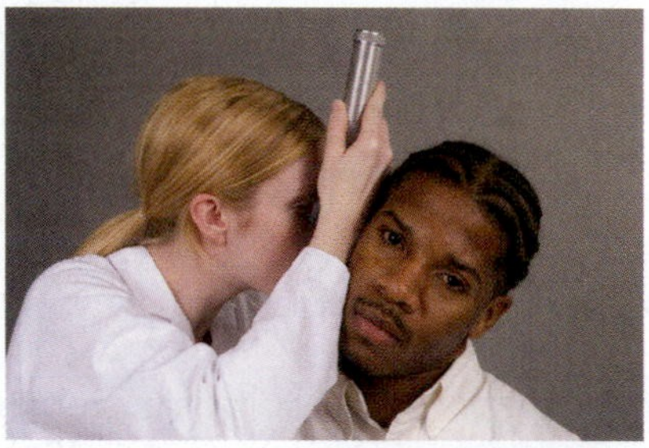

Otoscope insertion with handle up

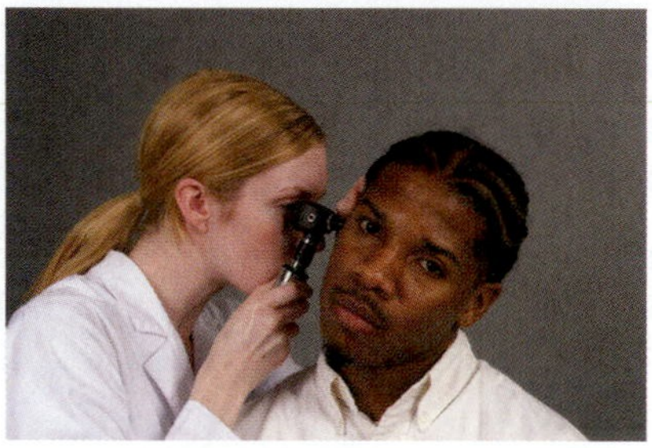

Otoscope insertion with handle down

   e. Look through the magnifying lens.
      (1) Observe the ear canal.
      (2) Observe the tympanic membrane.
   f. Test the mobility of the tympanic membrane by using the otoscope's pneumatic tube to gently "puff" air into the external ear canal while observing movement of the cone of light.

NOTE: The ears are mirror images, with the cone of light at the 7 o'clock position in the left ear and at the 5 o'clock position in the right ear.

Developmental Modifications

Children—many young children fear the otoscopic exam. Demonstrating the procedure on a parent or a doll may relieve anxiety.

   g. Carefully remove the otoscope from the ear canal, being careful not to traumatize the delicate tissue.

Expected findings: The ear canal is light in color and patent, with a small amount of yellow cerumen (color may vary). The tympanic membrane (TM) is shiny and pearly gray, with a cone of reflective light on the nasal aspect (this would be 7 o'clock in the left ear and 5 o'clock in the right ear). Bony landmarks are visible. The TM is mobile. No bulging or retraction of the TM. ▼

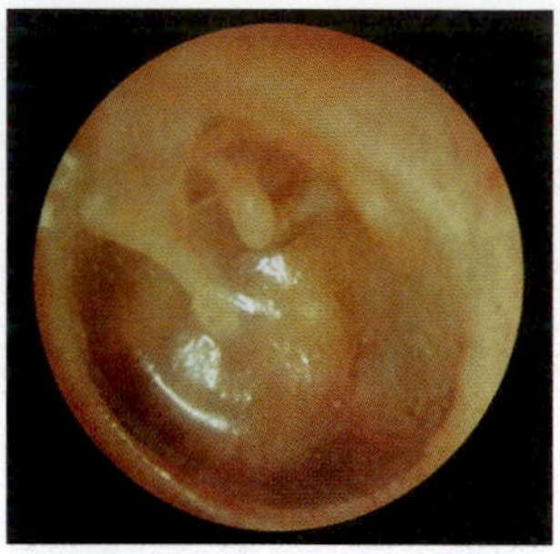

Normal TM left ear

Developmental Variations

Older adults—may have dry ear wax. The TM is translucent, and the light reflex may be diminished.

Abnormal findings: Excessive wax may occlude the canal. TM that is red, with a distorted light reflex, suggests otitis media. A change in the position or shape of the cone of light reflex indicates an imbalance in middle ear pressure. ▼

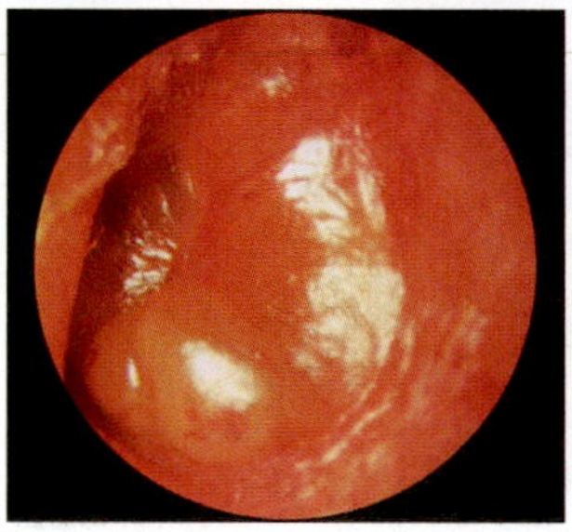

Otitis media

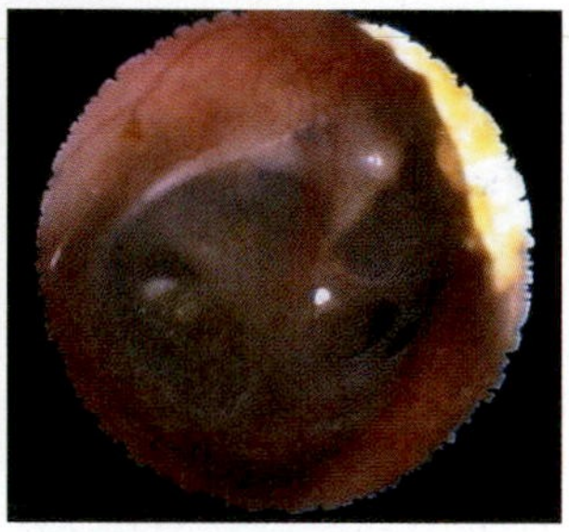

Perforated TM

4. **Test gross hearing.**
   a. Stand 1 to 2 ft behind the patient. Have the patient cover one ear as you whisper some words. Repeat on the other side. Have the patient repeat the words she heard.
   A test of hearing also indicates CN XIII is intact.
   b. Have the patient occlude one ear. Hold a ticking watch next to the patient's unobstructed ear. Slowly move it away until the patient says she can no longer hear the sound. Repeat for the opposite ear.

Developmental Modifications

Infants—for infants younger than 3 months of age, clap your hands loudly behind the infant, and observe whether he startles. After age 3 months, the infant should turn his head or eyes toward a sound, for example, when the parent stands behind the infant and calls his name.

Expected Findings: The patient is able to hear you whisper on both sides. The patient hears the watch at a distance of about 12 to 13 cm (5 in.).

Developmental Variations

Older adults—often have a generalized loss of hearing. It first occurs in the high-frequency sounds (*f, s, sh,* and *ph*) and then progresses to include all frequencies.

Abnormal findings: Problems detected in the whisper test indicate low-tone hearing loss. Problems found in the watch-tick test indicate a high-pitch deficit.

---

5. **Perform the Weber test.** Place a vibrating tuning fork on top of the patient's head. Ask the patient whether the sound is the same in both ears or louder in one ear.

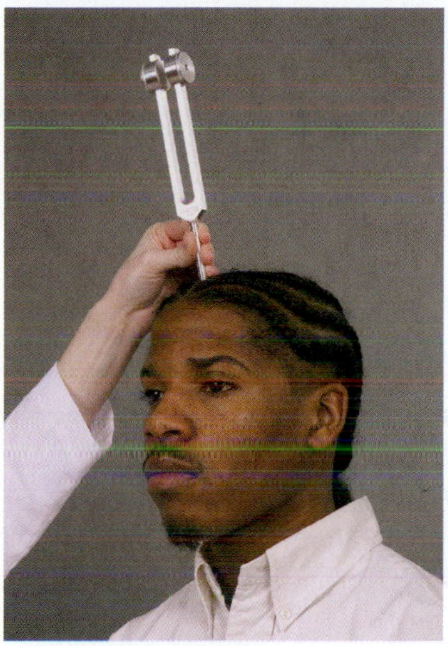

Weber test

Expected findings: The patient hears the sound equally in both ears.

Abnormal findings: Sound is louder in one ear.

- If there is a *conductive hearing loss*, the vibration will be louder in the impaired ear. Conductive hearing loss may be caused by external or middle ear problems, such as infection, blockage of the canal by cerumen, or trauma to the TM.
- If there is a *sensorineural hearing loss*, the sound will be louder in the unaffected ear. Sensorineural loss may result from inner ear problems or from some medications.

---

6. **If the Weber test is positive: Perform the Rinne test.**
   a. Strike a tuning fork on the table. While it is still vibrating, place it on the patient's mastoid process.
   Tests bone conduction of sound.
   b. Measure the elapsed time in seconds that the patient hears the vibration.
   c. Move the tuning fork to 2.5 cm (1 in.) in front of the ear, and measure the elapsed time until the patient can no longer hear the vibration.
   Tests air conduction of sound.

Expected findings: Normally, sound transmission through air (step 6c) is twice as long as transmission through bone (step 6b); that is,

$$AC = 2 \times BC.$$

The ratio of AC to BC is similar in both ears.

(continued on next page)

Procedure 22-7 ■ Assessing the Ears and Hearing (continued)

d. Repeat for the opposite ear.

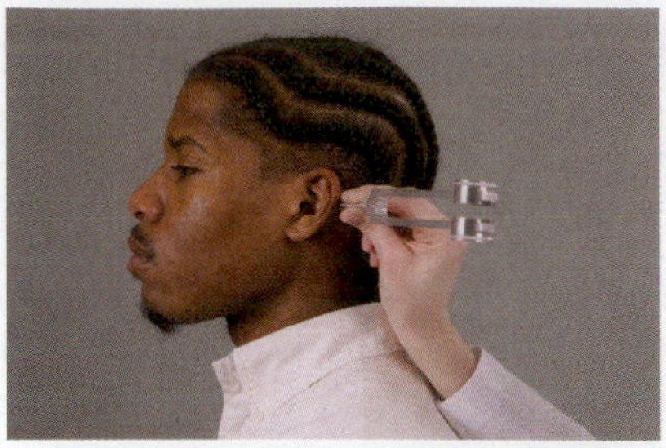

Rinne test

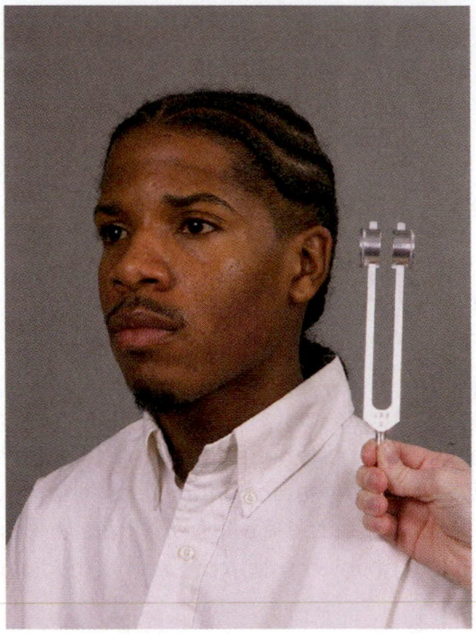

Step 6c

Abnormal findings:

- *Conductive loss:* AC is < 2 × BC.
- *Sensorineural loss:* AC is > BC but not 2 × longer; or the patient is unable to hear the tuning fork through BC.
- A difference between ears indicates unilateral hearing loss.
- Inability to hear the tuning fork through BC indicates sensorineural hearing loss.

7. **Perform the Romberg test.** Have the patient stand with feet together, hands at side, with eyes opened and then with eyes closed. Note the patient's ability to maintain balance.

Stand nearby in case the client loses his balance.

Tests for balance. Strictly speaking, it does not assess the ears, but the vestibular nerve and other parts of the central nervous system. Therefore, you may prefer to perform the test during the neurological exam.

Expected findings: The patient maintains balance with minimal sway.

Abnormal findings: Positive result on the Romberg test (swaying) is seen with vestibular and cerebellar disorders.

Patient Teaching

Teach the patient the importance of routine hearing exams.

Documentation

- If you need more information about documenting your findings, review Caring for the Nguyens, and

Go to Chapter 22, **Documenting Physical Examination Findings (Nam Nguyen),** in Volume 1.

Procedure 22-8 ■ Assessing the Nose and Sinuses

➤ For steps to follow in *all* procedures, refer to the Universal Steps for All Procedures found on the inside back cover.

Equipment

- Nonlatex procedure gloves (if exposure to body fluids is a possibility)
- Penlight
- Nasal speculum or otoscope with a wide-tipped speculum
- Pen and record form

Positioning

Have the patient seated, if possible.

Focused History Questions

- Do you have any nasal congestion?
- Do you have a history of nose or sinus problems?
- Do you have problems with seasonal or environmental allergies?
- Do you have a history of sinus headaches?
- Do you experience nose bleeds (epistaxis)?
- Have you ever broken your nose?
- Have you had any changes in your sense of smell?
- Do you use any nasal sprays or allergy medications?

➤ When performing the procedure, always identify your patient according to agency policy, using two identifiers, and be attentive to standard precautions, hand hygiene, patient safety and privacy, body mechanics, and documentation.

Procedure Steps

1. **Position the client for the exam.** Sitting is the preferred position.

2. **Inspect the external nose.** Note the position, shape, and size. Observe for discharge and flaring.

Findings:

Expected findings: The nose is midline and symmetrical. No discharge or flaring.

Abnormal findings:
- Asymmetry suggests congenital deformity or trauma.
- Flaring suggests respiratory distress (especially in infants, who cannot breathe through the mouth).
- Clear drainage suggests allergy; yellow or green drainage suggests upper respiratory infection; bloody drainage may result from trauma, hypertension, or a bleeding disorder.

3. **Check for patency of the nasal passages.** Ask the patient to close her mouth, hold one naris closed, and breathe through the other naris. Repeat with the opposite naris.

Expected findings: The client breathes freely through both nares.

4. **Inspect the internal structures.**
   a. Use a nasal speculum or an otoscope with a large speculum (or a penlight with a speculum) to assess the internal structures.
   b. Tilt the patient's head back to facilitate speculum insertion and visualization.
   c. Brace your index finger against the patient's nose as you insert the speculum.

Expected findings: Nasal mucosa is pink and moist. Septum is intact and midline. No lesions

Developmental Variations

Older adults—the sense of smell diminishes in older adults because of a gradual decrease in and atrophy of the olfactory nerve fibers.

(continued on next page)

Procedure 22-8 ■ Assessing the Nose and Sinuses (continued)

d. Insert the speculum about 1 cm into the nares. Use the other hand to position the client's head and to hold the penlight if you do not have a lighted scope.

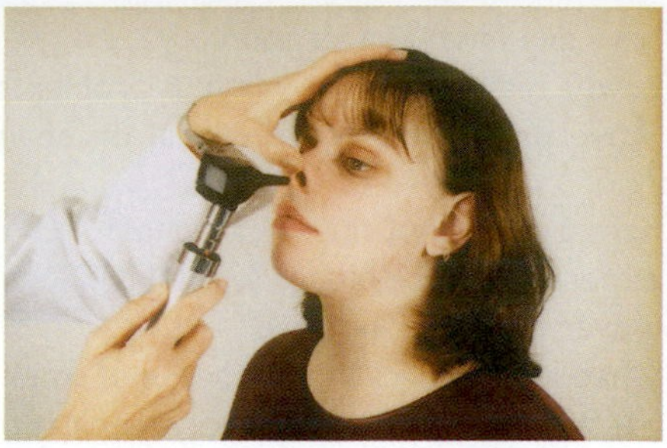

Step 4d

e. Observe the nasal mucosa for color, edema, lesions, erosion or ulceration, blood, and discharge. Inspect the septum for position and intactness.

f. Check for sense of smell using commonly recognized objects, such as a lemon or vanilla. Do not use a noxious odor. You can defer this test until the sensorineurological part of the exam if you choose, but keep the same order for every exam.

CN I is intact when the patient shows the ability to detect odor.

Abnormal findings: Deviated septum; polyps.

- Pale boggy mucosa is seen with allergies; bright red mucosa is associated with rhinitis, sinusitis, and cocaine use.
- Clustered vesicles suggest herpes infection.
- Erosion of nasal mucosa should signal you to investigate further for other signs or history of crack/cocaine use.
- Blood in the nasal passage indicates trauma, nose bleeds, or polyps.

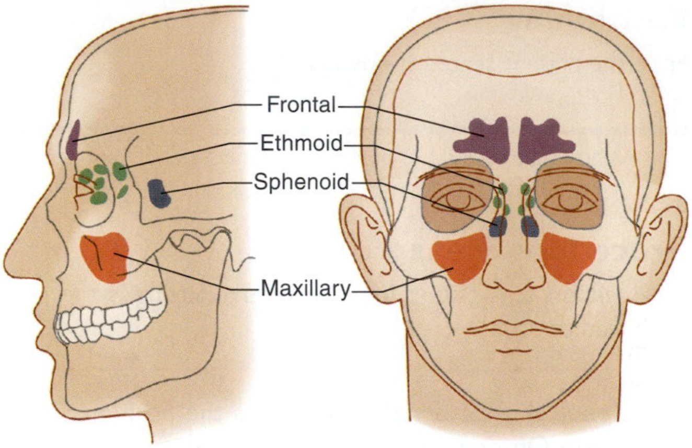

Paranasal sinuses frontal, ethmoid, sphenoid, and maxillary.

Developmental Modifications

Infants and children: You will not need a speculum to examine internal structures. Push the tip of the nose upward with your thumb, and direct a penlight into the nares.

---

5. Transilluminate the frontal and maxillary sinuses. First, darken the room.

a. *Frontal sinuses:* Shine a penlight or the otoscope with speculum below the eyebrow on each side.

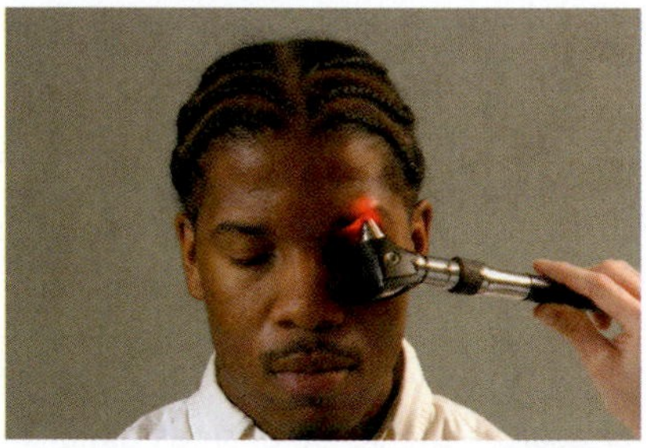

Step 5a

a. **Expected findings:** A red glow is seen above the eyebrow, indicating that the frontal sinus is patent.

b. *Maxillary sinuses:* Place the light source below the eyes and above the cheeks. Look for a glow of red light at the roof of the mouth through the client's open mouth.

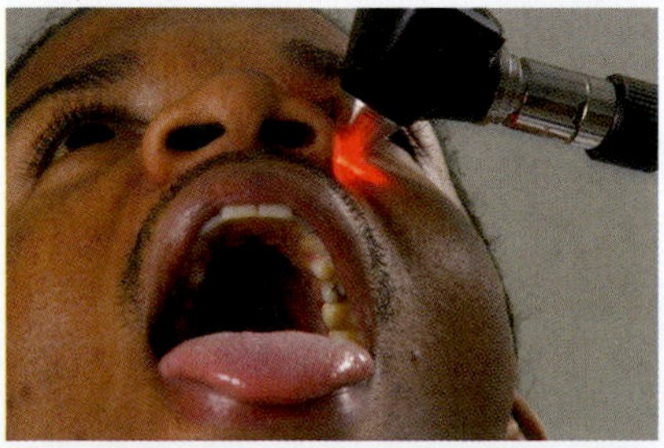

Step 5b

b. **Expected findings:** A red glow may be (but is not always) seen in the roof of the mouth, indicating that the maxillary sinus is patent.

Abnormal findings: Absence of transillumination may result from mucosal thickening or sinusitis.

6. Palpate the external structures.

Expected Findings: No tenderness, lesions, or deformity.

7. Palpate the frontal and maxillary sinuses.

Expected findings: No tenderness.

Abnormal findings: Tenderness may indicate infectious or allergic sinusitis.

Documentation

- If you need more information about documenting your findings, review Caring for the Nguyens, and

Go to Chapter 22, **Documenting Physical Examination Findings (Nam Nguyen),** in Volume 1.

Procedure 22-9 ■ Assessing the Mouth and Oropharynx

➤ For steps to follow in *all* procedures, refer to the Universal Steps for All Procedures found on the inside back cover.

Equipment

- Nonlatex procedure gloves
- Penlight
- Tongue blade
- Small gauze pad
- Pen and record form

Positioning

Have the patient seated, if possible.

Focused History Questions

- Do you have any problems with your mouth or teeth?
- When was your last dental exam?
- Do you have any discomfort in your mouth or throat?
- Have you had any recent changes in your mouth or teeth?
- How often do you brush your teeth? Floss?
- Do you smoke or chew tobacco?
- Do you have any sores or irritation in your mouth? If so, when did you first notice this?

➤ When performing the procedure, always identify your patient according to agency policy, using two identifiers, and be attentive to standard precautions, hand hygiene, patient safety and privacy, body mechanics, and documentation.

Procedure Steps

1. **Inspect the mouth externally.** Locate the placement of the lips and their color and condition. Ask the client to purse her lips.

Findings

Expected findings: The lips are midline, symmetrical, moist, and intact with no lesions. Coloring is consistent with ethnic group/race. The client can purse her lips.

Abnormal findings:

- Asymmetry—may be caused by congenital deformity, trauma, paralysis, or surgical alteration
- Pallor; cyanosis; redness
- Inability to purse lips—may indicate facial nerve damage
- Lesions—may be caused by bacteria, viruses, or trauma

(continued on next page)

Procedure 22-9 ■ Assessing the Mouth and Oropharynx (continued)

2. **Note the color and condition of the oral mucosa and gums.**
   a. **Don procedure gloves.**
   b. **Inspect and palpate the lower lip.** Pull the lower lip away from teeth, and inspect the inner side of the lip. Palpate any lesions for size, mobility, and tenderness.

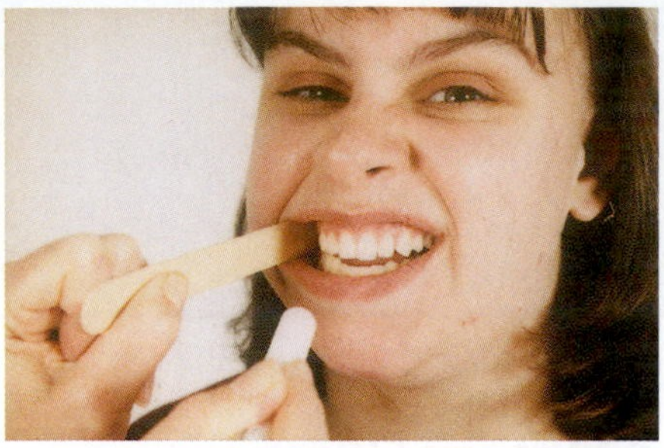

Step 2b

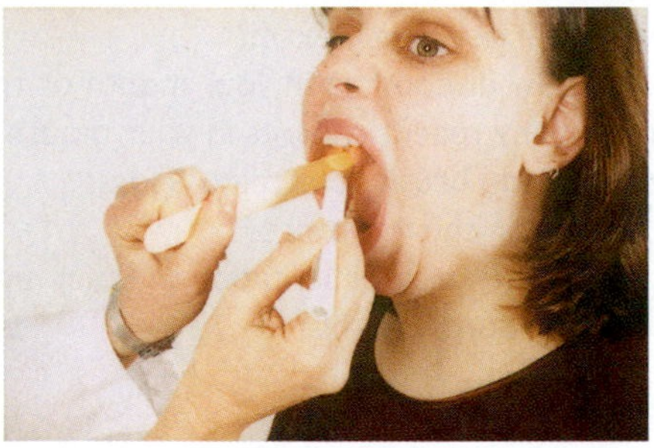

Step 2b

   c. **Inspect the buccal mucosa**, top to bottom and back to front.
      - Ask the client to open her mouth. Use a tongue depressor to retract the cheek, then shine a penlight onto the mucosa.
      - Using a tongue blade and penlight, inspect the Stensen's duct openings to the parotid glands.
      - Finally, **palpate inside each cheek** by placing a finger inside and thumb outside. Grasping the cheek between them, move the finger about. Repeat on both sides.

Expected findings: *Oral mucosa* is pink, moist, and intact; no lesions. *Gingiva* is consistent in color with the other mucosae and is intact, with no bleeding. *Buccal mucosa* is pink and moist, with no lesions. Mucosa is darker in dark-skinned clients.

Developmental Variations

Older adults—mucosa is drier than in young adults because of decreased salivary gland activity; brownish pigmentation of gums may be seen, especially in dark-skinned people.

Abnormal findings: Pallor may indicate anemia or inadequate oxygenation. The following are types of abnormal lesions.

- ***Gingivitis*** is a sign of periodontal disease. You will see red, swollen, or spongy, bleeding gingiva and receding gumlines. The gums may be tender.
- ***Parotitis*** is an inflammation of the parotid salivary gland.
- ***Stomatitis*** is inflammation of the oral mucosa.
- ***Leukoplakia*** (thick, elevated white patches) that do not scrape off may be precancerous lesions; white, curdy patches that scrape off and bleed indicate ***thrush*** (a fungal infection).
- ***Redness or abrasions*** of the gingiva may be caused by poorly fitted dentures.
- ***Aphthous ulcers*** are small, painful vesicles with a reddened periphery and a white or pale-yellow base.
- ***Canker sores*** are a benign type of aphthous ulcers believed to be caused by viral infection, allergies, stress, or trauma. So-called *major* aphthous ulcers may be caused by herpes simplex virus, HIV, and bacterial infections.

d. Also **examine the gums** as you are inspecting the buccal mucosa. Check for color, bleeding, edema, retraction, and lesions. Press gum tissue gently with gloved finger or tongue blade to assess firmness. ▼

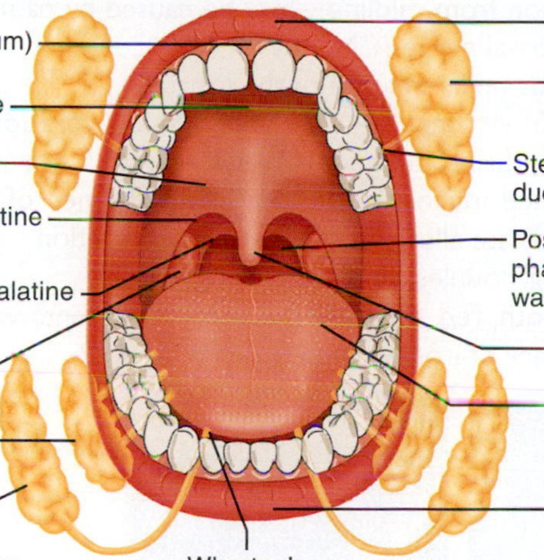

Structures of the mouth and oropharynx

3. **Inspect teeth.** You can do this while you are inspecting the oral mucosa and gums, in step 2.
   a. Observe the number, color, and condition of the teeth. Note the occlusion ("bite") and any loose teeth.
   b. If the client wears dentures, ask her to remove them. Inspect for cracked or worn areas; assess the fit. ▼

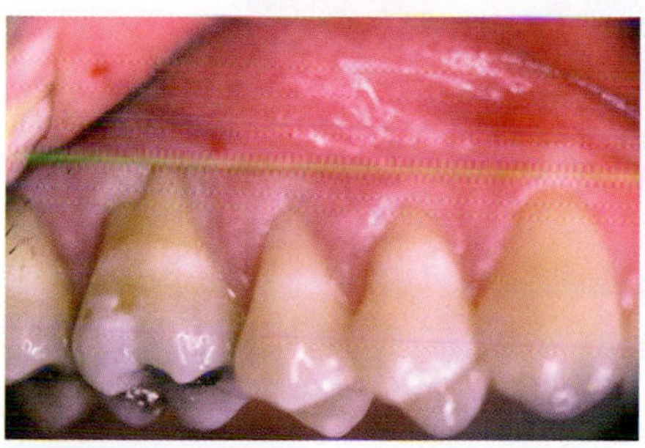

Gingival recession

Expected findings: Most adults have 28 teeth, or 32 if the wisdom teeth have erupted. Children have 20 teeth. Teeth should be white, be in good repair, have no caries, and have good occlusion. The top front teeth should slightly override the lower ones.

Developmental Variations

Older adults—may have receding gums, so teeth appear longer. Teeth may be chipped, eroded, or stained.

Abnormal findings: Missing or poorly anchored teeth, misalignment, and brown or black enamel (indicative of dental caries or staining (e.g., from taking tetracycline). White spots may indicate excessive fluoride intake.

4. **Inspect the tongue and the floor of the mouth.**
   a. Ask the client to "stick out" her tongue. Examine the upper surface for its color, texture, position, and mobility.
   b. Ask the client to roll her tongue upward and move it side to side.
   c. Have the client place the tip of her tongue on the roof of her mouth, as far back as possible. Using the penlight, inspect the underside of the tongue, the frenulum (which fastens the tongue to the floor of the mouth, in the center), and the floor of the mouth.
   d. Inspect the two Wharton's duct openings to the submaxillary glands, on either side of the frenulum.

Expected findings: Tongue is moist, with rough surface; coloring is consistent with the client's race. Mucosa has no lesions or discoloration. Papillae are intact. Tongue is midline with full mobility. The base of the tongue is smooth with prominent veins. No tenderness; no palpable nodules. A "geographic tongue" is a common normal variant.

Developmental Variations

Older adults—May have varicosities under the tongue.

(continued on next page)

Procedure 22-9 ■ Assessing the Mouth and Oropharynx (continued)

e. Use a tongue blade or gloved finger to move the tongue aside and examine the lateral aspects of the tongue and the floor of the mouth bilaterally. Use caution when placing your finger into the mouth of a noncompliant client.

Abnormal findings:
- Limited mobility
- Deviation from midline—may be caused by damage to the hypoglossal nerve (CN XII)
- ***Glossitis*** (inflammation of the tongue)
- A dry, furry tongue—associated with dehydration
- A black, "hairy" tongue—associated with fungal infections
- Reddened mucosa, ulcerations, and absence of papillae—may indicate allergy, inflammation, or infection
- Swelling, nodules, or ulcers
- A smooth, red tongue—may occur in clients who have a deficiency of iron, vitamin B_{12}, or vitamin B_3

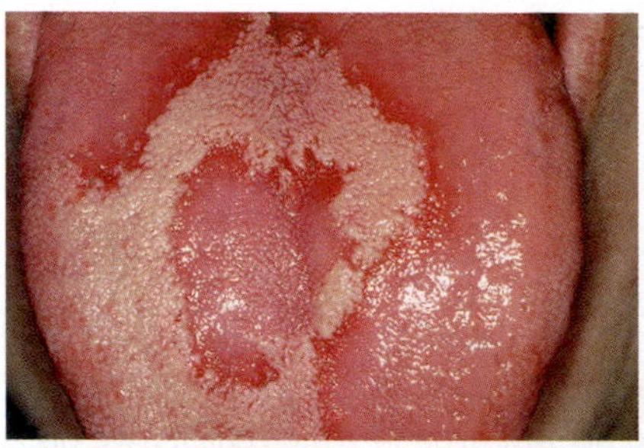

Geographic tongue

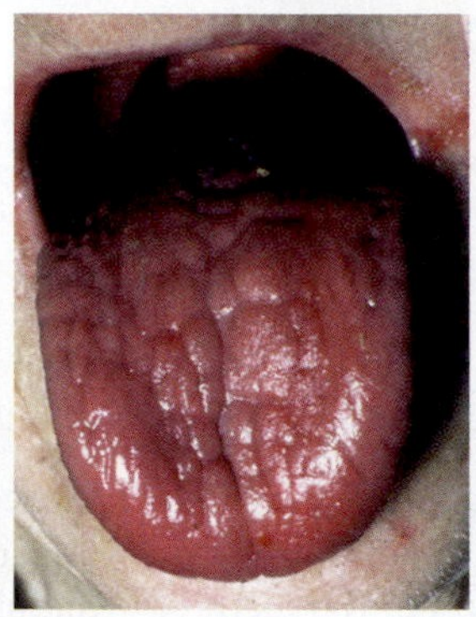

Red, beefy tongue

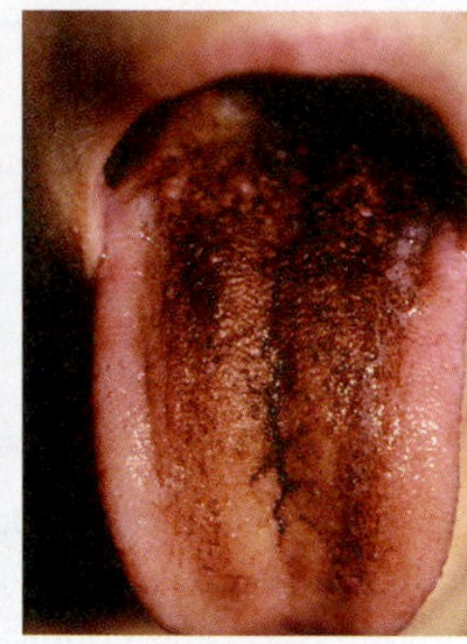

Black, hairy tongue

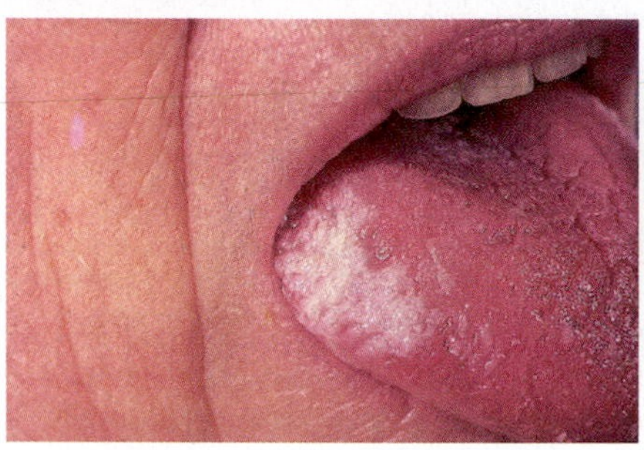

Leukoplakia

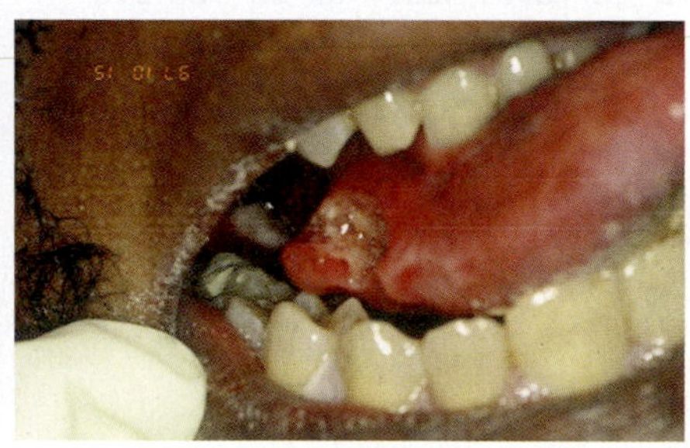

Cancer of the tongue

5. **Palpate the tongue and floor of the mouth.** Stabilize the tongue by grasping it with a gauze pad. Palpate the top, bottom, and sides with your other index finger.

6. **Inspect the oropharynx (hard/soft palate, tonsils, and uvula).** Note the color, shape, texture, and condition.
   a. **Have the client tilt her head back** and open her mouth as widely as possible. Depress the tongue with a tongue blade, and shine a penlight on the areas to be inspected.
   b. **To inspect the uvula**, ask the client to say "ah," and watch the uvula as the soft palate rises.
   c. **Inspect the oropharynx** by depressing one side of the tongue at a time, about halfway back on the tongue.
   d. **Note the size and color of the tonsils;** note any discharge, redness, swelling, or lesions.
   e. **Look and palpate for cleft palate**, especially in infants.

Expected findings: Hard and soft palates are pink and smooth. Uvula is midline and rises symmetrically. Tonsils are pink, symmetrical, and without lesions or exudate.

Developmental Variations

Children—until about age 12 years, the tonsils may extend beyond the palatine arch.

Abnormal findings:
- Redness, edema, lesions, plaques, drainage; yellow or greenish streaks on the posterior wall of pharynx (indicate postnasal drainage).
- Tonsils that are red, edematous, or enlarged or have white or pale patches of exudates.
- Asymmetrical rise of the uvula may indicate a problem with CN IX or X.

7. **Test the gag reflex** by touching the back of the soft palate with a tongue blade.

Expected findings: Positive gag reflex is present.

Developmental Variations

Older adults—may have a slightly slower gag response.

Abnormal findings:

- Absence of a gag reflex is seen with extreme sedation, head injury, or damage to CN IX and X.
- Inability to articulate the specified words indicates CN XII is not intact.

8. **Ask the client to repeat the following words:** *Light, tight, dynamite.* Again, you may defer this test to the sensorineurological portion of the exam if you choose.

Patient Teaching

Instruct the patient in the importance of dental care and the need for regular checkups.

Documentation

- If you need more information about documenting your findings, review Caring for the Nguyens, and

Go to Chapter 22, **Documenting Physical Examination Findings (Nam Nguyen),** in Volume 1.

Procedure 22-10 ■ Assessing the Neck

➤ For steps to follow in *all* procedures, refer to the Universal Steps for All Procedures found on the inside back cover.

Equipment

- Stethoscope and antiseptic wipe
- Pen and record form

Positioning

- Have the client seated, if possible.
- Place infants and children in the supine position.

Focused History Questions

- Do you have any difficulty swallowing?
- Do you have any neck pain or stiffness?
- Do you have any neck masses or lumps?
- Do you have any history of thyroid disease?
- Do you have any difficulty swallowing?

➤ When performing the procedure, always identify your patient according to agency policy, using two identifiers, and be attentive to standard precautions, hand hygiene, patient safety and privacy, body mechanics, and documentation.

Procedure Steps

1. **Inspect the neck.** Note symmetry, range of motion (ROM), and the condition of the skin.
   a. Inspect the neck when it is in the neutral position.
   b. Inspect the neck when it is hyperextended.
   c. Inspect the neck when the patient swallows water.

Findings

Expected findings: Neck is erect, midline, and symmetrical with full ROM. No masses are present; skin is intact. Larynx and trachea rise with swallowing. Thyroid is not visible.

Abnormal findings:

- Asymmetrical head position may result from damage to the muscles, swelling, or masses.
- Painful or erratic movement may be caused by a benign condition, such as muscle spasm, or by significant problems, including meningitis, neurological injuries, or chronic arthritis.
- Swollen lymph nodes may be visible.
- An enlarged thyroid may be visible in the lower half of the neck.

(continued on next page)

Procedure 22-10 ■ Assessing the Neck (continued)

2. **Palpate the cervical lymph nodes.** Note the size, shape, symmetry, consistency, mobility, tenderness, and temperature of any palpable nodes.
   a. Use light palpation with one or two fingerpads in a circular movement.
   b. Palpate the cervical nodes in the following order:
      (1) *Preauricular*—in front of the ear
      (2) *Posterior auricular*—behind the ear
      (3) *Tonsillar*—at the angle of the jaw
      (4) *Submandibular*—halfway up the lower jaw
      (5) *Submental*—under the tip of the chin
      (6) *Occipital*—at the base of the skull in the occipital area
      (7) *Superficial cervical*—below the tonsillar node over the sternocleidomastoid muscle
      (8) *Deep cervical*—under the sternocleidomastoid muscle
      (9) *Posterior cervical*—in posterior triangle along trapezius muscle
      (10) *Supraclavicular*—above the clavicle

NOTE: Use the same sequence every time so that the steps will become automatic and you will not omit any area.

Expected findings: Lymph nodes are supple and nontender; no masses are palpable. ▼

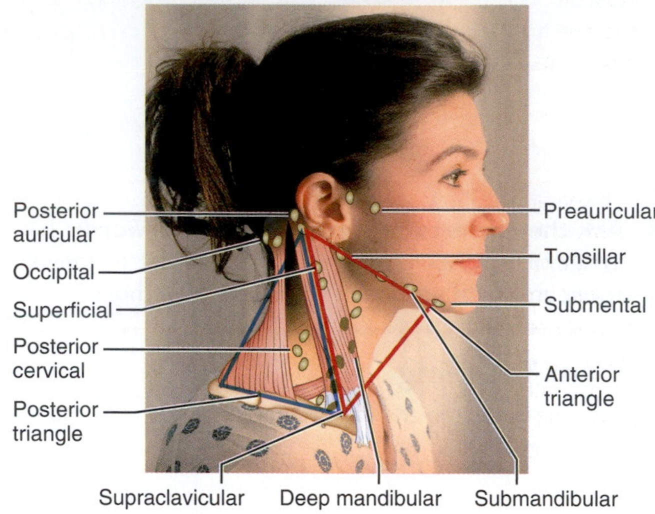

Abnormal findings: Lymphadenopathy (palpable nodes 1 cm or greater). Immobile nodes may indicate malignancy, inflammation, or infection in the area they drain.

3. **Palpate the thyroid.**

To use the posterior approach:

a. Stand behind the client, and ask her to flex her neck slightly forward and to the left.
b. Position your thumbs on the nape of the client's neck.
c. Using the fingers of your left hand, locate the cricoid cartilage, which is located below the thyroid cartilage. Push the trachea slightly to the left with your right hand as you palpate just below the cricoid cartilage and between the trachea and sternocleidomastoid muscle.
d. Ask the client to swallow (have her swallow small sips of water, if necessary), and feel for the thyroid gland as it rises up.
e. Reverse and repeat the same steps to palpate the right thyroid lobe (use the fingers of your left hand to displace the trachea to the right, while using the fingers of your right hand to palpate the thyroid to the right of the trachea).

To use the anterior approach:

f. Stand in front of the client, and ask her to flex the neck slightly forward and in the direction you intend to palpate.
g. Place your hands on the neck, and apply gentle pressure to one side of the trachea while palpating the opposite side of the neck for the thyroid as the client swallows.
h. Reverse and repeat the same steps on the opposite side.

Expected findings: The thyroid is generally nonpalpable. If some tissue is palpable, the consistency is firm and smooth. There is no nodularity, enlargement, or tenderness.

Abnormal findings: An enlarged thyroid may signify a tumor or goiter (hypo- or hyperthyroidism). A tender thyroid is associated with inflammation. ▼

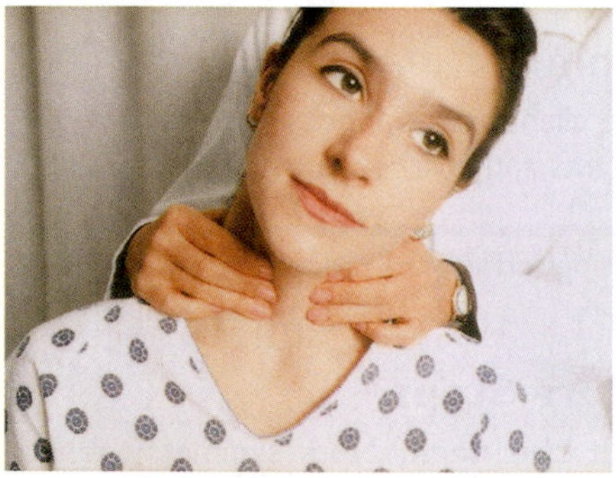

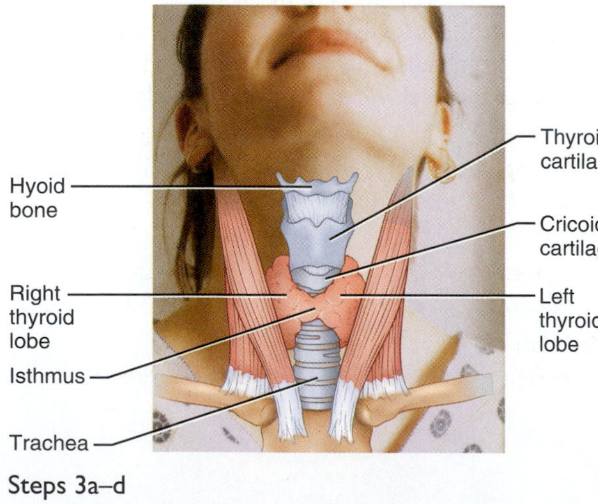

Steps 3a–d

? What if . . .

- **The thyroid gland is enlarged or there is a mass?**
  Auscultate the thyroid for bruits using the bell portion of the stethoscope. Ask the client to hold her breath as you auscultate. There should be no bruits.

Patient Teaching

Teach the patient how to perform a "neck check"—self-check the thyroid with a glass of water and a handheld mirror. Tell the patient: "Hold the mirror in your hand and focus on your neck just below the Adam's apple and above your collarbone. Tip your head back, take a drink of water, and swallow. As you swallow look at your neck. Check for any bulges in this area as you swallow." To download Neck Check instructions, and for more information about thyroid health,

Go to **http://www.thyroidawareness.com/.**

Documentation

- Describe enlarged nodes (> 1 cm in diameter) according to their location, size, shape, consistency, mobility, and tenderness.
- If you need more information about documenting your findings, review Caring for the Nguyens, and

Go to Chapter 22, **Documenting Physical Examination Findings (Nam Nguyen),** in Volume 1.

Procedure 22-11 ■ Assessing the Breasts and Axillae

➤ For steps to follow in *all* procedures, refer to the Universal Steps for All Procedures found on the inside back cover.

Equipment

- Nonlatex procedure gloves, if exposure to body fluids is possible
- Glass slide
- Culturette
- Pen and record form

Positioning

The patient must assume several positions during the breast exam (see step 1).

Focused History Questions

- Do you have a lump or thickening in your underarm or breasts that persists throughout your menstrual cycle?
- Do you have any breast pain or discharge?
- Have you noticed any changes in the skin on your breasts, nipples, or underarms?
- Have you had any changes in your nipples?
- Have your breasts changed in size, shape, or contour?
- Do you perform breast self-examination (BSE)?
- Are you taking any medications or hormones?
- If you are premenopausal, when was your last period?

➤ When performing the procedure, always identify your patient according to agency policy, using two identifiers, and be attentive to standard precautions, hand hygiene, patient safety and privacy, body mechanics, and documentation.

Procedure Steps

1. **Inspect the breasts.** Note size, shape, symmetry, and color. Inspect with the client in each of the following positions:
   a. Sitting or standing with arms at her side
   b. Sitting or standing with arms raised slightly but not over her head
   Aids in detecting dimpling or retraction of breast tissue
   c. Seated or standing with her hands pressed on her hips
   Aids in detecting dimpling or retraction of breast tissue
   d. With the client leaning forward
   Helpful when examining large, pendulous breasts

Findings

Expected findings: The breasts are symmetrical; however, the dominant side may be more developed, resulting in a slightly asymmetrical appearance. Skin color is lighter than exposed areas, and there are no lesions, redness, or edema. Texture is smooth, with no dimpling or retraction. Striae are a normal variation.

Developmental Variations

Newborns: You may see breast enlargement and watery, white discharge from the nipples during the first 2 weeks of life.

Children: Breasts typically begin to develop at about age 13 years; the breasts may not develop at equal rates.

(continued on next page)

Procedure 22-11 ■ Assessing the Breasts and Axillae (continued)

e. With the client supine, and a pillow placed under the shoulder of the breast being examined
Helps spread the breast tissue over the chest wall

Pregnancy: Breast size increases; areolae and nipples darken; superficial veins become prominent; stretch marks may be present; colostrum (a thick, yellow precursor to breast milk) can sometimes be expressed as early as the second trimester.

Older adults: Breasts lose firmness and become flaccid and pendulous.

Abnormal findings:
- Asymmetry warrants further investigation.
- Swelling or erythema may be seen in infection (mastitis).
- ***Peau d'orange*** (dimpled skin texture) skin changes may be seen with lymphatic obstruction that is present in some forms of breast cancer.
- Puckering, lesions, and retraction may also be seen with breast cancer.
- ***Gynecomastia*** (enlargement of breasts in males) may indicate hormone imbalance.

---

2. **Inspect the nipples and areolae.** Note color, shape, and symmetry. Observe for any discharge.

Expected findings: The areolae and nipples are darker in color than breast tissue. Nipples are everted and point in the same direction. No discharge is present, except in newborns and during pregnancy and lactation. No lesions or erosion is present.

Abnormal findings:
- Nipple discoloration that is not associated with pregnancy
- Nipples pointing in different directions. Such findings warrant follow-up as a potential sign of an underlying mass.
- Flat or inverted nipples, which are caused by shortening of the mammary ducts. May make breastfeeding difficult.
- Any nipple discharge not associated with newborns, pregnancy, or breastfeeding requires a thorough evaluation
- Cracks and nipple redness, which may occur with breastfeeding

---

3. **Inspect the axillae.** Note the color, condition of the skin, and hair distribution.

Expected findings: Skin is intact with no lesions or rashes. Presence of hair depends on the age of the client and personal preference. Axillary hair develops with puberty. Some women may choose to shave the hair, whereas others will allow it to grow.

Abnormal findings:
- Rashes, redness, or unusual pigmentation may indicate infection or allergy to deodorants.
- Dark-pigmented, velvety skin may be seen with ***acanthosis nigricans,*** a condition associated with obesity and type 2 diabetes mellitus.

---

4. **Palpate the breasts; wear procedure gloves, if necessary.** Using the fingerpads of your three middle fingers, make small circles with light, medium, and deep pressure.

Begin at an imaginary line drawn straight down the side from the underarm; move across the breast to the middle of the sternum. Check the entire breast area, moving down until you feel only ribs and up to the clavicle.

Expected findings: Breasts are soft and nontender with no lesions or masses.

Developmental Variations

Consistency depends on age; premenopausal women have firm and elastic tissue, whereas postmenopausal women have softer tissue that may be stringy or cord-like.

Follow one of the following three patterns (evidence suggests the vertical strip method is best).

a. ***Vertical strip method:*** Start at the sternal edge, and palpate the breast in parallel lines until you reach the midaxillary line. Go up one area and down the adjacent strip (like "mowing the grass").

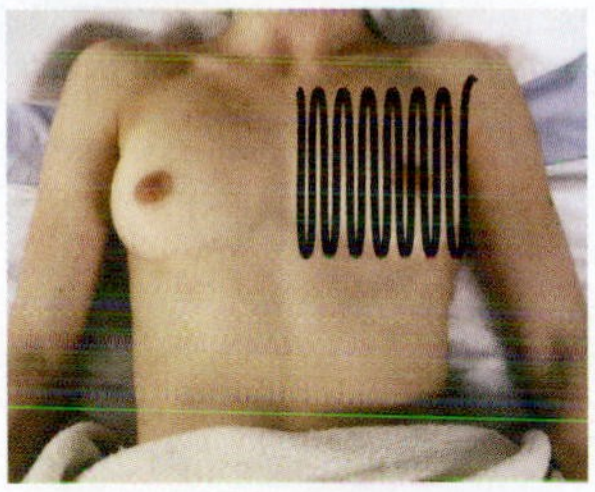

Vertical strip method

b. ***Pie wedge method:*** This method examines the breast in wedges. Move from one wedge to the next.

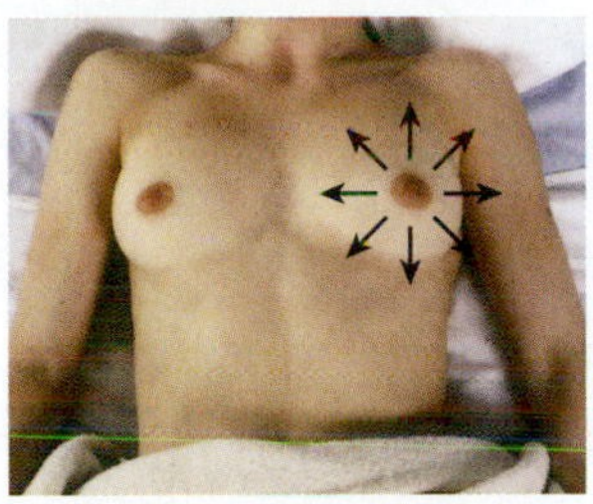

Pie wedge method

c. ***Concentric circles method:*** Start at the outermost area of the breast at the 12 o'clock position. Move clockwise in concentric, ever smaller, circles.

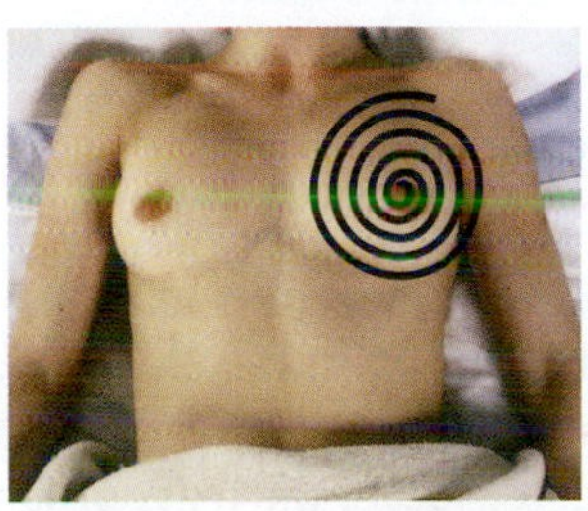

Concentric circle method

Abnormal findings: Breast lumps or masses may be benign or malignant and require follow-up.

Technique Hints

- Do not remove your fingers from the skin surface once you have begun palpating. Move from area to area by sliding the fingers along the skin.
- Most breast lesions in women are found in the upper outer quadrant.
- Most breast cancer in men occurs in the areola.

---

5. Palpate the nipples and areolae. Wear procedure gloves, if necessary.

a. If the woman is supine, place a small pillow or folded towel under the shoulder of the breast you are examining.
b. Squeeze the nipple gently between your thumb and finger to check for discharge.
c. Note tissue elasticity and tenderness.

Expected findings: Nipples are elastic and nontender. No discharge is present.

Developmental Variations

Nipple tenderness is normal when establishing breastfeeding.

Abnormal findings: Loss of elasticity may indicate underlying malignancy. Bloody, purulent discharge may indicate infection. Other forms of drainage may indicate malignancy.

---

6. Palpate the axillae and clavicular lymph nodes.

a. Have the woman seated, with her arms at her sides, or in the supine position.

Expected Findings: Nodes are nonpalpable.

(continued on next page)

Procedure 22-11 ■ Assessing the Breasts and Axillae (continued)

b. Using your fingerpads, move your fingers in circular fashion.
   - *Central nodes*—located high in the midaxillary region
   - *Anterior pectoral nodes*—located on the lower border of the pectoralis major in the anterior axillary fold
   - *Lateral brachial nodes*—located high in the axilla on the inner aspect of the humerus
   - *Posterior subscapular nodes*—located high in the axilla on the lateral scapular border
   - *Epitrochlear nodes*—located above the elbow
   - *Infraclavicular nodes*—located below the clavicle
   - *Supraclavicular nodes*—located above the clavicle

Abnormal findings: Palpable nodes may be seen with infection or malignancy. Enlarged lymph nodes caused by infection are tender.

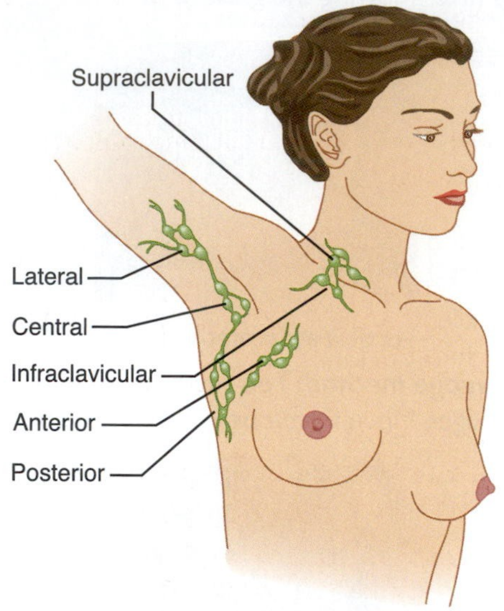

Location of normal lymph nodes

? What if . . .

- **There is a nipple discharge?**

If there is nipple discharge in a woman who is not pregnant or breastfeeding, obtain a specimen by placing a glass slide up to the breast to capture a drop of discharge. Transport the slide to the laboratory as soon as possible. If there is ample discharge, obtain a swab of the discharge with a culturette.

Patient Teaching

You should demonstrate BSE procedure as part of client teaching for self-care, if the patient chooses to perform BSE. Instruct clients that clinical breast exams should be done annually in women age 40 years and older, and every 1 to 3 years in women age 20 to 39 years (American Congress of Obstetricians and Gynecologists, 2012, reaffirmed 2014). Guidelines vary as to the age at which women should start having clinical breast exam (CBEs) and mammography to screen for breast cancer. Annual or biennial mammography or breast thermography most commonly begins after age 40 years or at a younger age and more often for those at high risk (American Cancer Society, n.d.b, revised 2018; 2017). Evidence at present does not support the need for a CBE if mammography is performed (Agency for Healthcare Research and Quality, 2014).

Documentation

- If you palpate a mass or lump, document its size, shape, symmetry, mobility, tenderness, and skin color changes. To document the location, divide the breast into four quadrants by intersecting vertical and horizontal lines. With the nipple as the center, locate the mass or lump as though the breast were a clock; state the distance in centimeters from the nipple (e.g., 4 o'clock, 2.5 cm from nipple).
- If you need more information about documenting your findings, review Caring for the Nguyens, and

Go to Chapter 22, **Documenting Physical Examination Findings (Nam Nguyen),** in Volume 1.

Practice Resources

Agency for Healthcare Research and Quality (2014); American Cancer Society (n.d.b, last revised 2018, 2017); American Congress of Obstetricians and Gynecologists (2012, reaffirmed 2014); Radhakrishnan, Nowak, Parker, et al. (2017); Takkar, Kochhar, Garg, et al. (2017)

Procedure 22-12 ■ Assessing the Chest and Lungs

➤ For steps to follow in *all* procedures, refer to the Universal Steps for All Procedures found on the inside back cover.

Equipment

- Stethoscope and antiseptic wipe
- Felt-tipped marker and ruler
- Pen and record form

Clean stethoscope and rulers before and after use unless they are only used for one patient.

Positioning

- Have the client sitting, if possible, and leaning forward for the posterior approach.
  If the client is unable to sit up, findings will be distorted.
- If the client is lying down, findings are more evident on the dependent side; help him change positions so that you can assess with each side being dependent.

Focused History Questions

- Do you have fatigue or activity intolerance?
- Do you have any current respiratory problems?
- Have you had any recent respiratory problems?
- Do you have a cough?
- Do you have any difficulty breathing?
- What, if anything, causes you to be short of breath?
- Have you had any chest pain?
- Do you have a history of allergies or asthma?
- Do you smoke? If so, how much and for how long?
- If you smoke, have you tried to quit? Would you like to quit?
- Are you exposed to air pollutants at home or at work?

➤ When performing the procedure, always identify your patient according to agency policy, using two identifiers, and be attentive to standard precautions, hand hygiene, patient safety and privacy, body mechanics, and documentation.

Procedure Steps

1. **Count the respiratory rate, and observe the rhythm and depth; observe the symmetry of chest and respiratory movements.**
   (See Chapter 20 if you need more information about counting respirations.)

Findings

Expected findings:

- Respirations are quiet with a regular rhythm and depth; rate 12 to 20 breaths/min for adults.
- Chest movement is symmetrical, rising and falling with each respiration.

Developmental Variations

Infants and children: The normal respiratory rate varies by age. A newborn may have a respiratory rate of 40 to 90 breaths/min. The rate gradually declines as the child matures. Newborns breathe abdominally, so you will see little chest movement. The chest in young children is apple shaped.

Older adults: Rate changes very little; however, respirations decrease in depth as muscles become weakened.

Abnormal findings:

- Chest asymmetry may be seen with musculoskeletal disorders of the spine, such as kyphosis or scoliosis.
- Asymmetrical movement during breathing is seen in rib fractures, pneumothorax, and atelectasis; affected chest area may not move at all with respiration.
- Sternal and intercostal retractions are seen with hypoxia, respiratory distress, and airway obstruction.
- Respiratory rate may be increased with activity, smoking, fever, pain, or anemia.

(continued on next page)

Procedure 22-12 ■ Assessing the Chest and Lungs (continued)

2. Inspect the chest.

a. Inspect the anteroposterior (AP)-to-lateral ratio.

a. **Expected findings:** Normal adult AP-to-lateral ratio is 1:2.

Developmental Variations

Infants: AP is equal to the lateral diameter.

Older adults: Kyphosis (excessive curvature of the thoracic spine), scoliosis (lateral curvature of the spine), and osteoporosis change the size and shape of the chest; weakening thoracic and diaphragm muscles allow the chest to widen and become more barrel-shaped, as does chronic obstructive pulmonary disease (COPD).

Abnormal findings: AP-to-lateral ratio is increased in COPD (barrel chest).

b. Inspect the costal angle. ▼

b. **Expected findings:** The costal angle is < 90°.

Abnormal findings: Costal angle is > 90° in COPD.

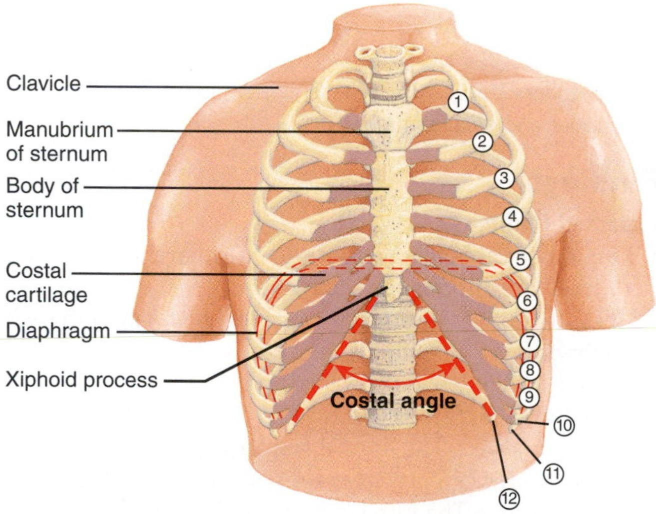

c. Identify any spinal deformities. ▼

c. **Expected findings:** The spine is straight without lateral curvatures or deformity.

Abnormal findings: Scoliosis is lateral curvature of the spine. Kyphosis is excessive thoracic curvature.

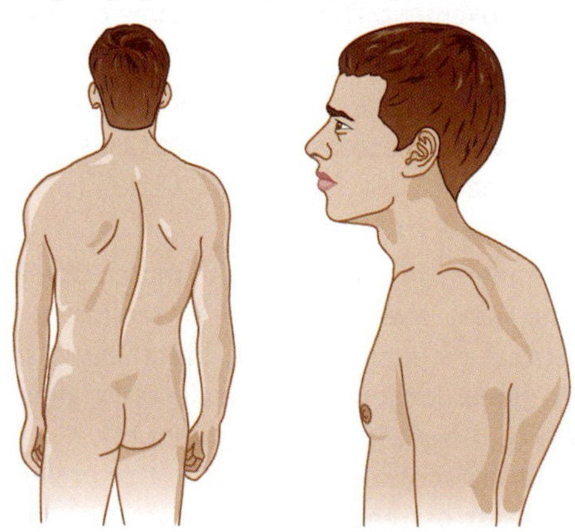

d. Observe the effort required to breathe.

d. **Expected findings:** Respirations appear effortless. No retraction or use of accessory muscles.

Abnormal findings: Sternal and intercostal retractions are seen in severe hypoxia or respiratory distress.

e. Note the color and condition of skin.

e. **Expected findings:** Skin color and hair distribution are consistent with the client's gender, ethnicity, and exposure to the sun. The skin is intact with no scars.

Abnormal findings: Cyanosis of the chest wall (caused by extreme hypoxia or cold temperature).

---

3. **Palpate the trachea.** Place your fingers and thumb on either side of the trachea and note its position. (In a comprehensive exam, you may have already done this with the neck exam.)

Developmental Modifications

Infants: Neck is short, so it may not be possible to palpate the trachea.

Expected findings: Trachea is in the midline.

Abnormal findings: Tracheal deviation may occur from a mass in the neck (e.g., thyroid enlargement) or from excess pressure in the lungs (e.g., ***tension pneumothorax***).

---

4. **Palpate the chest.**
   - Observe for tenderness, masses, or ***crepitus*** (crackling skin caused by air in the subcutaneous tissue).
   - Palpate the anterior, posterior, and lateral chest by placing your hands on the chest wall.

Expected findings: The chest is nontender. No masses or crepitus present.

Abnormal findings:
- Pain in the chest wall may be caused by fracture, inflammation, or trauma.
- Crepitus results from air leaking into the subcutaneous tissue. It is most likely to occur around wounds, central intravenous (IV) line sites, chest tubes, or a tracheostomy.

---

5. **Palpate chest excursion** (expandability).
   a. Place your hands at the base of the client's chest with fingers spread and thumbs about 5 cm (2 in.) apart (at the costal margin anteriorly and at the 8th to 10th rib posteriorly).
   b. Press your thumbs toward the client's spine to create a small skinfold between them.
   c. Have the client take a deep breath, and feel for chest expansion. This may be performed on the anterior or posterior portion of the chest, or both.

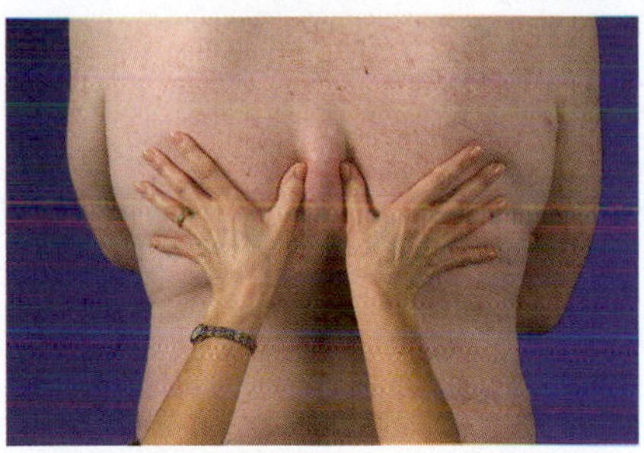

Expected findings: Chest excursion is symmetrical on the anterior and posterior aspect of the chest (you should feel equal pressure on your hands; thumbs should move apart equal distances).

Abnormal findings:
- Limited chest excursion may occur with shallow breathing, restrictive clothing, or restrictive airway disease.
- Asymmetrical excursion may result from airway obstruction, pleural effusion, or pneumothorax.

(continued on next page)

Procedure 22-12 ■ Assessing the Chest and Lungs (continued)

6. **Follow the same pattern and sequence** for palpating fremitus, percussing, and auscultating the chest. See the accompanying diagram. ▼

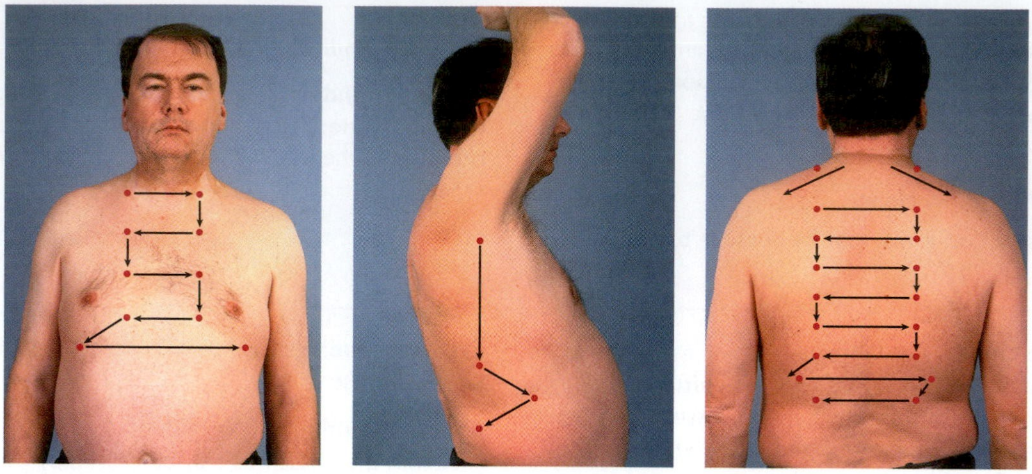

7. **Palpate the chest for tactile fremitus.**
   a. Use the palmar surface of your hands, but raise the fingers off the client's chest so that you palpate with the bony metacarpophalangeal joints of your hands.
   Bony prominences are best for detecting vibrations.
   b. Palpate for vibrations as the client says "99." ▼

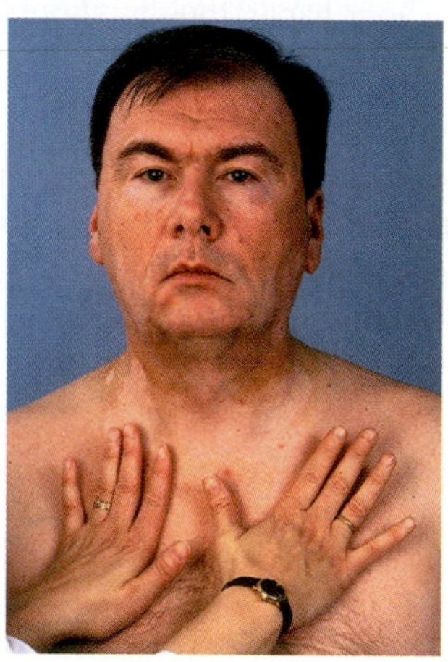

Developmental Modifications

Infants: Place your hand over the chest while the infant is crying.

Expected Findings: Tactile fremitus is equal bilaterally on the anterior and posterior chest; it is diminished at midthorax. Fremitus is normally diminished if the chest wall is very thick or the voice very soft.

Developmental Variations

Children and thin adults—may have increased fremitus.

Abnormal findings:
- Increased fremitus occurs with conditions that cause fluid in the lungs (e.g., pulmonary edema).
- Decreased or absent fremitus occurs when there is decreased air movement or tissue consolidation (e.g., emphysema, asthma).

8. **Percuss the chest.** Compare the right side to the left side.
   - Percuss over the intercostal spaces (ICS), rather than over the ribs.
   Percussion over bone produces less resonance.
   - Use the indirect percussion method on the anterior, posterior, and lateral chest, following the diagram in step 6.

Expected findings:
- The anterior chest is resonant to the 2nd ICS on the left and to the 4th ICS on the right.
- The lateral chest is resonant to the 8th ICS.
- The posterior chest is resonant to T12.

Abnormal findings: Dullness is heard with fluid or masses in the lungs. Hyperresonance is heard with air trapping that occurs with emphysema.

9. Percuss the posterior chest for diaphragmatic excursion.

a. Percuss the level of the diaphragm on full expiration. Have the client exhale completely and hold his breath while you percuss (beginning just below the scapula) from resonance over the lung downward toward the diaphragm. The sound will become dull at the diaphragm. Mark the area with a pen.

b. Percuss the diaphragm level on full inspiration. Have the client take a deep breath and hold it as you percuss again. Mark the location.

c. Measure the distance between the two marks. ➤

Expected findings: Diaphragmatic excursion (the distance between the two marks) is normally 3 to 6 cm.

Abnormal findings: Decreased excursion may indicate paralysis, atelectasis, or COPD with overinflated lungs.

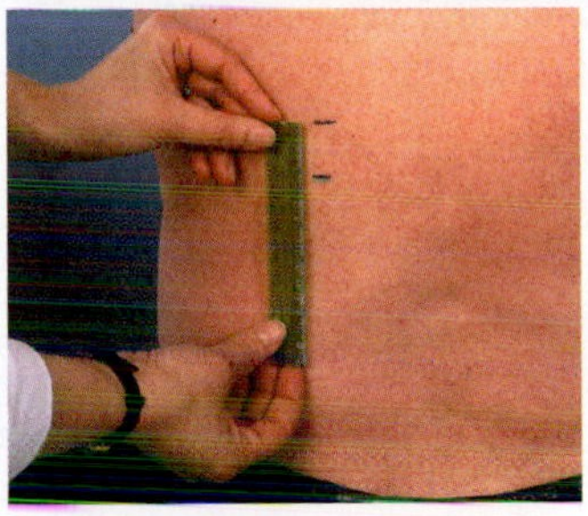

10. Auscultate the chest.

a. ***Routine daily assessment:*** Follow the pattern in step 6, using fewer locations.

b. ***For a focused assessment***, auscultate more areas while still following the pattern in step 6.
Following a "pattern" allows you to compare findings side to side.

c. Use the diaphragm of the stethoscope.

d. Have the client take slow, deep breaths through his mouth as you listen at each site through one full respiratory cycle.

To review lung sounds, refer to the tables at the end of this procedure.

Expected findings: No abnormal or adventitious sounds are heard. Lung fields are clear to auscultation.

- *Bronchial* breath sounds are heard over the trachea.
- *Bronchovesicular* breath sounds are heard over the sternum anteriorly and between the scapulae posteriorly.
- *Vesicular* breath sounds are heard over most of the lung fields.

Developmental Variations

Infants: Breath sounds are louder than in adults.

Abnormal findings: Crackles or rales, rhonchi, wheezing, stridor, friction rub, grunting

- **Diminished breath sounds** are heard with poor inspiratory effort, in the very muscular or obese, or with restricted airflow.
- **Misplaced breath sounds** (e.g., bronchial breath sounds heard over the lung fields) indicate constriction of flow.
- **Adventitious breath sounds,** such as wheezes, rhonchi, and rales, are sounds heard over normal breath sounds. **Key Point:** *If an abnormal sound is heard, have the client cough and listen again.*

11. Auscultate for abnormal voice sounds if there is evidence of lung congestion. Follow the pattern in step 6.

a. Assess for *bronchophony* by having the client say "1, 2, 3" as you listen over the lung fields.

b. Assess for *egophony* by having your client say "eee" as you listen over the lung fields.

c. Assess for *whispered pectoriloquy* by having your client whisper "1, 2, 3" as you listen over the lung fields.

Expected findings: No abnormal voice sounds are heard.

Abnormal findings:

a. ***Bronchophony*** is present if the words are clearly heard over the lungs.

b. ***Egophony*** is present if the sound you hear is "ay."

c. ***Whispered pectoriloquy*** is present if you hear, "one, two, three" clearly.

Patient Teaching

Instruct the patient about the dangers of tobacco use, especially smoking; exposure to air pollutants and environmental pollutants, such as radon or asbestos; and the signs and symptoms of lung cancer.

Home Care

- Instruct clients or caregivers to identify pollutants within the home, such as radon, dirty heating/air-conditioning systems, or mold, which may cause respiratory problems.
- Instruct caregivers or patients with allergies and/or asthma to eliminate potential allergens, such as cigarette smoke, dust, feathers, and pet dander.

Documentation

If you need information about documenting your findings, review Caring for the Nguyens, and

Go to Chapter 22, **Documenting Physical Examination Findings (Nam Nguyen),** in Volume 1.

(continued on next page)

Procedure 22-12 ■ Assessing the Chest and Lungs (continued)

Normal Lung Sounds

NORMAL LUNG SOUNDS	LOCATION	DESCRIPTION	ILLUSTRATION
Bronchial or Tubular	Heard over the trachea	Blowing, hollow sounds; inspiration is shorter than expiration and lower-pitched	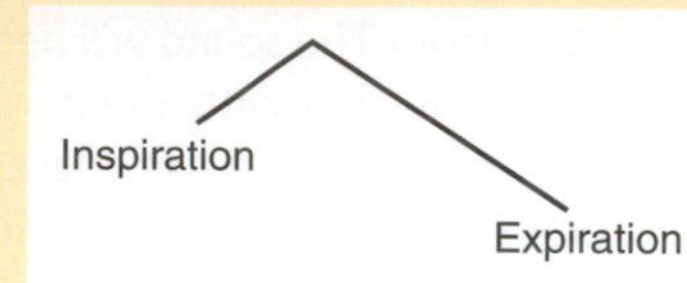
Bronchovesicular	Heard over the 1st and 2nd ICS anteriorly and over the scapula posteriorly	Medium-pitched, medium intensity, blowing sounds; inspiration and expiration are equal length and similar pitch	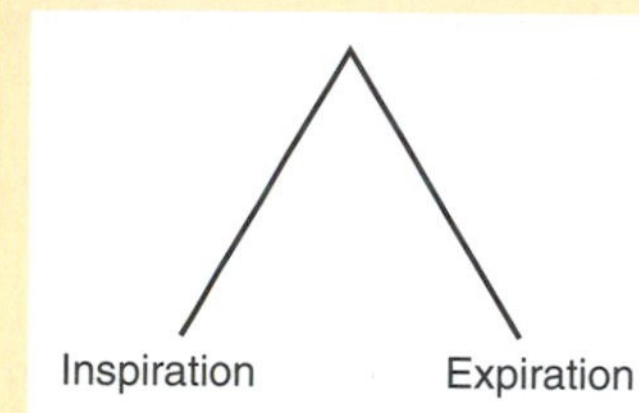
Vesicular	Heard over the lung periphery	Soft, low-pitched sounds; inspiration is longer, louder, and higher-pitched than expiration	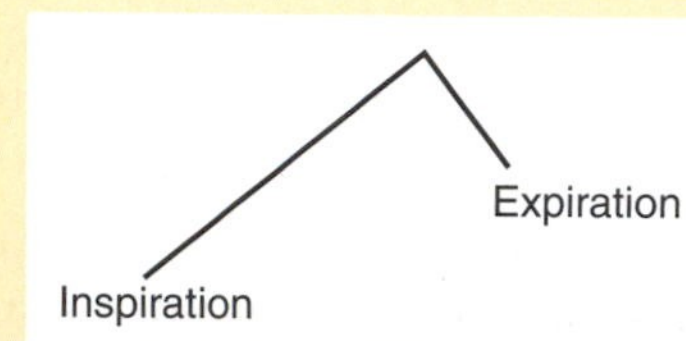

Abnormal Lung Sounds

ABNORMAL LUNG SOUNDS	CAUSE	CHARACTERISTICS	EXAMPLES
Crackles (sometimes called *rales*)	Air bubbling through moisture in the alveoli	Bubbling, crackling, popping. Soft, high-pitched, and very brief sounds, usually heard during inspiration	Pneumonia Congestive heart failure (CHF) Bronchitis Emphysema
Rhonchi	Mucous secretions in the large airways	Coarse, snoring, continuous low-pitched sounds heard during inspiration and expiration. May clear with coughing	Bronchitis Emphysema Narrowed airways Fibrotic lungs
Wheezes	Narrowing of small airways by spasm, inflammation, mucus, or tumor	High-pitched musical or squeaking sounds heard during inspiration or expiration	Acute asthma Emphysema
Stridor*	Partial upper airway obstruction or tracheal or laryngeal spasm	High-pitched, continuous honking sounds heard throughout the respiratory cycle but most prominent on inspiration	Acute respiratory distress Foreign body in airway Epiglottitis

Abnormal Lung Sounds—cont'd

ABNORMAL LUNG SOUNDS	CAUSE	CHARACTERISTICS	EXAMPLES
Friction Rub	Rubbing together of inflamed pleural layers	A high-pitched grating or rubbing sound that may be heard throughout the respiratory cycle. Loudest over lower lateral anterior surface	Pleuritis
Grunting	Retention of air in the lungs	A high-pitched tubular sound heard on expiration	Emphysema

*Patients with stridor need immediate medical evaluation.

Procedure 22-13 ■ Assessing the Heart and Vascular System

➤ For steps to follow in *all* procedures, refer to the Universal Steps for All Procedures found on the inside back cover.

Equipment

- Combination stethoscope with bell and diaphragm
- Alcohol or other antiseptic wipes
- Two rulers
- Pen and record form

Clean stethoscope and rulers before and after use unless they are only used for one patient.

Positioning

Place the client in three positions: sitting, supine, and left lateral (to facilitate hearing specific sounds).

Focused History Questions

- Have you experienced any fatigue or activity intolerance?
- Do you have a history of high blood pressure or stroke?
- Have you ever passed out or felt light-headed?
- Do you have any problems with your heart or circulation?
- Do you ever experience chest pain? If so, describe the circumstances that triggered the pain.
- What was the pain like? What did you do to relieve it?
- Do you ever experience palpitations or a rapid heartbeat?
- Do you ever feel short of breath?
- Do you ever get swelling in your feet?
- What medications are you taking?

➤ When performing the procedure, always identify your patient according to agency policy, using two identifiers, and be attentive to standard precautions, hand hygiene, patient safety and privacy, body mechanics, and documentation.

Procedure Steps

1. Inspect the neck.

a. With the patient supine, *inspect the carotid and jugular venous system* in the neck for pulsations.

b. *Assess jugular flow:* Compress the jugular vein below the jaw. The vein collapses, and the jugular wave is more prominent at the supraclavicular area. ▼

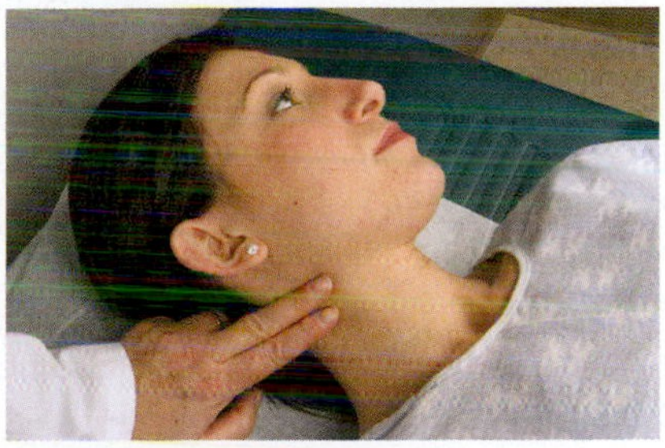

Assessing jugular flow

The jugular venous pulse is easily obliterated with gentle pressure.

Findings

Expected Findings: Carotid pulsation is easily visible. A slight pulsation in the supraclavicular area or suprasternal notch indicates jugular venous pressure (JVP). The pulsation should be easily obliterated when you apply pressure to the area.

Abnormal findings: Significant jugular vein distention suggests right-sided heart failure.

(continued on next page)

Procedure 22-13 ■ Assessing the Heart and Vascular System (continued)

c. *Assess jugular filling*: Compress the jugular above the clavicle. The vein distends and the jugular wave disappears.

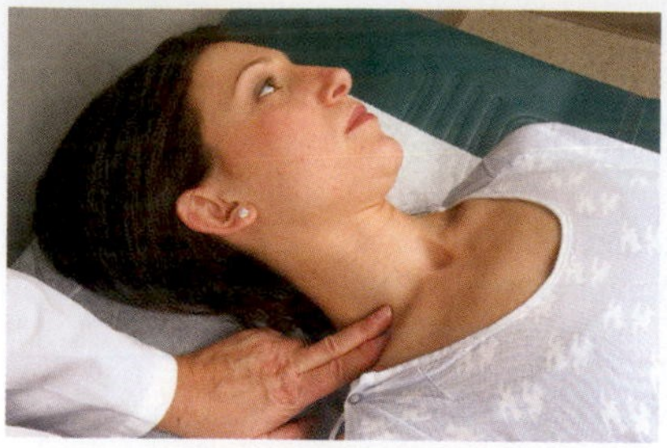

Assessing jugular filling

2. Measure jugular venous pressure (JVP).

a. Elevate the head of the bed to a 45° angle.
b. Identify the highest point of visible internal jugular filling.
c. Place a ruler vertically at the sternal angle (where the clavicles meet).
d. Place another ruler horizontally at the highest point of the venous wave.
e. Measure the distance in centimeters vertically from the chest wall.

Expected findings: Normal JVP is < 3 cm.

Abnormal findings: Elevated JVP (in congestive heart failure [CHF] or constricted flow into the right side of the heart); low JVP (in hypovolemia)

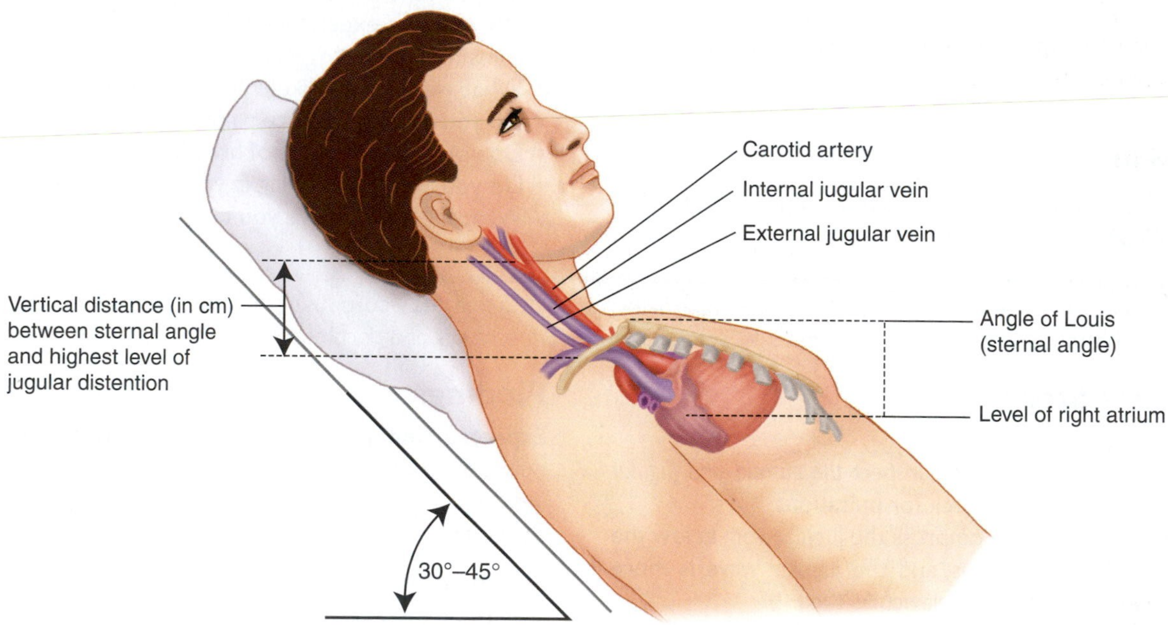

Measuring jugular venous pressure

3. Inspect the precordium for pulsations. (Place the patient in the supine position, under tangential lighting.)

Developmental Modifications

Children: Look for the PMI more medially and at about the 4th ICS in children younger than age 8 years.

Expected findings: Visible pulsation at the point of maximal impulse (PMI; the 5th ICS in the midclavicular line).

Developmental Variations

In thin adults and children, a pulsation may also be visible over the base of the heart.

Abnormal findings:

- A pulsation (a heave or lift) displaced toward the axillary line indicates left ventricular hypertrophy.
- Pulsations to the right of the sternum may indicate an aortic aneurysm.

4. **Very gently palpate the carotid arteries.** Note: this step is not done in all patients. It is a part of a thorough cardiovascular assessment and is done only when indicated.
   a. Palpate each side separately; never at the same time.
   Bilateral pressure may impair cerebral blood flow.
   b. Avoid massaging the carotid artery as you palpate.
   Increased pressure on the carotid will lead to a drop in the heart rate and blood pressure.
   c. Note the rate, rhythm, amplitude, and symmetry of the pulse.
   d. Note the contour, symmetry, and elasticity of the arteries.
   e. Note any thrills.

Expected findings:
- *Rhythm* is regular with +2 amplitude.
- *Contour:* There should be a smooth upstroke with less acute descent.
- *Symmetry:* Pulses are equal bilaterally.
- *Elasticity:* Carotids are soft and pliable.

Developmental Variations

Pulse rate is age dependent.

Older adults: The carotids may be stiff and cord-like.

Abnormal findings: A thrill indicates turbulent flow.

---

5. **Palpate the precordium.**
   a. For this part of the examination, have the patient sit up and lean forward. If he is lying down, have him turn to the left side.
   Brings the apex of the heart closer to the chest wall.
   b. Palpate in all five areas: apex, left lateral sternal border, epigastric area, base left, and base right.
   c. Feel for pulsations, lifts, heaves, and thrills.

Helpful Hint: *Perform cardiac palpation and auscultation from the patient's right side, whenever possible.*
This allows you to stretch the stethoscope during auscultation so that you minimize interference and "static."

Expected findings: PMI is palpable at the apex over a 1-cm to 2-cm area. Slight pulsation from the abdominal aorta may be felt at the epigastric area. No pulsations, lifts, heaves, or thrills are palpable.

Abnormal findings: A pulsation, lift, or heave may be seen with left ventricular hypertrophy.
- A ***lift*** is a pulsation that is forceful enough to seem to lift the examiner's fingers with palpation.
- A ***heave*** is a pulsation that feels rolling under your fingers.
- A ***thrill*** indicates turbulent flow and feels like a vibration over the PMI.

---

6. **Auscultate the carotids.**
   a. Place the bell portion of the stethoscope over the carotid artery to listen for bruits.
   Bruits are low-pitched sounds, best heard by the bell portion.
   b. Have the patient hold his breath as you listen.
   Breath sounds over the trachea are loud and could interfere with the ability to hear a bruit.

NOTE: If you hear a bruit, lightly palpate the neck for thrills (pulsations or vibrations), which further confirm turbulent flow.

Expected findings: No audible bruit is present.

Developmental Variations

Children: Bruit may be heard because of a high-output state.

Abnormal findings: In adults, a bruit suggests carotid stenosis, increased cardiac output secondary to fluid overload, use of stimulants, or hyperthyroidism.

---

7. **Auscultate the jugular veins.**
   a. Place the bell portion of the stethoscope lightly over the jugular veins to listen for a low-pitched venous hum.
   b. Have the patient hold his breath as you listen.

Expected findings: No venous hum is audible.

Developmental Variations

Children: A venous hum may be heard. This is a benign condition wherein blood travels to the brain and back down again to the heart, causing the vein walls to vibrate.

---

8. **Auscultate the precordium.** To review heart sounds, do the following:
   Key Point. *Be systematic. To keep from missing important parts of the exam, always auscultate in the same order to all the areas.*
   - Ask the patient to sit upright and lean forward a bit.
   This will position the heart closer to the chest wall for clearer auscultation.

Expected findings: No extra sounds are heard. No murmurs, clicks, or rubs are present.

An S_4 sound is normal in athletes.

Developmental Variations

Infants: You may hear a split S_2 when the child takes a deep breath.

(continued on next page)

Procedure 22-13 ■ Assessing the Heart and Vascular System (continued)

- Listen for the S_1, S_2, S_3, and S_4 sounds.
- Listen for murmurs.
- Listen with both the bell and the diaphragm at the sites in the following figure:

These sites are located along the pathway the blood takes as it flows through the atria, ventricles, and valves of the heart.

Children: The chest wall is thinner, so heart sounds are louder than in adults. An S_3 is normal in young children and adolescents when they are sitting or supine, but it disappears when they stand or sit up.

Pregnancy—An S_3 is a normal variant in the third trimester of pregnancy.

Older adults: An S_4 sound is considered normal; extra systoles per minute are considered normal. ▼

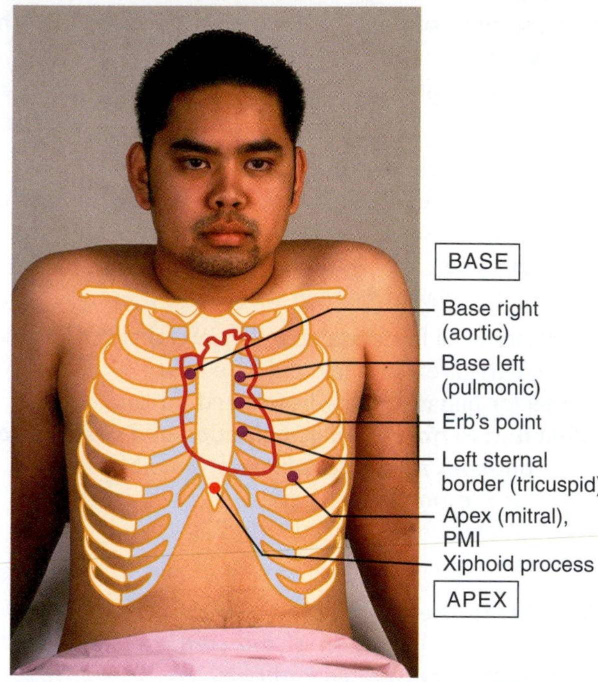

Cardiac auscultation sites

Abnormal findings:

- A split sound at either S_1 or S_2 may occur if there is a delay in closure of one of the valves.
- An S_3 that does not disappear with position change is abnormal and represents heart failure or volume overload.
- An S_4 may be heard in adults with coronary artery disease, hypertension, and pulmonic stenosis.

a. *Base right (aortic valve).* Locate the angle of Louis (the prominence on the sternum, two to three fingerbreadths below the suprasternal notch). Slide your fingers laterally until you feel the 2nd ICS.

The right 2nd ICS is the best place to auscultate the aortic valve.

a. **Expected findings:** $S_1 < S_2$

b. *Base left (pulmonic valve).* Locate the angle of Louis (the prominence on the sternum, two to three fingerbreadths below the clavicular notch). Slide your fingers laterally until you feel the 2nd ICS.
The left second ICS is the best place to auscultate the pulmonic valve. ▼

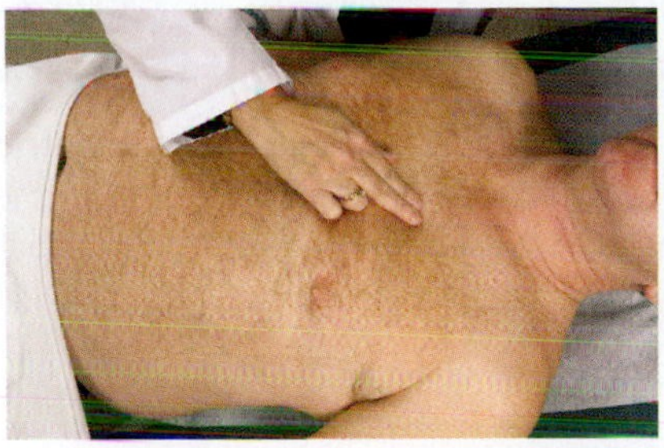

b. **Expected findings:** $S_1 < S_2$

c. *Apex (mitral valve).* You may be able to locate the apex by observing the pulsation at the PMI. It is at the 5th ICS in the midclavicular line.

c. **Expected findings:** $S_1 > S_2$

Developmental Variations

Children: You will hear S_3 at the apex in about 30% of children.

d. *Left lateral sternal border (LLSB) (tricuspid valve).* From the apex, *slide* your finger up to the 4th ICS, then move close to the sternum.

d. **Expected findings:** $S_1 \geq S_2$. You may hear a split S_1.

Abnormal findings: Extra sounds (S_3 or S_4), murmurs, clicks, or rubs.

NOTE: A diastolic murmur or a murmur greater than grade $^3/_6$ is never innocent.

Developmental Variations

A split S_2 sound during normal respirations may indicate an atrial–septal defect.

Assessing Murmurs

Auscultating murmurs is an advanced technique that requires practice and experience. However, if you hear a murmur, assess its:

- Location
- Quality
- Frequency (high, medium, or low pitch)
- Intensity (loudness)
- Timing (in relation to S_1 and S_2)
- Duration
- Configuration (constant or crescendo/decrescendo)
- Radiation (can you hear this in other locations?)
- Respiratory variation (does it change with breathing?)

Classifying Murmurs

Grade

$^1/_6$ Very faint, comes and goes

$^2/_6$ Quiet, but heard immediately

$^3/_6$ Moderately loud

$^4/_6$ Loud, associated with a thrill

$^5/_6$ Heard with stethoscope half off the chest wall; thrill present

$^6/_6$ Heard with stethoscope entirely off the chest wall; thrill present

9. Inspect the periphery for color, temperature, and edema. (You will probably already have done this when examining the integumentary system.)

Expected findings: Skin is warm. No edema is present. Color is appropriate for race.

Abnormal findings: Pallor, cyanosis, coolness, shininess, sparse hair growth, and clubbing of the nails (may indicate pulmonary oxygenation problems or impaired central or peripheral circulation)

(continued on next page)

Procedure 22-13 ■ Assessing the Heart and Vascular System (continued)

10. Palpate the peripheral pulses: radial, brachial, femoral, popliteal, dorsalis pedis, and posterior tibial.

- Using the distal pads of your second and third fingers, firmly palpate pulses.
- Palpate firmly but not so hard that you occlude the artery.
- If you have trouble finding a pulse, vary your pressure, feeling carefully at the correct anatomical location.
- Assess pulses for rate, rhythm, equality, amplitude, and elasticity.
- Describe pulse amplitude on a scale of 0 to 4:
  0 = *Absent:* Pulse cannot be felt.
  1 = *Weak (thready):* Pulse is barely palpable and can be easily obliterated by finger pressure.
  2 = *Normal quality:* Pulse is easily palpated, not weak or bounding, obliterated by finger pressure.
  3 = *Full:* Pulse is easily felt with little pressure; not easily obliterated.
  4 = *Bounding:* Forceful, obliterated only by strong finger pressure.

Expected findings: All pulses are regular, strong, and equal bilaterally. Pulse amplitude is +2.

Developmental Variations

Older adults: Arterial pulses may be difficult to palpate because of decreased arterial perfusion.

Abnormal findings: Weak, absent, or asymmetrical pulses may indicate partial or complete occlusion of the artery. Other signs of arterial occlusion include pain, pallor, cool temperature, paresthesia, or paralysis.

11. Inspect the venous system. If a client has varicosities, assess for valve competence with the manual compression test:

a. With the client standing, compress the distal portion of the vein.
b. Still holding the distal portion, compress the proximal portion.
c. Feel for a pulsation with your lower (distal) hand.
   - **If the valves are competent,** you will not feel backflow when you compress the vein.
   - **If the valves are incompetent,** you will feel a wave pulsation with your lower hand as a result of backflow when you press on the proximal segment.

Expected findings: Veins are not distended. Superficial spider-like veins, especially on the lower extremities, may occur with normal aging.

Developmental Variations

Older adults—often have peripheral edema as a result of chronic venous insufficiency.

Abnormal findings: Ropelike, distended, tortuous, or painful veins **(varicosities)**

? What if . . .

- **The patient is obese and heart sounds are difficult to hear?**

  The larger the body mass over the heart, the more difficult it is to hear heart sounds clearly. However, it may help to have the patient sit upright and lean forward as you auscultate.

- **Findings from inspecting and palpating peripheral pulses are abnormal?**

  If inspection or palpation findings are abnormal, perform the tests in the table (see More Extensive Tests for Abnormal Findings, at the end of this procedure).

Patient Teaching

Educate the patient about the risk factors for heart disease and stroke and about the signs and symptoms of heart disease.

Documentation

If you need information about documenting your findings, review Caring for the Nguyens, and

Go to Chapter 22, **Documenting Physical Examination Findings (Nam Nguyen),** in Volume 1.

If you need more information about assessing apical and peripheral pulses and measuring blood pressure,

The video, **Vital Signs,** along with questions and suggested responses, on the ***Davis's Nursing Skills Videos*** Web site on FADavis.com.

More Extensive Tests for Abnormal Findings

TESTS	EXPECTED FINDINGS
1. **Perform the capillary refill test** anywhere you note signs of diminished blood flow. a. Press the skin with sufficient pressure to produce blanching. b. Release the pressure, and observe for the return of color.	1. Color returns in < 3 seconds.
2. **Perform Allen's test** to assess abnormal pulse findings and arterial flow in the hands. a. Have the client form a tight fist with one hand. b. With her fist still clenched, compress her radial and ulnar arteries. c. Ask the client to open her hand; observe for pallor. d. Release the ulnar artery and watch for natural color to return. e. Then, repeat the process, but release the radial artery.	2. In a healthy individual skin color returns rapidly with each maneuver. Failure to return to normal color indicates impaired flow through the open artery. Normally pallor resolves in 3 to 5 seconds.
3. **Check the ankle–brachial index (ABI)** to assess circulatory impairment of the feet. a. Use a Doppler device (handheld ultrasonic device) to measure blood pressure at the posterior tibialis or dorsalis pedis pulse sites. b. Compare that pressure with blood pressure obtained over the brachial artery. c. To calculate the ABI, divide the systolic pressure at the ankle by the systolic pressure at the brachial site.	3. Normally ankle pressure is higher than brachial pressure. The following is a summary of ABI findings: Normal: 1 or greater Minimal disease: 0.80–0.95 Moderate disease: 0.79–0.40 Severe disease: 0.39–0.00 *Example:* If the systolic pressure at the ankle is 75 and at the brachial artery is 100, the ABI is 75/100, or 0.75. This indicates moderate peripheral vascular disease.
4. **Perform the color change test** to assess arterial circulation in the legs. a. While the client is lying supine, elevate the legs to increase venous return. b. Have the client quickly move to a sitting position with the feet dangling.	4. Normal color should return to the feet in < 10 seconds. Pallor with the legs elevated and dependent ***rubor*** (reddish-purple color) are signs of arterial insufficiency.

Procedure 22-14 ■ Assessing the Abdomen

➤ For steps to follow in *all* procedures, refer to the Universal Steps for All Procedures found on the inside back cover.

Equipment

- Stethoscope and antiseptic wipe
- Felt-tipped marker
- Tape measure and ruler
- Penlight or examination light
- Pen and record form

Clean stethoscope and other equipment before and after use unless they are only used for one patient.

Positioning

Begin with the client in the supine position, arms at sides, with small pillows under the head and knees.

Relaxes the abdominal muscles, allowing for more effective palpation.

Focused History Questions

- What types of foods do you typically eat?
- Are there any foods that you cannot eat? If so, why?
- How many cups of coffee, tea, cola, or caffeinated beverages do you drink per day?
- Do you smoke? If so, how much, and at what age did you start?
- Do you drink alcohol? If so, how many drinks per day? Per week?
- Do you use any drug for nonmedical purposes?
- Do you have any abdominal pain?
- How often do you have a bowel movement (BM)?
- Have you noticed any changes in your BMs?
- Are you having any problems with constipation, diarrhea, or getting to the bathroom in time to use the toilet?

(continued on next page)

Procedure 22-14 ■ Assessing the Abdomen (continued)

(continues from preceding page)

- Have you ever seen blood in your stool or noticed blood when you wipe after a BM?
- Have you ever had black, tarry stools?
- How often do you use antacids, laxatives, enemas, aspirin, or anti-inflammatory medicines, such as Anaprox or Motrin?
- What home remedy, herbal, or over-the-counter medicines do you use?
- What prescription medicines do you use?
- Have you ever been immunized for hepatitis?
- Have you ever had a blood transfusion?
- What is your occupation?
- Have you ever been diagnosed with an ulcer, hemorrhoids, hernia, bowel problem, cancer, hepatitis, liver problems, cirrhosis, or appendicitis?
- Have you ever had abdominal surgery? If so, when, what type, and what if any follow-up was done for the problem?
- Do you have any family history of abdominal problems, such as ulcers, gallbladder disease, bowel disease, or cancer?
- Do you ever have trouble with swallowing, heartburn, nausea, vomiting, diarrhea, bloating, excess gas, yellowing of the skin?

Developmental Modifications

For older adults, recall that "Problems with eating" is a part of the SPICES (Sleep problems, Problems with eating and feeding, Incontinence, Confusion, Evidence of falls, and Skin breakdown) assessment. Ask clients, for example:

- Do you have difficulty chewing or swallowing your food?
- How is your appetite?
- Are you able to shop for and prepare your food?

➤ When performing the procedure, always identify your patient according to agency policy, using two identifiers, and be attentive to standard precautions, hand hygiene, patient safety and privacy, body mechanics, and documentation.

Procedure Steps	Findings
1. Have the client void before the exam. *Empties the bladder so that you do not mistake a full bladder for a mass.*	
2. Position the client supine, with the knees slightly flexed. *Relaxes the abdominal muscles for more effective palpation.*	
3. Inspect the abdomen. a. Observe the size, symmetry, and contour of the abdomen. (1) Stand at the client's side and view across the abdomen. (2) If distention is present, use a tape measure to measure girth at the level of the umbilicus. (3) Have the client raise her head and check for bulges. *Accentuates hernia, if present.*	a. **Expected findings:** Abdomen is flat, slightly rounded, scaphoid (concave), or slightly protuberant; sides are symmetrical. No visible masses or distention are present. ***Developmental Variations*** *Infants and toddlers:* Protuberant abdomen is normal. **Abnormal findings:** ■ Asymmetry may be caused by tumors, cysts, or scoliosis. ■ Distention may be caused by gas, fluid retention, or bowel obstruction.
b. Observe the condition of skin and skin color. Look for lesions, scars, striae, superficial veins, and hair distribution (if you have not already done this in your examination of the integumentary system).	b. **Expected findings:** Skin color is consistent with ethnicity but is usually lighter in color than in exposed areas. No lesions are present. Hair distribution is appropriate for age and gender. Striae, superficial veins, and scars are common variations. **Abnormal findings:** ■ Skin color changes may be associated with bruising, internal bleeding, or jaundice. ■ Striae occur after periods of rapid growth or weight gain. Pink striae are new. Older striae are silver-white in color. ■ Dilated veins are associated with liver disease and obstruction of the vena cava.

c. Note abdominal movements.

c. **Expected findings:** On a thin client, peristalsis and aortic pulsations may be visible. Men tend to use their abdominal muscles for breathing.

Developmental Variations

Infants and children—Peristaltic waves are often visible. Abdominal breathing is common in infants and young children.

Older adults: Abdomen may be more rounded because of decreased muscle tone.

Abnormal findings:

- Peristaltic waves may be seen if there is intestinal obstruction.
- Abnormal respiratory movements may be seen with respiratory distress.
- Pulsations (in clients who are not thin) may indicate an aortic aneurysm.

d. Note the position, contour, and color of the umbilicus.

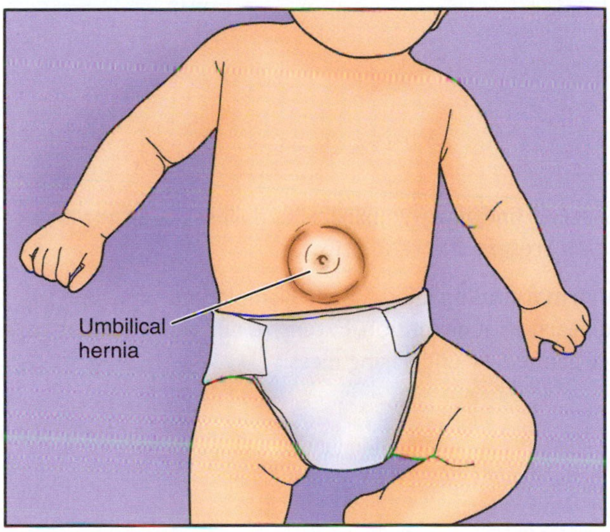

d. **Expected findings:** Umbilicus is inverted and in the midline. No discoloration or discharge is present.

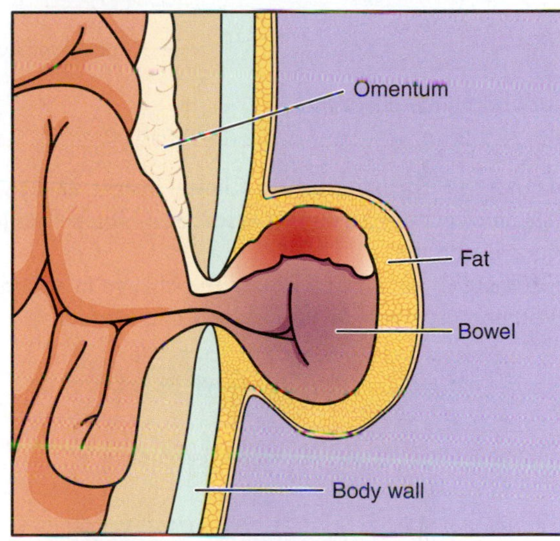

Abnormal findings: Protrusion of the umbilicus may result from a hernia or an underlying mass.

4. Auscultate the abdomen.

a. Ask the client when she last ate.
Bowel sounds are loudest 5 or 6 hours after the person eats, when the small intestine contents empty through the ileocecal valve into the large intestine. They also increase immediately after eating.

b. Listen for bowel sounds.

(1) Using the stethoscope diaphragm, listen in several areas in all four quadrants (see the figure).
The diaphragm of the stethoscope is used because bowel sounds are high-pitched.

(2) If bowel sounds are infrequent or difficult to hear, listen to the right of the umbilicus over the ileocecal valve.

(3) Listen for up to 5 minutes before concluding that bowel sounds are absent.

b. **Expected findings:** Audible bowel sounds, occurring every 5 to 15 sec or 5 to 30 times per min.

Abnormal findings:

- ***Hyperperistalsis*** (hyperactive)— > 2 or 3 sounds per sec or > 30 sounds per min
- ***Hypoperistalsis*** (hypoactive)— < 5 sounds per min
- ***Absent bowel sounds***—none after listening for 5 minute

(continued on next page)

Procedure 22-14 ■ Assessing the Abdomen (continued)

c. Use the stethoscope bell to listen for bruits over the aorta and the renal, femoral, and iliac arteries. ▼

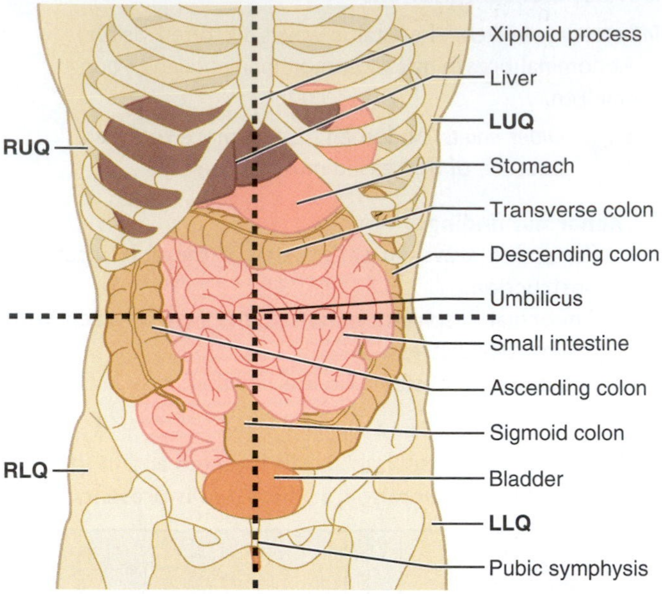

The four abdominal quadrants

c. **Expected findings:** No audible bruits are present.

Abnormal findings: A bruit is abnormal and may indicate an aneurysm or altered blood flow. ▼

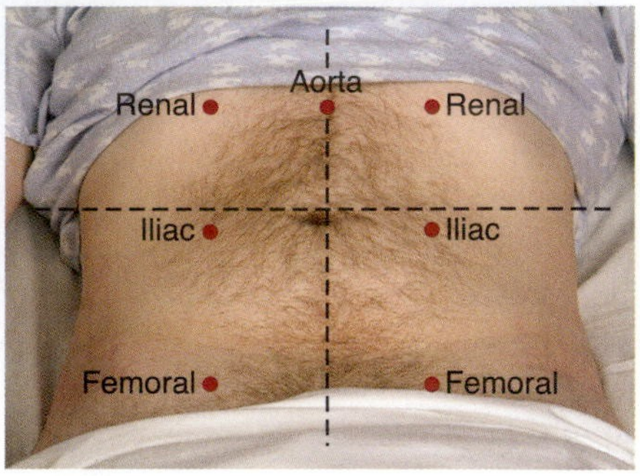

Locating abdominal arteries

5. **Percuss the abdomen.** (See Clinical Insight 22-1.)
   a. Use indirect percussion to assess at multiple sites in all four quadrants.
   b. Estimate organ size by noting the change in sounds as you percuss over the liver, spleen, and bladder. ▼

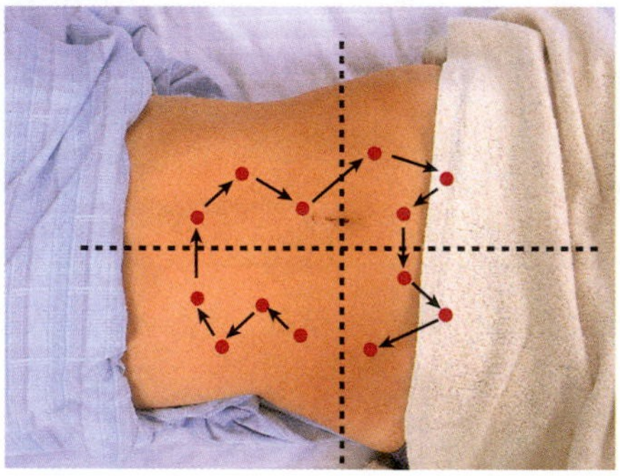

Expected findings: Tympany, with dullness over organs or fluid, is present. No tenderness.

Abnormal findings: Extremely high-pitched tympanic sounds are heard with distention. Extensive dullness indicates organ enlargement or underlying mass.

6. **Using fist or blunt percussion, percuss the costovertebral angle** (where the end of the rib cage meets the spine) bilaterally to assess for kidney tenderness. ▼

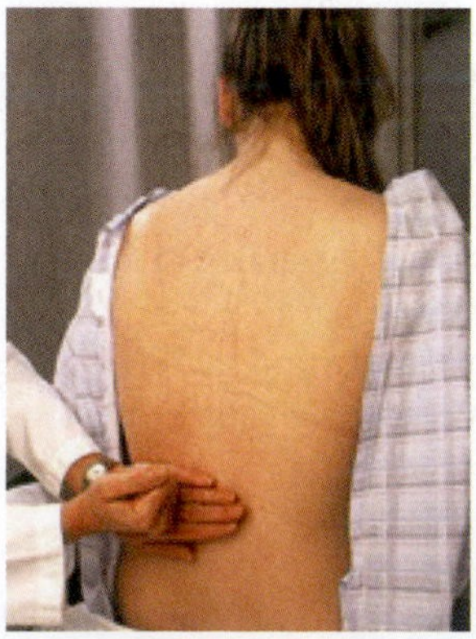

Expected findings: No costovertebral angle tenderness is present.

Abnormal findings: Pain or tenderness is associated with kidney infection or musculoskeletal problems.

7. Palpate the abdomen.

a. **Begin with light palpation** throughout the abdomen. Identify surface characteristics, tenderness, muscular resistance, and turgor.

(1) If the client is having pain in one area of the abdomen, palpate that area last.

A guarding response to pain from palpation can interfere with your assessment of the other areas.

(2) Using your fingertips, press down 1 to 2 cm in a rotating motion.

(3) Lift your fingers and move to the next site.

(4) Palpate the entire abdomen, if possible.

(5) Proceed in an organized fashion through all quadrants, using the same sequence in every examination.

(6) Observe for grimacing, guarding, or verbal statements of tenderness or pain.

a. **Expected findings:** The abdomen is soft and nontender, with no masses. Muscles are easily palpated; no guarding is present.

Abnormal findings: Guarding and rigidity may indicate peritonitis. Tenderness on light palpation indicates the need for further evaluation.

Developmental Modifications

Encourage a child to place her hand lightly over yours as you palpate.

Caution: Do not palpate the abdomen if the client has a Wilms' tumor, a large diffuse pulsation, or a history of organ transplantation.

b. **Use deep palpation** to palpate organs and masses. See the table Deep Palpation Techniques at the end of this procedure.

b. **Expected findings:** Tenderness may be noted in a normal adult near the xiphoid process and over the cecum and sigmoid colon.

Developmental Variations

Older adults—may have a higher pain threshold, so they may not react to palpation even if there is an abnormality in the abdomen.

Abnormal findings: A mass indicates the need for further evaluation.

c. **Palpate the liver.**

(1) Stand at the client's right side.

(2) Place your right hand at the client's right midclavicular line under the costal margin.

(3) Place your left hand under the client's back at the lower (11th to 12th) ribs, and press upward. This elevates the liver toward the abdominal wall.

(4) Ask the client to inhale and deeply exhale while you press in and up, gently but deeply, with your right fingers.

Alternative approach: Hooking technique. Place your hands over the right costal margin, and hook your fingers over the edge. Have the client take a deep breath, and feel for the liver's edge as the liver drops down on inspiration and then rises up over your fingers during expiration.

c. **Expected findings:** The liver is not normally palpable unless the client is very thin. If it is palpable, the edge should be smooth and nontender.

Developmental Variations

Children: Liver is relatively large and can be palpated 1 to 2 cm (0.5–1 in.) below the right costal margin.

Abnormal findings: Palpation below the costal margin indicates enlargement.

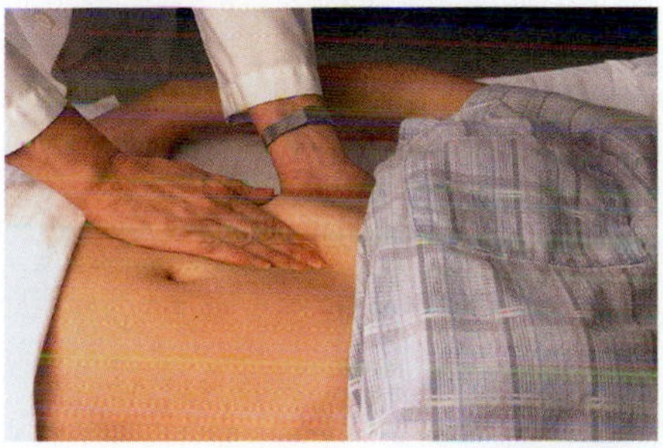

(continued on next page)

Procedure 22-14 ■ Assessing the Abdomen (continued)

d. **Palpate the spleen.**
   (1) Stand at the client's right side.
   (2) Reach across the client to place your left hand under the costovertebral angle, and pull upward to move the spleen anteriorly.
   (3) Place your right hand under the left anterior costal margin, and have the client take a deep breath.
   (4) During exhalation, press your hands together (inward) to try to palpate the spleen.

d. **Expected findings:** The spleen is not normally palpable.

Abnormal findings: Splenic enlargement or tenderness may result from infection, trauma, or cancer.

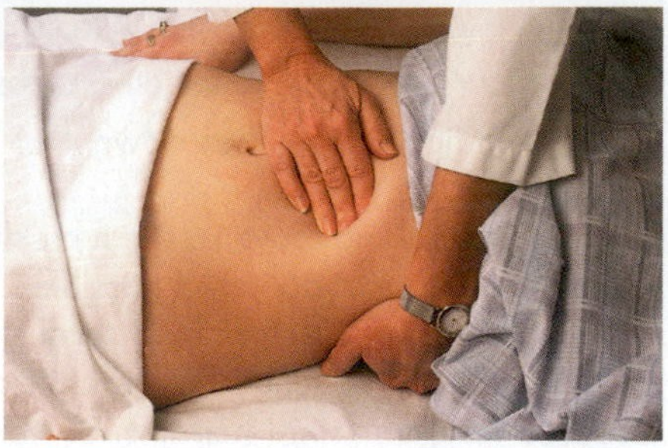

? What if . . .

- **The patient has a nasogastric (NG) tube attached to suction?**

  Discontinue suction or clamp the tube while auscultating so that you will not mistake the sound of suction for bowel sounds.

- **The patient is ticklish or guarding when you palpate the abdomen?**

  Distract the person by giving her a task, such as "Count aloud to 10" or "Count backward from 100." Alternatively, have the client place her hand on her abdomen; place your hand on hers and begin light palpation. When she begins to feel more relaxed, slip your hand underneath hers and continue.

- **The patient complains of abdominal pain?**

  Check for rebound tenderness: Place your hand perpendicular to the abdomen. Press firmly and slowly then release quickly.

  If pain increases when you remove your hand, this indicates peritoneal irritation. Rebound tenderness in the right lower quadrant may be a sign of appendicitis.

Patient Teaching

Instruct the patient in the importance of proper diet, the signs and symptoms of colorectal cancer, and the importance of screening colonoscopy.

Documentation

If you need more information about documenting your findings, review Caring for the Nguyens, and

Go to Chapter 22, **Documenting Physical Examination Findings (Nam Nguyen),** in Volume 1.

Deep Palpation Techniques

DEEP PALPATION: ONE-HANDED TECHNIQUE

- Using your fingertips, press down 4 to 6 cm in a dipping motion.
- Proceed in an organized fashion through all four quadrants.

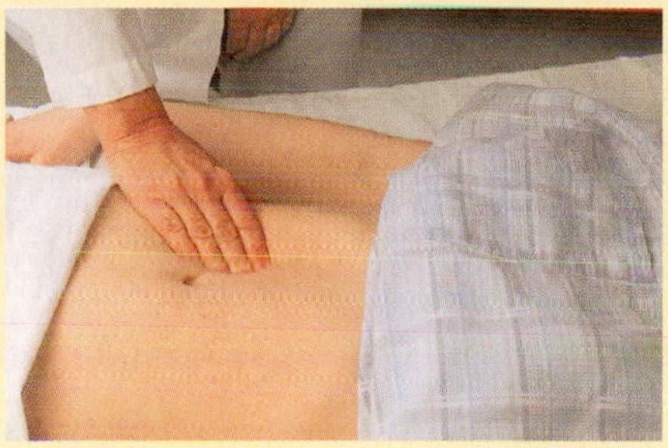

DEEP PALPATION: BIMANUAL TECHNIQUE

- This technique is useful when palpating a large abdomen.
- Place your nondominant hand on your dominant hand.
- Depress your hands 4 to 6 cm (1.5–2 in.) in a dipping motion.
- Proceed in an organized fashion through all four quadrants.

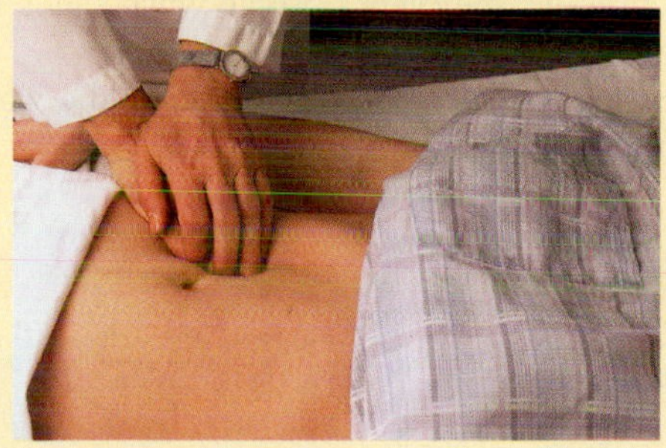

? What if . . .

- **You palpate a mass?**

  Have the client tighten her abdominal muscles.

  If the mass is in the abdominal wall, it will become easier to palpate. If it is deep in the abdomen, it will be difficult to palpate.

Procedure 22-15 ■ Assessing the Musculoskeletal System

➤ For steps to follow in *all* procedures, refer to the Universal Steps for All Procedures found on the inside back cover.

Equipment

- Tape measure
- Goniometer
- Pen and record form

Developmental Modifications

For older adults, recall that "Problems with falls" is a part of the SPICES assessment. If your facility has a falls assessment tool, perform that focused assessment.

Focused History Questions

- Do you have any difficulty with coordination (e.g., folding clothes, brushing your teeth)?
- Do you now have, or have you ever had, musculoskeletal problems, pain, or disease? If so, what medications or treatments are you using?
- Have you ever injured your bones or joints?
- Do your joints, muscles, or bones limit your activities?
- Do you lose your balance or fall?
- Do you have any occupational hazards that could affect your muscles and joints?

➤ When performing the procedure, always identify your patient according to agency policy, using two identifiers, and be attentive to standard precautions, hand hygiene, patient safety and privacy, body mechanics, and documentation.

Procedure Steps	Findings
1. Assess posture.	
a. Note the body and head position.	a. **Expected findings:** Posture is erect, with the head in the midline.
b. Check the alignment and symmetry of the shoulders, scapula, and iliac crests. Inspect from the front, back, and side.	b. **Expected findings:** The shoulders, scapula, and iliac crests are symmetrical.

(continued on next page)

Procedure 22-15 ■ Assessing the Musculoskeletal System (continued)

Developmental Modifications

Newborns: Palpate clavicles for fractures that may have occurred at birth. Check for congenital hip dysplasia (dislocation) by examining for asymmetry of the gluteal folds or shortening of the femur.

c. Assess the spinal curvature by:
   (1) Observing the client's profile while she is standing erect.
   (2) Having the client bend forward at the waist with arms hanging free at the sides. ▼

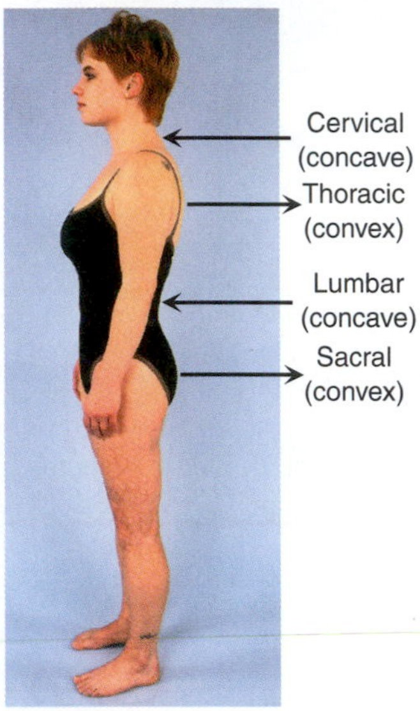

Assessing for normal curves

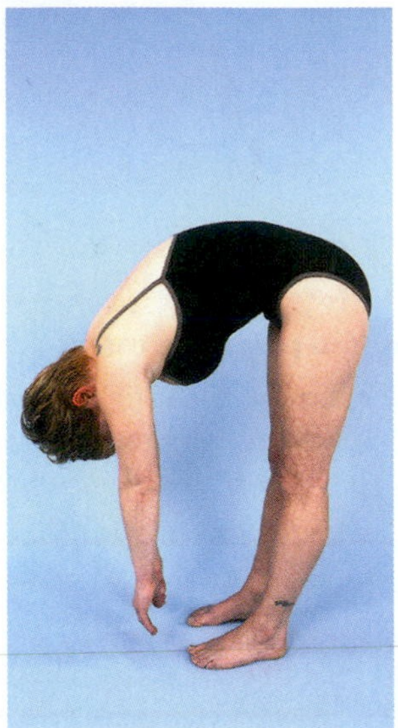

Assessing for kyphosis and scoliosis

c. **Expected findings:** Cervical and lumbar curves are concave; thoracic and sacral curves are convex.

Developmental Variations

Children: ***Lordosis*** (exaggerated lumbar curve) is normal before age 5 years.

Abnormal findings: Kyphosis, scoliosis, lordosis

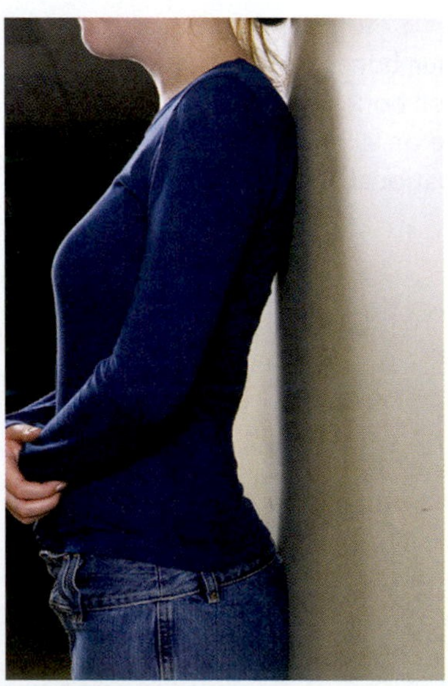

Lordosis

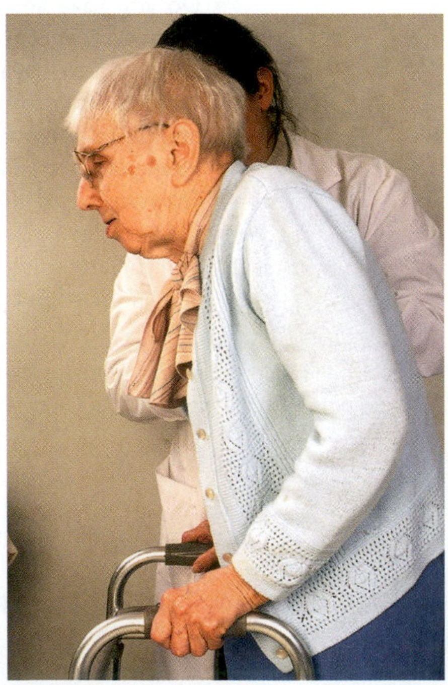

Kyphosis

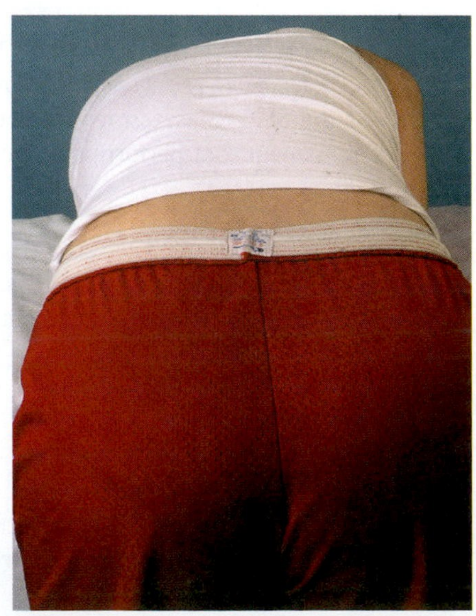

Scoliosis

d. Have the client stand upright with the feet together. Note the position of the knees.

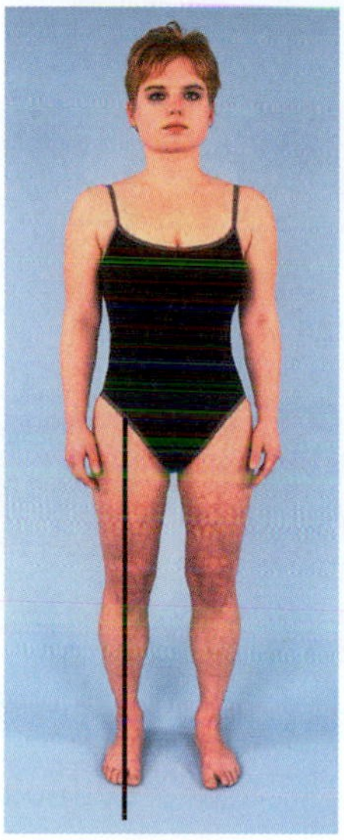

d. **Expected findings:** Patella is in the midline on an imaginary line drawn from the anterior superior iliac crest to the feet.

Developmental Variations

Children: ***Genu varum*** (bowlegs) is normal for 1 year after a child begins to walk.

2. Assess gait by observing the client walking.

Developmental Modifications

Children: Observe them at play.

a. Pay attention to the base of support (distance between the feet) and stride length (distance between each step).

a. **Expected findings:**

Average base of support for an adult is 5 to 10 cm (2–4 in.).

Average stride length is 30 to 35 cm (12–14 in.).

The longer the legs, the longer is the stride length.

Abnormal findings:

- *Abnormal gait* can be caused by muscle weakness, joint stiffness, pain, deformities, lumbar disk problems, central nervous system dysfunction, muscle atrophy or hypertonicity (e.g., from stroke or brain tumor), Parkinson's disease, cerebral palsy, multiple sclerosis, and spinal tumors.
- A *wide base of support and shortened stride length* reflect a balance problem, placing the client at risk for falls.

b. Observe the phases of the gait.

b. **Expected findings:** Movements are smooth and coordinated, weight is evenly distributed, arms swing in opposition, and toes point forward.

Abnormal findings: Toeing in or out, jerky or shuffling movements, touching the floor first with the toe rather than the heel, arms held out to the side or front.

(continued on next page)

Procedure 22-15 ■ Assessing the Musculoskeletal System (continued)

Stance Phase

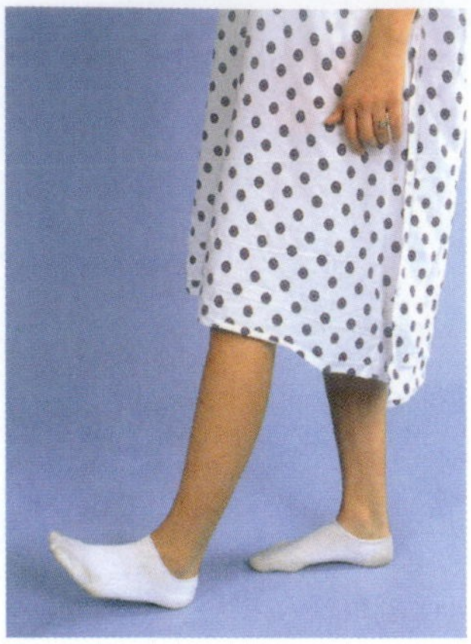
Heel strike

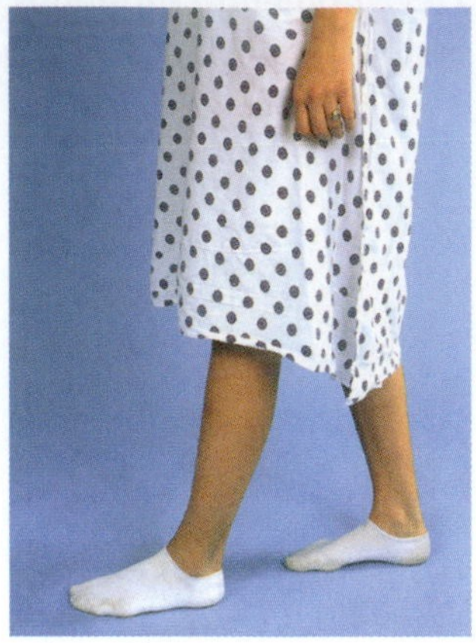
Foot flat

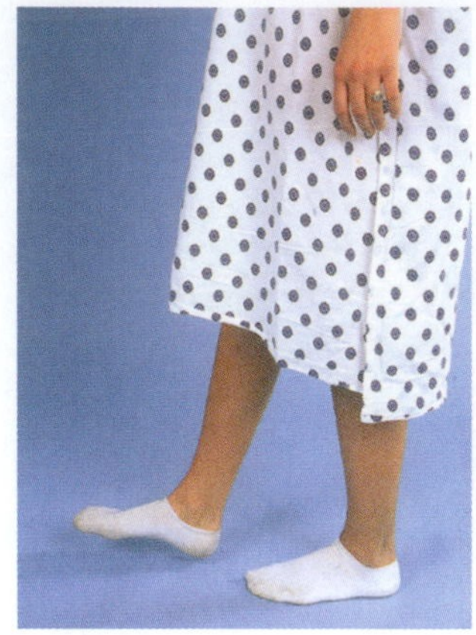
Midstance

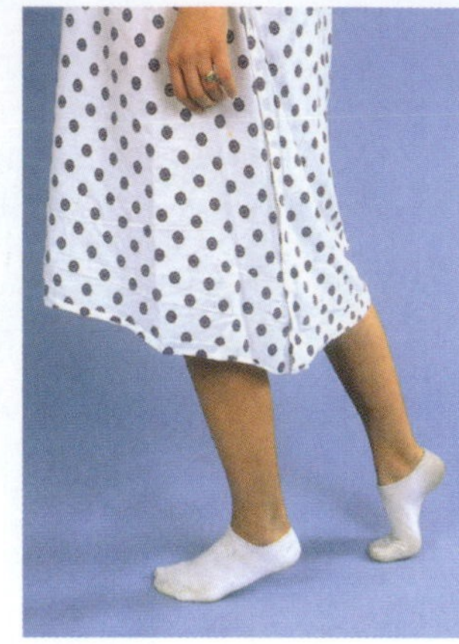
Push-off

Swing Phase

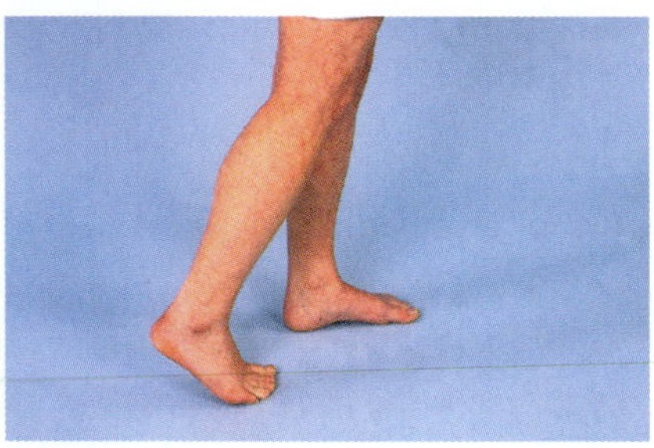
Accelerate

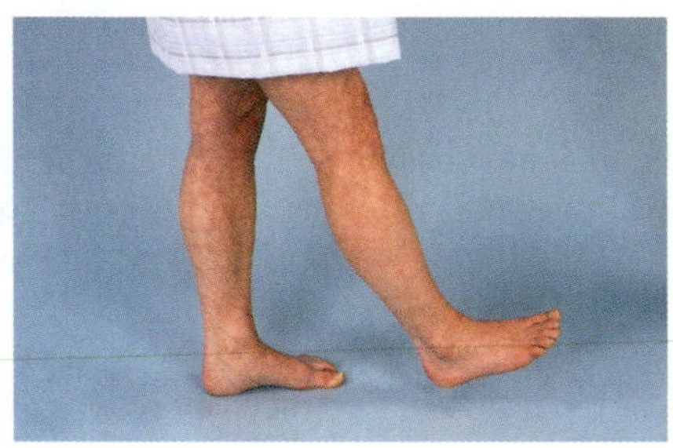
Swing-through

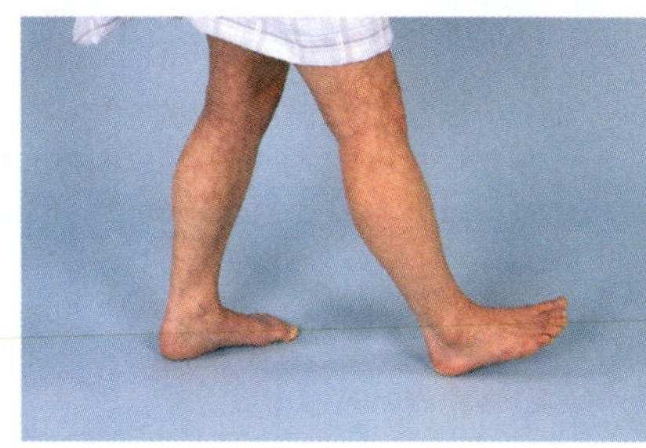
Decelerate

Abnormal Gaits

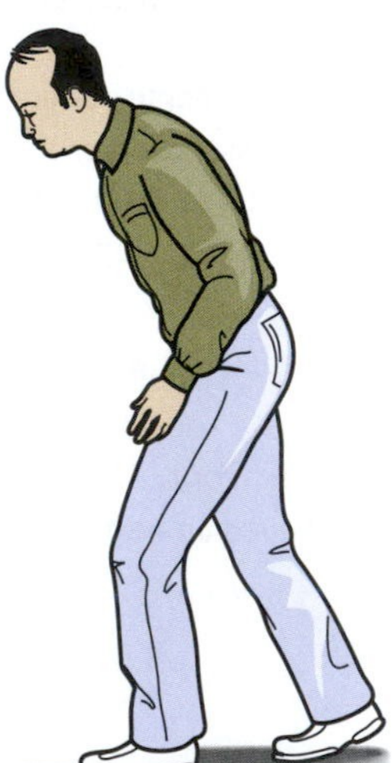
Propulsive gait

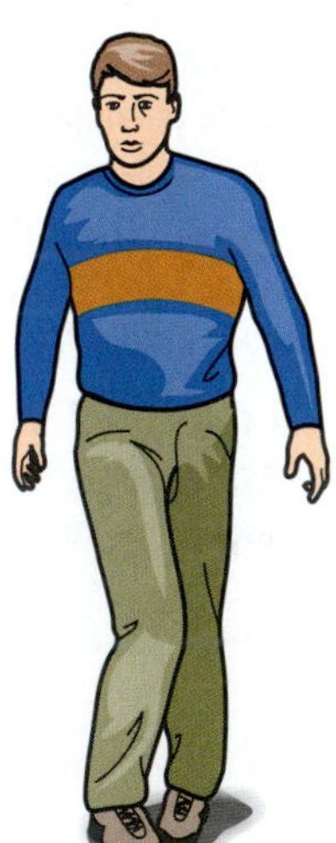
Scissors gait

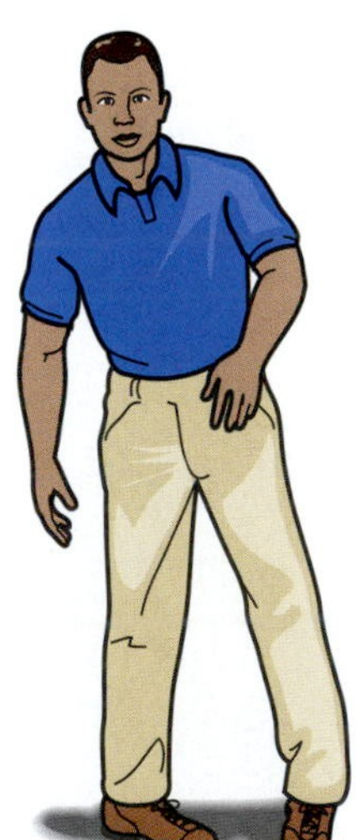
Spastic gait

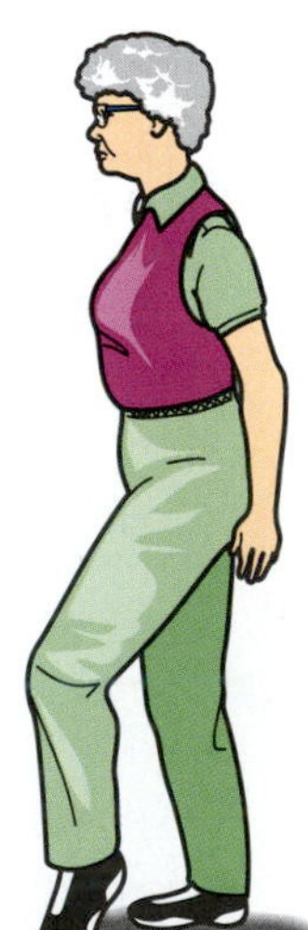
Steppage gait

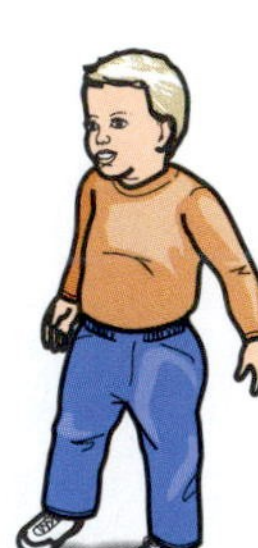
Waddling gait

3. Assess balance.

Key Point: *If the client was unsteady when walking, do not complete this portion of the exam. Proceed only if the gait is steady; stand nearby in case the client loses her balance.*

a. Have the client tandem walk heel to toe.
b. Have the client walk alternately on heels and toes.
c. Ask the client to do a deep knee bend.
d. Ask the client to hop in place on each foot several times.
e. Perform the Romberg test (if you did not already do so when examining the ears): Have the client stand with feet together and eyes open. Then, have her close her eyes and stand still.

Expected findings:

- The client is able to perform each of these maneuvers smoothly.
- The Romberg test (see Procedure 22-7) is negative—the client is able to maintain balance with minimal sway with eyes open and closed.

Developmental Variations

Infants—should be able to sit alone by age 8 months.

Abnormal findings: Balance problems may indicate a cerebellar disorder, an inner ear problem, or muscle weakness.

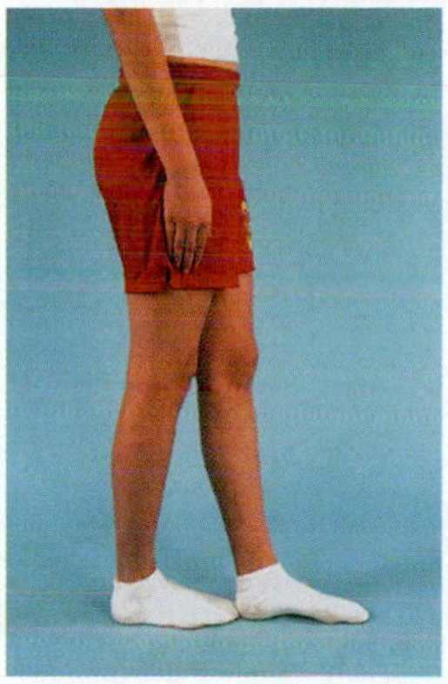

Step 3a. Walking heel-to-toe

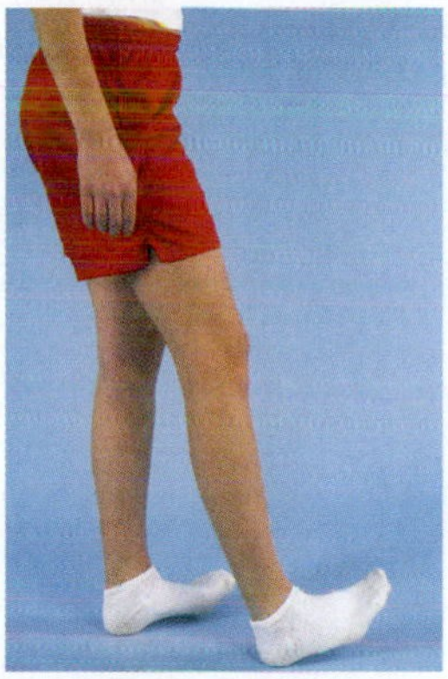

Step 3b. Walking on heels

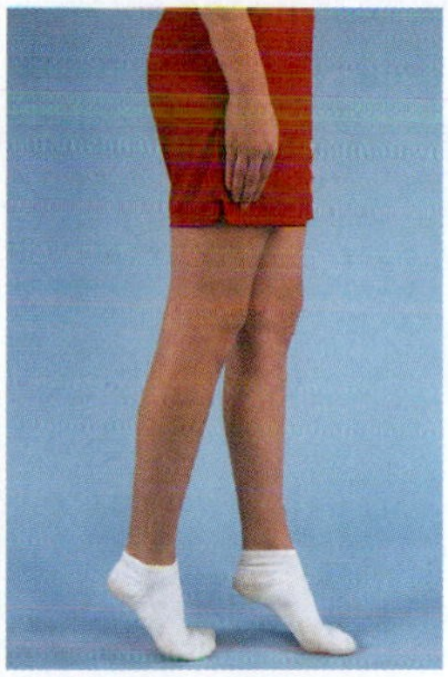

Step 3b. Walking on toes

Developmental Modifications

Infants: Observe sucking, swallowing, and kicking movements.

Children: To assess a child's movement, coordination, ROM, and so on, watch the child at normal play. Cerebellar function cannot be tested on infants and toddlers because of their immature neuromuscular system.

4. Assess coordination while the client is seated.

a. Test upper extremity coordination by having the client perform finger–thumb opposition. Test one side and then the other.

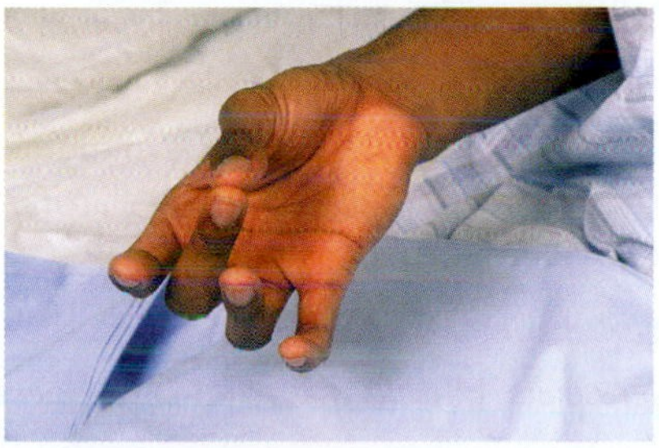

b. Test rapid alternating movements by having the client alternate between supinating and pronating her hands.
c. Assess lower extremity coordination by having the client perform rhythmic toe-tapping, one side at a time.
d. Have the client run the heel of one foot down the shin of the other leg. Repeat on the opposite side.

Expected findings: The client is able to perform these movements smoothly and in a coordinated fashion. The dominant side (usually the right) may be slightly more coordinated.

Developmental Variations

Older adults: Decreased coordination and reaction time may result from slower nerve conduction and loss of muscle tone.

Abnormal findings: Slowness or awkwardness with movement may indicate a cerebellar disorder or muscle weakness.

(continued on next page)

Procedure 22-15 ■ Assessing the Musculoskeletal System (continued)

5. **Test accuracy of movements.** Have the client touch her finger to her nose with her eyes open. Have her repeat with her eyes closed.

Expected findings: The movement is accurate with eyes open or closed.

Abnormal findings: Inaccurate movements indicate cerebellar dysfunction.

6. **Measure the limbs.**
   a. Measure arm length from the acromion process to the tip of the middle finger.
   b. *Apparent leg length:* Measure from the umbilicus (a nonfixed point) to the medial malleolus.
   c. *True leg length:* Measure from the anterior superior iliac crest, crossing over the knee to the medial malleolus ▼

Expected findings: The differences in length between the right and left arm and leg are 1 cm or less.

Abnormal findings: Leg length discrepancies may cause back and hip pain and gait problems. An *apparent leg length* discrepancy may result from a pelvic tilt or flexion deformity of the hip; a *true leg length* discrepancy results from unequal bone length.

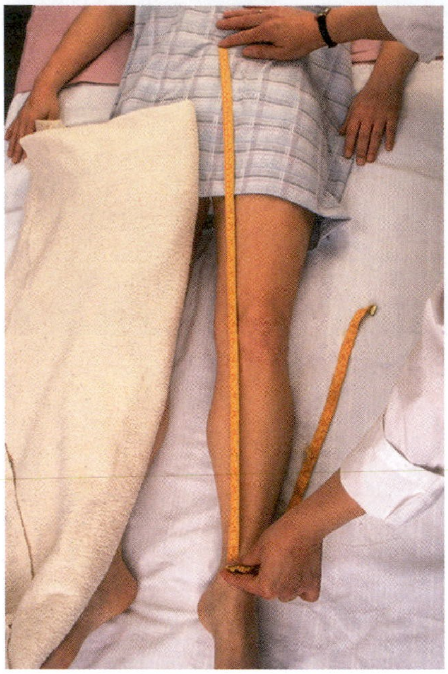

Apparent leg length

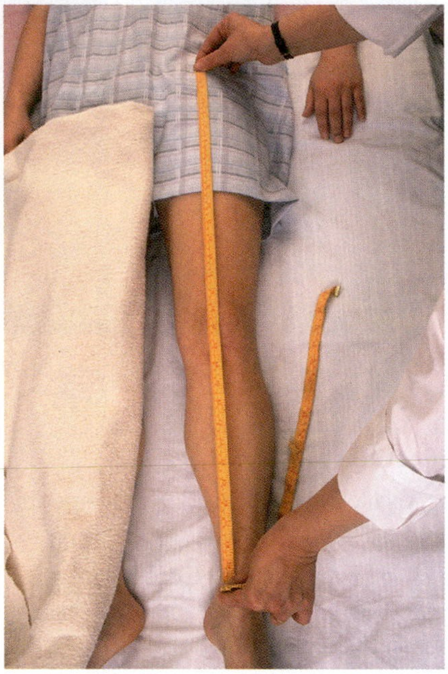

True leg length

   d. Measure the circumference of the forearms, upper arms, thighs, and calves.

d. **Expected findings:** The differences in circumference between the right and left arm and leg are 1 cm or less.

Abnormal findings: Circumference differences > 1 cm may reflect atrophy or hypertrophy.

7. **Inspect muscles and joints bilaterally for symmetry and shape.**

Developmental Modifications

Older adults: Observe for surgical scars indicating joint replacement or joint surgeries.

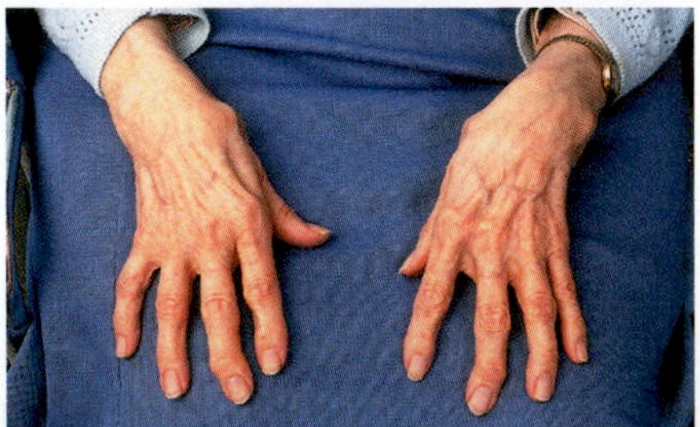

Degenerative joint disease (Heberden's nodes)

Expected findings: Size and shape are symmetrical. Muscles and joints are smooth, nontender, and similar in color and temperature to surrounding tissue.

Developmental Variations

Older adults: Muscle mass and tone decrease.

Abnormal findings:

- Hot, red, swollen, stiff, or painful joints may indicate injuries, arthritis, gout, bursitis, or other inflammatory diseases.
- ***Heberden's nodes*** are hard, painless nodules over the distal interphalangeal joints—usually seen with degenerative joint disease (DJD), but they may be seen with rheumatoid arthritis (RA).
- DJD most commonly affects weight bearing joints (lower back, hips, knees, feet), causing deformity, pain, and stiffness. Crepitus may be heard in DJD.

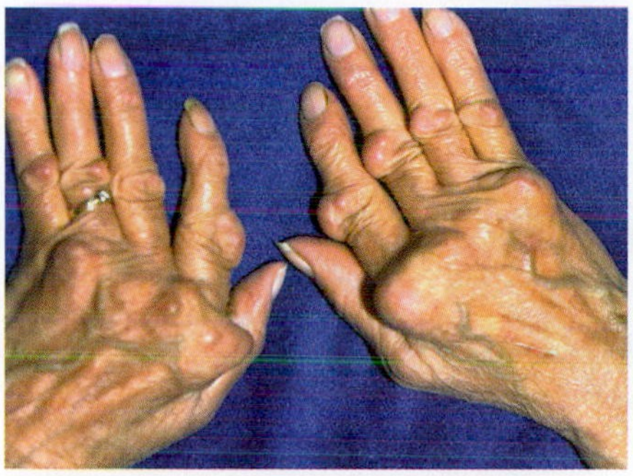

Rheumatoid arthritis

- RA most often involves the small joints of the hands and feet but can involve other joints, including the jaw, causing misalignment and deformity. The joint involvement is usually *symmetrical.*

---

8. Test active ROM by asking the client to move the following joints through ROM:

Expected findings:

a. Temporomandibular joint (TMJ)

TMJ—able to flex, extend, move side to side, protrude, and retract the jaw.

b. Neck

Neck—flexes, extends, hyperextends, bends laterally, and rotates side to side.

c. Thoracic and lumbar spine

Spine—able to bend at the waist, stand upright, hyperextend (bend backward), bend laterally, and rotate side to side.

d. Shoulder

Shoulder—able to move the arm forward and backward, abduct, adduct, and rotate internally and externally.

e. Upper arm and elbow

Upper arm and elbow—able to bend, extend, supinate, and pronate the elbow.

f. Wrist

Wrist—flexes, extends, hyperextends, and moves side to side.

g. Hands and fingers

Hands and fingers—able to:

Spread the fingers (abduct)

Bring them together (adduct)

Make a fist (flex)

Extend the hand (extend)

Bend fingers back (hyperextend)

Bring thumb to index finger (palmar adduction).

h. Hip

Hip—able to:

Extend the leg straight

Flex the knee to the chest

Abduct and adduct the leg

Rotate the hip internally and externally

Hyperextend the leg.

i. Knee

Knee—able to flex and extend the knee.

j. Ankles and feet

Ankles and feet—able to dorsiflex, plantar flex, evert, invert, abduct, and adduct the feet and ankles.

Key Point: *If a patient cannot move the limb, put the joint through passive ROM. Never force a joint against resistance or if it causes discomfort.*

(continued on next page)

Procedure 22-15 ■ Assessing the Musculoskeletal System (continued)

Joint Movements

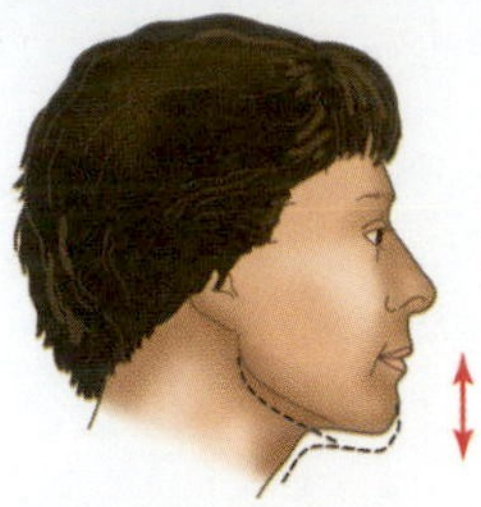

Depression: lowering a body part
Elevation: raising a body part

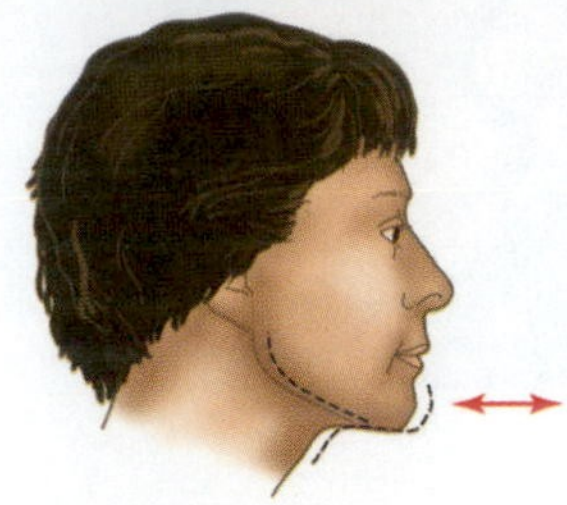

Retraction: moving backward
Protraction: moving forward

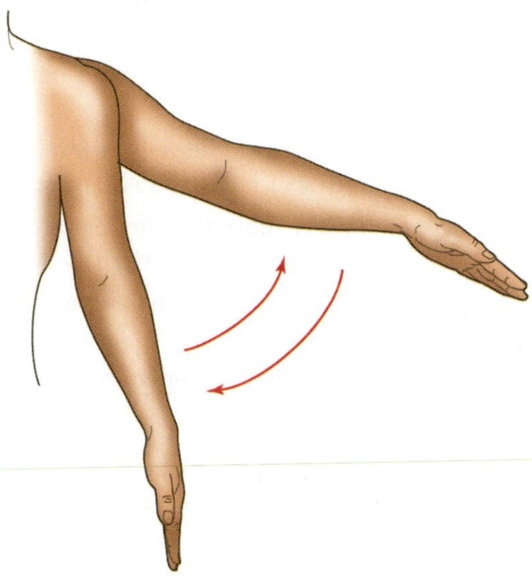

Abduction: moving away from midline
Adduction: moving toward midline

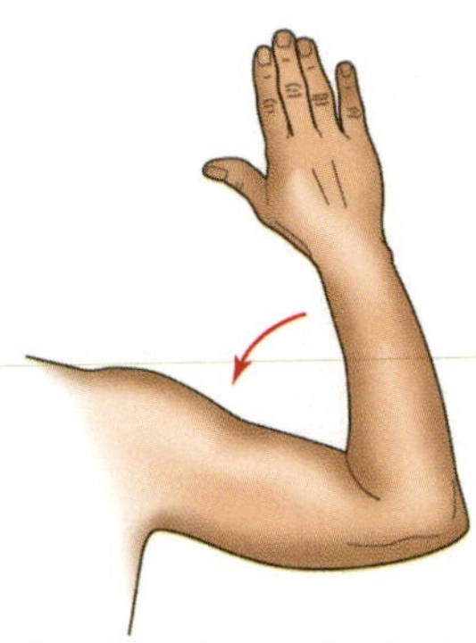

Flexion: bending, decreasing joint angle

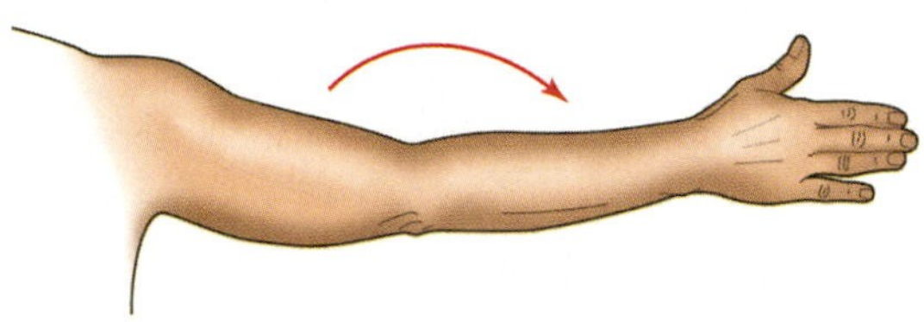

Extension: straightening, increasing joint angle

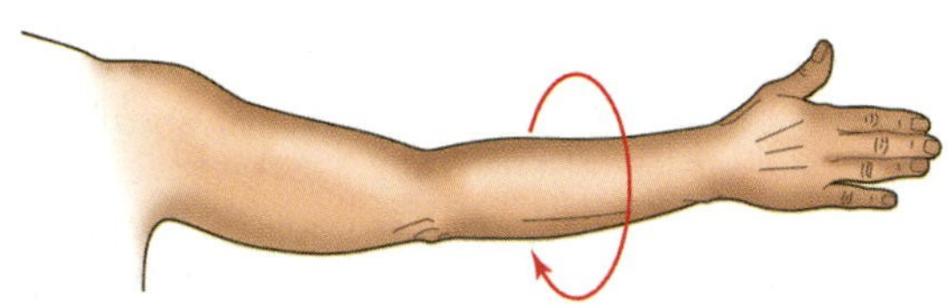

Circumduction: moving in a circular fashion

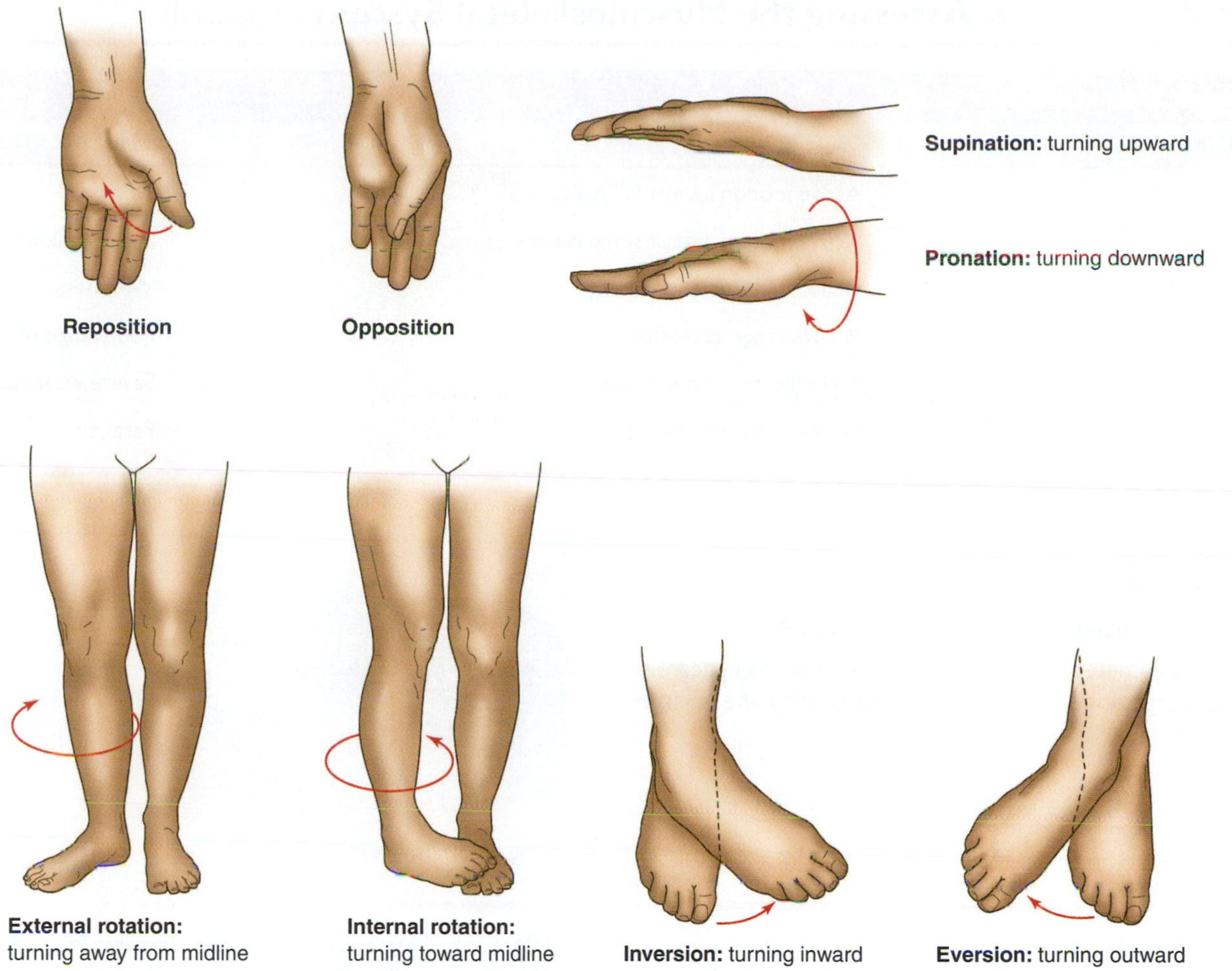

9. **Test muscle strength by repeating ROM against resistance.** Use the rating scale at the end of this step.
   a. **Test hand grip** by crossing your middle and index fingers and asking the patient to squeeze. (*Tip: If you are wearing rings, a strong hand grip on those fingers can be painful.)*
   b. **Test biceps strength.** Place one hand on the client's biceps and have the patient raise the forearm (flex the elbow) as you apply resistance at the wrist.
   c. **Test triceps strength** by having the client straighten the arm at the elbow (extend the elbow) as you apply resistance at the wrist.
   d. **Test leg strength** by having patient raise leg (straighten the knee) against your hand as you apply resistance.
   e. **Test ankle strength** by asking the patient to point the toes downward (plantar flexion) at the ankle while you apply resistance to the plantar surface of the foot.
   f. **Test ankle strength** by having the client point the toes toward the knee (dorsiflexion) as you apply resistance to the top of the foot.

Expected findings: Expect active motion against full resistance. There should be no crepitus (clicking) or pain with joint movement. ▼

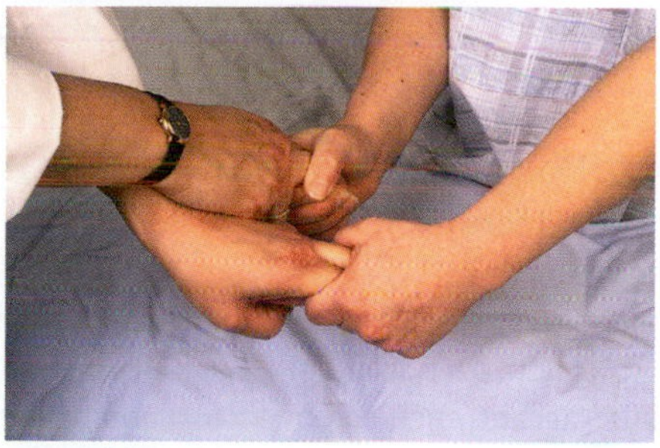

(continued on next page)

Procedure 22-15 ■ Assessing the Musculoskeletal System (continued)

Muscle Strength Rating Scale

RATING	CRITERIA	CLASSIFICATION
5	Active motion against full resistance	Normal
4	Active motion against some resistance	Slight weakness
3	Active motion against gravity	Weakness
2	Passive range of motion	Poor range of motion
1	Slight flicker of contraction	Severe weakness
0	No muscular contraction	Paralysis

? What if . . .

- **There is limited range of motion in a joint?**

  Use a goniometer to measure the limited motion in degrees. Place the goniometer over the joint, matching the angle of the joint.

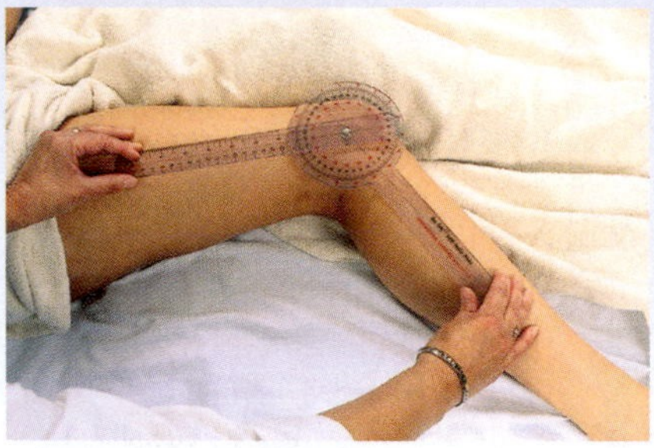

Using a goniometer

Documentation

If you need information about documenting your findings, review Caring for the Nguyens, and

Go to Chapter 22, **Documenting Physical Examination Findings (Nam Nguyen),** in Volume 1.

Procedure 22-16 ■ Assessing the Sensory–Neurological System

➤ For steps to follow in *all* procedures, refer to the Universal Steps for All Procedures found on the inside back cover.

➤ *Note:* This procedure provides guidelines for performing a comprehensive neurological exam. Steps 1 through 10 assess cognitive status, and the box at the end of the procedure contains questions that are useful for screening cognitive status.

Equipment

- Pen and record form
- Wisp of cotton
- Sharp object, such as a toothpick or sterile needle
- Objects to touch, such as a coin, button, or key
- Something fragrant, such as coffee or rubbing alcohol
- Something to taste, such as sugar, salt, or lemon
- Tongue blade
- Two test tubes
- Reflex hammer
- Ophthalmoscope

Developmental Modifications for Children

- For children younger than 5 years of age, use the Denver Developmental Screening Test II to assess neurological and motor functions.
- Check the child's ability to understand and follow instructions.

Developmental Modifications for Older Adults

You may need to perform the sensorineurological exam over several sessions. The full exam is lengthy, and older adults fatigue easily. If the client seems to be getting tired, stop the test and finish at a later time.

Focused History Questions

- Do you have any neurological ("nerve") problems?
- Have you ever had head trauma, loss of consciousness, dizziness, headaches, or seizures?
- Do you have memory problems, forgetfulness, or inability to concentrate?
- Have you noticed any changes in your ability to see, smell, taste, hear, feel, or maintain balance?
- Do you have any weakness, numbness, or paralysis?
- Do you have any problems performing activities of daily living (ADLs)?

- Do you have any problems walking?
- Do you have mood problems or depression?
- Do you use alcohol or drugs for nonmedical purposes? If so, how much, and how often?
- Have you ever been treated for neurological or psychiatric issues?
- Do you have a history of hypertension, diabetes, stroke, or circulation problems?

➤ When performing the procedure, always identify your patient according to agency policy, using two identifiers, and be attentive to standard precautions, hand hygiene, patient safety and privacy, body mechanics, and documentation.

Procedure Steps

1. Assess behavior. Note the client's facial expression, posture, affect, and grooming.

Findings

Expected findings: The client is well groomed, with an erect posture, pleasant facial expression, and appropriate affect.

Abnormal findings: Inappropriate behavior may result from neurological or psychological problems, as well as from a variety of medications, alcohol, and street drugs.

---

2. Determine level of arousal (LOA):

a. Note the client's response to ***verbal stimuli***.

b. If the client does not respond to verbal stimuli, try ***tactile stimulation***: Gently shake the client's shoulder. **Key Point:** *Clients who have hearing deficits lip-read to compensate. Catch the client's attention by combined auditory and visual stimuli (e.g., touch his hand).*

c. If the client does not respond to tactile stimuli, try ***painful stimuli***: Squeeze the trapezius muscle, rub the sternum, apply pressure on the mandible at the angle of the jaw, or apply pressure over the "moon" of the nail.

NOTE: Clients who respond to painful stimuli withdraw when pressure is applied.

The Glasgow Coma Scale and the FOUR Scale at the end of this procedure provide standard references for assessing LOA for a patient with head injury.

Expected findings: The patient is awake and alert and readily responds to verbal stimuli.

Abnormal findings: Lethargy, stupor, or coma may result from trauma, neurological disorder, hypoxia, or chemical substances

A changing level of arousal (along with forgetfulness, restlessness, or sudden quietness) is one of the earliest indicators of increased ICP, which can be life threatening.

---

3. Determine the level of orientation.

a. *Orientation to time:* Ask the client to state the year, date, and time of day.

b. *Orientation to place:* Ask the client to state where he is (i.e., city, state, where he lives).

c. *Orientation to person:* Ask the names of family members. Ask, "Do you know who I am?" If the client cannot answer these questions, ask him to state his name. *Self-identity remains intact the longest.*

Expected findings: The client is awake, alert (see step 2), and oriented to time, place, and person (AAO × 3).

a. **Expected findings:** Hospitalized patients commonly lose track of date and time of day, but they easily reorient. As a rule, they should at least know the year.

Abnormal findings: Older adults who become disoriented to time usually think it is an earlier date. If a client offers a bizarre time or futuristic date, consider psychiatric concerns as the cause of disorientation.

b. **Expected findings:** Interpret data carefully. In some situations (e.g., after an automobile accident away from home), the patient may know he is in the hospital but not know which hospital or which city.

c. **Expected findings:** Patient should know you are a healthcare worker, but not necessarily your name.

Developmental Variations

Older adults: The stress of an unfamiliar situation can create confusion in an older adult.

Abnormal findings: Disorientation may result from physical or psychological disorders. Bizarre responses are usually associated with psychiatric disorders.

(continued on next page)

Procedure 22-16 ■ Assessing the Sensory–Neurological System (continued)

4. Assess memory.

a. Assess *immediate memory* by asking the client to repeat a series of three numbers that you say slowly (e.g., 1, 5, 8). Gradually increase the length of the series until the client cannot repeat the series correctly. Record the length of the last correct series (e.g., "Successfully repeats a series of 7 numbers correctly.")

b. *Repeat the test,* beginning with a series of three numbers, but ask the client to repeat them back to you in reverse order.

c. Assess *recent memory* by naming three items (e.g., "mirror, truck," and "the letter X") and asking the client to recall them later during the exam. Alternatively, you can ask such questions as, "How did you get to the hospital? What did you have for breakfast?" However, you will need to verify the patient's answers.

d. Assess *remote memory* by asking the client his birth date or the date of a major historical event.

Developmental Modifications

Children Assess memory by using names of toys (e.g., truck, ball, puzzle), names of people in his family, or names of familiar cartoon characters.

Expected findings: Immediate, recent, and remote memory are intact. Average series recall is 5 to 8 numbers in sequence and 4 to 6 numbers in reverse order.

Developmental Variations

Children: Number of objects recalled is usually fewer than the child's age in years.

Older adults: Loss of immediate and recent memory is common; long-term memory is usually not impaired.

Abnormal findings: Memory problems may be benign or may signal underlying neurological problems. Temporary memory loss may occur after trauma.

---

5. Assess mathematical and calculation skills.

a. Have the client solve a simple mathematical problem, such as "3 + 3 = ?."

b. If he is able to solve that problem, present a more complex example, yet simple enough that regardless of math skills the client could still determine the appropriate response, such as, "If you have $3 and you buy an item for $2, how much money will you have left?"

c. To assess both calculation skills and attention span, ask the client to count backward from 100.

d. A more difficult test is to have the client perform serial threes or serial sevens. Ask him to begin at 100 and keep subtracting 3 (or 7).

Consider the person's language, education, and culture in deciding whether this test is appropriate for him.

Expected findings: Mathematical and calculation ability is appropriate for the patient's age, education level, and language ability. The average adult can solve simple mathematical problems and can complete serial sevens in about 90 seconds with 3 or fewer errors.

Abnormal findings: Inability to calculate at a level appropriate for age and educational level may indicate neurological impairment or developmental delay.

---

6. Assess general knowledge.

You can ask questions directly or work this into the overall interaction with the client.

NOTE: Ask the client how many days are in a week or months in a year.

Expected findings: Vocabulary and general knowledge are intact.

---

7. Evaluate thought processes. Assess throughout the exam. Notice attention span, logic of speech, ability to stay focused, and appropriateness of responses.

Expected findings: Thought processes are clear, client responds appropriately, and speech is coherent and logical.

Abnormal findings: Alteration in thought processes may be caused by physical disorders, such as dementia; psychiatric disorders, such as psychosis; or alcohol and drugs.

8. **Assess abstract thinking.** Ask the client to interpret a maxim (or saying), such as "A penny saved is a penny earned" or "A rolling stone gathers no moss."

Expected findings: Abstract thinking is intact.

Abnormal findings: Inability to think abstractly is associated with dementia, delirium, mental retardation, and psychoses.

Developmental Modifications

Children: The ability to think abstractly does not develop until the late school-age years or adolescence. To assess a child under age 12 years, ask the child to describe things that are like and unlike a named object (e.g., "Tell me something that is like a cup").

9. **Assess judgment.** Ask the client to respond to a hypothetical situation, such as, "If you were walking down the street and saw smoke and flame coming from a house, what would you do?"

Expected findings: Judgment is intact.

Abnormal findings: Impaired judgment may be associated with dementia, psychosis, or substance abuse.

10. **Assess communication ability**.

a. **Listen to the client's speech.** Note the rate, flow, choice of vocabulary, and enunciation.

Expected findings: Speech flows easily, and patient enunciates clearly. Vocabulary is consistent with the client's age, education, and language fluency.

Abnormal findings: Problems with flow (e.g., halting speech, stuttering, very rapid speech, slurred words) may be caused by language problems, nervousness, anxiety, or neurological problems.

b. **Test spontaneous speech:** Show the client a picture, and have him describe it.

Expected findings: Spontaneous speech is intact.

Abnormal findings: Impaired spontaneous speech is associated with cognitive impairment.

c. **Test motor speech** by having the client say "Do, re, mi, fa, so, la, ti, do." Assess ability to swallow. Observe for clarity of speech, facial mobility, drooling, and oral hypotonia. Ask the client to repeat a short phrase two or three times and observe for lack of coordination.

Expected findings: Motor speech is intact.

Abnormal findings: Impaired motor speech is associated with problems with CN XII or with coordination of speech muscles.

d. **Test automatic speech** by having the client recite the days of the week.

Expected findings: Automatic speech is intact.

Abnormal findings: Cognitive impairment or memory problems cause difficulty with automatic speech.

e. **Test sound recognition** by having the client identify a familiar sound, such as clapping hands.

Expected findings: Sound recognition is intact.

Abnormal findings: Temporal lobe problems may be the cause of impaired sound recognition.

f. **Test auditory–verbal comprehension** by asking the client to follow simple directions (e.g., "Point to your nose; rub your left elbow").

Expected findings: Auditory–verbal comprehension is intact.

Abnormal findings: Temporal lobe problems affect reception. Frontal lobe problems affect expression.

g. **Test visual recognition** by pointing to objects and asking the client to identify them.

Expected findings: Visual recognition is intact.

Abnormal findings: Impaired visual recognition indicates parieto-occipital lobe problems.

h. **Test visual–verbal comprehension** by having the client read a sentence and explain its meaning.

Expected findings: Visual–verbal comprehension is intact.

Abnormal findings: Impaired visual–verbal comprehension indicates cognitive impairment.

(continued on next page)

Procedure 22-16 ■ Assessing the Sensory–Neurological System (continued)

i. **Test writing** by having the client write his name and address.

Expected findings: Writing ability is intact.

j. **Test ability to copy figures** by having the client copy a circle, the letter "X," a square, a triangle, and a star.

Expected findings: The client is able to copy figures.

11. Test cranial nerve I—olfactory nerve.

NOTE: You can assess CN I with your examination of the nose and sinuses (see Procedure 22-8).

a. Before testing, check the patency of the nostrils by gently occluding each nostril and having the client sniff.
b. Have the client occlude one nostril, hold an aromatic substance (e.g., lemon, coffee, vanilla, alcohol) under the nostril, and have the client identify the substance.
c. Repeat with a different substance under the other nostril. ▼

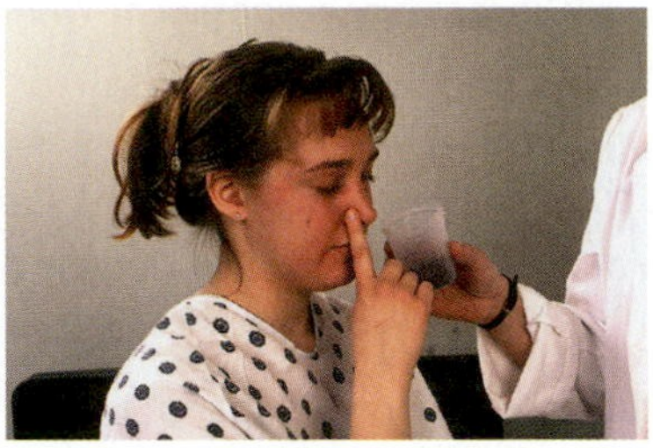

Developmental Modifications

Children: Select a substance that you are certain the child is familiar with (e.g., bananas or apples).

Expected findings: The client can identify the substances.

Developmental Variations

Older adults—may have a decreased sense of smell.

Abnormal findings: Anosmia is the loss of the sense of smell. It may be genetic, related to chronic nose or sinus problems, heavy tobacco use, snorting cocaine, or zinc deficiency.

12. Test cranial nerve II—optic nerve.

NOTE: You can assess CN II with your examination of the eyes (see Procedure 22-6).

a. Test visual acuity by asking the client to identify the smallest print readable on the Snellen chart.

Expected findings: Visual acuity is 20/20 in the right eye, left eye, and both eyes.

Abnormal findings: Many visual deficits are correctable with eyeglasses or contact lenses. They are not necessarily caused by optic nerve damage.

Developmental Modifications

Use picture chart for small children and the Snellen E chart for school-age children.

b. Identify visual field by having the client describe the boundaries of the visual field while her eye is in a fixed position.

Expected findings: Peripheral vision range is approximately 50° in the superior field, 70° in the inferior field, 60° in the nasal field, and 90 to 110° in the temporal field.

c. Perform a funduscopic exam. (See Procedure 22-6.)

Expected findings: Disk margins are sharply demarcated. The cup is half the size of the disk or less.

Abnormal findings: CN II deficits may be caused by a tumor or a cerebrovascular accident (CVA).

13. Test cranial nerves III, IV, and VI—oculomotor, trochlear, and abducens nerves.

a. Test EOMs by having the client move the eyes through the six cardinal fields of gaze while holding her head steady. ▼

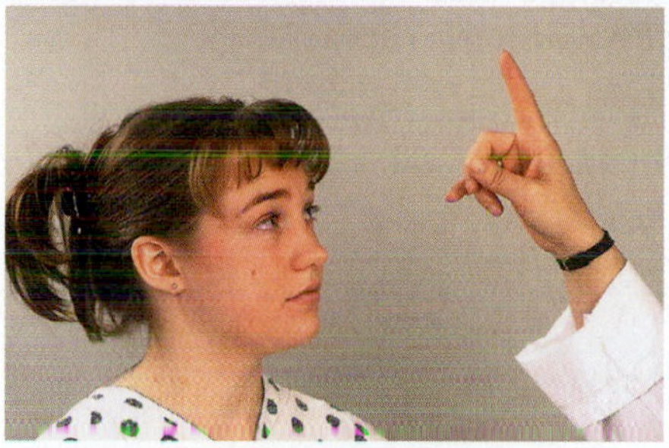

b. Test pupillary reaction to light and accommodation.

NOTE: See Procedure 22-6 for further details on each of these tests.

Expected findings: Client can move the eyes through the six cardinal fields of gaze. Pupils are equal in size and react to light and accommodation.

Abnormal findings: Changes in ICP may affect EOMs and pupillary reaction.

---

14. Test cranial nerve V—trigeminal nerve.

a. **Test motor function** by having the client move her jaw from side to side, clenching the jaw, and biting down on a tongue blade.

NOTE: You can assess this function in your examination of the mouth and oropharynx (see Procedure 22-9).

b. **Test sensory function** by having the client close her eyes and identify when you are touching her face at the forehead, cheeks, and chin bilaterally—first with your finger and then with a toothpick.

c. **Test the corneal reflex** by touching the cornea with a wisp of cotton or puffing air from a syringe over the cornea.

The corneal reflex is not usually tested on a conscious person because the procedure is unpleasant and a corneal abrasion can occur. A conscious person can blink intentionally, so there is no need to stimulate the blink.

NOTE: You can assess the corneal reflex in your examination of the eyes (see Procedure 22-6).

Expected findings: The client is able to perform all motor functions and can perceive light touch and superficial pain bilaterally; corneal reflex is intact.

Abnormal findings: Inability to perceive light touch and superficial pain may indicate peripheral nerve damage. An absent corneal reflex is an ominous neurological sign.

---

15. Test cranial nerve VII—facial nerve.

a. Test motor function by having the client make faces, such as smile, frown, or whistle.

NOTE: You can assess this function in your examination of the head and face (see Procedure 22-5).

b. Test taste on the anterior portion of the tongue by placing sweet (sugar), salty (salt), or sour (lemon) substance on the tip of the tongue. Do not use pungent, bitter, or markedly unpleasant flavors.

NOTE: You can assess this function in your examination of the mouth and oropharynx (see Procedure 22-9).

Expected findings: The client is able to perform all movements and can distinguish sweet, salty, and sour tastes.

Developmental Variations

Older adults—Have decreased taste sensation, especially sweet and salty, due to taste bud atrophy and diminished sense of smell.

Abnormal findings: Asymmetrical movement may be seen with nerve damage from a CVA or Bell's palsy. Impaired taste may be associated with nerve damage, chemotherapy, or radiation to the face or neck.

(continued on next page)

Procedure 22-16 ■ Assessing the Sensory–Neurological System (continued)

16. Test cranial nerve VIII—acoustic nerve.

NOTE: You can assess this function in your examination of the ears (see Procedure 22-7).

a. Perform watch-tick test for hearing by holding a watch close to the client's ear.
b. Perform the Weber and Rinne tests to assess air and bone conduction.
c. Test balance with the Romberg test, if it has not already been performed.

See Procedures 22-7 and 22-15 for further details on these tests.

Developmental Modifications

Children: The Romberg test is appropriate only after age 3 years.

Expected findings: Hearing is intact. The Romberg test is negative.

Abnormal findings: Hearing loss, loss of balance, or vertigo may result from acoustic nerve damage.

17. Test cranial nerves IX and X—glossopharyngeal and vagus nerves.

a. Observe ability to talk, swallow, and cough.
b. Test motor function by asking the client to say "ah" while you depress a tongue blade and observe the soft palate and uvula.
c. Test sensory function by taking a tongue blade and gently touching the back of the pharynx to induce the gag reflex.
d. Test taste (sweet, salty, and sour) on the posterior portion of the tongue. Avoid bitter or repulsive tasting substances.

Expected findings: Swallow and cough reflexes are intact. Speech is clear. The uvula and soft palate rise symmetrically, and the gag reflex is intact. Taste on the posterior tongue is intact.

Developmental Variations

Older adults—have decreased taste sensation, especially sweet and salty, as a result of atrophy of the taste buds and a diminished sense of smell.

Abnormal findings: Damage to CNs IX and X impairs swallowing. Damage to CN X changes voice quality.

18. Test cranial nerve XI—accessory nerve.

NOTE: You can assess this motor nerve function with your examination of the musculoskeletal system (see Procedure 22-15).

a. Place your hands on the client's shoulder, and have her shrug the shoulders against resistance.
b. Have the client turn her head from side to side against resistance.

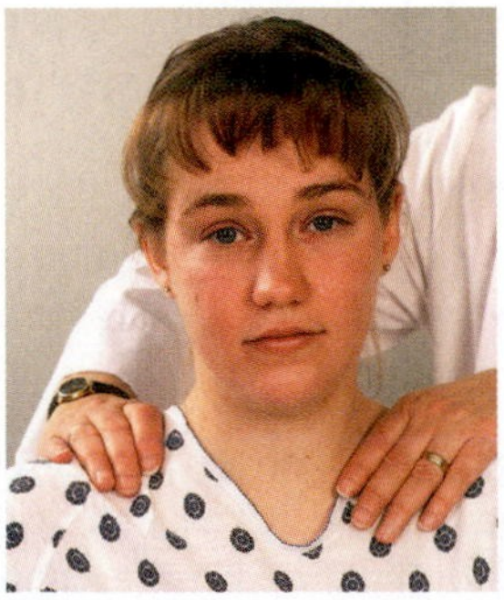

Expected findings: Movement is symmetrical and pain-free. Full ROM of the neck with +5 strength.

Abnormal findings: Asymmetrical movement, pain, or absent movement indicates CN XI disorders.

19. Test cranial nerve XII—hypoglossal nerve.

a. Ask the client to say "d, l, n, t."
b. Have the client protrude the tongue and move it from side to side.

Expected findings: The client can articulate the sounds and move the tongue easily.

Abnormal findings: Tongue paralysis

20. Test superficial sensations.

- Begin with the most peripheral part when testing the limbs (e.g., test the foot before the leg). ➤
  If the client can feel sensation in the most peripheral part, you can assume the sensory nerve is intact to that point.
- If the client does not perceive the touch in an area, determine the boundaries of the dysfunction by testing at about every inch (2.5 cm). Sketch the area of sensory loss.
- Wait about 2 seconds before moving to each site.
  Wait so that you can be sure that the patient is perceiving each stimulus separately.

a. *Light touch:* With the patient's eyes closed, brush a cotton wisp on various areas of the body, comparing sides. Ask the client to say, "Now," when she feels your touch and to point to the spot you are touching.

b. *Pain:* Have the patient close her eyes; use a toothpick (or sterile needle) with dull and sharp ends, and touch various areas of her body (except the face). Have the patient identify whether the sensation is dull or sharp. Alternate the dull and sharp ends as you move from spot to spot. Compare both sides of the body.

c. *Temperature sensation:* Test only if the patient's perception of pain is abnormal. Use test tubes filled with hot and cold water. Touch the tube to various areas of the body, comparing sides; have the client say "Hot," "Cold," or "Don't know."
If pain sensation is intact, temperature will be, too, because sensations for pain and temperature are transmitted along the same tracts.

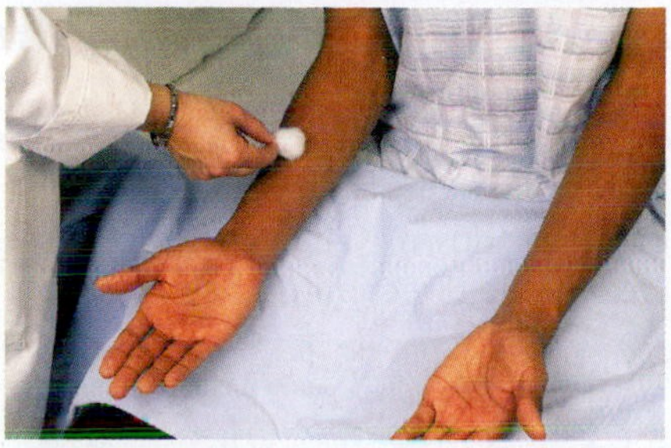

Testing light touch

a. **Expected findings:** Able to identify areas of light touch.

Abnormal findings: Diminished sensation or areas of absent perception

b. **Expected findings:** The client is able to identify the areas stimulated and the type of sensation.

Abnormal findings:

- Hyperalgia—increased pain sensation
- ***Analgesia***—no pain sensation
- Paresthesia—numbness and tingling

Developmental Variations

Older adults—may have a decreased perception of temperature and deep pain.

21. Test deep sensations.

Assess vibratory sensation by placing a vibrating tuning fork on a metatarsal joint and distal interphalangeal joint. Have the patient identify when he feels the vibration and when it stops. ▼

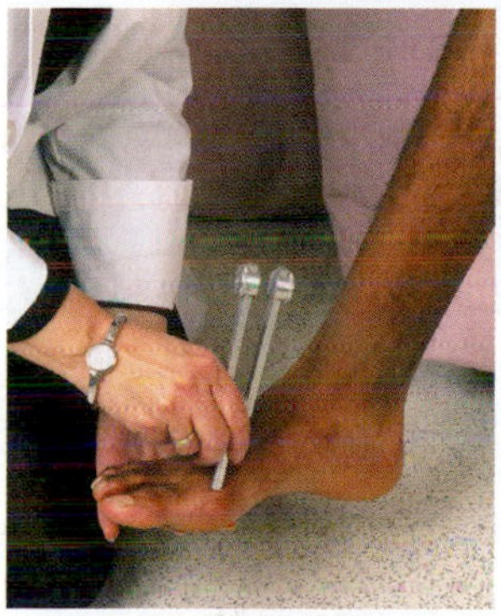

Expected findings: Vibratory sense is intact bilaterally in the upper and lower extremities.

Abnormal findings: Diminished or absent vibration sense is seen with peripheral nerve damage from vascular disease, diabetes, alcoholism, or damage to the posterior column of the spinal cord.

(continued on next page)

Procedure 22-16 ■ Assessing the Sensory–Neurological System (continued)

22. Test kinesthetic sensation (position sense). By holding the client's finger or toe on the sides and moving it up or down. Keeping his eyes closed, have the client identify the direction of the movement.

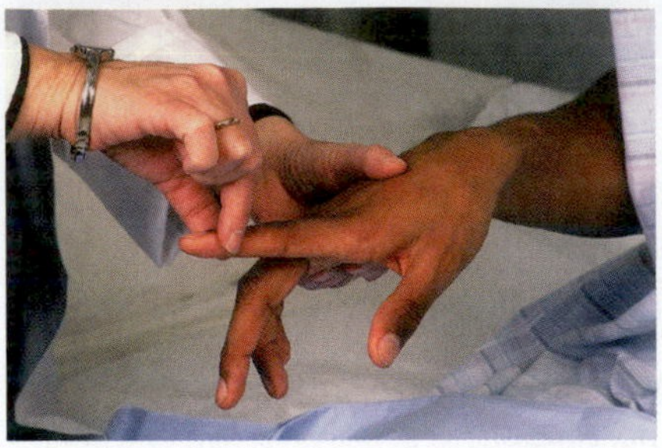

Expected findings: Position sense is intact bilaterally in the upper and lower extremities.

Developmental Variations

Older adults—may lose position sense in the great toes.

Abnormal findings: Diminished or absent position sense indicates nerve or spinal cord damage.

23. Test discriminatory sensations.

a. *Assess stereognosis* by placing a familiar object (e.g., a coin or a button) in the palm of the client's hand and having him identify it.
b. *Assess graphesthesia* by drawing a number or letter in the palm of your patient's hand and having him identify what was drawn.
c. *Test two-point discrimination* with toothpicks. Have the patient close his eyes. Touch him on the finger with two toothpicks simultaneously. Gradually move the points together, and have the patient say, "One," or "Two," each time you move the toothpicks. Document distance and location at which he can no longer feel two separate points.

a. **Expected findings:** ***Stereognosis*** (the ability to recognize the form of solid objects by touch) is intact bilaterally.

b. **Expected findings:** ***Graphesthesia*** (the ability to recognize outlines, numbers, or symbols written on the skin) is intact bilaterally.

c. **Expected findings:** ***Point discrimination*** (recognizing being touched in one area or two areas of the skin). Discriminates between two points on fingertips no > 0.5 cm apart.

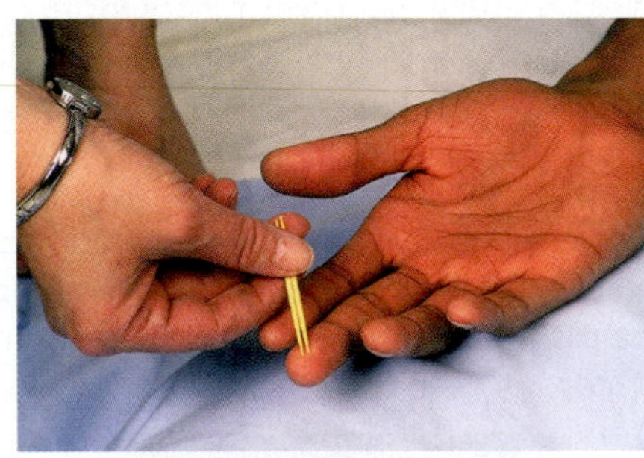

d. *Test point localization* by having the patient close the eyes while you touch him. Have the patient point to the area you touched. Repeat on both sides and the upper and lower extremities.
e. *Test sensory extinction* by simultaneously touching the patient on both sides (e.g., on both hands, both knees, both arms). Have him identify where he was touched.

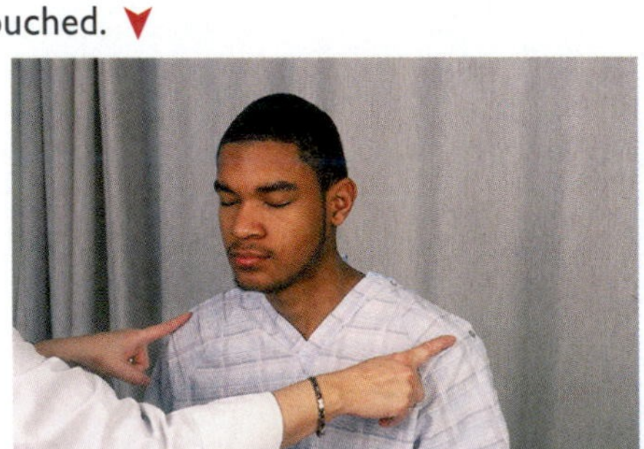

Developmental Modifications

Older adults—may need more time to respond to a stimulus, as reaction time may be slower.

d. **Expected findings:** ***Point localization*** (the ability to identify where one is being touched) is intact bilaterally in the upper and lower extremities.

e. **Expected findings:** Extinction is intact: Client should feel the sensation on both sides of the body.

Abnormal findings: Abnormalities in any of the discriminatory sensation tests may indicate a lesion or disorder of the sensory cortex or disorder of the posterior column of the spinal cord.

Developmental Variations

Older adults: Reflex responses may not be as strong as in young adults. Reaction time is slower as well.

24. Test deep tendon reflexes.

Use the accompanying scale to grade responses.

Deep Tendon Reflex Grading Scale

0	No response detected
+1	Diminished response
+2	Response normal
+3	Response somewhat stronger than normal
+4	Response hyperactive with ***clonus*** (involuntary contractions that continue after the first contraction is elicited by the hammer)

a. ***Biceps reflex*** (spinal cord level C5 and C6). Rest the patient's elbow in your nondominant hand, with your thumb over the biceps tendon. Strike the percussion hammer to your thumb.

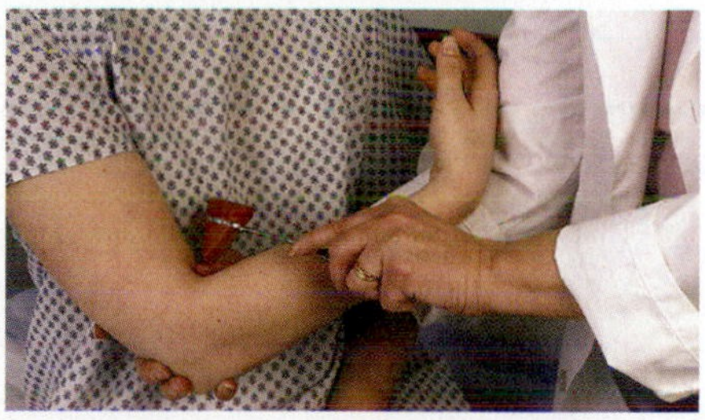

a. **Expected findings:** +2 response: You can feel the biceps contract with your thumb; slight flexion of the elbow.

b. ***Triceps reflex*** (spinal cord level C7 and C8). Abduct the patient's arm at the shoulder, and flex it at the elbow. Support the upper arm with your nondominant hand, letting the forearm hang loosely. Strike the triceps tendon about 2.5 to 5 cm (1–2 in.) above the olecranon process.

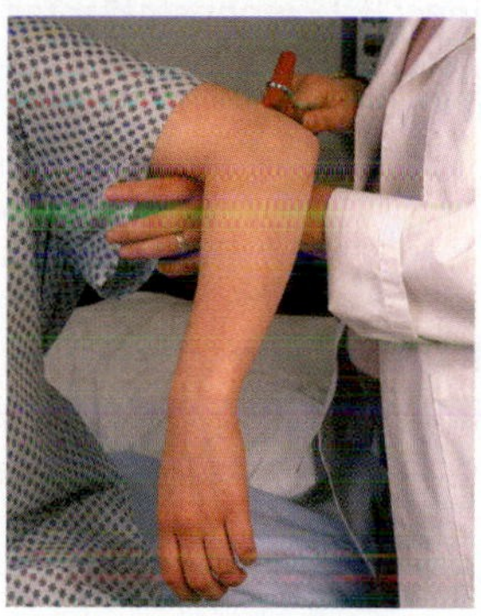

b. **Expected findings:** +2 response: Contraction of triceps with slight extension at elbow.

(continued on next page)

Procedure 22-16 ■ Assessing the Sensory–Neurological System (continued)

c. *Brachioradialis reflex* (spinal cord level C3 and C6). Rest the client's arm on her leg. Strike with the percussion hammer 2.5 to 5 cm (1–2 in.) above the bony prominence of the wrist on the thumb side. ▼

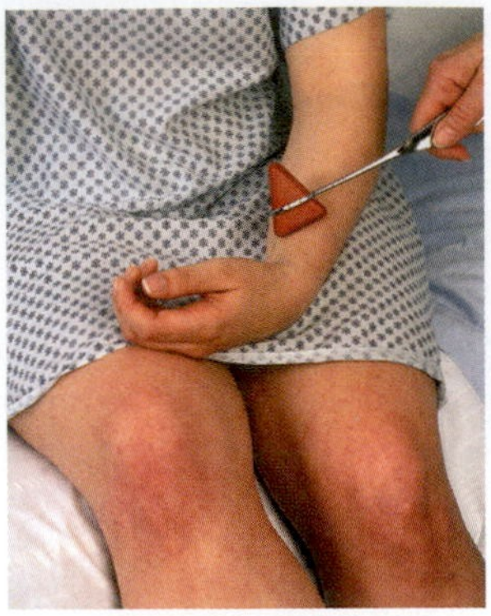

c. **Expected findings:** +2 response: Flexion at elbow and supination of forearm

d. *Patellar reflex* (spinal cord level L2, L3, and L4). Have the client sit with legs dangling. Strike the tendon directly below the patella. ▼

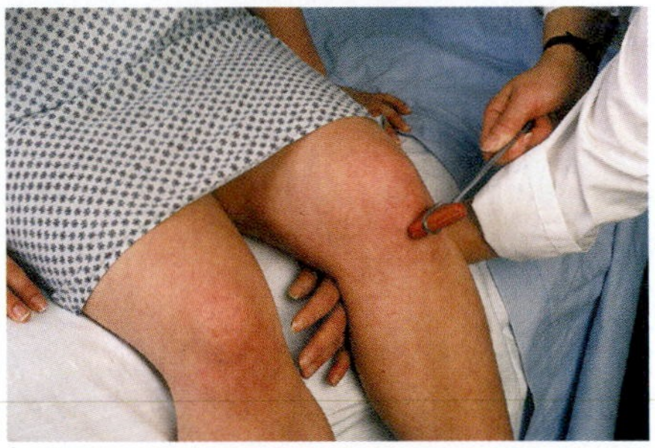

d. **Expected findings:** +2 response: Contraction of quadriceps with extension of leg

e. *Achilles' reflex* (spinal cord level S1, S2). Have the patient lie supine or sit with legs dangling. Hold the patient's foot slightly dorsiflexed, and strike the Achilles' tendon about 5 cm (2 in.) above the heel with the percussion hammer. ▼

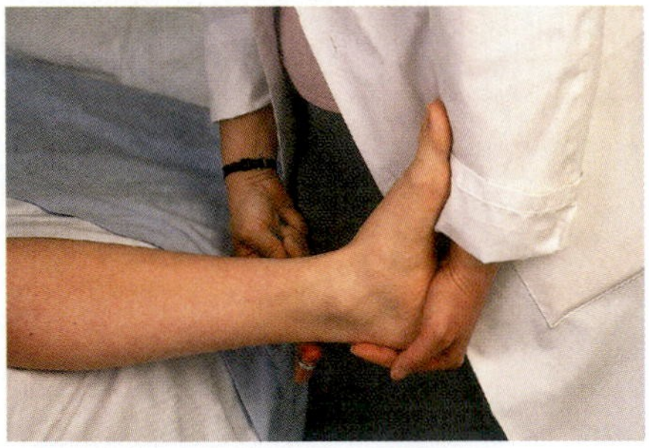

e. **Expected findings:** +2 response: Plantar flexion of foot.

Developmental Variations

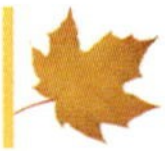

Older adults—may lose this reflex.

Abnormal findings:

- Absent or diminished responses are seen with degenerative disease, nerve damage, or lower motor neuron disease.
- Hyperactive reflexes are seen with spinal cord injuries and upper motor neuron disease.
- Rooting, palmar grasp, and tonic neck reflexes present after age 6 months.

Developmental Modifications

Newborns: Test the following reflexes:

- ***Rooting reflex:*** Stroke the cheek; the head should turn to the side you touched.
- ***Palmar grasp:*** PLACE one finger in the baby's hand; the baby's fingers should curl around your finger.
- ***Tonic neck reflex:*** Position the baby supine; turn his head to one side. The arm and leg on that side should extend, and those on the other side will flex.

25. Test superficial reflexes.
Plantar reflex (Babinski response): With your thumbnail or pointed object, stroke the sole of the client's foot in an arc from the lateral heel to medially across the ball of the foot. Record response as negative (normal) or positive (abnormal).

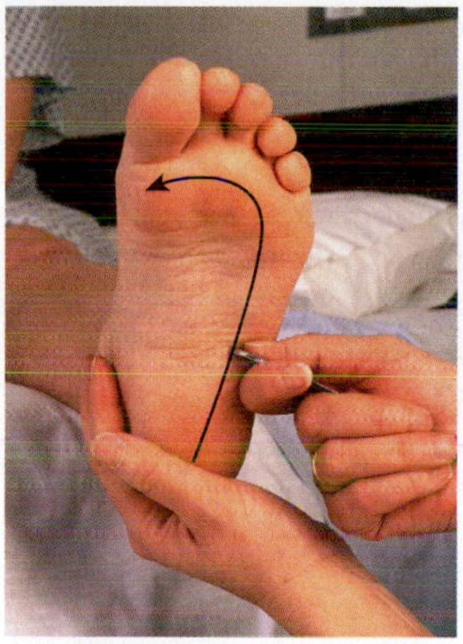

Developmental Modifications

Older adults: This reflex may be difficult to elicit.

Expected findings: Babinski response is negative. All the toes curl downward or there is no response.

Developmental Variations

Infants and children: Positive Babinski is normal until age 2 years or until the child begins walking.

Abnormal findings: A positive Babinski response: dorsiflexion of the great toe and fanning of the other toes. Seen with drug or alcohol intoxication or upper motor neuron disease.

26. Mental status screening.
The following questions may be used for a rapid evaluation of cognitive status. You may have already assessed for some aspects of mental status (e.g., orientation to time).

Questions for Evaluating Cognitive Status

This complete set of questions is included so that you can use them for a mental status exam that is not part of a comprehensive assessment. In a comprehensive assessment, do not repeat questions you have already covered in other portions of the assessment.

QUESTION	FUNCTION ASSESSED
What is today's date?	Orientation to time
What time is it?	Orientation to time
Where are you?	Orientation to place
What is the reason for your visit? (If the patient is hospitalized, modify the question as: Why are you in the hospital?)	Communication, vocabulary, thought processes, recent memory
Ask the patient to count backward from 100.	Word comprehension, abstract reasoning
Ask the patient to name several objects that you point to. Be sure to use common objects, such as a pen, shoe, or window.	Vocabulary, general knowledge, and word comprehension
Write a brief command, such as "Clap your hands," on a slip of paper. Hand the paper to the patient and ask him to follow the instructions.	Reading comprehension
Ask the patient to write the names of his family members, along with their relationship to him.	Writing, thought processes, memory, sound recognition
Ask the patient to name three things that begin with the letter D.	Auditory comprehension, thought processes
Ask the patient to draw a circle, a square, and a triangle next to each other on a sheet of paper.	Word comprehension, mathematical and calculation skills, communication (naming
Difficulty with any of these questions requires further evaluation.	

(continued on next page)

Procedure 22-16 ■ Assessing the Sensory–Neurological System (continued)

? What if . . .

■ **The patient is an older adult?**

For a mental-status exam for older adults, you may wish to use the following sites:

The Mini-Cog (mental status assessment of older adults)

https://mini-cog.com

Mini-Mental State Examination

https://www.ihpa.gov.au/what-we-do/standardised-mini-mental-state-examination-smmse

You should also assess older adults for dementia, which is characterized by these four features:

- Mental status change of sudden onset, or fluctuating course
- Difficulty focusing attention, distractible
- Disorganized, illogical thinking
- Increased or decreased level of consciousness (e.g., hyperalert, lethargic)

  Delirium occurs in 15% to 60% of older hospitalized patients. You should assess them frequently to facilitate prompt identification and management of delirium.

  For a reliable tool for assessing confusion and dementia in older adults, go to the following Web site or search in your browser for the Confusion Assessment Method Instrument: https://consultgeri.org/try-this/general-assessment/issue-13.pdf

Home Care

Instruct caregivers in home safety if the client has cerebral function deficits or sensory or motor deficits.

Documentation

If you need more information about documenting, review Caring for the Nguyens, and

Go to Chapter 22, **Documenting Physical Examination Findings (Nam Nguyen)**, in Volume 1.

Glasgow Coma Scale

EYE RESPONSE	SCORE	MOTOR RESPONSE	SCORE	VERBAL RESPONSE	SCORE
Opens spontaneously	4	Obeys verbal commands for movement	6	Oriented and converses	5
Opens to verbal commands	3	Reacts purposefully to localized pain	5	Disoriented but converses	4
Opens to pain	2	Withdraws in response to pain (generalized body response)	4	Uses inappropriate words	3
No response	1	Assumes flexor posture (decorticate posturing—arms flexed to chest, hands clenched and internally rotated) in response to pain. Indicates problem is at or above the brainstem	3	Makes incomprehensible sounds	2
		Assumes extensor posture (decerebrate posturing—arms extended, hands clenched and hyperpronated). Indicates problem at the brainstem level	2	No response	1
		No response	1		
Totals	___		___		___

Full Outline of UnResponsiveness (FOUR)

Eye Response

4—Eyelids open or opened, tracking, or blinking on command

3—Eyelids open, but not tracking

2—Eyelids closed, but open to loud voice

1—Eyelids closed, but open to pain

0—Eyelids remain closed with pain

Motor Response

4—Thumbs-up, fist, or peace sign

3—Localizing to pain

2—Flexion response to pain

1—Extension response to pain

0—No response to pain or generalized myoclonus status

Brainstem Reflexes

4—Pupil and corneal reflexes present

3—One pupil wide and fixed

2—Pupil or corneal reflexes absent

1—Pupil and corneal reflexes absent

0—Absent pupil, corneal, and cough reflexes

Respirations

4—Not intubated, regular breathing pattern

3—Not intubated, Cheyne-Stokes breathing pattern

2—Not intubated, irregular breathing

1—Respirations greater than ventilator rate

0—respirations at ventilator rate or apnea

Note: Education is necessary to use this scale properly.

To see how to use it,

Go to Mayo Clinic Proceedings, Wolf, Wijdicks, Bamlet, et al., 2007. Further validation of the FOUR Score Coma Scale by intensive care nurses, figure 1, is found at http://www.ncbi.nlm.nih.gov/pmc/articles/PMC2719522/

Sources: Hanrahan, K., Wagner, M., Matthews, et al. (2015). Sacred cow gone to pasture: a systematic evaluation and integration of evidence_based practice. *Worldviews on Evidence_Based Nursing, 12*(1), 3–11.; Okasha, A. S., Fayed, A. M., & Saleh, A. S. (2014). The FOUR Score predicts mortality, endotracheal intubation and ICU length of stay after traumatic brain injury. *Neurocritical Care, 21*(3), 496–504; Wijdicks, E. F., Kramer, A. A., Rohs, T., Jr., et al. (2015). Comparison of the Full Outline of UnResponsiveness Score and the Glasgow Coma Scale in predicting mortality in critically ill patients. *Critical Care Medicine, 43*(2), 439–444.

Procedure 22-17 ■ Assessing the Male Genitourinary System

➤ For steps to follow in *all* procedures, refer to the Universal Steps for All Procedures found on the inside back cover.

Equipment

- Nonlatex procedure gloves
- Penlight
- Pen and record form

Developmental Modifications for Children

- Obtain parental permission to perform this assessment.
- Explain to the child what you are going to do, and expect some resistance or embarrassment.
  Children are taught to not let strangers touch their genitals, and many children are modest.

Developmental Modifications for Older Adults

- Assess for incontinence.
  Incontinence is one of the elements of the SPICES assessment model for older adults.

Focused History Questions

- Have you noticed any redness, swelling, discharge, or odor in your genital area?
- Have you noticed asymmetry, lumps, or masses in your genitals? If so, describe them, and show me where they are.
- Have you ever been told you have a hernia?
- Have you ever had trauma to your genitals?
- Are you having any problems urinating?
- Are you sexually active? If not, have you ever been?
- Do you have sex with men, women, or both?
- What types of sexual activity do you engage in? Oral, anal, genital?
- Do you have more than one partner? How many partners have you had in the past 6 months?
- Do you use birth control? If so, what type, and how often?
- Have you ever been treated for a sexually transmitted infection (STI)? If so, what type?
- Are you concerned about STIs or HIV infection?
- Do you take any precautions to avoid infections?

(continued on next page)

Procedure 22-17 ■ Assessing the Male Genitourinary System (continued)

- Do you have any concerns about your sexual function?
- Do you have any difficulty achieving or maintaining an erection?
- Have you been taught to examine your testicles?
  In spite of the low prevalence of testicular cancer, men should be aware that a lump in the testicle and/or a feeling of heaviness or swelling in the scrotum could be a sign of testicular cancer and should report these findings to his healthcare provider immediately (American Cancer Society, n.d.a).
- How often do you do testicular self-examination?
- Have you had any surgery of your reproductive tract?

➤ When performing the procedure, always identify your patient according to agency policy, using two identifiers, and be attentive to standard precautions, hand hygiene, patient safety and privacy, body mechanics, and documentation.

Procedure Steps / Findings

1. Instruct the client to empty his bladder and undress to expose the groin area.

2. Have the patient stand while you sit at eye level to the genitalia; alternatively, the patient can lie supine on the exam table with his legs slightly apart.

3. Inspect the external genitalia.

a. ***Hair*.** Note the hair distribution pattern and condition of pubic hair. See the table discussing Tanner's staging, at the end of this procedure.
The appearance of the external genitalia depends on the client's developmental stage.

Expected findings: Hair distribution is triangular and appropriate for age. No pediculosis is present.

Abnormal findings: Sparse or absent hair may result from genetic factors, aging, or local or systemic disease.

b. ***Skin*:** Inspect the condition of the skin of the penis. Observe for the presence or absence of the foreskin. Note the position of the urethral meatus and any lesions or discharge.

Expected findings: Skin is intact with no lesions or discharge. Color is consistent with ethnicity. The urethral meatus is midline. The foreskin may be absent (circumcised); if present, it covers the glans and easily retracts.

Developmental Variations

Infants: Foreskin is difficult to retract in the uncircumcised male until about age 3 months.

Older adults: Penis and testes decrease in size.

Abnormal findings: Ulcerations or lesions (may be seen with a number of STIs, such as genital warts and genital herpes); ***phimosis*** (foreskin cannot be retracted and becomes swollen).

c. ***Scrotum*:** Observe the condition, size, position, and symmetry of the scrotal sacs.

Expected findings: The skin should be free of lesions, nodules, swelling, rash, and erythema. The skin is rugated and deeper in color than the rest of the body. Size and shape vary greatly. The left scrotal sac is usually lower than the right.

Abnormal findings:
- A rash may be caused by ***tinea cruris,*** a fungal infection often called "jock itch."
- Swelling may indicate hernia, tumor, or infection.

d. ***Inguinal area***: Note the condition of the inguinal areas. Look for swelling or bulges. The best way to do this is to have the client bear down while you palpate the inguinal canal.

Expected findings: The inguinal area should be free of swelling or bulges.

Abnormal findings: A bulge may indicate a hernia or enlarged lymph node.

Abnormalities: Male Genitourinary System

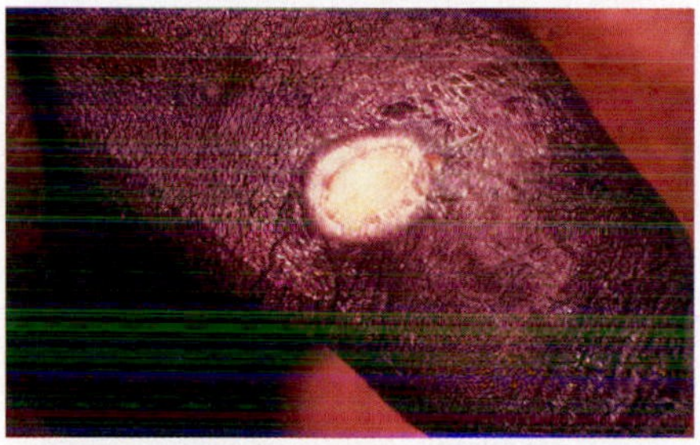

Syphilitic chancre

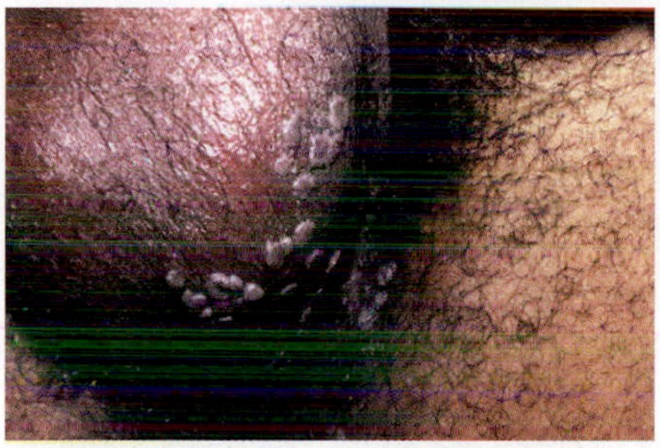

Genital warts

4. Palpate the penis.

a. With a gloved hand, use your thumb and fingers to palpate the shaft of the penis. Note consistency, tenderness, masses, or nodules.
b. Retract the foreskin, if present.

Expected findings: The penis is nontender with no masses or nodules. Pulsations are present on the dorsal side. The foreskin, if present, easily retracts.

Abnormal findings:

- Inability to palpate a pulse may indicate vascular insufficiency.
- Difficulty retracting the foreskin or problems with its return to position need further evaluation.

5. Palpate the scrotum, testes, and epididymis.

a. Don a procedure glove, and use your thumb and fingers to palpate. ▼

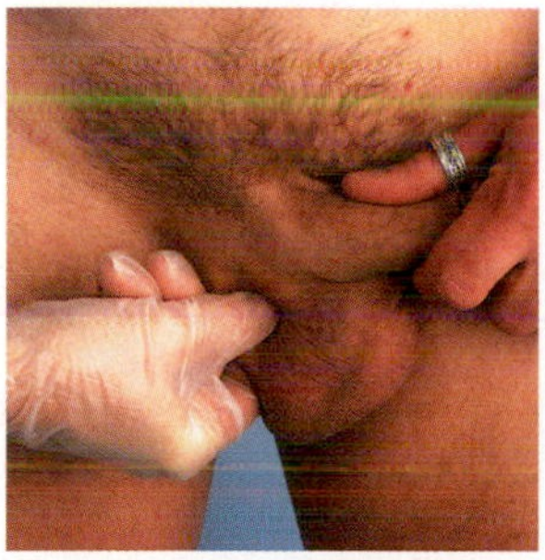

b. Note size, shape, consistency, mobility, masses, nodules, or tenderness.
c. Transilluminate any lumps, nodules, or edematous areas by shining a penlight over the area in a darkened room. ▼

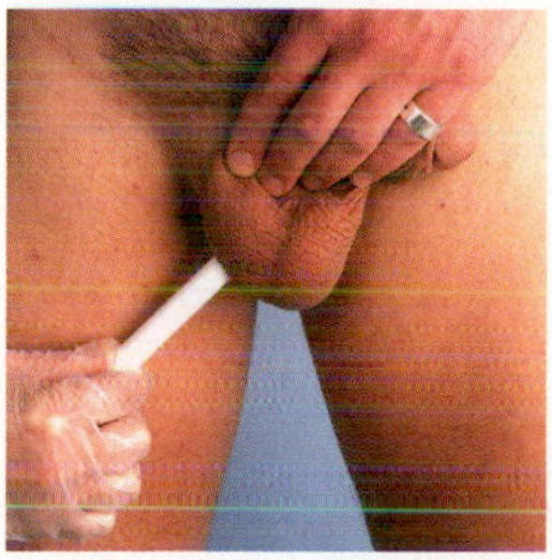

Expected findings:

- The scrotal skin is rough but without lesions.
- Each testicular sac contains a testicle and epididymis.
- The testes are rubbery, round, movable, and smooth. They are sensitive to pressure but nontender.
- The epididymis is comma shaped.
- The spermatic cord is smooth and round.
- There is no swelling or nodules.
- The left scrotal sac is usually lower than the right.

Abnormal findings:

- A unilateral mass
- Painless intratesticular masses may represent testicular cancer.
- A testicle that is swollen or tender may indicate infection or torsion.

(continued on next page)

Procedure 22-17 ■ Assessing the Male Genitourinary System (continued)

6. Palpate the inguinal and femoral area for hernias.

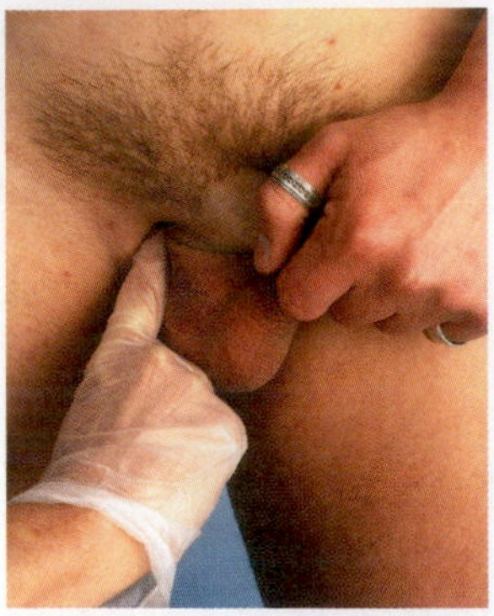

a. Assess for inguinal hernias with a gloved hand. Have the patient hold his penis to one side. Place your index finger in the client's scrotal sac above the testicle, and invaginate the skin. Follow the spermatic cord until you reach a slitlike opening (Hesselbach's triangle). Ask the client to cough or bear down as you feel for bulges.
b. Palpate for femoral hernias by palpating below the femoral artery while having the client cough or bear down.

Expected findings: No bulges or palpable masses are present in the inguinal or femoral area.

Abnormal findings: A bulge or mass often represents a hernia.

Direct hernia—protrusion through the abdominal wall

Indirect hernia—protrusion into the inguinal canal or into the scrotum

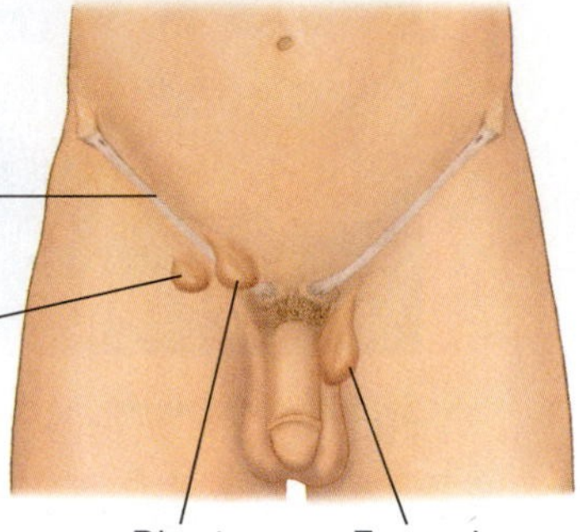

Locations of direct and indirect hernias

7. Palpate the lymph nodes in the groin area and the vertical chain over the inner aspect of the thigh.

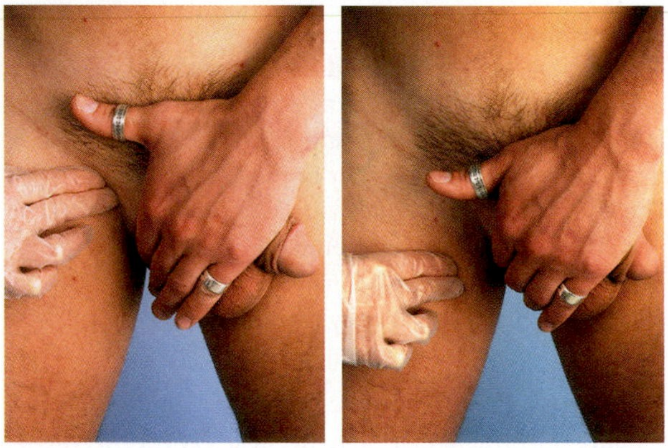

Expected findings: Nodes should be < 1 cm in size and freely mobile.

Abnormal findings: Enlarged or tender lymph nodes may indicate local or systemic disease.

Documentation

If you need more information about documenting your findings, review Caring for the Nguyens, and

Go to Chapter 22, **Documenting Physical Examination Findings (Nam Nguyen),** in Volume 1.

Tanner Staging

STAGE	PUBIC HAIR	PENIS	TESTES AND SCROTUM
Stage 1: Preadolescent 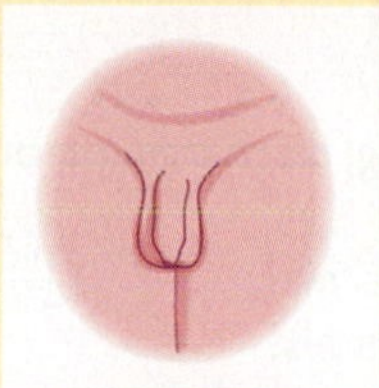	No pubic hair except for fine body hair similar to that on abdomen	Same size and proportions as in childhood	Same size and proportions as in childhood
Stage 2 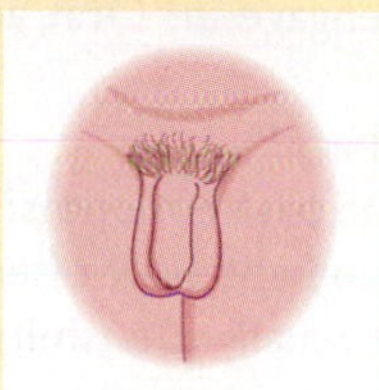	Sparse growth of long, slightly pigmented, downy hair, straight or only slightly curled, chiefly at base of penis	Slight or no enlargement	Testes larger, scrotum larger, somewhat reddened and altered in texture
Stage 3 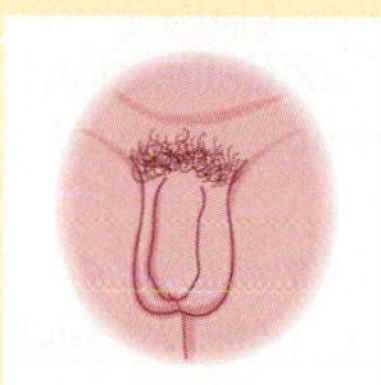	Darker, coarser, curlier hair spreading sparsely over pubic symphysis	Larger, especially in length	Further enlarged
Stage 4 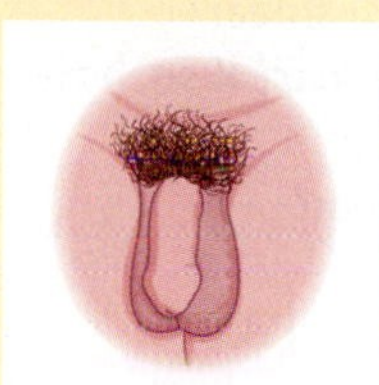	Coarse and curly hair, as in adult; area covered greater than in stage 3, but not as great as in adult	Further enlarged in length and breadth, with development of glans	Further enlarged; scrotal skin darkened
Stage 5 Adult 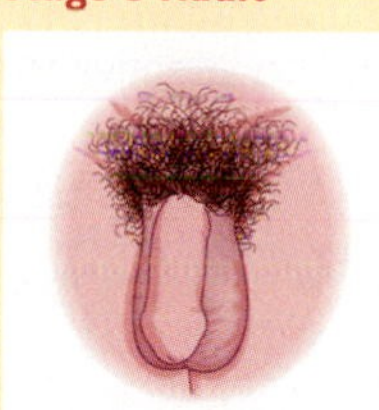	Hair same as adult in quantity and quality, spreading to medial surfaces of thighs, but not up over abdomen	Adult in size and shape	Adult in size and shape

Adapted from: Tanner, J. (1962). *Growth at adolescence* (2nd ed.). Oxford: Blackwell Scientific.

Procedure 22-18 ■ Assessing the Female Genitourinary System

➤ For steps to follow in *all* procedures, refer to the Universal Steps for All Procedures found on the inside back cover.

Equipment

- Patient drape
- Additional light source
- Nonlatex procedure gloves (if exposure to body fluids is a possibility)
- Pen and record form

Positioning

Lithotomy position, if possible.

Developmental Modifications for Older Adults

- Assess for incontinence.

Incontinence is one of the elements of the SPICES assessment model for older adults.

- Older women may have arthritis, which, along with muscle weakness, may make it difficult for them to assume the lithotomy position. You may need to use Sims' position and/or provide support for them to maintain a position.

Developmental Modifications for Children

- Obtain parental permission for this examination.
- Explain to the child what you are going to do, and expect some resistance or embarrassment.

Children are taught to not let strangers touch their genitals, and many children have a heightened sense of modesty.

Key Point: ***Do not perform internal assessment of an adolescent female unless the individual is sexually active.***

Focused History Questions

- Are you having any problems urinating?
- Have you noticed any redness, swelling, discharge, or odor in your genital area?
- Have you ever been told you have a hernia?
- Have you ever had trauma to your genitals?
- Are you sexually active? If not, have you ever been?
- Do you have sex with men, women, or both?
- What types of sexual activity do you engage in? Oral, anal, or genital?
- How many partners do you currently have?
- How many partners have you had in the past 6 months?
- Do you use birth control? If so, what kind and how often?
- Have you ever been treated for a sexually transmitted infection (STI)? If so, what type?
- Are you concerned about STIs or HIV infection?
- Do you take any precautions to avoid infection?
- Do you have any concerns about your sexual function?
- Have you had any surgery of your reproductive tract?
- When was your last menstrual period?
- What is the frequency of your periods?
- Do you have any problems with your periods, such as cramping, breast pain, or heavy flow?
- How often do you have a gynecological health examination?
- When was your last Pap (Papanicolaou) smear?
- Have you ever had an abnormal Pap smear? If so, how was it treated?
- How many times have you been pregnant?
- How many children do you have?
- Have you ever had a miscarriage? An abortion?

➤ When performing the procedure, always identify your patient according to agency policy, using two identifiers, and be attentive to standard precautions, hand hygiene, patient safety and privacy, body mechanics, and documentation.

Procedure Steps	Findings
1. Instruct the client to undress; assist her to assume the lithotomy or Sims' position, providing support, as needed.	
2. Inspect the external genitalia. a. Note the hair distribution pattern and the condition of pubic hair. See the table Maturation Status in Females at the end of this procedure. *The appearance of the external genitalia depends on the developmental stage of the client.*	a. **Expected findings:** Hair distribution in the pubic region is inverse triangular. Some hair may extend onto the abdomen and upper thighs. Hair distribution is appropriate for age. **Abnormal findings:** Sparse or absent hair (may result from genetic factors, aging, or local or systemic disease). ***Pediculosis pubis*** (lice), ***nits*** (white lice eggs), or flecks of dried blood on the skin.

b. Inspect the condition of the skin of the mons pubis and labia. Observe for color, condition, lesions, and discharge.

b. **Expected findings:** Skin is intact with no lesions or discharge. Labia majora and minora are symmetrical, with smooth to moderate wrinkling. Skin color is consistent with ethnicity. No ecchymosis, excoriation, nodules, edema, rash, or lesions are present.

Developmental Variations

Older adults: Labia and vulva are atrophied.

Abnormal findings: Ulcerations or lesions may occur with a number of STIs.

---

3. Inspect the clitoris, urethral meatus, and vaginal introitus.

a. Wearing gloves, use your thumb and index finger to separate the labia and expose the clitoris. Observe the clitoris for size and position.

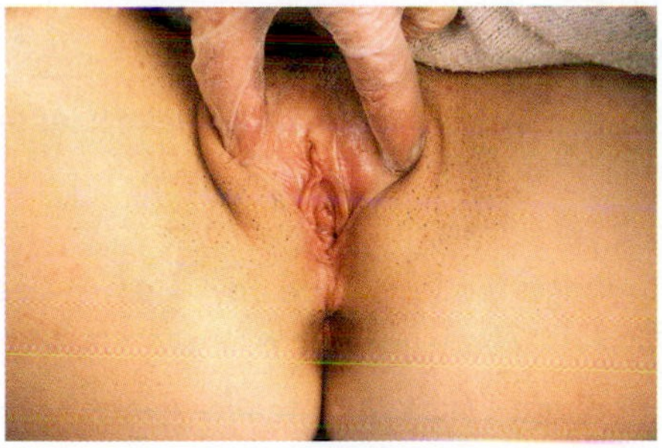

a. **Expected findings:** The clitoris is about 2 cm long and 0.5 cm in diameter. No redness or lesions are present.

Abnormal findings: Enlargement of the clitoris may result from androgen excess or swelling related to trauma. Absence of the clitoris, along with parts of the labia, is seen with female circumcision.

b. With the labia separated, observe the urethral meatus and vaginal introitus. Observe for color, size, and presence of discharge or lesions.

b. **Expected findings:** The urethral meatus is slitlike, midline, and free of discharge, lesions, swelling, or erythema. The mucosa of the introitus is pink and moist. Some clear to white discharge may be present and is odor-free.

c. Have the client bear down while you observe the introitus.

c. **Expected findings:** The introitus is patent, and there is no bulging or discomfort with bearing down.

Abnormal findings:

- Discharge, redness, or swelling may result from infection.
- Pale and dry mucosa may result from aging or use of topical steroids.
- Bulging may indicate prolapse of the uterus, bladder, or rectum.

---

4. Palpate Bartholin's glands, the urethral glands, and Skene's ducts.

a. Lubricate the index and middle fingers of your dominant hand with water-soluble lubricant.

b. To palpate Bartholin's glands, insert your lubricated fingers into the vaginal introitus, and palpate the lower portion of the labia bilaterally between your thumb and fingers.

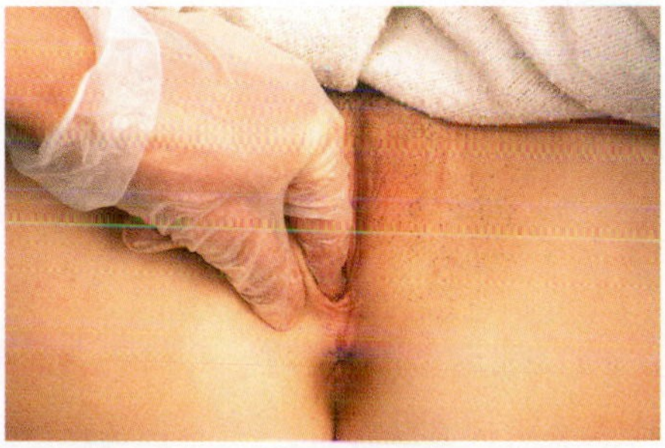

Expected findings:

- No swelling, masses, or tenderness of the glands is present.
- No urethral discharge.
- Labia are uniform in texture, no discharge or pain with palpation.
- Perineum is smooth and firm in ***nulliparous*** women (women who have had no children), thinner in ***parous*** women (women who have had children).

Abnormal findings:

- Pain or discharge from the glands may indicate infection.
- Fissures or tears in the perineum are painful and require treatment.

(continued on next page)

Procedure 22-18 ■ Assessing the Female Genitourinary System (continued)

c. To palpate Skene's ducts, rotate your internal fingers upward, and palpate the labium bilaterally.

d. To milk the urethra, apply pressure with your index finger on the anterior vaginal wall, and observe for urethral discharge. Culture any discharge you see. ➤

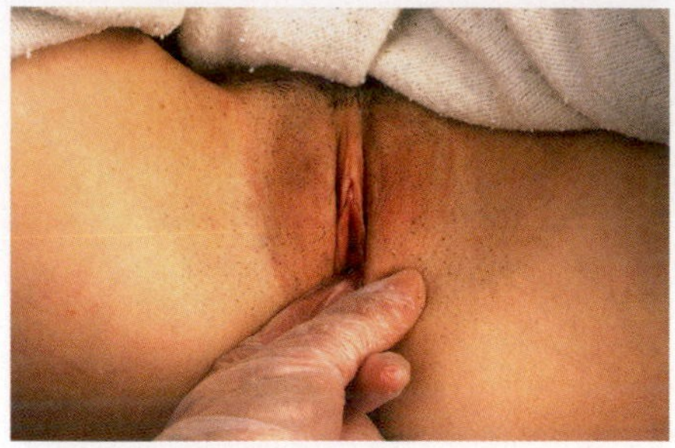

5. **Assess vaginal muscle tone and pelvic musculature.**
   a. Insert two gloved fingers into the vagina.
   b. Ask the woman to constrict her vaginal muscles and then to bear down as though she were having a bowel movement.

Expected findings: Muscle tone should be strong in women who have never given birth. With increasing ***parity*** (number of births), pelvic muscle tone diminishes. Diminished tone may also result from injury, age, or medication. No bulges should be noted.

6. **Palpate the inguinal and femoral area for hernias.**

Expected findings: No bulges or palpable masses are present in the inguinal or femoral area.

7. **Palpate the lymph nodes** in the groin area and the vertical chain over the inner aspect of the thigh.

Expected findings: Nodes should be < 1 cm in size and freely mobile.

Abnormal findings: Enlarged or tender lymph nodes may indicate local or systemic disease.

Documentation

If you need more information about documenting your findings, review Caring for the Nguyens, and

Go to Chapter 22, **Documenting Physical Examination Findings (Nam Nguyen),** in Volume 1.

Maturation Status in Females

STAGE OF DEVELOPMENT	BREASTS	PUBIC HAIR
Stage 1. Prepuberty	Elevation of papilla. 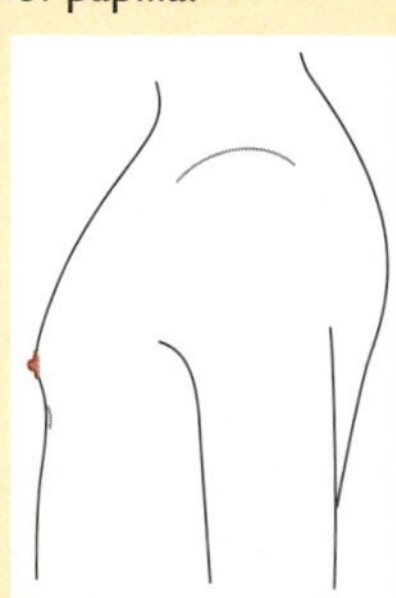	No pubic hair except for fine body hair similar to hair on abdomen. 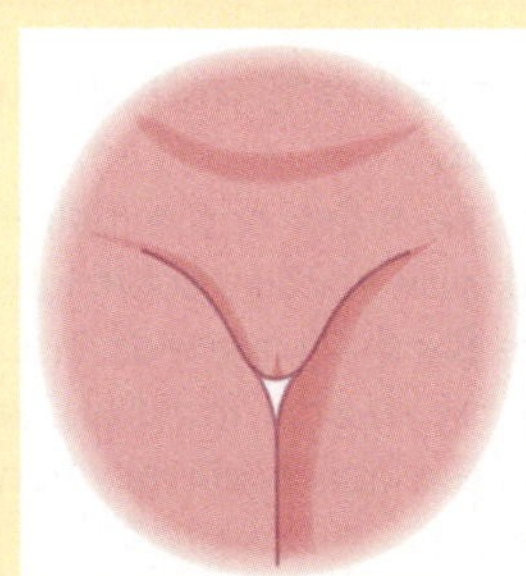

Maturation Status in Females—cont'd

STAGE OF DEVELOPMENT	BREASTS	PUBIC HAIR
Stage 2	Breast bud. Elevation of breast and nipple and increased diameter of areola. 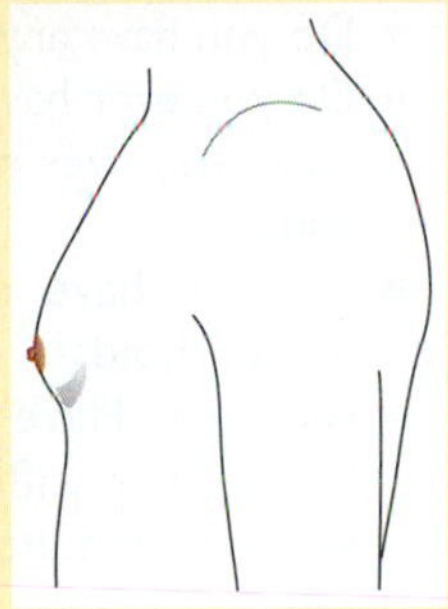	Sparse growth of long, slightly pigmented, downy hair, straight or only slightly curled, mostly along labia. 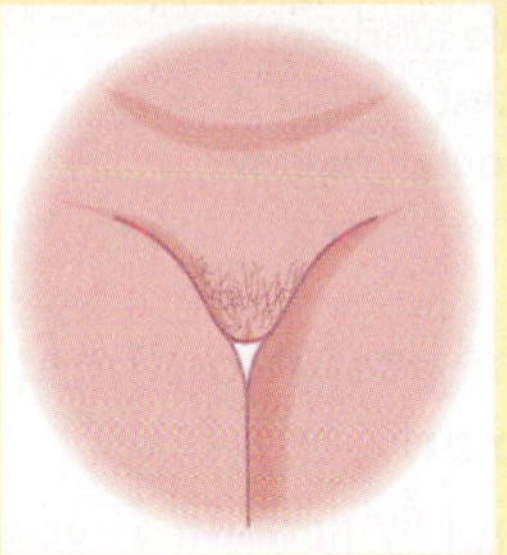
Stage 3	Areola deepens in color and enlarges further. Glandular tissue begins to develop beneath areola. 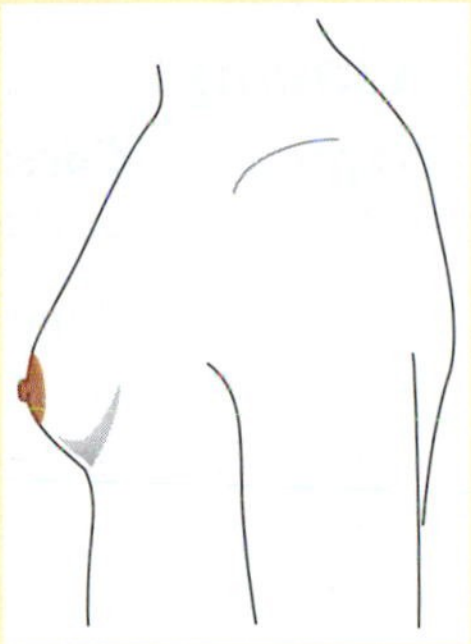	Hair becomes darker, coarser, and curlier and spreads sparsely over pubic symphysis. 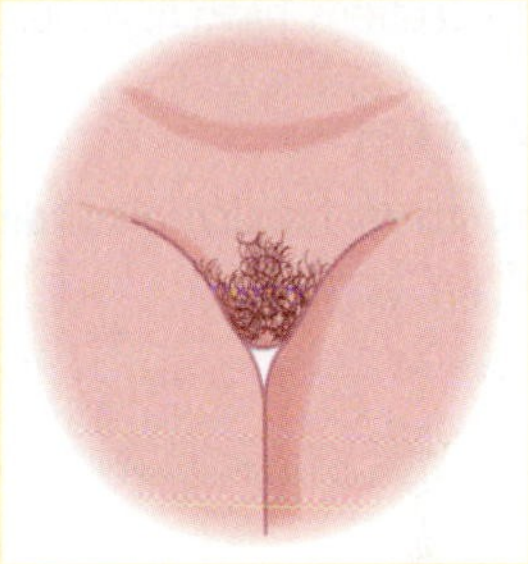
Stage 4	Areola appears as a mound; breast appears as a mound; papilla and areola form a secondary mound. 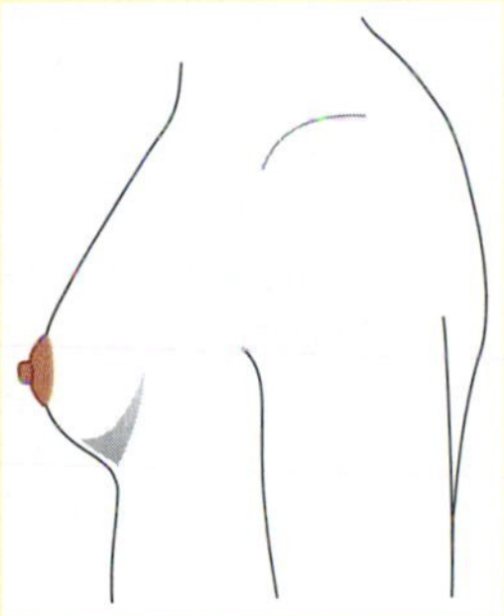	Pubic hair is coarse and curly as in adults. It covers more area than in stage 3 but does not extend to the medial thighs. 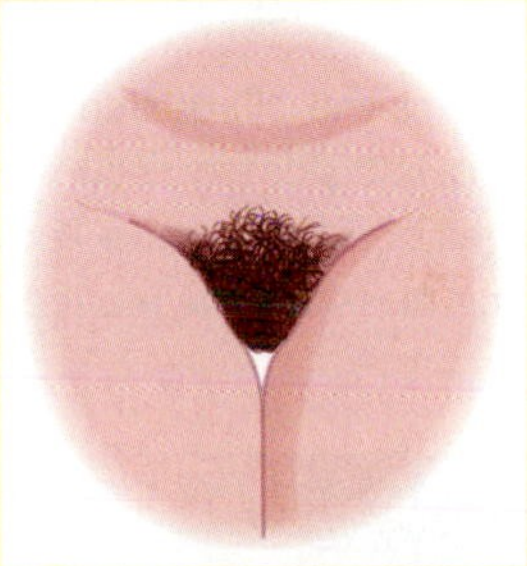
Stage 5. Adult	Mature breast. Areola recesses to general contour of breast; nipple projects forward. 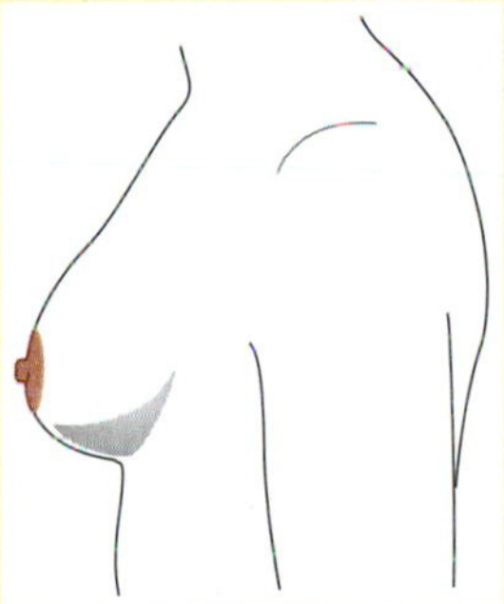	Quality and quantity are consistent with adult pubic hair distribution and spread over medial surfaces of thighs but not over abdomen. 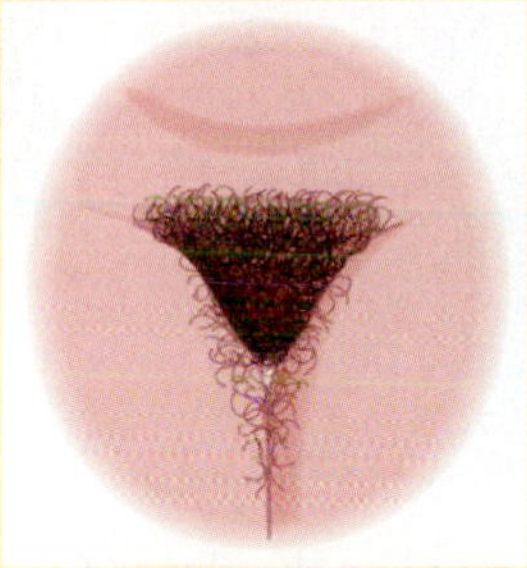

Adapted from: Tanner, J. (1962). *Growth at adolescence* (2nd ed.). Oxford: Blackwell Scientific.

Procedure 22-19 ■ Assessing the Anus and Rectum

➤ For steps to follow in *all* procedures, refer to the Universal Steps for All Procedures found on the inside back cover.

Equipment

- Water-soluble lubricant
- Hemoccult test
- Nonlatex procedure gloves
- Pen and record form

Developmental Modification for Infants and Children

You will not usually perform a rectal exam on infants and children.

Focused History Questions

- Do you have any pain or discomfort around your anus?
- Do you ever have difficulty passing stool?
- Have you ever noticed blood on your stool or when you wipe?
- Do you have or have you ever been told you have hemorrhoids?
- *For men:* Have you ever had a prostate exam or a prostate-specific antigen (PSA) blood test? If so, what were the results?

➤ When performing the procedure, always identify your patient according to agency policy, using two identifiers, and be attentive to standard precautions, hand hygiene, patient safety and privacy, and body mechanics.

Procedure Steps

1. **Inspect the anus.** Note the condition of the skin and the presence of any lesions.

Findings

Expected findings: Anal area is intact, with no inflammation or lesions. Anus is a darker color than surrounding tissue.

Abnormal findings:

- A fissure or tear may be caused by trauma, severe constipation, or an abscess.
- External hemorrhoids or skin tags may be visible.

---

2. **Palpate the anus and rectum.**
   a. *For women:* Change gloves to prevent cross-contamination. Insert a lubricated index finger gently into the rectum. Palpate the rectal wall, noting masses or tenderness.
   b. *For men:* Have the client bend over the exam table or turn on his left side to recumbent. Insert a lubricated index finger gently into the rectum. Palpate the rectal wall, noting masses or evidence of tenderness. ▼

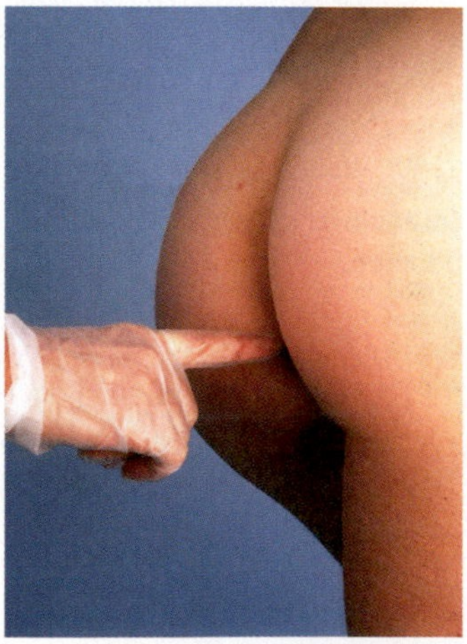

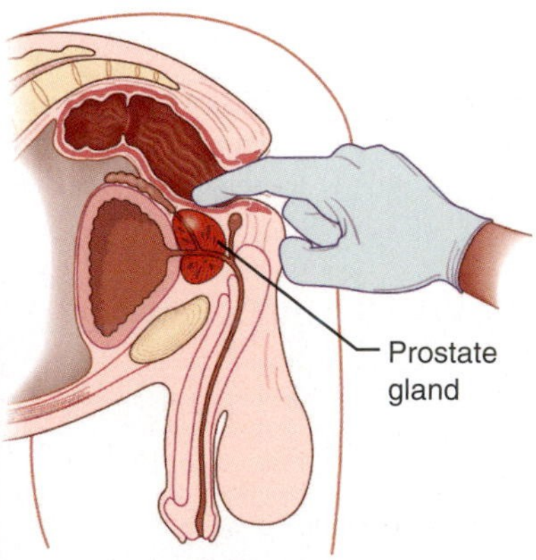

   c. Test any stool on the gloved finger for occult blood. See Procedure 29-1

Expected findings: Good sphincter tone. Rectum is nontender. No palpable masses or hard stool. The stool is brown and negative for occult blood.

Abnormal findings:

- Hard stool in the rectum indicates impaction.
- Positive occult blood indicates bleeding in the gastrointestinal (GI) tract.
- A palpable mass or enlarged prostate gland requires further evaluation.
- Internal hemorrhoids may be present.

Patient Teaching

Instruct the client in the importance of colonoscopy and prostate exam.

Documentation

If you need more information about documenting your findings, review Caring for the Nguyens, and

Go to Chapter 22, **Documenting Physical Examination Findings (Nam Nguyen)**, in Volume 1.

Procedure 22-20 ■ Brief Bedside Assessment

NOTE: This assessment is not as detailed as in Procedures 22-1 through 22-19. You might perform such an assessment when admitting a patient to a hospital unit. You can also use it for ongoing assessments. For daily patient assessments, you will modify the procedure to fit the patient's health status. You may be able to omit some portions, and you may need to add in-depth, focused assessments of some body systems. The entire assessment should take no more than 15 minutes after you become skilled.

➤ For steps to follow in *all* procedures, refer to the Universal Steps for All Procedures found on the inside back cover.

Equipment

- Thermometer, stethoscope, sphygmomanometer
- Procedure gloves

Focused History Questions

- Ask about any health problems, allergies, or medications.
- Ask your patient how she feels currently and during the previous month and year.
- Ask other questions as you assess each body system.

➤ When performing the procedure, always identify your patient according to agency policy, using two identifiers, and be attentive to standard precautions, hand hygiene, patient safety and privacy, body mechanics, and documentation.

Procedure Steps

1. **Greet the patient and explain what you need to do.** Ask the patient to state his name and confirm by checking his identity band.
   Ensures that you have the correct patient and also allows you to assess mental status and communication.

2. **Observe the environment** (e.g., IV lines, oxygen, urinary catheter) and patient's general appearance (including signs of distress).
   This allows you to identify any immediate actions you may need to take before performing the assessment.

3. **Begin by measuring the vital signs (patient supine or sitting):**
   a. Temperature, pulse, respirations, blood pressure
   b. Pain status
   c. Pulse oximetry

4. **Now assess each body system.**
   a. Use a systematic approach, such as from head to toe.
   b. As you assess each system, observe for mobility, ROM, balance, and coordination.
   c. As you talk with the patient, observe his thought processes and level of consciousness.

5. **Assess the integument.**
   a. Ask about any hair, nail, or skin changes, including rashes.
   b. With each body system, inspect skin color, rashes, and lesions; and palpate for temperature, turgor, and texture. Also inspect the hair and nails in that area (e.g., when assessing the legs and feet).
   c. Assess wounds—appearance, size, drainage, dressings, drains.
   d. Inspect and palpate the hair and scalp.

6. **Assess the head and neck.**
   a. Ask the patient about any problems with the head and neck.
   b. **Key Point:** ***Remember to continue assessing mental status and orientation to time, place, and person.***
   c. Inspect the external ears; observe for apparent hearing deficit.
   d. Check the eyes for pupil reaction and cardinal fields of gaze. Ask about and observe for any problems with vision.
   e. Inspect the color of the lips, mucous membranes, and conjunctiva.
   f. Inspect the tongue and oropharynx.
   g. Inspect for hydration, color, and lesions of the mucous membranes.
   h. Lightly palpate the carotid pulse (only if indicated by patient's condition), and listen for carotid bruits.

> Do not palpate both carotid arteries at the same time. See Procedure 22-13.

7. **Assess the heart.**
   a. Have the patient sit up and lean forward a bit.
   b. Ask about any cardiovascular problems.
   c. Auscultate heart sounds. Note rate, rhythm, S_1, S_2, and extra sounds.

(continued on next page)

Procedure 22-20 ■ Brief Bedside Assessment (continued)

8. **Assess the back while patient is in the sitting position.**
   a. Inspect the skin.
   b. Auscultate breath sounds; compare side to side and apex to base.
   c. Assess respiratory rate, rhythm, and effort.
   d. Note cough, secretions, how many pillows used to sleep on, and whether head of bed is elevated for breathing.
   e. Check oxygen saturation (SaO_2); ability to use incentive spirometer.

9. **Assess the anterior chest.**
   a. Ask about any respiratory problems.
   b. Palpate skin turgor, temperature, and PMI.
   c. Auscultate breath sounds.

10. **Assess the abdomen, with the patient supine.**
    a. Inspect the size, shape, symmetry, and condition of the abdominal skin.
    b. Observe abdominal movements, including respirations, pulsations, and peristalsis.
    c. Auscultate bowel sounds in all four quadrants, and the aorta for bruits.
    d. Palpate all four quadrants for tenderness, guarding, and masses; and inspect for rebound tenderness.
    e. Ask the patient about any weight changes, GI complaints, a change in appetite or diet.
    f. Review the pattern for bowel movements, and when examining a woman, ask about her last menstrual period.

11. **Assess urinary status.**
    a. Review voiding pattern with the patient (including frequency and dysuria).
    b. If there is an indwelling catheter, observe for patency, kinks in the tubing, and color of urine; monitor intake and output.
    c. Palpate for bladder distention.

12. **Assess the upper extremities.**
    a. Ask about any problems with the hands and arms, such as weakness, arthritis, and changes in sensation, temperature, or color.
    b. Inspect the condition of the skin and nails.
    c. Palpate skin temperature and bilateral brachial and radial pulses.
    d. Check capillary refill.
    e. Note any stiffness or limited ROM of the hands and arms.
    f. Test muscle strength by having the patient grip your hands or two fingers.
    g. Note whether the patient has any casts, traction, splints, or slings.
    h. Observe for edema.

13. **Assess the lower extremities.**
    a. Ask about any problems with the legs, such as weakness, numbness, tingling, arthritis, edema, change in sensation, and temperature or color.
    b. Observe ROM and ability to ambulate or move about in bed.
    c. Inspect the condition of the skin and nails.
    d. Palpate skin temperature and pedal pulses; check capillary refill.
    e. Test for leg strength by asking the patient to raise the leg against your counterpressure. (This is more easily done with the patient sitting.)
    f. Check sensation through light touch, proceeding to pain, as needed.
    g. Observe for such problems as paralysis.
    h. Observe for edema.

14. **Ask the patient to stand, and inspect for:**
    a. Gross spinal deformities
    b. Balance and coordination of movements
    c. ROM and gait

15. **With the patient seated in bed, legs extended, check for:**
    a. Babinski reflex
    b. Homans' sign

Documentation

- Document your findings and report any significant changes or findings to the primary care provider. As a student, report your findings to the instructor and the patient's assigned registered nurse (RN) for validation and action.
- If you need more information about documenting your findings, review Caring for the Nguyens, and

Go to Chapter 22, **Documenting Physical Examination Findings (Nam Nguyen)**, in Volume 1.

Thinking About the Procedure

The video, **Brief Bedside Assessment,** along with questions and suggested responses, is available on the ***Davis's Nursing Skills Videos*** Web site on FADavis.com.

CLINICAL INSIGHTS

Clinical Insight 22-1 ➤ Performing Percussion

Direct Percussion

Tap lightly with the pads of the fingers directly on the skin.

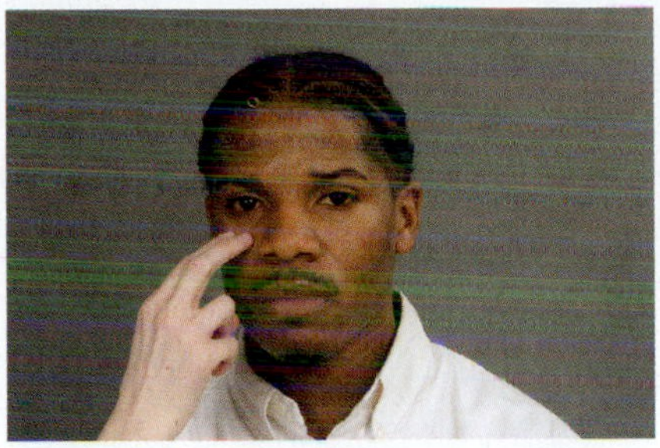

Direct percussion over the sinuses

Indirect Percussion

- Keep your fingernails short.
- Strive for a quiet environment: Turn off all entertainment media and music, shut the door, and so on.
  This allows you to better perceive the subtle differences in percussion notes.
- One hand is considered the stationary hand; the other is the striking hand.
- Hyperextend the middle finger of your stationary hand, and place its distal portion firmly against the client's skin over the area you wish to percuss.
- Lift the rest of your fingers off the patient's skin.
  Prevents dampening the sounds produced.
- Be sure both of your hands are relaxed to best perform the technique.
  Stiff hands will not effectively produce the percussion sounds for assessment.
- Use the middle finger of your dominant hand as the striking finger ***(plexor)***, and tap the distal portion of the middle finger of the stationary hand using a quick motion from your wrist.

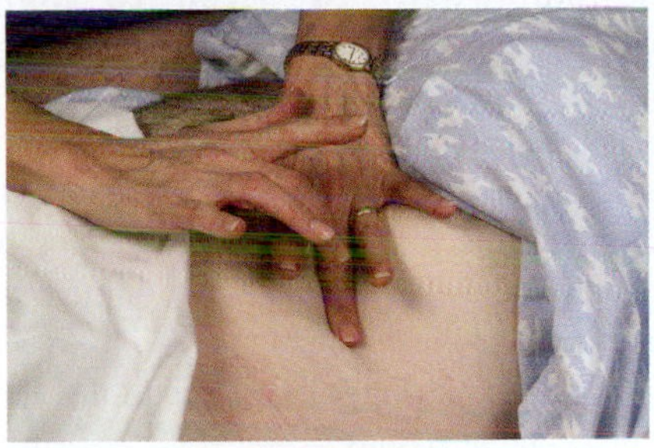

Indirect percussion

- Use enough force to elicit a clear sound.
- Percuss two times over each location, then move to a new body location, and repeat.

Describing Sounds

Use the terms in the following list to describe the sounds you hear. The terms are based on the components of the sounds produced by percussion:

- ***Amplitude***—the loudness or softness of a sound
- ***Pitch***—the number of vibrations per second; either high or low in nature
- ***Quality***—a distinctiveness about the sound produced
- ***Duration***—how long the sound lingers

Percussion Notes

SOUND	AMPLITUDE	PITCH	QUALITY	DURATION	EXAMPLE
Resonant	Medium-loud	Low	Hollow	Medium	Normal lung
Hyperresonant	Louder	Lower	Booming	Longer	Hyperinflated lung (as in emphysema)
Dull	Soft	High	Muffled thud	Short	Liver/spleen
Flat	Very soft	High	Absolute dullness	Very short	Thigh or tumor
Tympany	Loud	High	Musical	Longest	Gastric air bubble, intestinal air

Clinical Insight 22-2 ➤ Performing Auscultation

- Provide a quiet environment to facilitate auscultation.
- **Clean your stethoscope** with a 70% alcohol or benzalkonium chloride wipe before and after using it to examine a patient. Most stethoscopes are colonized by bacteria, although only a small percentage are pathogenic. Cleaning can reduce the bacterial count by 94% to 100%.
- **Use the diaphragm to listen to high-pitched sounds** that normally occur in the heart, lungs, and abdomen. Press the diaphragm hard enough to produce an obvious ring on the patient's skin.
- **Use the bell to hear low-pitched sounds**, such as extra heart sounds (murmurs) or turbulent blood flow (bruits). Apply the bell lightly with just enough pressure to produce an air seal with its full rim.
- Place the earpieces facing forward. *Seals the ear canal and improves detection of sounds.*
- Warm the stethoscope before you place it on the client's skin.
- Place the stethoscope directly on the client's skin. Do not listen through clothing. *Clothing can create artifact or reduce the quality of auscultation.*
- If body hair prevents good contact with the skin, dampen the hair before you listen.
- Close your eyes as you listen through the stethoscope. This helps improve your focus.
- Concentrate on one sound at a time. Do not try to evaluate breath and heart sounds at the same time. This improves the quality of the data.

Practice Resources

Centers for Disease Control (2009, updated 2016); Holleck, Merchant, Lin, & Gupta, (2017); Messina, Rosadini, Burgassi, et al. (2017)

Clinical Insight 22-3 ➤ Assisting With a Speculum Exam

Equipment

- Patient drape
- Nonsterile gloves
- Vaginal speculum (see accompanying figure)
  - The speculum may be plastic or metal.
  - The size of the speculum depends on the patient's history. Use a small speculum for a woman who has never been sexually active or an older woman who is not sexually active.
  - If a culture or a Pap smear is to be obtained, lubricate the speculum with warm water. Otherwise, use a water-soluble lubricant.
- Lubricant
- Pap smear slide, spatula, brush, or specimen broom and container with solution
- Fixative, if the smear technique is used
- Genital culture supplies
- Additional light source

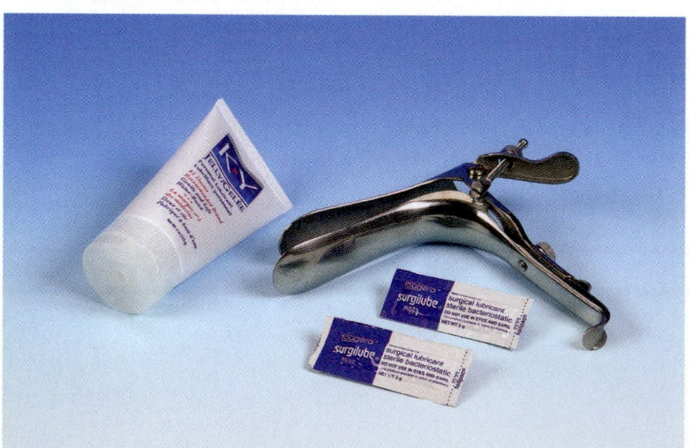

Equipment. A vaginal speculum

Preparing the Patient

iCare ▪ Explain to the patient that an internal examination of her vagina and pelvic organs will be performed. The examination usually takes only a few minutes, and although it might not be comfortable, it should not be painful.

- Have the woman urinate before the examination, if needed. *Emptying the bladder helps the patient feel more comfortable during the examination.*
- Provide privacy, and keep the patient warm during the procedure.
- Assist the woman to the lithotomy position, and cover her with a drape.

Inserting the Speculum

The speculum is inserted into the vagina to visualize the cervix (see accompanying figure). Once the speculum is inserted, you may need to adjust the light source for the examiner.

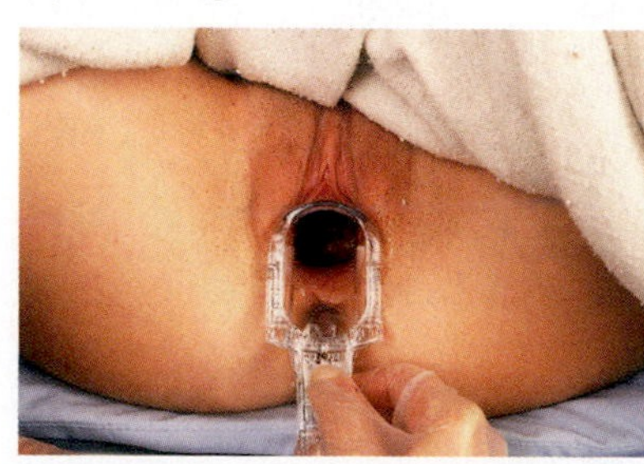

A, A vaginal speculum examination. Placement of the speculum in the vagina.

Clinical Insight 22-3 ➤ Assisting With a Speculum Exam—cont'd

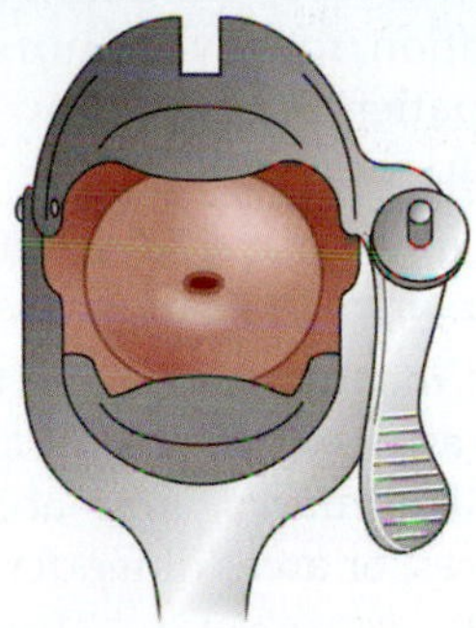

B, View through the speculum

Collecting Specimens

If a routine screening for cervical and uterine cancer is being done, a specimen will be collected. Additional cultures or screens may be required if there is unusual discharge or risk of STIs. Genital cultures are endocervical smears.

Pap Smear Procedure

Most commonly, the examiner inserts a small brush through the cervical os and rotates it to obtain cells from within the cervical canal (endocervical smear). The brush is then rolled onto the slide.

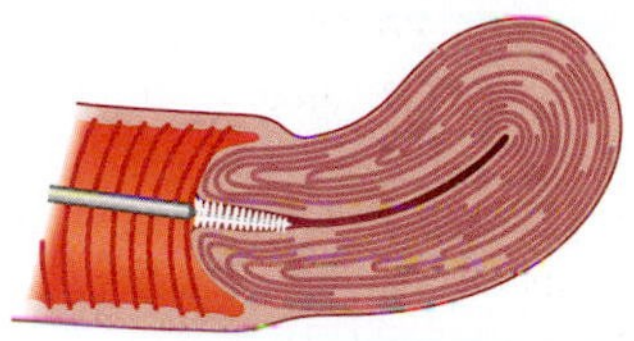

Using a specimen broom to obtain endocervical cells

A second specimen may be obtained by lightly scraping the cervix with a wooden spatula to obtain cells from the ectocervix (the lowest portion of the cervix that protrudes into the vagina).

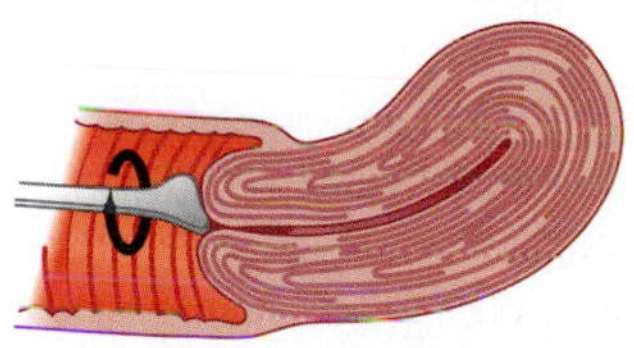

Using a spatula to obtain ectocervical cells

The spatula is then smeared on the slide. Some examiners use both specimen sources and then apply a fixative, usually a spray or liquid, on top of the specimen to preserve it for examination. After the samples are obtained, the speculum is removed.

Pap Smear, Alternative Method

The examiner inserts a specimen broom into the cervical os and rotates it. The broom is then inserted into a fixative solution and rotated to disperse cells into the solution. This technique is gaining popularity because it is considered more sensitive for detection of cervical changes. After the samples are obtained, the speculum is removed.

Bimanual Exam

After removing the speculum, the examiner inserts lubricated gloved fingers into the vagina while pressing down on the lower abdomen and suprapubic area. This is known as a ***bimanual exam.*** It is used to assess the consistency of the cervix and the size of the uterus, and to detect tenderness over the ovaries, fallopian tubes, or with movement of the cervix.

Postprocedure

- Assist the woman to a sitting position at the end of the exam.
- You may need to assist the woman with perineal care.
- If there is any bleeding or discharge, provide a perineal pad.
- Document the date and time of the procedure, the name of the examiner, the patient's tolerance of the procedure, and any nursing assessments or interventions performed.

Practice Resources

American Congress of Obstetricians and Gynecologists (2014); Bibbins-Domingo, Grossman, Curry, et al. (2017).

What Are the Main Points in This Chapter?

- A physical examination may be conducted to obtain data about the patient, to further investigate an identified health problem, to monitor a client's health status, or to screen for health problems.
- A comprehensive physical assessment includes a complete head-to-toe examination of every body system. Data from a comprehensive physical assessment provide guidance for care and determine the need for further assessment.
- A focused physical assessment is performed to obtain data about an actual, potential, or possible problem that has been identified. A focused examination adds to the database created from the comprehensive assessment.
- An ongoing assessment is appropriate for periodic reassessment of the client and reflects the dynamic state of the client. This is a less detailed examination than a comprehensive assessment.
- Before a physical assessment, you will need to gather equipment, prepare the environment, review the skills you will use, familiarize yourself with the patient situation, review the nursing plan of care, and assist the patient to relax by taking the time to develop a rapport.
- *Inspection* is the use of sight to gather data. Inspection begins the moment you meet the client.
- *Palpation* is the use of touch to gather data. Use palpation to assess temperature, skin texture, moisture, anatomical landmarks, and abnormalities, such as edema, masses, or areas of tenderness.
- *Percussion*, tapping on the skin with short strokes from your fingers, produces vibrations that allow you to determine the location, size, and density of underlying structures.
- *Auscultation* is the use of hearing to gather data. Direct auscultation is unassisted listening. Indirect auscultation is listening to the sounds produced by the body with the help of a stethoscope.

Knowledge Map

PHYSICAL EXAMINATION

Health Assessment → Physical Assessment

PURPOSE:
- Obtain baseline data
- Identify nursing diagnoses, PCs, Wellness dx
- Monitor status of identified problems
- Screening

TYPES:
- Comprehensive:
  - interview
  - head-to-toe
- Focused:
  - data gathered on particular topic, body part/functional ability
- Ongoing:
  - prn with every pt. contact

APPROACHES:
ways to gather data
- Head to toe
- Body systems

PREPARATION

SELF
- Know A&P
- Know purpose of exam
- Know pt. situation & plan of care
- Be familiar with equipment
- Exam technique
- Therapeutic communication
- How to document

ENVIRONMENT
- Provide privacy
- Decrease extraneous noise
- Adequate lighting
- Comfortable temperature

PATIENT
- Promote relaxation
- Develop a rapport
- Position patient properly
- Have patient void prior
- Alert patient to touch
- Attend to cultural preferences

AGE MODIFICATIONS:

Infant: have parent hold

Toddler:
- allow to sit on parent lap
- allow choices; use praise
- invasive assessments last

Preschooler:
- demo assessment on doll
- let child help
- give reassurance

School-age Child:
- develop rapport
- allow independence
- demo equipment

Adolescent:
- no parent/sibling present
- respect privacy during exam
- emphasize healthy lifestyle habits
- assess for suicide potential

Young/Middle-Aged Adult:
- no specific modifications unless acute/chronic disease

Older Adult:
- tailor exam to energy and mobility levels
- adapt techniques for vision & hearing changes

ASSESSMENT SKILLS:

Inspection:
- use of sight/observation

Palpation:
- use of touch: fingertips, dorsum/palm of hand, finger/thumb grasp

Percussion:
- vibrations elicited through tapping
- sound indicates location, size, density of underlying structure

Auscultation:
- use of hearing
- direct via stethoscope

Olfaction: not a formal skill
- use of sense of smell

GENERAL SURVEY:
- Appearance/behavior
- Body type; posture
- Dress; grooming; hygiene
- Mental status
- Vital signs/height/weight assessment

Proceeding to: Assessment of all body systems

CHAPTER 23

Promoting Asepsis & Preventing Infection

STUDENT RESOURCES

The questions and exercises in this book allow you to practice the kind of thinking you will use as a full-spectrum nurse. Critical-thinking questions usually have more than one right answer, so we do not provide "correct answers" for these features. Try to answer these questions yourself. It is more important to develop your nursing judgment than to just cover content. You will learn more by discussing the questions with your peers. If you are still unsure, see the Davis Advantage chapter resources for suggested responses.

To explore learning resources for this chapter,

Go to Davis Advantage and find:

Answers and Suggested Responses for all questions in this chapter
Concept Map
Knowledge Map
References and Bibliography
Lists of NOC Outcomes and NIC Interventions

Key Concepts

Body defenses
Infection
Infection prevention and control
Medical asepsis
Surgical asepsis

Related Concepts

See the Concept Map on Davis Advantage.

Example Problems

Multidrug-Resistant Organism (MDRO) Infections

Caring for the Nguyens

Mrs. Nguyen works as a preschool teacher in her community. Kim, her grandchild, has been attending the preschool since he came to live with his grandparents. Mrs. Nguyen tells you at a recent visit to the clinic that Kim has had "a lot of problems with colds and a runny nose since he started preschool."

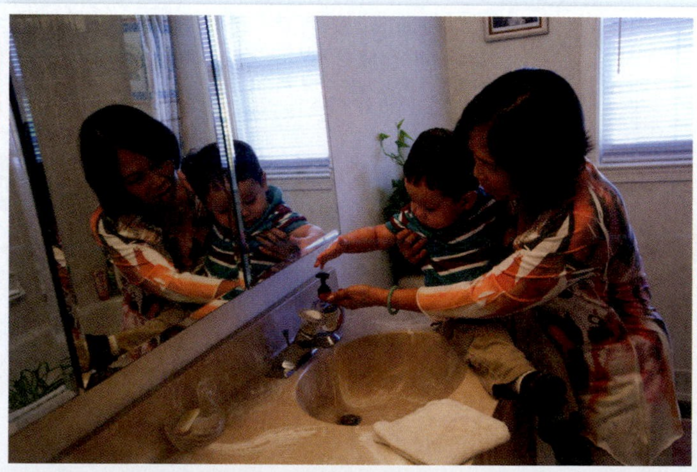

Caring for the Nguyens (continued)

A. Based on your theoretical knowledge of asepsis and immunity, what is the most likely explanation for Kim's symptoms?

B. Do you have enough patient data to make any conclusions? If not, what other information should you gather?

C. Identify three alternatives that may explain what is happening.

D. What strategies could you recommend that Mrs. Nguyen implement at the preschool to help limit the number of infections? Identify at least two strategies.

PracticalKnowledge clinical application

As a nurse, you play a vital role in preventing the transmission of infection. Most infection control measures are independent nursing activities that do not require a medical prescription. You do need to have theoretical knowledge and follow scrupulous medical and surgical asepsis techniques. The Procedures and Clinical Insights in this volume provide the guidance you will need to implement your infection-control concepts in providing safe, effective nursing care.

PROCEDURES

Procedure 23-1 ■ Hand Hygiene

➤ For steps to follow in *all* procedures, refer to the Universal Steps for All Procedures found on the inside back cover. For this procedure, also refer to Clinical Insight 23-1.

Equipment

- Liquid soap
- Paper towels
- Warm, running water
- Hand moisturizer (recommended)

Pre-Procedure Assessments

- Check your hands for breaks in the skin.
  Breaks in the skin provide a route for microbial entry.
- Inspect the condition of your nails.
  —Nails should be no longer than one-quarter inch from the fingertips.
  —Do not wear artificial nails or extensions.
  —Nail polish should not be chipped.
  —Preferably, do not use nail polish.
  The area under the nails, artificial nails/extensions, and chipped polish act as reservoirs for microorganisms. If your gloves were to tear or perforate, microorganisms could enter into the surgical wound.

Procedure 23-1A ■ Using Soap and Water

➤ When performing the procedure, always identify your patient according to agency policy, using two identifiers, and be attentive to standard precautions, hand hygiene, patient safety and privacy, body mechanics, and documentation.

Procedure Steps

1. **Bare your hands and forearms.** Push your sleeves above your wrists; remove your wristwatch and rings.
   Moist clothing facilitates transfer of microorganisms; jewelry harbors bacteria and creates a moist area on the skin, which facilitates bacterial growth.

2. **Turn on the water. Use electronic faucet, when possible.** Adjust water to warm, not hot.
   Hands-free electronic faucets lessen the risk of recontamination of hands after washing because there is no need to turn off the water manually. Warm water opens pores and helps remove microorganisms without removing skin oils. It also reduces chapping of the skin. Hot water increases the risk for skin breakdown.

(continued on next page)

Procedure 23-1 ■ Hand Hygiene (continued)

3. **Wet your hands and wrists.** Keep your hands below your wrists and forearms.
Prevents water from running from hands to the wrists and forearms. Hands are considered more contaminated than the wrists and arms.
   a. Avoid splashing water onto clothing.
   b. Avoid touching the inside of the sink.
   Microorganisms travel in moisture. The inside of the sink is considered contaminated.▼

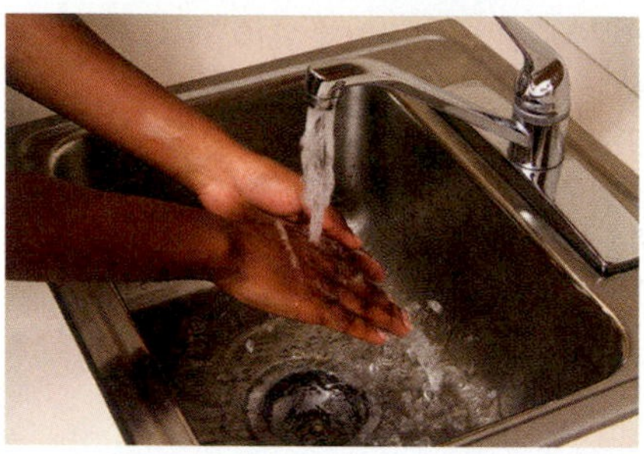

4. **Apply enough liquid soap to cover all hand surfaces** (typically 3 to 4 pumps from a dispenser).
About 3 to 5 mL of liquid soap provides adequate amounts to completely cover the hands for maximum effectiveness to remove transient microorganisms.

5. **Vigorously rub your hands together** for at least 15 seconds. Lather all surfaces, interlacing fingers, rubbing around each finger and thumb, rubbing the backs and palms of the hands in a circular motion.
It takes at least 15 seconds for mechanical removal of microorganisms and for antimicrobial products to be effective. The areas of the hands most often missed are the thumb, the wrist, and the areas between the fingers.▼

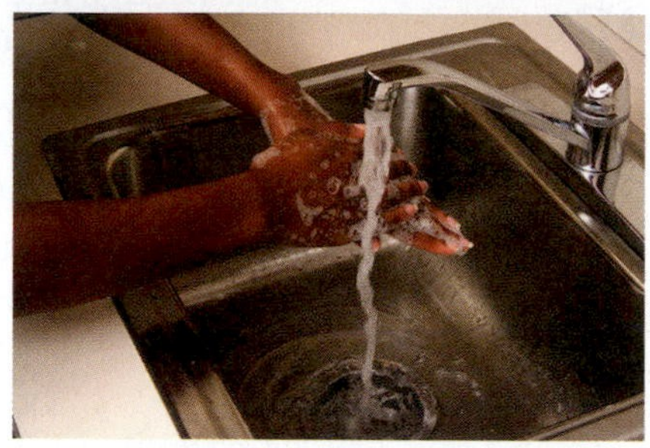

6. **Clean under your fingernails,** if needed, using a disposable nail cleaner.
Areas under the nails harbor high concentrations of microorganisms.

7. **Rinse your hands thoroughly.** Keep your hands below your wrists and forearms.

8. **Dry your hands thoroughly,** moving from your fingers up to your forearms and blotting with paper towel.
Move from the area you wish to keep cleanest (hands). Blotting decreases skin irritation.

9. **Turn off the faucet.** If the faucet is not hands-free, hold a dry paper towel in your hand to turn it off. Do not handle the paper towel with the opposite hand.
A paper towel acts as a barrier to prevent contamination of hands from the faucet. After the towel has contacted the contaminated faucet, it can transfer microorganisms to your clean hand. Many pathogens can live on faucets and countertops.

10. **Apply a hand moisturizer** at least twice daily; use hand care products recommended by infection preventionists. (Many agencies use soaps that contain moisturizers.)
Hand moisturizer helps prevent skin from drying and chapping, which may lead to transmission of infection. Petroleum-based products compromise latex gloves, resulting in permeability.

Procedure 23-1B ■ Using Alcohol-Based Handrubs

➤ When performing the procedure, always identify your patient according to agency policy, using two identifiers, and be attentive to standard precautions, hand hygiene, patient safety and privacy, body mechanics, and documentation.

Procedure Steps

1. **Use alcohol-based handrubs** when hands are not visibly soiled and when certain pathogens are suspected.
Antiseptic solutions are not effective when organic material or dirt from hands is present. Alcohol-based handrubs cannot remove spores and, therefore, should not be used for hand hygiene when Clostridium difficile or Bacillus anthracis is suspected of being present.

2. **Bare your hands and forearms.** Push your sleeves above your wrists. Remove your jewelry and wristwatch.

3. **Apply antiseptic solution** in a quantity sufficient (at least 3 mL) to cover the hands and wrists.
All surfaces must be covered with sufficient product to effectively remove microorganisms.▼

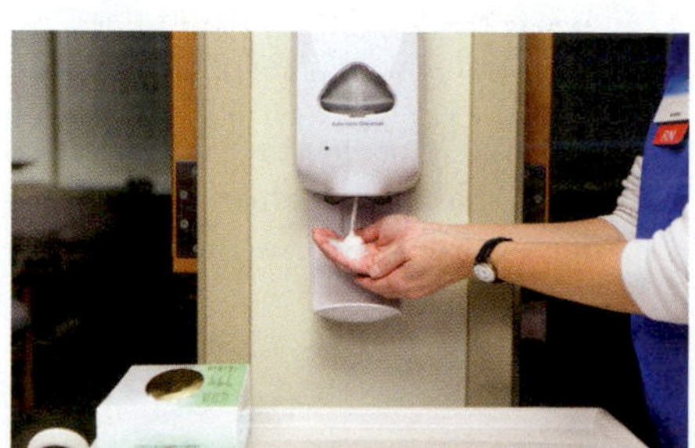

4. **Vigorously rub antiseptic solution** into your hands for 20 to 30 seconds (or as long as it takes to sing "Happy Birthday" if no clock is available). Cover all surfaces of the hands: interlacing fingers, rubbing around each finger and thumb, and rubbing the backs and palms of the hands in a circular motion, including under the nails, until the solution is completely dry.
A period of 20 to 30 seconds is required for effective disinfection by alcohol handrubs (World Health Organization, 2009). All surfaces must be thoroughly covered with product to effectively remove microorganisms.

Evaluation

Hands are free of handrub and dry.

Documentation

Hand hygiene is a responsibility of all healthcare providers. It usually does not require documentation.

Practice Resources

Association of periOperative Registered Nurses (AORN) (2016); Boyce, J., & Pittet, D. (2002); Centers for Disease Control and Prevention (CDC) (2017, March 17, updated); CDC (2013, October 25, updated); Siegel, J., Rhinehart, E., Jackson, M., et al. (2007).

Thinking About the Procedure

The videos **Hand Hygiene: Using Soap and Water** and **Using Alcohol-Based Handrubs,** along with questions and suggested responses, are available on the ***Davis's Nursing Skills Videos*** Web site on FADavis.com.

Procedure 23-2 ■ Donning Personal Protective Equipment (PPE)

➤ For steps to follow in *all* procedures, refer to the Universal Steps for All Procedures found on the inside back cover.

Equipment

Following CDC recommendations, you will usually use some combination of gloves, gown, mask, and eye protection, depending on the organism and level of precaution. In certain situations, you may need hair covers and shoe covers (e.g., when full barrier precautions are needed). Determine the availability of appropriate PPE.

- Disposable gloves of the proper size
- Disposable isolation gown
- Face mask (or N-95 respirator mask, as indicated)
- Face shield or goggles
- Hair cover (if needed)
- Shoe covers (if needed)

➤ When performing the procedure, always identify your patient according to agency policy, using two identifiers, and be attentive to standard precautions, hand hygiene, patient safety and privacy, body mechanics, and documentation.

Procedure Steps

1. Assess the need for PPE.

a. **Gloves:** When you may be exposed to body secretions directly or indirectly.
Gloves provide a barrier against body fluids. All patients are considered potentially infected per Standard Precautions (see Clinical Insight 23-3).

b. **Gowns:** When your uniform (e.g., scrubs) may become exposed to potentially infective secretions. **Key Point:** ***Do not substitute a patient gown for a disposable isolation or protective gown. Isolation gowns must be made of moisture-repelling materials to prevent contamination of underlying clothing and skin.***
Examples of such situations include excessive wound drainage, fecal incontinence, or other discharges from the body or when fluids may be splashed (as in eye irrigation).

c. **Face mask:** When splashing may occur during close contact (3 ft or less) and potentially contaminate your mouth or nose.
Surgical masks provide a barrier to large-particle droplets (>5 microns in diameter), helping prevent transmission of pathogens to the nurse's mucous membranes.

d. **Face shield or eye goggles:** When splashing might occur and fluids enter your eyes (e.g., blood splashes, respiratory droplets, or wound debridement). To protect the entire facial area, wear a face shield (for maximum protection, it should protect the crown and chin and wrap around the face to the ear).
Helps prevent pathogens from entering the conjunctiva directly or indirectly.

e. **N-95 respirator:** When caring for clients infected with airborne organisms (<5 microns), such as the tuberculosis bacillus.
This device prevents the airborne transmission of the tuberculosis bacterium. The respirator mask shown is disposable; some are reusable. ▼

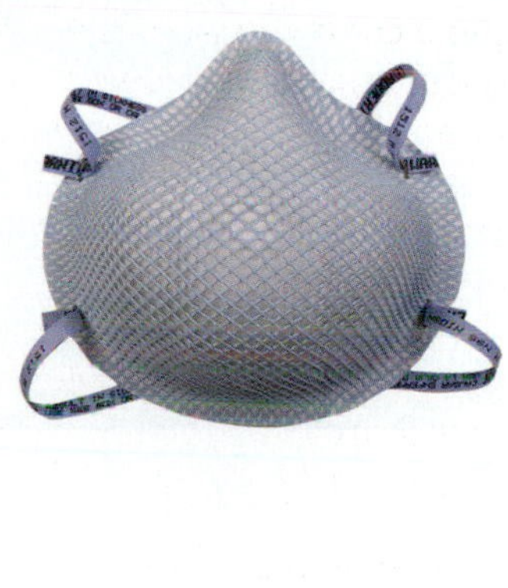

(continued on next page)

Procedure 23-2 ■ Donning Personal Protective Equipment (PPE) (continued)

f. **Hair covers:** When there is a potential for spraying or splashing of body fluids.
Although this is not included in the CDC report (Siegel, Rhinehart, Jackson, et al., 2007), agency policy may recommend the use of hair covers in certain situations.

g. **Shoe covers:** When there is a potential for contamination of shoes with body fluids.
The floor (and anything in contact with it) is considered contaminated. However, certain categories of pathogens require full protective gear, and in those circumstances, shoe covers are necessary.

2. Don the isolation gown.

a. Pick up the gown by the shoulders, allowing the gown to fall open without touching the floor or other surfaces.
Touching the floor or other surfaces will contaminate the gown with environmental pathogens. ▼

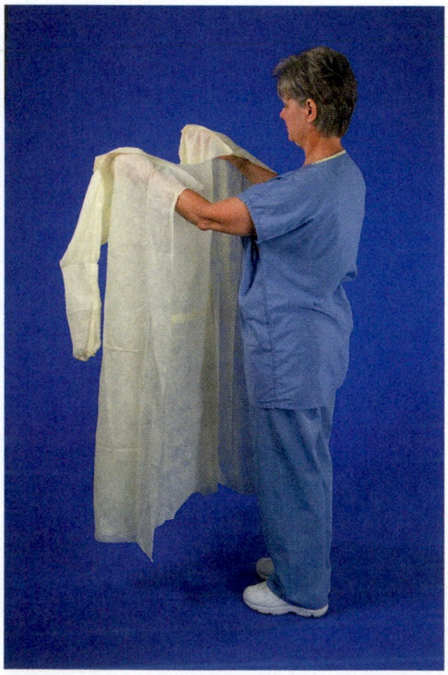

b. Slip your arms into the sleeves. ▼

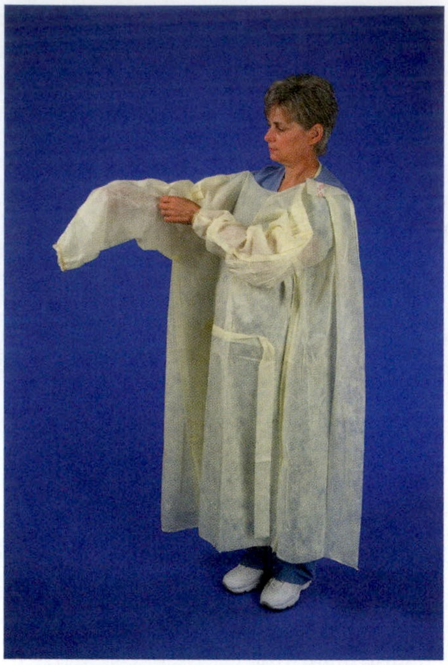

c. Fasten ties at the neck.

d. Position the gown so that it covers the back, and fasten the ties at the waist. Do not bring ties around to the front of the gown.
The front of the gown is considered contaminated after you enter the patient's room. If the ties are at the front of the gown, they will become contaminated, making it difficult to remove the gown safely.

e. If the gown does not completely cover your clothing in the back, wear two gowns.
- Don the first gown so that the opening is in the front.
- Then place the second gown over the first so that the opening is in the back.

3. Don the face mask or N-95 respirator.

a. Determine how the mask is secured. Identify the top edge of the mask by locating the thin metal strip (nosepiece) that goes over the bridge of the nose.
Surgical masks may be secured with ties at the back of the head and neck, loops around the ears, or elastic bands.

b. Pick up the mask with the top ties or ear loops. Place the mask over your nose, mouth, and chin. Press the flexible metal strip so that it conforms to the bridge of your nose.
The mask must fit snugly to the face for maximum barrier protection. Correct positioning will also keep your glasses or goggles from fogging. ▼

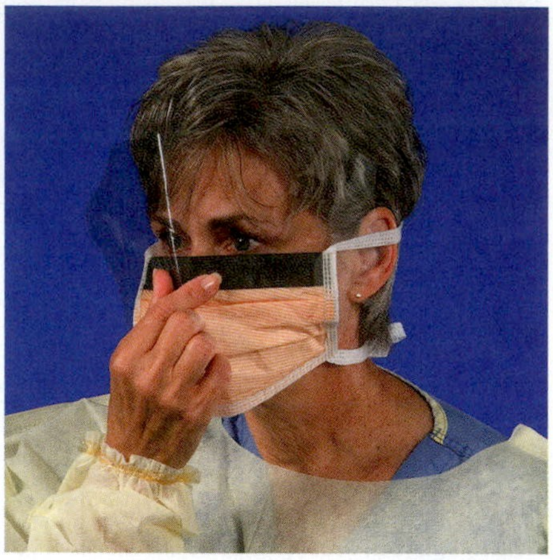

c. Tie the upper ties to the back of your head and the lower ties to the back of your neck or slip the loops around your ears or place the elastic bands as with the ties.

d. Place the lower edge of the mask below your chin, and tie the lower ties.
Covering the nose and mouth creates a barrier to prevent droplet pathogens from entering through the nasal and oral mucous membranes or the respiratory system.

4. Don the face shield or goggles.

a. *Face shield:* Place the shield over your eyes, adjust the metal strip over the bridge of your nose, and tuck the lower edge below your chin. Secure the straps behind your head.

b. *Safety glasses or goggles:* Set them over the top edge of the mask.
See Step 1c, d, and e for the rationale.

5. Don hair cover, if indicated.
Hair covers can be worn to protect from contamination when you anticipate sprays or airborne exposure.

6. Don shoe covers, if indicated.

7. **Don gloves.**
   a. Select nonsterile disposable gloves of the appropriate size. See Clinical Insight 23-3.
   The correct size will prevent gloves from falling off or ripping while you are working with the client.
   b. If you are wearing a gown, make sure that the glove cuff extends over the cuff of the gown. If skin is visible between the gown and the glove, tape the glove cuff to the gown cuff, covering all visible skin.
   To provide complete protection of hands and wrists, no skin should be visible between the glove and the gown.

Patient Teaching

Answer questions the patient may have and provide education about the need for PPE, the disease process, and the purpose of isolation.

Home Care

- Identify the type of PPE needed, and ensure that the necessary supplies are available.
- Develop a plan with the client and the family for using and disposing of PPE and contaminated items.
- Teach family members to don PPE, as needed.
- Obtain referral for a home health agency to provide support.

Documentation

The use of PPE is generally assumed and does not require documentation.

Practice Resources

AORN (2016); CDC (n. d.); Cowperthwaite, L., & Holm, R. L. (2015); Ortega, Bhadelia, Obanor, et al. (2015); Siegel, J. D., Rhinehart, E., Jackson, M., et al. (2007).

Thinking About the Procedure

The video **Donning Personal Protective Equipment (PPE)**, along with questions and suggested responses, is available on the ***Davis's Nursing Skills Videos*** Web site on FADavis.com.

Procedure 23-3 ■ Removing Personal Protective Equipment (PPE)

➤ For steps to follow in *all* procedures, refer to the Universal Steps for All Procedures found on the inside back cover. For this procedure, also refer to Clinical Insights 23-2 and 23-3 if you need more information.

Key Point: ***Considered contaminated: front areas, sleeves, mask, and gloves of the PPE, and head and shoe covers, if you are wearing them.***

Key Point: ***Considered clean: inside of the gown, gloves, the ties on the mask, and ties at the back of the gown, and the inside of the head and shoe covers, if you are wearing them.***

➤ When performing the procedure, always identify your patient according to agency policy, using two identifiers, and be attentive to standard precautions, hand hygiene, patient safety and privacy, body mechanics, and documentation.

Procedure Steps

1. **Remove gloves first** (unless the gown ties in front; in that case, see, "What If . . .").
   Gloves are the most contaminated PPE and must be removed first to avoid contamination of clean areas of the PPE during their removal.
   a. **Remove the first glove:**
   - Grasp the outside cuff of the glove with the opposite gloved hand.
   - Pull downward so that the glove turns inside out.
   - Do not touch the skin of your wrist or hand with your gloved hand.
   The outside of both gloves is contaminated. To prevent contamination, touch only the outside (contaminated) surface of first glove to outside (contaminated) surface of second glove. "Dirty touches dirty" and "clean touches clean."

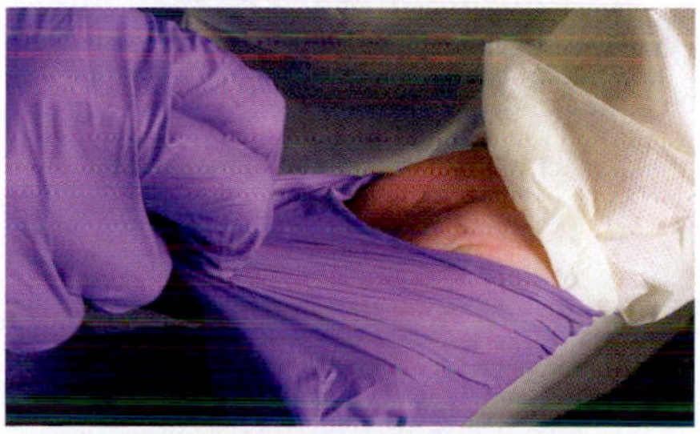

   b. **Remove the second glove:**
   - Hold the removed glove in the palm of your gloved hand.
   - Slip two ungloved fingers inside the cuff of the remaining glove.
   - Pull the glove off, inside out, over the glove that hand is holding. Do not touch the outside of the soiled glove with your bare fingers.
   The insides of gloves are considered "clean" because they have not been in contact with client or contaminated surfaces. Therefore, you can touch the insides with your bare hands.

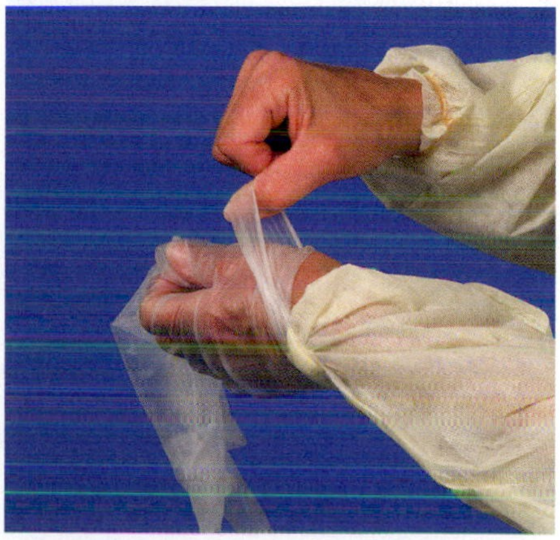

(continued on next page)

Procedure 23-3 ■ Removing Personal Protective Equipment (PPE) (continued)

c. **Dispose of gloves** in a designated waste container, keeping them away from your body.

2. **Remove the gown**:
   a. **Release the waist ties** and the neck ties of the gown, bending slightly forward to allow the gown to fall forward.
   Allowing the gown to fall forward exposes the clean area for the hands to grasp more readily.
   b. **Slip your hands inside the neck** and peel the gown away from the shoulders.
      - Reach inside to pull off the cuff and remove your arm from the sleeve.
      - Repeat the maneuver to remove the second sleeve.
      - Do not touch the front of the gown, even if it is not visibly soiled.
      The inside of the gown is clean and will not contaminate your hands. The front of the gown and the sleeves are considered contaminated.

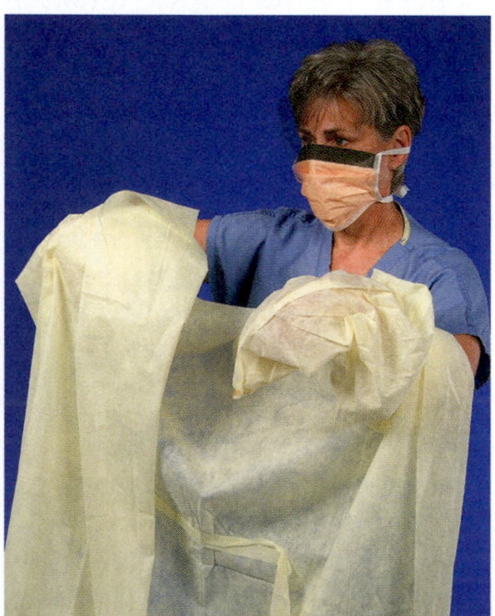

3. **Fold the gown so the inside of the gown is to the outside.** Holding the gown away from your uniform, roll it up with the contaminated front and sleeves in the center, and place in the designated waste container.
Folding the gown prevents contamination of your hands, the clothing, and the environment.

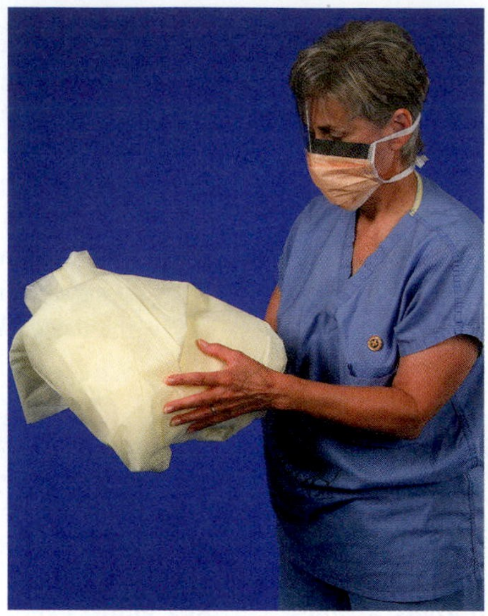

4. **Remove goggles.**
   a. Grasp only the earpieces (or head band) of the goggles and pull them off the face.
   b. If the goggles are not disposable, place them in the container provided for disinfection.
   Earpieces are considered clean. Some goggles are cleaned and reused.
5. **Remove your mask or face shield,** unless the mask is a respirator. In that case, remove it after leaving the patient room and closing the door.
   a. Untie the lower ties first.
   b. Untie the upper ties next, being careful not to let go of the ties.
   c. Touch only the ties; do not touch the front of the mask.
   d. Dispose of the mask by holding on to the ties and placing it in a designated waste container.
   Ties are considered clean. Touching the outside of the mask would contaminate your hands.
6. **Remove your hair covering.**
   a. Slip your bare fingers under the edge of the hair cover, being careful not to touch the outside of it.
   b. Lift it up and away from your hair.
   c. Touching only the inside of it, place it in a designated waste container.
   The inside of the hair covering is considered clean, so you may touch it with your bare hands.
7. **Remove shoe covers.** Be careful to touch only the insides of the covers.
8. **Perform hand hygiene** immediately after removing PPE.
Even if gloves are worn, hands may become contaminated.
9. **Close the door.**
Keeping the door closed contains contaminants and makes signage more visible.

? What if . . .

- **The gown is tied in front?**
  Untie the front gown ties before removing your gloves; then remove the gloves, and untie any back ties (e.g., at the neck). (This would be an unusual circumstance.)
  Because the front of the gown (including a front tie) is considered contaminated, once you remove your gloves, you could not use your bare hands to untie a front tie.
- **You are wearing two gowns (top one tied in back, inner one tied in front)?**
  Remove gloves; untie waist ties of outer gown, remove the gown, and fold it inside out. Remove the inner gown by untying it in front. Fold inner gown inside out. Take off goggles and face mask or shield.

Patient Teaching

See Procedure 23-2.

Home Care

See Procedure 23-2.

Documentation

The removal of PPE is generally assumed and does not require documentation.

Practice Resources

AORN (2016); CDC (n. d.); Ortega, Bhadelia, Obanor, et al. (2015); Siegel, J., Rhinehart, E., Jackson, M., et al. (2007); World Health Organization (2014).

Thinking About the Procedure

The video **Removing Personal Protective Equipment (PPE)**, along with questions and suggested responses, is available on the ***Davis's Nursing Skills Videos*** Web site on FADavis.com.

Procedure 23-4 ■ Surgical Handwashing: Traditional Method

➤ For steps to follow in *all* procedures, refer to the Universal Steps for All Procedures found on the inside back cover. For this procedure, also refer to Clinical Insights 23-2, 23-3, and 23-4 if you need more information.

Equipment

- Antimicrobial soap (FDA–approved for surgical hand asepsis)
- Soft, nonabrasive scrub sponge
- Disposable single-use nail cleaner
- Deep sink with foot or knee controls
- Surgical shoe covers, cap, and face mask
- Sterile gloves of the correct size
- Surgical pack containing a sterile towel

➤ When performing the procedure, always identify your patient according to agency policy, using two identifiers, and be attentive to standard precautions, hand hygiene, patient safety and privacy, body mechanics, and documentation.

Procedure Steps

1. **Determine that sterile gloves,** gown, and towel are set up for use after the scrub.
To maintain sterility, the sterile towel, gown, and gloves must be ready for use immediately after you scrub. If you need to gather supplies after the scrub, you must start the scrub procedure over again.

2. **Determine the agency policy for** the duration of the surgical scrub and the type of cleansing agent used.
The type of cleansing agent determines how long to scrub. Typically, an alcohol-based antimicrobial soap requires 2 to 6 minutes.

3. **Avoid nail polish and artificial nails.** Trim so nails do not extend beyond fingertips. Remove rings, watches, and bracelets.
Rings are a substantial risk factor for harboring moisture and gram-negative bacilli and Staphylococcus aureus; artificial nails and chipped polish are more likely to carry gram-negative pathogens, including Pseudomonas, because water collects between the artificial and natural nails.

4. **Don surgical shoe covers, cap, and face mask** before the surgical scrub.

5. **Perform a prewash** before the surgical scrub (see Procedure 23-1).
The prewash removes any visible soil, reduces the number of microorganisms on your skin, and allows you to begin the surgical scrub with clean hands. (Boyce & Pittet, 2002; Ellingson, Haas, Aiello, et al., 2014; Wood & Conner, 2018; World Health Organization [WHO], 2009).

6. **Remove debris from under your nails** using a single-use nail file under running water.
Decreases the number of microorganisms.

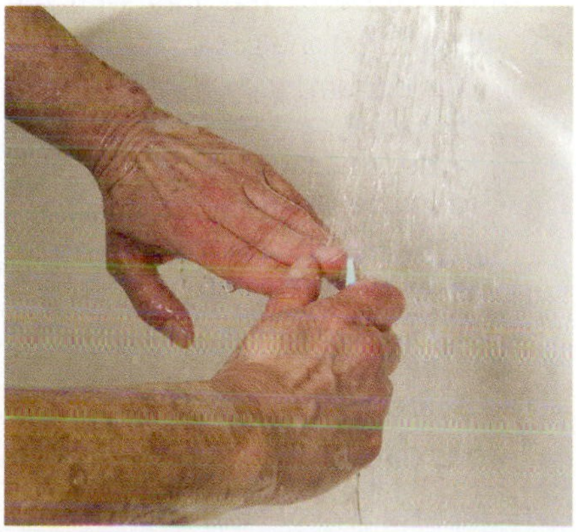

7. **To begin the surgical scrub**, turn on the water, using the knee or foot controls or motion sensors. Adjust the temperature so that the water is warm.
Hot water removes the skin's protective oils. Knee and foot controls help prevent contamination of the hands. Do not touch any unsterile surface once you begin the surgical hand wash.

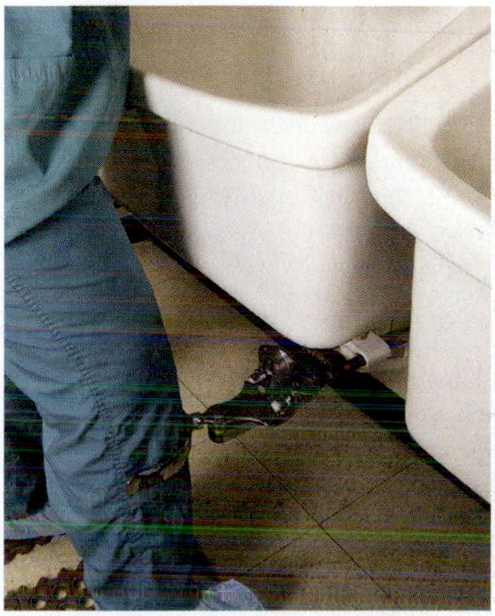

(continued on next page)

Procedure 23-4 ■ Surgical Handwashing: Traditional Method (continued)

8. **Wet your hands and forearms** from elbows to fingertips, keeping hands above elbows and away from your body. If using a scrub sponge, wet the sponge.
Prevents water running down from your "dirty" elbows and forearm over "clean" rinsed hands.

9. **Apply antimicrobial soap, a liberal amount** onto your hands and the sponge.
   - Lather well to 2 inches above the elbow.
   - Do not touch the inside of the sink with your fingers, hands, or elbows.
   - Avoid splashing your surgical attire.
   Scrub brushes are harsh on the skin. Soft, nonabrasive sponges are recommended instead. Antimicrobial soap reduces the number of microorganisms.

10. **Scrub one hand and arm,** all surfaces, using a circular motion.
   - Start at the fingers. Scrub at least 10 strokes each on nail, all four sides of each finger, hands, and arms.
   - When scrubbing the arm, use 10 strokes each for the lower, middle, and upper areas of the forearm.
   - Keep hands higher than elbows.
   Cover all surfaces to remove maximum number of microorganisms from the skin. Keep hands higher than elbows so that water from the area nearest the unscrubbed skin does not run downward and contaminate the hands.

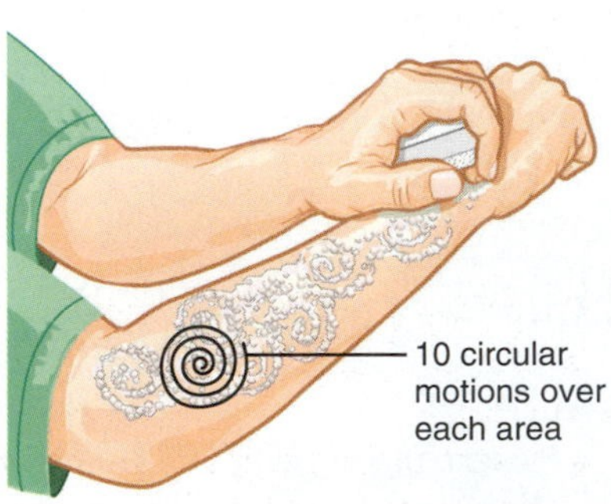

11. **Rinse the brush and reapply** antimicrobial soap. Repeat the scrub on the second hand and arm. Normally the scrub takes at least 2 to 6 minutes.
The length of the scrub depends on the time needed for the particular scrub agent to be effective in removing microorganisms on the hands.

12. **Rinse your hands and arms,** keeping your fingertips higher than your elbows.
Prevents contamination of hands from water running from the upper arm down onto hands.

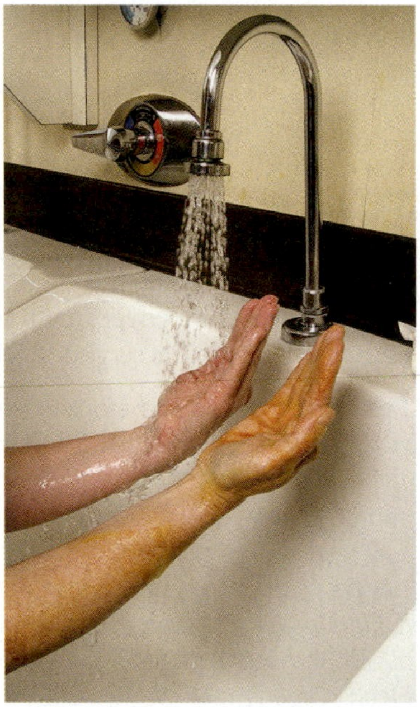

13. **Repeat Steps 8 through 12** if directed to do so by the soap manufacturer or agency policy.

14. **With arms flexed and your hands** held higher than your elbows, move to the area with the sterile towel and gown.
Avoids contamination of hands from water runoff.

15. **Grasp the sterile towel,** and step back while not turning your back or your eyes from the sterile field.
Backing away keeps the sterile field dry and prevents you from inadvertently brushing against the table, which would contaminate the field.

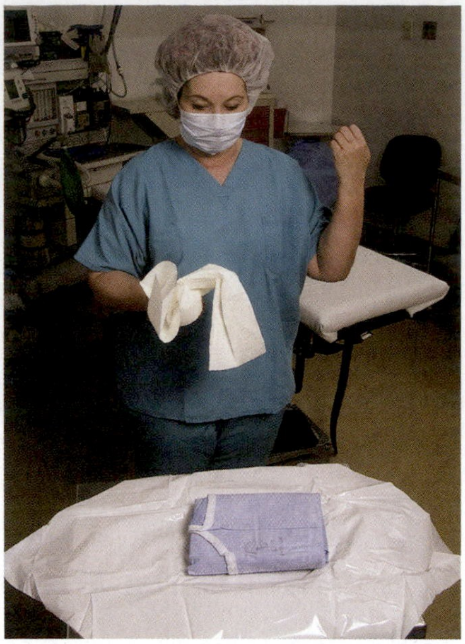

16. **Lean forward slightly,** and allow the towel to fall open, being careful not to let it touch your clothing.
The towel would be contaminated if it brushed against your clothing.

17. **Use one end of the towel** to dry one hand and arm. Use the opposite end to dry the other hand and arm. Be certain your skin is thoroughly dry before donning sterile gloves.
Drying skin prevents maceration and allows gloves to go on much more easily. Use a separate section of the towel to prevent rewetting the skin or contaminating an already clean area.

? What if . . .

- **The agency uses an alcohol-based surgical hand-scrub product?**
  a. Perform Steps 1 through 6. Omit Steps 7 through 17.
  b. Using the indicated amount of handrub, rub all surfaces of the hands, including the nails and up the arm to 2 inches above the elbow, according to the manufacturer's recommendations and agency policy.
  Many different products are available. Be careful to follow the manufacturer's guidelines for use for maximum effectiveness.
  c. Allow the handrub to dry completely before you don sterile gloves.

Patient Teaching

If the patient is able to observe the procedure, explain the purpose of the surgical scrub and sterility.

Documentation

A surgical hand scrub does not require documentation. Instead, chart the procedure (or surgery) and how the patient tolerated it.

Practice Resources

AORN (2016); AST (2008); Boyce, J., & Pittet, D. (2002); CDC (n. d.); Siegel, J., Rhinehart, E., Jackson, M., et al. (2007; 2006, updated 2017, February 15).

Procedure 23-5 ■ Surgical Handwashing: Brushless System

➤ For steps to follow in *all* procedures, refer to the Universal Steps for All Procedures found on the inside back cover. For this procedure, also refer to Clinical Insights 23-2 and 23-3 if you need more information.

Equipment

- Antimicrobial soap (60% to 95% alcohol, or other FDA-approved product for surgical hand asepsis)
- Disposable single-use nail cleaner
- Deep sink with foot or knee controls
- Surgical shoe covers, cap, and face mask
- Sterile gloves of the correct size
- Surgical pack containing a sterile towel

➤ When performing the procedure, always identify your patient according to agency policy, using two identifiers, and be attentive to standard precautions, hand hygiene, patient safety and privacy, body mechanics, and documentation.

Procedure Steps

1. **Determine agency policy** for the type of cleansing product to be used and for duration of the surgical scrub (typically 2 to 6 minutes).
   Policies vary from institution to institution, although all should be based on sound principles for infection control designed in accordance with the CDC and AORN guidelines and follow manufacturer's directions for product use. The type of cleansing agent determines how long to scrub. Typically, alcohol-based handrub is rubbed onto hands and arms until dry.

2. **Before starting the scrub,** gather supplies and set up sterile gloves, gown, and towel for use after the scrub.
   To maintain sterility of the hands after the scrub, the sterile gloves, gown, and towel must be ready before washing.

3. **Observe recommended hygiene.**
   a. Do not wear artificial nails. Nails should be free of polish and not extend beyond the end of the fingers.
   Especially important when in direct contact with patients or in high-risk situations, such as the perioperative setting or among those receiving immunosuppressant therapy. Artificial nails have been shown to harbor more pathogenic organisms in the subungual area compared with natural nails, particularly gram-negative bacilli (especially Pseudomonas) and various strains of yeast. Long nails can tear gloves.
   b. Remove rings, watches, and bracelets before starting the scrub.
   Hand jewelry can prevent the handrub from reaching all skin areas and increase the spread of potential pathogens. Risk of infection from microorganisms increases exponentially in relation to the number of rings worn.

4. **Don shoe covers, a cap, and a mask.** Tuck hair completely under the cap.
   Masks filter out possible airborne pathogens carried in the nose or mouth, preventing contamination of sterile areas. Covering the hair reduces the transmission of pathogenic organisms that adhere to the hair shaft or the scalp.

5. **Perform a prewash** before the surgical scrub. Use a pick to remove dirt and debris from under the nails; discard.
   Prewash removes any visible soil, reduces the number of microorganisms on your skin, and allows you to begin the surgical scrub with clean hands. The area under the nails harbors dirt, debris, and microorganisms.

6. **Turn on the water,** using the knee or foot controls or motion controls. The temperature usually adjusts automatically in a surgical scrub sink. If it does not, adjust to warm.
   Water temperature that is too hot can cause injury to the skin, making it prone to disruption in skin integrity. It can also remove the skin's normal flora and natural oil, which has a protective effect.

7. **Wet hands and forearms** from the fingertips to elbows, keeping hands above the elbows and away from the body at all times.
   Prevents water running down from your elbows and forearm over washed and rinsed hands.

8. **Dispense a palm full of** antibacterial cleansing solution into your dominant hand.
   a. Insert the fingertips of your nondominant hand into the cleansing solution using a twisting motion to apply the product to the fingertips and nails.

(continued on next page)

Procedure 23-5 ■ Surgical Handwashing: Brushless System (continued)

b. Then, rub the hands together to distribute the soap over the hands.

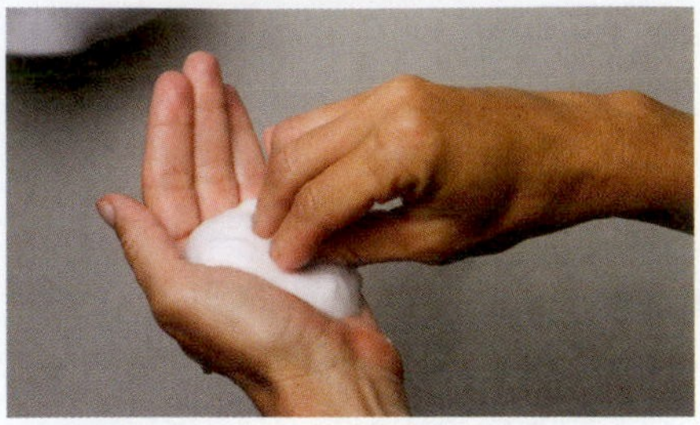

9. Vigorously rub all surfaces of your nondominant hand and fingers, adding water as needed.

- Be sure to rub each finger on all sides.
- Do not touch the inside of the sink during the cleansing procedure.

Complete contact and friction are necessary for removal of microorganisms adherent to the skin's surface. The inside of the sink is considered contaminated with microbes. Incidental contact necessitates repeating the cleansing procedure.

a. Rub the hands together, palm to palm.
b. Using your dominant palm, clean the back of your nondominant hand.
c. Then, rub your nondominant palm over your dominant hand.
d. Then, rub your palms together with your fingers interlaced.
e. Rub the back of your fingers on your closed right hand back and forth across your nondominant palm, with your curved fingers interlaced. Do the same with your other hand.

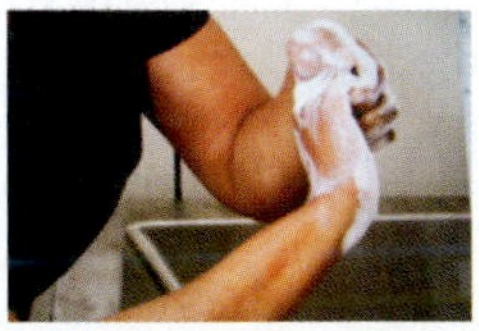

f. With your nondominant hand, clasp your dominant thumb, and make rotational movements to cleanse the thumb. Repeat on the other hand.
g. Hold your fingers together on the dominant hand, and move them back and forth and in a circular pattern against your other palm, and vice versa.

Although the palmar surface carries more organisms compared with the back side of the hands and arms, this area nonetheless should be cleansed thoroughly to reduce the microbial count.

10. Rinse using deep basin sink with knee-, foot-, or motion-operated controls. Dispense soap into the hands each time when cleansing a new area.

Improved adherence to sterile technique commonly results from use of motion- or foot/knee-operated or motion controls for faucets.

11. Next, cleanse the remaining two-thirds of the arms, beginning at the wrist, to 2 inches above the elbow. Cover every aspect of the middle and upper third of the forearm.

12. Dispense cleansing solution into the hands each time you cleanse a new area.

13. First, scrub the nondominant arm, wrist to elbow. Then, repeat the wrist-to-elbow scrub on the dominant arm. Rinse each arm thoroughly and independently.

14. This completes one washing cycle.

a. Using the same motions, beginning with Step 8, perform a 2nd cycle.
b. Then, finish with a third cycle, in which you scrub only the hands (Steps 8–11). The scrub is complete after cleansing every aspect of the hands and forearms for 3 full minutes.

The AORN promotes a 2- to 3-minute scrub time with use of an antiseptic detergent to achieve maximal microbicidal activity while avoiding irritant contact dermatitis associated with use of an abrasive sponge. Reduced time required to perform the surgical scrub often results in increased compliance with the prescribed technique.

15. With arms flexed and hands held higher than the elbows away from the body, move to the area with the sterile towel and gown.

This position prevents water running down from your elbows and forearm over rinsed hands.

16. Grasp the sterile towel, and back away from the sterile field. Lean forward slightly, and allow the towel to fall open, being careful not to let it touch clothing or gown.

This motion is performed to maintain a dry sterile field and prevent inadvertent brushing against the table and contaminating the field.

17. Use one end of the towel to dry one hand and arm using a dabbing motion. Dry the other hand and arm with the opposite end of the towel.

Use of a separate section of the towel guards against inadvertently rewetting the skin or contaminating an already clean area.

18. Allow time for the skin to dry thoroughly before donning sterile gloves.

Dry skin prevents maceration and allows the gloves to go on more easily. Moisture left on the skin can be a source of further microbial contamination.

19. Once the brushless scrub is complete, keep your hands in front of your body and above the waist. It may be necessary to enter backward through the door of the surgical suite.

These actions help prevent contamination of the hands and forearms when moving from the scrub sink.

Documentation

A brushless surgical hand scrub does not require documentation in the patient's medical record, although there may be a checklist. However, you must adhere to the institution's policy for performing the technique.

Patient Teaching

If the patient is able to observe the procedure, explain the purpose of a diligent approach to surgical scrub for promoting a low-risk environment for infection.

Home Care Adaptations

Sinks in the home environment typically do not have knee- or foot-operated controls or motion-sensor on/off devices. Therefore, when scrubbing for a sterile procedure in the home, keep a barrier object (e.g., a paper towel or a sterile towel for a sterile scrub) between your clean hands and the environmental surface.

Practice Resources

AORN (2018); AST (2008); CDC (2002); Cowperthwaite, L., & Holm, R. L. (2015).

Thinking About the Procedure

The video **Surgical Handwashing: Brushless System**, along with questions and suggested responses, is available on the ***Davis's Nursing Skills Videos*** Web site on FADavis.com.

Procedure 23-6 ■ Sterile Gown and Gloves (Closed Method)

➤ For steps to follow in *all* procedures, refer to the Universal Steps for All Procedures found on the inside back cover. For this procedure, also refer to Clinical Insights 23-2 and 23-3 if you need more information.

Equipment

- Sterile gloves of the right size
- Sterile gown

NOTE: You should find these items placed on a sterile field. If they are not, you will need to create a sterile field to place them on.

➤ When performing the procedure always identify your patient according to agency policy, using two identifiers, and be attentive to standard precautions, hand hygiene, patient safety and privacy, body mechanics, and documentation.

Procedure Steps

1. **Grasp the gown at the neckline.**
   a. Hold the gown up, and allow it to fall open as you step back from the table.
   b. Do not allow the gown to come into contact with nonsterile areas while you are lifting it off the table and opening it.
   The gown will be contaminated if it touches unsterile objects. ➤

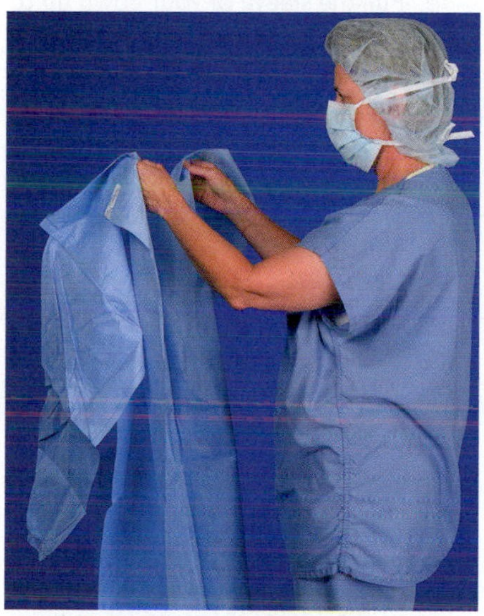

2. **Slide both arms into the sleeves,** but do not extend your hands through the cuffs.
   Sleeve cuffs are considered unsterile when your hands pass beyond the cuff (they are sterile if you don gloves using the closed method).

3. **Keep the sleeves of the gown** above waist level.
   Hands will contaminate the sleeve edge if allowed to pass through the cuff. ▼

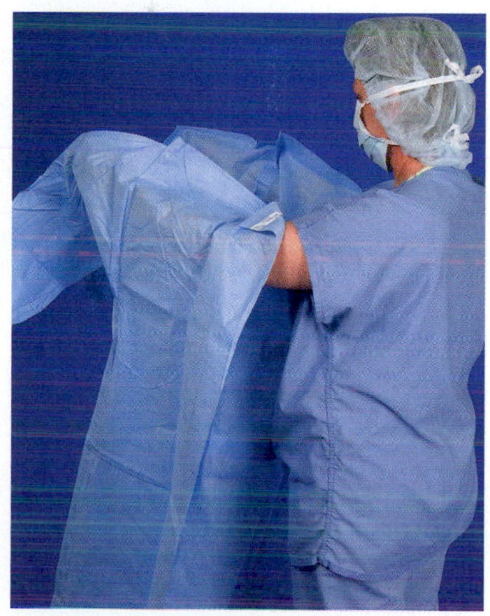

(continued on next page)

Procedure 23-6 ■ Sterile Gown and Gloves (Closed Method) (continued)

4. **Have a coworker** (or the circulating nurse, if you are in the surgical suite) stand behind you and pull the shoulders of the gown up and tie the neck tie. The coworker touches only the inside of the gown while pulling it up. *Touching only the inside prevents contamination of the gown with the nurse's hands.*

5. **Don sterile gloves** using the closed method. Open the sterile glove wrapper, keeping your fingers inside the sleeve of the gown. The outer wrapper has already been discarded.

Glove the dominant hand first:

a. With your nondominant hand, keeping your hands inside the gown sleeves, grasp the cuff of the glove for your dominant hand. Turn your dominant hand palm up. *Keeping the hand inside the cuff ensures that you are making contact with the sterile gown; sterile is touching sterile.*

b. Lay the glove on the dominant gown cuff, thumb side down, with the glove opening pointed toward the fingers and the thumb of the glove positioned over the thumb side of the dominant hand. ▼

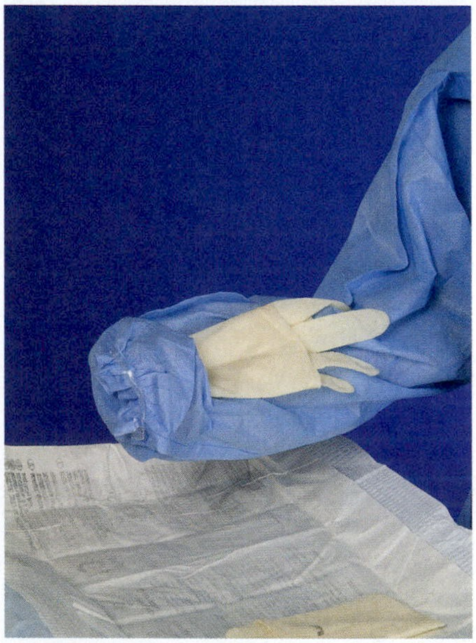

c. Keeping your dominant hand inside the sleeve, grasp the inside of the glove cuff. ▼

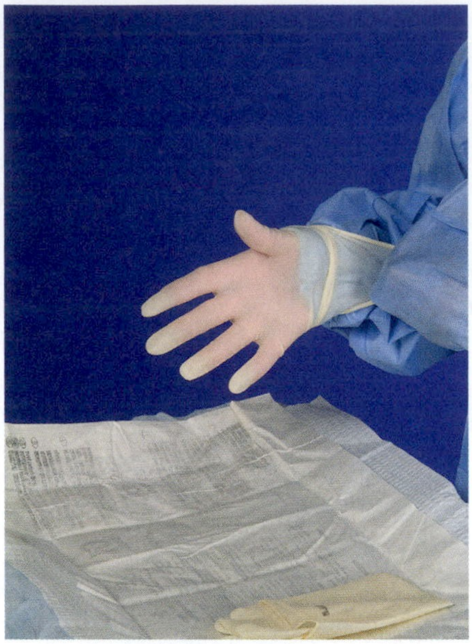

d. With your other hand (inside its sleeve), grasp the upper side of the glove cuff, and stretch it over the gown cuff.

e. Pull the sleeve of your gown up to pull the glove cuff over your wrist as you move your fingers into the glove fingers.

Glove the nondominant hand:

f. Place the fingers of your gloved hand under the cuff of the second glove.
   - Lay the glove on the forearm of your nondominant hand, thumb side down, with glove opening pointing toward the fingers.
   - Grasp and anchor the inside glove cuff with your nondominant (ungloved) hand through the gown, being careful to keep fingers inside the gown.

g. With your dominant (gloved) hand, pull the glove cuff over the cuff of the gown as you move your fingers into the glove. ▼

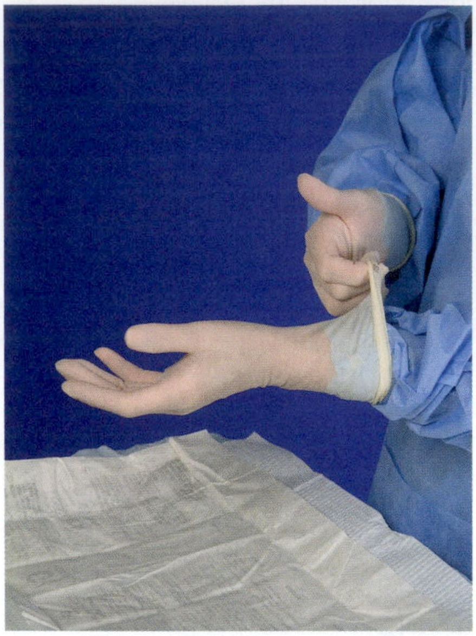

h. **Adjust the fingers in both gloves for a snug fit over the fingers.** *Maintains sterility of the gown and gloves by maintaining a closed system. The final adjustment of the gloves is done when both gloves are in place to prevent contaminating the gloves. Taut gloves, especially over the fingertips, allow for better feel and dexterity.*

6. **Grasp the waist tie on the gown**; then hand the tie to the circulating nurse or a coworker who is wearing a hair cover and mask. Your coworker will grab the tie with sterile forceps. *The tie is considered sterile. You will need help to pull it around you. A coworker can help you. Using sterile forceps keeps the tie sterile.* ▼

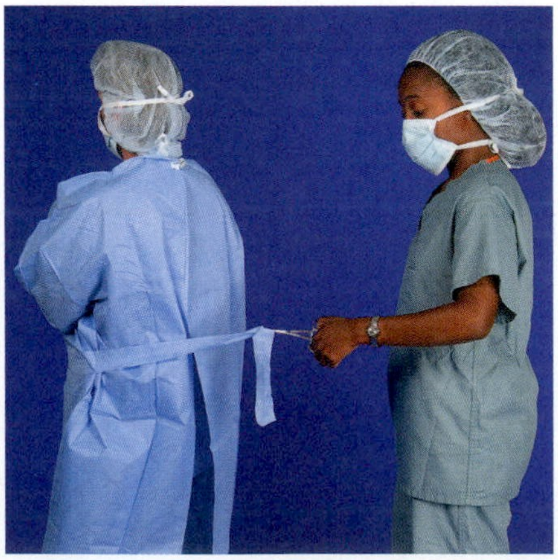

7. **Make a three-quarter turn**; then, receive the tie from your coworker.
Because only areas within your field of vision are considered sterile, a coworker must pull the waist tie around your waist.

8. **Secure the waist tie.**
Ensures that the gown is secured and will not expose a sterile field to your clothing.

Patient Teaching

If the patient is alert during the procedure, explain:

- The need for the sterile procedure
- Why he must not touch the drapes
- Why he must not move or talk once the drapes are in place
- Any special precautions during the procedure

Documentation

- Donning sterile gown and gloves does not require documentation.
- You will need to chart the procedure performed and how the patient tolerated it.
- In the surgical suite, the circulating nurse charts about the surgery and the patient's response.

? What if . . .

- **Your hand inadvertently comes through the cuff opening when putting on the gown?**

  Change gowns. The cuff would have been contaminated and would then contaminate your glove.

Practice Resources

AORN (2016, 2018); CDC (2002); Cowperthwaite, L., & Holm, R. L. (2015).

Thinking About the Procedure

The video **Sterile Gown and Gloves (Closed Method),** along with questions and suggested responses, is available on the ***Davis's Nursing Skills Videos*** Web site on FADavis.com.

Procedure 23-7 ■ Sterile Gloves (Open Method)

➤ For steps to follow in *all* procedures, refer to the Universal Steps for All Procedures found on the inside back cover. For this procedure, also refer to Clinical Insights 23-2, 23-3, and 23-4 if you need more information.

Equipment

- Sterile gloves of the correct size

➤ When performing the procedure, always identify your patient according to agency policy, using two identifiers, and be attentive to standard precautions, hand hygiene, patient safety and privacy, body mechanics, and documentation.

Procedure Steps

1. **Determine the correct size** of sterile glove. The gloves should be snug, but not tight.
Gloves that are too loose are more easily contaminated and make handling equipment or supplies difficult. Gloves that are too tight are uncomfortable and may tear during use.

2. **Assess the glove package** for intactness and expiration date. Do not use the gloves if the package is torn, has become moist, or is past the expiration date.
Torn packaging may allow the gloves to become contaminated. Moisture allows wicking and may cause contamination. Expired gloves are not considered sterile. ➤

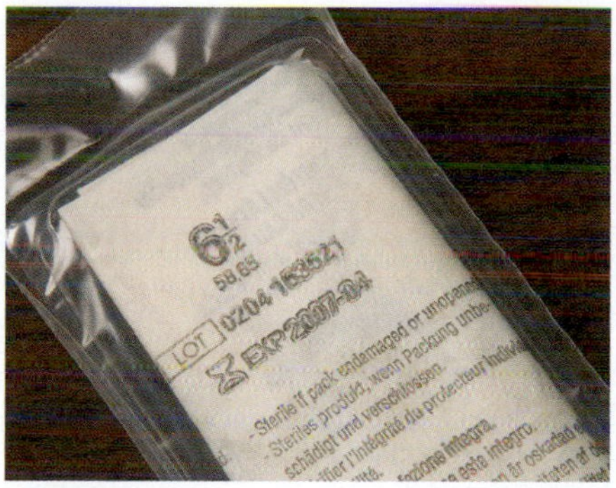

3. **Assess the patient's environment** for a clean, flat space with enough room to allow you to open the glove package. Don the gloves without touching a nonsterile item.
Inadvertently touching a nonsterile item will contaminate the gloves.

4. **Open the outer wrapper,** and place the inner glove package on a clean, dry surface.

5. **Open the inner glove package** so that the glove cuffs are closest to you. Be careful to fully open the flaps of the package so that they do not fold back over and contaminate the gloves.
The outer 1-inch border of the glove package is considered contaminated.

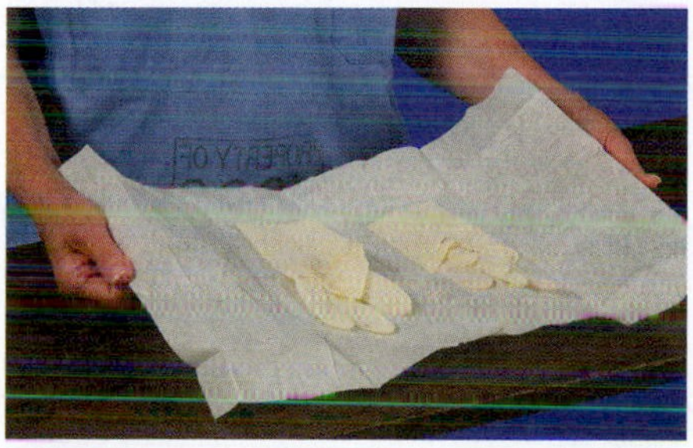

(continued on next page)

Procedure 23-7 ■ Sterile Gloves (Open Method) (continued)

6. **With your nondominant hand,** grasp the inner surface of the glove for the dominant hand.
   - Lift the glove up and away from the table, keeping it away from your body.
   - Do not touch anything else on the sterile field.

   The inside of the glove is not considered sterile because it is in contact with your skin. Lifting the glove up and away from the table prevents you from accidentally touching the table or your clothing while donning it.

7. **Slide your dominant hand** into the glove, keeping your hand and fingers above your waist and away from your body.

   The area below the waistline is considered contaminated. Keeping gloves away from your body prevents accidental contamination.

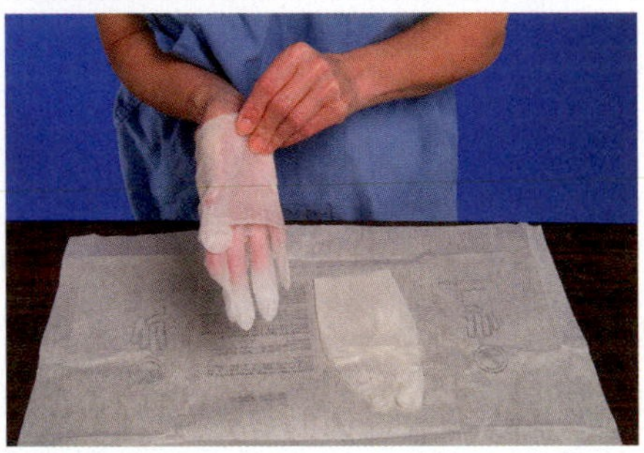

8. **Slide your gloved fingers under the cuff** of the glove for the nondominant hand, keeping your gloved thumb well away from your ungloved hand. Lift the glove up and away from the table and away from your body.

   The outside of the glove is sterile and may be touched with your sterile gloved hand.

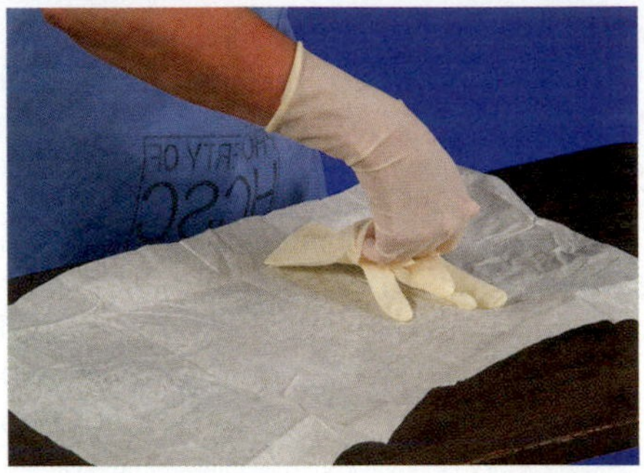

9. **With gloved fingers still under the cuff,** slide your nondominant hand into the glove and pull it on, being careful to avoid contact with your gloved hand, especially the thumb.

   As a general rule, when applying the second glove, touch glove to glove and skin to skin. The already-gloved hand may touch any of the sterile surfaces of the second glove. The second hand may touch only the inside of the glove—the portion that will have contact with the skin.

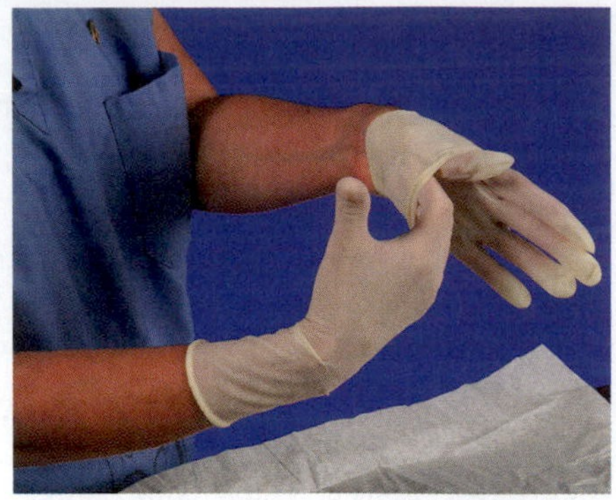

10. **Adjust both gloves to fit your fingers.** If necessary, pull the fingers of the gloves down so that no excess is at the fingertips.

    Adjusting your gloves after both have been donned decreases the risk of contamination and allows for greater dexterity during the procedure.

11. **Keep your hands between shoulder and waist level** in front of you.

    Keeps the gloves within your field of vision and helps avoid contamination.

NOTE: To remove soiled gloves after the procedure, refer to Procedure 23-3.

Patient Teaching

Explain why sterile gloves are needed for the procedure.

Home Care

- Many home care procedures are clean, rather than sterile. The client is in her own environment and not surrounded by other patients, who may serve as hosts for infection.
- You may need to teach caregivers how to apply sterile gloves for some procedures. No modifications are required. Demonstrate the procedure, and have the caregiver do a return demonstration.

Documentation

- No special documentation is needed for sterile gloving.
- Chart the procedure you performed and the patient's response to the procedure.

Practice Resources

AORN (2016, 2018); CDC (n.d.); Cowperthwaite, L., & Holm, R. L. (2015).

Thinking About the Procedure

The video **Sterile Gloves (Open Method)**, along with questions and suggested responses, is available on the ***Davis's Nursing Skills Videos*** Web site on FADavis.com.

Procedure 23-8 ■ Sterile Fields

➤ For steps to follow in *all* procedures, refer to the Universal Steps for All Procedures found on the inside back cover. For this procedure, also refer to Clinical Insights 23-2 and 23-3 if you need more information.

Equipment

- Package of sterile supplies required for the procedure
- Sterile gloves of the correct size

Procedure 23-8A ■ Setting Up a Sterile Field

➤ When performing the procedure, always identify your patient according to agency policy, using two identifiers, and be attentive to standard precautions, hand hygiene, patient safety and privacy, body mechanics, and documentation.

Procedure Steps

- **Close doors, and limit the number of people in the area.**
  Air currents can carry dust and microorganisms.
- **Prepare a sterile field as close as possible to the time of use.**
  To minimize the opportunity for contamination via air currents.

1. **Check all packaging of supplies and equipment** to be sure all are intact and expiration dates are current.
   Only sterile items should enter a sterile field. Any compromise in packaging means that the item is assumed not to be sterile.

2. **Arrange the environment** for performing the sterile procedure.
   a. Remove all items from the surface you will use to set up the sterile field.
   Inadequate space causes inadvertent contamination during sterile procedures.
   b. Position the patient as needed for the procedure before setting up the sterile field.
   Allows you to efficiently proceed with the procedure. Once the sterile field is established, air movement can create contamination of the sterile items.

Procedure Variation. Using Sterile Packaged Equipment

3. **Place the sterile package** on a clean, dry surface.
   Prevents contamination of the sterile item. If a surface is damp, strike-through may occur, making the item unsterile. ➤

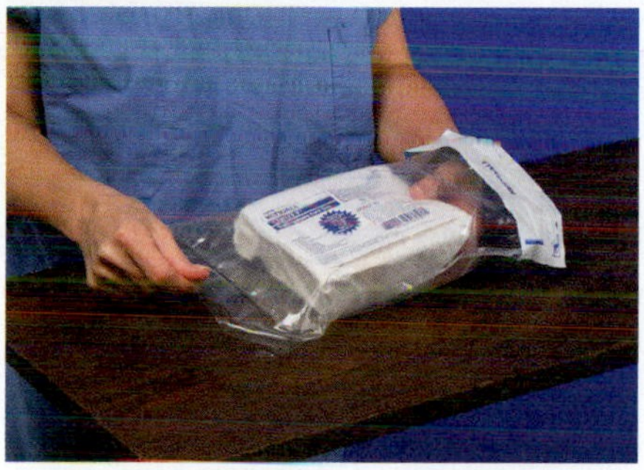

4. **Open the flap away from you first** to prevent passing an unsterile arm over the sterile items.
   If you move an unsterile item over a sterile field, the field is no longer considered sterile. ▼

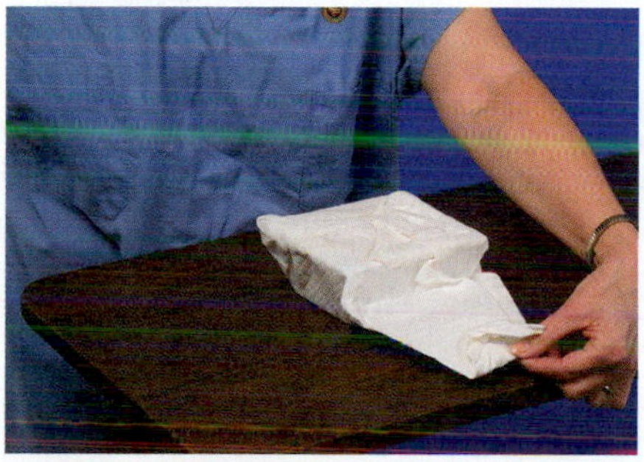

5. **Open the side flaps.** ▼

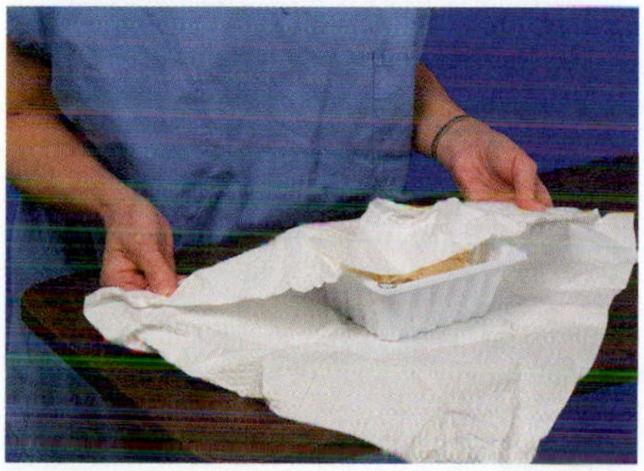

6. **Pull the final flap toward you.** The wrapper is now the sterile field. Touch the inside of the wrapper only after you don sterile gloves.
   - The area 1 inch from the edge of the wrapper and 1 inch from the table edge is considered unsterile.
   - Do not readjust the sterile area after the package has been opened.
   Only the horizontal surface of the draped area is considered sterile. Any part of the sterile wrapper that falls below the level of the sterile area (e.g., top of the table) is considered unsterile. If you move the field after opening, the field shifts and places unsterile areas of the wrapper on the surface. ▼

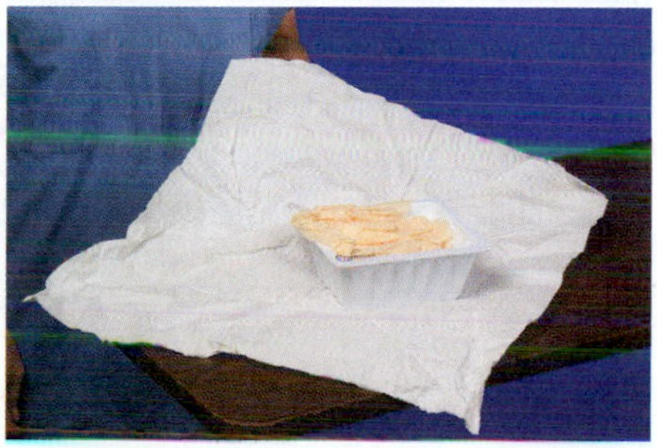

Procedure Variation. Opening a Fabric- or Paper-Wrapped Sterile Package

7. **Check and remove** the chemical indicator strip.
   Confirms that the package was sterilized. The package usually is also dated.

8. **Remove the outer wrapper,** and place the inner wrapped package on a clean, dry surface.
   The outer wrapper is not considered sterile and is discarded.

(continued on next page)

Procedure 23-8 ■ Sterile Fields (continued)

9. **Open the inner wrapper** following the same technique described in Steps 3 through 6.

Procedure Variation. Using a Sterile Drape
Omit Steps 3 through 6.

10. **Place the package on a clean, dry surface:**
    a. With the outer wrapper still on the package, hold the edge of the package flap down toward the table.
    b. Grasp the top edge of the package, and peel back.
    The sterile drape is inside the outer wrapper. This maneuver helps open the package without contaminating the sterile drape.

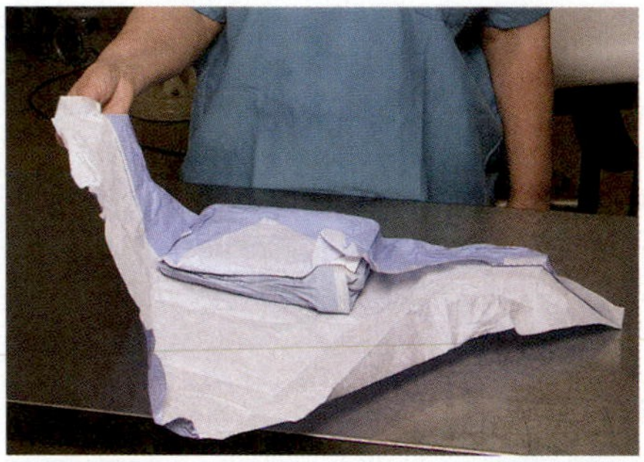

11. **Pick up the sterile drape by the corner.**
    - Allow the drape to fall open, away from your body and away from unsterile surfaces.
    - Place it on a clean, dry surface by touching only the edge of the drape.
    - Do not fan the drape.

    A 1-inch border around the sterile drape is considered unsterile.

12. In some situations, when placing a sterile drape (e.g., under a patient), you may need to protect your gloved hands by cuffing the drape over your hands.

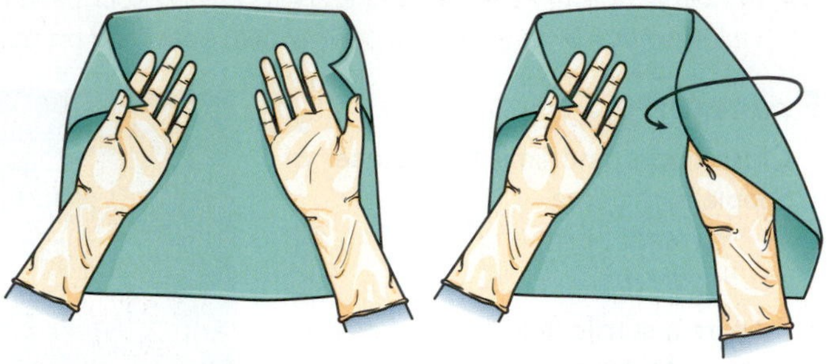

Protecting gloved hands

Procedure 23-8B ■ Adding Supplies to a Sterile Field

➤ When performing the procedure, always identify your patient according to agency policy, using two identifiers, and be attentive to standard precautions, hand hygiene, patient safety and privacy, body mechanics, and documentation.

Procedure Steps

1. **Before adding items to a sterile field,** inspect them for proper packaging, integrity, and inclusion of a sterilization indicator. Never assume an item is sterile. If there is any doubt about its sterility, consider it contaminated.

2. **Hold the sterile package in your dominant hand.** Grasping the corner of the wrapper, peel each corner back with your nondominant hand.
The inside of the wrapper is sterile and will be used as a barrier when placing the sterile item onto a sterile field.

3. **Holding the contents several inches above the field,** allow the supplies to drop onto the field inside the 1-inch border of the sterile field. Do not let your arms pass over the sterile field.
By holding the package upside down, you ensure that the sterile part of the package is facing the sterile field and that you deposit the item onto the sterile field.

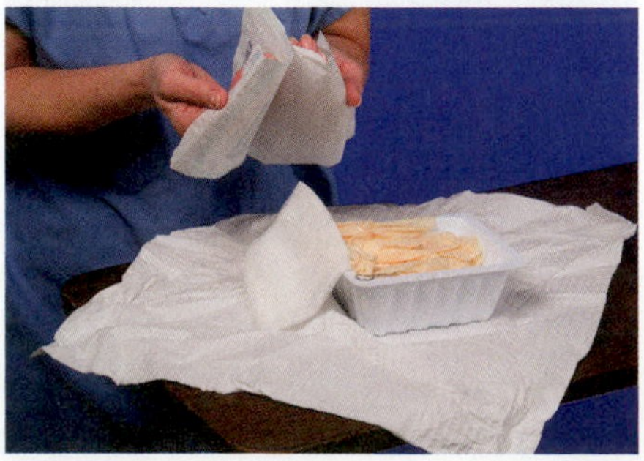

4. **Dispose of the wrapper**; then, continue opening any needed supplies for the procedure.

Key Point: *Once sterile gloves are on, you will not be able to add items without contaminating the gloves.*

Procedure 23-8C ■ Adding Sterile Solutions to a Sterile Field

➤ When performing the procedure, always identify your patient according to agency policy, using two identifiers, and be attentive to standard precautions, hand hygiene, patient safety and privacy, body mechanics, and documentation.

Procedure Steps

1. **Use a sterile bowl or container.** Place it on the side of the sterile field closest to you.
   Prevents you from reaching over and thereby contaminating the field.

2. **Check that the sterile solution** is correct; then, confirm that the solution concentration is correct and that the expiration date has not passed.

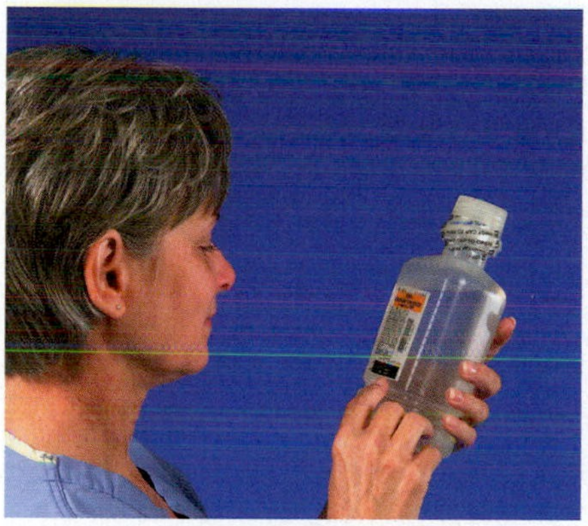

3. **Remove the cap from the solution bottle** by lifting it directly up. Throw the cap away.
   The edge of the container is considered contaminated after the contents have been poured and the sterility of the contents cannot be ensured if the cap is replaced.

4. **Hold the bottle 4 to 6 inches above the bowl,** and pour the needed amount of the solution into the bowl.
   Prevents you from inadvertently touching the sterile bowl with the bottle and thereby contaminating the bowl. Limited height reduces the risk of splashing, which strikes through and contaminates a cloth or permeable sterile field. A disposable sterile drape generally has a plastic membrane in the middle to prevent strike-through.

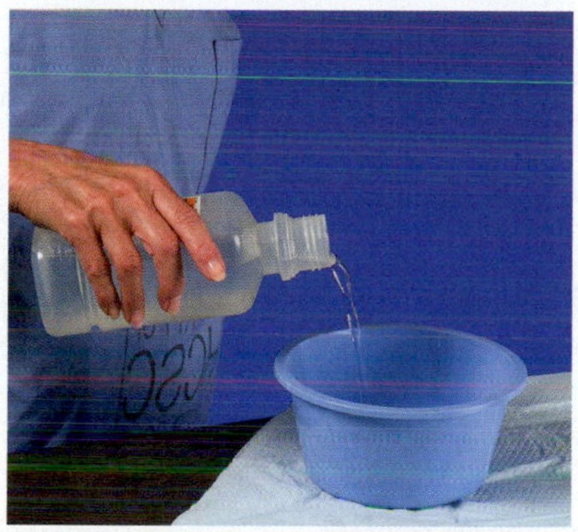

5. **Discard the remaining solution.**
   Reusing open containers may cause contamination as a result of drops contacting the unsterile areas and running back over the container opening.

6. **Before donning sterile gloves** to perform the procedure, double-check that all supplies have been added to the field using sterile technique.
   - Do not leave the sterile field unattended.
   - Do not turn your back to the sterile field.

   If a sterile item is out of your field of vision, it is no longer considered sterile because airborne particles, insects, or liquids could contaminate the field.

Home Care

- Most sterile procedures in the home are done by visiting nurses.
- Procedures performed by clients or family members are usually clean, rather than sterile.

Documentation

- You will not document the actual setting up of the sterile field.
- Document the procedure, your assessment of the patient's tolerance for the procedure, and your assessment of the area being treated by the procedure.

? What if . . .

- **The nurse observes a breach in sterility by the surgeon?**
  The nurse's duty is to protect the patient above all else, even when the situation is uncomfortable with the healthcare provider. The nurse is obligated to follow the institution's policy and advocate for patient safety.

Practice Resources

AORN (2016, 2018); Simko (2012).

Thinking About the Procedure

The videos **Setting Up a Sterile Field; Adding Supplies to a Sterile Field;** and **Adding Sterile Solutions to a Sterile Field,** along with questions and suggested responses, are available on the ***Davis's Nursing Skills Videos*** Web site on FADavis.com.

CLINICAL INSIGHTS

Clinical Insight 23-1 ➤ Guidelines for Hand Hygiene

Handwashing

When to Wash

- When hands are visibly dirty or soiled with blood or body fluids
- When arriving on and leaving the patient care unit
- Before direct contact with a patient, even if you intend to wear procedure gloves
- Before donning gloves (either procedure or sterile)
- When gloves are changed during a procedure
- After removing gloves
- After contact with a patient's intact skin (e.g., when lifting a patient or taking a blood pressure)
- After contact with body fluids, mucous membranes, non-intact skin, and wound dressings even if hands are not visibly soiled
- When moving from a contaminated body site to a clean body site during patient care
- Before and after contact with objects and equipment in the patient's immediate vicinity
- Before eating and after using a restroom (Use soap and water.)
- Before and after touching any area on your face and hair

What to Use

- Use alcohol-based handrub (at least 60% alcohol) for routine hand hygiene and if hands are not visibly soiled.
- Use soap and water:
  When hands are dirty or visibly soiled.
  After using a restroom.

If there is potential for exposure to *Bacillus anthracis* (or other spore-producing bacteria, such as *C. difficile*). *Alcohol-based solutions are not effective against spores.*

- Use warm, not hot, water.
- Use disposable paper towels.

How to Wash

Refer to Procedure 23-1: Hand Hygiene.

Fingernails

- Keep natural fingernails short (one-quarter inch or less) and avoid wearing fingernail polish or artificial nails in the perioperative setting (AORN, 2018; WHO, 2009). *Chipped nail polish can contaminate a sterile environment when gloves are not worn or are punctured or torn. Artificial nails, including gels, acrylics, and resins harbor microorganisms and impede proper hand hygiene.*
- Scrub the undersides of fingernail with soap and water and nail brush every time you wash your hands.
- Clean nail grooming tools before use.
- Avoid biting or chewing nails or cuticles. Never rip a hangnail; instead, trim with a sanitized nail trimmer (CDC, 2009b).

Jewelry

- Remove all jewelry before beginning hand hygiene, or surgical hand scrub. CDC (2013). *Hand jewelry may make donning gloves more difficult and cause gloves to tear more readily.*
- The WHO (2009) prohibits any jewelry or watches on the hands of the surgical team. *Skin underneath rings is more heavily colonized than comparable areas of skin on bare fingers.*
- We recommend that you not wear a watch or rings in the clinical setting, especially rings with stones. If your agency permits you to wear jewelry, clean it thoroughly and often.

Practice Resources

AORN (2016, 2018); Boyce, J., & Pittet, D. (2002); CDC). (2017, March 17, updated); Pittet., D., Boyce, J. M., & Allegranzi, B. (eds.) (2017); Rupp, M., Fitzgerald, T., Puumala, S., et al. (2008); Siegel, J., Rhinehart, E., Jackson, M., et al. (2007); WHO (2009).

Clinical Insight 23-2 ➤ Providing a Clean Patient Environment

Use the following guidelines along with standard precautions for all patients.

Supplies and Equipment

- Do not stock rooms with unnecessary supplies.
- Consider supplies that are brought into a patient's room contaminated. Do not return them to the linen or supply cart; instead, handle them according to agency policy.
- Items brought from the patient's home and gifts from visitors are considered unclean.
- Mobile devices should be cleaned (e.g., pagers, smartphones, point-of-care keyboards, and medication administration devices). Be sure to perform hand hygiene after using such a device.
- Wipe stethoscopes with alcohol before use on a patient.
- Disinfect reusable equipment that is soiled with blood or body fluids according to agency policy—typically, autoclaving, ethylene oxide gas, or dry heat.
- Do not reuse equipment for the care of another patient until it has been cleaned and processed appropriately.
- Dispose of single-use equipment that is soiled with blood or body fluids in appropriate biohazard containers.
- Wear gloves when handling equipment that is visibly contaminated. Perform hand hygiene.

Linens

- While wearing gloves, handle contaminated linens carefully.
  To prevent skin and mucous membrane exposure, contamination of clothing, and transfer of microorganisms to other patients or the environment.
- Bag and remove soiled linens from the room immediately.
  Linens may harbor microorganisms that may transfer to your clothing, open skin, or mucous membranes and could then be carried to other clients or the environment.

Uniforms and Lab Coats

- Do not wear a uniform (e.g., scrubs) or a lab coat for more than a day without laundering.
  Care provider clothing is often contaminated when moving from patient to patient. The traditional lab coats are considered vehicles for the transfer of pathogens (AST, 2008; CDC, updated 2015).
- Visibly soiled, wet, and/or contaminated scrub attire must be changed as soon as possible (Scott, Goodyear, Nicoloro, et al., 2015).
- If you wash your scrubs at home, use warm or hot water and detergent. However, exposure to multidrug-resistant organisms is possible, so add bleach.
- Home laundering of surgical attire is not recommended.

Spills and Waste

- Empty and clean bedpans, urinals, and emesis basins immediately after use.
- Place soiled dressings, drains, and so forth in appropriate waterproof bags for disposal and *never* in an open trashcan.
- Wipe up small spills from tabletops and floors. Notify the housekeeping or environmental services department for large spills.

Needles and Sharps

Do not recap, bend, break, or hand-manipulate used needles. If recapping is necessary, use a one-handed "scoop" technique. Place used sharps in puncture-resistant containers.

Practice Resources

AST (2008); AORN (2016); CDC (2002); Siegel, J. D., Rhinehart, E., Jackson, M., et al. (2007).

Clinical Insight 23-3 ➤ Following CDC Standard Precautions

Key Point: *Standard precautions (Tier 1) apply to all clients and should be used whenever there is a possibility of coming in contact with blood, body fluids (except sweat), excretions and secretions, mucous membranes, and breaks in the skin.*
These precautions are designed to protect you from exposure to potential pathogens, to decrease the likelihood that you will transmit pathogens among patients, and to protect the patient from microorganisms that you may carry.

Assume that every person may be infected or colonized by an organism that could be transmitted to others.

STANDARD PRECAUTIONS	RECOMMENDATIONS
Hand Hygiene	■ Perform hand hygiene after touching blood, body fluids, secretions, excretions, contaminated items; immediately after removing gloves; between patient contacts. Refer to Clinical Insight 23-1 for details.
Respiratory Hygiene/ Cough Etiquette (for Patients)	■ Instruct symptomatic persons to cover mouth/nose when sneezing/coughing. ■ Provide and use tissues and dispose in a no-touch container. ■ Perform hand hygiene after soiling hands with respiratory secretions or after using a tissue or covering the mouth/nose. ■ Wear a surgical mask if tolerated or do not come within 3 feet of another person, if possible. Some patients may not be able to tolerate the decreased oxygen that is available when breathing room air through a mask.
Masks and Eye Protection (for Nurses)	■ Wear a mask and eye protection or a face shield to protect mucous membranes of the eyes, nose, and mouth during patient care activities that are likely to generate splashes or sprays of blood, body fluids, secretions, and excretions.
Patient Placement	Place the patient in a single-patient room if: ■ The patient is at increased risk of transmitting or acquiring infection ■ Does not maintain appropriate hygiene ■ Is likely to contaminate the environment ■ Is at increased risk of developing adverse outcome following infection
Gowns	■ Wear a clean, nonsterile, nonpermeable gown during procedures and activities when you anticipate contact of clothing or exposed skin with blood or body fluids, secretions, and excretions (e.g., when there is a risk of spray or splash onto clothing). ■ Promptly remove the gown once it is soiled. Avoid contaminating clothing when removing the gown. ■ Perform hand hygiene after removing the gown. ■ See Procedures 23-2 and 23-3, Donning PPE and Removing PPE.
Needles and Sharps	■ Never recap, bend, or break used needles, or otherwise manipulate them using both hands, or use any other technique that involves directing the point of a needle toward any part of the body. Instead, use either a one-handed "scoop" technique or a mechanical device designed for holding the needle sheath (see Procedure 26-10, Recapping Needles ...). ■ Use safety features, when available. ■ Place "sharps" in puncture-resistant containers for disposal.
Patient Resuscitation	■ Use one-way valve mouthpieces, resuscitation bags, or other ventilation devices as an alternative to mouth-to-mouth resuscitation methods in situations where there is a predictable need for resuscitation. *To prevent contact between the rescuer's and the client's mucous membranes and airflow, thus preventing transmission of microorganisms.*

Clinical Insight 23-3 ➤ Following CDC Standard Precautions—cont'd

STANDARD PRECAUTIONS	RECOMMENDATIONS
Soiled Patient Care Equipment, Environment, Textiles, and Laundry	▪ Wear gloves if the equipment or laundry is visibly contaminated. ▪ Handle equipment, textiles, and laundry in a manner to prevent transfer of microorganisms to others and the environment. ▪ Perform hand hygiene. ▪ Develop procedures for routine care, cleaning, and disinfection of environmental surfaces, especially frequently touched surfaces in patient care areas.
Gloves	***When to Wear*** ▪ If you have an area of irritation or a break in the skin, wear gloves or apply an occlusive dressing during patient contact. ▪ Wear gloves when contact with blood or other potentially infectious materials, mucous membranes, and nonintact skin could occur. ***When to Remove or Change*** ▪ Remove gloves immediately after caring for a patient. Avoid touching clean items, environmental surfaces, or another patient. ▪ Do not wear the same gloves for care of more than one patient; do not wash gloves and reuse gloves between patient contacts. ▪ Change gloves during patient care if moving from a contaminated site to a clean site on the body. ▪ Change gloves between tasks or procedures on the same patient if you have made contact with material that may contain a high concentration of microorganisms. ***Use and Storage*** ▪ When preparing for a procedure, first, collect equipment, and place at the bedside ready for use; then, perform hand hygiene, and don gloves just before performing the procedure. Donning gloves ahead of time increases the risk for contamination before the procedure. ▪ Do not carry gloves in your pocket. Keep them in their original box and remove them when and where required. ▪ Do not store gloves on top of trash containers or on windowsills. ▪ Handwashing or disinfection is required regardless of whether gloves are used or changed. Gloves are not completely impermeable to microorganisms; furthermore, they may leak or tear. Hands can also be easily contaminated when removing gloves.

Practice Resources

Boyce, J., & Pittet, D. (2002); CDC (n. d.); CDC (2017, February 28, updated); CDC (2017, January 16, updated); CDC. (2017, March 17, updated); Pratt, R., Pellowe, C., Wilson, J., et al. (2007); Siegel, J., Rhinehart, E., Jackson, M., et al. (2007).

Clinical Insight 23-4 ➤ Following Transmission-Based (Tier 2) Precautions

When to Use Transmission-Based Precautions

Use when the routes of transmission are not completely interrupted using Standard Precautions alone. Refer to Clinical Insight 23-3 if you need to review standard precautions. *Pathogens may be transmitted by contact, droplet, or air. Each mode of transmission requires a different approach to prevent infection and has a different set of precautions.*

Contact Precautions

When to Use: Use contact precautions when **direct contact** with the patient or the patient's environment (e.g., draining wounds, dressings, patient supplies, and secretions) can lead to spread of the pathogen. **Indirect contact**, or contact with fomites, can also transmit pathogens that spread by this method.

Patient Placement and Transport

- Consult with an infection preventionist for patient placement.
- Place in a private room, when possible.
- If no private room is available, place patient in a room with a patient with an active infection caused by the same organism and no other infections.
- When transporting the patient, ensure that infected or colonized areas of the body are contained and covered.
- *Ambulatory care:* Place the patient in an examination room or cubicle as soon as possible.

Personal Protective Equipment

- Don clean, nonsterile gloves for any contact with the patient's intact skin. Put them on when entering the room.
- Wear a clean gown if you anticipate your clothing may contact the patient or any contaminated items in the room.
- Remove PPE, and observe hand hygiene before leaving the room. Be careful that your skin and clothing do not contact environmental surfaces on the way out of the room.

Equipment, Supplies, and Environment

- Keep contact precaution supplies just outside the patient's room on a cart.
- Double-bag all linen and trash (or use a single waterproof bag), and clearly mark as contaminated.
- Use disposable equipment (e.g., blood pressure cuffs), if possible; otherwise, clean and disinfect the equipment according to institutional policy before removing them from the room and before use on another patient.
- Ensure that the patient room is cleaned and disinfected at least daily.
- *Home care:* Limit the amount of nondisposable equipment brought into the home. If possible, leave the equipment in the home until discharge from home care. If not, disinfect items, or place them in a plastic bag for sanitation and transport to a reprocessing area.

Other

- Follow any additional precautions specific to the microorganism.
- Discontinue contact precautions according to pathogen-specific recommendations.

Droplet Precautions

When to Use: Droplets can spread infection by direct contact with mucous membranes or through indirect contact—for example, suctioning or touching a bedside table that was contaminated with droplets and then rubbing your eyes. Use droplet precautions when pathogens can be spread via moist, large droplets (e.g., sneezing, coughing, talking).

Patient Placement and Transport

- If no private room, ensure that the patients are physically separated by more than 3 feet. Keep the privacy curtain closed. Consult with an infection preventionist for patient placement. *A private room provides the most effective protection.*
- Limit transport outside the room to medically necessary purposes; if transport is necessary, the patient should wear a mask.

Personal Protective Equipment

- Keep droplet precaution supplies just outside the patient's room on a cart.
- Wear a mask when working within 3 feet of the patient. Don the mask on entry into the room. The need to wear goggles remains an unresolved issue. Follow agency policy.
- Change PPE, and perform hand hygiene between contacts with patients in the same room, regardless of one or both patients being on droplet precautions.

Other

- Instruct patients to observe respiratory hygiene/cough etiquette.
- Discontinue droplet precautions according to pathogen-specific recommendations.

Airborne Precautions

When to Use: Use airborne precautions to control the spread of infections that are transmitted person to person through air currents (e.g., ventilation system, fanning sheets, sweeping the floor).

Patient Placement and Transport

- Place the patient in an airborne infection isolation room (AIIR)—one with negative pressure that discharges and exchanges the air outside or through a high-efficiency particulate air (HEPA) filtration system. Monitor air pressure daily (usually this is via an electronic device with an alarm).
- If such a room is not available, transfer the patient to a facility where one is available.
- Keep the room door closed when not required for entry and exit. *To maintain the negative pressure and contain the airborne organisms.*
- In the event of an outbreak involving large numbers of patients who require airborne precautions, consult with infection preventionists for patient placement.
- Limit moving the patient out of the room only for medically necessary purposes. If transport is necessary, cover any infectious skin lesions, and have the patient wear a mask. Notify the receiving department to take airborne precautions.

Clinical Insight 23-4 ➤ Following Transmission-Based Precautions—cont'd

- *Ambulatory or emergency care*: Triage and identify patients with suspected airborne precautions upon entry to the agency. Place the patient in an AIIR as soon as possible. If one is not available, place a mask on the patient, and place him in an exam room. Do not reuse the room for at least 1 hour after the patient leaves it, or according to agency policy.

Personal Protective Equipment

- Keep airborne isolation supplies just outside the patient's room on a cart.
- Don a mask on entering the room. Wear a special, fit-tested, approved mask (e.g., N-95 respirator) if the patient is suspected of having pulmonary tuberculosis or smallpox.
- Remove your respirator/mask outside the room after closing the door. If the respirator is not disposable, clean and store it according to the manufacturer's instructions.
- When using a respirator mask, check the seal. Hold your hands over the respirator and exhale. If you feel air around your nose, adjust the nosepiece; if you feel air at the edges, adjust the straps.
- When the patient has rubeola, chickenpox, or disseminated zoster, the CDC does not recommend use of PPE if, based on your history of vaccination or disease, you presume you are immune to the disease. If a hospitalized patient has or is suspected of having rubeola or varicella, only immunized caregivers should provide care to that patient.

Other

- Discontinue airborne precautions according to the pathogen-specific recommendations of the CDC.
- Tape a waterproof bag to the bedside. *To facilitate proper disposal of tissues.*

Practice Resources

Centers for Disease Control and Prevention (CDC) (2017, February 28, updated); CDC (2017, March 17, updated); Pratt, R. J., Pellowe, C. M., Wilson, J. A., et al. (2007); Siegel, J. D., Rhinehart, E., Jackson, M., et al. (2007; 2006, updated 2017, February 15).

DIAGNOSTIC TESTING

Diagnostic Testing

Common Tests for Evaluating the Presence of or Risk for Infection

TEST	DESCRIPTION
White blood cell (WBC) count with differential	A breakdown of the number and types of WBCs; normal WBC count is 5,000–10,000/mm^3.
Blood cultures	A sample of blood placed on culture media and evaluated for growth of pathogens. Normally, should show no growth of infectious microorganisms.
Urine cultures	Urine is normally sterile, with no microorganism growth.
Throat cultures, wound cultures	Presence of microorganisms is normal, but there should be no growth of infectious microorganisms. For the most reliable results, blood cultures should be obtained from peripheral sites, using venipuncture performed by trained phlebotomists, unless a culture is specifically ordered from a central catheter or peripherally inserted central catheter.
Disease titers	Blood tests for specific disease immunity (e.g., to rubella).
Panels to evaluate specific disease exposure	Blood tests to evaluate exposure to specific diseases (e.g., HIV, hepatitis).
Immunoglobulin (IgG, IgM) levels	Blood tests to evaluate humoral immunity status.
Cross-reactive protein (CRP)	A blood test to measure inflammatory change or bacterial infection.
Agglutinins, warm or cold	Used to diagnose atypical infections by detecting antigens in the blood.
Erythrocyte (red blood cell [RBC]) sedimentation rate (ESR, or sed rate)	A measure of inflammatory changes. Sed rate increases with inflammation. Normally it is at 15 mm/hr for men and <20 mm/hr for women.
Iron level	Normally 60–90 g/100 mg. Lower in chronic infection.

CLINICALJUDGMENT

Applying the Full-Spectrum Nursing Model

PATIENT SITUATION

Mr. Long, a frail elderly man, is in the hospital because he has become dehydrated and needs intravenous fluids and other supportive care. The nurse administered intravenous fluids. Mr. Long also has a fairly large pressure injury (bedsore), which was cultured recently and found to be infected with *Staphylococcus aureus*. The nurse wore gloves to treat the ulcer. While doing so, she noticed that the IV was infusing too fast and, without thinking, regulated the IV without removing her soiled gloves. The next nurse to regulate the IV did so with her bare hands, and then, without realizing it, rubbed her neck. Later, the nurse developed a boil on her neck, which was infected with *S. aureus*.

THINKING

1. *Theoretical Knowledge:*
   a. What are the six links in the chain of infection?
   b. Why do you think the *S. aureus* was able to thrive in Mr. Long's pressure injury?
   c. What are the three modes of transmission of microorganisms? Which one is the most frequent mode of transmission?
2. *Critical Thinking (Reflecting):*
   a. What was the reservoir for the *S. aureus*?
   b. What was the exit from Mr. Long?
   c. What was (were) the fomite(s) for transmission to the nurse?
   d. What was the portal of entry into the nurse?

DOING

3. *Nursing Process (Implementation):* In addition to wearing gloves, what other PPE (if any) does the nurse need if she is performing decubitus care and changing Mr. Long's bed linens?

CARING

4. *Self-Knowledge and Ethical Knowledge:* Think of one instance in the clinical setting in which you did *not* follow standard precautions. Why do you think that happened?

Critical Thinking and Clinical Judgment

1. You notice that your clinical instructor is not washing his hands between patients. What should you do?
2. As you are gowning and gloving for your first experience in the operating room, you become nervous and forget the proper procedure for applying sterile surgical garb. How should you handle this situation?
3. What action should you take if you contaminate yourself while gowning and gloving?
4. Refer to Procedure 23-7, the open method for donning sterile gloves. In the photograph at Step 7, you can see that the nurse has a sterile glove on her right hand and is touching the glove with her bare left hand. Is the nurse breaking the "sterile-touches-sterile" principle? Explain your thinking.

5. Refer to Procedure 23-6, the closed method of donning a sterile gown and gloves. Examine the very last photograph, in which one nurse is preparing to turn and receive her gown tie from a coworker. The gowned nurse has already donned sterile gloves, using the closed method. When the gowned nurse turns to receive the tie, what must she take care to not touch? What can she touch?

6. For each of the following concepts, use critical thinking to describe how or why it is important to nursing, patient care, or promoting asepsis and preventing infection. Note that these are *not* to be merely definitions.

Chain of infection	Standard precautions
Pathogens	Transmission-based precautions
Asepsis	Protective isolation
Healthcare-related infections	Sterile
Multidrug-resistant organisms (MDROs)	Medical asepsis
Contamination	Surgical asepsis

What Are the Main Points in This Chapter?

- The chain of infection consists of six links that must all be present for infection to be transmitted from one individual to another: infectious agent, reservoir, portal of exit, mode of transmission, portal of entry, and susceptible host.
- Pathogens are strains of bacteria, viruses, fungi, protozoa, helminths, and prions that cause disease.
- Drug-resistant and multidrug-resistant organisms (MDROs) have mutated to develop resistance to one or more classes of antimicrobial drugs. They are a serious problem because (1) options for treating MDRO infections are limited; (2) they are associated with serious illness, increased hospitalization, and higher death rates; and (3) they are associated with serious illness and increased mortality.
- Many emerging pathogens are airborne and widely spread before the carrier shows any symptoms. They have the potential for causing epidemics and pandemics.
- Infectious illnesses typically follow five predictable stages: incubation, prodromal stage, illness, decline, and convalescence.
- Primary body defenses, such as intact skin and mucous membranes, block entry of pathogens into the body.
- Invading microorganisms trigger the body's secondary defenses, which include phagocytosis, the complement cascade, the inflammatory response, and fever.
- The humoral immune response results in the production of antibodies that neutralize pathogens or trigger their destruction.
- The cell-mediated immune response results in the production of T cells that destroy infected body cells.
- Nutrition, hygiene, rest, exercise, stress reduction, and immunization protect the body against infection.
- Anything that weakens the body's defenses or increases the person's exposure to pathogens makes the person more susceptible to infection. Such factors include illness, injury, medical treatment and certain medications, infancy or advanced age, frequent public contact, and various lifestyle habits.
- Medical asepsis requires that objects and surfaces in the healthcare environment be disinfected.
- Thorough handwashing markedly decreases the transmission of infection and is the most important aspect of medical asepsis.
- Standard precautions are used with all clients whenever there is a possibility of contact with blood, body fluids (except sweat), excretions and secretions, mucous membranes, and break in the skin.
- Transmission-based precautions are added to standard precautions when there is concern about transmission of infection via contact, droplets, or air currents.
- Isolation precautions are designed to prevent the spread of disease, not to isolate the person who has the disease.
- Surgical asepsis reduces patient contact with *any* microorganisms.
- Sterile technique is required in many patient treatments, such as administering an injection, starting an intravenous line, or performing a sterile dressing change.
- Exposure to blood, body secretions, or body tissues containing blood or secretions requires immediate action. Minimize the exposure by washing hands or flushing the area thoroughly. Contact the infection preventionist or employee health nurse as soon after the exposure as possible, complete an incident report, and seek medical care.
- The task of the infection preventionist is to minimize the number of infections in the healthcare facility.
- A key factor in minimizing infectious outbreaks is recognizing unusual disease patterns.

Knowledge Map

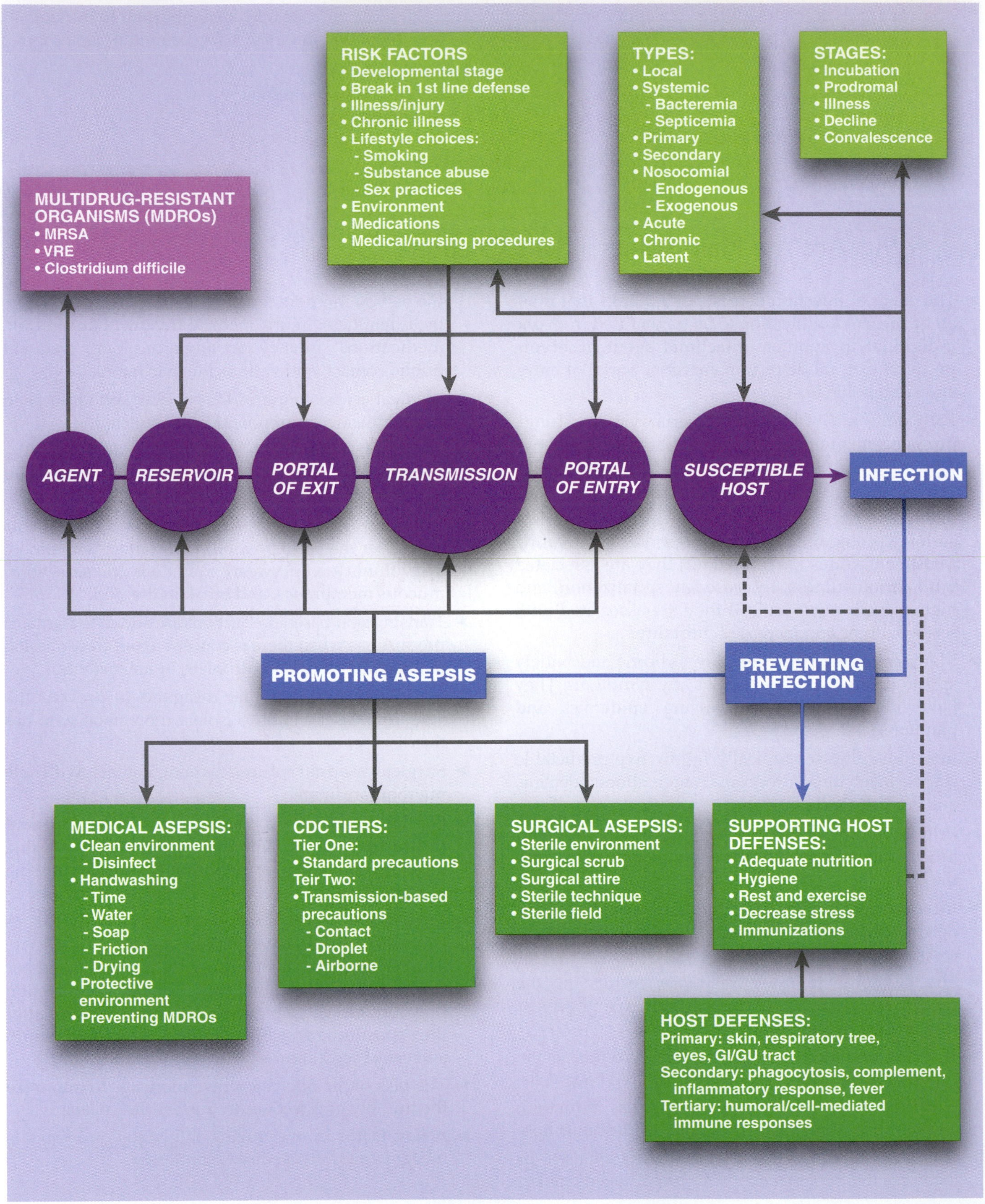

CHAPTER 24

Promoting Safety

STUDENT RESOURCES

The questions and exercises in this book allow you to practice the kind of thinking you will use as a full-spectrum nurse. Critical-thinking questions usually have more than one right answer, so we do not provide "correct answers" for these features. Try to answer these questions yourself. It is more important to develop your nursing judgment than to just cover content. You will learn more by discussing the questions with your peers. If you are still unsure, see the Davis Advantage chapter resources for suggested responses.

To explore learning resources for this chapter,

Go to Davis Advantage and find:

Answers and Suggested Responses for all questions in this chapter

Concept Map

Knowledge Map

References and Bibliography

Lists of NOC Outcomes and NIC Interventions

Key Concepts

Safety

Patient safety

Related Concepts

See the Concept Map on Davis Advantage.

Example Problem

Falls

Caring for the Nguyens

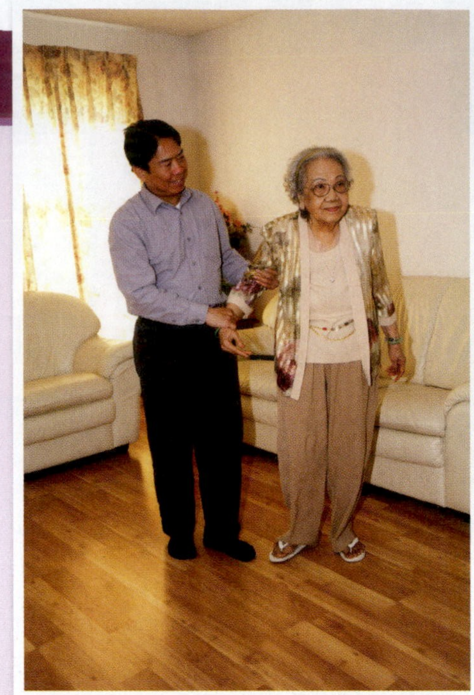

Refer to the assessment data for Nam Nguyen in Volume I of this book. Use full-spectrum thinking to identify safety hazards for Mr. Nguyen, his 3-year-old grandchild (Kim Phan, who lives with him), and his widowed mother, Mai Nguyen, who lives alone.

A. Without even using any of the Nguyen's patient assessment data (except ages), what theoretical knowledge do you have that will help you identify risks that commonly occur in the developmental stages represented by these three clients?
   Mr. Nguyen
   Mr. Nguyen's 3-year-old grandchild, Kim
   Mr. Nguyen's widowed mother, Mai

B. From Mr. Nguyen's assessment, what data can you put with your theoretical knowledge to identify the most likely safety risks for him? What are those risks?

C. From the risks and possible risks you have identified, for which one do you definitely need more data before deciding whether it increases his risk for accidents? That is, which piece of data is especially vague? What do you need to find out?

D. You know the theoretical (or possible) risks for Mr. Nguyen's mother. What data do you need in order to determine her *actual* safety risks?

E. What, if any, data do you have that would help you to identify any *actual* safety risks for Mr. Nguyen's grandchild? What, if any, are those risks?

F. What would you want to assess at the child's preschool to be sure that safety measures exist for preventing falls?

PracticalKnowledge clinical **application**

Nursing interventions to promote safety in the home focus mainly on patient teaching. In inpatient facilities, however, you will take a more proactive role in preventing injury to patients. You will need skills and techniques to prevent falls and to apply and manage restraints safely.

PROCEDURES

Procedure 24-1 ■ Using Bed and Chair Monitoring Devices

➤ For steps to follow in *all* procedures, refer to the Universal Steps for All Procedures found on the inside back cover.

Equipment

Bed or chair exit monitoring device

At least four types of notification systems are used to warn caregivers that a patient is leaving a bed or chair: (1) pressure sensitive, (2) posture indicators, (3) motion sensors, and (4) pull-cord and combination alarms.

Delegation

As a nurse, you must determine whether a monitoring device is needed. You must also select the appropriate device and provide ongoing evaluation of its effectiveness. You may delegate to an unlicensed assistive personnel (UAP) the installation of the device, after verifying the UAP has the necessary knowledge and skill.

Pre-Procedure Assessments

Assess for intrinsic factors that increase the risk for falls:

- Older than age 75 years
- History of falling
- Bowel and bladder incontinence (particularly urge bladder incontinence)
- Cognitive impairment
- Mood changes, lability
- Dizziness
- Functional impairment
- Medications (especially new medications or changes)
- Comorbidities (e.g., dementia, hip fracture, type 2 diabetes, Parkinson's disease, arthritis, and depression)
- Identify factors that increase risk for more severe injury in the case of a fall. These include use of anticoagulants (e.g., Coumadin, Plavix, or aspirin) and osteoporosis.

Assess for extrinsic (environmental) factors that increase the risk for falls:

- Use of an assistive device
- Equipment in the room
- Wet or uneven floors
- Use of physical restraints
- Poorly fitting footwear
- Poor lighting
- Lack of grab rails and bars in the bathroom
- Furniture and adaptive aids that are in disrepair or unstable (e.g., bed rails, IV poles)
- Clothing that may cause tripping
- Alarm on the monitoring device to be checked to ensure that it is working properly

➤ When performing the procedure, always identify your patient according to agency policy, using two identifiers, and be attentive to standard precautions, hand hygiene, patient safety and privacy, body mechanics, and documentation.

Procedure Steps

1. **Apply the device.**

Variation: Bed or Chair Monitor

Place sensor pads under the patient's buttocks.

The sensor will trigger the alarm when the patient attempts to get out of the bed or chair; it does so when there is no weight on it for more than a few seconds. With some devices, you may need to set the alarm sensitivity. For example, you may set the system to trigger the alarm when the patient exits the bed, when the patient attempts to exit the bed, or even when the patient moves in the bed.▼

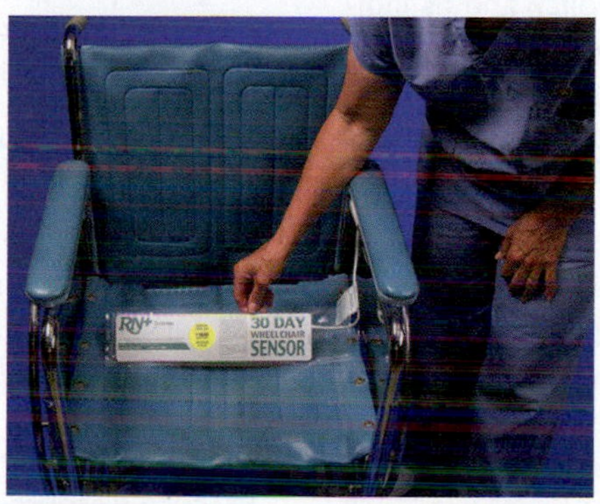

Variation: Leg Sensors

Place sensors on the patient's thigh.

The alarm will sound when the leg assumes a near-vertical position.▼

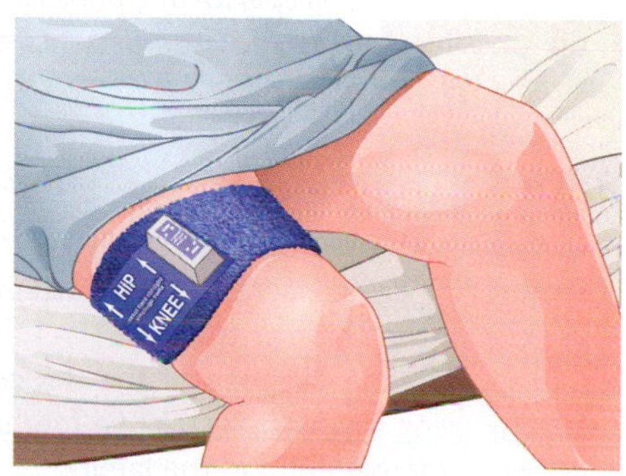

(continued on next page)

Procedure 24-1 ■ Using Bed and Chair Monitoring Devices (continued)

Variation: Infrared Beam Detector

Attach next to the bed or on the wall.

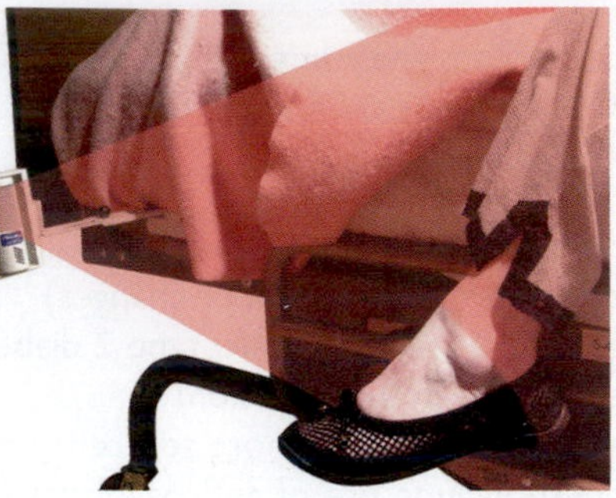

Variation: Cord-Activated Sensor

Attach one end of the cord (clip) to the patient's garment. Attach the other end to the control unit. The cord should be long enough to allow moderate movements but short enough to prevent false alarms. Be sure the cord is free to pull straight out from the monitor and is not blocked by pillows, bedding, or bedrails.
The alarm is activated when the patient's movement causes the cord to be detached from the control unit. Some patients may deactivate the alarms, including removing the alarms clipped to their garments.

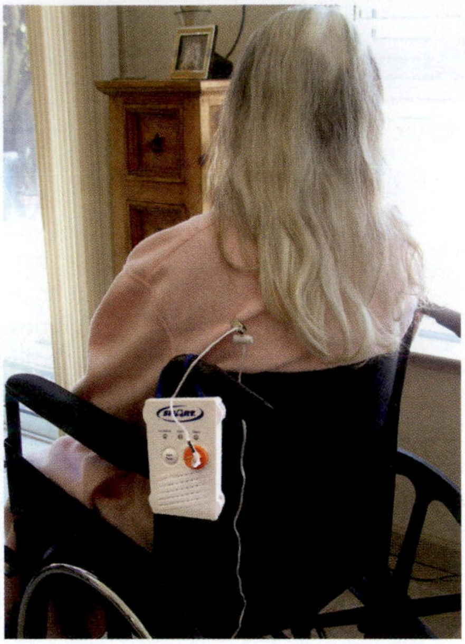

2. **Connect the control unit to the sensor pad.**

Variation: Bed or Chair Monitor

Mount the control unit on the bed or chair.

Variation: Leg Sensor

Mount the control unit directly on the leg sensor.

Variation: Infrared System

Mount the control unit next to the bed or on the wall.

Variation: Cord-Activated System

Mount the control unit next to the bed or on the wall.

3. **Connect the control unit** to the nurse call system, if possible.
Allows for a quicker response; however, not all call systems will accommodate this.
4. **Before assisting the patient out of the bed** or the chair, disconnect or turn off the alarm.
Prevents false alarms. Some systems have a standby setting to allow the alarm to be temporarily suspended.
5. **Reactivate the alarm** after assisting the patient back to the bed or the chair.
Helps improve timeliness of staff response, which may prevent patient falls.
6. **Be sure the patient can access** the nurse call light easily.

Evaluation

- Assess the sensitivity of the monitoring device, and adjust, as needed, to ensure that the alarm is activated if the patient tries to get out of the bed or the chair.
- Continue to assess fall risk per agency policy and as indicated by the patient's physical and/or mental status.
- In the event of a fall, perform a post-fall assessment to identify possible causes. Monitor patients closely for 48 hours after a fall.

Patient Teaching

- Explain to the patient and family that a bed or chair exit monitoring device alerts the staff when the patient tries to get out of the chair or the bed.
- Explain that the purpose of the device is to help prevent falls by using the least restrictive method possible; this will reassure the patient and the family.
- Explain to the patient that she will need to call for assistance when she wants to get up.
Calling for assistance will prevent the alarm from sounding and can prevent falls.

Documentation

- Document the initial sensor placement, including type of sensor used and the location of placement.
- After documenting initial placement, follow agency policy for documenting the use of bed exit monitor. Usually, the minimum documentation for exit monitors is every 8 hours.
- Place the patient on fall risk precautions, according to agency policy.
- Document on the fall risk assessment sheet, restraint flowsheet, and nursing notes, according to agency policy.

Sample documentation

9/14/20 1230. Continues to be confused and to stand up without assistance. Wheelchair exit alarm placed on wheelchair and monitoring clip attached to back of client's gown. Notified client's daughter, June Kennedy, via telephone. Daughter agreed the exit alarm would help keep her mother from falling. ———— Mary Clinton, RN

Practice Resources

Gray-Micelli, D., & Quigley, P. (2016); Lipsitz, Tchalla, Iloputaife, et al., (2016); National Guideline Clearinghouse (2016).

Thinking About the Procedure

The video **Using Bed and Chair Monitoring Devices,** along with questions and suggested responses, is available on the ***Davis's Nursing Skills Videos*** Web site on FADavis.com.

Procedure 24-2 ■ Using Restraints

➤ For steps to follow in *all* procedures, refer to the Universal Steps for All Procedures found on the inside back cover.

➤ Caution: This procedure describes Medicare standards, but state and agency policies may be more restrictive.

Equipment

- Restraint of the appropriate size: belt, vest, wrist or ankle, or mitt
- Soft gauze or cotton padding for bony prominences

Delegation

As the nurse, you must determine whether restraints are needed in each specific situation. You must also select the least restrictive type of restraints, evaluate their effectiveness, and continue to assess for complications that may occur. You may delegate to UAPs the application and periodic removal of ordered restraints, after verifying that the UAP has the knowledge and skill to do so.

Pre-Procedure Assessments

- Assess the patient's risk for falls, including mobility status and level of awareness.
- Assess for need for restraints: The immediate physical safety of the patient, a staff member, or others is threatened.
  If a patient must be temporarily restrained so that a procedure may be performed, this is not considered "restraint."
- Determine that all less restrictive interventions have been tried and have failed.
- Identify the appropriate restraint:
  - The least restrictive possible
  - Does not interfere with care or exacerbate patient's medical condition
  - Does not pose a safety risk to the patient
  - Can be changed easily to keep it clean

➤ When performing the procedure, always identify your patient according to agency policy, using two identifiers, and be attentive to standard precautions, hand hygiene, patient safety and privacy, body mechanics, and documentation.

Procedure Steps

1. **Determine whether dangerous** behaviors continue despite attempts to eliminate causal factors using less restrictive interventions.

2. **Obtain a physician's prescription** for restraint, including type of restraint, indications for use, site of restraint application, and duration. Determine if the restraint is being used for medical–surgical or behavioral reasons.
   Federal and state regulations and laws permit healthcare facilities to use restraints only when they are medically needed. Restraints can be used only with a physician's or advanced practice nurse's order for a specified and limited time. When you apply restraint in an emergency, obtain the order as the restraint is being applied or as quickly as possible afterward. When the restraint prescription expires (maximum 24 hours), physician assessment and a new prescription are needed.

3. **Notify the family of the change** in patient status and the need for restraints. Obtain patient and family consent when clinically feasible.
   Patients have the right to refuse treatment. Consent may not be necessary if there is an immediate threat to patient safety; however, as a rule, the family must be notified of the use of restraints if the patient has cognitive impairment. Many times family members prefer to sit with the patient as an alternative to the use of restraint.

4. **Pad bony prominences** and apply the appropriately sized restraint, using appropriate knotting techniques.
   - Use a quick-release knot, such as the half-bow, when tying restraints to the bed frame or wheelchair.
   - Do not tie restraints to the siderails. ➤

   A quick-release knot is used to prevent patient injury and for ease of caring for the patient. Tie the knot on an immovable part of the bed to prevent injuring the patient if the siderails or head of bed is lowered. A quick-release knot will not tighten or slip when the patient moves about but unties quickly when you pull on the loose end.

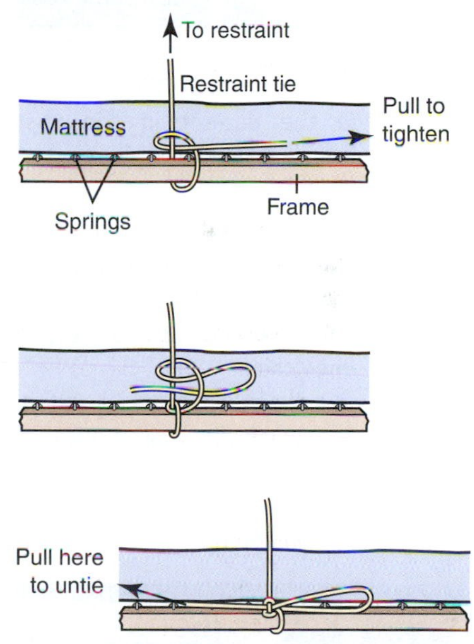

Variation: Belt Restraint

a. Place the belt restraint at the patient's waist, removing any wrinkles.
b. Make sure that the belt is snug but does not constrict the patient's waist.

(continued on next page)

Procedure 24-2 ■ Using Restraints (continued)

c. Some belts have a key-locked buckle to prevent slipping.

A belt restraint is used mainly to prevent a patient from falling when getting up from a chair or a wheelchair and may be used to remind a patient not to get out of bed unassisted.

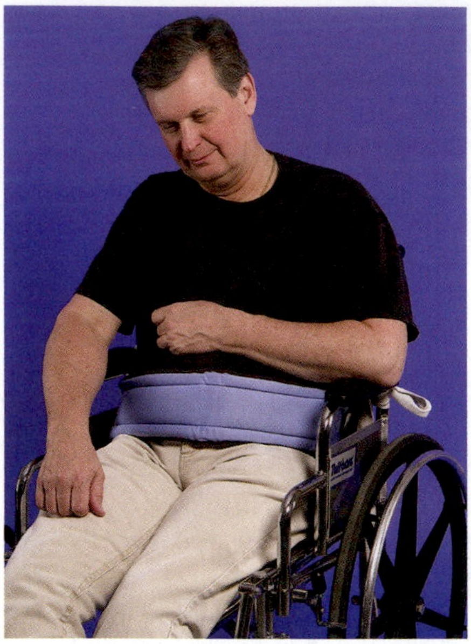

Variation: Vest or Jacket Restraint

d. Place the patient in the vest restraint. A zipper-style vest is preferred.

A vest restraint with a rear zipper is less likely to accidentally strangle the patient.

e. Attach the vest straps to the bed or wheelchair.

A vest restraint is used mainly to prevent a patient from falling out of a chair or a wheelchair and sometimes to prevent a patient from getting out of bed unassisted.

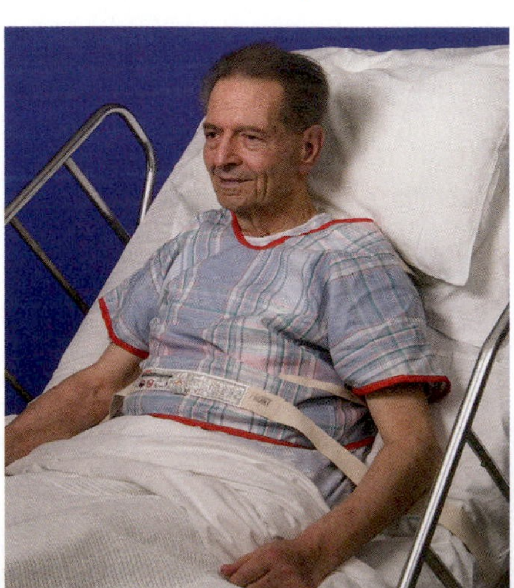

Variation: Wrist or Ankle Restraint

f. Apply the padded portion of the wrist or ankle restraint around the patient's wrist or ankle.

g. Make the restraint snug enough to prevent the patient from being able to slip it off, but not tight enough to impair circulation.

h. Attach the restraint strap to the bed frame. Do not attach to bed rails.

A wrist restraint is used mainly to prevent an agitated patient from pulling at tubes, such as IV sites and nasogastric tubes.

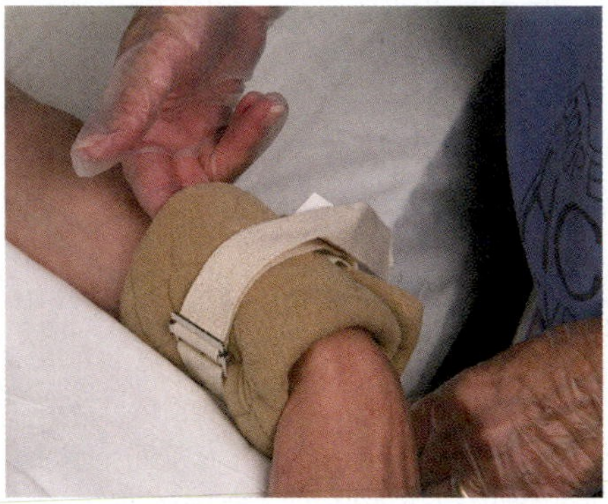

Variation: Mitt Restraint

i. Place patient's hand in the mitt restraint, ensuring that fingers are slightly flexed in the mitt.

j. Attach restraint strap to the bed frame, if necessary.

A mitt restraint is used mainly to prevent a patient from pulling at tubes, such as IV sites and nasogastric tubes. Mitt restraints limit the use of the fingers, which may be enough to prevent the patient from grasping the tube. If this is the case, mitts that are not tied to the bed frame are the least restrictive restraint.

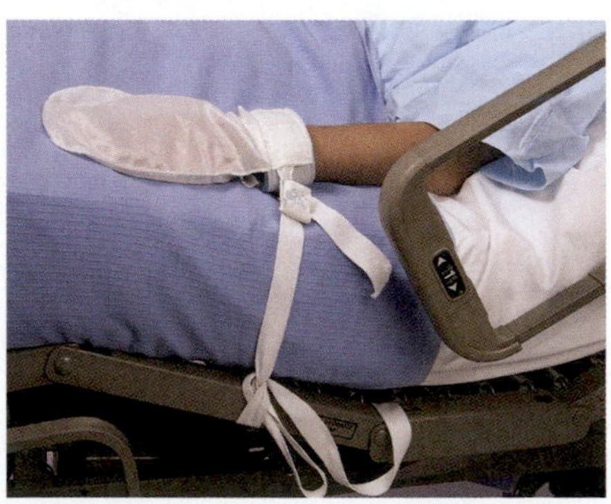

Variation: Enclosed Bed

k. Place the patient in the bed, and zip all sides. Be sure zippers are completely closed and that the zipper tabs are positioned in the upper aspects of the net panels out of the patient's reach.

l. Adhere to the manufacturer's minimum height and weight recommendations.

m. Never leave the bed in the high position with the patient unattended.

An enclosed bed is a canopy-like padded bed that is used mainly to keep a patient from wandering or from falling out of bed. The bed has nylon netting on all four sides, with zippered panels that can be opened to provide care. The patient has full freedom of movement and access to all parts of his body. Patients in enclosed beds have a higher risk of becoming entrapped between the bed rails and the mattress risking suffocation. The dangers are greater for smaller patients and when the bed is left in a high position.

5. **Adjust the restraint** to maintain good body alignment, comfort, and safety. You should be able to slide two fingers under a wrist or ankle restraint.

The restraint should be snug enough to prevent it from slipping off, but not tight enough to impair circulation.

6. **Release restraints at least** every 2 hours to provide skin care, passive and active range of motion (ROM), ambulation, toileting, hydration, and nutrition. Assess for the continued need for restraint.

Prevents impaired circulation and injury. Medicare- and Medicaid-certified healthcare agencies must ensure that a patient's abilities do not decline unless the decline cannot be avoided because of the patient's medical condition. Patients often lose the ability to bathe, dress, walk, toilet, eat, and communicate when they are regularly restrained. If restraints are necessary, they must be used in a way that does not cause these functional losses.

7. **Place the patient on fall risk** precautions, according to agency policy.
Patients who are restrained have a higher risk of falls.

? What if . . .

- **I must apply a restraint in an emergency, for the safety of the patient or others?**

In such an emergency, an RN may initiate a restraint. When you apply restraint in an emergency, obtain the physician's order as the restraint is being applied or as quickly as possible afterward.

Evaluation

- Assess the initial restraint placement, circulation, and skin integrity. Observe for pallor, cyanosis, and coolness of extremities when extremities are restrained.
- Check the restraint every 30 minutes (more often for a behavioral restraint).
- Reassess the restraint, circulation, the patient's response to the intervention, and the need for continuing the use of the restraint every 2 hours; remove it when it is no longer needed.

Key Point: ***Patients in behavioral restraints require more frequent monitoring and, in some circumstances, require continual observation.***
Ensures that the restraint is still functioning as intended. Monitoring and reassessment are critical components of caring for patients in physical restraints. Frequency of monitoring is determined by the type of restraint (behavioral versus medical–surgical).

- Check every 24 hours to see that the restraint prescription has been renewed.
- Remove the restraint as soon as possible.
- Modify the plan of care to reflect the application of restraints and the plan for monitoring.

Patient Teaching

- Explain to the patient and the family the need for the restraints.
- Explain that the restraints will be removed as soon as possible.

Home Care

- The same guidelines apply to clients in the home.
- Evaluate caregivers' knowledge and skill in using restraints, and provide teaching as needed (e.g., regarding padding bony prominences and the need to periodically release the restraints).
- If an enclosed bed is used in the home, instruct the caregiver in its safe use.

Documentation

Document the following:

- All nursing interventions that were done to eliminate the need for the restraint (e.g., moving patient closer to the nurses' station, asking a family member to remain with the patient, reorienting the patient)
- Reasons for placing the restraint (e.g., patient behaviors)
- The initial restraint placement, location, circulation, and skin integrity
- The teaching session with the patient and family members
- Circulation checks, ROM, and restraint removal per agency protocol
- Entries on fall risk assessment sheet, restraint flowsheet, and nursing notes, according to agency policy

Sample documentation

12/24/20 1230. Continues to be confused, pulling at IV lines. Physician notified and evaluated patient. Mitt restraints ordered and placed on bilateral hands. Fall risk precautions initiated. Mitt restraints explained to patient and wife. Wife agreed that mitt restraints would help keep her husband from removing IV line. —— Mary Clinton, RN

Practice Resources

Centers for Medicare & Medicaid Services (2006, revised 2017); Springer, G. (2015).

Thinking About the Procedure

The videos **Using Restraints: Belt Restraint, Mitt Restraint, Vest Restraint, and Wrist/Ankle Restraint,** along with questions and suggested responses, are available on the ***Davis's Nursing Skills Videos*** Web site on FADavis.com.

CLINICAL INSIGHTS

Clinical Insight 24-1 ➤ Choking Rescue Maneuver

For Adults or Children Over Age 12 Months: If you suspect airway obstruction in an adult, do the following:

1. Determine whether the victim is able to speak or cough forcefully (other signs include noisy breathing, loss of consciousness, and dusky skin, lips, and nail beds).
2. Ask, "Are you choking?"
3. If the person cannot speak or indicates he is choking, perform the Heimlich or choking rescue maneuver.

Infants under 1 year: Management of choking is for adults and children. Do not use the Heimlich maneuver for infants under 1 year of age.

1. Determine that the infant is choking. Before performing the choking maneuver, be certain that the airway is completely blocked: the infant cannot cough, breathe, or cry. The infant might also have high-pitched, noisy breathing; rib and sternal retractions; and bluish lips or skin.
2. Call 911. Have someone do that for you, if possible.
3. Deliver back blows:
   - Sit, and rest your forearm on your thigh.
   - Place the infant facedown along your forearm, head lower than the body. Support the chest and jaw in your hand. Do not cover the infant's mouth.
   - With the heel of your other hand, deliver five rapid blows to the infant's back between the shoulder blades.

- For a summary and illustration of choking first aid for an infant under 1 year of age, go to MedlinePlus, at the following URL.

https://medlineplus.gov/ency/presentations/100221_1.htm

- You can obtain a summary and illustration of the Heimlich maneuver at the U.S. National Library of Medicine, MedlinePlus, at this URL:

https://medlineplus.gov/ency/imagepages/18152.htm

- There is also a YouTube video at:

https://www.youtube.com/watch?v=XOTbjDGZ7wg&feature=youtu.be

Clinical Insight 24-2 ➤ Preventing Needlestick Injury

Use needleless systems (e.g., retractable needles), when possible. *More than 80% of needlestick injuries can be prevented with the use of safe needle devices (ANA, 2002).*

For more discussion on how to handle needles safely,

Go to Chapter 26, **Procedure 26-10B: Recapping Sterile Needles,** in Volume 2.

Before beginning a procedure:

- Ensure adequate lighting and space to perform the procedure.
- Place the sharps container near the work area, if it is moveable.
- Obtain assistance if there is a risk the patient may be uncooperative, combative, or confused.
- Inform the patient about the procedure, and explain the importance of avoiding any sudden movement.

During the procedure:

- Be sure you can see the sharps container at all times.
- When handling a sharp, be aware of other persons in the immediate area.
- Do not hand-pass exposed sharps from one person to another.
- When using a safety needle, observe for audio or visual cues that the feature has engaged.

Handling needles:

- Do not shear or break contaminated needles.
- Avoid recapping, bending, or removing contaminated needles and other sharps unless there is no feasible alternative.
- When you must recap a sterile needle, use a mechanical recapping device or a modified "scoop" technique (see Procedure 26-10).
- Never carry syringes in your uniform pocket.

Sharps containers:

- Keep puncture-proof needle disposal containers in every room.
- Place sharps containers at eye level; do not overfill the container.
- Make sure the container is large enough to hold the entire sharp device.

Clinical Insight 24-2 ➤ Preventing Needlestick Injury—cont'd

- Dispose of sharps immediately. Do not wait until you have finished the procedure.
- Inspect sharps and waste containers for protruding sharps. If found, notify safety personnel for removal of the hazard.

If your agency does not use needleless systems or protective devices, you should do the following:

- Explain the Occupational Safety and Health Administration (OSHA) Bloodborne Pathogens Standard (BPS) to your employer, including the need to provide needleless systems or protective devices for blood products and parenteral medication administration.
- Refer your employer to the OSHA Web site at http://www.osha.gov/needlesticks/needlefaq.html
- OSHA requires worker involvement in evaluating, selecting, and implementing the use of safer needle products; volunteer to serve on that committee.
- Ask your agency for a copy of their exposure control plan, which is required by the BPS for monitoring compliance with the new law.
- Keep a record of needlestick injuries on your unit and of "near-misses" (e.g., overfilled sharps containers, sharps left on bed or overbed table).
- Submit your concerns in written form to your employer.
- If your employer refuses to purchase safety devices, you may want to file an OSHA complaint. If you do so, refer to whistleblowing in Chapter 44. Complaints can be filed anonymously.
- For complaint filing,

Go to http://www.osha.gov/as/opa/worker/complain.html

Practice Resources

Adapted from: American Nurses Association (ANA) (2002); Centers for Disease Control and Prevention (2011.); National Institute for Occupational Safety and Health (NIOSH) (n.d., updated 2018.); U.S. Department of Labor, Occupational Safety and Health Administration (OSHA) (n.d.).

{end Clinical Insight 24-2>

Clinical Insight 24-3 ➤ What You Should Know About Using Restraints

- **Agency policy,** *professional guidelines, and state laws should guide restraints use.*
- **Use restraints only for safety** *to ensure the immediate physical safety of the patient or others.*
- **You must obtain a medical prescription** *from a physician or other licensed care provider.*
- **No standing orders** *or "as needed" orders for physical restraint are allowed.*
- **You must renew restraint prescriptions every 24 hours** *(more often for behavioral restraints).*
- **You must modify the plan of care** *to reflect the application of restraints and the plan for monitoring.*
- **Explain the need for the restraints** *if you must use them.*
- **Obtain consent** *from the patient and family, when feasible.*
- **Medications are considered a restraint** *when they are used to restrict the patient's freedom of movement or to manage behavior.*
- **Physical holding of a patient is not always considered restraint.** *Sometimes it is necessary to use devices or methods that involve the physical holding of a patient for routine physical examinations or tests.*
- **Monitor and reassess.** *These are critical components of caring for patients in physical restraints. Assess restraints every 30 minutes (more frequently for patients with behavioral restraints, who may need continuous monitoring).*
- **Remove restraints for assessment, feeding, toileting, and skin care every 2 hours.** *Patients in medical–surgical restraints should be evaluated by an RN at least every 2 hours. Patients in behavioral restraints require more frequent monitoring.*
- **Always use the least restrictive restraint that ensures safety.**
- **Remove the restraint as soon as possible.**

ASSESSMENT GUIDELINES AND TOOLS

Focused Assessment

Safety Assessment Scale

CLSC CÔTE-DES-NEIGES

Name ______________________

S.A.S. SAFETY ASSESSMENT SCALE

CAREGIVER AND LIVING ENVIRONMENT (1)

a) This person lives on her own. Yes [1] No [0] ______

b) This person is alone at home.
Always [4] Most of the time [3] Occasionally [2] Never [1] ______

SMOKING (2)

This person leaves cigarette bum marks on the floor, furniture, or clothing.
Yes [1] No [0] ______

FIRE AND BURNS (3)

a) The stove on/off buttons are located...
on the front of the stove [1] on the top of the stove [2]
behind the hotplates [3] ______

b) This person is capable of turning on the stove him/herself
Yes [1] No [0] Doesn't know [1] ______

c) This person cooks his/her own food.
Always [4] Most of the time [3] Occasionally [2] Never [1] ______

d) This person forgets a pan on the stove.
Very often [4] Often [3] Sometimes [2] Never [1] ______

e) The heating system uses...
electricity [1] natural gas [2] wood [3] ______

NUTRITION (4)

a) This person receives meals-on-wheels or other prepared meals.
More than once a day [1] Once a day [2]
A few times a week (2 to 6 times a week) [3] Once a week or less [4] ______

b) This person's meals contain foods from different food groups
(dairy products, meat or fish, cereals, fruit and vegetables).
Always [1] Most of the time [2] Occasionally [3] Never [4] ______

FOOD POISONING AND TOXIC SUBSTANCES (5)

This person can tell the difference between food that is fresh and food that is spoiled. Yes [0] No [1] ______

MEDICATION AND HEALTH PROBLEMS (6)

a) This person takes, on a regular basis...*
1 to 3 medications [2] 4 to 6 medications [3]
7 medications or more [4] Does not take any medication [1]
*prescribed medications only ______

b) This person takes medication to help him/her sleep or relax.
Yes [1] No [0] ______

c) Does this person suffer from any physical health problem?
None [1] Minor [2] Moderate [3] Severe [4] ______

d) This person accepts treatment for his/her physical health problems.
Yes [0] No [1] Does not apply [0] ______

WANDERING AND ADAPTATION TO CHANGING TEMPERATURE (7)

a) This person gets lost in familiar surroundings.
Very often [4] Often [3] Sometimes [2] Never [1] ______

b) Has this person ever gotten lost? Yes [1] No [0] ______

c) Can this person find his/her way home? Yes [0] No [1] ______

d) Does this person dress appropriately according to the changing temperature, both indoors and outdoors?
Yes [0] No [1] ______

SCORE ____ / 47

Assessed by ______________________

An Affiliated University Centre
Affiliated with McGill University

Source: Dr. Louise Poulin de Courval ©CLSC Côte-des-Neiges. Used with permission.

Focused Assessment

"Get Up and Go" Test

As a nurse, you can perform this test. If the patient has difficulty or unsteadiness you will need to assess further, so

Go to **Example Problem: Falls,** in Volume 1.

Timed Up & Go

For more information about the Timed Up & Go Test,

Go to **Example Problem: Falls,** in Volume 1

You can also see this tool if you,

Go to the CDC website at https://www.cdc.gov/steadi/pdf/TUG_Test-print.pdf

STANDARDIZED LANGUAGE

Examples of NIC Interventions Related to Safety

INTERVENTIONS FROM THE SAFETY DOMAIN	
Abuse Protection Support (Child, Domestic Partner, Elder, Religious)	Fire-Setting Precautions
Allergy Management	First Aid
Area Restriction	Infection Control
Aspiration Precautions	Latex Precautions
Crisis Intervention	Physical Restraint
Dementia Management	Radiation Therapy Management
Elopement Precautions	Sports-Injury Prevention: Youth
Emergency Care	Suicide Prevention
Environmental Management: Safety	Surveillance: Community
Fall Prevention	Vehicle Safety Promotion
SAFETY INTERVENTIONS FROM OTHER DOMAINS	
Communicable Disease Management	Environmental Management: Worker Safety
Community Disaster Preparedness	Home Maintenance Assistance
Environmental Management: Community	Surveillance: Community
Environmental Management: Violence Prevention	

Source: Butcher, G., Bulechek, G., Dochterman, J., et al. (eds.). *Nursing Interventions Classification (NIC),* ed. 7. St. Louis, MO: Elsevier, 2018. Used with permission.

NOC Standardized Outcomes for Safety Problems	
DIAGNOSTIC LABEL	**ASSOCIATED NOC OUTCOMES (EXAMPLES)**
*Contamination	Community Disaster Response Gastrointestinal Function Immune Hypersensitivity Response Kidney Function Neurological Status Respiratory Status
*Risk for Contamination	Community Risk Control: Lead Exposure Personal Safety Behavior Risk Detection
Hyperthermia (Saba, 2017)	Thermoregulation
Hypothermia (Saba, 2017)	Thermoregulation: Newborn
Home Maintenance, Inadequate	Self-Care: Instrumental Activities of Daily Living (IADLs) Safe Home Environment
Skin Integrity Alteration	Tissue Integrity: Skin and Mucous Membranes
Skin Integrity Impairment Risk for Skin Integrity Impairment (Saba, 2017)	Sensory Function: Tactile
*Impaired Tissue Integrity Impaired Thermoregulation Risk for Impaired Thermoregulation	Wound Healing: Primary Intention Vital Signs Risk Control: Infectious Process
Impaired Airway Clearance (choking)	Swallowing Status Respiratory Status: Airway Patency Respiratory Status: Ventilation
Latex Allergy Response (Saba, 2017) Latex Allergy Response, Risk	Allergic Response: Localized Allergic Response: Systemic Tissue Integrity: Skin and Mucous Membranes
Aspiration Risk (Saba, 2017)	Respiratory Status: Airway Patency Swallowing Status
*Risk for Falls	Balance Fall Prevention Behavior Falls Occurrence
*Risk for Infection	Community Risk Control: Communicable Disease Immune Status Infection Severity Risk Control: Sexually Transmitted Diseases (STD)
*Risk for Injury	Personal Safety Behavior Physical Injury Severity Risk Control Safe Home Environment

NOC Standardized Outcomes for Safety Problems—cont'd

DIAGNOSTIC LABEL	ASSOCIATED NOC OUTCOMES (EXAMPLES)
Perioperative Positioning Injury Perioperative Positioning Injury, Risk (Saba, 2017)	Circulation Status Sensory Function Tissue Perfusion: Peripheral
*Risk for Poisoning	Safe Home Environment
Risk for Suffocation	Respiratory Status: Ventilation
Risk for Trauma	Personal Safety Behavior Physical Injury Severity Tissue Integrity: Skin and Mucous Membranes
*Risk for Sudden Infant Death	Parenting Performance: Infant/Toddler Physical Safety Risk Control: Tobacco Use
*Risk for Vascular Trauma	Allergic Response: Localized Tissue Integrity: Skin and Mucous Membranes

*To make safe and effective judgments using NANDA International (NANDA-I) nursing diagnoses, it is essential that nurses refer to the definitions and defining characteristics of the diagnoses listed in this work.

Sources: Butcher, H., Bulechek, G., Dochterman, J., et al. (Eds.). (2018). *Nursing Interventions Classification (NIC)*, ed. 7. St. Louis, MO: Elsevier; Johnson, M., Bulechek, G., Butcher, H., et al. (2012). *NANDA, NOC, and NIC Linkages*, ed. 3. St. Louis, MO: Elsevier; Moorhead, S., Swanson, E., Johnson, M., et al. (eds.) *Nursing Outcomes Classification (NOC)*, ed. 6. St. Louis, MO: Elsevier, 2018; *Herdman, T., & Kamitsuru, S. NANDA International, Inc. *Nursing Diagnoses: Definitions and Classification 2018–2020.* New York: Thieme, 2018. Used with permission.

CLINICALJUDGMENT
Applying the Full-Spectrum Nursing Model

PATIENT SITUATION

Recall your patient, Alvin Lin, from Meet Your Patient scenario in Volume 1. Mr. Lin is a 79-year-old man who was just transferred from a long-term care facility to your medical unit. His admitting diagnoses are dehydration and pneumonia. In the handoff report you were told he had rested well during the night and was alert and oriented. When you enter his room, you find that he is confused and does not know where he is. He is becoming combative and is trying to get out of bed.

THINKING

1. *Theoretical Knowledge:*
   a. What is the pathophysiology of pneumonia?
   b. When the oxygen level of the blood falls, what is the effect on the central nervous system? If you do not know the answer to this question, consult a reliable reference.
   c. What are the defining characteristics for the NANDA-I diagnosis, Deficient Fluid Volume?
2. *Critical Thinking (Considering Alternatives):*
   a. Which of the three defining characteristics (in 1c) may increase Mr. Lin's risk for falls? Why?
   b. What else may be increasing his confusion and his risk for falls?

DOING

3. *Practical Knowledge:* Suppose you have tried all the less restrictive restraints, but Mr. Lin still attempts to get out of bed. He has even pulled out his IV line. You decide you must apply restraints to keep him safely in bed. You have called the physician, but he has not returned your call. You cannot wait any longer because you have other patients who need you, and yet you must stay with Mr. Lin to keep him from falling. What should you do right now?

4. *Nursing Process (Diagnosis):* Which nursing diagnosis seems more useful to you in planning care for Mr. Lin?
   a. Confusion related to disease process
   b. Risk for Falls related to confusion and possibly r/t weakness

CARING

5. *Self-Knowledge:*
   a. Do you think having a restraint-free facility is a valuable goal, or not? Explain your thinking.
   b. How did you come to believe that?

6. *Ethical Knowledge:* Suppose Mr. Lin is too confused to give consent for restraints, and you cannot reach his family by telephone. How can you justify applying restraints, and what must you do later to follow up?

Critical Thinking and Clinical Judgment

1. Recall from Meet Your Patients, in Volume 1, the clients you encountered in the community setting. Teresa was caring for her 2-year-old daughter and her elderly grandmother. The grandmother has a fear of falling. In Volume 1, we addressed some of the issues related to child-proofing the home. You would like to suggest ways for Teresa to safe-proof the home for her frail grandmother.
   a. Refer to the critical-thinking model and questions on the inside back cover of Volume 1 of your textbook. What questions in the Inquiry section should you ask before making suggestions to Teresa?
   b. What specific information do you need about the grandmother? About the home?
   c. Once you have the necessary information, what suggestions could you make about home safety measures?
   d. Consider alternatives. What types of assistive devices might be helpful in preventing falls?
   e. Explore the alternatives. For example, are they practical? What do you need to know about this family to determine whether it is practical for them to obtain such devices?
   f. Think now about Teresa. Given the situation, what might create a safety risk for her?

2. Recall Alvin Lin (Meet Your Patients, in Volume 1), the 79-year-old man you were assigned to care for on your first day on the medical unit. The initial report you received was that he was alert and oriented, but you find that he is now confused and is becoming combative.
   a. What should be your first two priorities in this situation?
   b. What specific patient data do you need to determine what might have caused this change in behavior? How could you get that data?
   c. What alternatives to restraints might you consider?

3. A friend calls to tell you she thinks her 18-month-old daughter swallowed some of her sleeping pills. The child is very sleepy, and your friend is having difficulty arousing her. Your friend has ipecac in her medicine cabinet and wonders whether she should try to get her awake enough to take it.

   a. What is the first thing that you would recommend that the mother do?

   b. What is a major concern with inducing vomiting, given that you must assume from the mother's report that the child is very drowsy? What could go wrong if the child vomits?

   c. If the mother decides to take the daughter to the hospital instead of taking time to call the poison control center (PCC), what should you remind her to take with her?

4. An older couple has health problems, and both are taking several medications. The husband has assumed care for himself and his wife Ethyl because Ethyl has been exhibiting confusion at times. He says he sometimes becomes overwhelmed with everything he has to do, and he is not sure that he always gives the medicine at the right times.

   a. What information do you need to know to be able to help with this situation? About the medications? About resources? How would you obtain the information?

   b. What suggestions can you make to help the husband organize the medications?

5. You are caring for a patient 12 hours after surgery following an abdominal hysterectomy for cancer. She asks you to help her to walk to a chair. You note that she has IV fluids infusing and is receiving narcotics via a patient-controlled analgesia (PCA) pump. She states that she has not been out of bed since the surgery and that she has just self-administered some medication and would like to get up while she has pain relief. You also notice that there is a Foley (indwelling urinary) catheter connected to a bedside drainage.

   a. What environmental factors could be safety hazards when this patient gets out of bed?

   b. What assessments and other interventions would help to ensure safe ambulation despite those obstacles?

6. For each of the following concepts, use critical thinking to describe how or why it is important to nursing, patient care, or promoting safety. Note that these are *not* to be merely definitions.

Environmental hazard
Pathogens
Poisoning
Scald injuries
Falls
Teaching firearm safety to children
Pollution
Radiation
Restraint
Ambularm
Choking rescue maneuver
Refrigeration
Mosquito control
Rodent control
Reduce, reuse, recycle, respond
Back injuries
Needlestick injuries
Time, distance, and shielding
Gang culture
Morse Fall Scale

What Are the Main Points in This Chapter?

- Safety is a basic human need.
- Unintentional injuries are the fifth leading cause of death in the United States.
- Major causes of unintentional deaths in the United States are motor vehicle accidents, poisoning, and falls.
- The environment includes the physical and psychosocial factors that contribute to the life and well-being of each person. It may be identified as any setting where the nurse and client interact.
- A person's safety is influenced by developmental factors as well as individual factors, such as lifestyle, cognitive awareness, sensoriperceptual status, ability to communicate, mobility status, and sensory losses, particularly hearing and vision losses.
- The main safety hazards in the home are poisoning, carbon monoxide poisoning, scalds and burns, fires, falls, firearm injuries, suffocation and drowning, and take-home toxins.
- Most fatal home fires occur while people are asleep, and most deaths result from smoke inhalation.
- More than half of all falls occur in the home; about 80% involve people older than age 65 years.
- Community hazards include motor vehicle accidents, pathogens, improper sanitation, pollution (air, water, noise, and soil), and electrical storms.
- Safety hazards in the healthcare agency include falls, equipment-related accidents, fires and electrical hazards, restraints, mercury exposure, and biological hazards.
- When possible, nurses should use alternative interventions instead of restraints.
- Medical prescriptions for restraints must be renewed at least every 24 hours.
- Workplace hazards to nurses include back injuries, needlestick injuries, radiation injury, and violence.
- All inpatients should be assessed for their risk for falls.
- Identifying anxiety may allow the nurse to intervene before a patient becomes aggressive.
- The Heimlich maneuver differs from the American Red Cross's choking rescue maneuver in that the Heimlich does not include back blows.
- Nursing interventions for promoting safety in the home focus on client teaching.
- Nursing interventions for promoting safety in the healthcare facility focus on assessing for risk and creating a safe environment.

Knowledge Map

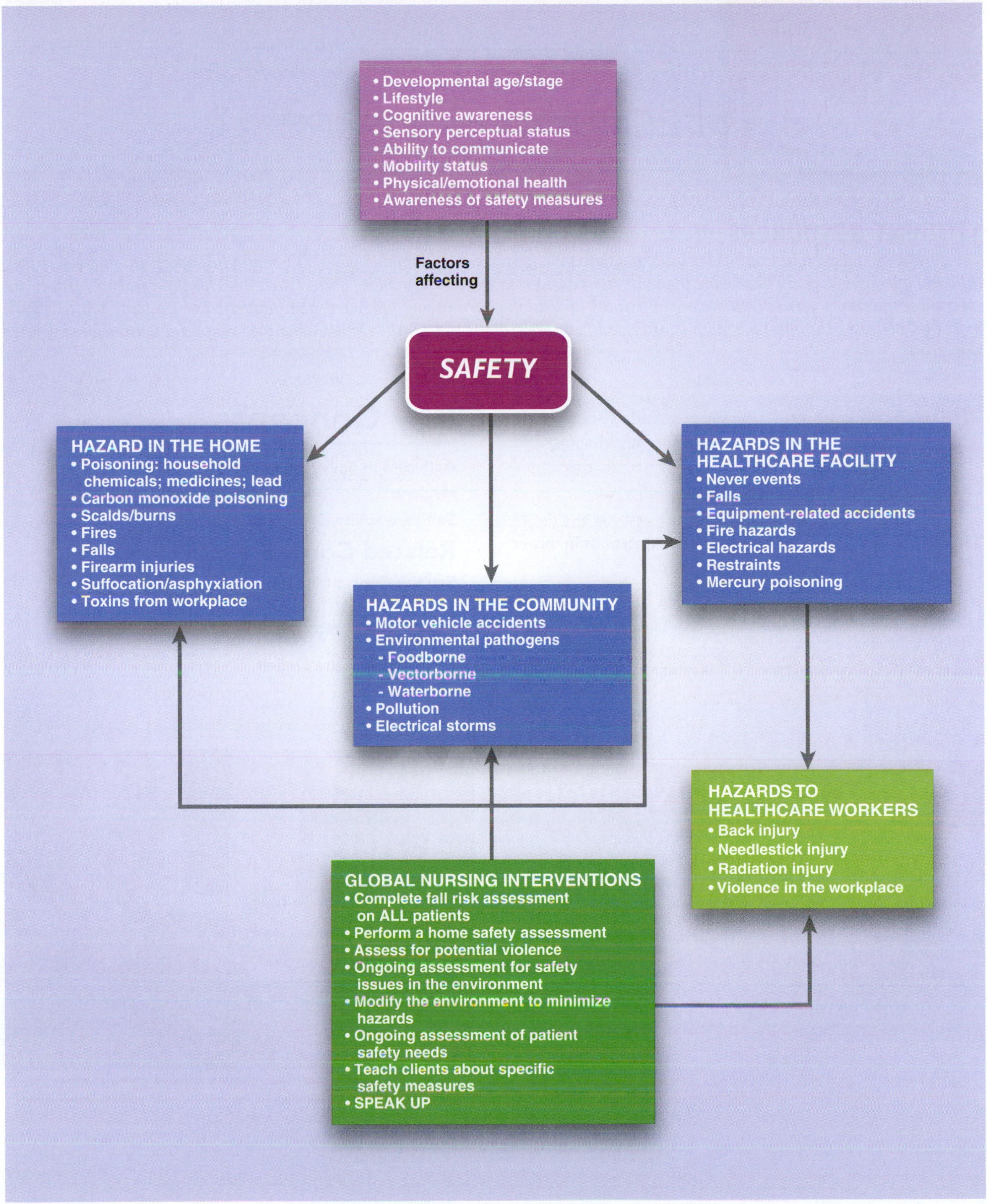

CHAPTER 25

Facilitating Hygiene

STUDENT RESOURCES

The questions and exercises in this book allow you to practice the kind of thinking you will use as a full-spectrum nurse. Critical-thinking questions usually have more than one right answer, so we do not provide "correct answers" for these features. Try to answer these questions yourself. It is more important to develop your nursing judgment than to just cover content. You will learn more by discussing the questions with your peers. If you are still unsure, see the Davis Advantage chapter resources for suggested responses.

To explore learning resources for this chapter,

Go to Davis Advantage and find:

Answers and Suggested Responses for all questions in this chapter
Concept Map
Knowledge Map
References and Bibliography
Lists of NOC Outcomes and NIC Interventions

Key Concepts

Activities of daily living
Hygiene
Self-care ability

Related Concepts

See the Concept Map on Davis Advantage.

Example Problem

Hygiene Self-Care Deficit

Caring for the Nguyens

Yen Nguyen works as a preschool teacher. She schedules a clinic visit to discuss a variety of concerns. For each of the concerns she mentions, answer the following four questions:

1. What theoretical knowledge do you need?
2. Where could you find it?
3. What, if any, additional patient information do you need?
4. How would you respond to Mrs. Nguyen's concerns?

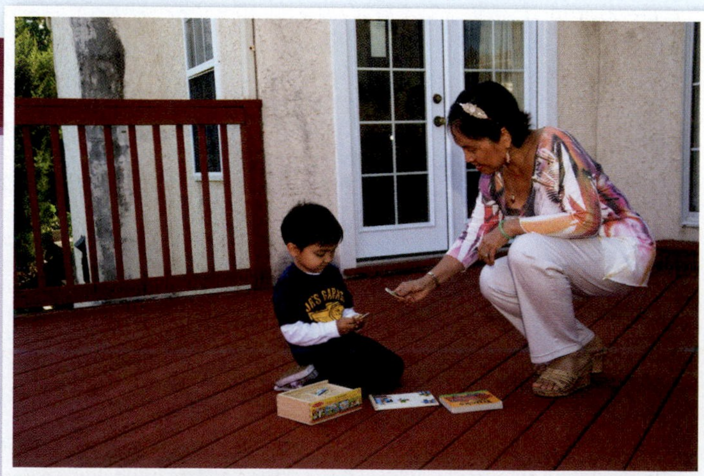

Caring for the Nguyens (continued)

A. Yen tells you that her skin is very dry and irritated.

B. Yen tells you that several of the children at the preschool have recently been diagnosed with head lice. She would like to know how to assess for pediculosis.

C. Yen tells you that her 3-year-old grandson, Kim, frequently refuses to bathe. She asks for advice on how to handle this.

PracticalKnowledge clinical application

The following procedures and clinical insights provide the practical knowledge you will need to assist patients with personal cleanliness and grooming. Patient Teaching and Home Care content in the procedures help you to promote increased activity and independence for patients.

PROCEDURES

Procedure 25-1 ■ Bathing: Providing a Complete Bed Bath Using a Prepackaged Bathing Product

➤ For steps to follow in *all* procedures, refer to the Universal Steps for All Procedures found on the inside back cover.

Equipment

- Prepackaged bathing product with disposable wipes (e.g., Comfort Bath)
- Bath blanket
- Clean patient gown (with shoulder snaps or Velcro closures if the patient has an intravenous [IV] line)
- Clean bed linen
- Orangewood stick
- Deodorant, lotion, and/or powder, as needed
- Emollient (if not included in prepackaged bathing product)
- Procedure gloves (for anal and perineal care)
- Bedpan or urinal
- Laundry bag
- Plastic trash bag for used wipes and other disposable soiled items ➤

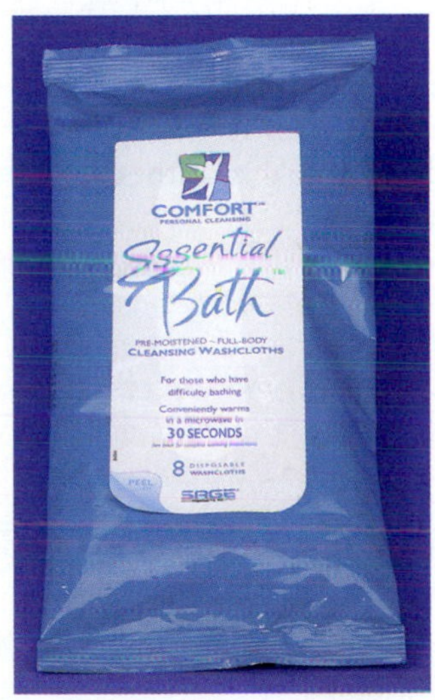

Delegation

You can delegate this procedure to the unlicensed assistive personnel (UAP) if you conclude that the patient's condition and the UAP's skills allow. Perform the pre-procedure assessments, and inform the UAP of the specific type of bath (e.g., packaged bath, towel bath); the amount of help the patient needs; any special considerations, such as IV lines, drains, and so on. Ask the UAP to report the condition of the patient's skin, level of self-care, and ability to tolerate the procedure.

Pre-Procedure Assessments

- Assess mobility, activity tolerance, type of bath needed, and level of ability to perform bathing self-care.
  A patient who has decreased activity tolerance or mobility (e.g., chest pain or shortness of breath with exertion) may have limited ability to assist with the bath. Having the patient assist as much as possible increases mobility and sense of control and comfort.

(continued on next page)

Procedure 25-1 ■ Bathing: Providing a Complete Bed Bath Using a Prepackaged Bathing Product (continued)

- Check for positioning or activity restrictions (e.g., maintaining hip abduction following a total hip replacement).
  Prevents injuring the patient during the procedure.
- Determine the number of people you need to safely bathe and reposition the patient.
  Helps prevent injury to the patient or the nurse.
- Assess for personal and cultural issues that may be of concern to the patient regarding the bath.
  Bathing may conflict with the patient's sense of privacy or modesty. Cultural norms and individual preferences must be considered.
- Assess for specific patient needs and preferences during a bath, such as lotions and extra wipes or towels.
  Advanced age, certain skin conditions, or skin breakdown may require special soaps and/or lotions. Incontinence or drainage may require additional wipes, towels, and precautions. Meeting patient preferences helps prevent depersonalization and promotes patient cooperation with the procedure.

➤ When performing the procedure, always identify your patient according to agency policy, using two identifiers, and be attentive to standard precautions, hand hygiene, patient safety and privacy, body mechanics, and documentation.

➤ *Note:* You may find that you need to adapt the bathing order and other steps to meet individual needs.

Procedure Steps

1. **Provide for patient privacy** and comfort.
   a. Close the door or privacy curtains, adjust room temperature, and assist the patient with elimination, as needed.
   b. Assist the patient with elimination before beginning the bath.
   Helps prevent interruptions during the procedure.
   c. Ask the patient if she wishes family members to assist with the bath, and discuss this with the family members.
   Bathing practices differ among cultures and individuals but are often private. The patient or family may wish to have a family member assist with the bath, or the patient may prefer that they leave the room.
2. **Peel open the label on the commercial bath** without completely removing it.
   Allows for steam to escape as contents heat to avoid spilling of the contents.
3. **Heat the package** in the microwave for no longer than 1 minute. The temperature of the contents should be approximately 105°F (41°C). This is controversial. Some references suggest that for safety, the contents of the commercial bag bath should be used at room temperature.
   Heating to 105°F (41°C) brings contents to a safe and comfortable temperature. This must be done with caution to prevent burning, especially in patients who have fragile skin.

If Using a Warmer Unit

You do not need Step 3 because the bags are always warm.

4. **Adjust the bed** to working height, lower the siderail nearest you, and position the patient supine close to the side of bed you will be working on.

   Raise the siderail before you leave that side of the bed.

   Prevents patient falls and keeps nurses from having to lean over the patient or reach across the siderail, which can cause back strain or injury.
5. **Remove the bedspread,** and spread the bath blanket over the top sheet; then ask the patient to hold the bath blanket in place while you remove the top sheet.
   Maintains the patient's modesty and prevents chilling. If no bath blanket is available, you can use the top sheet in its place. However, if the sheet becomes damp, it may chill the patient.

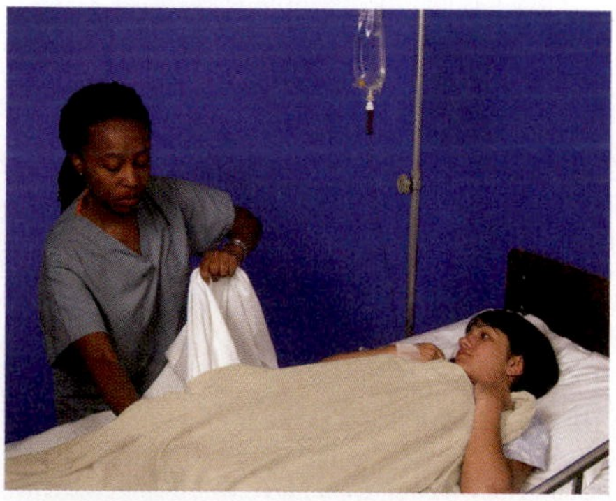

Note: Before proceeding, assist the patient with oral hygiene, as needed. See Procedures 25-6 and 25-7.

6. **Remove the patient's gown,** keeping the patient covered with the bath blanket. During the bath, expose just the part of the body you are bathing.
   Maintains the patient's modesty and prevents chilling.

Patient With an IV Line

If the patient has an IV line and is wearing a gown that has snap-open sleeves:

Some systems include a needle-free 2-way connector that allows you to disconnect the tubing while still maintaining a closed line. In that case, you simply open the connection, remove the gown, and then reconnect the tubing. After the bath, follow the same procedure to place the clean gown on the patient.

If there is no 2-way, needle-free connector on the tubing,

a. Remove the gown first from the arm without the IV line.
b. Lower the IV container, and pass the gown over the tubing and the container, taking care to keep the container above the level of the patient's arm.

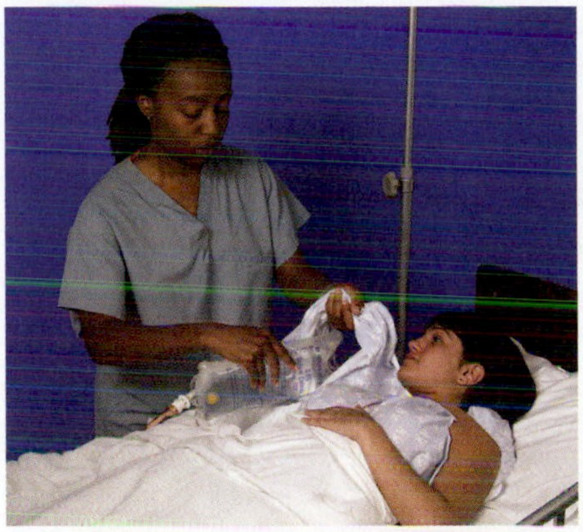

c. Never disconnect this type of IV tubing connection; this breaks the sterile system and provides a portal of entry for pathogens.

d. Rehang the container; check the flow rate.
Manipulating the IV equipment may change the flow rate; flow rate must be maintained as prescribed.

e. After the bath, replace the gown by threading the IV equipment from inside the arm of the gown and onto the affected arm. Then, place the unaffected arm through the other gown sleeve.

7. Don clean procedure gloves if exposure to body fluids is likely or if either you or the patient has any breaks in the skin.
Follows universal precautions; helps prevent transfer of microorganisms.

8. Wash the patient's face, neck, and ears.

a. Fold the wipe around the hand to make a mitt, tucking in loose corners.
Keeps loose ends from dragging across the skin. This is uncomfortable for the patient because loose ends cool quickly.

b. Wash the face using one wipe.

c. Use a different corner of the wipe to gently wipe each eyelid outward from the inner canthus.
Some wipes contain chlorhexidine gluconate (CHG), an antimicrobial that can be irritating to the eyes and mucous membranes. Use pH-balanced prepackaged wipes for the face, or use gauze squares moistened with agency-approved water or normal saline. **Key Point:** ***A major principle is cleaning from "clean to dirty" to prevent contamination of a cleaner area. The inner canthus is considered the cleanest area.*** *Prevents moving debris toward the nasolacrimal duct, which is located near the inner canthus.*

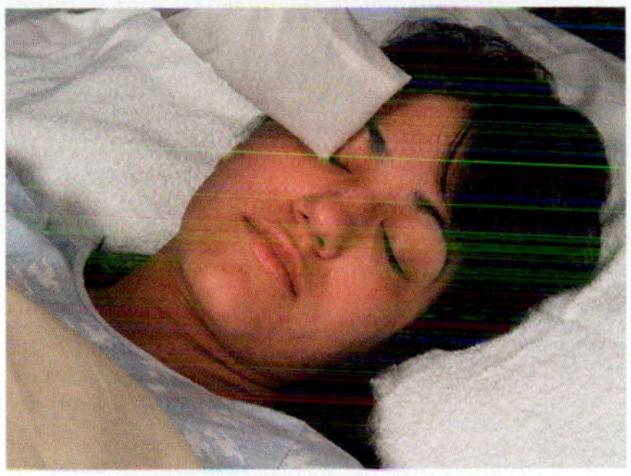

d. Wash the rest of the patient's face, neck, and ears.
Move sequentially through the bath to make it less tiring for the patient and more efficient for the nurse.

e. Allow areas to air dry. Do not rinse.
Prevents the emollient and surfactant skin protectants from being removed.

9. Discard each wipe after use.
Ensures following the "clean-to-dirty" principle.

10. Wash the patient's arms, using a new, clean wipe.

a. Fold the bath blanket off one arm at a time, and place a folded bath towel under the arm. Beginning with the patient's far arm, support the arm, and wash the arm from the hands upward using long strokes.
Long strokes increase circulation in the extremity. Washing from distal to proximal increases venous return from the periphery. Lifting the arm provides range of motion (ROM) to preserve joint mobility.

b. Continue to support the arm while washing the axilla.
Prevents potential injury to the joints. A sprain, subluxation, or dislocation of the joint can occur when an extremity is not properly supported, especially in older adults.

c. Allow the areas to air dry; do not rinse.
Prevents the emollient and surfactant skin protectants from being removed.

d. Apply deodorant and/or powder, if desired.
Follow patient preferences, whenever possible, to increase comfort.

e. Clean under the nails with an orangewood stick, as needed.

f. Repeat the preceding Steps 10a–d for the arm nearest you.

11. Wash the patient's chest, using a new clean wipe.

a. Cover the patient's chest with a bath towel, and lower the bath blanket to the patient's waist.
Maintains patient comfort and modesty.

b. For women, gently lift each breast to wash the skinfold, if needed. Keep the chest covered between the wash and the rinse.
Skinfolds are a source of odor and can become irritated because of skin-to-skin contact and dampness from perspiration.

c. Cover to maintain privacy and warmth.

d. Allow the areas to air dry; do not rinse.
Prevents the emollient and surfactant skin protectants from being removed.

12. Wash the abdomen, using a new, clean wipe.

a. Fold the bath blanket down to the perineal area, and cover the chest with a bath towel.

b. Wash the abdomen, including the umbilical area; allow to air dry. Pay special attention to skinfolds.
Perspiration and moisture do not evaporate well from skinfolds, predisposing them to maceration.

c. Cover the abdomen and chest with the bath blanket.
Prevents chilling, maintains privacy.

13. Wash the legs and feet, using a new, clean wipe for each leg.

a. Uncover one leg at a time, beginning with the leg farthest from you. Place the bath towel under the leg.
Keeps the sheet dry; prevents chilling.

(continued on next page)

Procedure 25-1 ■ Bathing: Providing a Complete Bed Bath Using a Prepackaged Bathing Product (continued)

b. Wash the leg from distal to proximal with long, gentle strokes. Allow the leg to air dry.

Do not massage the calves of the legs.

Washing from distal to proximal may help promote venous return. If a venous thrombus is present, massaging might dislodge the clot and cause an embolus.

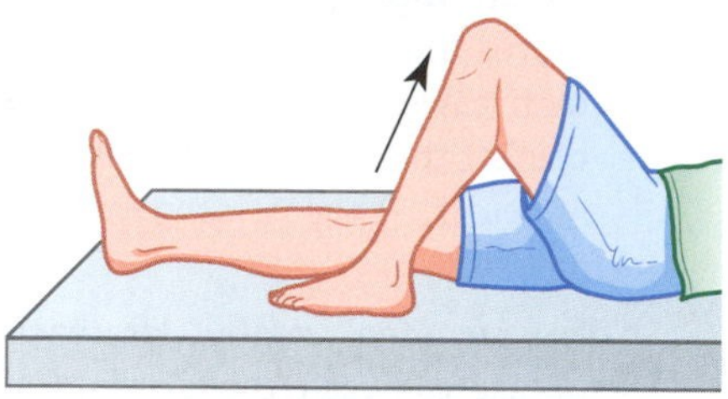

c. Thoroughly wash the foot and toes. Allow the foot to air dry. Apply lotion if the prepackaged bath product does not include emollient and as needed, but do not apply between the toes.
Disease processes frequently decrease circulation to the feet and lower legs, increasing the likelihood that minor skin irritations may become more severe. Applying emollient between the toes can lead to skin breakdown.

d. Repeat the procedure on the other leg and foot.

14. Wash the back and buttocks, using a new, clean wipe.

a. Position the patient on her side with her back facing you or in the prone position. Make sure the siderail on the far side of the bed, facing the patient, is still up.
Provides for clear visualization of back and access to the area.

b. Exposing only the back and buttocks, place the bath towel under the back and buttocks. Wash the back first and then the buttocks. Observe for redness and skin breakdown in the sacral area.
Maintains the principle of "clean to dirty." The sacral area is a common site of pressure injuries.

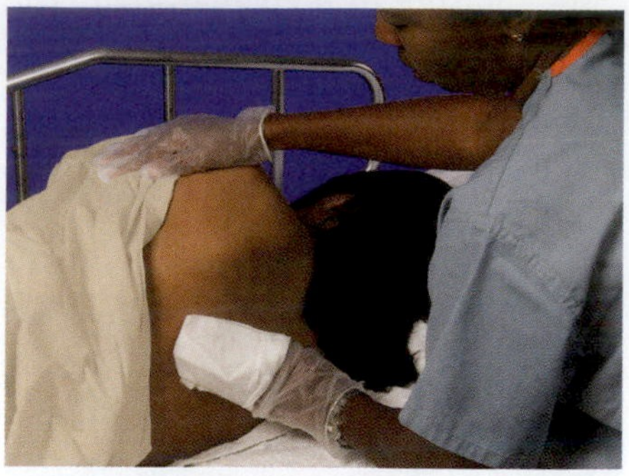

c. Unless contraindicated, give the patient a back rub, applying lotion to the back and buttocks (see Chapter 34, Procedure 34-1: Giving a Back Rub).
Stimulates circulation and maintains the health of the skin. Because the patient is in bed, he is at risk for skin irritation and breakdown from immobility and friction. A back rub may be contraindicated in patients with musculoskeletal injuries or cardiovascular disease.

d. Don procedure gloves if you have not already done so, and wash the rectal area, removing any fecal matter with tissues before washing with the wipe. Wash from front to back.
Washing the rectal area at this time removes the need for the patient to turn to her side again and helps prevent soiling clean linen when changing the linen in an occupied bed. Fecal matter usually contains microorganisms. Washing from front to back helps prevent transferring bacteria from the rectum to the vagina and urethra.

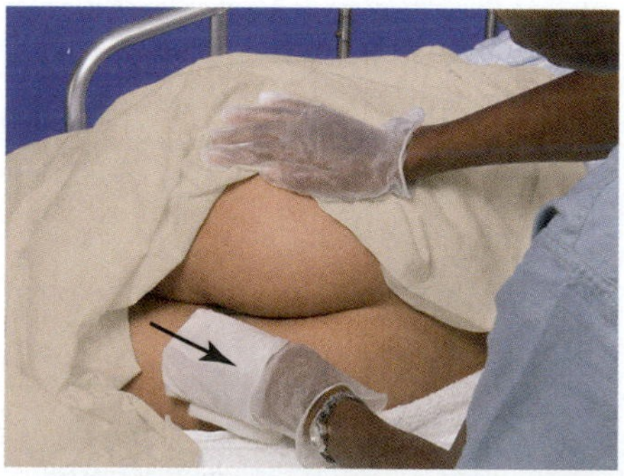

e. Discard the soiled wipe. If linens are soiled, cover them with a clean sheet before repositioning the patient.

f. Remove soiled gloves, and perform hand hygiene. Don new procedure gloves before providing perineal care.
Prevents transferring microorganisms from the anal area to the genital area—cleansing the gluteal and anal areas contaminates the wipe. Maintains standard precautions during the bath and prevents soiling of clean linens during bed change and cross-contamination to other body sites.

15. Cleanse the perineal area. See Procedure 25-4: Providing Perineal Care.

16. After providing perineal care, reposition and cover the patient with the bath blanket. Remove soiled gloves and perform hand hygiene. Help the patient put on a clean gown, and attend to other hygiene needs (e.g., hair grooming).
Prevents contaminating clean linen with soiled gloves. Ensures proper body position and warmth.

17. Change the bed linen, as needed, including soiled linen or linen that became damp during the bath. Properly dispose of soiled items by placing it in a linen bag. See Procedure 25-16: Making an Occupied Bed.
Ensures patient safety, comfort, and privacy.

? What if . . .

- **You are bathing the patient without assistance, or you are not tall enough to comfortably reach across the patient?**

These situations put you at risk for back strain. Thus, you may want to bathe one side of the body—that is, the right arm, trunk, right leg—and then move to the other side of the bed to bathe the opposite side of the body (instead of the order given in Steps 8 and 9). Move the patient close to you before beginning the bath.

- **You are bathing a patient in leg traction?**

  You may decide to bathe the arms and trunk first. Then, have the patient sit forward so that you can cleanse his back. Then, have the patient lift up slightly so that you can wash his buttocks. Finally, wash the lower extremities.

- **You are bathing a patient with dementia?**

  Use your knowledge of the person's bathing practices and preferences to determine a time of day and a routine the person will accept. Keep stimulation to a minimum. Turn on some calming music, speak softly and reassuringly, and do not rush. Keep the patient warm. If the patient becomes agitated and you cannot calm him, do not force him to bathe. You may wish to consider a towel bath (Procedure 25-2) for patients with dementia. Also,

Go to **iCare Box 25-2, Caring Tips for Bathing a Patient with Dementia**, in Volume 1.

Many steps in the bathing process may be misinterpreted or stressful for the person, who may become disruptive or agitated. If forced to bathe, the patient may be upset for hours. Towel baths are effective hygiene measures.

- **Your patient becomes agitated and uncooperative during the bath?**

  Speak calmly and softly. Give the patient a few minutes to calm down. Discontinue the bath if the patient continues to be upset.

- **Your patient is an older adult?**

  a. Some clinicians recommend bathing older adults every other day instead of daily, and it is generally agreed that they should not bathe more than once a day unless soiling occurs.
  Helps prevent skin dryness.

  b. Ensure that the wipes are warm prior to use, but not hot.
  Prevents burns (older adults may have decreased sensation in their extremities).

  c. If you are not using a commercial packaged bath, use antibacterial soap or a mild soap substitute. If you must use soap, it should be nonperfumed and should be rich in moisture. If you use soap, rinse the skin well.
  To avoid skin irritation.

  d. Pat the skin dry or air dry; do not rub.

  e. Immediately after drying, wash your hands and apply moisturizer while there is still moisture in the skin.

  f. Cleanse the skin immediately after every incident of soiling (e.g., when the patient has a bowel movement).
  Prevents maceration and irritation from enzyme activity.

Evaluation

- Assess how well the patient tolerated the procedure. Was there any discomfort, shortness of breath, and so on?
- Observe the patient's mobility, both ROM and ease of movement.
- Note the condition of the patient's skin, including redness and other abnormal findings, especially in skinfolds.
- Ask the patient whether she is comfortable and satisfied.
- If someone other than the nurse performs the procedure, the nurse must still evaluate the care to be certain that it was done and performed satisfactorily.

Patient Teaching

- Discuss the need for activity (e.g., moving about in bed) and the hazards of immobility.
- Discuss usual skin care and how to increase the health of the skin.
- Demonstrate bathing procedure to family or other caregivers.

Home Care

Note: (1) Many of the following apply to older adults and others with self-care deficits. (2) The following refer to all types of home bathing, not just to Procedure 25-1:

- Evaluate the home for bathing safety considerations (not limited to bed bath), such as the following:
  Safety bars in the bathroom?
  To facilitate transfers and provide support while washing.
  A safe water supply for bathing?
  Bathing supplies that are available and accessible?
  Nonskid mat or abrasive strips for shower or tub?
  Stool for shower; transfer bench or stool for getting into the tub?
  Handheld shower spray?
  Long-handled brush or sponge?
- Assess the client's ability to help with the bath or to bathe independently.
- Ask how the client usually bathes (e.g., shower, at the sink). Follow the client's preference as much as possible.
- Ask what supplies the client usually uses for the bath, and ask where they are stored. You will need to adapt the procedure, depending on the available equipment and supplies.
- Suggest the use of large plastic trash bags or a shower curtain to protect the mattress during a bed bath.
- Instruct caregivers to wear gloves when handling linens that are soiled with blood or other body fluids. Linens should be washed in cold water, separately from other household laundry, and then washed again, using hot water, detergent, and bleach.
  Hot water coagulates proteins in the blood and makes it more difficult to remove. Detergent and bleach are used to destroy pathogens.

Documentation

Chart the type of bath given, how much patient was able to help with the bath, how well the patient tolerated the procedure, the patient's mobility, and any abnormal findings. Hygiene care is charted on checklists and flowsheets in most agencies.

(continued on next page)

Procedure 25-1 ■ Bathing: Providing a Complete Bed Bath Using a Prepackaged Bathing Product (continued)

Sample documentation

0630 Complete bed bath given, pt. unable to assist in care. Patient tolerated procedure well, VSS, denied pain. Patient turned side to side with assist of one. Skin warm, dry, and intact. Emollient applied to dry areas. Encouraged patient to shift weight while in bed to prevent injury to skin. ——————— K. Barnett, RN

Practice Resources

Denny & Munro (2017); D'Hondt, A., Kaasalainen, S., Prentice, D., et al. (2012); Konno, Stern, & Gibbs (2013); Nøddeskou, Hemmingsen, & Hørdam (2015); Powers & Fortney (2014); Powers, J., Peed, J., Burns, L., et al. (2012); Siegel, J., Rhinehart, E., Jackson, M., et al. (2007).

Thinking About the Procedure

The videos, **Bathing: Providing a Complete Bed Bath Using a Prepackaged Bathing Product, Providing Perineal Care, Brushing and Flossing the Teeth,** and **Providing Foot Care,** along with questions and suggested responses, are available on the ***Davis's Nursing Skills Videos*** Web site on FADavis.com.

Procedure 25-2 ■ Bathing: Providing a Towel Bath

➤ For steps to follow in *all* procedures, refer to the Universal Steps for All Procedures found on the inside back cover.

➤ *Note:* Because the towel bath is a variation of the bed bath, only the steps differing from a bed bath are listed.

Equipment

- Large plastic bag containing a bath blanket (or a very large towel, about 3 × 6 ft), one standard bath towel, and two or three washcloths
- Dry bath blankets (two or more) and dry bath towels
- Pitcher and approximately 2 qt (2,000 mL) of warm distilled, sterile, or filtered water (105°F [41°C]), according to agency policy
- 30 mL of no-rinse liquid soap or commercial solution of soap, moisturizer, and disinfectant (preferably a CHG and water solution)
- Other supplies for a bed bath (see Procedure 25-1)

Delegation

You can delegate this procedure to the UAP if you conclude that the patient's condition and the UAP's skills allow. Perform the pre-procedure assessments and inform the UAP of the amount of help the patient needs and any special considerations, such as IV lines and drains. Ask the UAP to report the condition of the patient's skin, level of self-care, and ability to tolerate the procedure.

Pre-Procedure Assessments

- Assess the patient's mobility and activity tolerance to determine whether she will be able to assist with the bath, whether a towel bath is appropriate, and the amount of help you will need.
  Decreased activity tolerance or mobility (e.g., because of chest pain or shortness of breath with exertion) may limit the patient's ability to assist with the bath, making a towel bath the most appropriate choice. For severely compromised patients, having two nurses give the bath will make the procedure much quicker and less demanding on the patient.

➤ When performing the procedure, always identify your patient according to agency policy, using two identifiers, and be attentive to standard precautions, hand hygiene, patient safety and privacy, body mechanics, and documentation.

Procedure Steps

1. Prepare the towel bag.

a. Fold the bath blanket.
   Allows for organized application and ease of handling the blanket.

b. Fill a large pitcher with 2,000 mL warm water (approximately 105°F [41°C]). Distilled, sterile, or filtered water is recommended; follow agency policy.
   - Tap water exposes patients to pathogens if biofilm is present in the water lines or faucets. This differs among agencies.
   - The amount of water varies, depending on the size of the bath blanket and bath towel. Use enough water to saturate them.
   - Hot water can injure the patient and removes more of the skin's protective oils, but if the water is too cool, the patient may become chilled.

c. Add 30 mL of no-rinse soap or commercial solution to the water, according to the manufacturer's instructions.
   Adding a prescribed amount of soap to the water before pouring into the bag prevents excessive sudsing.

d. Pour the about 2,000 mL of the solution into the bag, over the bath blanket, bath towel, and wash cloths. Ensure even distribution.

2. **If you do not plan to change** the linen, work one dry bath blanket under the patient.
   Protects the linen and provides warmth.

3. **Spread a dry bath blanket** over the patient; remove the patient's clothing, working underneath the blanket.
   Protects privacy and prevents chilling.

4. **Replace the dry blanket with** the wet blanket:
   a. Take the wet bath blanket or towel out of the bag, squeezing out excess water so that it does not drip.
   b. Push the dry bath blanket down to the patient's waist, and place the wet bath blanket on the patient's chest.
   c. Continue to unfold the wet bath blanket until it covers the patient, pushing the dry bath blanket out of the way as you do so.
   The wet bath blanket will feel warm and relaxing. You will use the dry bath blanket to dry the patient.
   d. If necessary, place yet another dry blanket on top of the wet one.
   This helps hold in the warmth if the patient is chilled or the room is cool.

5. **Bathe the patient**, beginning at the feet and working toward the head.
   a. Keeping the patient covered, use the wet bath blanket to wash the legs, abdomen, and chest.
   b. As you work, replace the wet bath blanket with the dry one.
   Keeps the patient from getting chilled.

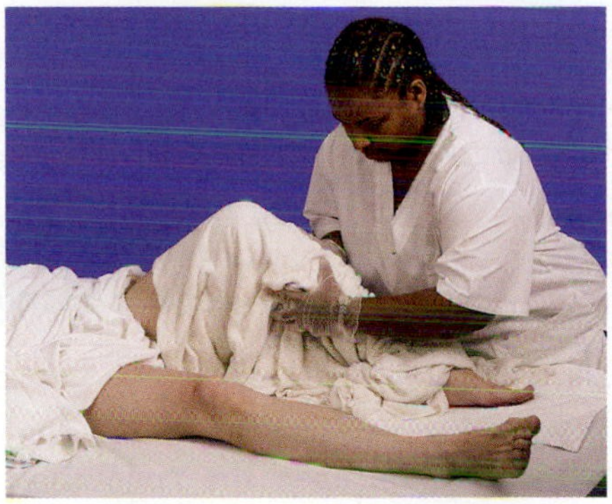

   c. Fold the wet bath blanket as each area is bathed, allowing only clean surfaces to contact clean surfaces.
   Prevents contamination of the clean side of the wet bath blanket.
   d. Use one of the wet washcloths to wash the patient's face, neck, and ears.
   Note that this varies from the order of most baths, which proceed from head to toe. However, this is the most efficient way to accomplish a towel bath. It does not really compromise the "clean to dirty" principle because the legs, abdomen, and chest are usually equally "clean," and you are washing those before the back, buttocks, and perineum.

6. **Don procedure gloves.** Roll the client to one side, unfold the wet bath towel so the clean surface covers the patient, and use the wet bath towel to wash the back and then the buttocks.

7. **Remove procedure gloves,** wash your hands. Don clean procedure gloves and wash the perineal area with a washcloth. See Procedure 25-4: Providing Perineal Care.

8. **Finish the bath** as in Procedure 25-1. Follow patient preferences, whenever possible, to increase feelings of comfort.

9. **Change linen as needed,** including soiled linen or linen that became damp during the bath. You will almost certainly need to change the linen if you have not padded the bottom sheet well before the bath.
   Ensures patient safety and comfort. Because the bath is finished rapidly, there is no real need to pad the bottom sheet if you know that you will have time to change the linens after the bath.

? What if . . .

- **Your patient becomes agitated and uncooperative during the bath?**

  Speak calmly and softly. Give the patient a few minutes to calm down. Discontinue the bath if the patient remains upset.

For Evaluation, Documentation, and Patient Teaching, see Procedure 25-1: Bathing: Providing a Complete Bed Bath Using a Prepackaged Bathing Product.

Practice Resources

Gallagher, M., & Hall, G. R. (2014); Konno, R., Stern, C., & Gibbs, H. (2013); Wilson, M., (2018); Wolf, Z. R., & Czekanski, K. E. (2015).

Procedure 25-3 ■ Bathing: Using a Basin and Water

➤ For steps to follow in *all* procedures, refer to the Universal Steps for All Procedures found on the inside back cover.

Key Point: ***Evidence indicates that (1) bath basins can become a reservoir for microorganisms and for cross-contamination of the immediate environment and healthcare personnel; and (2) biofilm is commonly present in hospital water lines and faucets. Use this method only when a patient is grossly contaminated or refuses other types of bath.***

Equipment

- Disposable water basin for single-patient use
- Tap, distilled, filtered, or sterile water (depending on facility policy)
- CHG and water solution (for bathing the patient and cleaning the basin)
- Lotion, deodorant, and/or powder, as needed
- Bath blanket
- Clean patient gown (gown with shoulder snaps or Velcro closures if the patient has an IV line)
- Clean linen
- Procedure gloves

(continued on next page)

Procedure 25-3 ■ Bathing: Using a Basin and Water (continued)

Delegation

You can delegate this procedure to the UAP if you conclude that the patient's condition and the UAP's skills allow. Perform the pre-procedure assessments, and inform the UAP of the amount of help the patient needs and of any special considerations, such as IV lines and drains. Ask the UAP to report the condition of the patient's skin, level of self-care, and ability to tolerate the procedure.

Pre-Procedure Assessments

Assessments are the same as in Procedure 25-1: Bathing: Providing a Complete Bed Bath Using a Prepackaged Bathing Product.

➤ When performing the procedure, always identify your patient according to agency policy, using two identifiers, and be attentive to standard precautions, hand hygiene, patient safety and privacy, body mechanics, and documentation.

Procedure Steps

1. **Fill the disposable basin** with warm water (approximately 105°F [41°C]). Check the temperature with a thermometer or your hand. If possible, ask the patient to test the water temperature to ensure that it can be tolerated.
   Using tap water for bathing exposes patients to waterborne pathogens; use distilled, filtered, or sterile water, if available. This differs among institutions, so follow agency requirements. Use water that is comfortable for the patient. Hot water removes protective skin oils and can injure the patient. If the water is too cool, the patient may become chilled.
2. **Prepare a solution of 60 mL CHG** solution diluted in 3 qt (2.85 L) of water for bathing the patient (Petlin, Schallom, Prentice, et al., 2014).
   Evidence indicates that use of CHG is effective in preventing the bath basin from becoming a reservoir for microorganisms and in preventing hospital-associated infections (HAIs).
3. **Prepare the patient for the bath** by doing the following (refer to Procedure 25-1 for rationales):
   a. Adjust the bed to working height.
   b. Remove the bedspread and spread bath blanket over top sheet.
   c. Remove the patient's gown, keeping the patient covered with the bath blanket.

   Patient With an IV Line:
   - For a needle free 2-way connector, open the connection, remove the gown, and reconnect the tubing.
   - If there is no 2-way, needle-free connector, remove the gown first from the arm without the IV line, lower the container, and pass gown over the container and tubing, taking care to keep the container above the level of the patient's arm. Rehang the container, and check the flow rate.
   - After the bath, replace the gown by threading the container from inside the arm of the gown and onto the affected arm. Then, place the unaffected arm through the other gown sleeve.

   d. Don clean procedure gloves if exposure to body fluids is likely or if either you or the patient has any breaks in the skin.
4. **Using a clean, rinsed washcloth, wash the patient following the following sequence:**
   Face, neck, ears
   Eyes
   Chest
   Abdomen
   Legs and feet
   Back and buttocks
   Perineum
   Rectal area
   Rinse and wring water from the washcloth as you move from each body area. Change water and use a clean washcloth to wash the perineal area.
   Rinsing keeps washcloth warm and clean. Changing water prevents cross-contamination and contamination of wounds with dirty bath water.
5. **Rinse body areas, as needed** (e.g., if you use soap), and pat dry.
   Preserves skin integrity by preventing the drying effect of the soap on the skin.
6. **Apply deodorant, lotion, and/or powder, as desired or as needed.**
7. **Put used washcloths in the laundry** for future use.
8. **Help patient don a clean gown.**
9. **Provide a back rub**, if not contraindicated.
10. **Reposition patient**, as needed.
11. **Change linens**, as needed, and bag soiled linen for laundering.
12. **Clean and dry the basin** according to agency policy.
   Evidence supports single-patient use of a disposable basin, cleaning it with chlorhexidine solution, drying the basin after each use, storing it upside down, not storing anything (e.g., bathing supplies) in it, and not reusing it (Powers, Peed, Burns, et al., 2012).

For Evaluation, Documentation, and Patient Teaching, see Procedure 25-1: Bathing: Providing a Complete Bed Bath Using a Prepackaged Bathing Product.

Practice Resources

Doughty, D., Junkin, J., Kurz, P., et al. (2012); Petlin, Schallom, Prentice, et al., (2014); Powers, J., Peed, J., Burns, L., et al. (2012); Ritz, J., Pashnik, B., Padula, C., et al. (2012); Wolf, Z. R., & Czekanski, K. E. (2015).

Procedure 25-4 ■ Providing Perineal Care

➤ For steps to follow in all procedures, refer to the Universal Steps for All Procedures found on the inside back cover.

Equipment

- Procedure gloves
- Prepackaged bathing product (i.e., Comfort Care)
- Bedpan or portable sitz tub (optional)
- Bath towel
- Toilet paper
- Plastic trash bag for used wipes and other disposable soiled items
- Perineal ointment or lotion, if needed

If prepackaged bathing product is not available:

- Sterile, filtered, distilled, or tap water according to agency policy
- Disposable basin or perineal wash bottle, if needed
- Perineal cleansing solution or no-rinse soap
- Wash cloths

Delegation

You can delegate perineal care to the UAP if the patient's condition and the UAP's skills allow. Perform the pre-procedure assessments, and inform the UAP of the amount of help the patient needs and any special considerations (e.g., presence of a urinary catheter, vaginal drainage). Ask the UAP to report the condition of the patient's perineum (skin, drainage), level of self-care, and ability to tolerate the procedure.

Pre-Procedure Assessments

- Assess the patient's mobility and activity tolerance.
  Determine whether the patient will be able to assist with the perineal care. Doing as much self-care as possible increases the patient's sense of independence and maintains modesty.
- Check for positioning or activity restrictions, such as maintaining hip abduction following a total hip replacement.
  Prevents injuring the patient during the procedure.
- Assess for psychosocial issues related to perineal care.
  Consider personal and cultural norms to ensure that the perineal care is appropriate for the patient. For example, in some cultures a woman would find it completely unacceptable for a male nurse to provide perineal care (pericare).
- Assess for any specific patient needs, such as presence of a urinary catheter, perineal surgery, lesions, incontinence, or skin breakdown.
  You may need to adapt the procedure (e.g., clean around an indwelling urinary catheter or surgical incision, use special soaps). Incontinence requires assessment and follow-up to prevent Impaired Skin Integrity.

➤ When performing the procedure, always identify your patient according to agency policy, using two identifiers, and be attentive to standard precautions, hand hygiene, patient safety and privacy, body mechanics, and documentation.

Procedure Steps

1. **Adjust the room temperature,** and assist with elimination, as needed.
   Assisting the patient with elimination before perineal care helps prevent interruptions during the procedure and allows for thorough cleansing. Adjusting room temperature prevents chilling.

2. **Warm the perineal bathing** product (disposable wipes).

Variation: If Using a Microwave

Heat the package in the microwave for no longer than 1 minute. The temperature of the contents should be approximately 105°F (41°C). This step is controversial. Some authors suggest that for safety, the commercial bag bath should be performed at room temperature.

Variation: If Using a Warmer Unit

You do not need Step 2 because the bags are always warm.

3. **Prepare the patient.**
   a. Position the patient on her back (supine). Place waterproof pads under the patient if they are not already in place. You may wish to place the patient on a bedpan or portable sitz tub, especially if the perineum is grossly soiled. Place a waterproof bag within reach to discard wipes.
   Placing the patient on a bedpan raises the hips to increase visualization and allows for more thorough cleansing. A bedpan also allows for using water when needed.
   b. Wear procedure gloves (and other protective wear, as needed) when providing perineal care. If you are using a basin and water you may wear a procedure gown and goggles if you are concerned about splashing (e.g., if the patient is confused and may be unable to follow instructions).
   When providing perineal care there is a possibility of coming in contact with urine, vaginal secretions, or fecal material.
   c. Drape the patient to protect privacy.

Variation: For Female Patients

- Drape the bath blanket so that one point faces the patient's head (drape it in the shape of a diamond).
- Take one of the side points of the diamond, and wrap it around the patient's leg. Anchor the end of the blanket under the patient's foot.

(continued on next page)

Procedure 25-4 ■ Providing Perineal Care (continued)

- Repeat on the other leg with other point of the diamond.

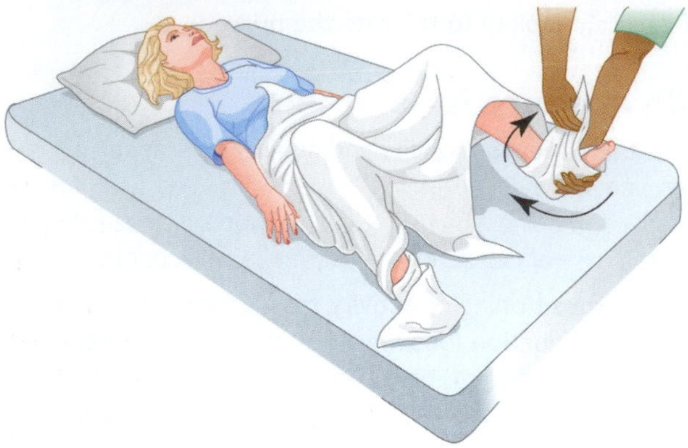

- Fold the center lower point of the diamond up to expose the patient's perineum.

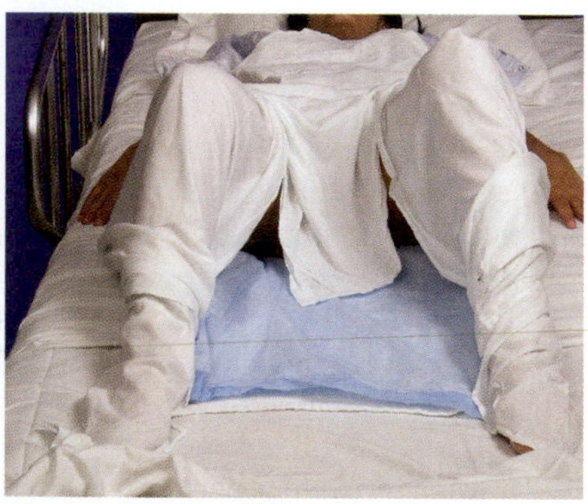

This draping technique covers the patient as much as possible, which helps maintain privacy and prevents chilling during the procedure. The patient can also relax her legs against the bath blanket.

Variation: For Male Patients

- Place the bath blanket over the patient's chest.
- Fold the bed linens down to expose only the patient's groin.

d. Remove any fecal material with toilet paper.
Prevents contamination of the perineum with feces, which can lead to bladder or incisional infections. If you are providing perineal care as part of a bed bath, you will have cleaned the anal area when the patient was in the lateral position.

4. **Wash the perineum,** using a warm disposable wipe. In both males and females, cleanse the skinfolds of the groin area thoroughly. Examine the skin creases for redness or excoriation.

Variation: For Female Patients

Wash the perineum from front to back, using a clean portion of the wipe for each stroke. Cleanse the labial folds and around the urinary catheter, if one is in place.
Prevents contaminating the urethra with fecal material. Any fecal particles that are left can cause skin breakdown as a result of enzyme activity and may increase the risk of a urinary tract infection because of the presence of Escherichia coli in the feces.

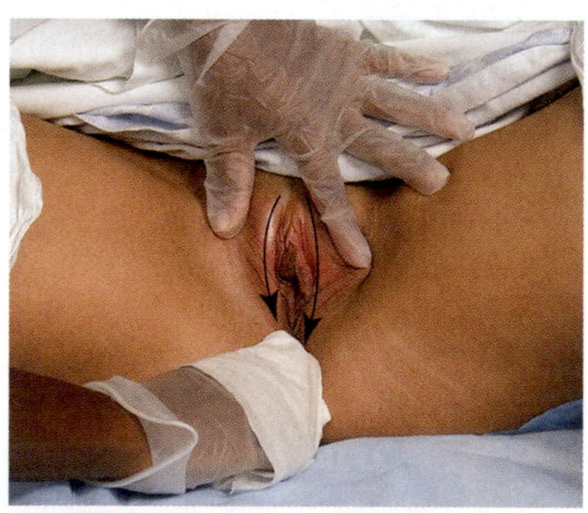

Variation: For Male Patients

Retract the foreskin, if present, and gently cleanse the head of the penis using a circular motion. Replace the foreskin, and finish washing the shaft of the penis, using firm strokes. Then, wash the scrotum, using a clean portion of the wipe with each stroke. Handle the scrotum with care because the area is sensitive.
To adequately clean the head of the penis in an uncircumcised male, you must retract the foreskin. After cleaning, replace the foreskin to prevent constriction and edema of the penis. Firm strokes may help to prevent an erection. Using a clean portion of the wipe for each stroke prevents fecal contamination of the urethra and perineum.

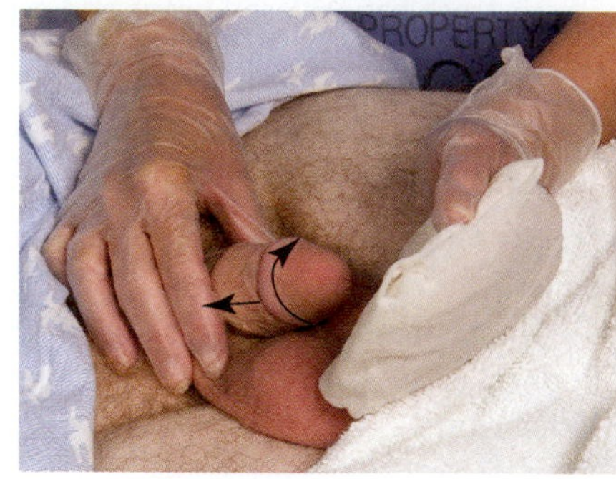

Detects and prevents excoriation in skinfold areas, where moisture accumulates.

5. **Allow body areas to air dry**; do not rinse.
Prevents the emollient and surfactant skin protectants from being removed.

6. **Discard each wipe after use**, or place on the waterproof pad to discard when finished.
Ensures following the "clean-to-dirty" principle.

7. **If perineal care is not being done** as part of the bath, also clean the anal area. Ask the patient to turn to the side, and wipe the buttocks and anal area, as needed.
Fecal contamination of the perineum can lead to urinary tract infections and skin irritation. Therefore, the anal area is cleansed last.

8. **Apply skin protectants,** as needed. Powder only if the patient requests it.
If urinary or fecal incontinence is present, skin barriers may be used to prevent urine, feces, or other drainage from contacting the skin. This helps prevent skin breakdown. For female patients, powder is a medium for bacterial growth. In the presence of moisture, it also creates a paste, which irritates the skin.

9. **If the patient has an indwelling** catheter and if agency policy requires special catheter care, you will usually provide the care at this point. Don clean gloves before providing catheter care, and follow the agency's procedure. For more information about catheter care, see Clinical Insight 28-1: Caring for a Patient With an Indwelling Catheter.

10. **Reposition and cover the patient** with the bath blanket. Remove soiled gloves, discarding in a waterproof bag.
Prevents contaminating clean linen with soiled gloves.

11. **Change linen, as needed**, including soiled linen or linen that became damp during perineal care.
Ensures patient safety, comfort, and privacy.

? What if . . .

- **The patient is unable to control bowel and/or bladder?**

Gently cleanse the perineal/perigenital area after each incontinence/soiling episode, and apply a moisture barrier, according to agency protocols.
Minimizing contact with irritants, such as moisture, urine, and stool, can decrease the development of incontinence-associated dermatitis.

Use a spray, no-rinse cleanser and soft wipes.
These aid in preventing irritation from friction and in reducing drying effects on the skin.

Follow agency policy, and use skin assessment tools (some geared particularly to perineal skin).

Assess for signs of secondary infection in addition to irritation and report, as needed.

Consider bowel and bladder retraining and scheduling to reduce frequency of incontinence.

- **Your patient is in postpartum status?**

Educate the patient about perineal care. Include the importance of handwashing before and after cleansing the perineum, measures to keep the perineum clean, frequent changing of sanitary pads, and checking for signs and symptoms of abnormal lochia. If the patient had an episiotomy, laceration, or tear, teaching should also include management of discomfort and signs of wound infection.

Evaluation

- Assess the patient's responses to the procedure (e.g., any discomfort?).
- Observe for difficulty with movement or ROM during the procedure.
- Note the condition of the skin, including redness and other abnormal findings.
- Ask the patient whether she feels comfortable now.

Patient Teaching

- Discuss adaptations to perineal care. For example, if the area is tender, (1) wash the area with warm moistened wipe after going to the bathroom, instead of using toilet paper; or (2) use a skin protectant on the area.
- Review the importance of handwashing after elimination.
- As needed, teach the caregiver how to provide perineal care, including the major concept of cleaning front to back ("clean to dirty"). Stress the importance of wearing gloves and washing hands.
- Advise women not to douche because it disturbs the balance of normal vaginal flora and can irritate or injure mucosal cells.
- Explain that scented and deodorant feminine hygiene products are not necessary for cleanliness and may even be harmful. Daily cleansing is the most effective means of odor control.

Home Care

- Evaluate the ability of the client or caregiver to provide perineal care.
- Determine the availability of supplies needed for perineal care.
- You will need to adapt the procedure, depending on the available equipment and supplies. Major issues involved in perineal care in the home are the lack of clean water and/or linens. In some instances, you may need to use bottled water or to boil water for the procedure. One option is to use prepackaged moistened towelettes to provide the care (e.g., Comfort Bath towelettes).

Documentation

Usually, perineal care is part of routine hygiene care and is charted on a flowsheet. If you need to write a narrative note, chart that perineal care was given, any patient responses to the procedure, and the condition of the perineal area.

Sample documentation

8/16/20 1430 Perineal care given. Patient had no complaint of discomfort. No redness or discharge noted.—————— Nora Noyes, RN

Practice Resources

Martin, Haider, Palleschi, et al., (2017); Pather, P., & Hines, S. (2016).

Thinking About the Procedure

The video, **Providing Perineal Care**, along with questions and suggested responses, is available on the ***Davis's Nursing Skills Videos*** Web site on FADavis.com.

Procedure 25-5 ■ Providing Foot Care

➤ For steps to follow in *all* procedures, refer to the Universal Steps for All Procedures found on the inside back cover.

➤ *Note:* This procedure describes foot care using a basin and water. It may also be done with prepackaged wipes, along with the bath.

Equipment

- Procedure gloves (if there are open lesions)
- Pillow (if procedure is done with the patient in bed)
- Disposable basin for water (distilled, sterile, or filtered tap water, per agency requirements)
- Liquid no-rinse soap
- Bath towel and washcloth
- Waterproof pad
- Orangewood stick
- Toenail clippers and nail file
- Lotion or prescribed ointment or cream

Delegation

You can delegate foot care to the UAP if the patient's condition and the UAP's skills allow. For example, as a rule, you should not delegate care if the patient has impaired peripheral circulation or foot ulcers. Perform the following pre-procedure assessments, and inform the UAP of the amount of help the patient needs and any special considerations (e.g., ability to sit in a chair). Ask the UAP to report the condition of the patient's skin and nails, level of self-care, and ability to tolerate the procedure.

Pre-Procedure Assessments

- As you assess the feet and toenails, compare the findings for both feet.
- Assess bilateral dorsalis pedis pulses, capillary refill, skin color, and warmth. Compare right and left feet. Palpate pulses at the same time bilaterally to determine whether one side is weaker than the other.
  Decreased circulation to the feet increases the risk for tissue injury and infection. A variety of diseases can cause poor circulation. For example, cardiac or renal disease may cause pedal edema, which impairs circulation to the skin, and diabetes causes vascular changes leading to poor circulation to the lower extremities.
- Assess for diseases (e.g., diabetes mellitus and peripheral vascular disease) that create risks for foot problems.
- Thoroughly assess all areas of the feet for skin integrity, edema, condition of toenails, and any abnormalities. Check carefully between the toes.
  Decreased circulation in the feet commonly causes such problems as thickened toenails, dry skin, and increased risk of infection. Changes in vision and mobility can increase the risk for injuries to the feet. Patients with diabetes also may have neuropathy, which prevents them from knowing when they have injured their feet. Identifying abnormalities enables you to provide interventions to help prevent potential problems. ▼

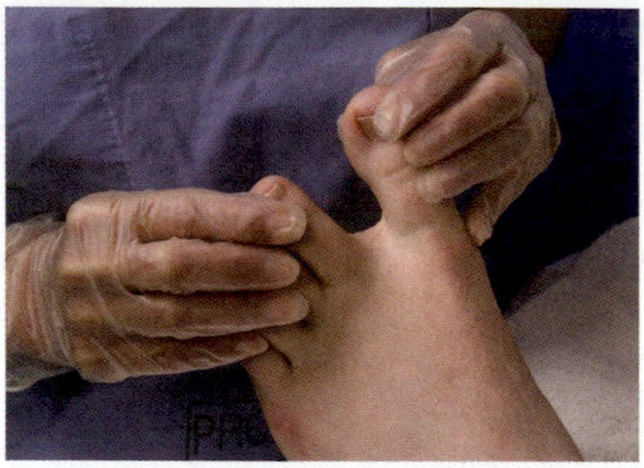

- Check institutional policy to verify whether a nurse is allowed to trim nails. Obtain a primary provider's prescription for trimming the patient's nails, if necessary.
  Patients who have diabetes or impaired circulation to the lower extremities require a prescription for trimming their nails. Refer the patient to a podiatrist if the circulation is severely compromised or if edema would make the procedure difficult.
- Assess the patient's usual footwear.
  Improperly fitting shoes, especially if they are too tight, are a common cause of foot problems (e.g., bunions, ingrown toenails).
- Assess the patient's self-care ability to provide foot care. Evaluate the need for a referral. Determine whether the patient has the necessary vision and mobility to be able provide his own foot care.
- Assess the patient's knowledge about foot care, including usual foot care practices.

Identify potential deficits in understanding that may require additional teaching or referral to a podiatrist, general practice physician, or advanced practice nurse.

Many home remedies for foot problems can damage the tissue. For example, corn pads can increase pressure on the tissue, compromising circulation and causing local tissue ischemia. Cutting the sides of the toenails can lead to ingrown toenails.

➤ When performing the procedure, always identify your patient according to agency policy, using two identifiers, and be attentive to standard precautions, hand hygiene, patient safety and privacy, body mechanics, and documentation.

Procedure Steps

1. **Wear procedure gloves** and other protective wear, as needed, when providing foot care.
   Follows standard precautions. The heel is a common place for skin breakdown, so use gloves if you are unable to see the area without lifting the foot. If the patient has significant drainage to the area, such as a draining wound, you may need to wear a protective gown.
2. **Ask the patient to sit in a chair** with a waterproof pad or bath towel under the feet, if possible. If the patient is unable to sit in a chair, place him in semi-Fowler's position in bed; place a pillow under his knees.

It is easier to perform the procedure with the patient in a chair. The pillow supports the knee joints and prevents muscle fatigue.

3. **Fill the basin halfway** with warm water (approximately 105°F to 110°F [40°C to 43°C]).
Recent research recommends the use of filtered, distilled, or sterile water. Using tap water for bathing exposes patients to waterborne pathogens that may be contained in biofilm in water lines and faucets. Hot water can injure the skin. Warm water promotes circulation. Filling the basin halfway prevents spilling when the patient places his foot in the water.

4. **Help the patient place one foot** in the water, first checking with the patient that the temperature is comfortable.
   a. If the patient is in a chair, place the basin on the floor (on the waterproof pad).
   b. If the patient is in bed, place the basin near the foot of the bed on the waterproof pad; pad the basin with a towel.
   The waterproof pad keeps the bed dry. Padding the basin prevents pressure on the back of the leg, which could cause discomfort and interfere with circulation.

5. **Allow the foot to soak** for 5 to 20 min, depending on the patient's tolerance and the condition of his feet.

Soaking is not recommended for patients with diabetes or peripheral vascular disease (PVD).

Soaking softens the skin and helps relax the patient. For patients who have diabetes or PVD, soaking is not recommended because it may remove natural oils, cause cracking of the skin, and may cause burns even if the water is at the recommended temperature.

6. **Cleanse the foot** with mild or no-rinse soap.
Removes loose debris. No-rinse soaps do not dry the skin.

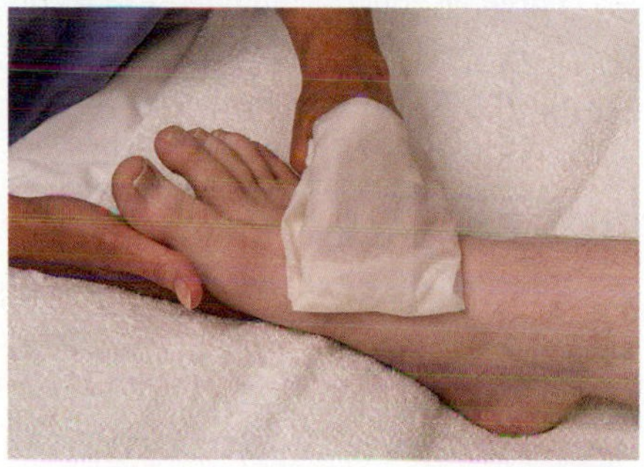

7. **Clean under the nails** with the orangewood stick while the foot is still in the water.
Water softens the nails and makes cleaning easier.

8. **Remove the foot from** the water, and dry it gently and thoroughly.
Remaining moisture, especially between the toes, can cause maceration and promotes development of fungal infections.

9. **Change the water.**
Ensures proper temperature and prevents cross-contamination.

10. **Soak the opposite foot** while performing Steps 11 through 14 for the first (clean) foot.
Efficient use of time.

11. **Gently push the cuticles back** with the orangewood stick or towel.
Increases cuticle health. Do not damage the cuticle; doing so can increase the risk of infection.

12. **Trim the nails straight across** with toenail clippers, if not contraindicated by the patient's condition and if permitted by agency policy. Note whether the nail has cut into the skin of the toe being trimmed or the adjacent toes. If the nails are brittle or thick, allow the foot to soak for 10 to 20 minutes before trimming.
Trimming straight across prevents ingrown toenails. Early recognition and treatment of problems will prevent further complications, such as infection.

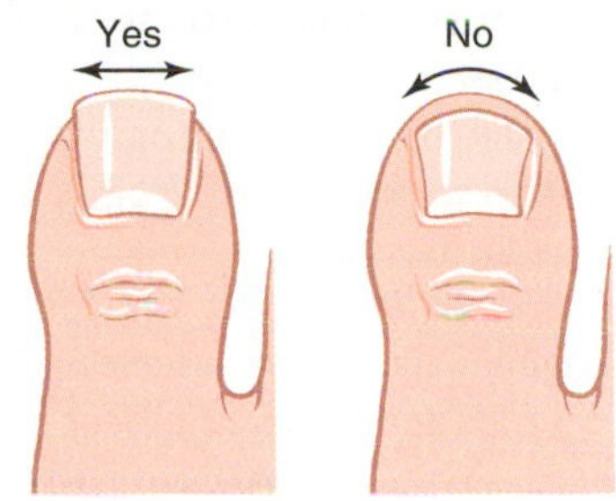

13. **File the nails** with an emery board.
Smooths the edges to prevent scratching the skin with the toenails.

14. **Apply cream, lotion,** or foot powder lightly to the feet and toes.
Cream hydrates the skin; however, excess cream can cause maceration. Foot powder absorbs moisture and functions as a nonirritating deodorant for patients whose feet perspire heavily.

15. **Repeat Steps 11 through 14** with the second foot.

16. **Check the patient's footwear** for rough edges that may injure feet.

? What if . . .

- **My patient has Impaired Bed Mobility?**
  Apply protective devices (e.g., lamb's wool), as needed.
- **My patient has an injury, lesions, or pain?**
  You may need to use a bed cradle to keep the pressure of the bedding off the patient's feet. Refer to Chapter 35 for other measures to preserve skin integrity.
- **My patient has diabetes mellitus?**
  In addition to controlling blood glucose levels, adhering to a specific foot care plan is essential for people with diabetes. Include the following in your teaching:
  - The importance of inspecting the feet daily
  - Ways to protect the feet (e.g., by wearing shoes when out of bed)

(continued on next page)

Procedure 25-5 ■ Providing Foot Care (continued)

- Potential complications involving the feet
- Management of symptoms
- When to seek advice from a health-care professional
- What to include in the foot care regimen (apply moisturizing lotion on tops and bottoms of feet but not between toes)—and what not to do (cut corns and calluses, use topical corn removers, or soak the feet)

- Elderly patients with diabetes are especially at risk for development of foot-related complications. Visual changes and loss of flexibility could make it challenging to bend and visualize the feet. Plastic mirrors may be helpful in this regard.

Early detection and treatment of problems can minimize foot-related complications.

Evaluation

- Observe that feet are clean, smooth, and intact; nails are trimmed and smooth; and the skin is pink and warm.
- Ensure that foot problems are identified and interventions provided.
- Ask the patient to demonstrate or describe correct foot care.

Patient Teaching

For patient teaching,

Go to the **Self-Care box, Teaching Your Client About Foot Care,** in Volume 1.

Home Care

The procedure does not vary in the home. The nurse must:

- Work with the client and the caregiver to determine the availability of supplies needed for foot care (clean water and so on).
- Identify home care practices, and teach the client and/or the caregiver proper foot care techniques. Influencing older adults can be especially difficult if they have usual routines (e.g., walking barefoot) that put them at risk for injury. For clients with diabetes, the biggest risk to foot health is inadequate regulation of their blood glucose levels.

Documentation

In most agencies, you will not document routine foot care (except, perhaps, on a checklist) unless there are problems. If you do document, chart that foot care was given, and chart assessment findings.

Sample documentation

09/25/20 0900. Foot care given. 2 cm circular reddened area on right heel. Skin abrasion outer lateral aspect of 5th toe, left foot —bioocclusive dressing applied. —————————— Ann Hopkins, RN

Practice Resources

Bonner, T., Foster, M., & Spears-Lanoix, E. (2016); National Guideline Clearinghouse (2015); Powers, J., Peed, J., Burns, L., et al. (2012); Siegel, J., Rhinehart, E., Jackson, M., et al. (2007, updated 2017).

Thinking About the Procedure

The video, **Providing Foot Care,** along with questions and suggested responses, is available on the ***Davis's Nursing Skills Videos*** Web site on FADavis.com.

Procedure 25-6 ■ Brushing and Flossing the Teeth

➤ For steps to follow in all procedures, refer to the Universal Steps for All Procedures found on the inside back cover.

Equipment

- Toothbrush or sponge toothettes
- Toothpaste
- Dental floss (two pieces, each about 10 inches long) and floss holder (optional)
- Tonsil-tip suction connected to suction source (if aspiration is a concern)
- Emesis basin
- Towel
- Glass of water (distilled, sterile, or filtered water, according to agency requirements)

Key Point: ***Recent studies recommend that hospitalized patients at high risk for infection avoid exposure to hospital water. Follow agency policy.***

- Mouthwash and/or lip moisturizer, if desired
- Procedure gloves; mask and goggles, if splashing may occur

Delegation

You can delegate oral hygiene to the UAP if the patient's condition and the UAP's skills allow. Perform the following assessments, and inform the UAP of the specific type of oral care and the amount of help the patient needs. Ask the UAP to report the condition of the patient's mouth, level of self-care, and ability to tolerate the procedure.

Pre-Procedure Assessments

- Assess the patient's ability to assist with oral care.
  Having the patient assist whenever possible promotes independence and supports a positive self-image.
- Determine whether the patient has dentures, bridgework, or partial plates.
  Determines how you will provide oral care.
- Assess general oral health, including gag reflex and the condition of teeth, gums, and mucous membranes. If a patient has dentures, examine the mouth with and without the dentures.
  (a) If the patient has a hypoactive or absent gag reflex, you will need a suction setup to prevent aspiration. (b) Inflammation or lesions in the mouth increase the patient's risk of infection and may make eating difficult or painful, leading to malnutrition. (c) Poorly fitting dentures can cause irritation of the gums.
- Assess the patient's usual oral care, including cultural practices.
  Helps determine the type of oral care you will provide and identifies areas of patient teaching needed.

- When performing the procedure, always identify your patient according to agency policy, using two identifiers, and be attentive to standard precautions, hand hygiene, patient safety and privacy, body mechanics, and documentation.

Procedure Steps

1. **Position the patient in a high-Fowler's** position or in a chair, if possible. Position the patient on her side if the head of bed cannot be elevated.
   Prevents aspiration and makes the procedure easier.

2. **Set up suction, if needed.** Attach suction tubing and tonsil-tip suction; check suction.
   Suctioning equipment may be needed to prevent aspiration of secretions during the procedure, especially if the gag reflex is decreased.

3. **If the patient is able to perform self-care:**
   a. Arrange supplies within the patient's reach.
      Promotes the patient's ability to perform self-care and, thus, independence.
   b. Assist the patient with brushing and flossing, as needed.
      Ensures that the teeth are thoroughly cleaned.

Procedure Variation: For Nurse-administered Brushing and Flossing

Follow the remaining steps.

4. **Place the towel across the patient's chest.**
   Prevents getting the patient's gown or linen wet during the procedure.

5. **Don procedure gloves, as needed.** Wear gown and goggles if splashing might occur, such as with a confused patient.
   Follows standard precautions.

6. **Adjust the bed to working height**; lower the siderail nearest you.
   Prevents you from having to lean over the patient or reach across the siderail, possibly causing back strain or injury.

7. **Moisten a small, soft toothbrush**, and apply a small amount of toothpaste. See Equipment for type of water to use.
   A small toothbrush fits more easily into the mouth and reaches more areas. The soft bristles can be used to brush the tongue and also the gums if the patient is edentulous. Excessive toothpaste does not increase the cleaning, and toothpaste residue has a drying effect on the mucosa. Moistening the toothbrush increases patient comfort because patients frequently experience dry mouth.

8. **Place, hold, or ask the patient** to hold the emesis basin under the chin.
   Collects oral secretions and protects clothing and linens.

9. **Brush the patient's teeth,** holding the bristles at a 45° angle to the gumline.
   a. Using short circular motions, gently brush the inner and outer surfaces of teeth, from the gumline to the crown of each tooth.
   b. Brush the biting surface of the back teeth by holding the brush bristles straight up and down to the teeth and brushing back and forth.
      This is the most effective technique for removing all food particles and plaque from the teeth and gums. Removing debris and subsequent plaque helps decrease microbial colonization.
   c. If the patient is frail, perform oral suctioning when fluid accumulates in the mouth.
      Prevents choking and aspiration.

Brush teeth, holding bristles at a 45° angle to the gumline. Using short circular motions, gently brush the inner and outer surfaces of the teeth, including the gumline.

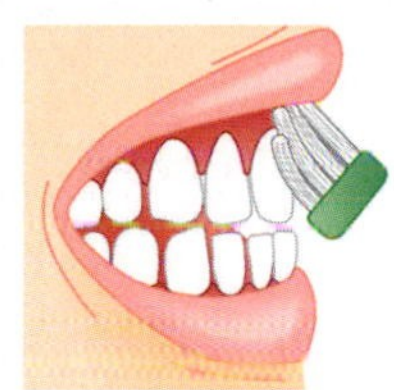
Clean front teeth.

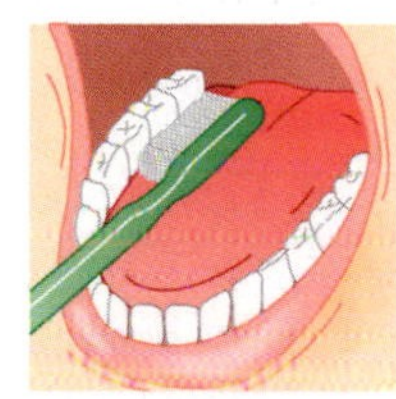
Clean both inner and outer surfaces of the teeth.

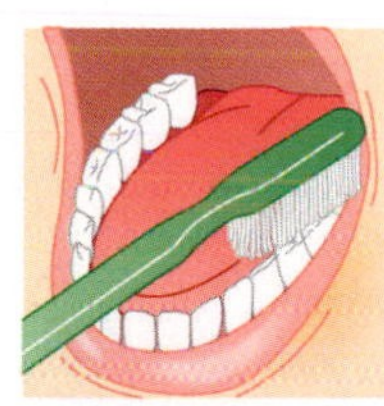
Brush the biting surfaces of the back teeth with the brush bristles straight up and down.

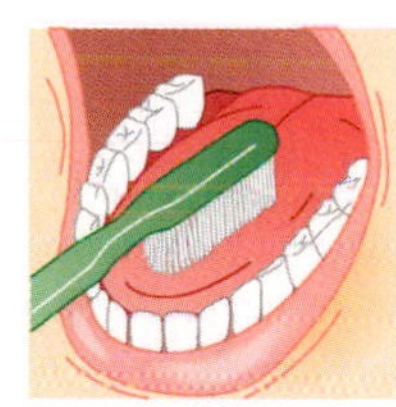
Brush the surface of the tongue.

10. **Gently brush the patient's tongue.**
    Removes coating and accumulated debris that can be a reservoir for bacteria. Brush gently to prevent gagging or vomiting.

(continued on next page)

Procedure 25-6 ■ Brushing and Flossing the Teeth (continued)

11. **Floss the teeth.** Grasp dental floss in both hands, or use a floss holder.

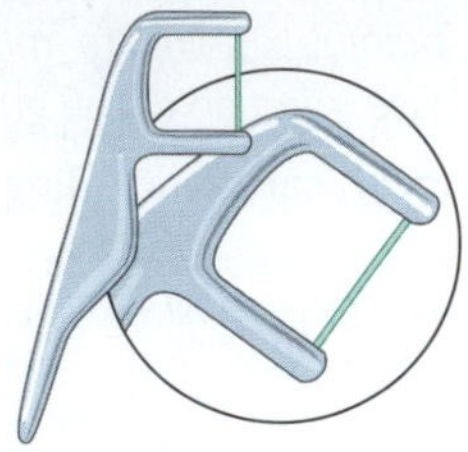

Variation: If you are not using a floss holder

a. Wrap one end of the floss around the middle finger of each hand.

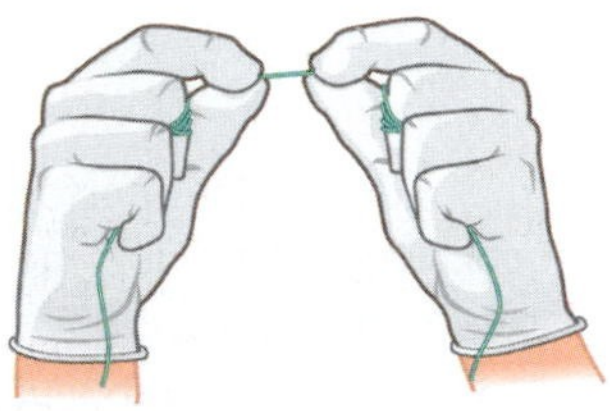

b. Stretch the floss between your thumbs and index fingers, and move the floss up and down against each tooth.

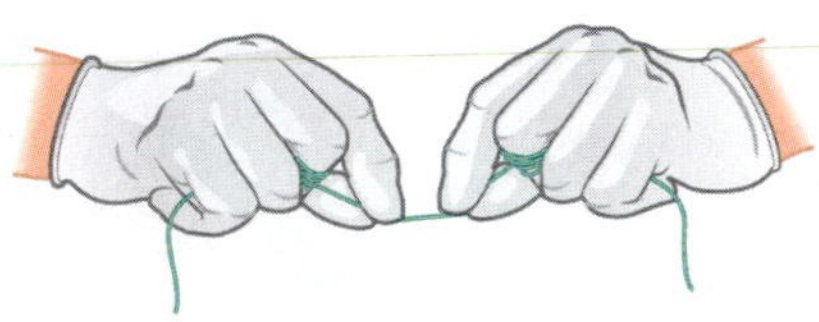

c. Floss between and around all teeth. *Moving the floss up and down instead of back and forth prevents damaging the gums.*

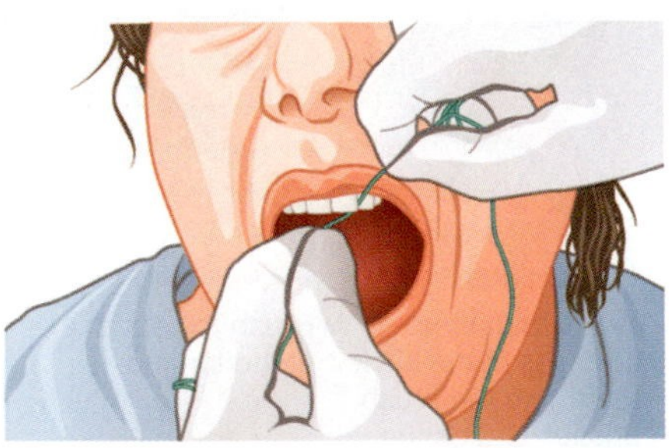

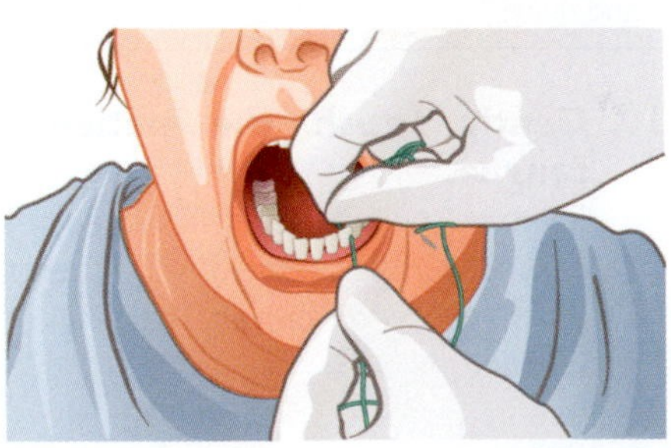

12. **Assist the patient in rinsing** his mouth, suctioning as needed. Or ask the patient to rinse vigorously and spit the water into the emesis basin. *Removes food particles from mouth. Suction if the patient has a decreased or absent gag reflex.*

13. **Offer a mild or dilute mouthwash,** and apply lip moisturizer, if desired. *Prevents irritation of the mucous membranes. Apply lip moisturizer for dry lips, for unconscious patients, or those on a ventilator, or per patient preference.*

14. **Reposition the patient,** as needed, and return the bed to the low position. *Ensures patient comfort and safety.*

? What if . . .

- **My patient has an excessively dry oral cavity?**

  You may need to use a saliva substitute. *Aging, adverse medication effects, and illness often lead to decreased salivary production.*

- **My patient has viscous (thick) mucus?**

  Use appropriately diluted sodium bicarbonate to dissolve viscous mucus.

- **My patient has a high risk of bleeding of gums (e.g., associated with thrombocytopenia), has painful mouth lesions, or toothbrushing is otherwise contraindicated?**

  You may use foam or cotton mouth swabs instead of a toothbrush. Do not use glycerin swabs, lemon glycerin swabs, or gauze squares. Use normal saline mouthwash. *Foam swabs are less effective in removing debris and plaque, so it is best to brush when not contraindicated. Lemon glycerin swabs are drying to the mucosa and may cause decalcification of tooth enamel. Mouthwashes may be painful.*

- **My patient has dementia or is uncooperative and agitated for other reasons?**

  Use dementia-focused behavior management strategies:

  Older adults with dementia frequently accumulate greater amounts of plaque and calculus, exhibit a higher incidence of periodontal gingival bleeding, and demonstrate a greater prevalence of denture-related oral mucosal lesions, and yet they often resist oral care.

  - Provide oral hygiene at the same time every day, not necessarily at bathing time.
  - Use as many staff members as necessary.
  - Give care in a quiet, distraction-free environment. Keep stimulation to a minimum, turn on some calming music.
  - Speak softly; give one-step directions in short, simple sentences.
  - Use a relaxed, slow approach; be sure your facial expression does not reflect tension.
  - Give reassuring body contact, and use gentle touch. *Promotes trust. Quick or forceful touch may frighten the patient.*
  - Provide diversion. *Occupies the patient's hands and prevents "grabbing."*
  - Never place your fingers between the teeth.
  - Try placing a spare toothbrush or a rolled facecloth in the patient's hands while you provide oral care. *Minimizes "grabbing."*
  - Use the "hand-over-hand" technique to gently guide the patient's own hand.
  - Try starting the task (e.g., brushing) and then having the resident help finish it.
  - If the procedure is not going well, find another care provider to come in and attempt the task.
  - Use modified equipment and aids, if available (e.g., mouth props, backward-bent and suction toothbrushes).

- **My patient is on a ventilator, is a frail older adult, or has undergone cardiac surgery?**

  Be certain that teeth are brushed twice a day.
  In addition to brushing, use moisturizer on lips and oral mucosa every 2 to 4 hours.
  Apply a 0.12% CHG solution twice daily to complement oral care.

- **My patient is receiving chemotherapy?**

  Stress the importance of good oral hygiene, including brushing teeth after meals and before going to bed. *Chemotherapy can cause neutropenia (reduced white blood cell count), predisposing the patient to infections. The oral cavity is a common site for infections in patients with neutropenia.*

  Routine rinses of mouthwashes with chlorhexidine are not recommended. Instead, use a bland rinse of diluted salt and/or sodium bicarbonate. Patients should swish for a minimum of 30 seconds and then expectorate the residue. *Chlorhexidine products have not proved superior to bland rinses in preventing or reducing either chemotherapy/radiation-induced mucositis or yeast colonization. In addition, chlorhexidine products may contain alcohol, may cause discomfort, may alter taste sensations, and may stain teeth. Bland rinses containing 1 teaspoon of salt or sodium bicarbonate per pint of water reduce the acidity of oral secretions, lessen mucus accumulation, and discourage yeast colonization.*

  An antifungal agent or a multiagent rinse (sometimes labeled "magic" or "miracle" rinse) may be used, followed by a short NPO (nothing by mouth) period of 30 to 60 minutes. If other mouthwashes or rinses are also being used, allow 30 minutes to pass between their use and the use of an antifungal agent.

  Multiagent rinses typically contain lidocaine. The resulting numbing effect may pose risks for a biting injury or aspiration. These rinses can neutralize antifungal agents.

Evaluation

- Inspect teeth, gums, and mucous membranes to verify that they are free of food particles.
- Inspect for abnormalities, such as bleeding, that may have been stimulated by the brushing or flossing.
- Observe for patient discomfort or gagging during the procedure.
- If the procedure was performed by the UAP, the nurse should still perform an evaluation of the care. This includes a physical assessment of the oral cavity as well as objective and subjective findings related to the patient's tolerance of and satisfaction with the care.

Patient Teaching

- Discuss the importance of daily oral care.
- Review any areas of brushing or flossing that the patient has not been performing adequately.
- Discuss any problems that need further follow-up, such as inflammation, bleeding, dryness, caries, missing teeth, or broken or missing dentures.

Home Care

The procedure does not vary in the home setting. The nurse must:

- Work with the client and care provider to determine supplies needed for the home.
- Determine whether suction is needed (e.g., if the client is unconscious or has a decreased gag reflex). Explain to the client and/or caregiver how to obtain a portable suction unit.
- Demonstrate how to position the client and perform the procedure if the height of the bed is not adjustable or if both sides of the bed are not accessible.

Documentation

Document that oral care was given, the patient's response, any abnormal findings, and nursing interventions. Oral care is usually charted on a flowsheet.

Sample documentation

12/16/20 0815 Oral care given. Mucous membranes intact, pink and dry. No choking or complaints of discomfort. Patient encouraged to increase fluid intake. ——————— Nancy Botha, RN

Practice Resources

AACN (2017); Berry, A. Davidson, P., Nicholson, L., et al. (2011); Coker, E., Ploeg, J., Kaasalainen, S., & Carter, N. (2017); Philip, P., Rogers, C., Kruger, E., et al. (2012); Weening-Verbree, L., Huisman-de Waal, G., van Dusseldorp, L., et al. (2013).

Thinking About the Procedure

The video, **Brushing and Flossing the Teeth,** along with questions and suggested responses, is available on the ***Davis's Nursing Skills Videos*** Web site on FADavis.com.

Procedure 25-7 ■ Providing Denture Care

➤ For steps to follow in *all* procedures, refer to the Universal Steps for All Procedures found on the inside back cover.

Equipment

- See Procedure 25-6: Brushing and Flossing the Teeth.
- Denture cup

Delegation

You can delegate denture care to the UAP if the patient's condition and the UAP's skills allow. Perform the pre-procedure assessments, and inform the UAP of the specific care and the amount of help the patient needs. Ask the UAP to report the condition of the patient's mouth and dentures, level of self-care, and ability to tolerate the procedure.

Pre-Procedure Assessments

See Procedure 25-6: Brushing and Flossing Teeth.

➤ When performing the procedure, always identify your patient according to agency policy, using two identifiers, and be attentive to standard precautions, hand hygiene, patient safety and privacy, body mechanics, and documentation.

Procedure Steps

1. **Don gloves, and remove dentures** (if the patient cannot do so).
   a. ***Upper denture:*** With a gauze pad, grasp the denture with your thumb and forefinger, and move it gently up and down. Tilt the denture slightly to one side to remove it, without stretching the lips. Place the denture in the denture cup.
   The gauze gives you a better grip. Breaking the seal on the top dentures can be difficult; movement breaks the suction. Always place dentures in a denture cup as soon as you remove them to prevent accidental breakage.▼

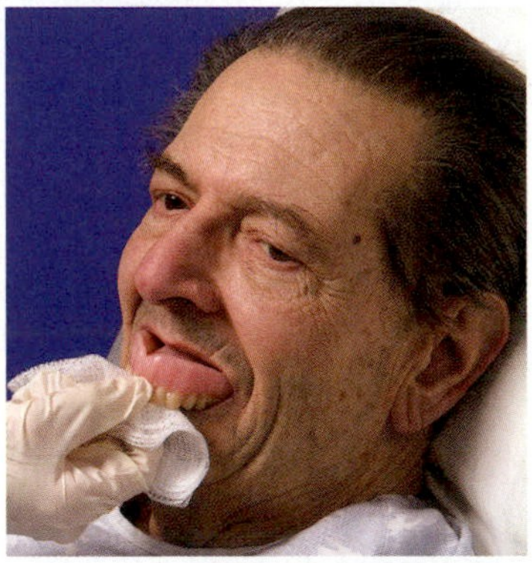

   b. ***Lower denture:*** Use your thumbs to push up gently on the denture at the gumline to release from the lower jaw. Grasp the denture with your thumb and forefinger, and tilt it to remove it from the patient's mouth. Place the denture in the denture cup.
   A gauze pad is not usually needed to grasp the lower dentures; however, you can use one if the dentures are difficult to grasp. Pushing up on the dentures breaks the seal. Rotating the dentures is necessary to remove the dentures from the patient's mouth.▼

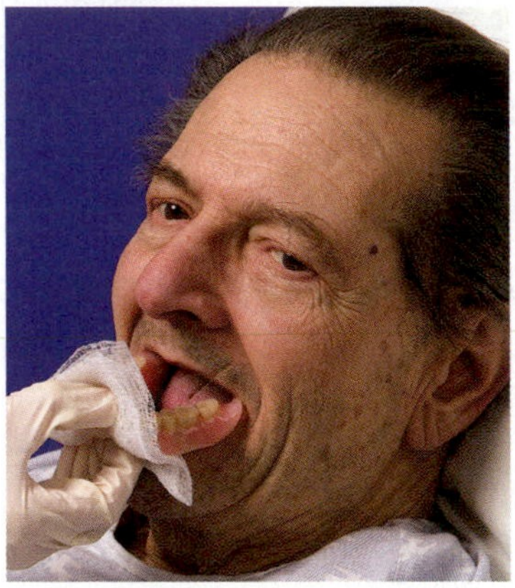

2. **Place the towel in the sink**, and pour cool water (in accordance with agency policy) over the dentures to cleanse them.
   Heat can damage some dentures. It is best to cleanse dentures in the sink, under running water, and over a plastic pan or towel. Running water facilitates cleansing; the towel/pan helps keep dentures from breaking. Dentures are expensive and usually not reimbursed by insurance. Institutions vary with regard to the existence of biofilm in the water lines.
   a. Apply a small amount of special denture paste to a soft-bristled toothbrush.
   Denture paste assists in cleaning. Toothpaste and stiff-bristled brushes may be too abrasive for dentures. However, follow the patient's preference in use of denture cleaner. Some patients prefer to soak their dentures in a cleanser overnight. If dentures have been soaking, rinse them well before placing them in the patient's mouth.
   b. Brush all surfaces of each denture.
   Loosens all food particles and any old denture adhesive.
   c. Rinse thoroughly with cool water.
   Removes loosened particles and the cleaning agent. Do not use hot water with dentures because hot water can react to make the denture material sticky. Hospitalized patients at high risk for infection should avoid exposure to hospital water and use distilled sterile or filtered water instead.

   Note: You can soak stained dentures in a commercial cleaner, following the manufacturer's instructions. Do not soak the denture overnight if the appliance has metal parts.

   Soaking can cause corrosion of the metal parts.

3. **Inspect dentures** for rough, worn, or sharp edges.
   These can irritate the tongue, gums, or mucous membranes of the mouth.

4. **Inspect the mouth** under the dentures for redness, irritation, lesions, or infection.
   If present, refer to a dentist to check the fit of the dentures or to make needed repairs.

5. **Apply denture adhesive,** as needed (ask the patient whether he uses denture adhesive).
   Adhesives are needed to "seal" some dentures and prevent slipping and irritation of the gums.

6. **Moisten the top denture,** if it is dry. Then, insert the top denture, at a slight tilt, and press it up against the roof of the mouth.
Moistening the dentures eases insertion. You can tell when you have securely seated the dentures by checking to feel for any slippage or to confirm that the dentures stay in place. Because the top denture is larger, it is removed first and inserted first for ease of insertion.

7. **Moisten the bottom denture,** if it is dry. Then insert bottom denture, rotating it as you put it in the patient's mouth.
Because it is smaller, the bottom denture is inserted after the top one.

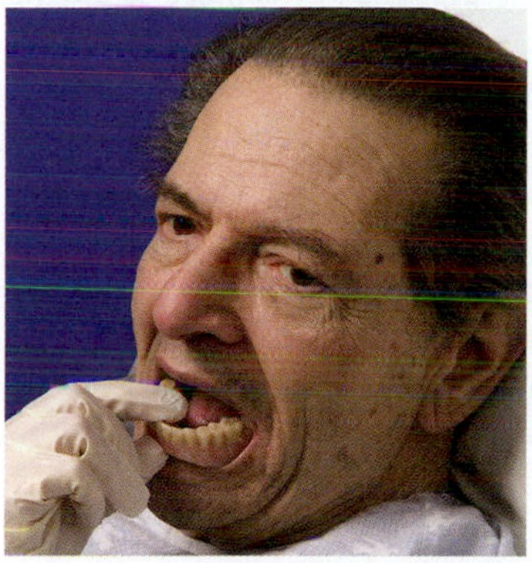

8. **Ask the patient whether** the dentures are comfortable.
Ensures that the dentures are properly placed.

9. **If the patient does not wish to** wear the dentures, keep them covered with water in a clean denture container with a lid. Label the container with the patient's name and the agency identifying number. Place denture container in bedside drawer, rather than on top of bedside table, for safekeeping.
Drying can cause dentures to warp. Hospitalized patients at high risk for infection avoid exposure to hospital water and use sterile water instead. Having the denture out of the mouth for several hours a day relieves pressure on the oral tissues, allows saliva to clean the tissues, and helps minimize gingival irritation.

10. **Offer mouthwash.**

? What if . . .

- **My patient develops *Candida*-related denture stomatitis?**

Follow agency protocols. Microwave disinfection of complete dentures has been documented as an effective treatment of *Candida*-related denture stomatitis and can reduce the recurrence of infections.
Denture stomatitis ranges in severity. Treatment includes good oral and denture hygiene and administration of antifungal agents. Recurrence of infection after treatment can result from colonization by Candida on the dentures.

Evaluation

- See Procedure 25-6: Brushing and Flossing the Teeth.
- Check to see that dentures are comfortable and fit properly.

Other

For Documentation, Patient Teaching, and Home Care, see Procedure 25-6: Brushing and Flossing the Teeth.

Practice Resources

Coker, E., Ploeg, J., Kaasalainen, S., & Carter, N. (2017); Siegel, J., Rhinehart, E., Jackson, M., et al. (2007, updated 2017); Silva, M., Mima, E., Colombo, A., et al. (2012).

Thinking About the Procedure

The video, **Providing Denture Care,** along with questions and suggested responses, is available on the ***Davis's Nursing Skills Videos*** Web site on FADavis.com.

Procedure 25-8 ■ Providing Oral Care for an Unconscious Patient

➤ For steps to follow in *all* procedures, refer to the Universal Steps for All Procedures found on the inside back cover.

Equipment

- Toothbrush with soft bristles or sponge oral swabs
- Toothpaste
- Denture cup, if the patient has dentures
- 4 × 4 in. gauze pad to remove dentures, if present
- Tonsil-tip suction connected to suction source (you may use a product that combines the toothbrush or oral swab with the suction device)
- Tongue blade (padded) or bite-block
- Towel

(continued on next page)

Procedure 25-8 ■ Providing Oral Care for an Unconscious Patient (continued)

- Waterproof linen protector
- Disposable emesis basin
- Water-soluble lip moisturizer
- Procedure gloves and goggles

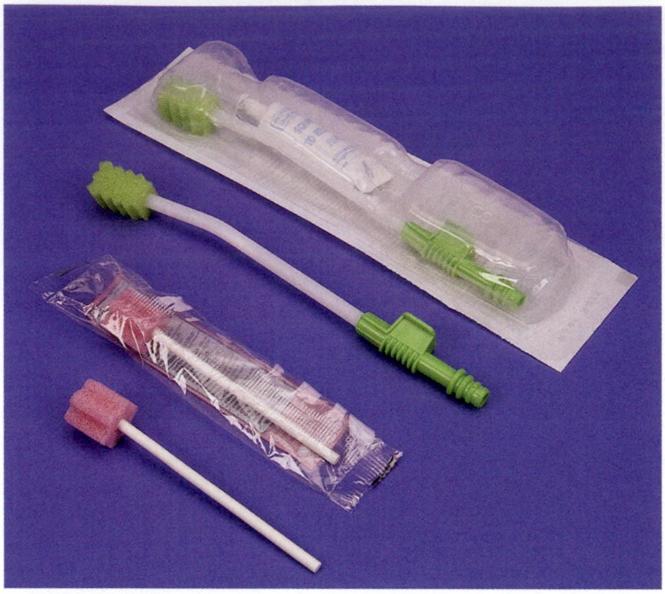

Delegation

As a rule, you probably should not delegate oral hygiene for an unconscious patient to a UAP. However, in some situations it may be acceptable—for example, when agency policy permits, when the UAP has a great deal of experience caring for unconscious patients, and when the UAP's ability to perform oral hygiene safely for them is documented. Perform the pre-procedure assessments, and inform the UAP of any special considerations for care (e.g., if the patient must have the head of the bed elevated to facilitate breathing). Ask the UAP to report the condition of the patient's mouth and the patient's ability to tolerate the procedure (e.g., ask the UAP to take vital signs before and after the procedure, or to note the oxygen saturation if it is being monitored).

Pre-Procedure Assessments

- Determine whether the patient has dentures or partial plates.
  The presence of these appliances determines how you will provide oral care.
  - *You may leave dentures out in the case of an unconscious patient to decrease the risk of damage to the dentures or blocking of the airway. However, when possible, keep the dentures in place to ensure that they will fit adequately later.*
  - *Remove partial plates in an unconscious patient to prevent the plate from causing aspiration or damage to the mouth if it becomes loosened.*
- Assess the patient's gag reflex.
  If the patient has an intact gag reflex, the risk of aspiration is lower.
- Assess the patient's general oral health, including the condition of the teeth and gums, and hydration of the mucous membranes. If the patient has dentures, examine the mouth with and without the dentures.
  Unconscious patients tend to breathe through the mouth, so the oral mucosa is often dry. Because the oral mucosa acts as a barrier against microorganisms, inflammation or lesions in the mouth increase the risk for infection. The lips, gums, and mucous membranes should be pink, moist, and intact. The teeth should be intact and clean. Assess the fit of dentures and the condition of the skin under the dentures to determine whether the fit is proper and whether any irritation is present. The condition of the mouth determines what you will use to provide oral care.

➤ When performing the procedure, always identify your patient according to agency policy, using two identifiers, and be attentive to standard precautions, hand hygiene, patient safety and privacy, body mechanics, and documentation.

Procedure Steps

1. **Place the patient** in the **side-lying** position, with the head turned to the side and, if possible, with the head of the bed down.
   Secretions will pool in the dependent side of the mouth. This position helps prevent aspiration and facilitates the removal of secretions by gravity.
2. **Don procedure gloves and eye goggles.**
   Follows standard precautions. Eye protection is needed when suctioning because of the risk of splashing.
3. **Place a waterproof pad** and then a towel under the patient's cheek and chin.
   The towel and pad will absorb water and keep the bed linens dry.
4. **Set up suction.** Attach suction tubing and tonsil-tip suction; check suction.
   Suctioning helps ensure that the patient does not aspirate oral secretions during mouth care.
5. **Brush the patient's teeth.**
   a. Use a padded tongue blade or bite-block, as needed, to hold the patient's mouth open.
   A padded tongue blade or bite block is used to hold the mouth open so you can visualize and reach the different areas of the mouth without injuring the oral mucosa. It also keeps the patient from biting the nurse's fingers.

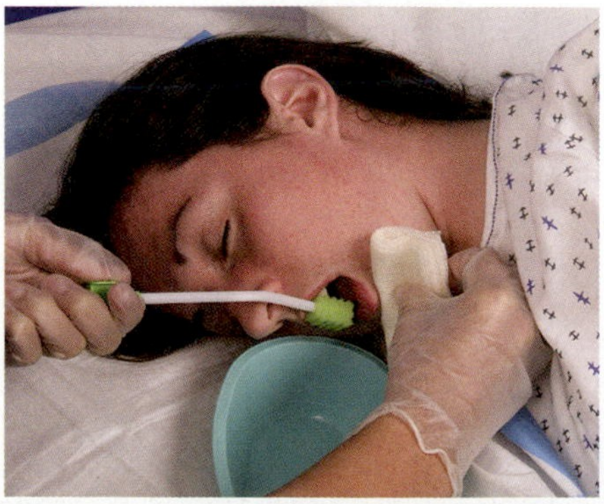

b. Place an emesis basin under the patient's cheek.
Catches the secretions draining from the patient's mouth.

c. Moisten the toothbrush, and apply a small amount of toothpaste. Use hospital-approved water (e.g., sterile, distilled, or filtered tap water).
Excessive use of toothpaste does not enhance cleaning. Brushing the teeth with a soft-bristled brush stimulates the mucosa, which promotes the health of the gums.

d. Brush the teeth, holding the bristles at a 45° angle to the gumline.
(1) Using short, circular motions, gently brush the inner and outer surfaces of the teeth, including the gumline.
(2) Brush the biting surface of the back teeth by holding the brush bristles vertical to the teeth and brushing back and forth.
(3) Brush the patient's tongue.
This is the most effective technique for removing plaque and debris from the teeth and gums. The tongue can be a reservoir for bacteria.

e. Perform oral suctioning when fluid accumulates in the mouth.
Removing fluid prevents choking and aspiration.

f. Draw about 10 mL of distilled, sterile, or filtered water or mouthwash (e.g., dilute hydrogen peroxide) into a syringe; eject it gently into the side of the mouth. Allow the fluid to drain out into the basin, or suction, as needed.
Removes any toothpaste residue, which may have a drying effect. Remove all fluid from the mouth to prevent aspiration into the lungs. Use a minimal amount of solution to prevent aspiration.

6. **Provide denture care**, if necessary. See Procedure 25-7: Providing Denture Care.

7. **Clean the tissues in the oral cavity,** according to agency policy. Use foam swabs or a moistened gauze square wrapped around a tongue blade. Use a clean swab for each area of the mouth: cheeks, tongue, roof of the mouth, and so on.
Oral tissues may be dry and sticky from mouth breathing. Using separate swabs prevents transfer of microorganisms from one area to another.

8. **Remove and dispose of the basin,** dry the patient's face and mouth, and apply water-soluble lip moisturizer.

Petroleum-based lip moisturizers (e.g., mineral oil, petroleum jelly) are not recommended because of the possibility of aspiration, which might cause pneumonia. Never use petroleum-based jelly for patients receiving oxygen therapy; it can cause burns.

9. **Remove the waterproof pad** and towel; turn off suction equipment; discard gloves and used supplies.

10. **Reposition the patient,** as needed.
Maintains good body alignment.

11. **Cleanse and store reusable** oral hygiene tools in clean containers, separate from other articles of personal hygiene.
Prevents possible contamination from the environment and other personal hygiene tools.

? What if . . .

- **You are providing oral care to a patient receiving mechanical ventilation?**

Provide oral cleansing, including subglottic suctioning, at least every 2 hours and prn. Brush the teeth at least twice a day.
Keeping the oral cavity clean and clear of secretions has been proven to decrease the incidence of ventilator-associated pneumonia (VAP). Pooled oral secretions become rapidly colonized with pathogens that contribute to VAP.

Avoid tap water. Use normal saline or a half-strength solution of saline for oral rinses.
Studies show hospital plumbing and tap water are often colonized with microbial organisms.

Apply a 0.12% CHG solution twice daily to complement oral care.

- **It is difficult to floss the patient's teeth, or the patient does not tolerate flossing?**

Handheld interdental tools may be used instead of floss. These devices are special small brushes, picks, or sticks.
Toothbrush bristles cannot reach between teeth to dislodge food particles and bacteria. Interdental cleaners can be as effective as floss in keeping these areas clean.

- **Oral tissues are dry and sticky?**

Use appropriately diluted sodium bicarbonate to dissolve viscous mucus.

Evaluation

- Inspect teeth, gums, and mucous membranes for cleanliness.
- Observe the oral mucosa and gums for hydration, inflammation, bleeding, or infection.
- Observe the patient's overall responses to the procedure (e.g., gagging, coughing, vital signs, skin color).

Patient Teaching

- Discuss with family members any problems that need further follow-up.
- Teach oral hygiene measures, as needed.

Home Care

The procedure steps do not vary in the home setting.

- Work with the client and the caregiver to determine supplies needed for the home.
- Determine whether suction is needed, and explain to caregivers how to obtain a portable suction unit.
- Demonstrate how to position the client and perform the procedure if the height of the bed is not adjustable or if both sides of the bed are not accessible.

(continued on next page)

Procedure 25-8 ■ Providing Oral Care for an Unconscious Patient (continued)

Documentation

Document that oral care was given, any abnormal findings, and nursing interventions. Typically, however, oral care is documented on a checklist or flowsheet.

Sample documentation

11/22/20 0730 Oral care given. Mucous membranes pink and moist. White coating on tongue—physician notified. Patient had no coughing during procedure. Gag reflex intact. Respiratory rate 18. ——— Pamela Giordano, RN

Thinking About the Procedure

The video, **Providing Oral Care for an Unconscious Patient**, along with questions and suggested responses, is available on the ***Davis's Nursing Skills Videos*** Web site on FADavis.com.

Practice Resources

AACN (2017); American Dental Association (n.d.); Ames, N., Sulima, P., Yates, J., et al. (2011); Berry, A., Davidson, P., Nicholson, L., et al. (2011); Karki, S., & Cheng, A. C. (2012).

Procedure 25-9 ■ Shampooing the Hair

➤ For steps to follow in *all* procedures, refer to the Universal Steps for All Procedures found on the inside back cover.

Delegation

You can delegate this procedure to the UAP if the patient's condition and the UAP's skills allow. Perform the preprocedure assessments, and inform the UAP of the specific type of procedure needed (e.g., in bed, at sink, disposable shampoo equipment) and the amount of help the patient needs. Inform the UAP of any special considerations, such as positions the patient cannot assume or presence of scalp lesions. Ask the UAP to report the condition of the patient's scalp and hair, level of self-care, and ability to tolerate the procedure.

Pre-Procedure Assessments

- Assess for contraindications to a shampoo (e.g., scalp sutures or limited head or neck movement). A rinse-free shampoo would be more appropriate in these cases.
- Determine the patient's ability to assist with the procedure.
  Promotes independence and provides active ROM.
- Assess the condition of the patient's hair and scalp. Note any dryness or irritation.
  Dry and brittle hair may indicate hypothyroidism or malnutrition and may require special shampoos or conditioners.
- Determine the need for special hair care products.
  Dandruff, lice, and dry hair are examples of conditions that require medicated shampoos or conditioners.
- Ask the patient how she normally cares for her hair.

Procedure 25-9A ■ Shampooing the Hair for a Patient on Bedrest—Using Rinse-Free Shampoo

➤ When performing the procedure, always identify your patient according to agency policy, using two identifiers, and be attentive to standard precautions, hand hygiene, patient safety and privacy, body mechanics, and documentation

Equipment

- Rinse-free shampoo (no water is needed); conditioner is optional
- Bath towel
- Brush or hair pick, and comb
- Procedure gloves (if scalp lesion or infestation present)

Procedure Steps

1. **Elevate the head** of the bed, if possible.
   Makes it easier to maintain good body mechanics during the procedure.
2. **Place a protective pad** or bath towel under the patient's shoulders.
   Prevents the linen from getting wet.
3. **Don procedure gloves** if lesions or infestations are present.
   Helps prevent transmission of disease.
4. **Work your fingers through the hair**, or comb the hair to remove tangles before washing. If the patient has her hair in small braids, do not take out the braids to wash the hair.
5. **Apply rinse-free shampoo.** Apply enough shampoo to thoroughly wet the hair. One application is usually sufficient to clean the hair.
6. **Work the shampoo through the hair**, from scalp down to ends.
   Helps prevent pulling on and damaging the hair.
7. **Dry the hair** with a bath towel.
   Removes the shampoo. Leaves the hair feeling clean and soft.

8. **Comb or brush hair** to remove tangles, starting at the ends and working toward the scalp.
Prevents excessive pulling on the patient's hair, which may cause breakage.

9. **Dry the hair** with a hair dryer at a medium temperature, if desired.
Use a medium temperature to avoid burning the patient.

10. **When you are finished**, be sure that the patient's clothing and bed linens are dry. Wash and store brushes and combs.

Procedure 25-9B ■ Shampooing the Hair Using Rinse-Free Shampoo Cap

➤ When performing the procedure, always identify your patient according to agency policy, using two identifiers, and be attentive to standard precautions, hand hygiene, patient safety and privacy, body mechanics, and documentation.

Procedure Steps

1. **Warm the shampoo cap** using a water bath or a microwave according to package instructions. Be careful to not overheat. Check the temperature before placing on the patient's head to prevent burns.
A commercial no-rinse shampoo cap is a microwavable cap that contains a no-rinse shampoo and conditioner. Different products are available. Be sure to follow the directions on the package.

2. **Place the cap on the patient's hair**, and gently massage.

3. **Remove the cap**, and towel-dry the patient's hair.
Removes the shampoo and excess water.

4. **Complete hair care** according to the patient's needs (see Procedure 25-9A, Steps 7–10, preceding).

Procedure 25-9C ■ Shampooing the Hair Using a Basin and Water

Key Point: ***The use of prepackaged shampoo products is recommended. However, some patients prefer the traditional shampooing technique or may have excessive soiling of the hair and scalp requiring the use of water and basin. This traditional method of hair hygiene can result in significant variation from caregiver to caregiver and increase the risk of HAIs from contaminated basins and/or tap water. Such techniques also take longer so they require more nursing time and may be more tiring for the patient.***

Equipment

- Shampoo; conditioner is optional
- Disposable shampoo tray or commercial system, if available
- Disposable washbasin, plastic pail, small easy-to-handle plastic container
- Towels (2), washcloth, bath blanket
- Waterproof pads or plastic trash bag
- Brush and comb
- Procedure gloves, if indicated by the presence of lesions or infestation
- Hair dryer
- For inpatients, filtered tap water, distilled, or sterile water are recommended (see Key Point above). Follow agency policy, as conditions vary among institutions.

➤ When performing the procedure, always identify your patient according to agency policy, using two identifiers, and be attentive to standard precautions, hand hygiene, patient safety and privacy, body mechanics, and documentation.

Procedure Steps

1. **If lesions or infestation is** present, don procedure gloves.
Observes standard precautions.

2. **Unless contraindicated** (e.g., by a neck condition), lower the head of the bed, take the pillow from under the patient's neck, and place it under her shoulders.
Hyperextends the neck and helps keep water from the eyes.

3. **Place the waterproof pad** or plastic trash bag under patient's shoulders, and cover with towels. A commercial system will have a drain hose to use.
Protects the bed from getting wet.

4. **Collect warm, not hot, water** (see Equipment) in a container, and bring to the bedside.

5. **Place the shampoo tray** under the patient's shoulders (or head, depending on the type of tray). If you are using a hard plastic tray, pad the neck area with a towel. An inflatable shampoo tray needs minimal padding, but you will need to inflate it before beginning the procedure, either by mouth or with an air pump.
Protects the patient from lying on a hard surface and prevents water from leaking out onto the bed.

6. **Ensure that the tray will drain** into the washbasin or plastic pail.
Prevents water draining onto the bed or floor.

7. **Fold the top linens down** to the patient's waist, and cover her upper body with a bath blanket.
Keeps the linen dry; keeps the patient warm.

8. **Work your fingers through** the patient's hair, or comb the hair to remove tangles prior to washing.
It is easier to remove tangles from dry hair. Note that very tangled or matted hair may sometimes indicate a lice infestation.

9. **Wash the hair.**
   a. Wet the hair, pouring warm water from the pitcher. Do not get water in the person's eyes or ears.

(continued on next page)

Procedure 25-9 ■ Shampooing the Hair (continued)

b. Next, apply shampoo and lather well, working from the scalp out and from the front to the back of the head.

c. Gently lift the patient's head to rub the back of the head.

10. Rinse thoroughly.
Shampoo is drying if left in the hair.

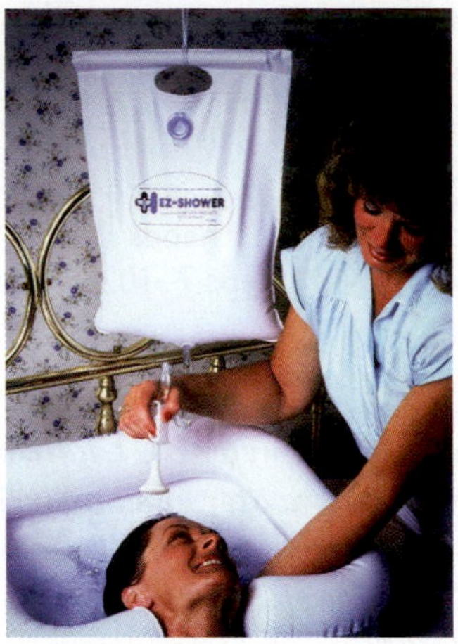

11. Apply conditioner to the hair, if desired, especially for patients with hair that tangles easily, such as dry, long, curly, or kinky hair. Rinse, if needed. Leave-in conditioner can be used and is recommended for curly hair.

12. Remove the tray, and blot-dry the hair with the towel. Do not use a circular motion to dry the hair.
Circular motion will increase tangles.

13. Comb or brush hair to remove tangles, starting at the ends and working toward the scalp.
Prevents excessive pulling on the patient's hair, which may cause breakage.

14. Dry the hair with a hair dryer at a medium temperature, if desired.
Use a medium temperature to avoid burning the patient.

15. When you are finished, be sure that the patient's clothing and bed linens are dry. Wash the shampoo tray and the brushes and combs.

Procedure Variation: Shampooing the Hair of African American Patients

16. If the hair is in cornrows or braids, do not take out the braids to wash the hair. You may need to apply a cloth or net cap to the head prior to shampooing.

17. Handle the patient's hair very gently, being careful not to pull on the hair.
Many African Americans have fragile hair that breaks easily. Because it is fragile, apply moisturizer, if needed, to untangle the hair.

18. When shampooing, thread your fingers through the hair from the scalp out to the ends. Do not massage the hair in a circular motion.

19. Rinse thoroughly, then apply a conditioner on the hair if the hair is dry and fragile.
A leave-in conditioner helps minimize tangles and breakage.

20. Comb through the hair.

a. Use a wide-toothed comb or hair pick. Do not use a brush or fine-toothed comb.

b. Part the hair into four sections, and begin combing near the ends of the hair, working through each section.

c. Use additional moisturizer to help soften and ease combing.
Never pull on the hair because it will break easily.

21. Apply a natural oil to the hair, if desired. Examples of natural oils are coconut, sweet almond, shea butter, and avocado. Many commercial products use these oils.
Mineral oil and Vaseline tend to clog pores and damage the hair, so use them only if the patient insists on using them even after receiving this information.

22. Let the hair air-dry if possible.
Prevents the hair from becoming frizzy. A high temperature, such as from a hair dryer, will also damage the hair.

? What if . . .

- **You discover head lice or nits as you begin the shampoo?**
  Stop the procedure. Discuss your findings with the patient, and offer reassurance. Leave the patient in a position of comfort and safety. Perform hand hygiene. Report the findings, and obtain an order for a prescription shampoo.
- **You do not have a shampoo tray?**
  Improvise by using a new bedpan, and reserve it only for washing hair. Pad it liberally with towels.

Evaluation

- Observe that the hair is clean, dry, and free of tangles.
- Observe for patient discomfort or fatigue during the procedure.
- Ask the patient how the hair and the scalp feel.

Patient Teaching

- Educate patients and their families about how bathing technology has changed to improve patient care and reduce the risk of infection. Special products, such as rinse-free shampoo or shampoo cap, can make shampooing easier to accomplish for a bedridden patient.
- Advise patients with coarse hair to wash it less frequently (every 3 to 7 days, depending on dryness). Leave-in conditioners are often recommended for dry, curly, or kinky hair.

Home Care

- In the home care setting, determine how the client usually washes her hair.
- If the client is confined to bed, work with the caregiver to develop an effective plan for washing the client's hair. For example, if a shampoo tray is not available, you can make one by using a plastic garbage bag and pillows or rolled towels.

- The newer rinse-free products or the inflatable shampoo tray may be good choices for the client.
- If the client cannot afford the adaptive equipment needed, refer the caregiver to the local resources, such as senior services.
- If the client is ambulatory, recommend a shower stool. The stool needs to fit into the shower or bathtub securely, without wobbling, to prevent falls.
- If the client has only a bathtub, an adaptor for the faucet can be used to attach a handheld showerhead. Using a shower stool will make the procedure easier.

Documentation

Chart that hair was shampooed, the condition of the hair and scalp, and the patient's responses to the procedure.

Sample documentation

mm/dd/yyyy 2045 Hair shampooed. Scalp without signs of irritation. Hair dry. Conditioner applied. No c/o discomfort. Pt states "My hair feels wonderful now, and my head doesn't itch anymore." ———— Alicia Nelson, RN

Practice Resources

EZ-Shampoo Instructions for Use (2015); Thompson Healthcare, Inc. (2018). (Caveat: These are not research articles; they are manufacturers' recommendations.)

Procedure 25-10 ■ Providing Beard and Mustache Care

➤ For steps to follow in *all* procedures, refer to the Universal Steps for All Procedures found on the inside back cover.

Equipment

- Scissors or beard trimmer
- Wide-toothed comb
- Mild shampoo; conditioner for coarse and/or dry hair
- Basin (single-patient use, disposable)
- Bath towel
- Procedure gloves (if skin nicks occur, contact with blood may occur)

Delegation

You can delegate beard and mustache care to the UAP if the patient's condition and the UAP's skills allow. Perform the pre-procedure assessments, and inform the UAP of the specific type of care needed (e.g., in bed, at sink, safety razor, electric razor). Inform the UAP of any special considerations, such as skin irritation or activity intolerance. Ask the UAP to report the condition of the patient's skin and beard, level of self-care, and ability to tolerate the procedure.

Pre-Procedure Assessments

- Ask the patient or family about preferences for beard and mustache care.
  Beards and mustaches may have personal and/or cultural meaning. Men in some cultures never cut or trim their beards. Some patients use a comb and scissors to do a slight trim of their beard and/or mustache, whereas others use a beard trimmer for a closer trim.
- Assess the patient's skin and hair condition.
  Determine whether the skin has any reddened or dry areas and whether skin treatments are needed.

➤ When performing the procedure, always identify your patient according to agency policy, using two identifiers, and be attentive to standard precautions, hand hygiene, patient safety and privacy, body mechanics, and documentation.

Procedure Steps

1. **Drape the towel around** the patient's shoulders.
   Protects the patient's clothing from falling pieces of hair and water from shampooing the beard or mustache.
2. **Trim the beard and mustache** when they are dry.
   The beard and mustache are often shorter when dry. If they are cut when wet, they may be shorter than desired after they dry.

Variation: If Using a Comb and Scissors

a. Comb through the beard, and cut the hair on the outside of the comb. Be conservative; cutting too little is better than cutting too much.
   Trimming too much off the beard can be upsetting for the patient, whereas if you cut too little, you can always trim off more.

b. Trim from the front of the ear to the chin on one side, and repeat on the other.
   Keeps the beard equal on both sides of the face.

Variation: If Using a Beard Trimmer

c. Select the trimming guide to the correct length. Adjust the guide to a longer length rather than a shorter length.
   Ensures that you do not cut the beard too short.

(continued on next page)

Procedure 25-10 ■ Providing Beard and Mustache Care (continued)

d. Trim from the front of the ear to the chin on one side, and repeat on the other.

3. **Trim the mustache.**

a. Comb the mustache straight down.
Cuts the length equally so that the mustache is just above the upper lip.

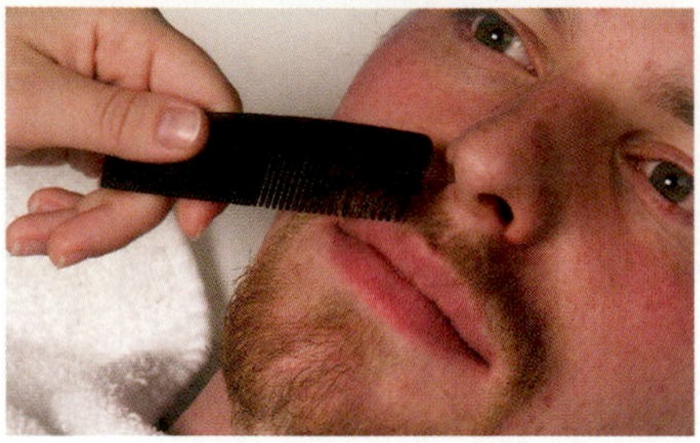

b. Using either scissors or a beard trimmer, start in the middle, and trim toward one side of the mouth and then toward the other. Do not trim the top of the mustache.
Trimming from the center out toward each side helps you cut both sides equally.

4. **Define the beard line** by one of the following methods:

a. Using either the scissors or a beard trimmer, trim the line of the beard so that it is well defined. Trim very little to ensure that you only define the beard and do not change the length.

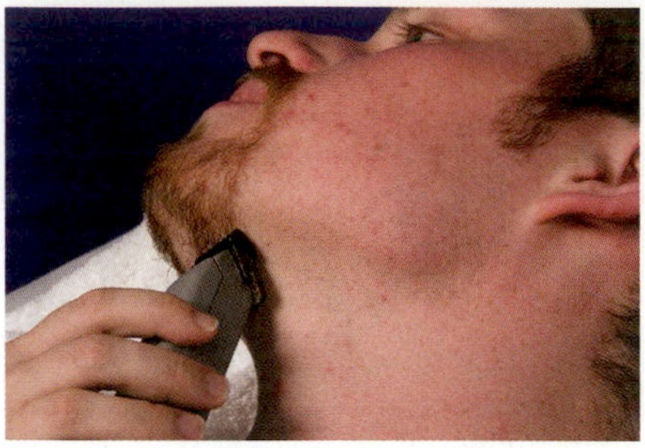

b. Shave the neck to define the beard line, particularly for short beards.

5. **Apply procedure gloves**, if needed, and shampoo the beard and mustache by using warm sterile, distilled, or tap water and a mild shampoo.
The skin under a beard or mustache can be tender, so treat it gently with a mild shampoo. Follow standard precautions because it is possible to nick the skin and cause bleeding. Policies about use of tap water vary among institutions.

6. **Rinse well, and pat and wipe** the beard and mustache dry with the towel.
Any shampoo left in can irritate the skin, as can rubbing motions with the towel.

7. **Apply conditioner**, if desired.

8. **Comb the beard and mustache** with a wide-toothed comb or a brush.
Do not use a fine-toothed comb because it will pull the hair.

Evaluation

- Make sure that the beard and mustache are trimmed to the desired length and are clean.
- Verify that skin problems are identified and treatment initiated.

Home Care

No adaptations are required in the home. The patient's usual supplies are sufficient, as a rule.

Documentation

Chart that beard and mustache were trimmed and shampooed; chart the condition of the skin.

Practice Resources

Procter & Gamble (n.d.). (Caveat: This is not an evidence-based practice article. It is a manufacturer's recommendation.)

Procedure 25-11 ■ Shaving a Patient

➤ For steps to follow in *all* procedures, refer to the Universal Steps for All Procedures found on the inside back cover.

Equipment

- Safety razor or electric razor
- Shaving cream or soap; after-shave lotion, if desired
- Shaving brush, if desired
- Warm water (sterile, distilled, or tap water, per agency policy)
- Face towel and bath towel
- Procedure gloves

Delegation

You can delegate shaving to the UAP if the patient's condition and the UAP's skills allow. Perform the pre-procedure assessments, and inform the UAP of the amount of help and specific type of care (e.g., safety or electric razor, in bed, or at the sink) the patient needs. Inform the UAP of any special considerations, such as skin irritation or activity intolerance. Ask the UAP to report the condition of the patient's skin, level of self-care, ability to tolerate the procedure.

Pre-Procedure Assessments

- Determine how much assistance the patient needs.
Aids you in promoting as much independence as possible.

- Assess the patient's skin and hair condition for redness, skin lesions, or moles.
  Identifies skin problems and determines whether skin treatments are needed or the procedure must be modified. To prevent abrading the skin, do not shave any areas that have skin lesions or moles.
- Assess the patient's usual shaving method, including use of electric razor or safety razor.
  When possible, follow the patient's routine. The patient may or may not use shaving cream or shaving soap, shaving brush, and after-shave lotion.
- Check for any contraindications to shaving, such as an increased risk of infection or bleeding (e.g., because of neutropenia, thrombocytopenia, or the administration of anticoagulants, such as warfarin or heparin).

➤ When performing the procedure, always identify your patient according to agency policy, using two identifiers, and be attentive to standard precautions, hand hygiene, patient safety and privacy, body mechanics, and documentation.

Procedure Steps

1. **Don procedure gloves.**
   To prevent exposure to blood if skin is nicked or scratched.
2. **Place a warm, damp face towel** on the patient's face for 1 to 3 minutes.
   Opens the pores and softens the beard to prevent pulling. Do not use hot water because it will dehydrate the skin and can burn sensitive skin.
3. **Apply shaving lotion** to the face with your fingers or a shaving brush. Lather well for 1 to 2 minutes.
   Lathering well helps to further soften the beard. Do not use shaving creams that contain numbing agents because they close the pores and stiffen the beard.
4. **Shave the patient.**
   a. Pull skin taut with your nondominant hand, and gently pull the razor across the skin. If you are using a safety razor, hold the blade at a 45° angle to the skin.
   b. Shave the face and neck in the same direction of hair growth (the direction is not the same for all people). Using short strokes, start shaving at the sideburns, and work down to the chin on each side and then the neck.
   c. Last, shave the chin and the upper lip areas.
   Usually, the hair on the face will grow down toward the chin and on the neck up toward the chin. The hair is generally thickest on the chin and upper lip, so shaving them last allows more time for the shaving cream to soften the hair. Shave in the same direction as the hair is growing to prevent skin irritation.

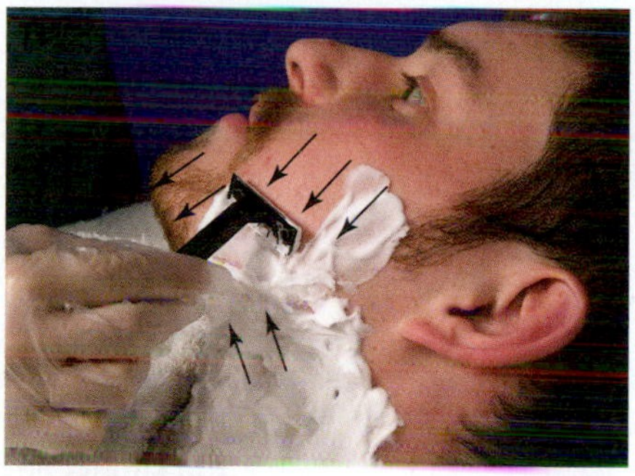

5. **Rinse the razor** frequently while you are shaving.
   Avoids clogging the blade.
6. **When you have finished shaving,** rinse the patient's face with cool water (per agency policy), and gently pat it dry.
   Cool water helps close the pores. Pat dry, do not rub, to avoid irritating the skin.
7. **Apply after-shave lotion,** if desired.
   After-shave lotions that contain alcohol are not recommended because alcohol stings and dries out the skin. A moisturizer is recommended.
8. **Dispose of the single-use razor** in the sharps container.
   Prevents cutting injury to others.

Variation: If Using a Multiuse Razor

Shake the razor to remove excess moisture. Do not bang the razor against objects or dry with a towel. Store the razor in a covered container.
Banging or wiping the razor edge will dull the razor and may damage the holding mechanism. A covered container protects others from a cutting injury.

? What if . . .

- **Your patient has a condition that predisposes him to bleeding (e.g., thrombocytopenia) or infection (e.g., neutropenia)?**

Such patients must be shaved carefully using an electric razor, if at all.
A razor scratch or cut causes a break in skin integrity, providing a portal of entry for pathogens. This could be especially serious for a patient with compromised defense against infection. For a patient with a delayed clotting time, a cut could cause excessive blood loss.

(continued on next page)

Procedure 25-11 ■ Shaving a Patient (continued)

Evaluation

- Inspect the patient's face, closeness of the shave, and for nicks or cuts.
- If the procedure was performed by the UAP, ask the patient about his satisfaction with and tolerance of the care.

Patient Teaching

Teach patients about changes that need to be made in their shaving technique as a result of changes in their health status. For example, a patient who has begun taking anticoagulants may need to change from a blade to an electric razor because of the increased risk of bleeding.

Home Care

The procedure does not vary in the home setting. The nurse must:

- Determine the availability of supplies
- Assess the client's or the caregiver's ability to perform the procedure.

Documentation

Chart that the patient was shaved and the condition of the skin. There will probably be a flowsheet or checklist for this information.

Practice Resources

Dunkley & McLeod, (2015); Procter & Gamble (n.d.); Men's Health (2016). (Caveat: The preceding are not evidence-based resources. They are information from manufacturers.)

Procedure 25-12 ■ Removing and Caring for Contact Lenses

➤ For steps to follow in *all* procedures, refer to the Universal Steps for All Procedures found on the inside back cover.

Equipment

- Contact lens wetting solution
- Contact lens soaking solution
- Sterile saline (optional)
- Contact lens case
- Contact lens remover (optional)
- Procedure gloves

Delegation

You can delegate this procedure if the patient's condition and the UAP's skills permit. For example, if the patient is unconscious, you must determine whether contact lenses are present, and you should not delegate their removal.

Pre-Procedure Assessments

- Determine whether the patient is wearing contact lenses. If the patient is unconscious, examine the eyes for the presence of contact lenses by shining a penlight across the eye. You should be able to see the edge of the lens.
- Determine the type of contact lenses in place.
  Hard lenses are smaller than soft lenses. Each type of contact lens has different care requirements. Hard lenses can be worn for only up to 18 hours. Rigid gas-permeable (RGP) lenses may be worn overnight or for about 7 days, depending on the kind. Soft contacts are used for either short or longer periods.
- Ask the patient whether he is able to remove his contact lenses.

➤ When performing the procedure, always identify your patient according to agency policy, using two identifiers, and be attentive to standard precautions, hand hygiene, patient safety and privacy, body mechanics, and documentation.

➤ *Note:* It is difficult to remove a contact lens when wearing procedure gloves. For hard lenses, you can use a suction cup device if one is available. If you must use ungloved hands (e.g., in an emergency situation), it is extremely important to wash your hands thoroughly before and after the procedure. *Do not* use your fingernails.

➤ *Note:* Lens cases are marked "L" and "R" to indicate left and right lenses. Clean, rinse, and place the lens you remove first into its designated cup before removing the second lens.

Procedure Steps

1. **Perform hand hygiene,** and don gloves.
2. **Instill one to two drops** of contact lens wetting solution to moisten the lenses.
   Aids in lens removal.
3. **Remove the lenses.**

Variation: For Hard or Gas-Permeable Contact Lens

- *Alternative 1:* If the lens is not centered over the cornea, place your finger on the patient's lower eyelid, and apply gentle pressure to move it into position. Place your index finger at the outer corner of the eye, and gently pull sideways toward the ear; position your other hand below the eye to "catch" the lens. Ask the patient to blink. As the skin tightens, the palpebral fissure narrows, the lids catch on the edge of the lens and pop it out.

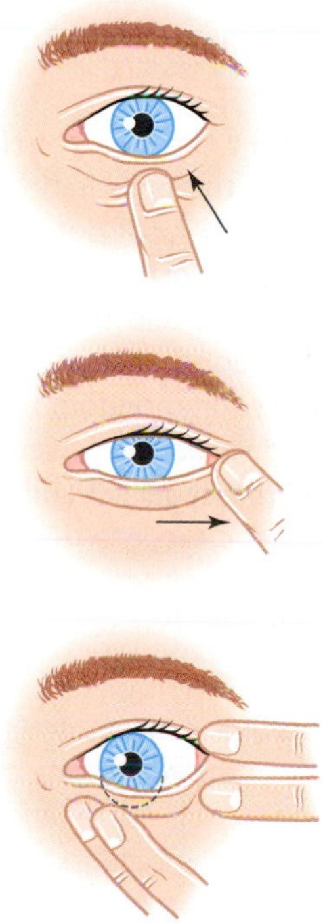

- *Alternative 2:* Use a small suction cup contact lens remover. Gently press the suction cup end of the remover onto the contact lens, and lift straight up off the eye.
- *Alternative 3:* Gently pull the top eyelid up and the lower lid down beyond the top and bottom edges of the lens. Then, gently press the lower eyelid up against the bottom of the lens. When the lens is slightly tipped, move the eyelids together. This should cause the lens to slide out.

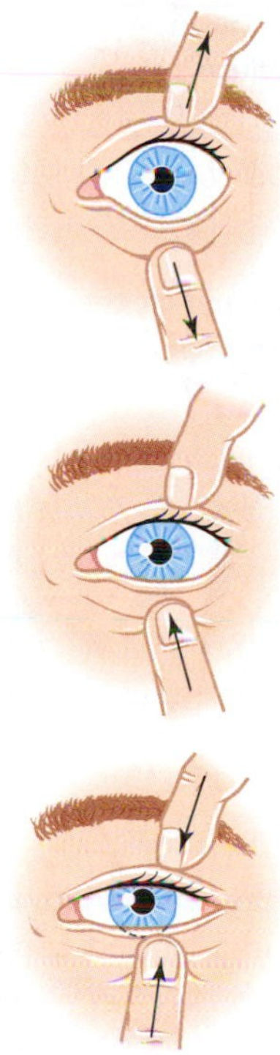

Variation: For Soft Contact Lens

a. Hold the eye open with your nondominant hand.
   Allows you to visualize the contact lens.

b. Gently place the tip of your index finger on the contact lens, and slide it down off the pupil to the white area of the eye.
   To prevent potential damage to the eye, do not pinch a lens directly over the pupil.

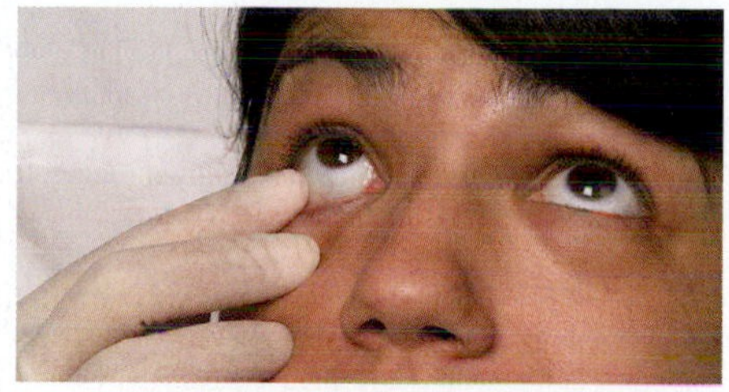

c. Using your thumb and index finger pads, gently pinch the lens, and lift it straight up off the eye. If the edges stick together, moisten with a few drops of wetting solution. Rub gently until edges separate.
   A soft contact lens is very flexible and pinches easily.

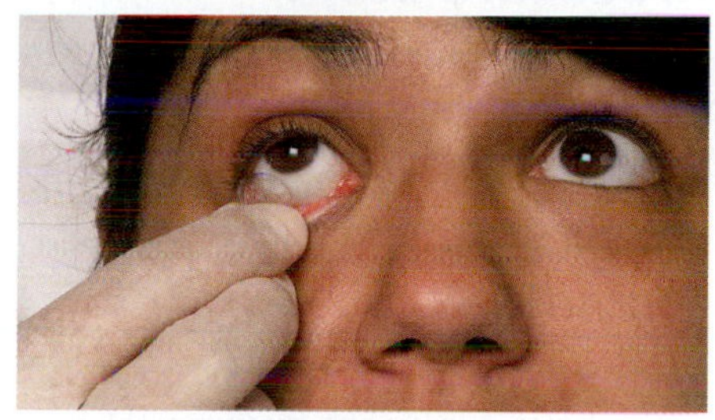

4. **Clean the lens** according to the instructions on the cleaning solution bottle. If there is no lens cleaner, use sterile saline. Be careful not to tear soft lenses.
5. **Rinse the lenses** with contact lens solution or sterile saline.
   Removes any particles from the lenses.
6. **Place the lenses in a contact** lens case containing soaking solution or sterile saline (see note above regarding lens cases). Never use water.
   Prevents bacterial growth on the contacts and keeps the lenses from drying out.

Evaluation

Examine the eyes for redness or irritation.

Patient Teaching

- Review with the patient and/or family the importance of keeping the contact lenses clean and moist.
- Teach the patient that contact lenses should not be worn or stored in water. If water touches the lens, remove and discard the lens.
- If hard contact lenses are used, they must be removed at bedtime to prevent hypoxia of the cornea.

Documentation

Chart that contacts were removed, what type of lenses they are, what solution they are stored in, and the condition of the patient's eyes.

Practice Resources

American Academy of Ophthalmology, (2015); Bausch & Lomb (2018a, 2018b); Massachusetts Eye and Ear Infirmary (2018).

Procedure 25-13 ■ Caring for Artificial Eyes

➤ For steps to follow in *all* procedures, refer to the Universal Steps for All Procedures found on the page facing the inside back cover.

Equipment

- Procedure gloves
- Normal saline solution
- Labeled container filled with saline or sterile, distilled, or filtered water
- Cotton balls

Delegation

You can delegate this procedure to the UAP if the patient's condition and the UAP's skills allow. Perform the pre-procedure assessments, and inform the UAP of any special considerations. Ask the UAP to report the patient's ability to tolerate the procedure.

Pre-Procedure Assessments

Assess the patient's activity tolerance and whether you will need another caregiver to assist.

➤ When performing the procedure, always identify your patient according to agency policy, using two identifiers, and be attentive to standard precautions, hand hygiene, patient safety and privacy, body mechanics, and documentation.

Procedure Steps

1. **Perform hand hygiene, and don gloves.**
2. **Position the patient lying down.**
   If you drop the eye when removing it, it will fall onto the bed instead of the floor.
3. **To remove the artificial eye:**
   a. Raise the upper eyelid with your nondominant hand, and depress the lower lid with your dominant hand.
   b. Apply slight pressure below the eye to release the suction holding it in place.
   c. Catch the eye in the palm of your dominant hand.
   d. Alternatively, you can use a small bulb syringe, place it directly on the eye, and squeeze to create suction and lift the eye straight up from the socket.

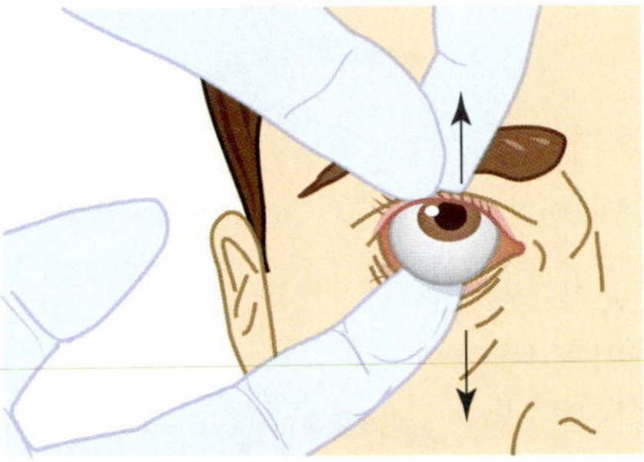

4. **Clean the eye with saline,** and store it in a labeled container filled with saline or sterile, distilled, or filtered water. Do not use solvents, disinfectants, or alcohol. These chemicals may irritate the socket or damage the artificial eye.
5. **Wipe the edge of the patient's** eye socket with a moistened cotton ball, wiping from outer canthus toward the nose.
6. **Inspect the socket** for redness, swelling, or drainage.
   Irritation or infection can occur if debris has entered the socket.
7. **To reinsert the prosthetic eye:**
   a. Remove the prosthetic eye from the container, but do not dry it.
   b. Hold the prosthetic eye between your thumb and the index finger of your dominant hand.
   c. With your nondominant hand, pull down on the lower lid while lifting the upper lid and guide the prosthetic eye into the socket.
   The prosthesis will slide into place more easily when it is wet.

Evaluation

- Observe that the prosthetic eye has been placed correctly in the socket.
- Ask the patient how the eye area feels.
- Observe the eye area for redness or irritation.

Patient Teaching

- Advise the patient to periodically inspect the eye area.
- Review the importance of hand hygiene and proper handling of the eye.
- If the eye wearer experiences dryness or irritation, a lubricant made for ocular prosthetics can be used.
- If the eye needs to be wiped but not removed, wipe from outer canthus toward the nose.
  Wiping outward may dislodge the prosthesis.
- Encourage the patient to sleep in the prosthesis at night and to remove it every 1 to 3 weeks for cleaning (follow prosthesis specialist's advice). Some patients do find that it is necessary to remove and clean the prosthesis every day.
  Frequent removal irritates the lining of the socket and increases the amount of discharge produced by the eye socket.
- The eye should be professionally polished every 6 to 12 months. Symptoms that may indicate the need for a polish are irritated or itchy lids, increased drainage or discomfort, or changes in the appearance of the artificial eye.

Home Care

- In the home care setting, determine how the client usually performs eye care.
- Discuss ways to promote the safety of the artificial eye.
- Work with the client or caregiver to develop a plan of care for cleaning the eye and care of the area associated with the socket.

Documentation

Chart that the artificial eye was cleansed, the condition of the socket, care given to the area around the socket, and the patient's responses to the procedure.

Practice Resources

Artificial Eyes (2018); Erikson Labs Northwest (n.d.); Peters, R. (n.d.).

Procedure 25-14 ■ Caring for Hearing Aids

➤ For steps to follow in *all* procedures, refer to the Universal Steps for All Procedures found on the page facing the inside back cover.

Equipment

- Face cloth, dry towel
- Damp cloth
- Cotton applicators
- Wax-loop and wax brush, if available
- Pipe cleaner or toothpick, if wax-loop and wax brush unavailable
- Procedure gloves (to prevent contact with earwax or ear drainage)

Delegation

You can delegate hearing aid care to the UAP if the patient's condition and the UAP's skills allow. Perform the pre-procedure assessments, and inform the UAP of the specific type of care needed (e.g., type of hearing aid) and the amount of help the patient needs. Inform the UAP of any special considerations, such as skin irritation or usual volume setting. Ask the UAP to report the condition of the patient's ears, level of self-care, ability to tolerate the procedure, and ability to hear in a normal conversation.

Pre-Procedure Assessments

- Determine how much assistance the patient needs.
  Aids you in promoting independence as much as possible.
- Determine the type of hearing aid in use. The three common types of hearing aids are (1) postaural hearing aid, (2) in-the-canal hearing aid, and (3) in-the-ear hearing aid.
  The cleaning procedure varies according to the type of hearing aid.

  To review the types of hearing aids,

  Go to Volume 1, **Figure 25-7**.
- Assess the patient's ear and outer canal for redness, skin lesions, earwax buildup, or drainage.
  Identify skin problems and determine whether any symptoms of infection exist. Earwax buildup increases with age and does not necessarily indicate a health problem.

➤ When performing the procedure, always identify your patient according to agency policy, using two identifiers, and be attentive to standard precautions, hand hygiene, patient safety and privacy, body mechanics, and documentation.

Procedure Steps

1. **Don procedure gloves.**
   The hearing aid may contain earwax buildup or drainage.
2. **Place a towel on a nearby table** or flat surface.
   The towel helps prevent the hearing aid from breaking if it is accidentally dropped. Hearing aids are expensive.
3. **To remove the hearing aid:**
   a. Turn the hearing aid off by applying slight pressure against the volume control wheel and turning it backward (away from the nose).
   Stops the hearing aid from whistling.
   b. Rotate the earmold slightly forward (toward the nose), and gently pull it out. Do not pull on the battery door or the volume wheel.
   Pulling on the battery door or the volume wheel may damage the faceplate.
   c. Place the hearing aid on the towel.
   The towel will prevent the hearing aid from rolling off the table or banging against the table.
4. **Clean the hearing aid.**
   a. Wipe all external surfaces with a damp cloth.
   b. Clean the canal portion of the hearing aid using the wax-loop and wax brush, cotton-tipped applicator, pipe cleaner, or toothpick. Clean the top portion only. Do not insert anything into the hearing aid itself.
   Poking utensils into any part of the hearing aid except for the canal portion may damage the hearing aid.

Variation: Detachable Earmold

c. Disconnect the earmold, and soak it in soapy water. Rinse and dry well, and then reattach it. Do not use alcohol. Never immerse a hearing aid in water; only the earmold should be immersed.
Detaching an earmold that is glued or fastened by a small metal ring will break the hearing aid. Alcohol will damage the earmold material.

(continued on next page)

Procedure 25-14 ■ Caring for Hearing Aids (continued)

d. Check the hearing aid and any tubings for cracks and loose connections.
A damaged hearing aid will be less effective and may cause injury to the ear. Early detection of hearing aid damage may allow for repair, rather than replacement, of the device.

5. **Cleanse the outer ear** using the corner of a washcloth or a cotton-tipped applicator. Inspect these areas for redness, abrasions, swelling, drainage, or other irregularities.
Poorly fitting or improperly positioned hearing aids may cause trauma to the ear.

6. **Insert the hearing aid.**
   a. Check that the battery is functioning. Hold the hearing aid in your hand. Close the battery compartment door if open. Turn the power on, turn the volume high, and listen for a whistling sound.
   Whistling indicates proper power level and functioning of the battery.
   b. Set the volume control to "Off."
   Prevents whistling during insertion and a sudden loud noise.
   c. Handle the hearing aid by the edges using your thumb and forefinger.
   Prevents whistling during insertion.
   d. Holding the hearing aid in your dominant hand, use your nondominant hand to gently pull the ear up and back.
   Opens the ear canal slightly for an easier insertion and better fit.
   e. Insert the canal portion of the hearing aid into the ear. Apply slight pressure, and gently rotate the hearing aid back and forth until the canal portion rests flat in the ear.
   Allows better fit and prevents hearing aid from falling out.

Variation: When Inserting a Postaural Hearing Aid

Insert the earmold first and then place the earmold over the ear.

Variation: When Inserting an In-the-Canal Hearing Aid

Insert with the volume control at the top. The canal should be facing away from your hand.

Variation: When Inserting an In-the-Ear Hearing Aid

Insert with the volume control at the bottom.

7. **Turn the hearing aid on,** and adjust the volume by turning the volume control wheel toward the nose. Set the volume control as low as possible.
Normal setting requires a one-third to two-thirds turn of the volume control wheel. A noisier environment requires less volume, or one-fourth turn.

8. **Protect the hearing aid** from curling irons, hair dryers, and hair spray and other hair products.
Heat and moist aerosols will damage the hearing aid.

Procedure Variation: Storing the Hearing Aid

9. **Open the battery compartment,** and place the hearing aid in a closed container labeled with the patient's name.
Saves battery power and allows any moisture to evaporate. Protects the hearing aid from accidental damage or loss.

10. **If the hearing aid is to be kept stored** and not worn for a week or more, remove the battery completely.
Prevents battery acid from leaking and damaging the hearing aid.

11. **Store the hearing aid** in a cool, dry place, preferably in the bedside drawer. Keep the hearing aid away from children and pets.
Moisture and heat will damage the hearing aid. Hearing aids and containers are easily lost. A child may choke on the hearing aid. Dogs and cats are attracted to the whistling noise and odor of the hearing aid and sometimes attempt to eat the device.

Procedure Variation: Replacing the Battery

12. **Use your finger** to swing the battery door open. Never force the door.

13. **Peel the tab off the new battery.**

14. **Hold the battery with the positive (+) side up,** and slide it into the door, not into the hearing aid itself.

15. **Gently close the battery door.** Never force the door.

16. **Dispose of the old mercury-free battery** in the regular trash.

Note: If the battery contains mercury, refer to the package for disposal instructions.

Guidelines for Care of the Batteries

- Always dispose of old batteries. Do not throw them into a fire.
Minimizes damage from leaking battery acid and prevents mistaking used battery for fresh battery. Heat and fire may cause the battery to explode.
- Store batteries in a cool, dry place. Do not place zinc-air batteries in the refrigerator.
Heat shortens the life of the battery. Cold batteries warming to room temperature are exposed to condensation and subsequent corrosion.
- Do not store batteries near coins or other metals.
Contact with other metals can short-circuit the batteries.
- Do not remove the tab from the battery until the battery is ready for use.
The tab keeps air out of the battery. Once the tab is removed, the battery is activated. Early removal decreases the life of the battery.
- Keep batteries away from children, confused adults, and pets.
Minimizes accidental swallowing.

? What if . . .

- **The hearing aid becomes wet?**
  If the hearing aid becomes exposed to moisture, dry it as thoroughly as possible. Remove the battery and throw it away. Keep the battery door open. Place the hearing aid in its container, and allow it to dry overnight. Do not place a new battery in the hearing aid until the next morning.
  Moisture will cause the battery to corrode.
- **The patient wears bilateral hearing aids?**
  Be sure to identify which hearing aid is for the left ear and which hearing aid is for the right ear. Most hearing aids have a color marking for easy identification: red = right ear; and blue = left ear.
  Attempting to force a hearing aid into the wrong ear may cause trauma to the ear.
- **The patient continues to have hearing difficulties despite hearing aids?**
  Hearing aids will not restore full hearing. General tips when communicating with a person with a hearing deficit are listed in Clinical Insight 30-2: Communicating With Hearing-Impaired Clients.
  Hearing aids will not block out background noise. A clear, distinct, low-pitched voice helps the client to understand what is being said.

Evaluation

- Assess how well the patient tolerated the procedure. Was there any discomfort, difficulty with insertion, and so on?
- Note the condition of the patient's skin, including pain, redness, and abnormal discharge.
- Note the condition of the hearing aid itself.
- Assess the patient's ability to hear normal speaking voices.
- Ask the patient whether he feels comfortable and hears satisfactorily.

Patient Teaching

- Discuss the importance of daily hearing aid care.
- Review any areas of care that the patient has not been performing adequately.
- Discuss any problems that need further follow-up, such as earwax build up, faulty or broken hearing aid, or ill-fitting hearing aid.

Home Care

- The procedure does not vary in the home setting. The issues are that the nurse must:
  - Work with the patient and care provider to determine supplies needed for the home.
  - Determine whether further knowledge is required (e.g., if the patient must expose hearing aids to prevailing weather conditions, uses a telephone extensively, or must make several adaptations from quiet to noisy environments throughout the day).
  - Provide a list of available resources (e.g., AARP, National Institutes of Health, Better Hearing Institute).

Documentation

Chart that the patient is wearing a hearing aid, the condition of the ear, and the ability to hear. There will probably be a flow sheet or checklist for this information.

Practice Resources

Department of Veterans Affairs (n.d.); National Institute on Deafness and Other Communication Disorders (2015); U.S. Food and Drug Administration (2018).

Procedure 25-15 ■ Making an Unoccupied Bed

➤ For steps to follow in all procedures, refer to the Universal Steps for All Procedures found on the inside back cover.

Equipment

- Bottom and top sheets, possibly drawsheet
- Pillowcase for each of the pillows
- Linen bag or hamper
- Procedure gloves (if exposure to body fluids is possible)
- Moisture-proof gown (if heavy soiling of linens with body fluids is possible)

Delegation

You can delegate this procedure to the UAP. You are responsible for supervising to ensure that the procedure is performed correctly.

Pre-Procedure Assessments

- Check to see whether the linens (including the mattress pad, blanket, and bedspread) need to be changed, and what linens are needed.
- Assess whether the patient is able to be out of bed during the linen change.
- Assess for drainage or incontinence to determine whether personal protective equipment, such as procedure gloves and gown, is needed.

Note: This procedure describes bed making by one person. It is more efficient for two people to work together on opposite sides of the bed.

(continued on next page)

Procedure 25-15 ■ Making an Unoccupied Bed (continued)

➤ When performing the procedure, always identify your patient according to agency policy, using two identifiers, and be attentive to standard precautions, hand hygiene, patient safety and privacy, body mechanics, and documentation.

Procedure Steps

1. **Assist the patient to a chair.** Provide a robe and/or blanket, if needed.
Ensures that the patient is comfortable and will be warm enough during the bed change.

2. **Prepare the environment:**
   - Position the bed flat, raise to appropriate working height, put the wheel brakes on, and lower the siderails.
   - Move the overbed table and other furniture, as needed.
   - Place the linen bag or hamper conveniently near the bed.
   Maintains good body mechanics and prevents back strain during the procedure.
   - Remove obstacles to allow easy access to the bed. Place all items so you can work efficiently, saving time and energy.

3. **Don protective gloves** and other gear, if necessary. Loosen all the bedding.
This observes Standard Precautions and reduces the risk of contaminating your clothing.

4. **If the blanket or bedspread** is clean, fold it, and place it on a clean area (e.g., on the back of a chair). Do not place on another patient's bed or furniture.
Reuse the blanket and/or bedspread if it is not soiled. Placing the item on a clean area prevents cross-contamination.

5. **Remove the bottom and top sheet**, draw sheet, and pillowcases.
   a. Do not shake the linens.
   Minimizes dispersal of dust, skin cells, and microorganisms into the environment.
   b. ✚ Holding the items away from your body, place them in a laundry bag or hamper. Never place linen on the floor. Place the pillows on a clean area (e.g., on a chair).
   Hold dirty linen away from your uniform to prevent contamination. Cross-contamination can occur if you place linens on the floor.▼

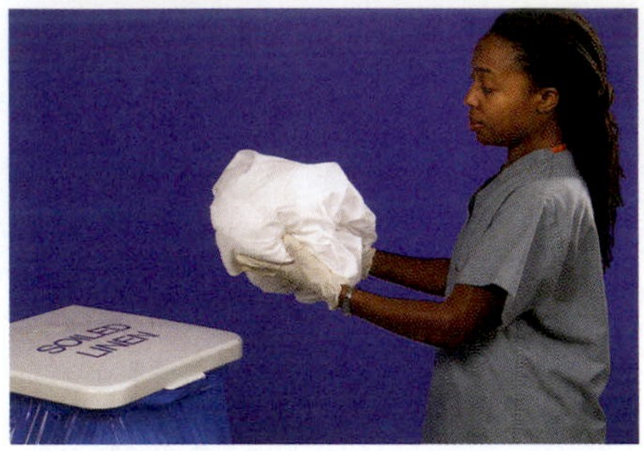

6. **Working from one side of bed,** to save steps:

Variation: For a Contour-Bottom Sheet

   a. Fit the contour-bottom sheet on one side of the bed, and smooth it out over half the mattress.

Variation: For a Flat-Bottom Sheet

   b. Fold the flat-bottom lengthwise with the center crease in the middle of bed, and unfold with the rough side facing down.
   c. Position the bottom sheet so that approximately 10 inches hang over at the top and sides. The hem of the bottom sheet should be just even with the bottom edge of the mattress.
   d. Tuck in the sheet, mitering the sheet at the top corner (see Step 11).
   When using a flat bottom sheet, having extra sheet at the top helps keep it in place when the head of the bed is raised and lowered. Unfold the sheet rather than shaking or fanning it to reduce dispersing microorganisms into the air. The sheet will not be long enough to tuck in at the bottom.

7. **Place the drawsheet with** the center fold in the middle of the mattress and unfold. Tuck the side in under the mattress, and smooth out over half of the mattress.
Ensures that all wrinkles are out of the bottom sheet and drawsheet.▼

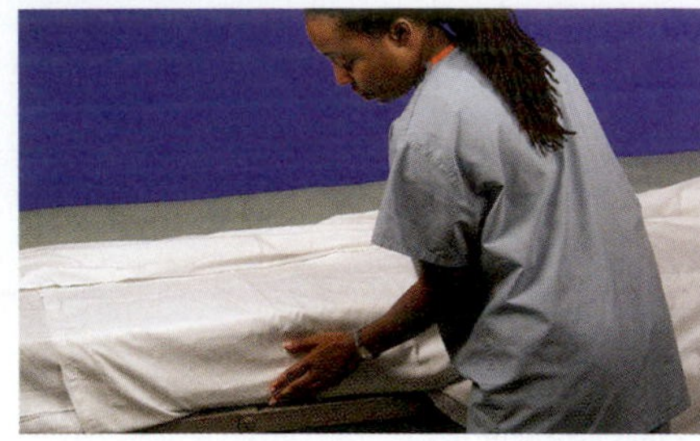

8. **Go to the other side of the bed,** straighten the linen, and finish tucking in the bottom sheet and drawsheet.
   a. Make the drawsheet tight, and smooth any wrinkles in the bottom sheet and drawsheet.
   Pulling the drawsheet tight helps prevent wrinkles from developing under the patient when she moves around in bed.▼

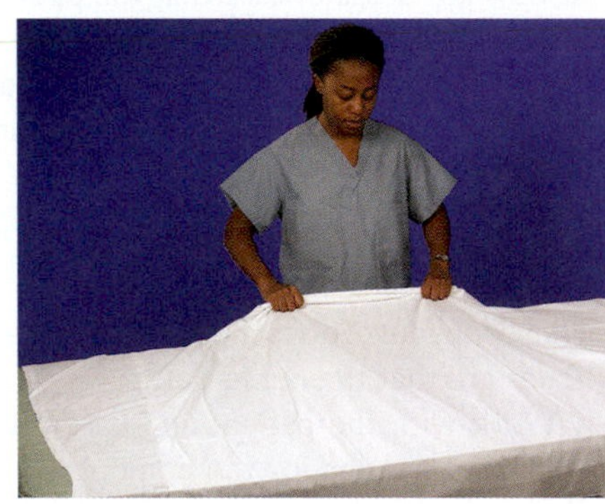

   b. If desired, place a waterproof pad on or under the drawsheet.

9. **Place the top sheet and bedspread** along one side of the mattress. Center the top sheet and bedspread so that when you straighten them from the other side of the bed, they fall equally over each side of the bed.
Putting the linen on one side of the bed saves steps.

10. At the foot of the bed, make a small pleat in the top sheet and bedspread.

Prevents the top covers from placing pressure on the patient's toes.

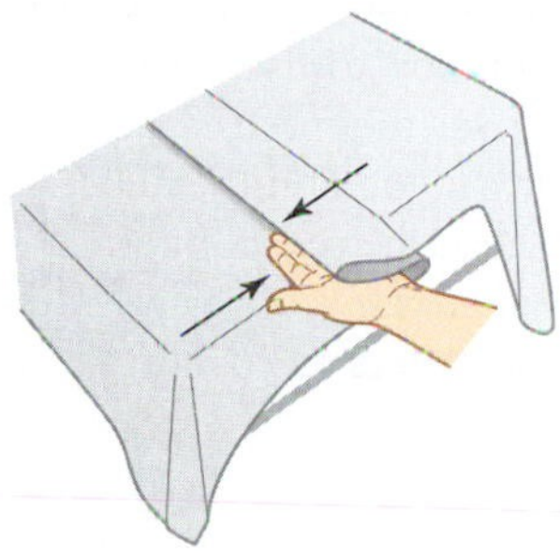

11. Tuck in the top sheet and bedspread at the same time, mitering the corners.

a. Tuck in the sheet and bedspread at the bottom of the mattress.

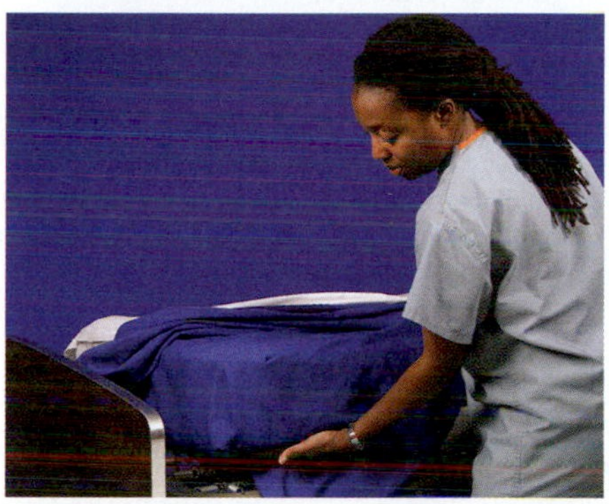

b. Bring the edge of sheet and the bedspread up to make a right angle.

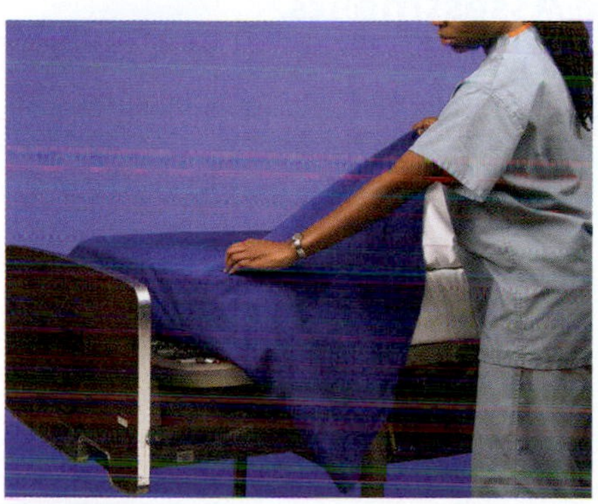

c. Tuck the lower edge of sheet and bedspread under the mattress.

Mitered corners help secure the linen at the foot of the bed.

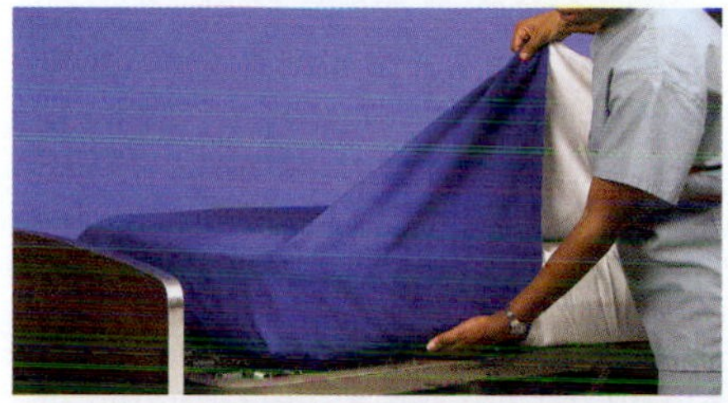

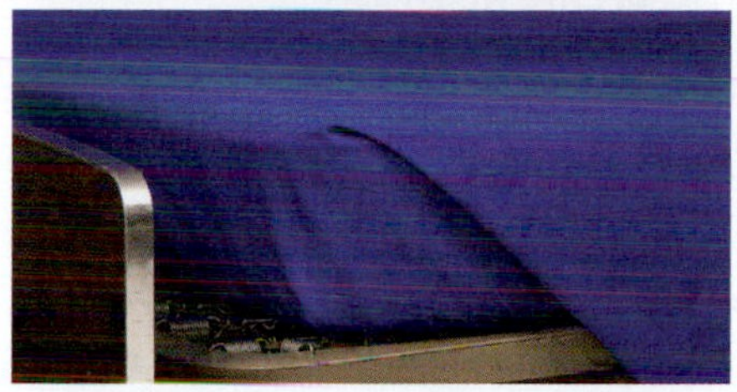

12. Move to the other side of the bed, smooth top linens, and repeat Step 11. At the head of the bed, fold the edge of sheet down over the bedspread.

Prevents the bedspread from rubbing against the patient's skin.

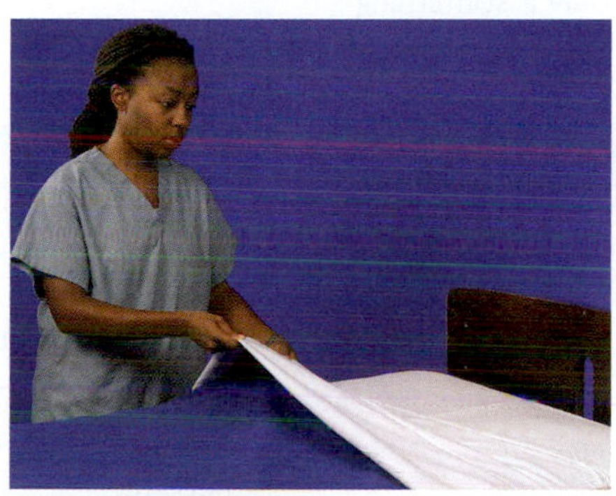

13. Fanfold the top sheet and bedspread back to the foot of the bed.

Makes it easier for the patient to get into bed.

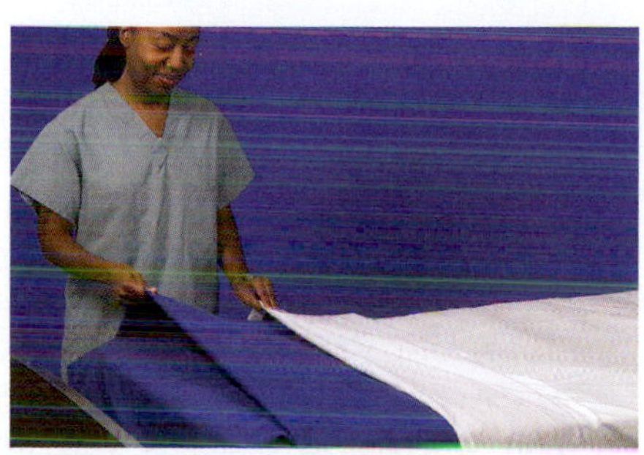

14. Change pillowcases.

a. Turn the pillowcase wrong side out.

b. Grasp the middle of the closed end of the pillowcase.

c. Reaching through the pillowcase, grasp the end of the pillow.

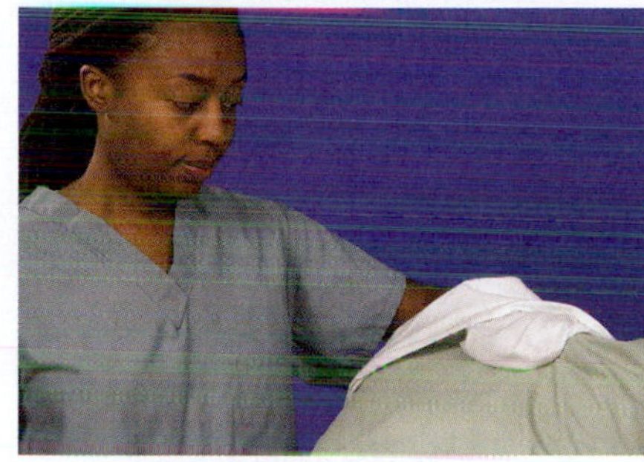

d. Continuing to grasp the end of the pillow, pull the pillowcase down over the pillow.

Do not hold the pillow under your arm or chin to put on pillowcase because contamination can occur.

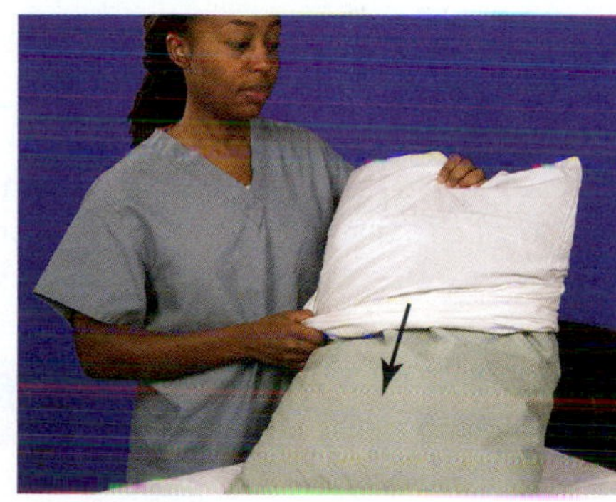

15. Assist the patient back to bed, return the bed to the low position, place the call signal within reach, and place the bedside table and overbed table so that they are accessible to the patient.

Provides for patient comfort and safety.

? What if . . .

- **The linens have been contaminated by body fluids?**

  Follow recommended infection control procedures for laundering of linens (e.g., wear procedure gloves, place linen in moisture-proof bags, and so on).

(continued on next page)

Procedure 25-15 ■ Making an Unoccupied Bed (continued)

- **The mattress has become contaminated by body fluids?**

  Follow agency policies for cleaning the mattress before putting on clean linens. This often involves notifying another department, such as housekeeping or environmental services, whose members are trained in this procedure.

- **The mattress cover is damaged or worn?**

  Regularly check each mattress cover for any visible signs of damage or wear, such as cuts, tears, cracks, pinholes, snags, or stains. Routinely remove the mattress cover, and check its inside surface for wet spots, staining, or signs of damage or wear. Check all sides and the bottom of the mattress. Remove any damaged, worn, or visibly stained medical bed mattress, according to the healthcare facility's procedures, and immediately replace any damaged mattress cover to reduce the risk of infection to patients.

- **The patient has a specialty bed or specialty mattress?**

  Several products are available with specific criteria to match patients' needs in terms of comfort, prevention, or treatment of pressure ulcers, and movement (e.g., specialty beds designed for bariatric patients). Follow the manufacturer's directions (e.g., a recommendation for a specific mattress may be to use only one layer of sheet over the mattress for maximum benefit). If you find the sheets are not large enough to accommodate a specialty mattress, you may need to use two flat sheets to cover it.

Home Care

The only adaptations at home depend on the type of bed the patient has. If the height of the bed is not adjustable or the bed is not accessible from both sides, the procedure may be more difficult.

Documentation

Linen changes are generally recorded on a checklist, if at all. Additional charting would need to be done only if something abnormal occurred, for example, "The drawsheet had a 20-cm circular area of serosanguinous drainage."

Practice Resources

Mitchell, B., Wilson, F., McGregor, A., et al. (2012); Sergent, A. P., Slekovec, C., Pauchot, J., et al. (2012); Siegel, J., Rhinehart, E., Jackson, M., et al. (2007, updated 2017); U.S. Food and Drug Administration (2017).

Procedure 25-16 ■ Making an Occupied Bed

➤ For steps to follow in *all* procedures, refer to the Universal Steps for All Procedures found on the inside back cover.

Equipment

- Bottom and top sheets; drawsheet
- Pillowcase for each of the pillows
- Bath blanket (as needed)
- Linen bag or hamper
- Procedure gloves (if exposure to body fluids is possible)
- Moisture-proof gown (if heavy soiling of linens with body fluids is possible)

Delegation

You can delegate this procedure if the patient's condition and the UAP's skills permit. For example, if the patient is very ill, in pain, or requires two people for turning and repositioning, you should assist with or perform the linen change yourself.

Pre-Procedure Assessments

- Determine the patient's ability to assist with the procedure and whether additional help or assistive devices are needed.
- Make other assessments listed in Procedure 25-15.

➤ When performing the procedure, always identify your patient according to agency policy, using two identifiers, and be attentive to standard precautions, hand hygiene, patient safety and privacy, body mechanics, and documentation.

➤ *Note:* If linen change is done at the same time as the bed bath, some of these steps will vary.

Procedure Steps

1. **Prepare the environment:** Move the overbed table and other furniture, as needed, to allow access to the bed. Place the linen bag or hamper conveniently near the bed.
To allow easy access to the bed and to work efficiently, saving time and energy.

2. **Don protective gloves** and other gear, if necessary.
This observes standard precautions and reduces the risk of contaminating your clothing.

3. **Position the bed flat** if possible, and raise it to working height. Lower the siderail nearest you.
Maintains good body mechanics and prevents back strain during the procedure. Having the head of the bed flat makes it easier to smooth the bottom sheet. To prevent the patient from falling out of bed, lower the siderails only on the side where you are standing.

4. **Disconnect the call device**, and remove the patient's personal items from the bed.
Prevents items from getting lost.

5. **Check that no tubes** (e.g., IV, nasogastric) are entangled in the bed linens.
Prevents dislodging tubes accidentally.

6. **If the blanket or bedspread** is clean, fold it, and place it on a clean area (e.g., the back of a chair); do not place it on another patient's bed or furniture.
Reusing the blanket and/or bedspread if it is not soiled conserves resources.

7. **Cover the patient** with a bath blanket, if available, or leave the top sheet over the patient.
Covering the patient prevents chilling and preserves modesty.

8. **Slide the patient to the far side** of bed, and place her in the side-lying position, facing the siderail. Place a pillow under her head. If needed for support, place a pillow between the patient and the siderail.
Placing the patient close to the side rail will allow you to place the clean linen over a larger area, making it easier to roll the patient back onto the clean linen. Patients who cannot maintain the side-lying position should have a pillow placed between the chest and the siderail to prevent them from accidentally rolling into the siderail.

9. **Roll or tightly fanfold** the soiled linens toward the patient's back. Tuck the roll slightly under the patient. Cover any moist areas with a waterproof pad.
Covering moist areas prevents contact with the clean linen or patient. ▼

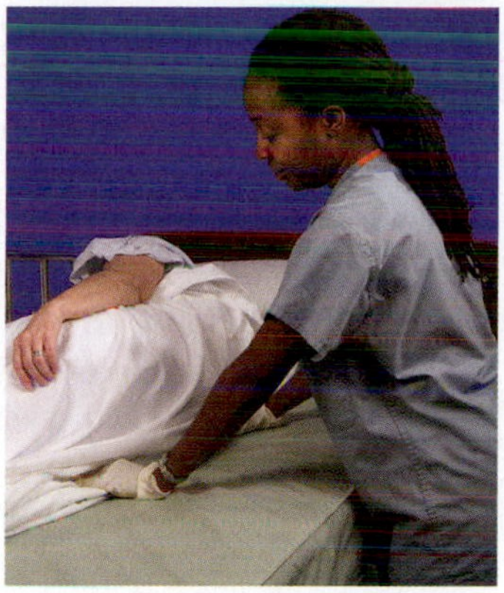

10. **Remove soiled gloves**, perform hand hygiene, and don clean gloves.

11. **Place the clean bottom sheet** and drawsheet (or pad) on the near side of the mattress, with the center vertical fold at the center of the bed. Fanfold the half of the clean linen that is to be used on the far side, folding it as close to the patient as possible and tucking it under the dirty linen. Tuck the lower edges of clean linen under the mattress. Smooth out all wrinkles.
Wrinkles under the patient can cause skin irritation. ▼

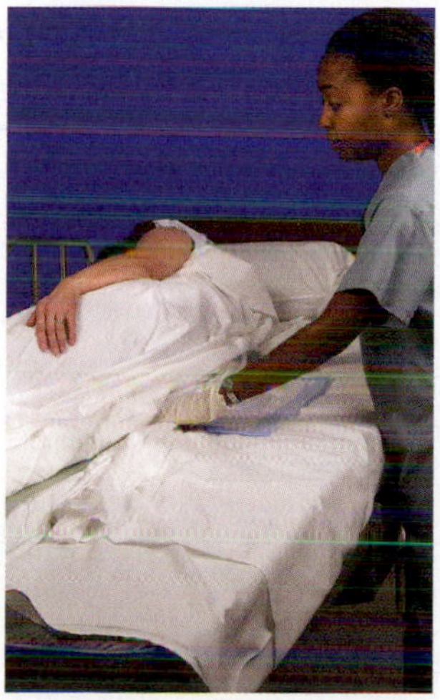

12. **Roll the patient over the clean and dirty linen**, turning him toward you. Explain to him that he will be rolling over a "lump," and then gently pull the patient toward you so that he rolls onto the clean linen. ▼

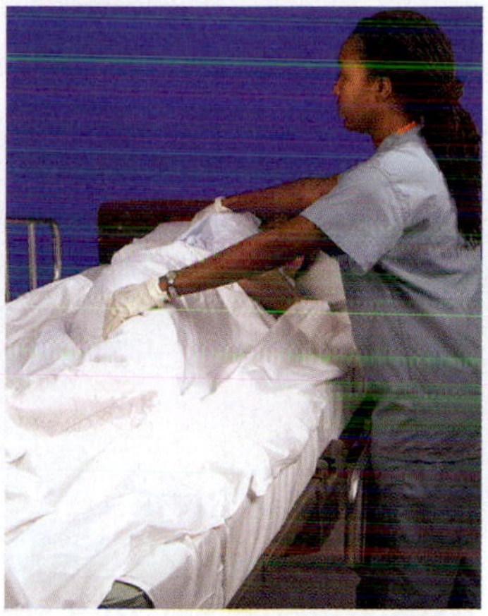

13. **Raise the siderail** on the clean side of the bed.
Prevents the patient from falling.

14. **Move the pillows** to the clean side. Position the patient comfortably on her side, near the siderail.
Always ensure patient comfort and safety before going to the other side of the bed.

15. **Go to the opposite side of bed**, and lower the rail. Pull the soiled linen away from under the patient and the clean linen, and place it in laundry bag or hamper. Never place linen on the floor.
Prevents cross-contamination. ▼

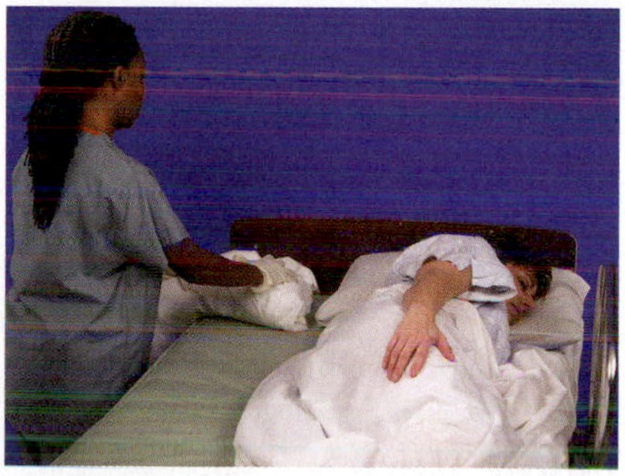

(continued on next page)

Procedure 25-16 ■ Making an Occupied Bed (continued)

16. Remove soiled gloves, and don clean gloves. Pull clean linens through, and tuck them in. Pull taut, starting with the middle section.
Ensures that no wrinkles will be under the patient.

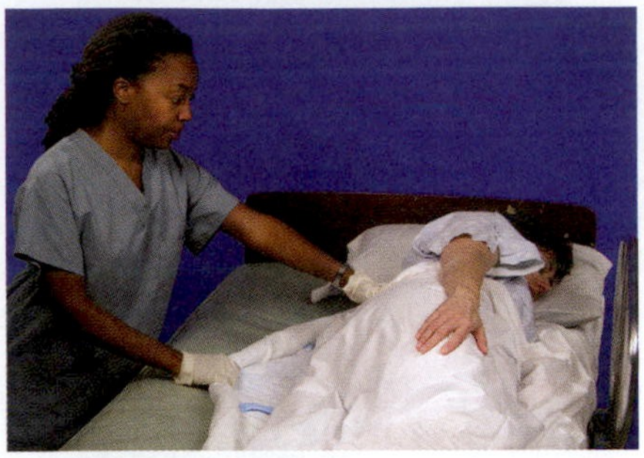

17. Assist the patient to a supine position close to center of the mattress.

18. Place the top sheet and bedspread along one side of the mattress, and continue making the bed as in Procedure 25-15, Steps 9 through 14, *except* remove the bath blanket from under the top linens before tucking them in.

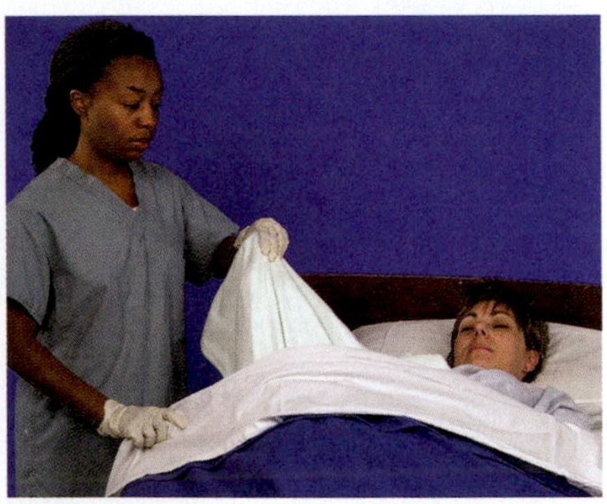

19. Return the bed to the low position, raise the siderails, and attach the call light within patient's reach. Position the bedside table and overbed table within patient's reach.
Ensures patient safety and comfort.

? What if . . .

- **You are making the bed with a patient in leg traction?**

It may be easier to make the bed from top to bottom, as follows:

- Loosen all bed linens, and bring the dirty linens from the top of the bed to the hip area. Put the clean bottom sheet on the top corners of the mattress, bring down to the hip level and tuck under the dirty linen. Cover any moist areas with a waterproof pad.
- Ask the patient to grasp the trapeze and raise his buttocks. If the patient is unable to raise his buttocks, use an assistive device, according to agency policy.
- Bring the dirty bottom sheet along with the clean bottom sheet toward the foot of the bed. Remove the dirty linen, and place it in the laundry bag.
- Tuck the clean sheet under the mattress. Cover with the top sheet. To accommodate traction equipment, do not tuck in the top sheet.

- **You need to move or reposition a patient in bed who is not able to assist or a patient who is obese?**

Before making the occupied bed, assess the patient's ability to move. Use assistive equipment, such as friction reducing devices, mechanical lifts, air powered mattresses, and/or lateral transfer devices.
These are essential tools in preventing work-related injuries. Limit the need to use your own strength while lifting, turning, or repositioning the patient in bed because of the stress placed on the weaker muscles in the arms and shoulders.

Follow agency policies and use of patient moving devices appropriately.
Many healthcare facilities have adopted safe lifting and patient-handling policies as a means to protect both the patient and the healthcare worker.

Evaluation

- Assess how well the patient tolerated the procedure. Was there any discomfort, shortness of breath, and so on?
- Ask the patient whether he feels comfortable.

Home Care

The only adaptations at home depend on the type of bed the client has. If the height of the bed is not adjustable or the bed is not accessible from both sides, the procedure may be more difficult.

Documentation

Linen changes are usually recorded on a checklist. Additional charting needs to be done only if something abnormal occurred.

Practice Resources

Centers for Disease Control and Prevention (2009); Pegram, A., & Bloomfield, J. (2015); Siegel, J., Rhinehart, E., Jackson, M., et al. (2007, updated 2017).

Thinking About the Procedure

The video, **Making an Occupied Bed,** along with questions and suggested responses, is available on the ***Davis's Nursing Skills Videos*** Web site on FADavis.com.

CLINICAL INSIGHTS

Clinical Insight 25-1 ➤ Assisting With a Shower or Tub Bath

Inpatient Care

- Assess the patient's self-care abilities: sensorimotor, musculoskeletal, and cognitive function; activity tolerance; level of knowledge.
- Ensure that the patient has the necessary supplies (e.g., soap, washcloth, towel, clean gown).
- If using prepackaged bath product, be sure to warm bathing products before use.
- Hang a sign on the door to ensure privacy, and place the call device within reach.
- Help wash and dry any areas that the patient cannot reach (e.g., feet, back).

Preventing Hospital-Associated Infections

- If using tap water for bath, check agency policy regarding the safety of the tap water for general use in bathing patients, including the following:
  - The hot water temperature is maintained above 55°C (131°F).
  - Routine sampling for bacterial contamination is done.
- Avoid showering and exposure to faucet water in the case of inpatients who are immunocompromised, the frail elderly, newborns, the critically ill, those having recent surgery or other loss of skin integrity, and patients requiring mechanical ventilation. Use prepackaged wipes instead.
- Verify water temperature for clients with impaired cognition or decreased sensory perception. Bath water should be 110°F to 115°F (43°C to 46°C) to avoid burns.
- Tubs should be stringently maintained and cleaned, preferably with a chlorhexidine gluconate (CHG)–based product, to prevent nosocomial infections related to the use of tubs (e.g., biofilm).

Preventing Falls

- Assist the patient to the shower or bathroom, as needed.
- Ensure that there is a nonskid surface or mat in the shower or tub.
- Use a shower chair in the shower or tub for patients who have impaired mobility or activity intolerance.
- Be sure that the shower or tub is safe (e.g., with grab bars and handrails).
- Provide a call device for the patient to obtain help, if needed; point out the emergency call device if there is one in the bathroom (usually it is a red button or cord on the wall).

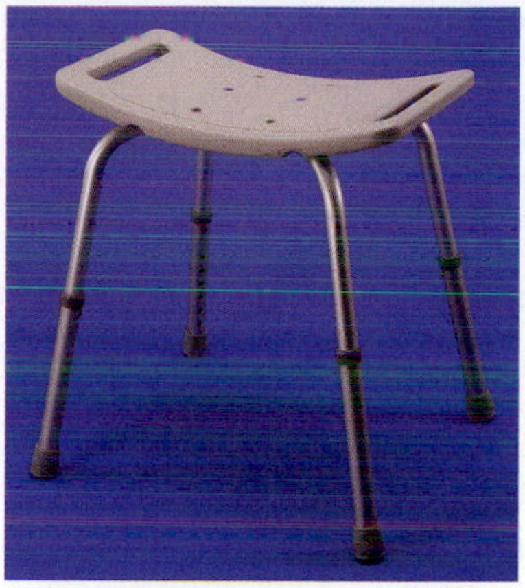

Shower chair

Home Care

- Encourage clients and families to install hand bars on the sides of the bathtub and on the wall next to the tub.
- Advise parents never to leave a child alone in the tub or shower and to have a way to unlock the bathroom door from outside the room.
- Advise older adults or those who are ill not to lock the bathroom door while bathing so that help can be summoned, if needed (e.g., if they fall).
- Help families to obtain benches for transferring into the bathtub, or have them use a plastic chair in the shower.
- Ensure that there is a nonskid surface or mat in the shower or tub.

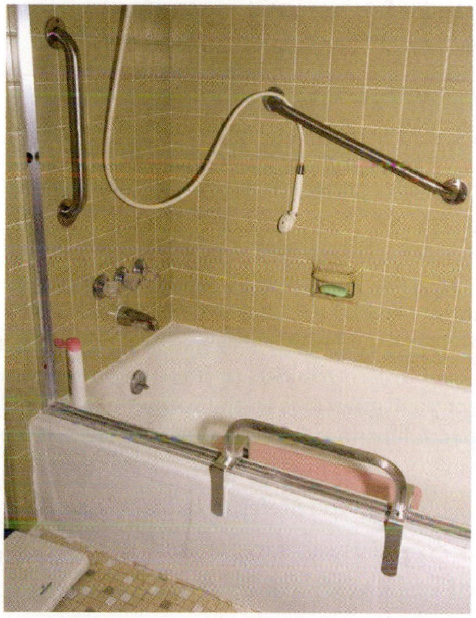

Bathtub with handrail and grab bars

ASSESSMENT GUIDELINES AND TOOLS

Focused Assessment

Guidelines for Assessing Hygiene

Assess Functional Status

Assessment of Functional Abilities for Activities of Daily Living

The Katz Index of Independence in Activities of Daily Living (ADLs) is used extensively to assess functional abilities in ADLs (bathing/hygiene, dressing/grooming, feeding, toileting). To use the Katz ADL Index,

Go directly to https://consultgeri.org/try-this/general-assessment/issue-2.pdf

Observe Self-Care Abilities

When bathing, dressing, eating, and toileting, which of the following best describes the patient's ability?

- Is completely independent; requires no assistance
- Requires a device or special equipment (e.g., a walker, a large-handle spoon)
- Requires help, supervision, or teaching from another person
- Requires help, from another person, as well as a device or special equipment
- Is totally dependent; does not participate in the activity (e.g., total bed bath)

The Environment

- Is the room temperature comfortable?
- Are the siderails up, when indicated? Is the bed in low position?
- Are bed wheels locked?
- Are bed linens clean and wrinkle free?
- Is the patient's call device within reach?
- Is the overbed table clean and uncluttered?
- Is the walking space uncluttered?
- Are there unpleasant odors?

Skin

Subjective Data

iCare Patients may be sensitive about skin problems or poor hygiene practices, so direct your questions to the patient in a nonjudgmental, respectful manner. General questions to ask include the following:

- How often do you prefer to bathe?
- How do you usually care for your skin?
- What soaps, lotions, or other skin care products do you use?
- Do you have difficulty controlling body odor?
- Have you ever had an allergic skin reaction to food, medications, plants, skin care products, or other materials?
- What problems have you had with your skin in the past?
- What problems are you having with your skin now?

For each problem identified, ask:

- What symptoms are you having (e.g., any rash or itching)?
- Where is the problem located?
- How long have you had this problem?
- What have you done to provide relief from the symptoms?
- Do you use any prescription, over-the-counter (OTC), or herbal remedies to treat this problem?
- Have you seen a healthcare provider about this problem?
- Was a diagnosis made? If so, what was it?
- How has this problem affected your life?
- How can I best help you with your skin care?

Also ask about the presence of diseases or other factors that are known to cause skin problems; for example, decreased mobility, decreased circulation, incontinence, inadequate nutrition, or deficient knowledge.

Objective Data

- Note the skin's overall cleanliness, condition, color, texture, turgor, hydration, and temperature.
- Observe for rashes, lumps, lesions, and cracking.
- Look for drainage from wounds or around tubes.
- Observe for four significant color changes: pallor, erythema, jaundice, and cyanosis.

Feet

Subjective Data

Ask the patient the following questions or obtain the data from his records:

- What is your normal foot care routine?
- What type of footwear do you usually wear? Observe what the patient is wearing.
- Have you had any foot problems; what treatments have you had for them?
- Do you examine your feet on a regular basis?
- Do you have diabetes mellitus or peripheral vascular disease?

Objective Data

Compare findings for both feet:

- Observe for cleanliness and skin integrity. Note open areas, drainage, or redness.
- Inspect for swelling, inflammation, or infection.

Focused Assessment

Guidelines for Assessing Hygiene—cont'd

- Palpate for edema.
- Check the skin between the toes for cracks or signs of a fungal infection.
- Note the color and temperature of the feet; are they the same bilaterally? The color and temperature provide data about circulation and oxygenation. For example, cold, dusky feet may indicate impaired circulation or tissue perfusion secondary to a peripheral vascular disease.
- Check capillary refill. How many seconds does it take for the color to return after you apply pressure?
- Note the presence of foot odors, if any.

Nails

Subjective Data
Ask about the patient's usual nail care practices, history of nail problems, and their treatments.

Objective Data
Inspect the nails for the following:

- Shape, contour, and cleanliness
- Presence of broken nails, hangnails, or cracked cuticles
- Hands: Do the fingernails appear neatly manicured, or does the patient bite the nails?
- Feet: Are the toenails trimmed appropriately, straight across?
- Presence of redness or swelling at the nail base or sides

Oral Cavity

Subjective Data

- Usual hygiene practices
- History of periodontal disease or other oral problems
- Financial or insurance problems that limit access to dental care
- Nutritional status and dietary habits (e.g., intake of refined sugars)
- Medications, such as anticonvulsants or diuretics
- Medical treatments, such as radiation therapy, oxygen therapy, and nasogastric tubes
- Other factors known to cause oral problems (smoking, alcohol use, NPO status, dehydration, mouth breathing)
- Self-care deficits (e.g., cognitive impairment, activity intolerance, impaired mobility, depression, lack of knowledge, lack of motivation)

Objective Data

- Observe the lips, which should be pink and moist without lesions.
- Inspect the oral mucosa and gums, which should also be pink, moist, smooth, and free of lesions.
- Healthy gums should have a well-defined margin at each tooth. There should be no visible bleeding.
- Instruct the patient to stick out his tongue and to move it around. It should move freely. The tongue should be symmetrical and pink, with a slightly rough surface.
- Assess the teeth for the presence of any loose, missing, or decaying teeth.
- Examine the hard and soft palates for color, lesions, patches, or petechiae.
- Note any unusual mouth odors or halitosis.

Hair

Subjective Data

- Use of special products or medicated shampoos
- History of hair problems or current conditions needing treatment (e.g., pediculosis)
- History or presence of disease or therapy that affects the hair (e.g., chemotherapy)
- Factors influencing the patient's ability to manage hair and scalp care (e.g., Impaired Mobility)
- Personal or cultural preferences for styling of the hair

Objective Data

- Note the condition, cleanliness, texture, and oiliness of the hair.
- Inspect the scalp for dandruff, pediculosis (head lice), alopecia (hair loss), secretions, or lesions.

Eyes

Subjective Data

- If the patient wears glasses, ask when he uses them (e.g., for reading, for driving) and ask how well he sees without them.
- If the patient wears contact lenses, determine:
  - The type of lens (hard, soft, long-wearing, disposable).
  - How often he wears them (daily, occasionally) and for how long at a time. Are they worn during sleep?
  - History of, or present, problems with lens usage (e.g., cleaning, removal).
  - Usual practices for cleaning and storage.
  - History of, or current, problems with the eyes (e.g., redness, tearing, irritation, dryness or "scratchy feeling").

Objective Data

- Inspect the eyes for redness, lesions, swelling, crusting, excessive tearing, or discharge.
- Check the color of the conjunctivae.

CLINICALJUDGMENT

Applying the Full-Spectrum Nursing Model

PATIENT SITUATION

Alice Baker is a frail elderly woman, 93 years old, who lives in a nursing home. She has almost total Self-Care Deficit related to her weakness, painful joints, and dementia. Her mental and physical conditions are not likely to improve. Imagine that your charge nurse has instructed you to provide a complete bed bath and other hygiene care for Ms. Baker. When you enter her room with bath supplies and say, "Good morning, Ms. Baker; it's time for your bath," she screams, "Go away from me. I just had a bath. I don't want a bath." You discuss this with the charge nurse, who says, "She has not had a bath, and she needs one today. You will need to do it whether she likes it or not." You tend to agree that Ms. Baker needs a bath because her clothing and linens have food stains, and she smells of urine and perspiration.

THINKING

1. *Theoretical Knowledge:*
   a. What benefits does a bath have for Ms. Baker?
   b. What are the disadvantages of bathing a patient with dementia who is resisting the bath?
2. *Critical Thinking (Considering Alternatives, Deciding What to Do):*
   a. What do you think Ms. Baker is feeling and experiencing, and how does that help you know what to do?
   b. What are some alternatives to a complete bed bath that would achieve the same purposes?

DOING

3. *Practical Knowledge:* Imagine that you have, indeed, decided that Ms. Baker needs a bath. Which type bath you will give her? What supplies will you need, and where will you find them in the clinical agency you have attended most recently?

CARING

4. *Self-Knowledge:* What is your greatest concern about bathing Ms. Baker? What is the cause of your concern?

Critical Thinking and Clinical Judgment

1. You are caring for Mrs. Little, a 57-year-old woman who has been experiencing severe arthritic pain for the past 2 years. She rates her pain at an 8 or 9 on a 10-point pain-rating scale. During your assessment, you notice that Mrs. Little has a moderate body odor, long and untrimmed fingernails and toenails, oily hair, and unshaven legs and axillae. Mrs. Little readily admits that she has neglected her hygiene practices.
   a. What is the first hygiene-related nursing diagnosis (problem and etiology) that comes to your mind for Mrs. Little?
   b. What data do you have to support a diagnosis of Self-Care Deficit: Bathing? What data do you have to support an etiology of "immobility secondary to pain"?
   c. With the information in the scenario, how would you rate her Self-Care Deficit: mild, moderate, severe, or total?
   d. Anything you could do to help relieve Mrs. Little's pain would facilitate her self-care abilities. However, to plan interventions in which you will assist with her hygiene care, what further patient data do you need?

e. Suppose you assess Mrs. Little further and determine that she has arthritis in multiple joints, including her hands, shoulders, back, knees, and feet. You also determine that she will need a complete bath, either tub or shower but that she can brush her own teeth if someone provides the necessary supplies. Could you delegate her a.m. hygiene care to an experienced UAP? If so, what instructions would you give the UAP?

2. Mr. Thomson is an 87-year-old African American man admitted 2 days ago after being found unconscious in his small apartment. Although Mr. Thomson denies being diabetic, his admission blood sugar was 653 mg/dL. His lower legs are swollen, red, and weeping a clear fluid. His toenails are long, thick, and yellow, and there is a small open sore on the great toe of his left foot. Mr. Thomson's skin is dry and scaly, his hair matted, and he has a strong odor of perspiration and urine. He is uncircumcised. He refuses help with hygiene, saying, "I've taken care of myself for 87 years, and I'll keep doing it. I take my bath once a week on Saturday evening. Now go away!"

   a. What theoretical knowledge will you need in order to know what to assess and how to provide his hygiene care?

   b. Self-knowledge is important in this case as well. What things in this situation would make caring for Mr. Thomson especially difficult for you? What biases, values, or attitudes might interfere with your ability to give your best care?

3. Recall the Meet Your Patients scenario in Volume 1 of your textbook. The remaining critical-thinking questions refer to that scenario:

   Scenario: Your instructor has assigned you to assist the following patients with their hygiene. You must assess the needs of each person, gather information on their bathing habits and preferences, plan nursing measures necessary to meet individual needs, and together with a UAP, provide care.

   The first person on your assignment is Mrs. Williams, a 76-year-old woman of Indian heritage, who was admitted yesterday after suffering a stroke that paralyzed her right side. Since the stroke, she has been unable to speak clearly and becomes frustrated as she attempts to communicate her needs. Her daughter says Mrs. Williams is a proud and tidy woman, who has been living alone and caring for herself independently since her husband's death last year, even maintaining the yard and garden. She wears eyeglasses for reading and driving and has a hearing aid.

   The second person on your assignment is Mr. Gold, a 68-year-old Orthodox Jewish man, admitted last week after a massive heart attack. Although his eyes are open, he does not respond to external stimuli. Because of Impaired Swallowing, Mr. Gold is unable to take food or fluid orally. A feeding tube was placed to ensure adequate nutrition and hydration. His oral mucous membranes and lips are dry and crusty. He is incontinent of urine and stool. Mr. Gold's son, Ira, tells you that Mr. Gold adheres to Orthodox Jewish law and requests that you respect this in his care.

   The following questions are about Mrs. Williams:

   a. To assess Mrs. Williams' self-care abilities, what important patient data do you still need?

   b. What problem has resulted from her stroke that will make it difficult for you to find out about Mrs. Williams' hygiene preferences and practices?

   c. From what you know of the patient situation, why do you think Mrs. Williams is becoming frustrated?

   d. How do you think you would react if this were to happen to you?

   e. How could you provide opportunities for Mrs. Williams to maintain her independence?

4. **The following questions are about Mr. Gold:**

   a. What additional theoretical knowledge do you need to meet Mr. Gold's religious and cultural needs when providing hygiene care?

   b. Where could you obtain such information?

   c. If you decide to delegate Mr. Gold's bed bath to a UAP, how could you incorporate his religious and cultural needs into your delegation decisions?

5. For each of the following concepts, use critical thinking to describe how or why it is important to nursing, patient care, or facilitating hygiene. Note that these are *not* to be merely definitions.

Personal hygiene
Delegation of tasks
Cultural differences
Skin integrity
Life span variables
Self-care deficits
The nursing process
Patient teaching
Bathing
Oral care
Environment and comfort
Hair care
Nail care

What Are the Main Points in This Chapter?

- Current guidelines are changing the way nurses provide hygiene. The long-held tradition of using a basin, soap, and water to bathe hospitalized patients is no longer the recommended standard of practice.
- Recent recommendations include (1) the use of disposable, single-patient-use basins to reduce risk of bacterial contamination and (2) avoiding the use of unfiltered tap water in hospitals, unless the water lines are known to not contain biofilm. Alternatives include prepackaged bathing products and the use of sterile or distilled water or filtered water from faucets.
- Personal hygiene contributes to physical and psychological well-being by promoting comfort, improving self-image, and decreasing infection and disease.
- Although a patient may need assistance with hygiene measures, the goal is to encourage as much independence with these tasks as possible.
- Numerous factors influence individual hygiene practices, including personal preferences, cultural/religious/spiritual values and beliefs, economic status, living environment, developmental or knowledge level, and physical and emotional health.
- Maintain a respectful, nonjudgmental attitude about cultural and spiritual differences. Avoid the temptation to impose personal values about hygiene practices onto patients.
- Consider patients' personal hygiene preferences, and incorporate them into the care plan, whenever possible. This reflects caring and promotes maximum participation and independence with ADLs.
- Although many hygiene measures can be delegated to the UAP, the nurse retains full responsibility for each patient and must instruct the UAP about the patient's limitations and restrictions, amount of assistance necessary, use of any assistive devices, any specific safety precautions to be undertaken, and any other factors influencing the patient's hygiene practices.
- The nurse should assess a patient's functional status regularly.
- Teaching patients about hygiene is a primary function of the professional nurse.
- Intact skin is the body's first line of defense to keep pathogenic microorganisms from entering the body and causing infection.
- Bathing removes perspiration and bacteria from the skin surface. It promotes relaxation and comfort, improves circulation, reduces odor, and enhances well-being by increasing self-image. However, it can be stressful for some patients.
- You should choose the type of bath to meet the patient's needs (e.g., assist bath, total bed bath, bag bath, and so on).
- Bathing is stressful to some patients (e.g., the frail elderly, people with dementia, people with morbid obesity). You should focus on the patient's needs for warmth, safety, and comfort, and adapt the bathing procedure to help reduce stress.
- Despite common myths, it does not take a lot of water to get a person clean, and not all patients need a complete bath every day.
- A complete bath includes perineal care.
- Careful assessment of the feet allows for early detection of common foot problems, such as calluses, corns, tinea pedis, ingrown toenail, or foot odor.
- Because dirt and debris can collect under the nails and serve as a source of infection, nail care is an important part of hygiene, especially in patients with diabetes mellitus or peripheral neuropathy.
- To maintain healthy mucous membranes, teeth, and gums, and to prevent tooth loss and gum disease, regular dental checkups and daily mouth care, including brushing and flossing teeth, are necessary.
- For critically ill and frail elderly patients, as well as those using ventilators, special attention to oral hygiene helps reduce the risk for pneumonia.

- Oral hygiene is challenging for patients with dementia, but it must not be neglected.
- The condition of the hair is a measure of an individual's overall health. Shampooing and daily brushing of the hair massages the scalp, stimulates the circulation, and distributes the natural oils in the hair.
- The eyes normally require very little care; however, when necessary, they may be gently cleansed from the inner canthus to the outer canthus.
- Unconscious or critically ill patients who no longer have a blink reflex may need eye care at least every 2 to 4 hours. Keeping the eyes lubricated protects them from corneal abrasions and drying.
- Some contact lenses can be worn for only about 12 hours at a time; others may be worn for up to 30 days. Some are disposable; some are not. All types must be cleaned carefully and regularly.
- Hearing aids are expensive and should be properly handled and stored. They should not be immersed in water.
- When reinserting an artificial (prosthetic) eye, first, be certain that it is wet.
- Usually, no special care is required for the nose. Excess secretions can be removed by gentle blowing with both nostrils open.
- Clean, wrinkle-free bed linens help promote comfort and a sense of well-being.
- Room temperature, adequate ventilation, low noise level, and neat and clean surroundings all contribute to a comfortable patient environment.

Knowledge Map

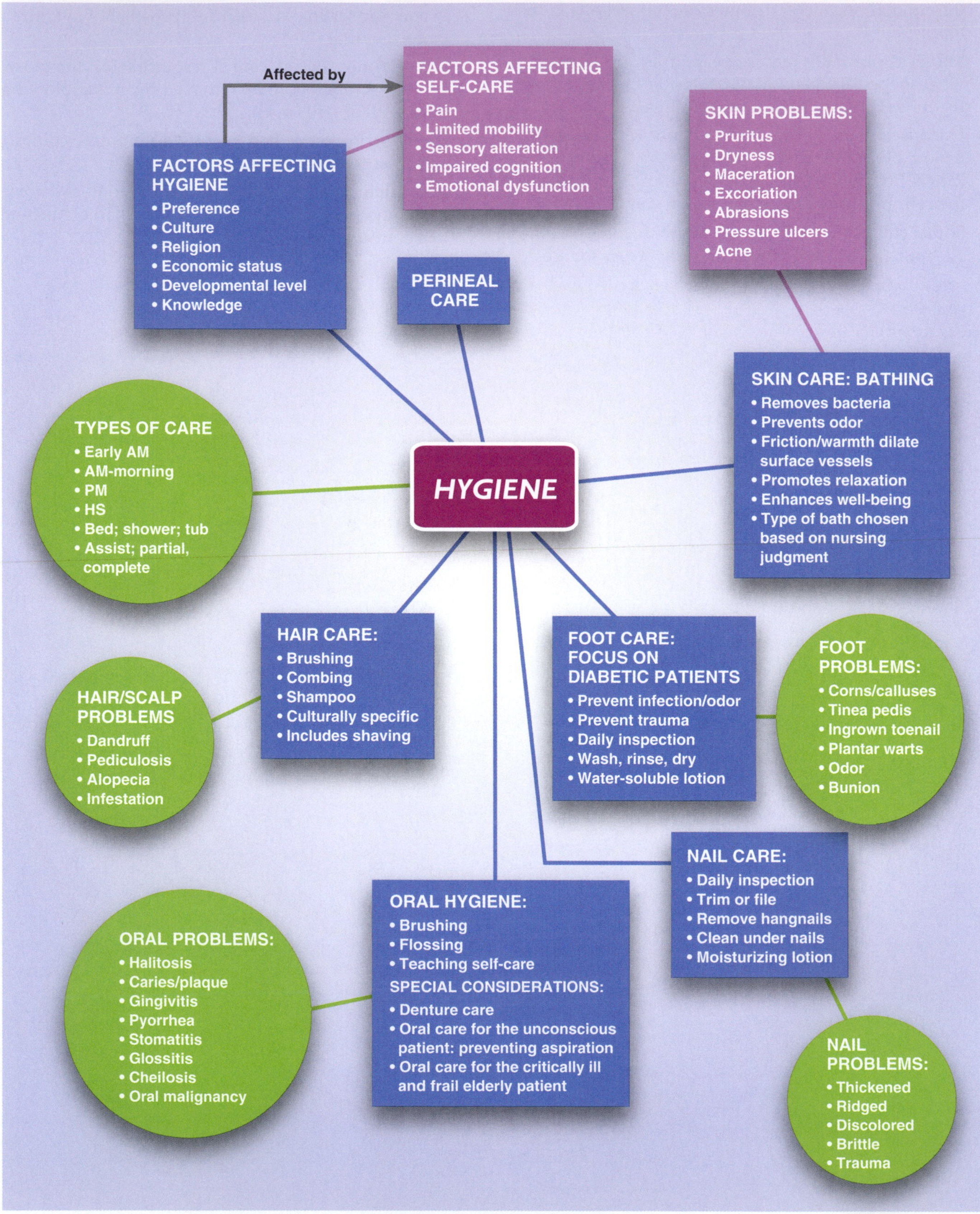

CHAPTER 26

Administering Medications

STUDENT RESOURCES

The questions and exercises in this book allow you to practice the kind of thinking you will use as a full-spectrum nurse. Critical-thinking questions usually have more than one right answer, so we do not provide "correct answers" for these features. Try to answer these questions yourself. It is more important to develop your nursing judgment than to just cover content. You will learn by discussing the questions with your peers. If you are still unsure, see the Davis Advantage chapter resources for suggested responses.

To explore learning resources for this chapter,

Go to Davis Advantage and find:

Answers and Suggested Responses for all questions in this chapter
Concept Map
Knowledge Map
References and Bibliography
Lists of NOC Outcomes and NIC Interventions

Key Concepts

Medication administration
Medication safety
Pharmacology

Related Concepts

See the Concept Map on Davis Advantage.

Caring for the Nguyens

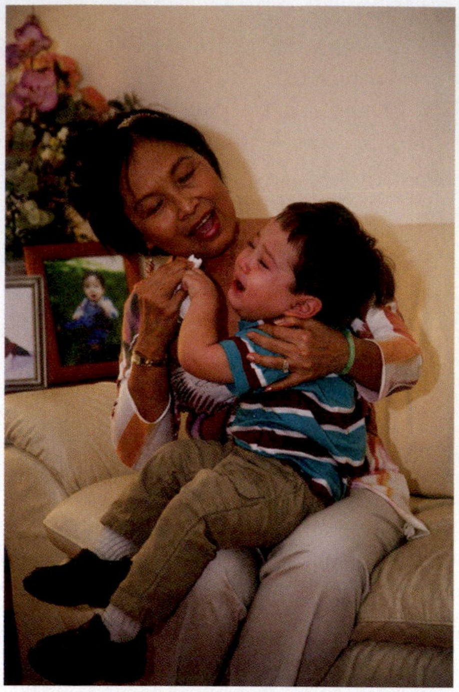

Kim Phan, the 3-year old grandson of Nam and Yen Nguyen, has been tired and observed to be sitting down a great deal at preschool. Last week, he developed coughing, wheezing, shortness of breath, nasal congestion, and extreme fatigue. The pediatrician at the Family Medicine Center diagnosed asthma. He prescribed a 5-day tapering course of prednisone, a leukotriene inhibitor (Singulair) 4 mg orally daily at bedtime, and periodic treatments with albuterol through a home nebulizer system.

Nam's mother, Mai Nguyen, became very upset when she saw the bottle of prednisone elixir. She was even more upset when she learned that Kim received an injection of the medicine in the office. She advised Yen not to give Kim the medicine because, she said, it causes weak bones and stunts growth. Yen has called the clinic asking for advice on how to handle this problem. (Look up the medications and use your knowledge of different routes of administration.)

A. What theoretical knowledge do you need to answer these concerns?

B. What are some reliable sources where you might find this information?

C. What rationale could you offer to Yen to explain the safety of the prednisone prescription? You will need to use a variety of references to answer this question.

D. Yen asks you to explain why Kim received both a shot and pills. How would you respond?

E. Why is Kim receiving a leukotriene inhibitor (Singulair) orally and albuterol by nebulizer?

PracticalKnowledge clinical **application**

The practical knowledge you will need to administer medications safely and effectively includes procedures, clinical insights, and guidelines for calculating and measuring dosages and administering medications by a variety of routes.

PROCEDURES

Procedures in this section will assist you to prepare, measure, and administer various types of medications, locate injection sites, and handle needles safely.

Use the following Medication Guidelines for all types and routes.

Medication Guidelines: ■ Steps to Follow for All Medications (Regardless of Type or Route)

➤ For steps to follow in *all* procedures, refer to the Universal Steps for All Procedures found on the inside back cover.

Key Point: *Regardless of the type or route of the medication you are giving, you should always follow the steps below.*

Equipment

- Medication administration record (MAR)
- Medication drawer or portable cart with, as needed, keys to the medication drawer
- Gloves for the procedure, as needed
- Other supplies and equipment needed for the specific procedure (e.g., water, antiseptic wipes)

Delegation

As a registered nurse (RN), you can usually delegate administration of medications (except for intravenous [IV] medications) to a licensed practical nurse/licensed vocational nurse (LPN/LVN). You cannot delegate this task to unlicensed assistive personnel (UAP). You can instruct a UAP in the therapeutic effects and side effects of medications and to report any effects observed.

Nurse practice acts (NPAs) governing medication administration vary from state to state, as do policies in healthcare agencies. In some states, with additional education and training, LPN/LVNs can administer IV medications and UAPs can administer some medications. You must know the scope of practice described in your state's NPA.

Key Point: ***The RN is always responsible for evaluating client responses, which include both therapeutic effects and side effects.***

Pre-Procedure Assessments

- Assess your knowledge of the medication (e.g., drug action, purpose, recommended dosage, time of onset and peak action, common side effects, contraindications, drug interactions, and nursing implications).
- Determine whether the prescribed dosage is appropriate for the patient's age and weight.
  Dosages are generally decreased for children because of both age and weight. Usually, dosing for older patients is not based on weight but on renal function. Both groups have less efficient liver and renal function compared with other age groups, increasing the length of time a drug stays in the body before being excreted.
- Check for any history of allergies to medications or food.
- At least the first time you administer medications to a patient, assess the his knowledge of the medications being given.
  The patient will be more likely to take the medication correctly if he understands the reasons for taking the medication.
- Assess for factors that could interfere with drug absorption (e.g., diarrhea, inadequate circulation, foods, impaired liver function, edema, inflammation, age-related changes, and other medication).
- Assess vital signs and check lab studies specific to the medication to determine whether the medication can be safely administered.
  Medications are metabolized more slowly in a person with decreased liver function.
- Assess for situations in which it would not be reasonable to administer the medication (e.g., oral medications prescribed for a patient who is NPO (nothing by mouth), vomiting, sedated, or has swallowing difficulties).
  If the medication does not seem reasonable, question the prescriber.

➤ When performing the procedure, always identify your patient according to agency policy, using two identifiers, and be attentive to standard precautions, hand hygiene, patient safety and privacy, body mechanics, and documentation.

Procedure Steps

1. **Check the MAR** for the patient's name and identification number, medication, dose, route, time, and drug allergies. The six rights of medication administration are the right patient, right drug, right dose, right route, right time, and right documentation. At the beginning of your shift, check the MAR to determine when medications are due **(first check).**
   Medication prescriptions may change even during your shift; checking the MAR helps ensure that you do not miss medication changes.

2. **Verify the prescription.** It should include the patient's name, patient identifier, medication name, dose, route, time, and patient allergies.
   You must note whether it has changed (e.g., since the last time you gave the drug). Clarify any discrepancies before giving the medication.

3. **Follow agency policies** for medication administration, including the time frame. Most agencies allow medications to be given 30 minutes before or 30 minutes after the time indicated on the MAR. Do not pre-pour medications.
   The time of administration is important for some medications. For example, if an anti-infective agent is given early or late, a therapeutic blood level may not be maintained.

4. **Perform hand hygiene.**
   Hand hygiene minimizes transmission of microorganisms.

5. **Access the patient's medication drawer,** unlock the medication cart, or log onto the medication dispensing computer.

6. **Obtain the narcotic cabinet key** (or code) when administering a narcotic or barbiturate and sign out the medication, including the patient's name, drug, dose, and other pertinent information, according to agency policy. Note the drug count when removing a narcotic.
   Federal law governs administration of controlled substances. All narcotics and barbiturates are counted and signed for by the outgoing nurse and the oncoming nurse every shift.

7. **Select the prescribed medication.** Read the label and compare medication with the MAR for the first five rights (patient, drug, dose, route, time); check for drug allergies:
   - An inpatient should be wearing an identification band with the drug allergies identified.
   - Allergies should be clearly marked in the medical record and on the MAR or in the electronic health record (EHR).
   - Ask the patient about allergies the first time you administer a medication and before giving a newly prescribed medication.
     These actions ensure that the correct drug is being given to the correct patient at the correct time in the correct dose by the correct route and that any allergies are identified. Do not

(continued on next page)

Medication Guidelines: ■ Steps to Follow for All Medications (Regardless of Type or Route) (continued)

administer the medication if the patient states an allergy to it.

Key Point: *Correct drug includes the correct form of the drug (e.g., oral, IV).*

8. **Calculate the medication dosage.** Double-check it. If you are unable to measure the dose exactly, contact the pharmacist.
9. **Check the expiration date** (on the label or on the box) of all medications.
   A medication that has expired is no longer guaranteed to be effective.
10. **Do a second check** after preparing the medications, to verify the correct patient medication, dose, route, and time **(second check).**
    Verifies the first five rights of medication administration.
11. **Lock the medication cart.** Never leave an unlocked medication cart unattended.
    This guards against pilferage and protects children, older adults with dementia, or anyone wanting to open the cart.
12. **Administer the medications.**
    a. Take the medication and MAR or a hand-held portable device with the EHR into the patient's room.
    You must be able to do the final check in the patient's room and verify that you are administering the correct medication to the correct patient.
    b. Identify the patient using two forms of identification, according to agency policy: Check the identification bracelet, have the patient state her name, compare the patient to her posted picture, and check the patient's date of birth against the MAR.
    Agencies have different means of identifying patients. The Joint Commission requires two forms of identification.

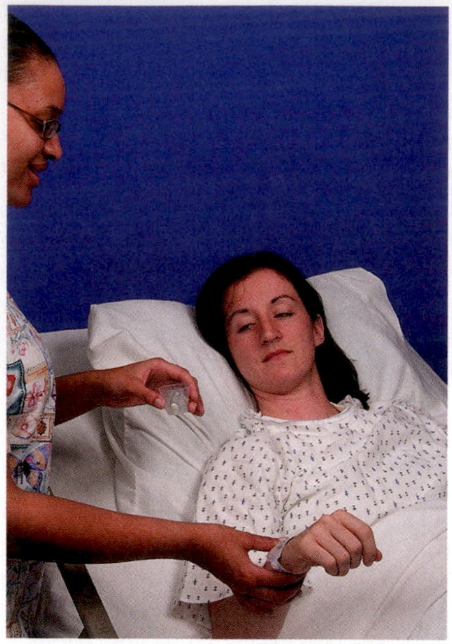

    c. Do a check of the rights of medication: right patient, right medication, right dose, right route, and right time **(third check).**
    Checks for the rights of medication are always required to prevent medication errors. Although it is not actually an "error" until the patient has taken a medication, you may be required to file a report for a "near miss" that was detected during the preadministration checking process.
    d. Perform any necessary assessments, such as checking the pulse or blood pressure.
    Some medications can be given only if physical findings or vital signs are within certain parameters. For example, antihypertensive medications may need to be held if the blood pressure is lower than the patient's normal baseline.
    e. Explain to the patient that you are there to administer the medication; teach the patient about the medication.
    Patient teaching increases understanding of and compliance with treatment. The patient may then be able to identify potential errors in medication administration.

If the patient questions a medication, double-check the medication to be sure you are giving the correct drug and dosage.

    f. Administer the medication using appropriate technique (see the procedures for administering medications by the specified route).
    g. Remain with the patient until you are sure that she has taken the medication.
    If you leave a medication at the bedside, someone else (e.g., another patient or a child) might take it, or the patient might discard it.
    h. Document the medication administered in the patient's medication record (date, dose, route, and your name).
    Your initials on the MAR means that you administered the medication to the patient. If the documentation is not in the patient's record, there is a risk that another nurse will assume the medication was not given and administer it again.

? What if . . .

- **The patient tells you the tablet you are ready to give him is a different color from what he normally takes of a certain prescribed medication?**

Determine why the tablet is different from what the patient normally takes to be sure you are administering the correct drug and dose. Always verify the identity of the drug, especially when it is called into question by the patient who is familiar with his usual routine medications.

Double-checking whenever you are uncertain about a medication you are about to administer helps prevent medication errors—it is possible you have the wrong drug or dosage.

- **The label on the medication shows an expiration date that has passed?**
  Do not give the medication. Send it back to the pharmacy for replacement.
  Expired medication can lose its potency.
- **The patient refuses to take the prescribed medication?**
  Discuss with the patient his concerns about the medication. Hold the dose and notify the prescriber of the patient's refusal, and explain the patient's concerns.
  The patient has a right to refuse medication. You must document the patient's reason for refusal.
- **You cannot decipher the prescriber's handwritten medication prescription?**
  Hold the dose and contact the prescriber for clarification. Never administer medication if you are unable to read the entire prescription.
  Handwriting that is hard to read is a common cause of preventable error. Electronic prescriptions can help to avoid this.
- **Your patient's medication is not available from the pharmacy at the time the dose is due?**
  Do not borrow the medication from another patient's supply. Administer only medication prescribed for that particular patient. Notify the pharmacy of the need to immediately dispense the medication.
  Using another patient's medication increases the risk for error because drug dilution or dosage might vary among patients; or the drug names might sound similar, but they might be different medications. Also, the safety system for charges and refills is bypassed when doses are borrowed from other patients, resulting in missing doses or erroneous charges.

Evaluation

- Evaluate the therapeutic effects of the medication (e.g., check blood pressure after administering an antihypertensive medication, or check pain level after an analgesic has been administered).
- Be alert for any adverse reactions, side effects, or allergic reactions. If present, notify the appropriate care provider.

Patient Teaching

- Describe how the drug is prescribed and when the patient should take the medication.
- Discuss the importance of taking the medication as prescribed.
- Explain the need for any laboratory tests for monitoring the medication, such as tests to measure drug level in the blood, if appropriate.
- Explain the purpose, common side effects, and drug interactions of the medications the patient is taking.
- Teach the patient to observe for side effects that signal the need to contact the prescriber.
- Discuss ways to minimize the side effects of a medication, such as avoiding the sun when taking a medication that causes photosensitivity or rising slowly when taking a medication that causes orthostatic hypotension.
- Discuss potential cultural issues related to taking the medication (e.g., in some Hispanic/Latino cultures, a patient may refuse a medication that is considered "hot" if she believes a "cold" treatment is needed).
- Teach the patient to self-administer medications (e.g., ear drops), as appropriate.

Home Care

- Assess the client's ability to safely self-administer medications.
- Determine the client's financial ability to obtain medications.
- Instruct the client about safe storage of medications.
- Provide instructions for use of each medication.
- Determine whether the client or caregiver has had past problems or present concerns about taking the medications as prescribed.
- If problems have occurred in the past or there are present concerns, discuss possible remedies. For example, you might teach the client or caregiver to use a medication storage container with compartments for the times and days of the week.

Documentation

- Document the medication, time, dose, and route given, preadministration assessments, and your signature.
- Do not document before giving the drug; do not document for anyone else; do not ask another nurse to document a drug you have given. Document only *after* administering the medication.
- Document all therapeutic and adverse effects of the medication. Also, document your nursing interventions and teaching of potential adverse effects.
- Record the scheduled medications on the MAR. Record prn (as needed) medications in the nursing notes and on the MAR, including the reason the medication was given and the patient's response to the medication.
- If the patient is unable or refuses to take the medication, document on the MAR that the medication was not administered and the reason, and inform the provider.
- For parenteral medications, document the site of injection.

(continued on next page)

Medication Guidelines: ■ Steps to Follow for All Medications (Regardless of Type or Route) (continued)

Sample EHR documentation

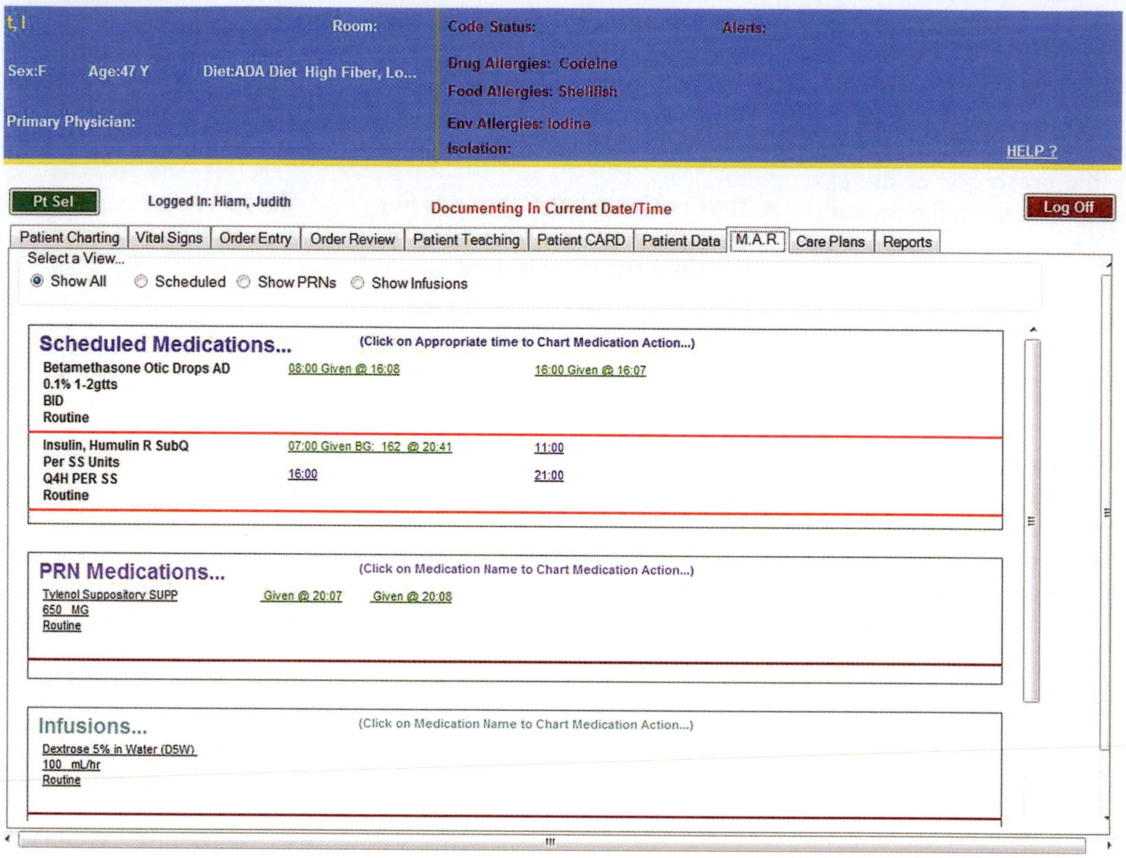

Practice Resources

Institute for Safe Medication Practices (2017); National Coordinating Council for Medication Error Reporting and Prevention (2015); U.S. Food and Drug Administration (2018b).

Thinking About the Procedure

The video **Medication Guidelines: Steps to Follow for All Medications (Regardless of Route),** along with questions and suggested responses, is available on the ***Davis's Nursing Skills Videos*** Web site on FADavis.com.

Procedure 26-1 ■ Administering Oral Medications

➤ For steps to follow in *all* procedures, refer to the Universal Steps for All Procedures found on the inside back cover. Also, refer to Medication Guidelines: Steps to Follow for All Medications (Regardless of Type or Route).

Equipment

- Desired liquid for swallowing medications
- Disposable medication cup
- Drinking straw, if needed
- Procedure gloves, if you will need to place a tablet in the patient's mouth
- For enteral medications:
  Water (for diluting and flushing the feeding tube)
  60-mL catheter-tip syringe
  Clean gloves
- Stethoscope
  For example, to check the apical pulse before administering some cardiac medications.

Delegation

- As a rule, you can delegate this skill to an LPN/LVN, depending on the medication, but not to a UAP, except under special policies and situations.

Pre-Procedure Assessments

- Assess the patient's condition to determine whether there are contraindications to oral medications or to the specific medication; for example, the ability to swallow.
  Impaired swallowing increases the risk for aspiration.
- Check fluid needs and restrictions. If the patient is NPO, check with the prescriber to determine whether the medication should be given by another route or can be given with small sips of water.
  A prescriber may decide it is medically necessary to administer oral medication to a patient who is NPO. If there is a fluid restriction, you need to consider how much fluid you can give with the medication. Give additional fluid to a patient with dehydration; offer only sips for the patient with a fluid restriction.
- For enteral medications, check that the nasogastric (NG) tube is in the stomach and is patent.

➤ When performing the procedure, always identify your patient according to agency policy, using two identifiers, and be attentive to standard precautions, hand hygiene, patient safety and privacy, body mechanics, and documentation.

Procedure Steps

1. **Prepare the medication** for administration.

For Tablet or Capsule

a. If you are pouring from a multidose container, do not touch the medication. Pour the tablet into the cap of the container and then into the medication cup.

b. If the medication is unit-dose, do not open the package. Place the entire unit-dose package into the cup.

c. Many institutions allow combining all tablets or oral caplets scheduled for the same time for the same patient into the same cup. However, even if the agency protocol permits dispensing from a single container, you will need separate cups for medications that require preadministration assessment (e.g., checking the apical pulse rate prior to administering digoxin).
If a medication is held because of a preadministration assessment finding, you can identify it more readily when it has been poured into a separate cup.

d. You may break scored tablets with a knife or a tablet cutter, if necessary.
Only scored tablets may be broken. Breaking an unscored tablet would deliver an imprecise dose.

e. If a patient has difficulty swallowing, check to see whether the medication can be crushed. If so, use a mortar and pestle to grind it. If the medication is in a unit-dose package, grind it while it is still inside the package. Mix the ground medication with a small amount of soft food, such as applesauce or pudding.
Crushing some medications (e.g., capsules, enteric-coated tablets, and sustained-release formulas) may alter their effectiveness or result in an overdose as a result of rapid absorption.

For Liquid Medications

f. Check to see whether you must shake the liquid before opening the container.
Some liquids, such as suspensions, will precipitate and need to be shaken to mix the active ingredient with the suspension liquid.

g. Remove the bottle cap, and place it flat side down on the cart or counter.

h. Hold the bottle with the label in the palm of your hand.
Keeping the label on the upward side of the bottle prevents the liquid from dripping down onto the label and obscuring it.▼

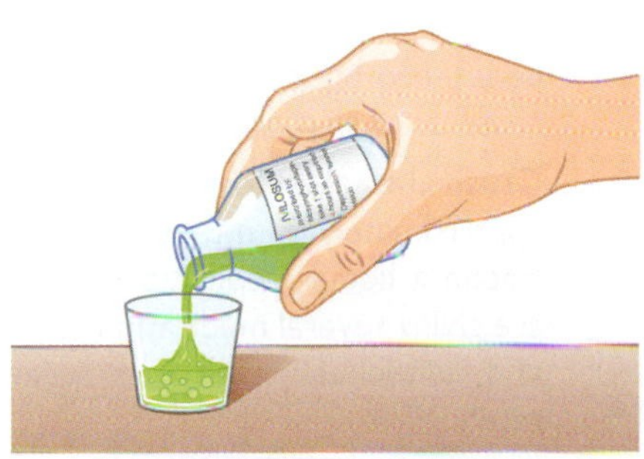

i. Place the plastic medication cup at eye level, and pour the desired amount of medication. Place the cup on a level surface and read the dosage where the lowest part of the concave surface (meniscus) of the fluid is on the line.
Measuring liquids above or below eye level will cause you to read the dose incorrectly and pour too much or too little medication.

j. As you finish pouring medication, slightly twist the bottle to prevent the medication from dripping down the lip of the bottle. If medication does drip down over the lip, wipe the outside of the lip with a tissue or paper towel.
Wiping the outside of the bottle helps prevent contamination, particularly for thicker solutions, such as elixirs or syrups containing sugar.

2. **Administer the medication.**

a. Assist the patient to a high-Fowler's position, if possible.
An upright position facilitates swallowing and prevents choking.

b. ***Powder:*** Mix with liquid at the bedside and give the mixture to the patient to drink.
Some powders thicken very quickly and must be mixed immediately before administration.

c. ***Lozenge:*** Instruct the patient not to chew or swallow it whole.
Medication is absorbed through the oral mucosa and is generally inactivated by the acidity in the stomach.

d. ***Tablet or capsule:***

1) If the patient is able to hold the medication in her hand, place the tablet or medication cup in her hand.
Promotes independence and is easier for the patient.

(continued on next page)

Procedure 26-1 ■ Administering Oral Medications (continued)

2) Give the patient water or other liquid.
Giving the medication with liquid moistens the mouth and helps the patient swallow the tablet or capsule.

3) If the patient is unable to hold the tablet, don procedure gloves and place the medication cup up to her lips, and tip the tablet or capsule into her mouth.
Encourage the patient to do as much as possible. Getting the tablet or capsule to the back of the mouth will assist in swallowing.

e. ***Sublingual medications:*** Have the patient place the tablet under the tongue and hold it there until it is completely dissolved.
Sublingual medications are made to be rapidly absorbed through the oral mucosa. The area under the tongue is very vascular, so sublingual medications act very rapidly. Sublingual medications, if swallowed are inactivated by gastric acid.

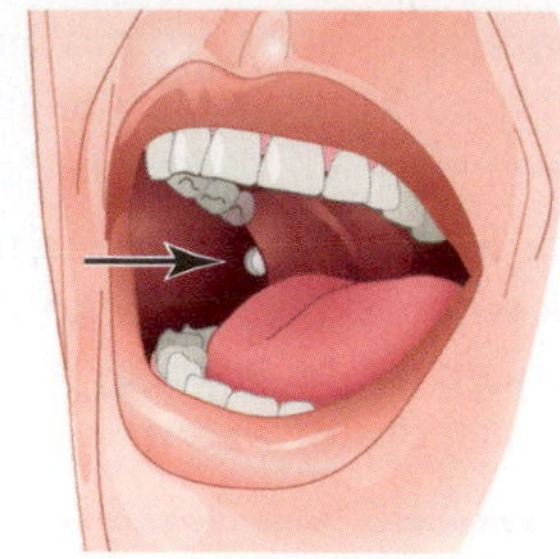

f. ***Buccal medications:*** Have the patient place the tablet between the cheek and gums.
Buccal medications act by being absorbed through the oral mucosa or by being dissolved and swallowed in the saliva.

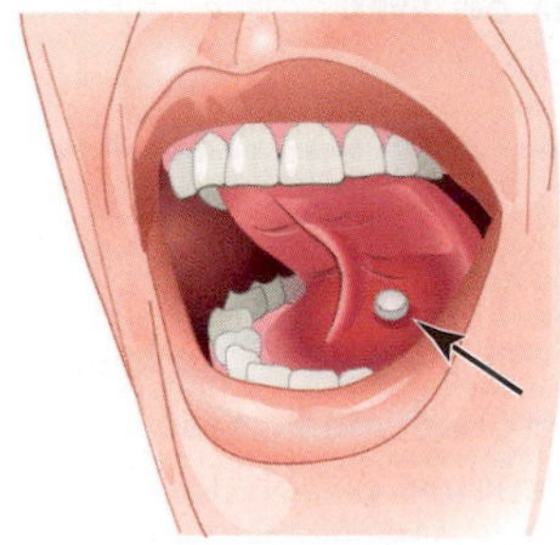

g. ***Liquid medications:*** Hand the medication cup to the patient. If she cannot hold the cup, don procedure gloves and bring it to her mouth and ask her to sip.

3. **Stay with the patient** until all medications have been swallowed or dissolved.
Some patients will "chipmunk" the medication in the side of the mouth without swallowing it, or spit it out. Staying at the bedside until the patient swallows oral medication ensures that the patient has received the dose.

Procedure 26-1A ■ Administering Medication Through an Enteral Tube

➤ For steps to follow in *all* procedures, refer to the Universal Steps for All Procedures found on the inside back cover. Also, refer to Medication Guidelines: Steps to Follow for All Medications (Regardless of Type or Route).

Preparation

- If the patient is receiving a continuous tube feeding, disconnect it before giving the medications. Leave the tube clamped for a few minutes after administering, according to agency protocol.
- If the enteral tube is connected to suction, you will usually discontinue the suction for 20 to 30 minutes after administration, and keep the tube clamped, to allow time for the drug to be absorbed.

➤ When performing the procedure, always identify your patient according to agency policy, using two identifiers, and be attentive to standard precautions, hand hygiene, patient safety and privacy, body mechanics, and documentation.

➤ *Note:* Follow Steps 1a through 1j of Procedure 26-1: Administering Oral Medication. Also, follow precautions for administering enteral medications.

Procedure Steps

1. **Prepare the medication.**
   a. Give the liquid form of medication, if possible. If the solution is hypertonic, be sure to dilute with 10 to 30 mL of sterile water before instilling through a feeding tube.
   Hyperosmolar substances administered too rapidly into the gut can cause bloating, nausea, and osmotic diarrhea.
   b. If tablets must be given, verify that the medication can be crushed and given through an enteral tube.
   Some tablets (e.g., sustained-release or enteric-coated tablets) should not be crushed or capsules opened because doing so changes their action.
   c. Crush the tablet and mix it with approximately 20 mL of water, or obtain a liquid medication. If you are giving several medications, mix and administer each one separately.
   If you are using a small-bore tube, such as a percutaneous endoscopic gastrostomy (PEG) tube, Keofeed NG feeding tube, or jejunostomy tube, always obtain the liquid form of the medication because small-bore tubes clog easily. Ensure that the medication is diluted enough to pass easily through the tube. Instilling drugs one at a time allows you to identify each medication.
2. **Don nonsterile procedure gloves.**
Gloving maintains standard precautions.
3. **Place patient in a sitting (high-Fowler's) position,** if possible.
An upright position reduces the risk for aspiration and choking.
4. **For NG tubes, check tube placement** (see Chapter 27, Clinical Insights 27-5 and 27-6) by x-ray, aspirating stomach contents or measuring the pH of the aspirate, if possible.

Other, less accurate methods are injecting air into the feeding tube and auscultating, or asking the patient to speak; however, these are not confirmatory methods (Fan, Tan & Ang, 2017). **Key Point:** ***Never rely on only one bedside method for checking tube placement; use a combination of methods.***
NG tubes can become displaced or positioned in the lungs. If medications are given through a misplaced NG tube, the patient may develop aspiration pneumonia.

5. **Check for residual volume** (see Chapter 27, Procedure 27-3).
6. **Flush the tube.** Depending on the type of tube, use a piston tip or luer-lock syringe (usually a 30- to 60-mL syringe). Remove the bulb or plunger, attach the barrel to the tube, and pour in 20 to 30 mL of water.
Flushing ensures patency of the tube and also clears the tube of feeding solution that could clump with medication.
7. **Instill the medication by depressing** the syringe plunger or using the barrel of the syringe as a funnel and pouring in the medication. A smaller tube or thicker medication will require instilling the medication with a 30- to 60-mL syringe, but when larger tubes are used, the medication can be poured.

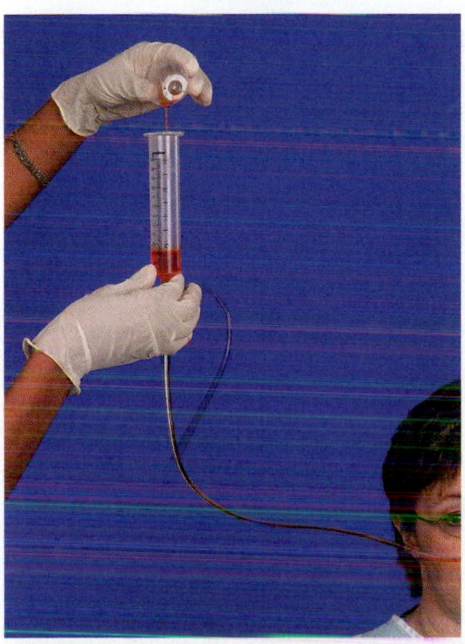

For Viscous Medication

Instill the medication by depressing the syringe plunger.

8. **Flush the medication through the tube** by instilling an additional 20 to 30 mL of water.
Flushing ensures that all the medication has been administered and prevents the tube from clogging.
9. **If there is more than one medication**, give each separately, flushing after each.
Some medications are less effective when given in combination, or there may be an additive effect if they have similar actions.
10. **Have the patient maintain a sitting position** for at least 30 minutes after you administer the medication.
An upright position minimizes the risk of aspiration. It takes at least 20 minutes for liquids to pass through the stomach.

? What if . . .

- **My patient vomits shortly after taking oral medication?**

Notify the prescriber for instructions about whether or not to repeat the dose.

- **My patient is unable to sit upright to take oral medication?**

Assist the patient into a side-lying position, and offer a straw to take water with capsules or tablets.

- **My patient has difficulty drinking from a cup?**

Use a syringe without a needle to place the medication in her mouth. Place the patient in a side-lying or upright position. Place the syringe between the gum and cheek in the back corner of the mouth, and slowly push the plunger to administer the liquid.

- **My patient is NPO?**

Check with the prescriber to determine whether the medication should be given by another route or can be given with small sips of water.

- **My patient is on fluid restriction?**

Use the smallest amount of water needed to swallow or dissolve tablets and to flush enteral tubes.

- **My patient is cognitively impaired?**

Request the patient open her mouth to see whether she has swallowed the medication; look under the tongue or side pocket near the inside of the cheek.

Check level of consciousness, mentation, or alertness. Check for potential aspiration risk by checking the patient's swallow and gag reflexes.

- **My patient is a child who is to receive medication through an enteral tube?**

Use only medications that are prepared in liquid form.
Helps prevent occlusion of the tube.

Position an infant in a prone, side-lying, sitting, or reverse Trendelenburg position for 30 minutes to 1 hour following medication administration.
These positions facilitate peristalsis and transport of medication through the intestine.

- **The prescribed medication should be given on an empty stomach?**

Stop the feeding 30 minutes before giving the drug. Resume 30 minutes later.
These periods allow for the stomach to empty and for drug absorption to occur before the feedings resume.

(continued on next page)

Procedure 26-1 ■ Administering Oral Medications (continued)

Evaluation

For medications administered orally:

- Note whether the patient has difficulty swallowing, gags, or coughs while swallowing oral medication.
- Evaluate for gastric discomfort, nausea, vomiting, or diarrhea.
- Assess for signs of drug allergy or intolerance to the medication.

For medications administered through a feeding tube:

- In addition to the preceding assessments, assess that the NG tube is correctly placed and patent before and after administering the medication.

Patient Teaching

- Refer to Medication Guidelines: Steps to Follow for All Medication (Regardless of Type or Route).
- Discuss drug safety measures with the patient, including use of child-safety caps (or using an easy-open cap for the elderly or those likely to have difficulty opening containers of this type); keeping the medication in its original container; discarding expired medications; avoiding transferring medication to another container; and carefully reading the label and directions for each medication.
- Discuss the relationship between food and the medication, if needed. For example, is the medication to be taken with food or not? Does taking medication on an empty stomach contribute to nausea or gastric irritation? Does the medication interact with any foods?

For Enteral Medications

Cover the preceding topics for patient teaching about oral medications, plus the do the following:

- Discuss the importance of upright positioning for 20 to 30 minutes after taking medication through an enteral tube.
- Instruct the patient to immediately notify his healthcare provider if he chokes or has difficulty breathing during or shortly after medication is given by enteral tube. The patient should stop the medication immediately, and emergency care might be necessary.

Home Care

Advise clients who are receiving enteral medication at home to do the following:

- Notify the healthcare provider (1) if any of the following lasts for more than a day: diarrhea, constipation, nausea, dark urine, bad-smelling urine, or dry mouth; (2) if the tube becomes clogged or seems to be moving farther out or in; or (3) if the feeding tube falls out or you cannot confirm that the end of the tube is in the stomach.
- To prevent a clogged feeding tube, flush the tube with water each time after administration of a medication or a feeding.
- Brush your teeth at least twice daily, if an NG tube remains in place continuously.
- Clean daily the area where the NG tube goes into the nostrils. Use a cotton-tip applicator moistened with warm water. If your nose is sore, apply a water-soluble lubricant.
- Change the nasal tape every other day or when it becomes loose or soiled.

Documentation

- Scheduled medications are often recorded only on the MAR.
- Document the drug, dosage, time, route, and your name as the healthcare provider administering the medication.
- Document any suspected drug reaction, intolerance, or patient response to the medication.
- For patients whose intake and output are being measured, document the amount of liquid medication and the water intake. Some patients may be on fluid restrictions, so record *all* intake. Follow your clinical facility protocol.

For Enteral Medications

Document the following:

- Patency, residual volume, and verification of placement.
- Any difficulty with administering the medications through the feeding tube.
- On the intake and output record, record the amount of liquid medication and the water used for flushing. Some providers prescribe a specific amount of water to flush with each medication administration or feeding. Some healthcare facilities use a protocol amount of water to flush gastrostomy tubes. Follow the protocol in your clinical facility.

Sample documentation for a prn oral medication

12/23/2021 1800 Placed client in Fowler's position. Administered Lasix 20 mg. PO tablet with 30 mL water. Patient tolerated medication with no swallowing difficulties. —————— S. Smith, RN

Sample documentation for an enteral medication

12/13/2021 1400 Placed client in Fowler's position. GT placement confirmed with pH of 4.5 gastric aspirate. Administered 10 mL of liquid medication and flushed with 20 mL of water. Tolerated medication with no complaints. —————— S. Smith, RN

Practice Resources

Fan, E., Tan, S., & Ang, S. (2017); Grissinger, M. (2013); Guenter, P., & Boullata, J. (2013); Morris, H. (2012).

Thinking About the Procedure

The videos **Administering Oral Medications: Tablet or Capsule, Administering Oral Medications: Sublingual, Administering Oral Medications: Buccal, Administering Oral Medications: Liquid Medications,** and **Administering Medication Through an Enteral Tube,** along with questions and suggested responses, are available on the ***Davis's Nursing Skills Videos*** Web site on FADavis.com.

Procedure 26-2 ■ Administering Ophthalmic Medication

➤ For steps to follow in *all* procedures, refer to the Universal Steps for All Procedures found on the inside back cover. Also, refer to the Medication Guidelines: Steps to Follow for All Medications (Regardless of Type or Route).

Equipment

- Eye drops or ointment
- Tissue

For irrigation, add:

- Prescribed eye irrigation solution (e.g., 500 to 1,000 mL of normal saline (NS) or lactated Ringer's solution are commonly used)
- IV tubing or eye irrigation insert, such as the Morgan lens (Follow manufacturer's directions for this specialized equipment.)
- Ocular anesthetic, according to protocol or provider's prescriptions
- pH paper
- Basin and towel

Delegation

An RN can usually delegate eye instillations to an LPN/LVN. You usually cannot delegate this task to a UAP, unless the UAP has special training for a specific, defined situation (e.g., "medication aides" in some long-term-care settings). See **Delegation,** in **Medication Guidelines: Steps to Follow for All Medication (Regardless of Type or Route).**

Pre-Procedure Assessments

- Assess the patient's eyes for redness, discharge, or other signs of irritation.
- Determine whether the eyes need to be cleansed before administration of the medication.
  Excess tearing, debris, or excess mucus in the eye could interfere with the absorption, and thus effectiveness, of the medication.

Check the prescription for where to instill medication.

*(NOTE: **We do not advise using these abbreviations**—they have been disallowed by The Joint Commission—but you may still see them written in prescriptions). Clarify with the provider the correct site.*

OD = right eye
OS = left eye
OU = both eyes

For irrigations, also assess the following:

- Determine the cause of the eye problem—acid, alkaline, or other chemical burn or body fluid splash; or non-embedded foreign body.
  Irrigations are generally used to remove chemical or physical irritants, but they may be done following surgery or to treat a severe infection. Normal saline (NS) or lactated Ringer's solution is the solution generally recommended for high-volume eye irrigations because the pH of 6 to 7.5 is closest to the normal tear pH of 7.1. Volumes of 500 to 1,000 mL are generally used.
- Assess the patient's eyes for swelling, redness, drainage, or complaints of pain.
  A baseline assessment is useful for determining the need for and effectiveness of irrigation. Sclera should be smooth, white, and glistening.
- Determine the patient's ability to cooperate with the procedure.
  Combative or otherwise uncooperative patients refusing instillation of medication can interfere with the efficiency of the procedure. If the patient cannot hold still for the procedure, he may need to be sedated.
- Assess the pain level.
  Debris, chemicals, and some liquids in the eye can be extremely painful. The eye may need to be anesthetized before irrigation or a general systemic pain medication given.

➤ When performing the procedure, always identify your patient according to agency policy, using two identifiers, and be attentive to standard precautions, hand hygiene, patient safety and privacy, body mechanics, and documentation.

Procedure Steps

1. **Assist the patient to a** high-Fowler's position with head slightly tilted back, if possible.

   Do not tilt the head back if the patient has a neck injury or other contraindication. The medication can be given with the patient supine.

   An upright position keeps eye drops in the eye and helps prevent eye drops from draining into lacrimal duct.

2. **Don procedure gloves.**
   Gloving complies with standard precautions.

3. **Cleanse the edges of the eyelid** from the inner canthus to the outer canthus, if needed.
   By following the principle of "clean to dirty," you avoid transferring debris into the nasolacrimal duct.

Procedure Variation: Instilling Eye Drops

(Follow Steps 1–3. Note, however, that some sources recommend that the patient lie supine for eye drops.)

4. **Gently rest your dominant hand** (the one with the eyedropper) on the patient's forehead.
   Stabilizes the hand in the event the patient moves—prevents accidental injury to the eye.

5. **With your nondominant hand,** pull the lower lid down to expose the conjunctival sac.
   Allows visualization of the area where you will administer the medication.

6. **Position the eyedropper** about 1.5 to 2.0 cm (½ to ¾ inch) above the patient's eye. Ask the patient to look up, and drop the prescribed number of drops into the conjunctival sac. Do not let the dropper touch the eye.

(continued on next page)

Procedure 26-2 ■ Administering Ophthalmic Medication (continued)

Keeping the dropper away from the globe of the eye reduces the risk of accidental injury to the eye and avoids contamination of the dropper. Having the patient look up helps to decrease the blink reflex.

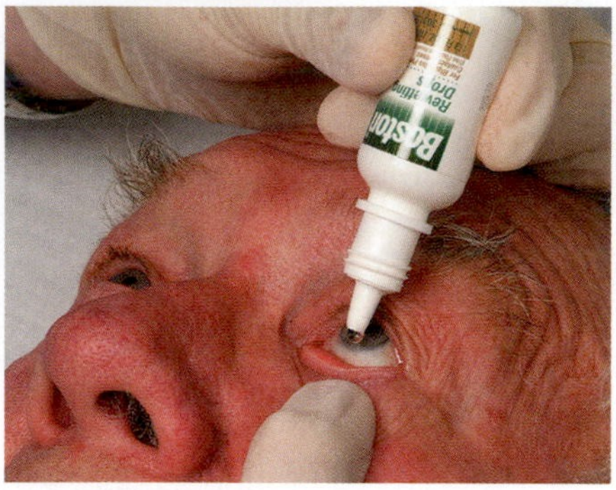

7. **Ask the patient to gently close his eyes.**
   Closing the eyes helps to distribute the medication.

8. **If the medication has systemic effects,** press gently against the same side of the nose for 1 to 2 minutes to close the lacrimal ducts.
   Reduces systemic absorption through the lacrimal duct.

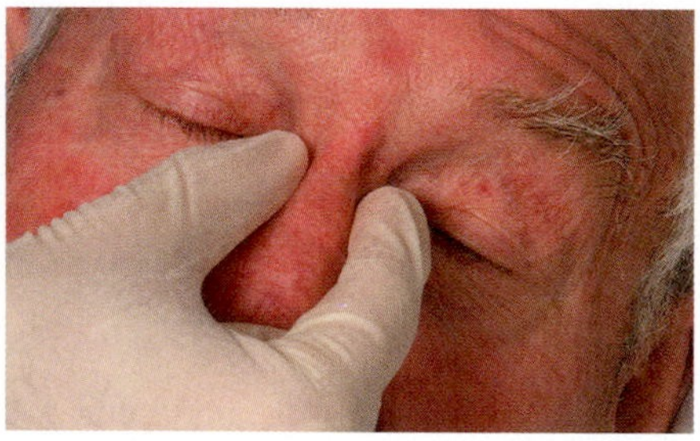

Procedure Variation B: Administering Eye Ointment

(Follow steps 1 to 3, then move to step 9.)

9. **Gently rest your dominant hand,** the one with the eye ointment, on the patient's forehead.
   Stabilizing your hand helps to prevent accidental injury to the eye.

10. **With your nondominant hand,** pull the lower lid down to expose the conjunctival sac.
    Allows visualization of area where you will administer the medication.

11. **Ask the patient to look up** as you apply a thin strip of ointment—usually about 2 to 2.5 cm (1 inch)—in the conjunctival sac; twist your wrist to break off the strip of ointment. Do not let the tube touch the eye.
    If the medication ribbon is not broken off, lifting the tube will pull the medication out of the conjunctival sac.

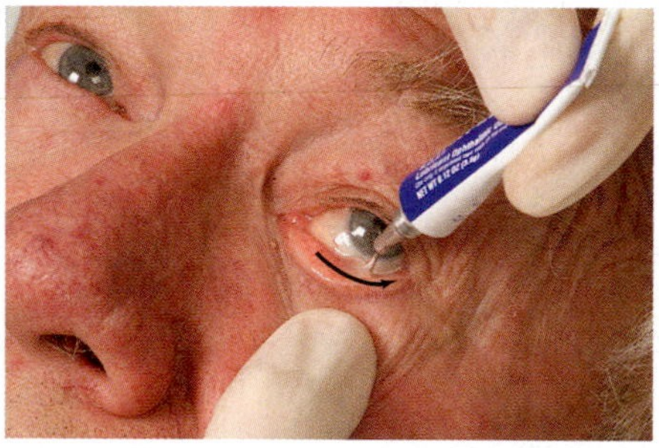

a. Ask the patient to gently close his eyes for 2 to 3 minutes. Alternatively, release the eyelids, and have the client blink several times.
   Helps to distribute the medication.

b. Explain to the patient that his vision will be blurred for a short amount of time after administration of the ointment.
   The viscosity of the ointment can cause blurring.

? What if . . .

- **My patient is a child who will not open the eye for the application?**

  Try distracting the child by turning on the television or offering an age-appropriate toy in view.
  Distraction and bribery are effective techniques for coaxing a child when cooperation is essential.

  Ask a family member to help you gain cooperation of the child.
  It might be fear or mistrust that is causing the child to be unwilling to open his eyes.

- **My patient wears soft contact lenses?**

  Have the patient remove contact lenses before administering the medication and wait at least 15 minutes after instilling eye drops before reinserting the lenses.

Procedure 26-2A ■ Irrigating the Eyes

➤ When performing the procedure, always identify your patient according to agency policy, using two identifiers, and be attentive to standard precautions, hand hygiene, patient safety and privacy, body mechanics, and documentation.

Procedure Steps

1. **Assist the patient to a low-Fowler's position,** with the head tilted toward the affected eye, if possible.
   This position helps to drain the irrigating solution from the eye and prevents contamination of the unaffected eye.

2. **Place the towel and basin** under the patient's cheek to absorb the drainage.
   The patient will be more comfortable when he is clean and dry.

3. **Check the pH** by gently touching the pH paper to secretions in the conjunctival sac.
   A litmus test determines the correct irrigating solution and whether the irritant is alkaline or acidic. The normal pH of tears is approximately 7.1.

4. **Follow agency protocol** or the prescriber's prescription for the use of ocular anesthetic drops.
   The ocular anesthetic will be washed out by the irrigation fluid, so it needs to be reinstilled every 2 to 3 minutes, or it can be added to the irrigation solution.

5. **Connect the solution and tubing,** and prime the tubing.
   Priming the tubing prevents blowing air across the cornea, which would be uncomfortable.

6. **Irrigate the eye.**
   a. Hold the tubing about 2.5 cm (1 inch) from eye.
   A safe distance helps prevent accidental trauma to the eye.
   b. Separate the eyelids with your thumb and index finger.
   It is easier to irrigate the cornea when the eyelids are separated.
   c. Direct the flow of solution over the eye from the inner canthus to the outer canthus.
   The inner canthus is considered clean, primarily because of the open duct in this area. Flowing irrigation solution in this manner follows the principle of "clean to dirty."

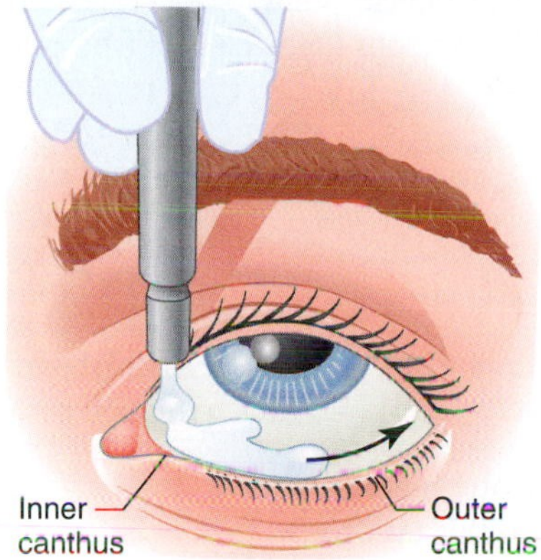

7. **Recheck pH, and continue** to irrigate the eye, as needed.
With alkaline or acidic chemical injuries, the pH of the eye needs to be returned to normal as soon as possible to prevent further eye injury.

Evaluation

- Examine the eyes for redness or drainage.
- Observe the patient's ability to follow instructions during the procedure.
- Observe the pain level during the procedure.
- After an irrigation, check for decrease in eye pain.

Patient Teaching

- Discuss how to prevent contaminating eye drops or ointment.
- Teach the best technique for instilling eye drops or ointment.
- Discuss the use of an eye drop guide, if the patient needs assistance with instilling drops.
- Discuss the signs and symptoms to report to the provider, including eye pain and increased redness or drainage.

For irrigations:

- Discuss the cause and prevention of eye injuries, including use of protective goggles.
- Discuss the need for follow-up treatment. If the patient will be instilling eye medications or applying eye patches, ensure that he demonstrates the correct technique.

Home Care

If a splash occurs to the eyes in the home, teach the client to immediately flood his eyes with cool water (as follows):

- Hold your eyelids open and put your head under a faucet or pour water from a clean container.
- Roll your eyes as much as possible while running water across your eyes.
- Flood your eyes for at least 20 minutes.
- Get medical help immediately after rinsing your eyes.

Documentation

- *For instillations:* Document assessment data before, during, and after instillation. Document the instillation on the MAR, as for all medications.
- *For irrigations:* Document the condition of the patient's eyes before the irrigation, including complaints of pain or burning. Document the eye pH, instillation of anesthetic drops, the type and amount of irrigation fluid used, the eye pH following irrigation, and the patient's response. Also document other treatment (e.g., instillation of lubricating and/or antibiotic ointment; application of eye patches).

Sample documentation

04/16/2021 1200. In preparation for discharge and after teaching, patient correctly self-administered garamycin eye drops 1 gtt in right eye as prescribed. Patient closed her eyes and gently pressed against the right side of the nose for 1 minute after instillation. Stated, "I will not have a problem doing this at home. Thank you for teaching me the right way." No redness, discharge, or complaints of pain. ——— S. Smith, RN

Practice Resources

Centers for Disease Control and Prevention (CDC) (2011); Glaucoma Research Foundation (n.d., reviewed 2017); Mason, I., & Stevens, S. (2010); Terrie, Y. (2012).

Thinking About the Procedure

The video **Administering Ophthalmic Medication**, along with questions and suggested responses, is available on the ***Davis's Nursing Skills Videos*** Web site on FADavis.com.

Procedure 26-3 ■ Administering Otic Medication

➤ For steps to follow in *all* procedures, refer to the Universal Steps for All Procedures found on the inside back cover. Also, refer to the Medication Guidelines: Steps to Follow for All Medications (Regardless of Type or Route).

Equipment

- Ear drops
- Dropper with flexible rubber tip
- Cotton-tipped applicators
- Cotton ball

Delegation

The RN can usually delegate administration of otic medications to an LPN/LVN. You usually cannot delegate this task to a UAP, unless allowed by the state's nurse practice act.

Pre-Procedure Assessments

- Assess the external ear and canal for erythema, drainage, and cerumen.
  You may need to clean the external ear to remove obstructions so that the medication can be distributed throughout the ear canal. Use the otoscope to evaluate the tympanic membrane if the drainage is bloody or the patient complains of pain or decreased hearing acuity. Use sterile technique if the tympanic membrane is ruptured.
- Assess for ear pain or hearing impairment.
  Establishes a baseline that can be used to evaluate the effects of treatment.

➤ When performing the procedure, always identify your patient according to agency policy, using two identifiers, and be attentive to standard precautions, hand hygiene, patient safety and privacy, body mechanics, and documentation.

Procedure Steps

1. **Hold the ear drop bottle** in your hand to warm it, or place it in warm water (not hot). Gently shake the bottle before using the drops.
   Warm solution is more comfortable than cool. Also, placing cool solutions in the ear can cause dizziness. Gently shaking the bottle disperses the medication throughout the solution.
2. **Assist patient to a side-lying** position (or turn her head to the side, if she cannot assume this position), with the appropriate ear facing up.
   Facilitates administering the drops and prevents drops escaping from the ear.
3. **Clean the external ear** with a cotton-tipped applicator, if necessary.
   Cleaning the ear allows ear drops to reach all areas of the ear canal without trauma. Be careful not to push cerumen further into the ear canal.
4. **Fill the dropper** with the correct amount of medication.
5. **For infants and young children,** ask a parent or another caregiver to immobilize the child while you administer the medication.
   Mobilization and restraint reduce the risk for injury in a child who is struggling during the procedure.
6. **Straighten the ear canal.**
   a. In a child younger than 3 years old, pull the pinna down and back. ▼

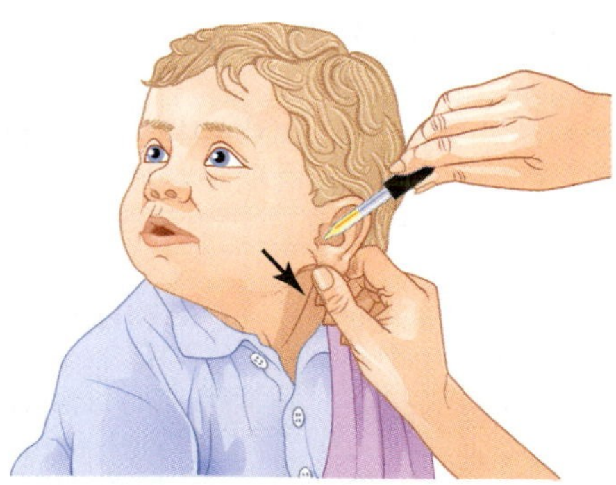

   b. In children 3 years and older and adults, pull the pinna up and back.
   These positions straighten the ear canal for proper channeling of the medication.

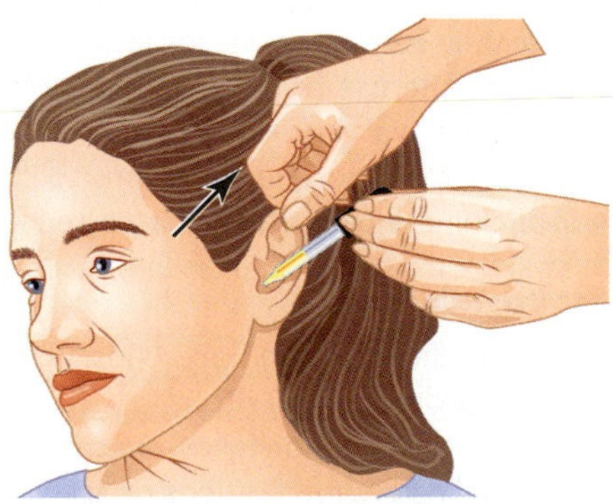

7. **Instill the prescribed number** of drops along the side of the ear canal, being careful not to touch the end of the dropper to any part of the ear.
   Avoiding contact between the dropper and the ear reduces the risk of contamination of the dropper.
8. **Gently tug on the external ear** after drops are instilled.
   Facilitates flow of medication into the auditory canal.
9. **Instruct the patient** to keep her head turned to the side for 5 to 10 minutes.

Assists in distributing the medication and prevents drops from escaping the ear canal.

10. Place a cotton ball, or a piece of it, loosely at the opening of the auditory canal for 15 minutes.
A cotton ball will absorb excess fluid and keep the medication from flowing out.

Keep in mind that cotton left near an infant can be a choking hazard and must be carefully supervised.

? What if . . .

- **My patient is a child and rolls over so most of the otic medication flows back out of the ear?**

Estimate the amount of the dosage that was lost. Replace it by repeating the procedure for instillation of the medication; however, the next time, position the child securely until you are confident that the medication has had time to penetrate the ear canal.

- **There is too much cerumen (ear wax) in the canal to instill otic drops?**

You can use special drops that soften the cerumen and allow for easier removal. Gentle irrigation with warm saline is effective, unless the patient has perforation of the tympanic membrane or myringotomy tubes.

You should not use a metal syringe (Pomeroy syringe) for the removal of cerumen because (1) this type of syringe is heavy and difficult to control and (2) because of the pressure exerted, it may be associated with a higher risk of perforations of the tympanic membrane.

Oral jet irrigators have been associated with some trauma, including tympanic membrane perforation.

You should not attempt to remove impaction by "ear candling," which is the application of hot candle wax.

Evaluation

- Assess for discomfort or pain during the procedure and for relief afterward.
- Evaluate for wax buildup, redness, swelling, or drainage.

Documentation

- Assess the amount, color, character, and odor of drainage, if present.
- Note any swelling or redness in the ear canal.
- Document pain or discomfort and hearing loss.

Thinking About the Procedure

The video **Administering Otic Medication,** along with questions and suggested responses, is available on the ***Davis's Nursing Skills Videos*** Web Site on FADavis.com.

Procedure 26-4 ■ Administering Nasal Medication

➤ For steps to follow in *all* procedures, refer to the Universal Steps for All Procedures found on the inside back cover. Also, refer to the Medication Guidelines: Steps to Follow for All Medications (Regardless of Type or Route).

Equipment

- Medication drops, spray, or aerosol
- Tissues

Delegation

As an RN, you can usually delegate administration of nasal instillations to an LPN/LVN. You usually cannot delegate this task to a UAP.

Pre-Procedure Assessments

- Check for nasal obstruction and congestion.
  Nasal obstruction or congestion can prevent the medication from reaching the nasal mucosa.
- Assess nasal discharge for color, consistency, and odor.
  The appearance of drainage is not always diagnostic of infection, especially for people with chronic sinus problems or polyps. Color can be indicative of the body's response to viral, bacterial, and allergic sources.
- Assess nasal mucous membranes for redness, color, moisture, excoriation, or trauma.
- Check the dropper tip to be sure it is not cracked or chipped.
  A cracked or chipped tip might interfere with drawing up the medication and scratch the nasal mucosa.

(continued on next page)

Procedure 26-4 ■ Administering Nasal Medication (continued)

➤ When performing the procedure, always identify your patient according to agency policy, using two identifiers, and be attentive to standard precautions, hand hygiene, patient safety and privacy, body mechanics, and documentation.

Procedure Steps

1. **Explain to the patient** that the medication may cause some burning, tingling, or unusual taste.
   The taste of nasal medications can cause nausea or vomiting. The medication is more likely to cause burning or tingling if the nasal mucosa is inflamed.

2. **Ask the patient to gently blow** her nose and perform hand hygiene afterward.
   Removing nasal discharge allows the medication to come into contact with the mucous membranes without traumatizing already inflamed mucosa.

3. **Don procedure gloves.**
   Prevents transmission of microorganisms.

4. **Position the patient.**

When Medicating the Frontal Sinuses With Spray

"Head down and forward." Remember: "To spray your nose, look at your toes!" If the patient can comfortably assume this position, ask her to lean forward or kneel on the bed with her head down. Administer the medication, and then ask her to tilt her head back to medicate the nasal passages.
Radionuclide studies have demonstrated that using nasal drops or sprays with the patient sitting and leaning the head back causes poor distribution of the medications into the nasal complex and sinuses. ▼

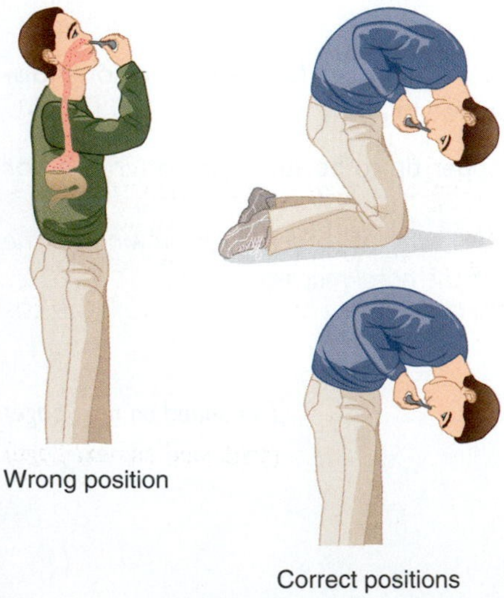

When Medicating the Ethmoid and Sphenoid Sinuses

Assist the patient into a supine position, tilt her head back over the edge of the bed. Support the patient's head. Alternatively, place a towel roll behind her shoulders, and allow the head to drop back.
These positions help to prevent straining of the neck muscles and facilitate distribution of the medication to the ethmoid and sphenoid sinuses. ▼

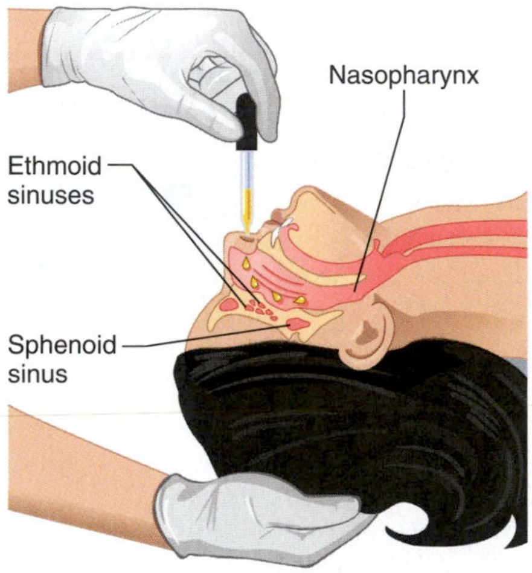

When Medicating the Frontal and Maxillary Sinuses With Drops

With patient supine, tilt the head back over the edge of the bed, or place a pillow under the head, and turn the head toward the affected side.
Titling the head promotes gravity to distribute the medication to the frontal sinuses. ▼

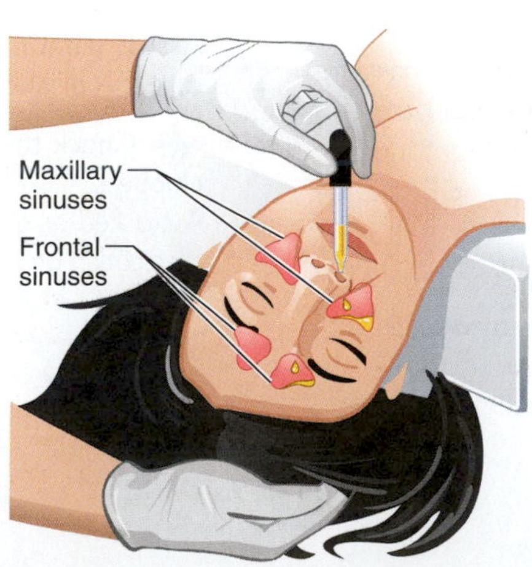

5. **Ask the patient to exhale** and then close one nostril.
   Blocking one nostril provides for deeper inhalation.

6. **Then, ask the patient to breathe in** deeply through the nose and while she is breathing in, press down firmly and quickly once on the applicator. Ask the patient to breathe out through the mouth. After spraying, lean the head backward for a few seconds. If a dropper is used, do not touch the sides of the nostril.
   Inhaling through the mouth prevents aspiration of the drops into the trachea and bronchi. Touching the dropper to the nostril will contaminate the dropper.

7. **Repeat for the other nostril.**

8. **If nose drops are used**, ask the patient to stay in the same position for 1 to 5 minutes (depending on the manufacturer's guidelines).
   Maintaining this position promotes better absorption by using gravity to disperse the medication throughout the nasal passages and sinuses instead of draining out the nose.

9. **Instruct the patient not to blow** her nose for several minutes.
   To prevent expelling the medication.

? What if . . .

- **My patient cannot assume the "head down and forward" position?**
  Help him to hold his head upright to administer the drops or spray.
- **My patient can taste the medicine after it is administered?**
  This means his head was not down enough or he did not inhale long enough. Instruct him to put his head back down and sniff again without the medicine.

- **My patient has an excoriated area on the inside septum?**

  Assess further, examining other areas of the nasal mucosa. Determine if the patient has a history of substance abuse or frequent nasal inhalations. Report the findings to the prescriber before administering nasal medication.

- **My patient begins to have nosebleeds after administration of the nasal medication?**

  First, control the nosebleed. Then, withhold the medication, and notify the prescriber. Assess for other signs of bleeding, bruising, or other petechiae.

Evaluation

Assess for a reduction of symptoms 15 to 20 minutes after administration.

Patient Teaching

- Teach the procedure for administering nasal drops or sprays, including proper positioning.
- Discuss the correct use of the medication and the adverse effects of overusing nasal decongestants.
- Explain the implications of the color of nasal secretions.

Documentation

Document according to Medication Guidelines: Steps to Follow for All Medication (Regardless of Type or Route). For example, document the administration of the medication on the MAR.

For nasal instillation, document:

- Premedication assessment
- Type and amount of solution administered
- Discomfort the patient experienced during the procedure
- Patient's report of response to nasal administrations, such as nasal discharge, obstruction of nasal passage, bleeding, or other complication following the procedure

Sample documentation

03/18/2021 1340 Client complained of nasal stuffiness. Administered mometasone furoate (Nasonex) 2 sprays per nostril, as ordered. Client noted nasal tingling following administration of this medication. Client left resting in recliner chair. ———————— H. Peratta, RN.

Practice Resources

Mundlia, J., Kumar, M., & Amardeep, A. (2015).

Thinking About the Procedure

The video **Administering Nasal Medication**, along with questions and suggested responses, is available on the ***Davis's Nursing Skills Videos*** Web site on FADavis.com.

Procedure 26-5 ■ Administering Vaginal Medication

➤ For steps to follow in *all* procedures, refer to the Universal Steps for All Procedures found on the inside back cover. Also, refer to the Medication Guidelines: Steps to Follow for All Medications (Regardless of Type or Route).

Equipment

- Medication: foam, jelly, cream, suppository, douche, or irrigating solution
- Applicator (if indicated)
- Perineal wash solution or wipes for perineal care, as needed
- Water-soluble lubricant
- Toilet tissue
- Perineal pad
- Bath blanket
- **For irrigation:** you will also need a waterproof pad, bedpan, vaginal irrigation set (consists of a solution container, nozzle, tubing, and clamp; may be disposable) and IV pole.

Delegation

An RN can usually delegate the administration of vaginal medications to an LPN/LVN. Delegation of this task to a UAP will vary, depending on the state's nurse practice acts and the healthcare facility policies. However, the RN is always responsible for evaluating patient responses, both therapeutic effects and side effects. You can instruct the UAP on the expected therapeutic effects and the side effects to be reported.

Pre-Procedure Assessments

- Assess for vaginal burning, pruritus, and pain.
  A baseline assessment helps to determine the patient's level of comfort and later the effectiveness of treatment. Infections can cause vaginal burning, itching, and pain.
- Inspect the labia and vaginal orifice for redness and lesions.
  This is a good time to assess the perineal area for signs of sexually transmitted infection or other findings requiring healthcare.
- Check for vaginal discharge, including color, amount, consistency, and odor.

(continued on next page)

Procedure 26-5 ■ Administering Vaginal Medication (continued)

➤ When performing the procedure, always identify your patient according to agency policy, using two identifiers, and be attentive to standard precautions, hand hygiene, patient safety and privacy, body mechanics, and documentation.

Procedure Steps

1. **Ask the patient to void** before you insert the vaginal medication.
   A full bladder could cause discomfort during the instillation of vaginal medications.

2. **Position the patient** in a dorsal recumbent or Sims' position; drape the patient with a bath blanket so that only the perineum is exposed.
   a. ***Dorsal recumbent position:*** Supine with knees flexed and legs rotated outward.
   b. ***Sims' position:*** Semiprone on the left side with the right hip and knee flexed.
   These two positions allow for visualization during administration and promote retention of the medication following administration. Draping respects the patient's modesty.

3. **Prepare the medication.**
   - *Suppository*: Remove the wrapper, and place the suppository on the wrapper or in a medication cup.
   - *Applicator*: Fill the applicator according to the manufacturer's instructions.
   - *For irrigation*: Use a warm solution of approximately 105°F (40.5°C).

   Some suppositories come with applicators. Using a warm irrigation solution promotes patient comfort and prevents injury to the vaginal tissue.

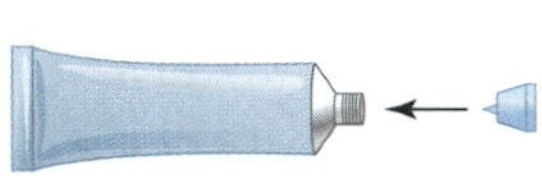

Invert cap and pierce end of medication tube

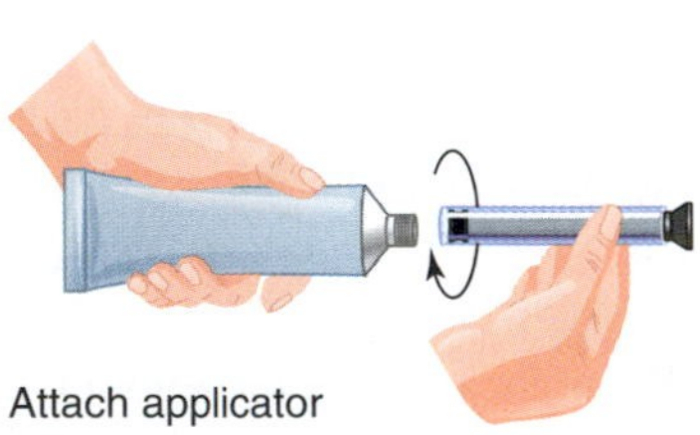

Attach applicator

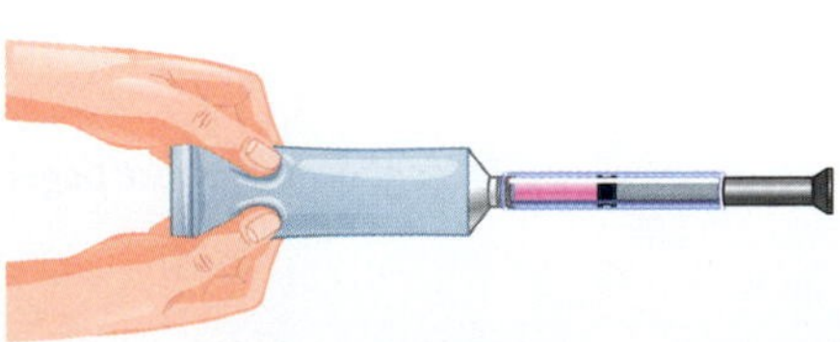

Squeeze medication into applicator

4. **Don procedure gloves.**
   Prevents contaminating your hands and spreading microorganisms.

5. **Inspect and clean around vaginal orifice.**
   Prevents the introduction of microorganisms into the vagina during medication administration.

6. **Administer the medication.**

For a Suppository

a. Apply water-soluble lubricant to the rounded end of the suppository and to your gloved index finger on your dominant hand.
   Eases insertion and prevents injury to the vaginal tissue.

b. Separate the labia with your nondominant hand.
   Allows visualization of the vaginal orifice.

c. Insert the suppository as far as possible along the posterior vaginal wall (about 8 cm [3 in.]) or as far as it will go. If using an applicator, insert the applicator into the vagina, and press the plunger.
   The posterior vaginal wall is about 2.5 cm (1 inch) longer than the anterior wall.

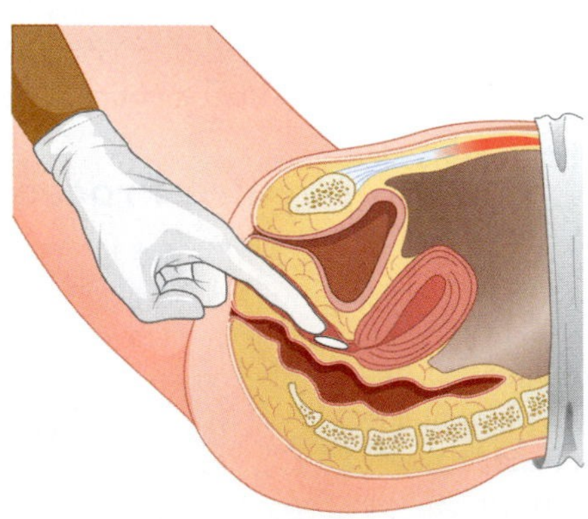

d. Ask the patient to remain in a supine position for 5 to 15 minutes. You may wish to elevate her hips on a pillow.
   Lifting the hips promotes retention and absorption of the medication.

For Applicator Insertion of Cream, Foam, or Jelly

e. Separate the labia with your nondominant hand.
f. Insert the applicator approximately 8 cm (3 in.) into the vagina along the posterior vaginal wall.
g. Depress the plunger on the applicator, inserting the medication into the vagina.
h. Dispose of the applicator, or place it on a paper towel if the applicator is reusable. You will later wash it in the appropriate solution.
i. Instruct the patient to remain in a supine position for 5 to 15 minutes.
   A flat position promotes retention and absorption of the medication.

For Irrigations

j. Hang the irrigation solution approximately 30 to 60 cm (1 to 2 ft) above the level of the patient's vagina.
   Uses gravity to create enough pressure for continuous irrigation without increasing the pressure so much that it causes the patient discomfort and possibly damages the vaginal tissue.

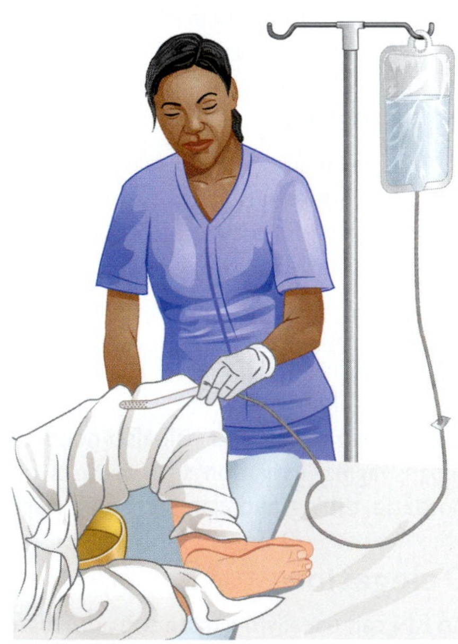

k. Assist the patient into a dorsal recumbent position, and position a waterproof pad and bedpan under the patient.
   Positioning the patient on the bedpan and using a waterproof pad protects the bedding.

l. If using a vaginal irrigation set with tubing, open the clamp to allow the solution to completely fill the tubing.
Flushing the tubing prevents introducing air into the vagina, which can cause discomfort.

m. Lubricate the end of the irrigation nozzle.
Lubrication reduces discomfort and irritation to the vaginal mucosa.

n. Insert the nozzle approximately 8 cm (3 in.) into the vagina, directing it toward the sacrum.

o. Start the flow of the irrigation solution, and rotate the nozzle intermittently as solution flows.
The rotation ensures even distribution of the solution throughout the vagina.

p. After all irrigating solution has been used, remove the nozzle.

q. Assist the patient to a sitting position on the bedpan.
Promotes removal of all the irrigating solution by gravity.

7. **Remove the bedpan and clean** the perineum with perineal wash solution and a washcloth or wipes. Dry the perineum.
Drainage could cause skin irritation.

8. **Apply a perineal pad** if necessary for excessive drainage.

? What if . . .

- **The labia are reddened?**

  Pour warm water (bottled or specially filtered tap water) over the labia with an irrigation bottle to soothe irritation and cleanse the area.

Evaluation

- Assess for complaints of vaginal burning, pruritus, or pain.
- Assess for purulent vaginal discharge.

Patient Teaching

- Discuss with the patient personal hygiene and pericare.
- Teach women that douching may be harmful because it disturbs the normal pH and healthy balance of microorganisms in the vagina. Research has revealed a relationship between douching and ovarian cancer (Gonzalez, O'Brien, Aloisio, et al., 2016).

Documentation

- **For vaginal medications**, chart according to Medication Guidelines: Steps to Follow for All Medication (Regardless of Type or Route).
- **For vaginal irrigations**, document your assessment; the type and amount of solution administered; discomfort the patient experienced during the procedure; and the patient's report of decreased vaginal pain, itching, and/or burning after the procedure.

Sample documentation

01/14/2021 1500 Explained medication and procedure. Client placed in dorsal recumbent position with knees flexed at 90° angle. Vaginal suppository lubricated with water-soluble lubricant and inserted using two fingers. Instructed client to retain suppository as long as possible. Tolerated procedure well with no voiced complaints of pain or discomfort.——————— S. Snider, RN

Practice Resources

Gonzalez, O'Brien, Aloisio, et al. (2016).

Procedure 26-6 ■ Inserting a Rectal Suppository

➤ For steps to follow in *all* procedures, refer to the Universal Steps for All Procedures found on the inside back cover. Also, refer to the Medication Guidelines: Steps to Follow for All Medications (Regardless of Type or Route).

Equipment

- Suppository
- Water-soluble lubricant
- Toilet tissue

Delegation

An RN can usually delegate administration of rectal medications to an LPN/LVN. Although in some institutions you can delegate the administration of a glycerin suppository (nonmedicated) to a UAP, you generally cannot delegate administration of rectal medications to a UAP.

Pre-Procedure Assessments

- Determine the presence of contraindications for rectal administration, such as recent rectal surgery, rectal bleeding, or cardiac disease.
- Assess the rectal area for hemorrhoids or irritation.

(continued on next page)

Procedure 26-6 ■ Inserting a Rectal Suppository (continued)

➤ When performing the procedure, always identify your patient according to agency policy, using two identifiers, and be attentive to standard precautions, hand hygiene, patient safety and privacy, body mechanics, and documentation.

Procedure Steps

1. **Ask whether the patient needs** to defecate before insertion of the suppository.
   Stool in the rectum interferes with insertion of medication against the rectal wall and therefore with retention of the medication.

2. **Assist patient to Sims' position**—lying on the left side with the right hip and knee flexed. Drape the patient, keeping her covered as much as possible.
   Sims' position allows visualization of the anus and promotes retention of the medication because the descending colon is on the left side. It also helps relax the external anal sphincter. Keeping the patient covered prevents chilling and maintains privacy.

3. **Don procedure gloves.**
   Gloving prevents exposure to feces and spread of microorganisms; maintains standard precautions.

4. **For an uncooperative patient,** such as a confused patient or a young child, ask someone to help immobilize the patient while you insert the suppository.
   Help holding the patient allows proper instillation of medication and prevents injury to the rectal mucosa.

5. **Prepare the suppository**: Remove the wrapper. Using a water-soluble lubricant, lubricate the smooth end of the suppository and the tip of glove on the index finger. If no lubricant is available, apply cool tap water to the rectal opening.
   Lubrication eases insertion and prevents friction damage to the rectal mucosa during insertion.

6. **Explain that there will be a cool feeling** from the lubricant and a feeling of pressure during insertion.
   The patient should not experience severe pain with the insertion of a suppository but will feel the coolness of the lubricant and pressure as the suppository is inserted past the rectal sphincter.

7. **Using your nondominant hand,** separate the buttocks.
   Separation of the buttocks allows you to visualize the anus.

8. **Ask the adult patient to take deep** breaths in and out through the mouth.
   Deep breathing helps relax the rectal sphincter. Pushing a suppository through a constricted sphincter produces discomfort.

9. **Insert the suppository**:
   a. Using the index finger of your dominant hand, gently insert the lubricated smooth end first, or follow the manufacturer's instructions.
   Lubrication eases insertion.

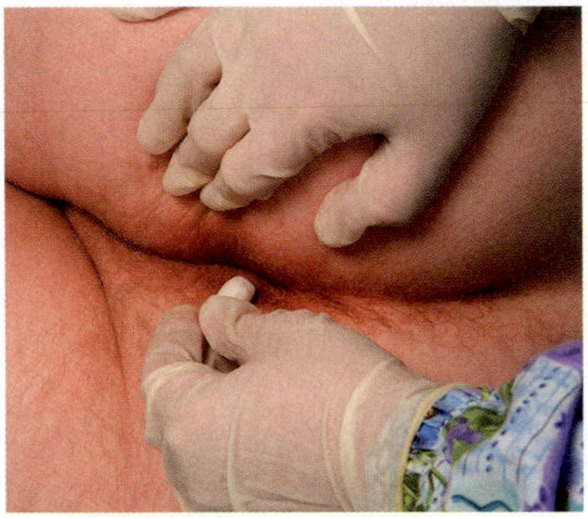

   b. Never force the suppository during insertion.
   Forcing the insertion of the suppository into a fecal mass would affect absorption. Forcing anything into the rectum may cause rectal irritation.

   c. Push the suppository past the internal sphincter and along the rectal wall (½ to 1 in. in infants and 1 to 3 in. in adults).
   The suppository must be in contact with the rectal wall for the medication to be absorbed. Inserting the suppository past the internal sphincter promotes retention. For a child, inserting the suppository too far could damage the rectal mucosa.

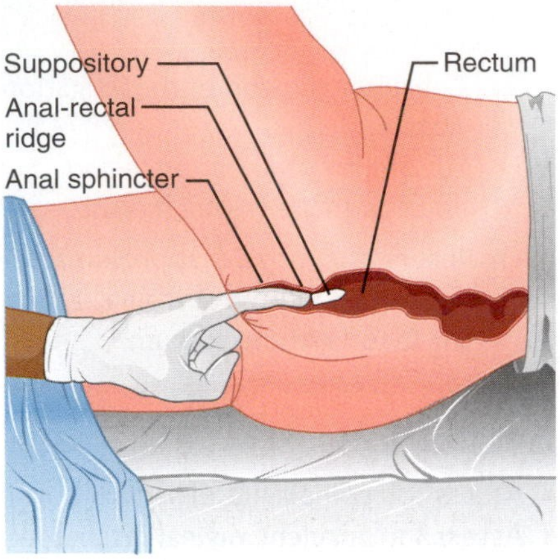

10. **Ask the patient to try to retain** the suppository if he is able. If he has difficulty retaining the suppository, hold his buttocks together for a short time.

11. **Wipe the patient's anus** with toilet tissue.
    Wiping maintains hygiene and comfort.

12. **Explain to the patient need** to remain in a side-lying position for at least 10 minutes, if possible.
    Sims' position promotes retention and absorption of the medication. Explanation promotes compliance.

13. **Discard used materials** into a biohazard receptacle, and wash hands thoroughly.

14. **Leave the call device within** reach and a bedpan handy, if the suppository was a laxative. Instruct the patient to call for assistance to get out of bed.
    In case the patient has a sudden urge to defecate or cannot retain the suppository for the recommended time, he can call for help. Providing assistance promotes safety.

? What if . . .

- **The prescribed dose is only half of the suppository?**
  Cut the suppository lengthwise with a clean, single-edge razor blade.

■ **My patient is a child. What is the best way to give a rectal suppository so the child does not expel it?**

For pediatric patients, it may be necessary to gently hold the buttocks together for 5 to 10 minutes.

■ **My patient is an older adult? Is there anything special I should know?**

Older adults may have difficulty retaining a suppository because of poor sphincter control. You may need to put the bedpan under the patient while you are inserting the suppository.

Evaluation

- Assess for pain or burning during and after insertion of the medication.
- Determine that the patient retained the suppository for the desired length of time after insertion (reinsertion may be required).

Patient Teaching

Explain that suppositories may take up to 30 minutes to be absorbed, depending on the medication.

Documentation

- Refer to Medication Guidelines: Steps to Follow for All Medication (Regardless of Type or Route).
- Document the condition of anal tissue if abnormalities are present, any complaints of discomfort that are outside of the expected feelings and experience, and the length of time that the suppository was retained.
- Document responses to medication (e.g., symptom relief, side effects).

Sample documentation

03/08/2021 1815 Patient temperature 103.2°F and complains of nausea. Tylenol grain X suppository given per rectum with patient in Sims' position. Instructed patient to remain in this position for 15 minutes. Voiced understanding. No rectal abnormalities observed. Tolerated procedure well with no complaints of pain or discomfort.——— J. Kinsley, RN

Practice Resources

Bartley, N. (2012b); Lowry, M. (2016).

Thinking About the Procedure

The video **Inserting a Rectal Suppository,** along with questions and suggested responses, is available on the ***Davis's Nursing Skills Videos*** Web site on FADavis.com.

Procedure 26-7 ■ Applying Medication to Skin

➤ For steps to follow in *all* procedures, refer to the Universal Steps for All Procedures found on the inside back cover. Also refer to the Medication Guidelines: Steps to Follow for All Medications (Regardless of Type or Route).

➤ *Note:* Follow agency policy or provider's prescription regarding use of prepackaged wipes or soap and water to cleanse the skin.

Delegation

An RN can usually delegate administration of most topical medications to an LPN/LVN. In some institutions, you can delegate the administration of an over-the-counter medication to a UAP. Refer to agency policy regarding administration of topical medication.

Pre-Procedure Assessments

- Assess for skin irritation, open lesions, area of hypersensitivity, or other skin abnormality.
- Determine the presence of contraindications for dermal application. Document and report these before administering medication.

Procedure 26-7A ■ Applying Topical Lotion, Cream, and Ointment

➤ When performing the procedure, always identify your patient according to agency policy, using two identifiers, and be attentive to standard precautions, hand hygiene, patient safety and privacy, body mechanics, and documentation.

Procedure Steps

1. **Don clean procedure gloves.**
   Complies with universal precautions and protects your skin from the topical medication.
2. **Cleanse the skin** with cleansing wipes or soap and water (according to agency policy), and pat dry before applying
   Clean skin enhances absorption. Moisture on the skin can interfere with adherence of topical ointment, depending on the product used to suspend the medication.
3. **Warm the medication** in your gloved hands.
   This will be more comfortable for the patient and make it easier to apply the preparation.

(continued on next page)

Procedure 26-7 ■ Applying Medication to Skin (continued)

4. **Use gloved hands or an** applicator to apply and spread the medication evenly, following the direction of hair growth when coating the area.
Excessive application may irritate the skin. Gloves will protect you so that you will not absorb the medication through your skin. ➤

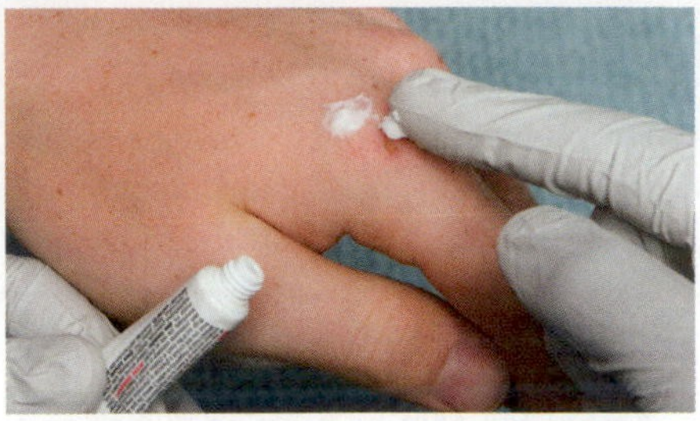

Procedure 26-7B ■ Applying Topical Aerosol Spray

➤ When performing the procedure, always identify your patient according to agency policy, using two identifiers, and be attentive to standard precautions, hand hygiene, patient safety and privacy, body mechanics, and documentation.

Procedure Steps

1. **Don clean procedure gloves.**
2. **Cleanse the skin** with cleansing wipe or soap and water (according to agency policy), and pat dry before applying to enhance absorption.
3. **Shake the container to mix** the contents.
To ensure that active ingredients are evenly distributed throughout the aerosolized suspension.
4. **Hold the container at** the distance specified on the label (usually 6 to 12 in.), and spray over the prescribed area.
Prevents excess application to a local area.
5. **Hold most containers upright** when spraying. If you are spraying near the patient's head, cover his face with a towel.
This will prevent him from inhaling the spray.

Procedure 26-7C ■ Applying Prescribed Powder

➤ When performing the procedure, always identify your patient according to agency policy, using two identifiers, and be attentive to standard precautions, hand hygiene, patient safety and privacy, body mechanics, and documentation.

Procedure Steps

1. **Don clean procedure gloves.**
2. **Cleanse the skin** with a cleansing wipe or soap and water and pat dry before applying to enhance absorption.
Powder applied to a moist surface creates a pasty solution, which may irritate the skin.
3. **Spread apart skinfolds**, and apply a very thin layer.
4. **Be careful that the patient does not inhale** the powder.
Particulate matter, such as powder, can irritate lung tissue and lead to pneumonitis or other inflammatory processes.

Procedure 26-7D ■ Applying Transdermal Medication

➤ When performing the procedure, always identify your patient according to agency policy, using two identifiers, and be attentive to standard precautions, hand hygiene, patient safety and privacy, body mechanics, and documentation.

Procedure Steps

1. **Don clean procedure gloves.**
Complies with universal precautions and protects your skin from the topical medication.
2. **Remove the previous patch**, folding the medicated side to the inside.
This helps prevent unintentional contact of the medication on a different area of the patient's skin.
3. **Dispose of the old patch** carefully in an appropriate receptacle, keeping it away from children and pets.
Even a used patch has some active medication on it. Proper disposal is important to prevent medication exposure to others.
4. **Cleanse the skin of traces** of remaining medication. Allow the skin to dry.
A clean, dry surface optimizes the effectiveness of adherence and absorption of the medication.
5. **Remove the new patch** from its protective covering, and then remove the clear, protective covering without touching the adhesive or the inside surface that contains the medication. ➤

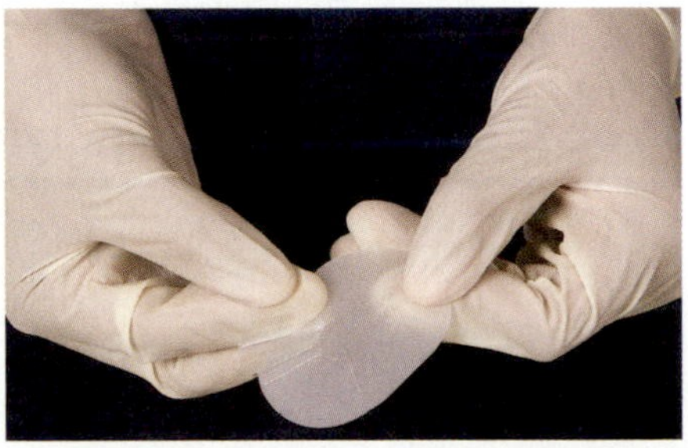

6. **Apply the patch** to a clean, dry, hairless (or little hair), intact skin area, pressing it down for about 10 seconds with your palm. Be sure

the area is free of scars, lesions, and irritation.
A smooth surface maximizes the contact between medication and the skin. Skin that is disrupted can become irritated by topical mediation. Lesions involving thickened layers of skin can compromise absorption.

7. **Rotate application sites** with each new application. Common sites are the trunk, lower abdomen, lower back, and buttocks.
Rotating sites prevents irritation to local areas of the skin.

8. **Advise the patient *not* to use** a heating pad over the area.
Heat can cause some ointments to irritate or even burn the skin.

9. **Write the date, the time, and your initials** on the new patch.
Complete documentation helps to reduce medication errors.

10. **Remove your gloves,** and perform hand hygiene.

11. **Observe for local side effects,** such as skin irritation, itching, and allergic contact dermatitis.
If an adverse response occurs at the local site, remove the patch, wipe the skin clean, and notify the prescriber.

What if . . .

- **The medication is packaged as an ointment form with calibrated paper?**
Wear gloves; apply the ointment in a continuous motion along those marks to measure the required dose. Fold the paper in half to distribute the ointment evenly on the patch.

- **My patient is a child who does not want the medication to be applied?**
Hold the child securely while medication is applied. Then, cover the site with a dressing to keep the child from disrupting the application of medication.

- **My patient is an older adult and has fragile skin?**
Avoid areas where penetration of the cream or ointment is likely to be reduced or cause irritation. Be gentle with application of anything to the skin and diligent with your assessment of the skin response to medication. Avoid using tape; use tape alternatives.

Evaluation

- Assess for rash, excoriation, hives, redness, swelling, or signs of allergy or skin sensitivity to topical medication.
- Ask the patient whether he feels burning, itching, pain, tenderness, or other sensation to skin where medication is applied.
- Assess for improvement in the patient's condition.

Patient Teaching

- Explain that topical medication may take up to 30 minutes to be absorbed, depending on the medication.
- Tell the patient to never ingest or inhale topical medication.
- Advise the patient to avoid touching his eyes after handling topical medication.
- Inform the patient not to use more medicine than prescribed or directed.

Documentation

- Refer to Medication Guidelines: Steps to Follow for All Medication (Regardless of Type or Route).
- Document the skin condition if abnormalities are present and complaints of discomfort during or after administration.
- Document responses to medication (e.g., symptom relief, side effects).

Sample documentation

06/18/2021 0835 Transdermal nitroglycerine 74.6 mg patch applied to upper chest. Pt instructed to leave patch intact for 12 hours. Pt reported mild, transient headache approximately 45 minutes after application of patch. No evidence of flushing, faintness, or dizziness. Pt denies chest pain.——— M. Finegold, RN

06/18/2021 0830 Fentanyl patch (dated 06/17/2021) removed from upper left arm. Skin intact, no irritation noted. Fentanyl patch applied to the left anterior chest wall below the clavicle. Pt stated, "This patch really helps my back feel better."——— M. Finegold, RN

Thinking About the Procedure

The video **Applying Transdermal Medication,** along with questions and suggested responses, is available on the ***Davis's Nursing Skills Videos*** Web site on FADavis.com.

Procedure 26-8 ■ Administering Metered-Dose Inhaler (MDI) Medication

➤ For steps to follow in *all* procedures, refer to the Universal Steps for All Procedures found on the inside back cover. Also, refer to the Medication Guidelines: Steps to Follow for All Medications (Regardless of Type or Route).

Equipment

- Metered-dose inhaler
- Spacer
- Tissues

Pre-Procedure Assessments

Assess the respiratory status before administration of medication to establish a baseline for evaluating the effects of treatment.

Delegation

An RN can usually delegate administration of MDI medications to an LPN/LVN. You usually cannot delegate this task to a UAP, unless the UAP has special training for a specific defined situation (e.g., "medication aides" in some long-term care settings in some states). If the patient is having respiratory distress, you should not delegate this task. Refer to Medication Guidelines: Steps to Follow for All Medications (regardless of Type or Route).

➤ When performing the procedure, always identify your patient according to agency policy, using two identifiers, and be attentive to standard precautions, hand hygiene, patient safety and privacy, body mechanics, and documentation.

Procedure Steps

1. **Determine the number** of remaining inhalations of medication in the canister based on the start date and instructions for use. **Key Point:** ***Do not use the old method of floating the canister in water, as it is not an accurate estimate.*** Replace the canister promptly when it is nearly empty.

Historically, patients have been instructed to float the canister in water to determine how much medication remains. However, propellants affect the weight of the canister and may lead to false reassurance that there is medication in an empty container.

Some MDI medications are used as rescue agents during asthma attacks or periods of dyspnea. It is important to always have medication available for use.

2. **Assist the patient to a seated** or high-Fowler's position if in bed.
   Facilitates the ability to take a deep inhalation when medication is administered.
3. **Ask the patient to rinse** out his mouth and spit the fluid out (not to swallow it).
   Helps prevent transfer of bacteria from the mouth to the inhaler.
4. **Shake the inhaler**. Then, remove the mouthpiece cap of the inhaler, and insert the mouthpiece into the spacer while holding the canister upright.
   A spacer is the most efficient method to deliver inhaled medications. It should be used if the patient has difficulty coordinating the use of the inhaler, is using a corticosteroid, or if it is prescribed.
5. **Remove the cap from the spacer.**
6. **Ask the patient to breathe out** slowly and completely. If a patient is unable to use the MDI independently, time the use of the device with the patient's own respirations.
   Deep breathing helps the patient to time the dose with his natural breathing.
7. **Place the spacer mouthpiece** into the patient's mouth and have him seal his lips around the mouthpiece. Press down on the inhaler canister sharply to discharge one puff of medication into the spacer.

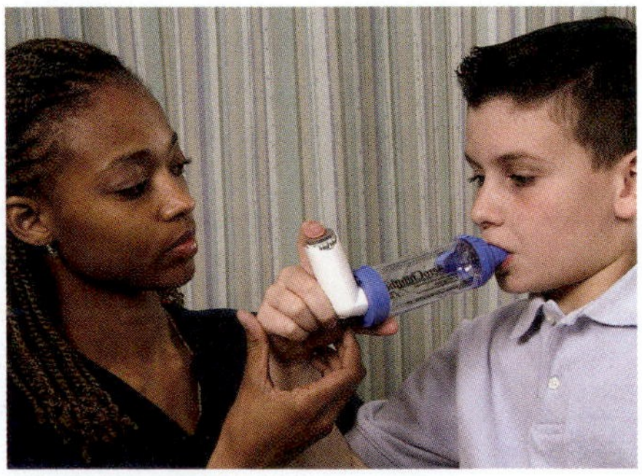

If No Spacer Is Used

If a spacer is not used, place the canister 2.5 to 5.0 cm (1 to 2 in.) from or directly into the mouth.
A good seal allows proper delivery of medication.

8. **Ask the patient to slowly inhale** and then hold his breath for as long as possible. Encourage the patient to hold his breath for 10 seconds, if possible.
   When the patient holds his breath, the medication can be delivered deep into the distal bronchioles of the lungs.
9. **If a second puff is needed**, wait at least 1 minute before repeating steps 6 through 8.
   Allows the medication to be absorbed and the canister to recharge.
10. **If a corticosteroid inhaler** was used, assist the patient to rinse out his mouth with water and spit out the rinse.
    Prolonged exposure of this medication to the oral mucosa is irritating and can lead to thrush in some patients.
11. **Wipe the mouthpiece** with a tissue or moist cloth, and replace the cap. Periodically rinse the spacer, mouthpiece, and cap with water.
    Proper cleaning of the MDI keeps the dispenser from clogging.

The following illustrations summarize the steps for using an MDI.

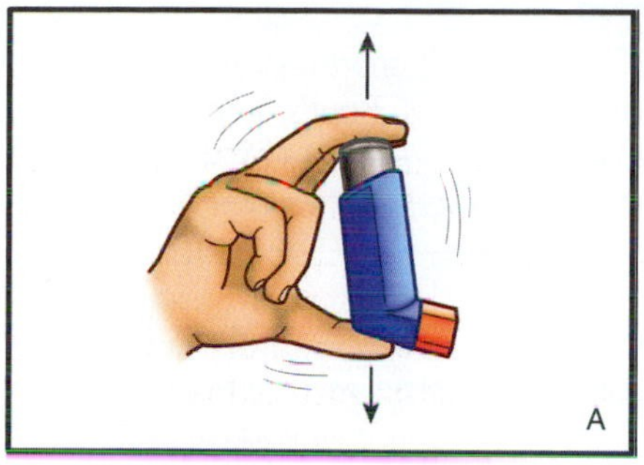

Shake canister.

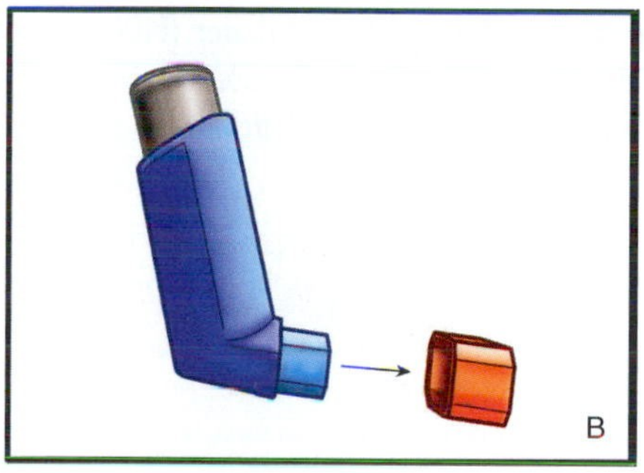

Remove cap. Discharge 2 puffs.

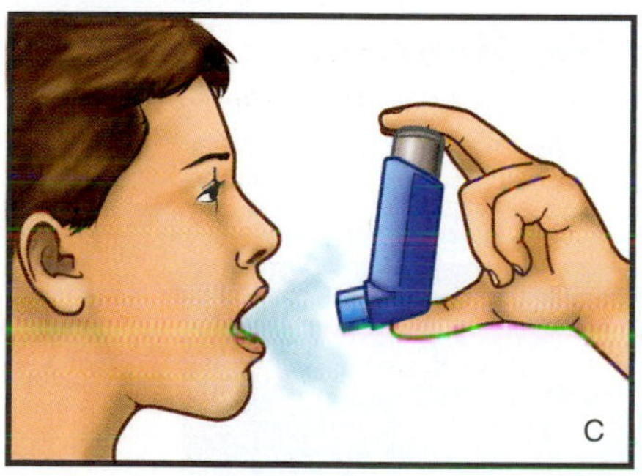

Deep breath out.

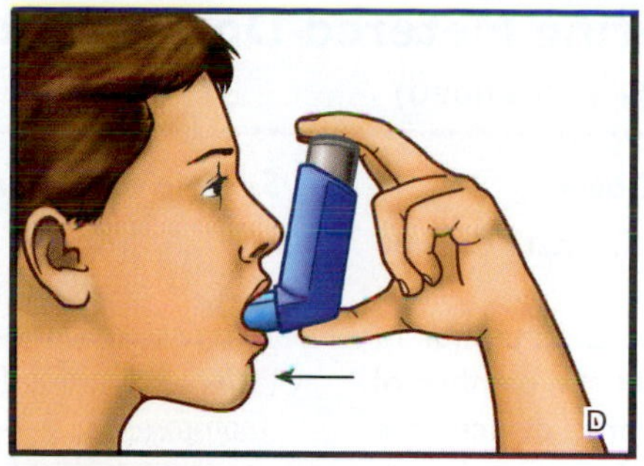

Press top. Inhale med slowly.

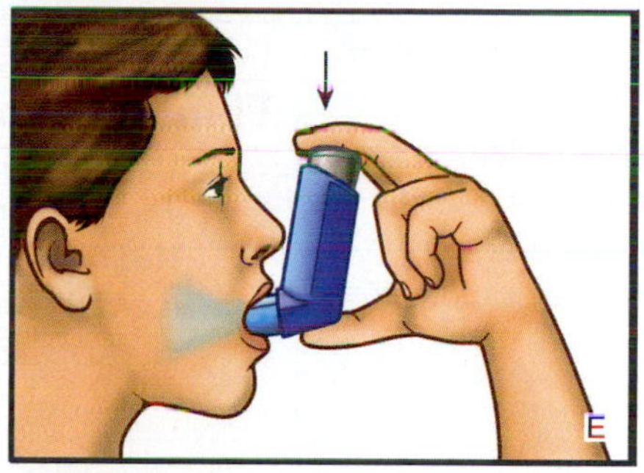

Hold breath. Exhale slowly.

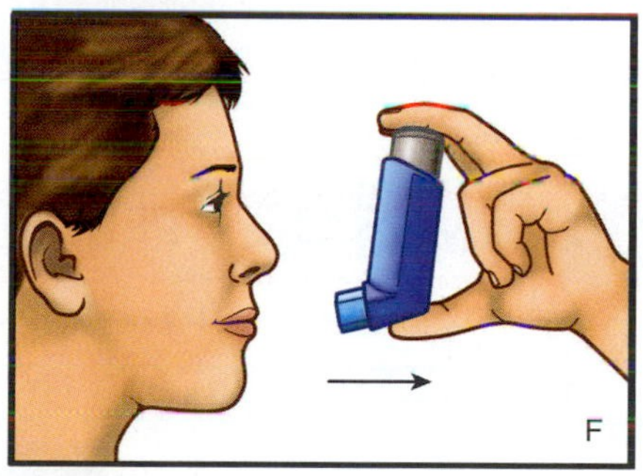

Remove inhaler from mouth.
Wait 1 minute before next puff.

? What if . . .

- **My patient is a small child or frail older adult who is unable to assist with taking medication from the inhaler?**

  You will need to time discharge of the medication with the client's inspiration if the patient is unable to administer the medication with his own deep breaths.

Evaluation

Assess for change in respiratory status after medication administration.

Patient Teaching

- Explain when to use the inhaler and what side effects to anticipate.
- Teach and demonstrate to patients how to correctly use a spacer and MDI.
- Explain how to determine if the MDI canister is nearly empty.
- Explain that some inhalers are used in combination with others and must be used in correct order to receive the desired effect.
- Be aware that many patients who have not been taught to use dry powder inhalers do not get any medication into their lungs.
- Errors in using dry powder inhalers increase with age and illness severity. Carefully supervise older adults and seriously ill patients.

Home Care

General Information for Patients

- Show your healthcare professional how you are using your MDI. If you are having trouble, ask for tips or for recommendation of another device.
- Never puncture or break the canister.
- Do not immerse the MDI in water.
- Keep the MDI where you can get it quickly when needed, but out of children's reach.
- Store the MDI at room temperature. If it gets cold, warm it by rubbing the canister between your palms. Never use anything else to warm it.

(continued on next page)

Procedure 26-8 ■ Administering Metered-Dose Inhaler (MDI) Medication (continued)

Determining the Number of Remaining Doses

- When you begin using a new MDI, write the start date on the canister.
- The only reliable method for determining the number of doses remaining in a canister is to subtract the number of doses used from the number available. Some devices are equipped with counters. Floating MDIs in water is not accurate for assessing remaining doses and often will clog the valve.

Cleaning the MDI

- Clean your apparatus regularly to avoid drug buildup that might keep the medication from reaching the lungs. Specific maintenance procedures may vary with the manufacturer.
- Remove the metal canister that contains the medication by pulling it out.

Documentation

- Refer to Medication Guidelines: Steps to Follow for All Medications (regardless of Type or Route).
- Document the response to medications.

Sample documentation

09/25/2021 0800 Pt. c/o shortness of breath. RR 26 and labored. Combivent MDI 2 puffs administered with spacer. —————— S. Smythe, RN
0815 RR 20, regular, even. Pt states he is comfortable. —————— S. Smythe, RN

Practice Resources

Gandhi, K., Dahiya, A., Taruna-Kalra, A., et al. (2012); Lareau, S., & Hodder, R. (2012)

Thinking About the Procedure

The video **Administering Metered Dose Inhaler (MDI) Medication,** along with questions and suggested responses, is available on the ***Davis's Nursing Skills Videos*** Web site on FADavis.com.

Procedure 26-9 ■ Preparing, Drawing Up, and Mixing Medication

➤ For steps to follow in *all* procedures, refer to the Universal Steps for All Procedures found on the inside back cover. Also, refer to the Medication Guidelines: Steps to Follow for All Medications (Regardless of Type or Route).

Equipment

- Medication vials, ampules, and/or prefilled syringe
- Alcohol prep pad (70% alcohol) or chlorhexidine gluconate (CHG)–alcohol product
- Syringe of the appropriate size for medication volume and viscosity
- Needle of the appropriate size for the site and viscosity to be aspirated through the vial access device (VAD)
- VAD, filter needle, or safety needle
- Gauze pad or ampule snapper, if you are using ampules

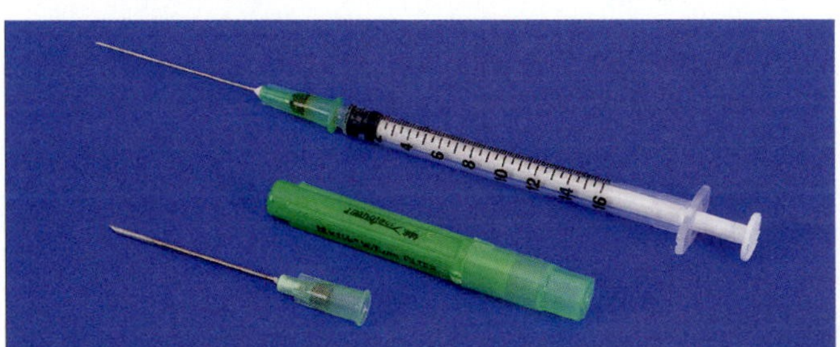

Top: Syringe with a regular needle.
Bottom: Filter needle.

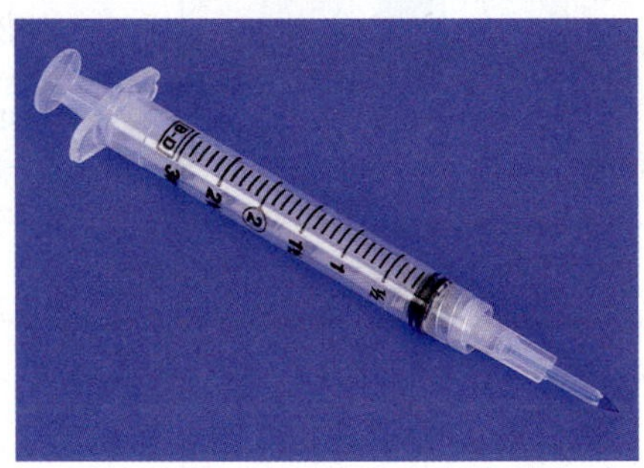

Vial access device.

Delegation

An RN can delegate administration of some parenteral medications to an LPN/LVN. You usually cannot delegate this task to a UAP. Nurse practice acts governing medication administration vary from state to state, and policies vary further among healthcare agencies. Nevertheless, the RN is always responsible for supervising and evaluating delegated care. You can instruct a UAP in the therapeutic effects expected from the medication.

Pre-Procedure Assessments

- **Check the ampule or vial for intactness, cloudiness, particles, and color.**
  A change in color, cloudiness, particles, or cracks indicate the medication is altered or contaminated and should not be used.
- **Check the compatibility of the medications to be mixed.**
  Some medications are either chemically or physically incompatible and cannot be mixed. Other medications may be compatible for only 20 to 30 minutes, so they must be given promptly after they are mixed. Although physically incompatible medications can frequently be identified by a change in appearance, such as precipitation, no such indication exists for chemically incompatible medications.
- **Determine the total volume of medications and whether the total volume is appropriate for the administration site.**
  Although the reason for mixing medications is to limit the number of injections a patient receives, the total volume of the injections must not be greater than what is appropriate for the site.

Procedure 26-9A ■ Drawing Up Medication From Ampules

➤ When performing the procedure, always identify your patient according to agency policy, using two identifiers, and be attentive to standard precautions, hand hygiene, patient safety and privacy, body mechanics, and documentation.

Procedure Steps

1. **Gently flick or tap the top** of the ampule with your index finger to remove medication trapped in the top of the ampule. *Alternative method:* Shake the ampule by quickly turning and snapping your wrist, like shaking down a mercury thermometer.
   Medication left in the top of the ampule may lead to administering an inadequate dose. All the medication must be in the bottom of the ampule before you open it.

2. Use an ampule snapper, if available. Alternatively, wrap a 2 × 2 inch gauze pad (or an unopened alcohol wipe) around the neck of the ampule. Snap the top off, breaking it away from you.
   Prevents you from accidentally cutting your fingers or spraying glass fragments toward you. Do not use an opened alcohol wipe to break the ampule because it is not thick enough to prevent injury.

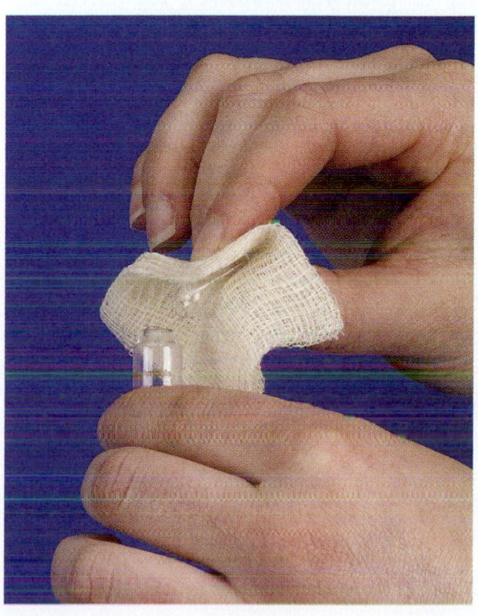

3. **Attach a filter needle** or filter straw to the syringe. If the syringe has a needle in place, remove both the needle and the cap, and place them on a sterile surface (e.g., a newly opened alcohol pad still in the open wrapper), and attach the filter needle or straw.
   Opening a glass ampule produces a spray of tiny fractured glass particles, which can enter the ampule and contaminate the contents. The filter needle or straw filters the solution drawn up from glass ampules to remove glass particles.

4. **Withdraw the medication** from the ampule with a filter needle by using one of the following techniques. Be careful not to touch the neck of the ampule with the filter straw or needle while withdrawing medication.
   Touching the neck of the ampule with the needle or straw increases the risk of contamination.
   a. *Invert the ampule*, place the filter needle or straw tip in the liquid, and withdraw the prescribed amount of medication. Be careful not to insert needle through the medication into the air at the top of the inverted ampule.
      This method is particularly useful with small ampules. The medication's surface tension prevents the liquid from leaking from the inverted ampule. However, if you insert the needle too far (into the air pocket above the medication), the medication will run out.

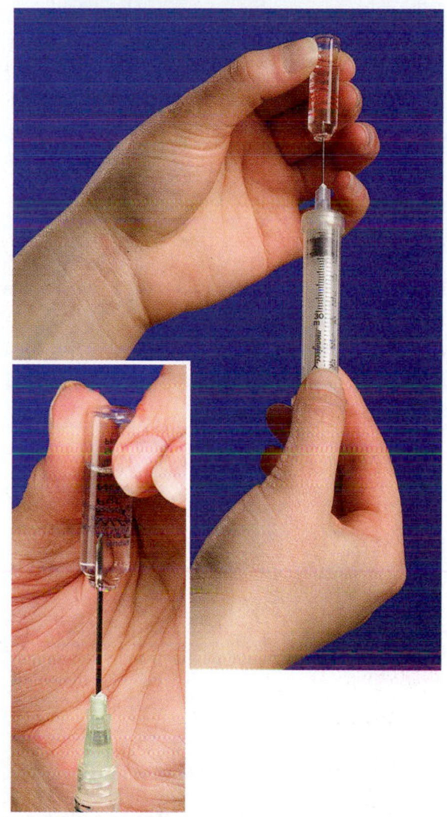

(continued on next page)

Procedure 26-9 ■ Preparing, Drawing Up, and Mixing Medication (continued)

b. *Alternatively, tip the ampule,* place a filter needle or straw in the liquid, and withdraw all medication. Reposition the ampule so that the needle or straw tip remains in the liquid.
This method allows for easier stabilization of the ampule while you withdraw the medication and may help prevent contamination of the needle on the edge of the vial opening.

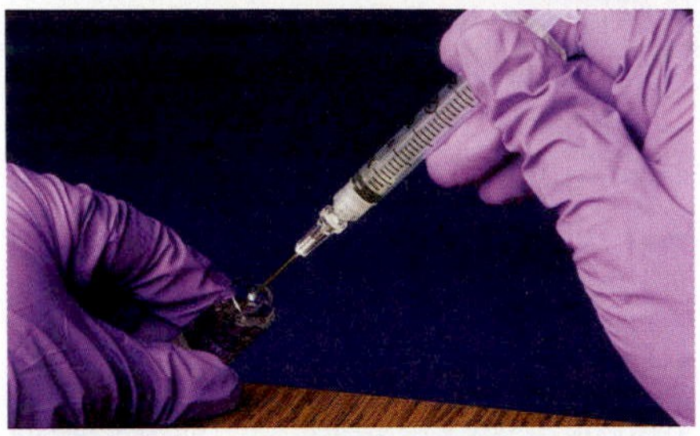

5. **Hold the syringe vertically**, and draw 0.2 mL of air into the syringe (also see Clinical Insight 26-5). Draw up and measure the exact medication dose, plus 0.2 mL of air (the syringe plunger should be at 0.2 mL more than the prescribed dose).
6. **Remove the filter needle** or straw, and reattach the "saved" needle for administering the injection.
7. **Eject the 0.2 mL of air, and read the dose.** After all of the air is removed, if you need to eject some medication to make the dose correct, tip the syringe until it is horizontal to push out the medication.
   - *Pulling air into the syringe allows for an exact dose when the medication is injected; the air will clear the needle (after the medication) so that the patient receives all the medication that is in the syringe.*
   - *The syringe must be vertical to eject air. However, if you eject the medication while holding the syringe vertically, the drug will run down the needle and then track through the patient's tissue during the injection.*

For a Filter Needle

Use a filter needle only to withdraw, not to measure, medication. Do not eject medication through it.
Pushing the medication out through the filter needle could cause the filter to break and release the glass fragments.

Key Point: ***This is not the old "air lock" technique; you will eject the air before administering the medication to the patient.***

For Medications that are Irritating to Tissues (e.g., Parenteral Iron)

You can leave the 0.2 mL of air in the syringe for injection. However, be sure to account for the air when you read the dose markings on the syringe.

8. **Dispose of the top and bottom** of the ampule and the filter needle in a sharps container.
Disposal into a puncture-proof container prevents accidental needlestick injury.

Procedure 26-9B ■ Drawing Up Medication From Vials

➤ When performing the procedure, always identify your patient according to agency policy, using two identifiers, and be attentive to standard precautions, hand hygiene, patient safety and privacy, body mechanics, and documentation.

➤ This procedure assumes you are using a vial access device (VAD) because that is preferred. Use a needle only when a filter needle is required.

Procedure Steps

1. **Mix the solution in the vial**, if necessary, by gently rolling the vial between your hands.
Aqueous suspensions will settle to the bottom of the vial, so they need to be mixed. Rolling the vial between your hands will mix the medication without forming air bubbles. Shaking the vial traps air in the medication.
2. **Place the vial on a flat work surface,** and thoroughly scrub the rubber top of the vial with an alcohol prep pad or CHG-alcohol product.
The alcohol prep pad removes dust, grease, and microorganisms.
3. **If a needle is attached** to the syringe, uncap it and place it on a sterile surface (e.g., sterile, opened alcohol pad).
   a. **If you are using a VAD,** uncap the VAD without touching the tip or shaft and attach the device to the syringe.
   VADs can be used only with single-use vials, unless the vial is designed for use with access pins, such as a Life-Shield vial.
4. **Place the VAD cap** on a clean surface, or hold the cap open-side out between two fingers of your nondominant hand.
This method prevents contamination of the cap and the needle during recapping.
5. **Draw air into the syringe** equal to the amount of medication to be withdrawn from the vial.
Injection of air into the vial makes withdrawing the medication easier. For small unit-dose vials, you may not have to instill air prior to withdrawing the medication, but you will need to maintain backward pressure on the plunger until the needle is completely withdrawn. If you release the plunger, the negative pressure in the vial will pull the medication back into the vial.
6. **Insert the VAD** into the vial without coring and while maintaining sterile technique. Use a needle *only* if for some reason (e.g., the type of medication) a filter needle is required.
   a. Place the tip of the VAD or filter needle in the middle of the rubber

top of the vial, with the bevel up at a 45° to 60° angle.

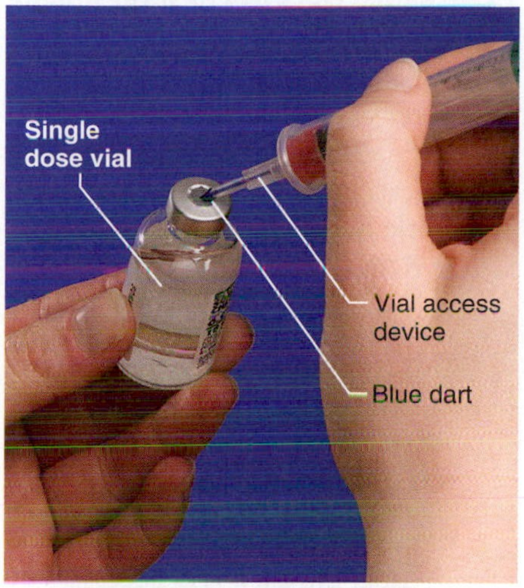

b. While pushing the VAD into the rubber top, gradually bring the syringe (and VAD) upright to a 90° angle.
This method helps prevent coring, which occurs when a small piece of the rubber top is trapped inside the VAD during insertion. Coring is more likely to occur with large-gauge needles and VADs.

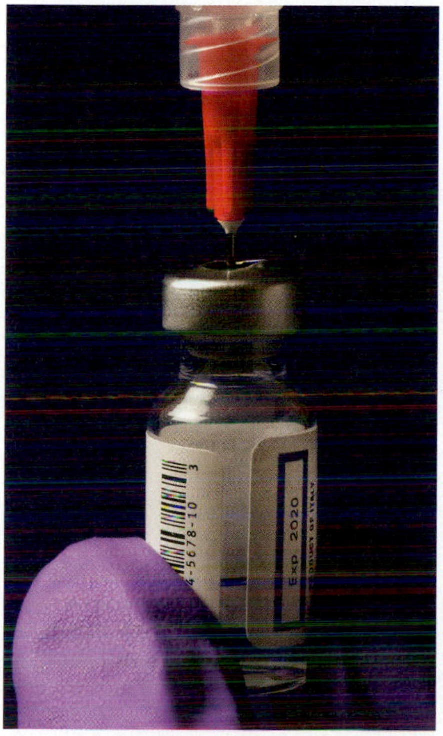

7. **With the tip of the VAD above the fluid line,** inject the air in the syringe into the air in the vial.
The air creates positive pressure in the vial, making the medication easier to withdraw. Injecting the air into the medication will create air bubbles, which interfere with dosage measurement.

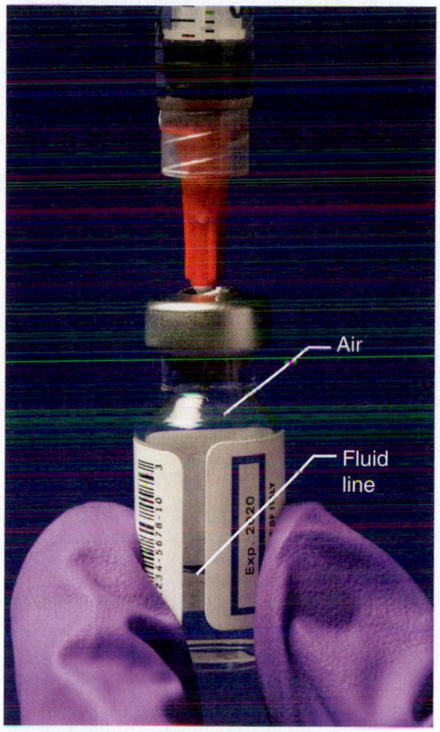

"Air to air."

8. **Invert the vial,** keep the VAD vertical in the medication, and slowly withdraw the medication.
The vial needs to be inverted so that all the medication can be withdrawn. Keeping the VAD in the medication and slowly drawing the medication will help prevent drawing of excess air into the syringe.

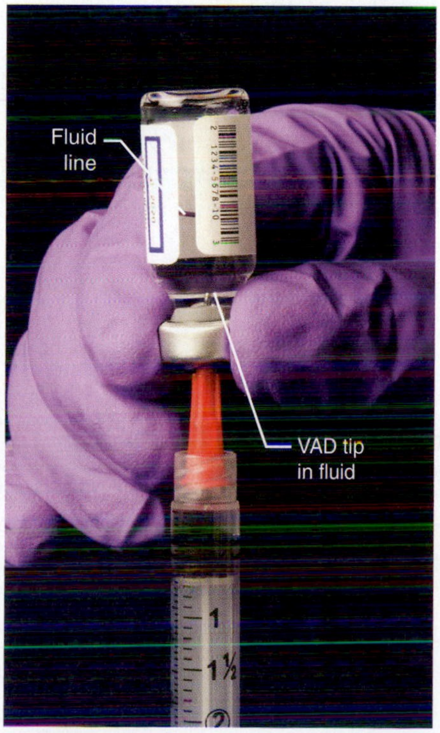

9. **Keeping the VAD in the vial,** remove any air from the syringe:
When the VAD is connecting the vial and syringe, a sterile unit is formed. The volume of air in the hub of the syringe and inside the needle/VAD, dead space, will be drawn back into the syringe. Air bubbles alter the dose of medication being administered, so they must be expelled. You can use a pen to tap the syringe if extra force is needed.

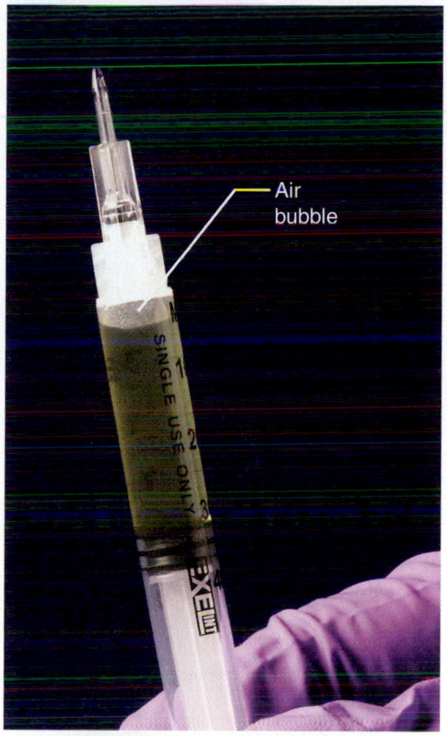

A, **Incorrect.** If syringe is not vertical, air is trapped near the hub.

(continued on next page)

Procedure 26-9 ■ Preparing, Drawing Up, and Mixing Medication (continued)

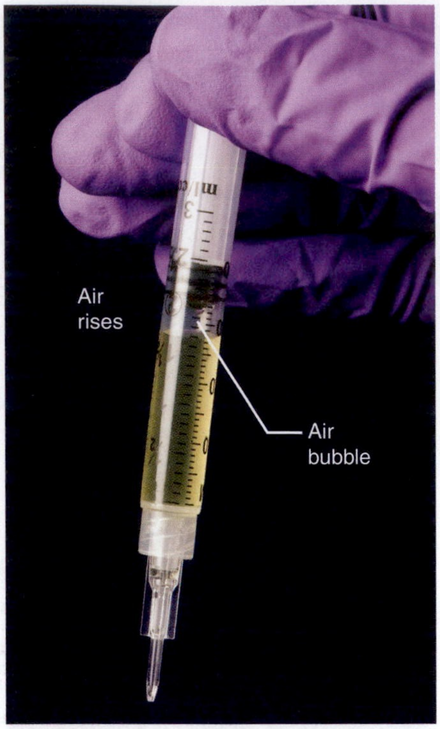

B, **Incorrect.** If tip is down, air is trapped at the plunger.

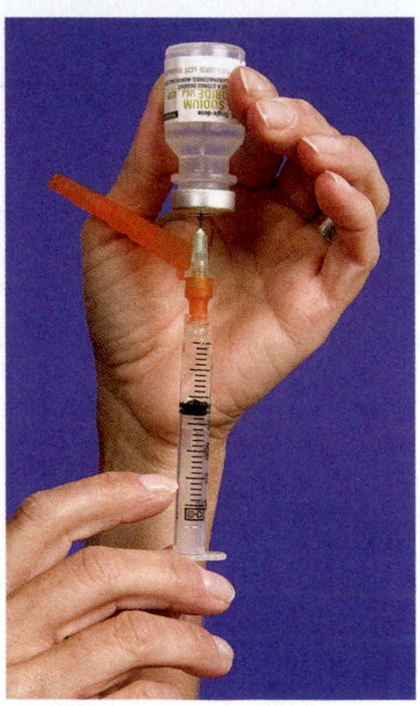

C, **Correct.** Syringe is vertical.

a. Carefully stabilize the vial and syringe, and firmly tap the syringe below the air bubbles. When air bubbles are at the hub of the syringe, make sure the syringe is vertical (straight up and down), and push the air back into the vial.
Remember that air rises, so if the syringe is tilted, air will be trapped in it.

b. If additional medication is necessary to obtain the correct dose, withdraw it before removing the VAD from the inverted vial.
When working with only one vial, you can withdraw and eject medication into the vial as many times as needed to expel bubbles from the syringe and obtain the correct dose.

10. **When the dose is correct,** withdraw the needle or VAD from the vial at a 90° angle.
A vertical angle prevents accidental contamination or bending of the needle.

11. **Hold the syringe upright** at eye level to recheck the medication dose.
Reading the syringe at an angle can result in inaccurate measurement.

12. **Recap the VAD** or vial access needle using a recapping device or the one-handed method. See Procedure 26-10.
Although recapping a sterile needle does not present a threat of exposure to bloodborne pathogens, using a mechanical recapping device or the one-handed method helps develop safe habits.

13. **Change the VAD or filter needle** before you inject the medication:
   a. Before changing the VAD or filter needle, draw back on the syringe plunger to remove all medication from dead space in the old needle (or VAD).
   b. Remove the old needle (or VAD), and reattach a sterile needle for injection (see Clinical Insight 26-5).
   You cannot eject medication through a filter needle; you cannot inject a patient with a VAD.
   c. Hold the syringe vertically and expel the air. If it is necessary to expel some medication, hold the syringe horizontally to do so.
   The difficulty with changing the needles is that you may slightly alter the dose. If you are planning to change the needles, draw slightly more than the prescribed dose unless you are combining in one syringe. After changing the needle, remeasure the dose. Holding the syringe horizontally prevents medication from running down the needle and tracking into the patient's skin.

14. **Dispose of the vial, VAD**, or any recapped needles in a sharps container.
This prevents sharps injury to healthcare workers or others in the vicinity. Proper disposal also reduces the risk of transmitting infectious organisms.

Procedure 26-9C ■ Mixing Medication From Two Vials

- First, review the Medication Guidelines: Steps to Follow for All Medications (Regardless of Type or Route); Procedure 26-9B (Drawing Up Medication From Vials); and Procedure 26-10A (Recapping Contaminated Needles).
- Always use a VAD instead of a needle, whenever possible. If you must use a needle, use a safety needle.
- When performing the procedure, always identify your patient according to agency policy, using two identifiers, and be attentive to standard precautions, hand hygiene, patient safety and privacy, body mechanics, and documentation.

Procedure Steps

1. **Scrub the tops of both vials** with an alcohol pad or CHG-alcohol product. *NOTE:* Some experts omit this step for single-dose vials.
   Not all pharmaceutical companies ensure the sterility of the rubber top on vials, even when they are first opened. However, be aware that once your fingers touch the alcohol pad, it is no longer sterile; therefore, you are not sterilizing but, rather, are cleaning the vial top.

2. **Draw air into the syringe** in the same amount as the total medication doses for both vials (e.g., if the prescription is for 0.5 mL for vial A and 1 mL for vial B, then draw up 1.5 mL of air).

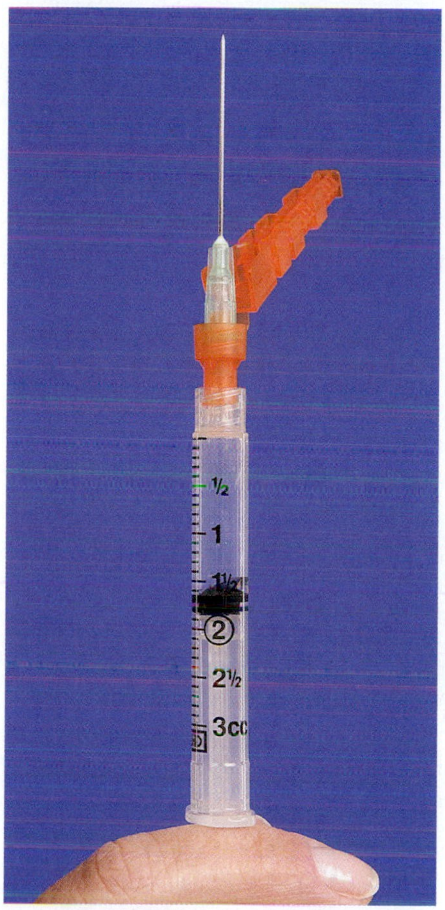

3. **Inject air into the vials.**
   a. Maintaining sterility, insert the vial access device or safety needle into the vial in the middle of the rubber top of the vial with the bevel up at a 45° to 60° angle. While pushing the VAD (or needle) into the rubber top, gradually bring the needle upright to a 90° angle.

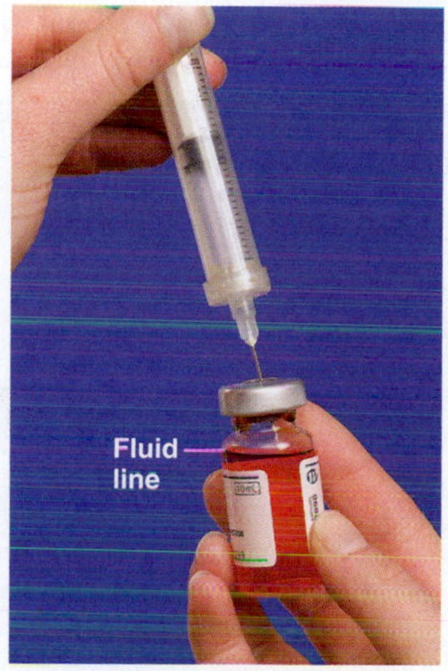

Vial A

This method helps prevent coring of the rubber top.

   b. Keeping the tip of the VAD (or safety needle) above the medication, inject an amount of air equal to the volume of drug to be withdrawn from the first vial (e.g., 0.5 mL for vial A in Step 2); then inject the rest of the air into the second vial (e.g., 1.0 mL for vial B). Take care to prevent coring.

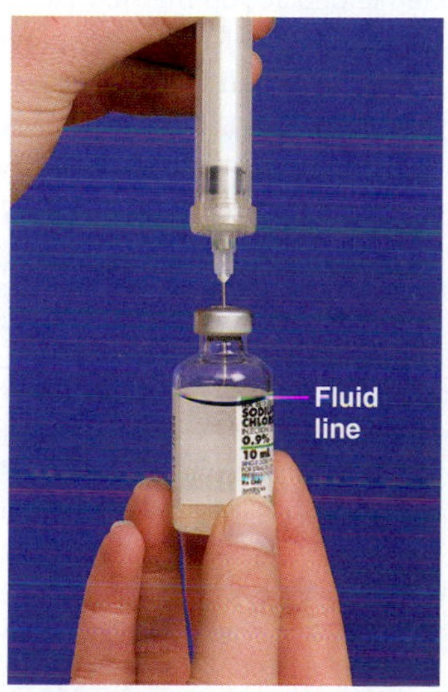

Vial B

Medication is easier to withdraw from a vial with positive pressure. For small unit-dose vials, it may be possible to withdraw the medication without instilling air, but you will need to maintain a slight backward pressure on the plunger until the needle is completely withdrawn. If you release the plunger, the negative pressure in the vial will pull the medication back in. Therefore, it is always safer to instill air.

Using One Multidose Vial and One Single-Dose Vial

You must withdraw medication from the multidose vial before withdrawing from the single-dose vial. However, the needle tip should stay above the medication at all times in steps 2 and 3.

This is an extra precaution to prevent contamination of the multidose vial with medication from the single-dose vial.

When Mixing Two Types of Insulin

If you are mixing two types of insulin at step 3, put air into the regular insulin last (see Clinical Insight 26-6 for mixing two types of insulin).

4. **Without removing the VAD,** or needle, from the second vial (B), invert it and withdraw the prescribed amount of medication. Expel any air bubbles, and measure the dose. Remove the VAD from the vial, then pull back on the plunger enough to pull all medication out of the VAD into the syringe (see Clinical Insight 26-5). Read the dose at eye level. Tip the syringe horizontally if you need to eject any medication.
   Allows you to withdraw all the medication. Keeping the needle in the medication and withdrawing the medication slowly helps prevent drawing excess air into the syringe and prevents bubbles.

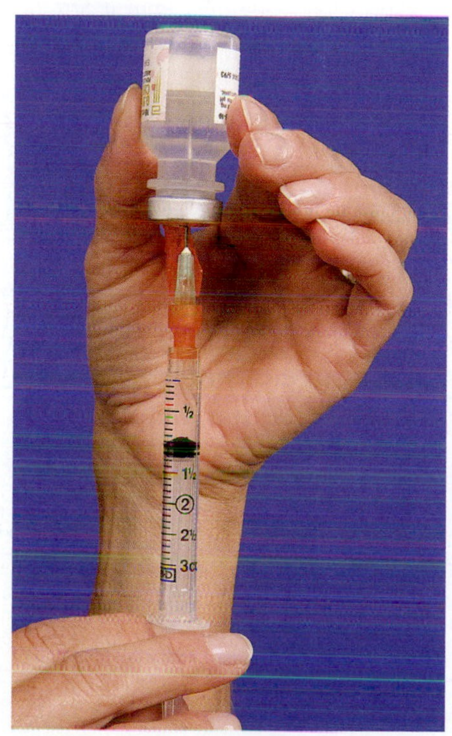

Vial B (Step 4)

(continued on next page)

Procedure 26-9 ■ Preparing, Drawing Up, and Mixing Medication (continued)

5. **Insert the VAD or needle** into the first vial (A), invert, and withdraw the exact prescribed amount of medication, holding the syringe vertical.
   - When finished, the plunger should be at the line for the total/combined dose for vials A and B. (Using the example in step 2, you would have 1.5 mL of the mixed medications in the syringe.)
   - Be very careful not to withdraw excess medication; keep your index finger or thumb on the flange of the syringe to prevent medication being forced back by pressure. If this occurs, you must discard the medication in the syringe and start over.

Because the medications are mixed, withdrawing extra from the second vial makes the entire mixture incorrect. If you draw up too much of the second drug or if your final measurement of the total for both drugs is incorrect you cannot eject medication because you cannot know how much of that is medication A and how much of it is medication B that you are ejecting. You must discard the syringe and medication and begin again.

You do not need to change the needle before step 5 because even if one vial is a multidose vial, you would have withdrawn the medication from it first (in step 4). It will not matter if you track medication into the single-dose vial.

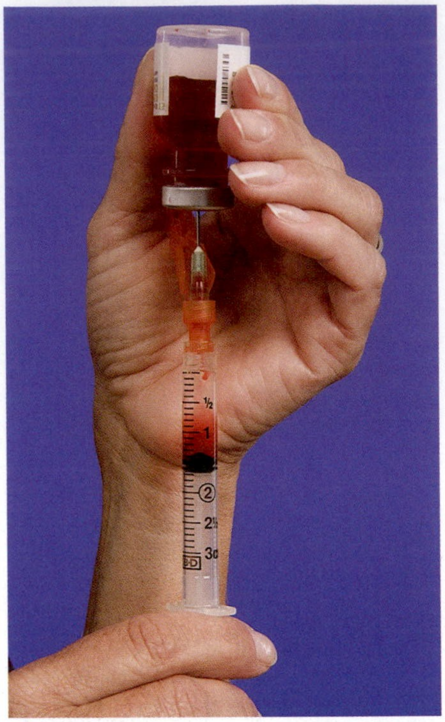

Vial A (Step 5)

6. **Recap the VAD or access needle,** using a needle-capping device or the one-handed scoop method (see Procedure 26-10: Recapping Needles Using a One-Handed Technique).
   Although recapping a sterile needle does not present a threat of exposure to bloodborne pathogens, using a mechanical recapping device or the one-handed method helps develop safe habits. As a rule, we do not recommend using the one-handed scoop for sterile needles; however, this needle will be discarded anyway, so if it is accidentally contaminated with a one-handed scoop, it will not be a major error.

7. **Remove the VAD** (or access needle), **and attach a new sterile needle on the syringe for the injection.**
   Obviously, you must replace a VAD with a needle for injection. In addition, if you used a needle instead of a VAD, by the time you are finished withdrawing both medications you will have put it through a rubber vial top at least three times. This dulls the needle. A sharp needle causes less trauma to the patient on injection. A new needle also prevents tracking of the medication through the skin and subcutaneous tissues.

8. **Hold the needle vertically** to expel all air and recheck the dosage (the total for both medications).
   Allows for more accurate accounting of the dose.

9. **If you have used a VAD or filter needle,** refer to Clinical Insight 26-5.

Procedure 26-9D ■ Mixing Medications From One Ampule and One Vial

➤ First, review the Medication Guidelines: Steps to Follow for All Medications (Regardless of Type or Route); Procedure 26-9A (Drawing up Medications from Ampules); Procedure 26-9B (Drawing Up Medication From Vials); and Procedure 26-10A (Recapping Contaminated Needles).

➤ When performing the procedure, always identify your patient according to agency policy, using two identifiers, and be attentive to standard precautions, hand hygiene, patient safety and privacy, body mechanics, and documentation.

Procedure Steps

1. **Begin with the vial.** Scrub the stopper of the vial, using an alcohol wipe or CHG-alcohol combination product.
   Protects against microbial contamination.

2. **Attach a VAD** and draw **the same volume of air** into the syringe as the dose prescribed for the medication in the vial.

3. **Keeping the tip of the VAD** (or safety needle) **above the medication, inject the amount of air equal to the volume of drug to be withdrawn from the vial. The needle should be injecting air to air within the vial.**
   Draw from the vial first because you do not need to add air to ampules before drawing up the medication. In addition, if it is a multidose vial, you would contaminate it with the medicine if you withdrew from the ampule first.
   Injecting air into the vial makes withdrawing the medication easier. For small unit-dose vials, it may be possible to withdraw the medication without instilling air, but you will need to maintain a slight backward pressure on the plunger until the needle is completely withdrawn. If you release the plunger, the negative pressure in the vial will pull the medication back into the vial. Therefore, it is safer always to instill air.

4. **Invert the vial.** Withdraw the prescribed volume (dosage) of medication, keeping the VAD tip in the fluid. See Procedure 26-9B.

5. **Expel any air bubbles,** and measure the dose at eye level. Recheck the dosage, and withdraw more or eject the drug as needed.
This prevents air from entering into the needle or the VAD.

6. **After safely recapping** the VAD, remove it from the syringe. You may place it on an opened, sterile alcohol pad if you need your hands to open the filter needle packaging.
Keeps the needle sterile, if you are using one; you will reuse it. **Key Point:** ***You would not reuse a VAD from this step on.***

7. **Attach a filter needle** or filter straw to the syringe.
The use of a 5-micrometer (μm) filter minimizes the possibility of withdrawing small glass fragments.

8. **Flick or tap the top** of the ampule (or snap your wrist) to remove medication from the neck of the ampule.
Flicking the neck of the ampule will help the fluid to drain down into the main part of the ampule, thus reducing waste.

9. **Open the ampule** by wrapping the neck with a folded gauze pad or an unopened alcohol wipe or use an ampule snapper. Snap open away from you.
Snapping outward prevents you from cutting your fingers or spraying glass fragments toward your face. Do not use an opened alcohol wipe to break the ampule, because it is not thick enough to prevent injury.

10. **Withdraw the exact prescribed amount** of medication from the ampule into the syringe (see Procedure 26-9A). **Key Point:** ***Be very careful in drawing up the second medication; if the total amount of the two medications is incorrect, you must discard the syringe contents and start over.***

11. **Draw 0.2 mL of air into the syringe.**
The extra bit of air clears the filter needle (see Clinical Insight 26-5).

12. **Confirm the dose is correct** by holding the syringe vertically and checking the dose at eye level.
Ensures the total volume in the syringe equals the prescribed amount of both medications plus 0.2 mL of air from the needle.

13. **Recap the filter needle,** using a needle capping device or the one-handed technique recommended in Procedure 26-10B.
Although recapping a sterile needle does not present a threat of exposure to bloodborne pathogens, using a mechanical recapping device or the one-handed method helps develop safe habits. Nevertheless, some scoop techniques pose a significant risk of contaminating the needle, so you must watch carefully that you maintain sterile technique.

14. **Remove the filter needle** or straw and discard it in a sharps container. Replace with a new sterile safety needle for administering the medication to the patient.
This needle-recapping method prevents accidental needlestick injury. You cannot measure the dose accurately with a filter needle. You should not eject medication through the filter needle because of risk of breaking the filter. See Clinical Insight 26-5.

15. **After placing the administration needle** on the syringe, eject the 0.2 mL of air, and check for the correct dose. If there is excess medication in the syringe, you must discard it and start over.

16. **Discard used needles and ampules** in a puncture-proof sharps container.

Procedure 26-9E ■ Using a Prefilled Cartridge and Single-Dose Vial—For Intravenous Administration

➤ *Note:* It is best not to use this technique with multidose vials because there is a risk of contaminating the multidose vial with the cartridge medication.

➤ First, review the Medication Guidelines: Steps to Follow for All Medications (Regardless of Type or Route). Review Procedures 26-9 and 26-10, as needed.

➤ When performing the procedure, always identify your patient according to agency policy, using two identifiers, and be attentive to standard precautions, hand hygiene, patient safety and privacy, body mechanics, and documentation.

Procedure Steps

1. **Scrub the rubber stopper** of the vial thoroughly with an alcohol prep pad or CHG-alcohol-based product.

2. **Assemble the prefilled cartridge** and holder (see Clinical Insight 26-3).

3. **Remove the needle cap** from the prefilled cartridge, expel the air, and measure the correct dose of medication.
You must confirm that the dose of the first medication is correct before you mix it with the second medication.

4. **Holding the cartridge with** the needle up, draw in an amount of air equal to the volume of medication you need from the vial.

5. **While continuing to hold** the syringe with needle straight up (vertically), invert the vial and insert the

(continued on next page)

Procedure 26-9 ■ Preparing, Drawing Up, and Mixing Medication (continued)

needle into it until the tip of the needle shows in the air above the medication. Then inject the air into the vial. Maintain counter-pressure on the plunger so that air and/or medication do not flow back into the syringe.
Injecting air into the vial makes it easier to withdraw the medication. ▼

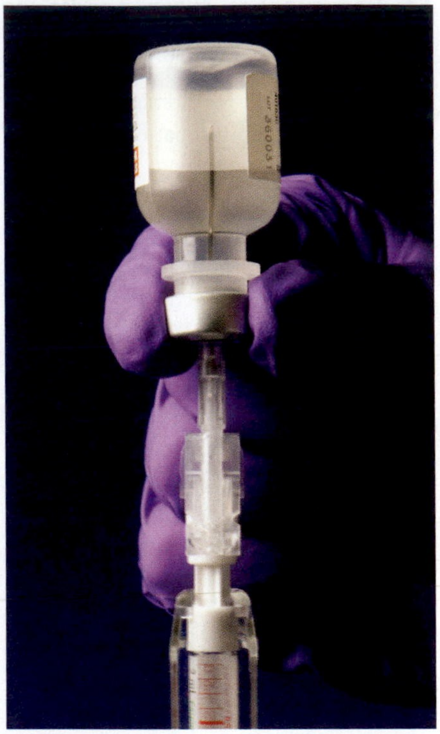

6. **While maintaining counterpressure** on the plunger, pull the needle down into the fluid, and allow the pressure in the vial to push the medication into the syringe. Withdraw the prescribed amount of vial medication, being careful not to withdraw any excess.
7. **The pressure will generally push** a little less than you need, so carefully withdraw the amount you need for a correct dose—again, do not withdraw any excess.
Withdrawing excess medication will result in an altered mixed dose, so you would need to discard the syringe and start over.
8. **Recap the needle** (use a one-handed method), and if possible, remove the needle from the prefilled syringe, and replace it with a sterile injection cannula for IV administration.

For an intramuscular (IM) injection, if the prefilled cartridge does not have a safety needle, you would need to transfer the medication to a new syringe with a sterile safety needle for injection.
VADs and injection cannulas prevent needlestick injury. Unless there is a needle safety device for the prefilled syringe, it is not recommended for IM injections.

? What if . . .

- **There is particulate matter in the ampule or vial?**

Discard the medication and obtain a new one.

Documentation

Document on the MAR.

Practice Resources

CDC (2017); Denholm, B. (2013)

Thinking About the Procedure

The videos **Drawing Up Medication From Ampules, Drawing Up Medication From Vials, Mixing Medication From Two Vials,** and **Mixing Medications From One Ampule and One Vial,** along with questions and suggested responses, are available on the ***Davis's Nursing Skills Videos*** Web site on FADavis.com.

Procedure 26-10 ■ Recapping Needles Using a One-Handed Technique

➤ For steps to follow in *all* procedures, refer to the Universal Steps for All Procedures found on the inside back cover. Also, refer to Medication Guidelines: Steps to Follow for All Medications (Regardless of Type or Route).

Equipment

- Mechanical recapping device, if available
- Needle cover
- Safety syringe, if available
- Other supplies depending on the method used.

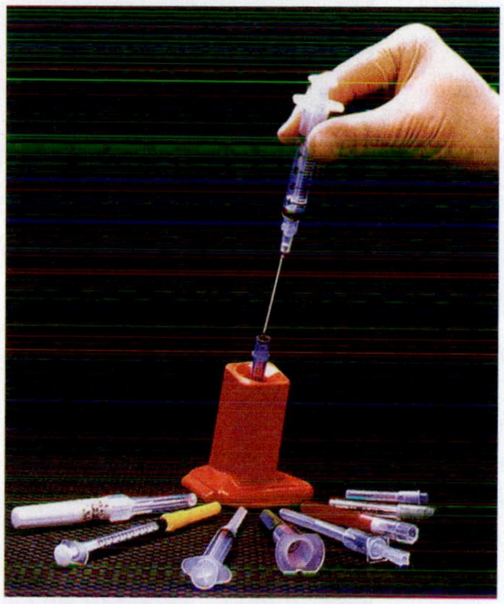

Needle recapping device.

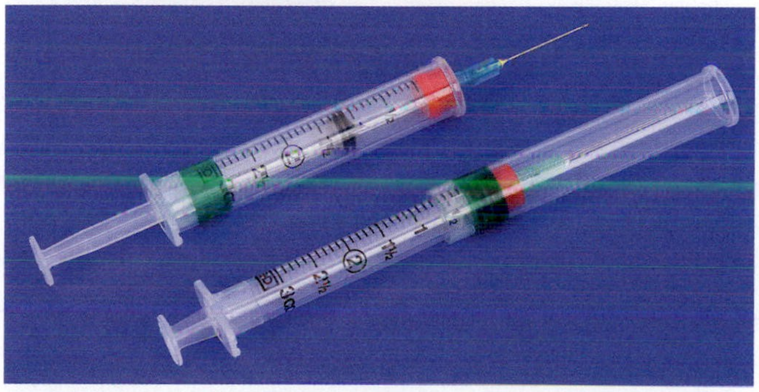

Safety syringe. *A*, Before injection. *B*, Cover slides up after injection.

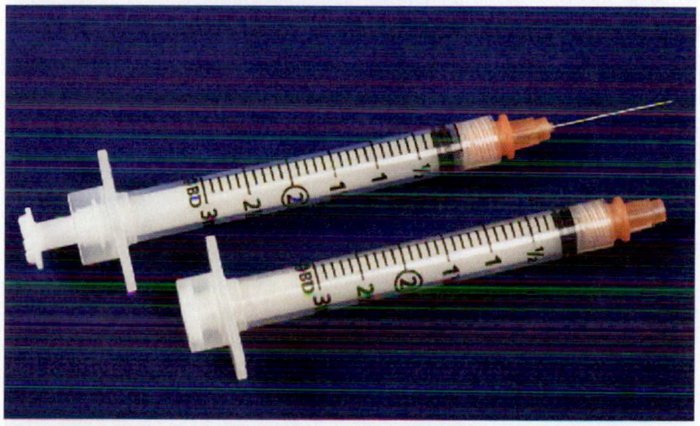

Safety syringe. *A*, Before injection. *B*, Needle retracted after injection.

Delegation

Delegation is not usually an issue because recapping needles is done in conjunction with administering parenteral medications, which you will usually not delegate. If you do delegate administration of parenteral medications to an LPN/LVN, you must supervise and evaluate recapping to ensure that the nurse uses proper technique.

Preparation

- **Assess the need to recap the needle.**
  Recap a contaminated needle only if doing so is absolutely unavoidable, according to Occupational Safety and Health Administration (OSHA) standards. As a rule, place a contaminated syringe and needle directly into a puncture-proof sharps container, without capping, bending, or breaking the needle.
- **Identify whether the needle is sterile or dirty.**
  Although a one-handed technique is used to recap both sterile and dirty needles, different considerations exist.
  Sterile needle: *When you use the one-handed method for recapping a sterile needle, it is easy to contaminate the needle without realizing it. You should modify the technique to prevent that—the main consideration is to "protect" the needle.*
  Contaminated Needle: *The danger in recapping a dirty needle is that you will stick yourself with it, exposing yourself to pathogens. The main consideration is to protect yourself.*
- **Determine the availability of a mechanical recapping device or safety syringe.**
  Key Point: ***Always use a mechanical recapping device or safety syringe, if one is available.***

(continued on next page)

Procedure 26-10 ■ Recapping Needles Using a One-Handed Technique (continued)

Procedure 26-10A ■ Recapping Contaminated Needles

➤ When performing the procedure, always identify your patient according to agency policy, using two identifiers, and be attentive to standard precautions, hand hygiene, patient safety and privacy, body mechanics, and documentation.

Procedure Steps

1. **If you are using a safety needle,** engage the safety mechanism to cover the needle. (See Equipment.)
   OSHA regulations require the use of safety syringes to prevent needlestick injuries. You must engage the safety mechanism before placing the needle and syringe into the sharps container.
2. **Alternatively, place the needle cap** in a mechanical recapping device, if one is available. (See Equipment.)
3. **If a mechanical recapping device** is not available, use the one-handed scoop method to recap the needle.
   a. Place the needle cover on a flat surface.
   Keeps the needle cover from rolling during the needle capping procedure.

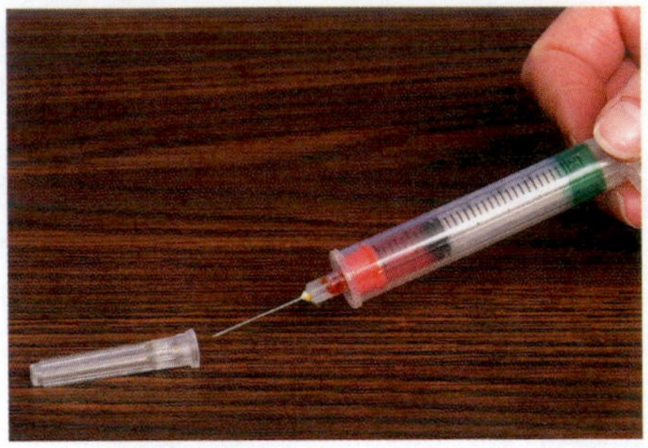

   b. Then, holding the syringe in your dominant hand, scoop the needle cap onto the needle. Tip the syringe vertically to slip the cover over the needle. Do not hold onto the needle cap with your nondominant hand while scooping.
   A mechanical recapping device protects against accidental needlestick injury. If it is unavailable, the one-handed method of recapping will prevent accidental injuries when your own safety or the patient's safety is a concern.

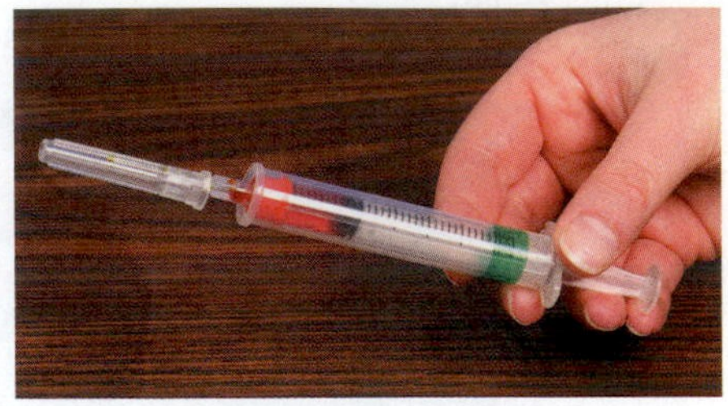

   c. Secure the needle cap by grasping it near the hub.
   Prevents an accidental stick if the needle goes through the needle cap. Needles are sharp enough to go through the needle cap if inserted at an angle.

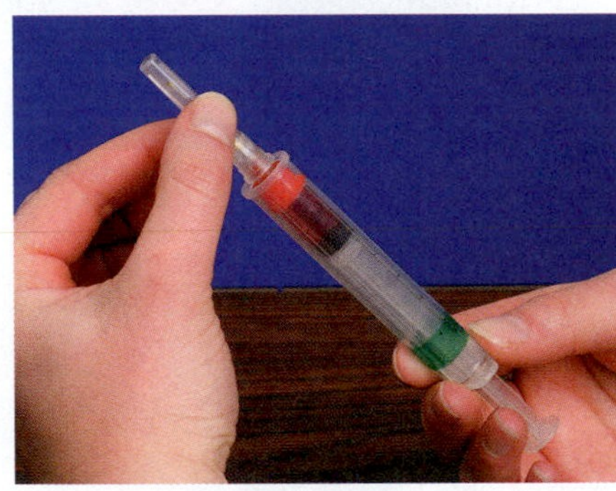

Procedure 26-10B ■ Recapping Sterile Needles

➤ When performing the procedure, always identify your patient according to agency policy, using two identifiers, and be attentive to standard precautions, hand hygiene, patient safety and privacy, body mechanics, and documentation.

Use one of the following techniques to ensure that you do not contaminate a sterile needle. If you contaminate the needle, microorganisms will be introduced with the injection.

Procedure Steps

1. **Place the needle cap** in a mechanical recapping device, if one is available.
   The device is specially developed to provide safe recapping.
2. **Alternative method: Medication cup.** Place the cap into a small liquid medication cup with the open end facing up. You can then insert the sterile needle into the cap, keeping your free hand well away from the cup.
   This step performs the same function as a mechanical recapping device. The needle and cover need to be taller than the cup you are using so that the open end of the cap protrudes above the cup. ➤

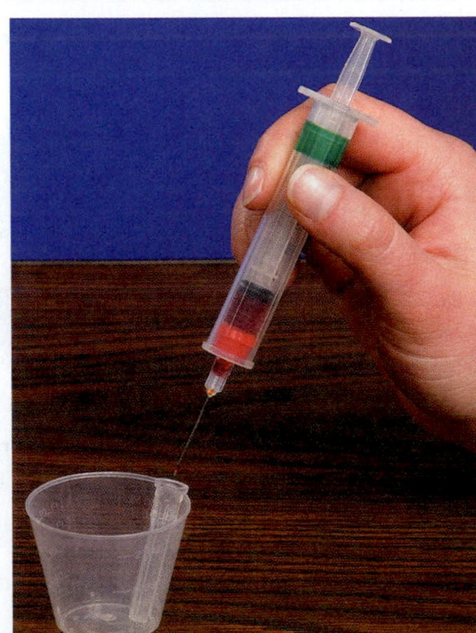

3. **Alternative method: Scoop technique.** Place the cap on a clean surface so that the end of the needle cap protrudes over the edge of the counter or shelf, and scoop with the needle; keep your free hand well away from the needle and cap as you are recapping.
This method prevents you from inadvertently hitting an unsterile surface with the needle.

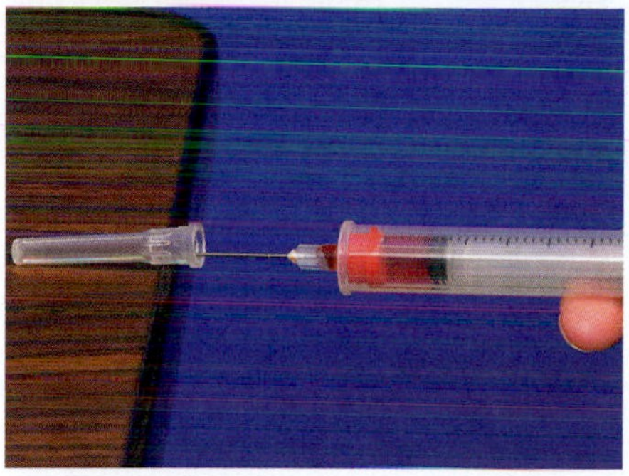

4. **Alternative method: Tubular container.** If the syringe is packaged in a hard plastic tubular container, stand the container on its large end; invert the needle cap; and place it in the top of the hard container. Insert the needle downward into the cap.

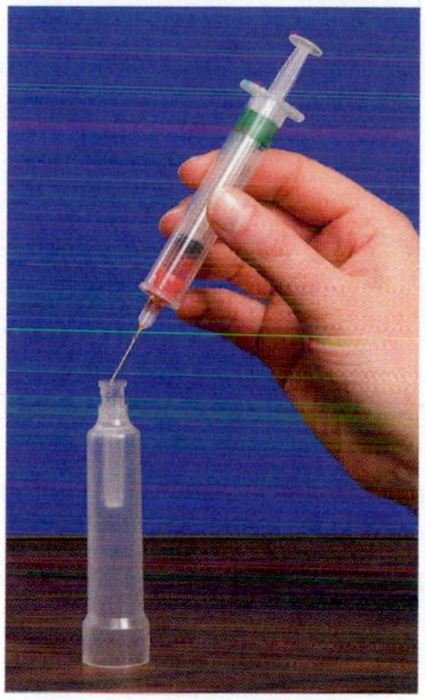

5. **Alternative method: Alcohol wipe.** Place the needle cap on a sterile surface, such as on an open alcohol prep pad, and use the one-handed scoop technique. Be very careful to ensure that the needle does not touch anything other than the inside of the needle cap.
The alcohol prep pad provides a sterile barrier. Because you must bring the needle parallel to the flat surface and because the alcohol pad is so small, it is easy to contaminate the needle when using this method.

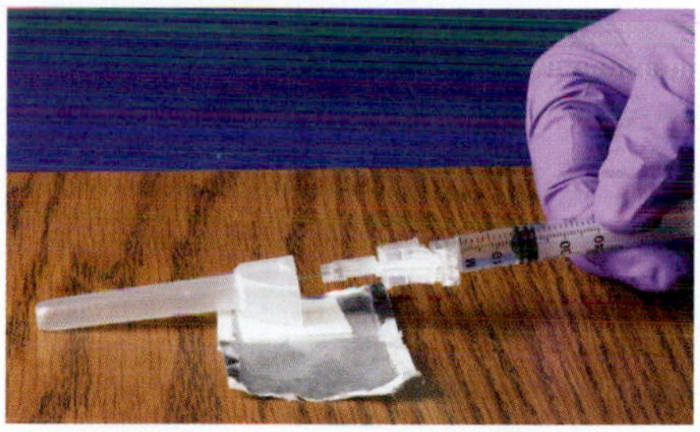

Documentation

No documentation needed for recapping needles.

Practice Resources

National Institute for Occupational Safety and Health (updated 2018); Waqar, S., Siraj, M., Razzaq, Z., et al. (2011).

Procedure 26-11 ■ Administering Intradermal Medication

➤ For steps to follow in *all* procedures, refer to the Universal Steps for All Procedures found on the inside back cover. Also, refer to Medication Guidelines: Steps to Follow for All Medications (Regardless of Type or Route).

Equipment

- Alcohol prep pad or CHG-alcohol product
- 2 × 2 inch gauze pad
- Pen (ink or felt)
- 1-mL syringe (tuberculin) with intradermal needle (25- to 28 gauge, ¼- to ⅝ inch with short bevel)

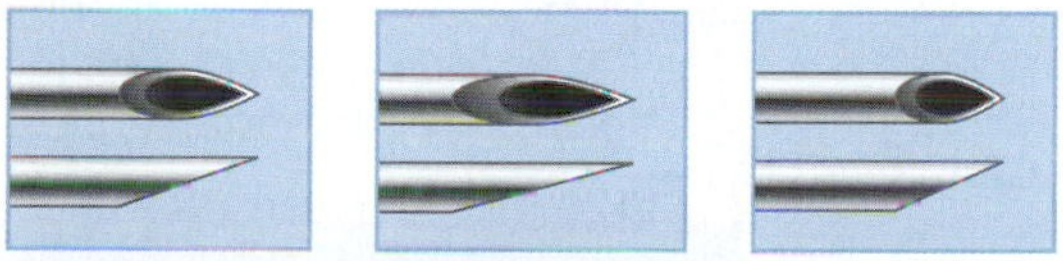

Delegation

As an RN, you can usually delegate administration of parenteral medications to an LPN/LVN. You usually cannot delegate this task to a UAP.

Pre-Procedure Assessments

- Assess for allergies, previous reactions to skin testing, and signs of irritation (e.g., bruising, swelling, tenderness).
Some skin tests, such as the tuberculin test, should not be repeated after positive test results. Do not administer intradermal skin tests if skin abnormalities are present. Also, avoid giving them in areas where reading the results may be difficult, such as areas of heavy hair growth.

Preparation

- Have appropriate antidotes (usually epinephrine hydrochloride, a bronchodilator, and an antihistamine) readily available before the start of the procedure.
Because many intradermal injections are used for allergy testing, this is an important consideration.
- Know the location of resuscitation equipment (artificial airway, Ambu bag, and code cart)
Allergic reactions can be fatal.

(continued on next page)

Procedure 26-11 ■ Administering Intradermal Medication (continued)

➤ When performing the procedure, always identify your patient according to agency policy, using two identifiers, and be attentive to standard precautions, hand hygiene, patient safety and privacy, body mechanics, and documentation.

Procedure Steps

1. **Draw up the medication** from the vial (see Procedure 26-9B). The usual dose is 0.01 to 0.1 mL.
Intradermal sites can only accommodate small volumes of medication.

2. **Select the site for injection.** Usual sites are the ventral surface of the forearm and upper back. The upper chest may also be used. If you need to review site locations,

Go to Chapter 26, Figure 26-23, in Volume 1.

Use areas where subcutaneous fat is less likely to interfere with administration and absorption. The forearm is the standard initial starting point because it has the least amount of subcutaneous tissue. The forearm and upper back usually have little hair, permitting easier visualization to interpret results accurately.

3. **Assist the patient to a comfortable position.** If you are using the forearm, instruct her to extend and supinate her arm on a flat surface. If you are using the upper back, ask the patient to lie prone or lean forward over a table or the back of a chair.
This method stabilizes the injection site. The procedure will be more comfortable if the patient is able to relax her muscles. Tension, in general, increases pain perception.

4. **Don procedure gloves.**
Procedure gloves are not required by OSHA for intradermal injections, but they are recommended by the CDC to prevent accidental exposure to bloodborne pathogens.

> Remember, gloves cannot prevent needlestick injuries.

5. **Scrub the injection site** with an alcohol prep pad or CHG-alcohol product pad. For an alcohol product, circle from the center of the site outward. For CHG products, use a back-and-forth motion. Allow the site to dry before administering the injection.
Cleansing to remove microorganisms follows the principle of "clean to dirty." Alcohol can interfere with the test results if a small amount is introduced during the injection. If the alcohol has not evaporated, it may cause the skin to sting during the injection.

6. **Grasp the syringe between the thumb and index finger** of your dominant hand, and uncap the needle.
Enables you to administer the solution at the correct angle.

7. **Hold the client's skin taut** with your nondominant hand by using one of the following methods:
   a. If using the forearm, you may be able to place your hand under the client's arm and pull the skin tight with your thumb and fingers.
   b. Stretch the client's skin between your thumb and index finger.
   c. Pull the client's skin toward the wrist or down with one finger.
   A downward motion while stretching the skin eases needle insertion. Holding the skin tight can be difficult because of the low angle of administration.

8. **Continuing to hold the client's skin taut** with your nondominant hand, hold the syringe in your dominant hand with the needle bevel up and parallel to the client's skin at a 5° to 15° angle. Slowly insert the needle. There is some controversy about whether it is better to have the bevel down or up; however, the CDC recommends bevel up.
The low angle of insertion is necessary to place the needle tip in the intradermal layer instead of the subcutaneous tissue. Having the bevel up likely decreases the chance of injecting the medication deeper into the subcutaneous tissue. Patients receiving intradermal injections report bevel up more comfortable.

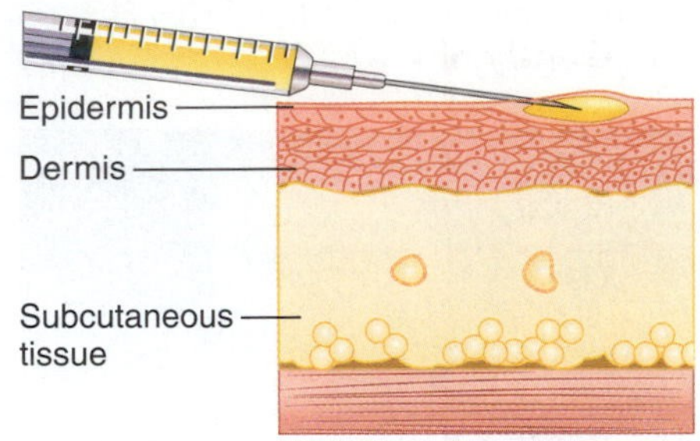

9. **Advance the needle** approximately 3 mm (1/8 inch) so that the entire bevel is covered. The bevel should be visible just under the skin.
If the entire bevel is not inserted, the solution will leak out of the tissue. If you can see the bevel under the surface of the skin, you can be sure that the bevel is not in the subcutaneous tissue.

10. **Do not aspirate.** Hold the syringe stable with your nondominant hand, and release the tightened skin.

11. **Slowly inject the solution.** You should feel firm resistance. A pale wheal, about 6 to 10 mm (1/4 inch) in diameter, will appear over the needle bevel.
The dermis does not have room to absorb the solution, so a wheal forms, stretching the skin. Slow administration gives you time to terminate the injection should a systemic reaction occur. If a bleb (wheal) forms, you have administered the drug properly. The size of the bleb depends on the amount of medication you injected.

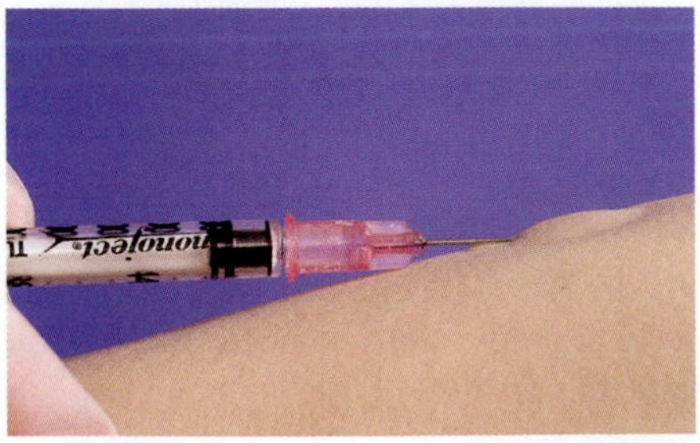

12. **Remove the needle** from the skin, engage the safety device, and dispose of the needle in a biohazard, puncture-proof container. If there is no safety device, place the uncapped syringe and needle directly in a biohazard, puncture-proof container.
Prevents needlestick injuries.

13. **Gently blot any blood** with a dry gauze pad. Do not rub the skin or cover it with an adhesive bandage.
Rubbing may cause the drug to leak out and alter absorption. An adhesive bandage can cause irritation and interfere with the skin test.

14. **With a pen, draw a 1-inch circle** around the bleb/wheal.
Marking the site helps you to identify any change in the size of the wheal at a later time.

? What if . . .

- **My patient has a history of a skin reaction to purified protein derivative (PPD) testing?**
Obtain details about the type and severity of the reaction. If the previous reaction involved ulceration at the site, further Mantoux testing is contraindicated. Report this to the prescriber.
- **My patient is pregnant, is receiving chemotherapy, or has severe eczema?**
Defer tuberculosis skin testing, and inform the prescriber.
- **My patient received a live vaccine at the time of tuberculosis skin testing?**
Tuberculosis skin testing should be deferred for 1 month after live viral vaccines or other major viral infection.
- **My patient has topical anesthetic cream on the skin?**
Use a site where the topical anesthetic cream was not applied, or reschedule tuberculosis skin testing for another date.

Evaluation

- Reassess the client 5 and 15 min after administration for allergic reactions that may subsequently occur.
- Read the site within 48 to 72 hours of injection, depending on the test.
- Observe that a wheal (about 6 to 8 mm in diameter) forms at the site and that it gradually disappears.
- Observe for minimal bruising that may develop at the site of injection.

Patient Teaching

- Explain when the patient needs to have the intradermal injection read to determine whether the result is positive or negative.
- Explain that mild itching, swelling, or irritation may occur at the injection site and is normal.
If the patient has antigens to the injected solution, a histamine response occurs, causing itching, swelling, or irritation. This response generally subsides within a week.
- Discuss the significance of a positive or negative skin test result. Explain that the appearance of some signs of irritation does not mean a positive test result.
- Instruct the patient not to scratch, apply lotions or creams, cover the site with a bandage, or scrub the site.
This might cause irritation and interfere with the test, which may produce false-positive results.

Documentation

- See the information in Medication Guidelines: Steps to Follow for All Medication (Regardless of Type or Route).
- Some medications require documentation of lot numbers (check agency policy).
- Document when the test is to be read.

Sample documentation

12/18/2021 0800 Explained purpose and procedure for Mantoux skin test. Client stated, "I need a PPD so that I can go to the long-term care facility." 0.2 mL of tuberculin purified protein placed in left forearm per physician prescription. No reaction noted 5 minutes after procedure. Will read test at 0800 on 12/20/2021 ——— M. Saleh, RN

Practice Resources

Diggle, J. (2014); Felicilda-Reynaldo, R. (2014); Garner, S. (2013); Tanizaki, H., Nakashima, C., Shimizuhira C., et al. (2015).

Thinking About the Procedure

The video **Administering Intradermal Medication,** along with questions and suggested responses, is available on the ***Davis's Nursing Skills Videos*** Web site on FADavis.com.

Procedure 26-12 ■ Administering Subcutaneous Medication

➤ For steps to follow in *all* procedures, refer to the Universal Steps for All Procedures found on the inside back cover. Also, refer to Medication Guidelines: Steps to Follow for All Medications (Regardless of Type or Route).

Equipment

- Syringe and needle appropriate for volume and site
- Alcohol prep pad or CHG-alcohol product
- Gauze pad (optional)

Delegation

As an RN, you can usually delegate administration of parenteral medications to an LPN/LVN. You usually cannot delegate this task to a UAP.

Pre-Procedure Assessments

- Check the selected site for inflammation, bruising, lumps, or other abnormalities that may contraindicate use of the site.
- Check the area for previous injection sites.
  Alternating among the arms, thighs, abdomen, and back changes the absorption rate of the medication. Absorption is fastest from the abdomen, then the arms, and lastly the thighs and back. Rotate sites within the same extremity or location, approximately 1 inch from the previous injection. Rotating the site helps prevent fat deposits and skin lumps.
- Do focused assessments for the specific medication being administered.

  Insulin: Check capillary blood sugar level, and determine when the patient will be having the next meal; check for signs of hypoglycemia or hyperglycemia.
  Insulin must be balanced with food intake to prevent the patient from developing hypoglycemia or hyperglycemia. Different insulins have specific rates of absorption, peak action, and duration. Some insulins, such as Humalog and regular insulin, are rapid acting. Before you administer rapid-acting insulin, the capillary blood sugar must be within the normal range or above, and the patient must be ready to eat. With Humalog, the patient's food tray should be in front of him before you administer the insulin.

  Heparin: Check activated partial thromboplastin time (aPTT) and for signs of overt bleeding (e.g., bleeding from gums, IV injection sites) and covert bleeding (e.g., blood in urine and stool)
  Heparin is an anticoagulant, so the major side effect is bleeding.

  NOTE: The aPTT will not be monitored as frequently with the low-molecular-weight heparins (LMWHs) because bleeding is less likely to occur.

➤ When performing the procedure, always identify your patient according to agency policy, using two identifiers, and be attentive to standard precautions, hand hygiene, patient safety and privacy, body mechanics, and documentation.

Procedure Steps

1. **Select an appropriate syringe and needle.**
   a. For insulin administration, you must use an insulin syringe—typically 0.3, 0.5, or 1.0 mL. Most insulin needles are 28 to 31 gauge. Needle length is often 3/16 to 1 inch. For more information about giving insulin, see Clinical Insight 26-6.

   Although both insulin and tuberculin (TB) syringes come in a 1-mL size, they are not interchangeable. Insulin syringes are calibrated in units; they have a permanent (nonremovable) needle and a very small amount of dead space.

   b. For other medications, for volumes less than 1 mL, use a tuberculin syringe with a 25- to 27-gauge, 3/8- to 5/8-inch needle.
   Because of the small increments on the tuberculin syringe, small doses can be measured more accurately.

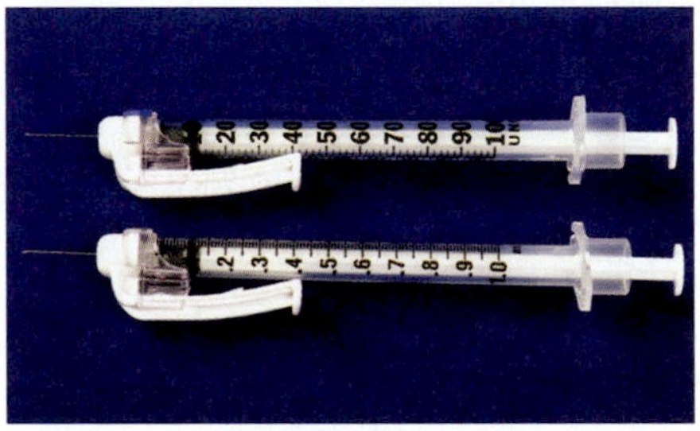

Top: Insulin syringe. *Bottom:* TB syringe.

   c. For administering a volume of 1 mL, you may use a 3-mL syringe with a 25- to 27-gauge, 3/8- to 5/8-inch needle.

   Subcutaneous injections are typically 1 mL or less.

   Although you can measure 1 mL with a tuberculin syringe, it will be difficult to handle the syringe because the plunger will be pulled back as far as it can go. It is easy to pull it inadvertently out of the end of the syringe. Some medications are supplied in prefilled syringes. Examples are enoxaparin sodium (Lovenox) and the other LMWHs.

2. **Draw up the medication.** See Procedure 26-9.
3. **Select an injection site** with adequate subcutaneous tissue. If you need to review site locations,

   Go to Chapter 26, Figure 26-25, in Volume 1.

   Helps avoid accidentally injecting into the muscle.
   a. The usual sites are the outer aspect of the upper arms, abdomen (at least 2 inches away from the umbilicus), anterior aspects of the thighs, and high on the buttocks near waist level.
   These areas usually have good circulation and are easily accessible. The buttocks are a more convenient site when the injection is administered by someone else, that is, when it is not self-administered.
   b. The anterolateral and posterolateral abdomen ("love handles") sites are the only subcutaneous

site used for administering heparin or LMWHs. For more information about giving heparin, see Clinical Insight 26-7.

The tissue 2 inches away from the umbilicus poses less risk of bleeding when an anticoagulant is administered.

4. **Position the patient** so that the injection site is accessible and the patient is able to relax the appropriate area. Check the site for inflammation, bruising, lumps, or other abnormalities.
Avoid areas with skin abnormalities, which may alter the absorption rates or increase patient discomfort during the injection.

5. **Don procedure gloves.**
To prevent exposure to bloodborne pathogens. You may prefer to don gloves before step 4.

6. **Scrub the injection site** with an alcohol prep pad or CHG-alcohol product. Allow the site to dry before administering the injection. For alcohol, circle from the site outward; for CHG, use a back-and-forth motion. Do not go back over already scrubbed areas.

7. **Remove the needle cap.**
The needle cap is more difficult to remove when using a one-handed technique.

8. **With your nondominant hand,** pinch the tissue at the injection site, and determine the angle at which to inject the needle. Insert the needle using a 45° to 90° angle, depending on the amount of adipose tissue (the less adipose tissue, the lower the angle). If the adipose tissue pinches 2 inches or more (client is obese), use a longer needle and spread the skin taut instead of pinching.
Grasping and lifting the tissue prevents you from accidentally injecting into the muscle. The subcutaneous injection must be given in the fatty tissue and not into intradermal layer. Traditionally, injections had been given using a 45° angle to ensure medication is deposited into the subcutaneous layer.

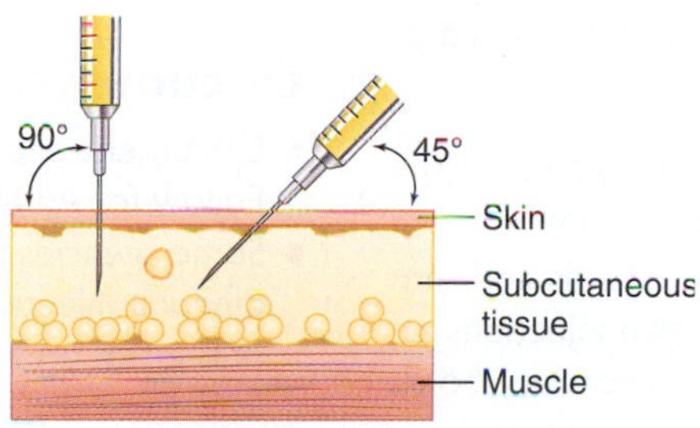

9. **Holding the syringe between the thumb and index finger** of your dominant hand like a pencil or dart, insert the needle at the appropriate angle into the skinfold.
Quickly inserting the needle through the skin minimizes discomfort.

10. **Using the thumb or index finger of your dominant hand,** press the plunger slowly to inject the medication while stabilizing the syringe with your other hand. Alternatively, after inserting the needle, you can continue to hold the barrel with your dominant hand and use your nondominant hand to depress the plunger.
Slow administration allows the medication to disperse and decreases discomfort. Subcutaneous injections do not need to be aspirated beforehand because accidental entry into a blood vessel is rare. Stabilize the syringe to avoid discomfort and tissue damage from the needle.

11. **Remove the needle** smoothly along the line of insertion.
Prevents pulling against the skin and tissue and thus minimizes discomfort.

12. **Gently blot the site with gauze,** if needed. Do not massage the site unless directed to do so by prescription or policy.
Occasionally, there will be blood at the site after the needle is removed. You might have nicked a surface blood vessel when you injected, and blood is following the needle track out to the surface. Massaging or rubbing the site will alter the rate of absorption of the medication.

13. **Engage the needle safety device,** and dispose of the needle in a biohazard container. If there is no safety device, place the uncapped syringe and needle directly into a biohazard, puncture-proof container.
A sharps container prevents needlestick injuries.

Evaluation

- Observe for minimal bruising that may develop at the site of injection.
- Reassess the patient for the anticipated response and any adverse reactions to the medication.

  For insulin, observe for signs that patient's blood sugar level has returned to normal and for signs of hypoglycemia.

  For heparin, observe for any signs of bleeding.

  For other medications, observe for side effects.

Patient Teaching

- Discuss possible lifestyle adaptations that the patient may need to undertake while receiving the medication (e.g., diet and exercise recommendations for managing diabetes mellitus).

Home Care

- Discuss with the client or caregiver the options for insulin administration to determine the most appropriate choice for the person administering the injections.
Many options are available, including specially designed syringes that are easier to handle and read, pen injectors, and prefilled syringes.
- In the home environment, the client might not routinely use an alcohol wipe to cleanse the site. This is acceptable as long as the skin is clean.
In the home environment, there is less risk for superinfection with resistant strains of organisms and other hospital-acquired infections.

(continued on next page)

Procedure 26-12 ■ Administering Subcutaneous Medication (continued)

- Do not encourage reusing needles and syringes. However, if the client or caregiver believes they need to reuse syringes and needles in the home, teach them how to safely do so. Teach them the guidelines in Clinical Insight 26-2.
- The very small insulin needles (30-gauge) bend very easily and are not recommended for reuse.

  Determine whether reusing syringes is appropriate for the patient. Contraindications include inadequate hygiene, immunocompromised status, and difficulty handling equipment to prevent contamination of the needle.

- Discuss safety concerns regarding subcutaneous medication administration in the home, such as how to dispose of biohazardous wastes correctly and where to obtain a puncture-proof biohazard container.

  The patient or caregiver may use a large plastic bottle or a coffee can. Local regulations regarding disposal must be followed.

- Discuss with the patient the need to rotate sites and the reasons for doing so. Recommend that he give injections at the same time of the day in the same body location about 1 inch from the previous injection site.
  Repeatedly giving the medication in the same site can cause abnormalities in the tissue and alter absorption rates.
- Remind the patient that when changing sites (thigh, arm, abdomen), the absorption rate may be altered.
- If the patient is receiving heparin or LMWHs, discuss the need to avoid nonsteroidal anti-inflammatory drugs (NSAIDs), such as acetylsalicylic acid (aspirin) and ibuprofen (Motrin, Advil).
  These drugs increase the risk of bleeding.
- For patients receiving heparin or LMWHs, discuss home safety measures and the need to avoid falls.
  The patient is at risk for bleeding and needs to follow safety guidelines to prevent injury. Research shows that older females are more susceptible to hematomas after administration of LMWH (Kim, Kang, Ryu, et al., 2014; Nourbakhsh, Anvari, & Nugent, 2011). Nurses should carefully assess for abdominal bruising and complaints of abdominal pain.

Documentation

- Document according to Medication Guidelines: Steps to Follow for All Medication (Regardless of Type or Route).
- Some agencies have a specific code for documenting subcutaneous injections, which allows for exact documentation of the site on an outline of the body.
- In the nursing notes, document any related patient assessment findings, such as capillary blood sugar, signs of hypoglycemia or hyperglycemia, bruising, and so on.
- Document in the nursing notes as well as MAR any medication that was given prn.

Sample EHR documentation

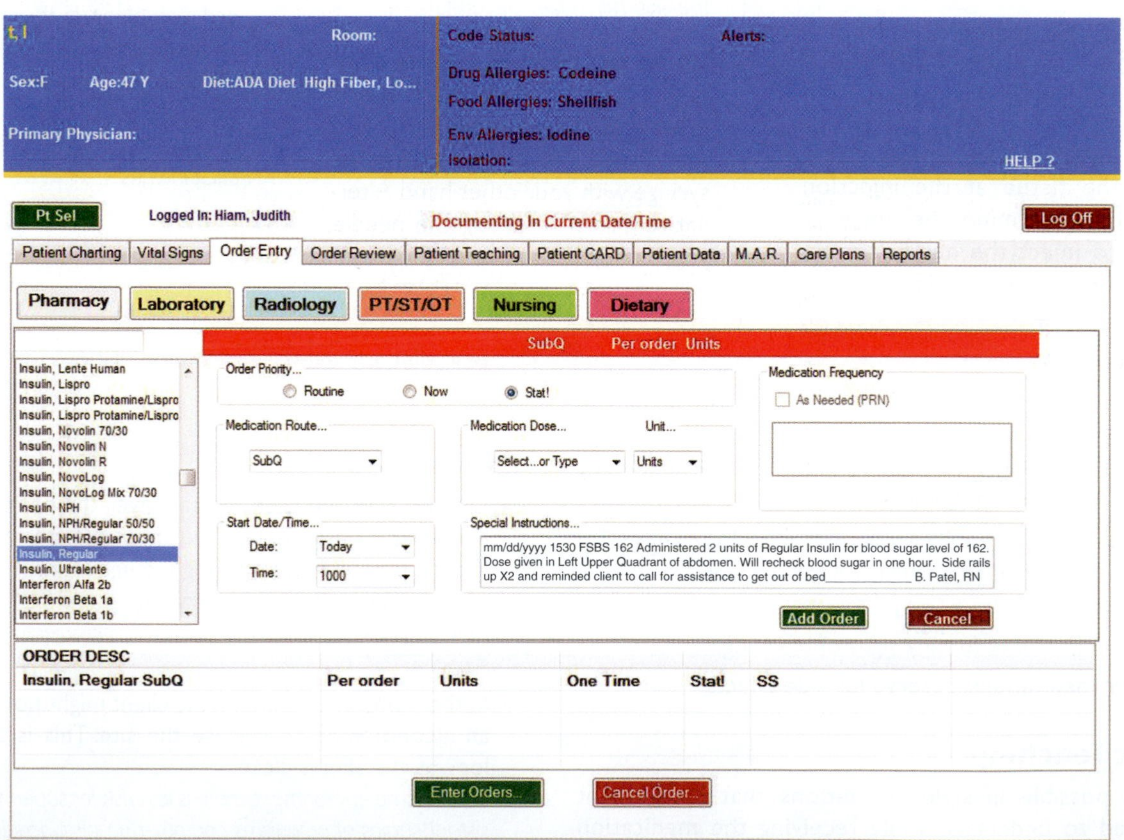

Practice Resources

Kim, H., Park, H. & Lee, S. (2017); Ogston-Tuck, S. (2014b); Pourghaznein, T., Azimi, A.V., & Jafarabadi, M. A. (2014); Sexton, K., Lindauer, A. & Harvath, T. (2016).

Thinking About the Procedure

The video **Administering Subcutaneous Medication,** along with questions and suggested responses, is available on the ***Davis's Nursing Skills Videos*** Web site on FADavis.com.

Procedure 26-13 ■ Locating Intramuscular Injection Sites

➤ For steps to follow in *all* procedures, refer to the Universal Steps for All Procedures found on the inside back cover. Also, refer to Medication Guidelines: Steps to Follow for All Medications (Regardless of Type or Route).

Delegation

As an RN, you can usually delegate administration of parenteral medications (including locating injection sites) to an LPN/LVN. You usually cannot delegate this task to a UAP. If you delegate the skill, you are responsible for evaluating the LPN/LVN's ability to locate injection sites correctly.

Pre-Procedure Assessment

Always palpate the landmarks and the muscle mass to ensure correct placement of the needle. Because patients' body shapes vary, the site locations will differ slightly.

Procedure 26-13A ■ Locating the Ventrogluteal Site

➤ When performing the procedure, always identify your patient according to agency policy, using two identifiers, and be attentive to standard precautions, hand hygiene, patient safety and privacy, body mechanics, and documentation.

Procedure Steps

1. **Ask the patient to assume a side-lying position,** with the legs straight, if possible.
   This position makes the site easier to locate.

2. **Locate the greater trochanter,** anterior superior iliac spine, and the iliac crest.

3. **Place the palm of your hand** on the greater trochanter, your index finger on the anterior superior iliac spine, and your middle finger pointing toward the iliac crest. (Use your right hand on the patient's left hip; use your left hand on the patient's right hip.) Note that if your hands are very large or very small, the location of the "triangle" will be higher or lower on the hip. Be sure you locate it well in the muscle mass.

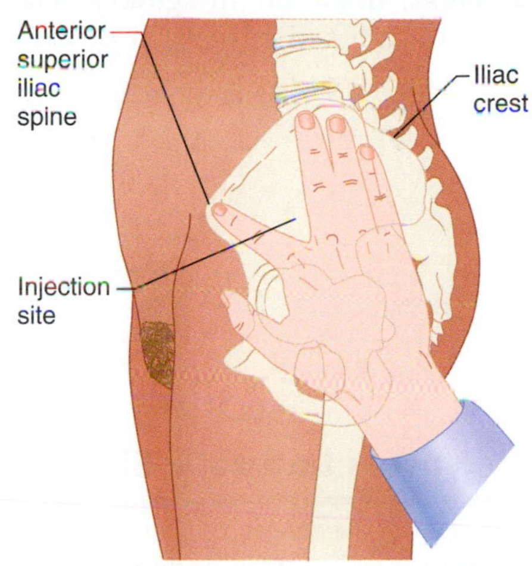

4. **The middle of the triangle** between your middle and index fingers is the injection site.
   This is a safe site for IM administration because it is not close to any major blood vessels or nerves. The landmarks are easy to find. This large muscle can take volumes up to 5 mL in the average adult. It is safe for patients of all ages and the preferred site for adults and children older than 7 to 12 months (there is some disagreement over the age; always palpate to assess adequacy of muscle mass, regardless of age).▼

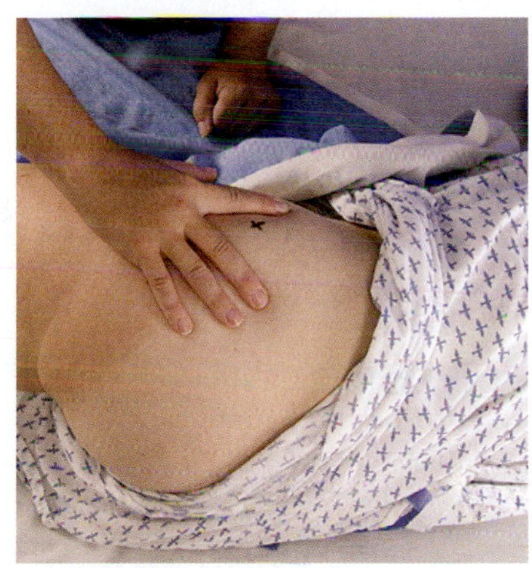

(continued on next page)

Procedure 26-13 ■ Locating Intramuscular Injection Sites (continued)

Procedure 26-13B ■ Locating the Deltoid Site

➤ When performing the procedure, always identify your patient according to agency policy, using two identifiers, and be attentive to standard precautions, hand hygiene, patient safety and privacy, body mechanics, and documentation.

Procedure Steps

1. **Completely expose the patient's upper arm.** Remove the garment; do not roll up the sleeve.
   Incomplete exposure of site and landmarks creates a risk of injecting into a site other than muscle tissue. This is a small site, and it is easy to make an error in location.

2. **Locate the lower edge** of the acromion process (knobby part of shoulder), and go two to three fingerbreadths down. Your bottom finger will form the base of an upside-down triangle. ▼

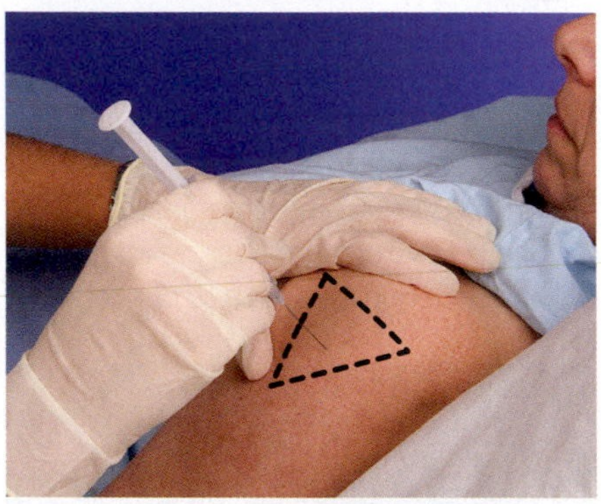

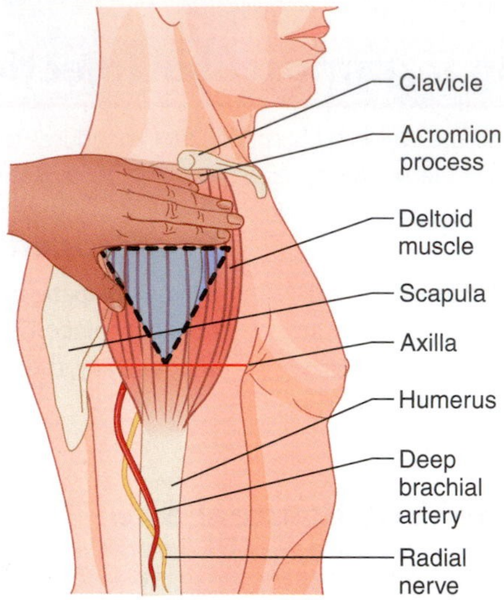

3. **Next, draw an imaginary line** from each end of the triangle base downward 3 to 5 cm (1 to 2 in.) to the midpoint of the lateral arm. The midpoint forms the apex of the triangle.

4. **The deltoid site is in the center** of the resulting inverted triangle.

5. **An alternative approach** is to place four fingerbreadths across the deltoid muscle, with your top finger on the acromion process. The injection goes three fingerbreadths below the process in the midline of the upper arm.
   Locates the appropriate site while avoiding the radial nerve and deep brachial artery. Because it is a fairly small muscle, only 0.5 to 1 mL of medication can be administered.

Procedure 26-13C ■ Locating the Vastus Lateralis Site

➤ When performing the procedure, always identify your patient according to agency policy, using two identifiers, and be attentive to standard precautions, hand hygiene, patient safety and privacy, body mechanics, and documentation.

Procedure Steps

1. **Position the patient** in a supine or sitting position.
   The patient may perceive the injection as less painful if supine because she cannot see the needle enter her leg. In some patients, seeing the injection may cause anxiety and intensify the pain.

2. **Locate the greater trochanter** and the lateral femoral condyle.

3. **Place your hands on the thigh,** with one hand against the greater trochanter and the other against the lateral femoral condyle.

4. **Visualize a rectangle** between your hands across the anterolateral thigh.
   - The index fingers of your hands form the smaller ends of the rectangle.
   - The long sides of the rectangle are formed by (a) drawing an imaginary line down the center of the anterior thigh and (b) drawing another line along the side of the leg, halfway between the bed and the front of the thigh.

- **This box marks the middle third of the anterolateral thigh, which is the injection site.**

  The rectus femoris lies on the top (or anterior) portion of the thigh and partially covers the edge of the vastus lateralis. Therefore, do not inject too near the midline of the anterior thigh. Because it is not near any major blood vessels or nerves, the vastus lateralis site is safe for patients of all ages and is the recommended site for children younger than 7 months of age.

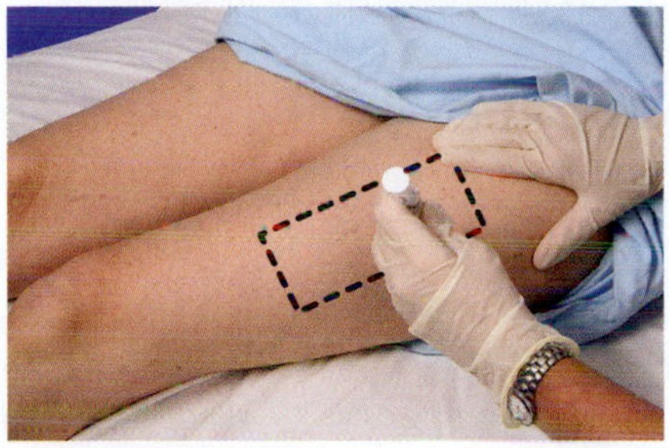

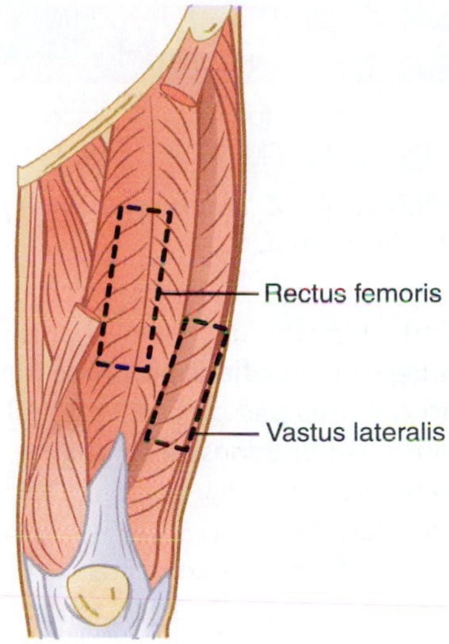

Procedure 26-13D ■ Locating the Rectus Femoris Site

➤ When performing the procedure, always identify your patient according to agency policy, using two identifiers, and be attentive to standard precautions, hand hygiene, patient safety and privacy, body mechanics, and documentation.

Procedure Steps

Key Point: ***Use this site only if no other sites are accessible and no other medication routes are feasible.***

1. **Position the patient** in a supine or sitting position.
2. **Divide the top of the thigh into thirds** from the groin to the knee, and identify the middle third.
3. **Visualize a rectangle** in the middle of the anterior surface of the thigh. This is the location of the injection site. Also, refer to the drawing of the adult thigh in Procedure 26-13C. ➤

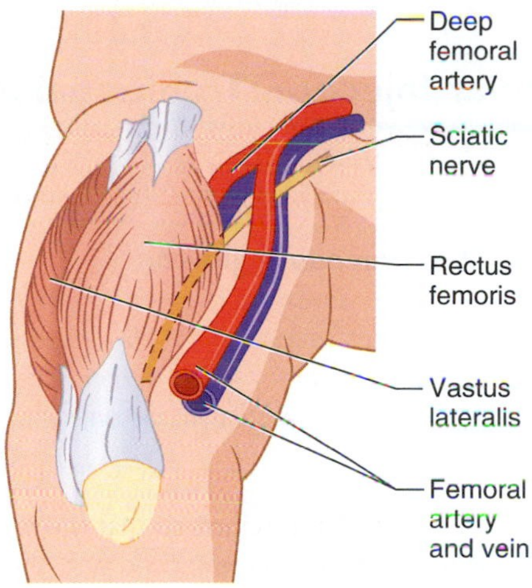

? What if . . .

- **My patient is a child? What is the best site to give an IM injection?**

  Because an infant's muscles are not fully developed, site selection is limited.

  For children who are walking, use the ventrogluteal site.

  For children who are not yet walking, use the vastus lateralis. Once the gluteal muscles have developed further, which occurs with walking, the ventrogluteal site can be used.

Thinking About the Procedure

The videos **Locating the Ventrogluteal Site, Locating the Deltoid Site,** and **Locating the Vastus Lateralis Site,** along with questions and suggested responses, are available on the ***Davis's Nursing Skills Videos*** Web site on FADavis.com.

Procedure 26-14 ■ Administering an Intramuscular Injection

➤ For steps to follow in *all* procedures, refer to the Universal Steps for All Procedures found on the inside back cover. Also, refer to Medication Guidelines: Steps to Follow for All Medications (Regardless of Type or Route).

Key Point: ***The Z-track method is preferred for all IM injections, except in the rare instance where it is contraindicated.***

Equipment

- Syringe and needle appropriate for volume and site
- Alcohol prep pad or CHG-alcohol product
- Gauze pad or adhesive bandage
- Medication
- Procedure gloves
- Biohazard (sharps) container
- Small piece of gauze or cotton ball
- Small adhesive bandage

Delegation

As an RN, you can usually delegate administration of parenteral medications to an LPN/LVN. You cannot delegate this task to a UAP.

Pre-Procedure Assessments

- Identify the site of the previous injection.
- Assess the site for adequate muscle mass, bruises, edema, tenderness, redness, or other abnormalities.
  Muscle mass must be large enough to absorb the amount of medication prescribed. Abnormalities at the site increase patient discomfort and alter the absorption rate of the medication.
- Assess for factors that might affect absorption of the medication, such as decreased intramuscular blood flow, as found in shock or muscle atrophy.
  Decreased peripheral circulation or muscle atrophy decreases the absorption of the medication.

Procedure 26-14A ■ Intramuscular Injection: Traditional Method

➤ When performing the procedure, always identify your patient according to agency policy, using two identifiers, and be attentive to standard precautions, hand hygiene, patient safety and privacy, body mechanics, and documentation.

Procedure Steps

1. Select the appropriate syringe and needle.

a. The usual syringe size is 1 to 3 mL, depending on volume of medication to be given. For doses less than 1 mL, you can use a tuberculin syringe with an intramuscular needle.

b. The needle size is usually 21- to 25-gauge, length is 1½ in. for adults (or 1 in. for the deltoid site), but if the patient is obese, a longer needle (3-in.) may be necessary to penetrate the muscle.
For IM administration, the needle gauge must be appropriate for the viscosity of the medication, and the needle must be long enough to deliver the medication into the muscle.

c. Some medications are supplied in prefilled syringes, which are used for administration.

2. Draw up the medication (see Procedure 26-9A), or obtain the prescribed unit dose, and verify the medication. If the volume for injection is more than 3 to 5 mL, divide the dose for separate injections.

3. Don procedure gloves.
Procedure gloves are required by OSHA to prevent exposure to bloodborne pathogens. You may prefer to don gloves at step 6, while waiting for the antiseptic to dry.

4. Position the patient so that the injection site is well exposed and the patient is able to relax the appropriate muscles. Ensure that the lighting is adequate.
When the patient's muscles are relaxed (and not tense), it is easier to perform the injection, and patient discomfort during injection is reduced. You must be able to fully visualize and safely access the site.

a. ***Deltoid site:*** Position the patient with the arm relaxed at the side or resting on a firm surface, and completely expose the upper arm.

NOTE: For small medication amounts only (0.5 to 1 mL).

b. ***Ventrogluteal site:*** Position the patient on the opposite side, with the upper hip and knee slightly flexed.
This position may cause the trochanter to become more prominent, making it easier to locate the site.

c. ***Vastus lateralis:*** Position the patient supine or sitting, as the patient prefers.

d. ***Rectus femoris:*** Position the patient supine. **iCare** Because this site often causes more discomfort than others, use it only if all other sites are inaccessible and no other route is feasible.

e. ***Dorsogluteal:*** Do not use this site because of the muscle's proximity to the sciatic nerve and major blood vessels.

5. Using appropriate landmarks, identify the injection site (see Procedure 26-13). If the client is to receive more than one injection, rotate sites.
Volumes of 1 to 5 mL may be given, depending on the muscle size (for adults, 0.5 to 1 mL in the deltoid; and typically 1 to 3 mL but up to 5 mL in the vastus lateralis site). If the volume for injection is more than 3 to 5 mL, then divide the dose for a separate injection. Rotating sites reduces discomfort and tissue trauma.

6. **Gently, but thoroughly scrub the injection site.** Do not "go back over" already cleansed areas.
   a. If using an alcohol prep pad, thoroughly clean the site by circling from the center of the site outward.
   b. If using a CHG-based antiseptic, use a back-and-forth motion.
   Cleanse to remove microorganisms; follow the principle of "clean to dirty."

7. **Place the wipe on the patient's skin** outside the injection site, with a corner pointing to the site. Allow the site to dry before administering the injection. Do not fan the site.
Leaving the antiseptic prep pad on the skin with a corner pointing to the injection site helps identify the location for the injection. If the antiseptic has not evaporated, it may cause the skin to sting during injection.

8. **Remove the needle cap.**

9. **With your nondominant hand,** spread the skin taut between your thumb and index finger.
It is quicker, easier, and less painful to insert a needle through the skin that is taut.

10. **Tell the patient what you are going to do** and that he will feel a prick as you insert the needle. Then, hold the syringe between the thumb and fingers of your dominant hand, like holding a pencil or dart, and insert the needle at a 90° angle to the skin surface. Insert fully.
Quickly inserting the needle through the skin minimizes discomfort. A 90° angle is needed for the needle to penetrate through the subcutaneous and adipose tissue to the muscle.

11. **Stabilize the syringe** with your nondominant hand.
This prevents the needle from moving around in the tissue, thereby causing discomfort and possible tissue trauma.

12. (If required by the agency policy) **Aspirate by pulling back on the plunger** and waiting for 5 to 10 sec. If you obtain a blood return, remove the needle, discard the syringe, and prepare the medication again. If there is no blood return, continue with step 13.
Aspirating blood indicates that the needle is in a blood vessel. Injecting would result in administering the medication intravenously instead of intramuscularly. If the needle is in a small vessel, it may take a few seconds for the blood to appear in the syringe. **Key Point:** ***There are variations in practice with regard to the requirement to aspirate for blood. Be sure to check with your instructor or the institution's protocol for the recommended method.***

13. **Using the thumb or index finger** of your dominant hand, press the plunger slowly to inject the medication (5 to 10 sec/mL).
Slow administration allows the medication to disperse and decreases discomfort.

14. **Remove the needle smoothly** along the line of insertion.
Removing the needle in this way prevents pulling against the skin and tissue and minimizes discomfort.

15. **Engage the safety device,** and dispose of the entire syringe in a biohazard container. If there is no safety device, place the uncapped syringe and needle directly into a biohazard puncture-proof container.
The biohazard sharps container prevents needlestick injuries.

16. **Gently blot the site** with a gauze pad, and apply an adhesive bandage, as needed.
Apply pressure to stop the bleeding, but do not massage or rub the site after an IM injection. This can cause the medication to disperse into the subcutaneous tissue where the needle was injected, which might be irritating to the tissue.

Procedure 26-14B ■ Intramuscular Injection: Z-Track Method

➤ When performing the procedure, always identify your patient according to agency policy, using two identifiers, and be attentive to standard precautions, hand hygiene, patient safety and privacy, body mechanics, and documentation.

Procedure Steps

1–8. Follow Procedure 26-14A, traditional method, preceding.

Step 5 Variation. For Z-Track Method, use the Larger Muscles:

a. ***Ventrogluteal site:*** Position patient on the side with upper hip and knee slightly flexed.
b. ***Vastus lateralis:*** Position patient supine or sitting.

9. **With the side of your nondominant hand,** displace the skin away from the injection site, about 2.5 to 3.5 cm (1 to 1.5 in.).
This displaces the skin and subcutaneous tissue over the muscle so that when it is released after the injection, the medication is sealed in the muscle.

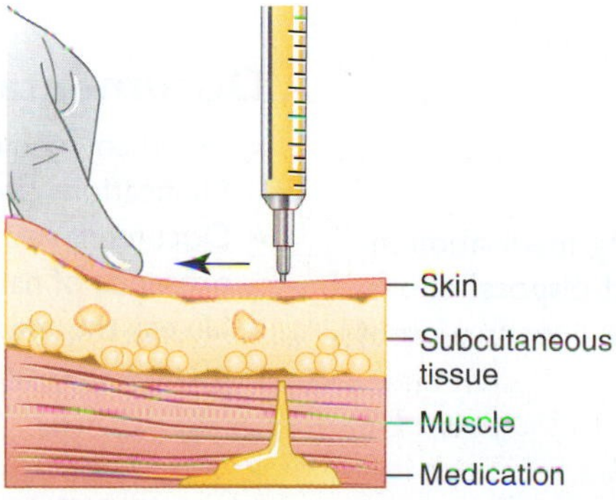

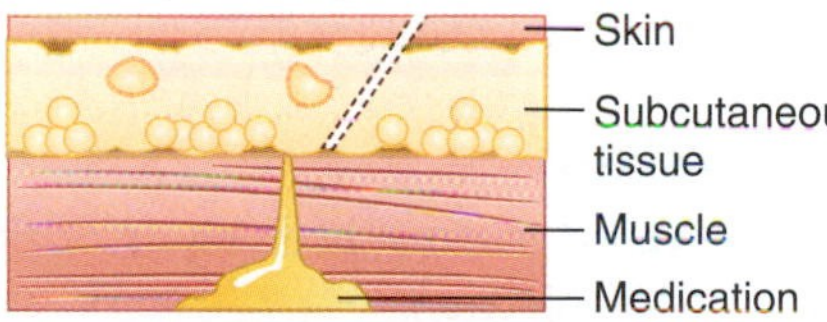

10. **Holding the syringe between the thumb and fingers of your dominant hand,** like holding a pencil or dart, insert the needle at a 90° angle to the skin surface. Insert smoothly, quickly, and fully.
Quickly inserting the needle through the skin minimizes discomfort. A 90° angle is needed for the needle to penetrate through the subcutaneous and adipose tissue to the muscle.

(continued on next page)

Procedure 26-14 ■ Administering an Intramuscular Injection (continued)

11. **Stabilize the syringe** with the thumb and forefinger of your nondominant hand while continuing to displace the skin with your other three fingers. Do not release the skin to stabilize the syringe.
Stabilizing the needle reduces discomfort and possible tissue injury. You must keep the skin retracted to create a seal after the medication is injected and the skin released.

12. **Aspirate by pulling back slightly** on the plunger for 5 to 10 seconds, if required by agency policy. If you obtain a blood return, remove the needle, discard the syringe, and prepare the medication again. You should follow your institution's policy regarding aspiration with parenteral injections.
Aspirating blood indicates that the needle has penetrated a vein. Continuing could result in administering the medication intravenously instead of intramuscularly.

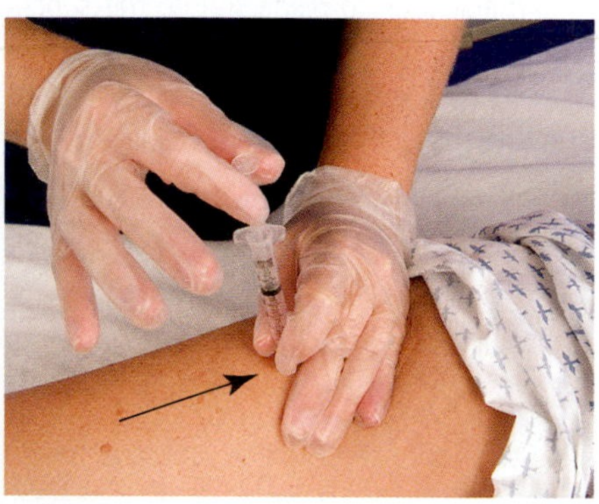

13. **Using the thumb or index finger** of your dominant hand, press the plunger slowly to inject the medication (5 to 10 sec/mL).
Slow administration allows the medication to disperse and decreases discomfort.

14. **Wait for 10 seconds**, then withdraw the needle smoothly along the line of insertion, then immediately release the skin.
Waiting before withdrawing the needle leaves a zigzag needle track that traps the medication in the muscle, preventing it from leaking up into the subcutaneous tissue.

15. **Engage the safety needle device**, and dispose of it in a biohazard container. If there is no safety device, place the uncapped syringe and needle directly in a biohazard puncture-proof container.

16. **Hold a cotton ball or gauze pad** with light pressure over the injection site. Do not massage the site. Apply an adhesive bandage, if necessary.
Light pressure will stop superficial bleeding at the injection site. Massaging and rubbing can force medication into the subcutaneous tissues.

? What if . . .

- **My patient is unable to cooperate during the procedure?**
Ask another healthcare provider or family member to help keep the patient from moving during the injection or to help position the patient.

- **My patient is a child? Is there anything different about giving an IM injection to a child?**
Adapt the following procedure to decrease pain: Apply topical anesthetic cream (e.g., EMLA [lidocaine–prilocaine]) or a topical cooling spray, if time permits. If not, distract the child with conversation, give him something to do, squeeze a hand, or apply a cold compress over the site.
Adapt the way you spread the skin to inject: In infants and small children, grasp the muscle with your thumb and index finger; in obese children, spread the skin and then grasp the muscle.
Adapt the medication volume: Inject no more than 1 mL in a single injection, 0.5 mL in a small infant.
The CDC recommends 1- and 1¼-inch needles for children 1 year old or younger. Follow agency procedures.

- **My patient is an older adult?**
Many older adults have decreased muscle mass, so use a shorter needle; spread the skin and grasp the muscle to localize and stabilize the site for injection.
Older adults tend to bleed from the site after injection because of reduced tissue elasticity. Apply a small pressure bandage, if needed.

Evaluation

- Observe for minimal bruising or oozing that may occur at the site of injection.
- Observe for local reactions at site (e.g., pain, swelling, redness).

Home Care

- Discuss safety concerns with administering medication intramuscularly in the home, such as correct disposal of biohazardous wastes, and where to obtain a puncture-proof biohazard container.
The caregiver or the patient can use a large plastic bottle. The local regulations must be followed for disposal.
- Discuss with the client the need to rotate sites.
Repeatedly giving the medication in the same site can cause abnormalities in the tissue and alter absorption rates.

Documentation

- Refer to Medication Guidelines: Steps to Follow for All Medications (Regardless of Type or Route).
- Document related assessment findings, such as pain level or presence of nausea.
- Unless the medication is given prn, you will typically document it only on the MAR.

Sample documentation for prn medication:

12/18/2021 1600 Client reports of nausea after ambulating 150 feet with assistive device. Phenergan 25 mg administered IM in right ventrogluteal site. No complaints of pain or discomfort. See MAR. ——— M. Santos, RN.

12-18-2021 1700 Client reports "I don't feel like I'm going to vomit anymore." ——— M. Santos, RN.

Practice Resources

Bartley, N. (2012a); Ogston-Tuck, S. (2014a); Sepah, Y., Samad, L., Altaf, A., et al. (2017); Strohfus, P., Paugh, O., Tindell, C., et al. (2018)

Thinking About the Procedure

The videos **Intramuscular Injection: Traditional Method** and **Intramuscular Injection: Z-Track Method,** along with questions and suggested responses, are available on the ***Davis's Nursing Skills Videos*** Web site on FADavis.com.

Procedure 26-15 ■ Adding Medications to Intravenous Fluids

➤ For steps to follow in *all* procedures, refer to the Universal Steps for All Procedures found on the inside back cover. Also, refer to Medication Guidelines: Steps to Follow for All Medications (Regardless of Type or Route).

Equipment

- Prescribed IV solution
- Syringe for measuring medication
- Needleless access device or safety needle (if a VAD is not available)
- Antimicrobial swab
- Label with medication, dose, date, time, and your initials

Delegation

As an RN, you would not usually delegate adding medications to IV fluids to LPN/LVNs. Nurse Practice Acts governing IV medication administration vary from state to state, and policies can further vary among healthcare agencies regarding which additives can be added by LPN/LVNs. Even if you delegate the skill, you are always responsible for evaluating the patient's responses, both therapeutic effects and adverse effects.

Pre-Procedure Assessments

- Assess the patency of the IV site.
- Assess the appearance of the IV site.
- Check the medication insert or the *Physician's Desk Reference (PDR)* for the appropriate time and rate for infusion and for compatibility.

➤ When performing the procedure, always identify your patient according to agency policy, using two identifiers, and be attentive to standard precautions, hand hygiene, patient safety and privacy, body mechanics, and documentation.

Procedure Steps

1. **Determine** whether the medications are compatible with the IV solution and with each other.
Not all medications or other additives can be mixed with the glucose or saline normally found in the primary IV bag. Multiple additives increase the risk of incompatibility.

2. **Calculate or verify the amount of medication** to be instilled into the IV solution, and the rate of administration.
Verifying the dose and the rate of infusion prevents medication errors.

3. **Remove any protective covers,** and inspect the bag or bottle for leaks, tears, or cracks. Inspect the fluid for clarity, color, and presence of any particulate matter. Check the expiration date.
Double-checking the IV solution reduces the risk of infusing contaminated or expired solutions.

4. **Using the appropriate technique,** draw up the prescribed medication (see Procedure 26-9, as needed). Alternatively, insert a VAD transfer device into the medication vial.
Medications can come in vials, ampules, or bags, with differences in administration techniques.

5. **Gently and thoroughly clean all surfaces of the IV additive port** with an alcohol or CHG-alcohol combination product.
Diligent cleaning with antimicrobial products reduces the transmission of microorganisms and helps maintain the sterility of the solution.

6. **Remove the cap from the syringe,** insert the needle or the needleless access device into the injection port, and inject the medication into the bag, maintaining aseptic technique. ▼

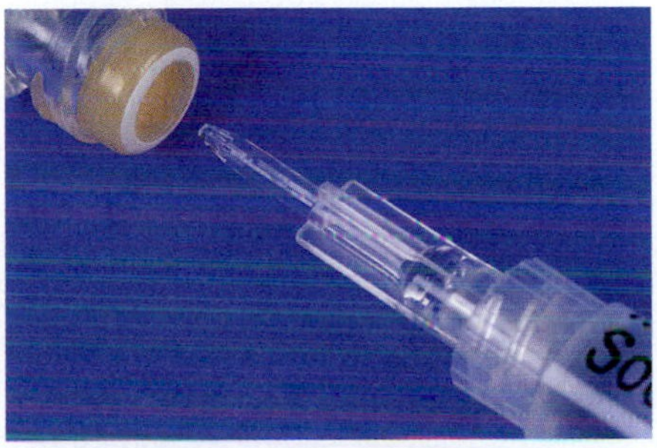

7. **Mix the IV solution and medication** by gently turning the bag from end to end.
Ensures even distribution of the medication or additive into the solution.

(continued on next page)

Procedure 26-15 ■ Adding Medications to Intravenous Fluids (continued)

8. **Place a label on the bag** so that it can be read when the bag is hung; include the medication name, dose, route, and your name. Be sure the label does not cover the solution label or volume marks.
   A label informs you and others of additives added to IV solutions. ➤

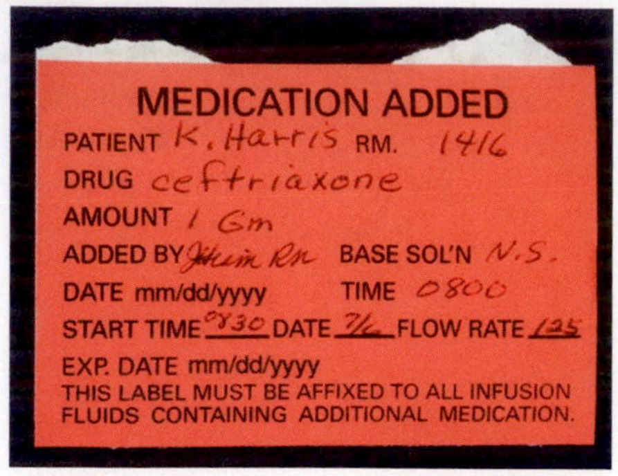

9. **Dispose of used equipment,** syringe, or VAD appropriately.

Evaluation

- Check the IV line at least once every hour to ensure that the ordered or calculated rate is maintained.
- Assess the patient for complaints of pain or signs of infiltration at the infusion site (e.g., redness, swelling).

Patient Teaching

- Discuss reasons the medication is being given intravenously.
- Explain whether it is a continuous or intermittent infusion.
- Explain the need to report immediately any reactions to the medication, such as breathing problems, rashes, or pain at the IV insertion site.

Documentation

- Document information according to Medication Guidelines: Steps to Follow for All Medications (Regardless of Type or Route).
- Document any findings on an IV flow record rather than in the nursing notes. Chart a nursing note only if there is something outside of the expected findings (e.g., if the IV has infiltrated).

Practice Resources

Gorski L.A., Hadaway L., Hagle M., et al. (2016)

Procedure 26-16 ■ Administering IV Push Medication

➤ For steps to follow in *all* procedures, refer to the Universal Steps for All Procedures found on the inside back cover. Also, refer to Medication Guidelines: Steps to Follow for All Medications (Regardless of Type or Route).

Equipment

- Syringe appropriate for medication volume and the type of line (e.g., peripheral IV, peripherally inserted central catheter [PICC])
- If you are administering through an intermittent device:
  - Two 5- to 10-mL syringes, or one 10-mL syringe with 2 to 10 mL of normal saline or heparin for flushing the line.
    Although either is acceptable, separate syringes pose less risk of contamination.
  - Depending on site and facility policy, one 5- to 10-mL syringe containing 2 to 5 mL of heparin flush (or saline) solution.
    Previous research indicated that heparin 100 units/mL, rather than saline solution, was recommended (Bertolino, Pitassi, Tinelli, et al., 2012); however, more recent research found little evidence to support that heparin was more effective than saline flush for central venous catheter (CVC) maintenance (López-Briz, E., Ruiz, G., Cabello, J., et al., 2018; Zhong, Wang, Xu, et al., 2017)
- Alcohol prep pad, or CHG-alcohol combination product and gauze pad
- Procedure gloves

Delegation

As an RN, you may, in some situations, be able to delegate administration of parenteral medications to an LPN/LVN. However, this is not a common practice.

Pre-Procedure Assessments

- Determine the type and amount of dilution needed for the medication.
- Check the compatibility of the medication with the existing IV solution, if it is infusing.
  Medications can be physically or chemically incompatible with the IV solution. Physical incompatibility is often obvious because precipitation may occur. Chemical incompatibility is not obvious and may result in the medication's having a weaker or a stronger effect than anticipated.
- Assess the patency of the IV line.
  If the line is occluded, you will not be able to instill the medication.
- Check the site for redness, swelling, tenderness, and other signs of infiltration or phlebitis.
  Some medications are irritating and may be toxic to the tissue. If the IV line is infiltrated, the medication may leak into the tissue and cause injury. IV medications can also irritate the veins and cause phlebitis. Do not infuse a medication into a compromised site.

Procedure 26-16A ■ Administering IV Push Medications Through a Primary IV Line

➤ When performing the procedure, always identify your patient according to agency policy, using two identifiers, and be attentive to standard precautions, hand hygiene, patient safety and privacy, body mechanics, and documentation.

Procedure Steps

1. **Determine how fast the medication may be administered** and whether the medication needs to be diluted for administration. Also, check to be sure the medication is compatible with the solution infusing.
IV push medications are frequently injected over 1 minute. Some must infuse over a longer time period, and some require diluting before administration. Giving an IV push medication too fast and/or undiluted can result in local or systemic adverse reactions.

2. **Prepare the medication** from a vial or ampule or obtain the prescribed unit dose and verify medication with the order (refer to Procedure 26-9). Dilute as needed. Temporarily pause the infusion pump to administer the medication. If the primary bag is infusing by gravity, simply clamp the tubing.

3. **Don procedure gloves,** and vigorously scrub all surfaces of the injection port closest to the patient with an alcohol prep pad or CHG-alcohol combination product (Gorski L. A., Hadaway L., Hagle M., et al., 2016).
   (a) *Scrub time: Follow agency policy. Some facilities require nurses to cleanse the port for 1 minute when accessing venous access devices.*
   (b) *The port: Using the port closest to the patient minimizes the distance the medication must travel and gets it into the patient's circulation faster. You must use an injection port, which is self-sealing because if you puncture the plastic IV tubing, it will leak.*
   (c) *Scrub agent: Use povidone-iodine solution (Betadine) only if the patient is sensitive to alcohol or CHG-alcohol combination.*

4. **Insert the medication syringe** into the injection port. If a needleless system is not available, use a syringe with a safety needle.
Using a needleless system prevents needlestick injuries.

5. **Pinch or clamp the IV tubing** between the IV bag and the port.
Occluding the tubing upline of the port prevents the medication from being injected back toward the IV bag.

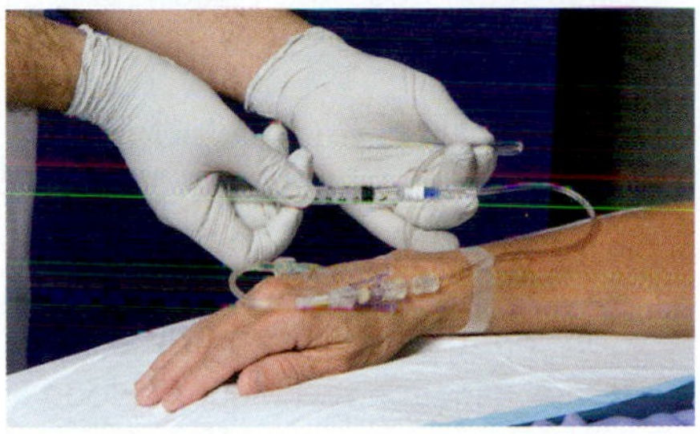

6. **Gently aspirate** by slowly pulling back on the plunger to check for a blood return.

   NOTE: Some newer connectors do not require or allow for aspiration. Follow institutional policy.

   (a) *A blood return is one indication that the IV catheter is in the vein. An IV site may still be patent if no blood is returned, and an infiltrated IV line may have a blood return. Use the blood return as one indication of patency (Phillips, 2015).*
   (b) *Injecting an IV medication into an IV site that is not patent administers the medication into the local tissue at the IV site. Some medications will cause tissue irritation and even necrosis if infused into the subcutaneous tissue. In addition, the patient would not receive the immediate therapeutic benefit from the drug.*

7. **If you have aspirated and obtained a blood return,** administer a small increment of the medication while observing for reactions to the medication.
Slow injection allows you to observe adverse reactions to the medication before all the medication has been injected. Administering IV push medications carries the highest potential risk to the patient because immediate, life-threatening reactions can occur.

8. **Administer another increment** of the medication (you may pinch the tubing while injecting medication and release it when not injecting; this is optional).

9. **Repeat steps 7 and 8 until** the full dose of medication has been administered over the prescribed amount of time.
Medications require different administration times. Follow agency guidelines, provider prescriptions, and pharmaceutical information regarding the need to dilute the medication and the rate of administration.

10. **If you clamped the IV tubing** during the infusion, open it now and reset the pump at the correct infusion rate, if necessary.

11. **Dispose of used supplies safely** and according to agency procedures.

(continued on next page)

Procedure 26-16 ■ Administering IV Push Medication (continued)

Procedure 26-16B ■ Administering IV Push Medications Through an Intermittent Device (IV Lock) When No Extension Tubing Is Attached to the Venous Access Device

➤ When performing the procedure, always identify your patient according to agency policy, using two identifiers, and be attentive to standard precautions, hand hygiene, patient safety and privacy, body mechanics, and documentation.

Procedure Steps

1. **Determine how fast the medication may be administered** and whether it needs to be diluted for administration.
IV push medications are frequently injected over 1 minute. Some medications must be administered over a longer period, and some medications must be diluted before administration. Giving an IV push medication too fast and/or undiluted can result in an adverse local or systemic reaction.

2. **Prepare the medication** from a vial or ampule. Dilute as needed. Refer to Procedure 26-9.

3. **Select the appropriate size of syringe** for flush solution.
Smaller syringes exert more pressure against the wall of the IV catheter than do larger syringes. Check with the IV catheter manufacturer for specific recommendations, and follow agency policy.

4. **Don procedure gloves.**

5. **Thoroughly scrub all surfaces** of the injection port closest to the patient with an alcohol prep pad or CHG-alcohol combination product (Gorski L.A., Hadaway L., Hagle M., et al., 2016).
Follow agency policy. Some facilities require nurses to scrub all surfaces of the port with an alcohol-based antimicrobial product for 1 minute when accessing venous access devices. (a) Port: Using the port closest to the patient minimizes the amount of medication in the IV line. (b) Scrub: Use povidone-iodine solution (Betadine) only when the patient cannot tolerate an alcohol-based disinfectant.

6. **Insert the flush syringe** into the injection port and gently aspirate by pulling back on the plunger to check for a blood return.
NOTE: Some newer connectors do not require or allow for aspiration. Follow institutional policy.
A blood return is an indication that the IV catheter is in the vein. An IV site may still be patent if no blood is returned; conversely, an infiltrated IV may have a blood return. Use the blood return as only one indication of patency.

7. **Administer a flush solution** (usually 1 to 3 mL) to clear the line if you aspirated and blood return was returned. Use a forward pushing motion on the syringe, with a slow, steady injection technique. If blood is not returned, see the What If . . . . ? section at the end of this procedure.
(a) Flush syringes may be prefilled; and in some cases, the amount to inject may be a part of agency policy. (b) Rapid flushing causes a jet effect that can cause the catheter tip to migrate to other venous locations; this should be avoided. (c) Injecting an IV medication into an IV site that is not patent administers the medication into the local tissue at the IV site. Some medications will cause tissue irritation and even necrosis if infused into the subcutaneous tissue.

8. **Continue to hold the injection port;** remove the flush syringe; and again scrub the port with the alcohol prep pad or CHG-alcohol combination product.
Cleansing the port reduces the risk of introducing microorganisms into the bloodstream. Scrub: Use povidone-iodine only when the patient is sensitive to alcohol-based disinfectants.

9. **Attach the medication syringe,** and inject the medication in small increments over the correct time interval. Use a slow, steady injection technique until the correct dose is instilled over the prescribed amount of time.
For example, if 1 mL of the medication is to be given over 1 minute, inject approximately 0.25 mL every 15 seconds.

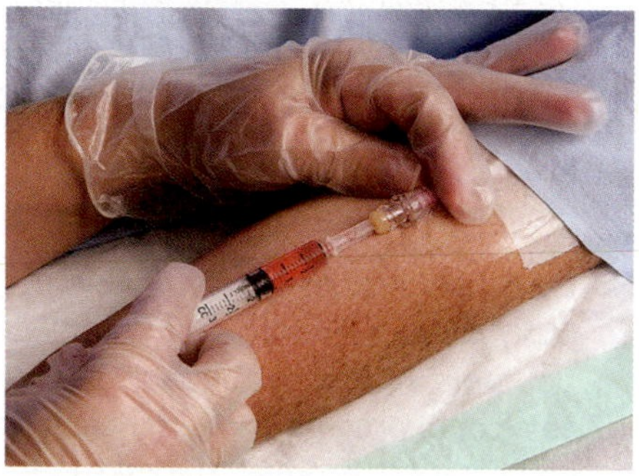

10. **Continuing to hold the injection** port, remove the medication syringe, and gently, but thoroughly scrub all surfaces of the port with alcohol prep pad or CHG-alcohol–based product for at least 15 seconds. Attach the flush syringe.
Gently, but thoroughly cleaning/scrubbing reduces the chance of contamination of the port.

11. **Administer the flush solution,** usually 1 to 3 mL, or according to prescription or agency policy.
Flushing ensures that all the medication has been administered and prevents occlusion of the IV catheter.

12. **Use a slow, steady injection pressure technique** when removing the syringe by placing your thumb or index finger to avoid movement of the plunger. (Follow equipment guidelines; you may not always need to do this.) Continue to administer the flush solution while withdrawing the syringe cannula from the injection port.
This positive-pressure technique prevents blood backflow into the IV catheter, which might cause an occlusion. Follow equipment guidelines because some injection ports maintain positive pressure by removing the syringe and then closing the clamp.

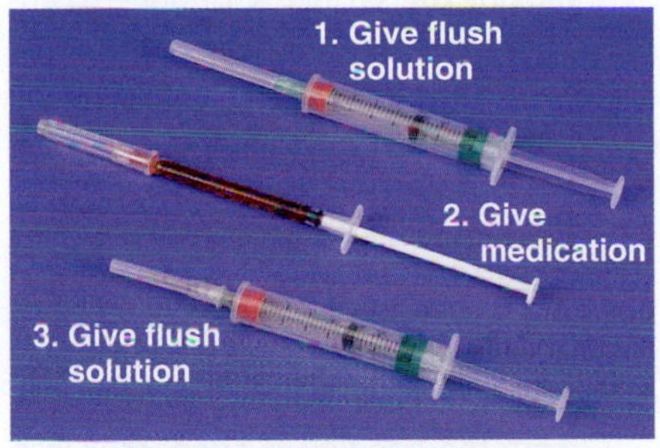

13. **Discard the flushing syringe** from the needleless connector into a safety disposal container.

Procedure 26-16C ■ Administering IV Push Medications Through an Intermittent Device With IV Extension Tubing

➤ When performing the procedure, always identify your patient according to agency policy, using two identifiers, and be attentive to standard precautions, hand hygiene, patient safety and privacy, body mechanics, and documentation.

Procedure Steps

1. **Determine how fast the medication** may be administered and whether the medication needs to be diluted for administration.
IV push medications are frequently injected over 1 minute. Some must be administered over a longer period, and some require diluting prior to administration. Giving an IV push medication too fast and/or undiluted can result in a local or systemic adverse reaction.

2. **Prepare the medication** from a vial or ampule. Dilute as needed. Refer to Procedure 26-9.

3. **Determine the volume of any extension tubing** attached to the access port.
The volume of extension sets can be greater than the IV push medication being given. If not accounted for, all the medication may be injected into the patient's bloodstream at once when the second flush solution is given.

4. **Don procedure gloves.**

5. **Clean/scrub all surfaces of the injection port** with an antiseptic wipe.

6. **Insert the flush syringe** into the injection port. If a needleless system is not available, use a syringe with a safety needle. Depending on the equipment, you may then need to aspirate for a blood return as one sign of vein patency. Some equipment does not require or allow aspiration.
(a) In tubing that allows for or requires aspiration, a blood return is a sign that the IV catheter is in the vein. However, an IV site may still be patent if no blood is returned. (b) Using a needleless system prevents needlestick injuries.

7. **Administer the flush** (commonly 1 to 3 mL) after establishing patency of the IV line. If blood appears in the tubing during aspiration, administer the rest of the flush. If blood is not returned, assess patency by administering a small amount of the flush solution and monitoring for ease of administration, swelling at the IV site, or patient complaint of discomfort at the site.

8. **Again clean/scrub the port.** Attach the medication syringe and inject a volume of medication equal to the volume of the extension set at the same rate as the flush solution.
   - When using a 5-mL syringe for peripheral lines and a 10-mL syringe for central lines, administer the flush solution briskly.
   - When you use a smaller syringe, use a slower rate to prevent excess pressure damaging the vein or shearing of the IV cannula.

   The medication clears the line of saline solution and fills it with medication; it also flushes the IV catheter with saline as the medication pushes the saline through the catheter.

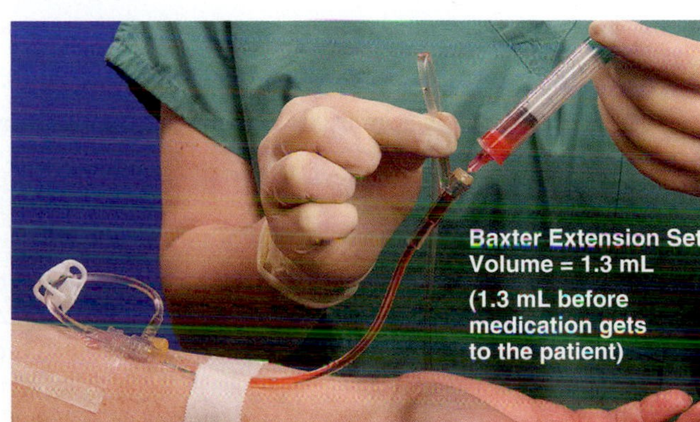

(continued on next page)

Procedure 26-16 ■ Administering IV Push Medication (continued)

9. **Using a slow, steady injection technique,** administer the remainder of the medication over the prescribed time interval for the specific medication.
   Rapid flushing can create a jet effect that can cause the catheter tip to migrate to an unintended venous location.

10. **Continuing to hold the injection port connector,** remove the medication syringe, gently but thoroughly scrub all surfaces of the connector for at least 15 seconds, then attach the flush syringe. **Key Point:** ***The only time you should open the catheter hub is when the needleless connector or primary continuous IV set must be changed, usually at 96-hour intervals or as otherwise prescribed.***

11. **Administer the same amount** of flush solution at the same rate as the medication, using a slow, steady injection technique. For example, if the extension tubing has a volume of 1.3 mL, give the first 1.3 mL of the flush solution at the same rate as the medication. Then, administer the remainder of the flush solution.
    (a) At this step, the extension tubing contains all the medication. Administering the flush solution all at once pushes the medication too fast (it will enter the vein all at once). (b) Once you have incrementally cleared the medication from the extension tubing and all the medication is already in the vein, then the rate no longer matters as far as the medication is concerned.

12. **Use a slow, steady injection pressure technique** when removing the syringe. Continue to administer the flush solution while withdrawing the syringe cannula from the injection port. Follow equipment instructions regarding the method and order of removing the syringe, closing the clamp, and maintaining positive pressure.

13. **Discard the flushing syringe** from the needleless connector into a safety disposal container.

? What if . . .

- **When using equipment requiring aspiration, no blood is returned?`**

  Do not give IV push medication until you can verify the patency of the IV site.

  If the patency of the IV site is questionable, restart the IV at another site.

  Further assess the patency of the IV line by administering a small amount of the saline flush and monitoring for ease of administration, swelling at the IV site, or patient complaint of discomfort at the site.

  Another technique to determine patency is to lower the IV bag below the level of the IV site—a blood return should occur.

  If the IV catheter is a small gauge, a blood return may not always be aspirated.

- **There is resistance when flushing the line?**

  Never force the flush solution into the VAD; look for a closed clamp on the catheter or tubing. Or you may check to see if an inline filter is clogged. Do not proceed with the medication infusion until you are sure the catheter is still correctly positioned and that the fluid pathway is unobstructed.

- **The IV infusing a dextrose solution infiltrates into the surrounding tissue of a peripheral catheter?**

  Immediately stop the intravenous infusion, and remove the catheter. Initially, apply a cool, moist compress to the site, and later use heat to promote comfort.
  Infiltration can cause tissue injury, inflammation, and edema and may even lead to tissue necrosis and sloughing.

  Some medications, such as vasopressors (e.g., dopamine), might need intradermal injection of an antidote, such as phentolamine (Regitine), to reverse the effects of extravasation.
  If the IV fluid contains dextrose at greater than 10% concentration, calcium salts, potassium salts, sodium bicarbonate, blood, and parenteral nutrition, contact the primary care provider, who will likely prescribe injection of hyaluronidase (Amphadase) into the surrounding tissue.

Evaluation

- Assess the patient for complaints of pain or discomfort at the site.

Patient Teaching

- Discuss why the medication is being administered intravenously.
- Explain the need to report immediately any reaction to the medication.

Home Care

- Discuss with the client and/or the caregiver how to care for the IV site, including flushing. Many IV push medications need to be administered by a nurse. However, cost-cutting efforts have led to short hospital stays, and some clients are now being taught to administer their own IV antibiotics at home.
- Explain how to identify problems with the IV site, such as infiltration and phlebitis.
- Determine whether the client has adequate facilities for storing the medication, such as refrigeration, if needed.
- Discuss safety issues, such as keeping medications and needles and syringes secure and away from children and pets.

Documentation

In addition to documenting according to Medication Guidelines: Steps to Follow for All Medications (Regardless of Type or Route), document related patient assessment findings, such as the appearance of the IV site and patient complaints of pain or discomfort during IV administration. You will usually document on an IV flow record and/or the MAR, rather than in the nursing notes. Document a nursing note only if there is a problem (e.g., if the patient experiences pain when you administer the medication).

Practice Resources

Gorski L.A., Hadaway L., Hagle M., et al. (2016); Phillips, L. (2015).

Thinking About the Procedure

The videos **Administering IV Push Medications Through a Primary IV Line, Administering IV Push Medications Through an Intermittent Device (IV Lock) When No Extension Tubing Is Attached to the Venous Access Device,** and **Administering IV Push Medications Through an Intermittent Device With IV Extension Tubing,** along with questions and suggested responses, are available on the ***Davis's Nursing Skills Videos*** Web site on FADavis.com.

Procedure 26-17 ■ Administering Medication by Intermittent Infusion

For steps to follow in *all* procedures, refer to the Universal Steps for All Procedures found on the inside back cover. Also, refer to Medication Guidelines: Steps to Follow for All Medications (Regardless of Type or Route). For step-by-step instructions in using volume-control devices (pumps), see Procedure 38-3.

Equipment

- Correct size syringe for measuring medication
- Needleless access cannula or safety needle
- Volume-control IV set (e.g., Buretrol, Volutrol, Soluset) or small bag of diluted medication with piggyback tubing
- Primary IV solution and tubing (unless one is already infusing)
- Antimicrobial swabs
- Labels for the IV tubing and medication administration system

Delegation

Nurse practice acts governing IV medication administration vary from state to state, and policies can further vary among healthcare agencies, regarding which medications or methods of administration the LPN/LVN may perform. You cannot delegate this procedure to a UAP.

Pre-procedure Assessments

- Check the compatibility of the medication with the IV solution.
  Medications can be physically or chemically incompatible with the IV solution. Physical incompatibility will be obvious if precipitation occurs. Chemical incompatibility is not obvious and may result in the medication having a weaker or a stronger effect than anticipated.
- Assess the patency of the IV line.
  If the line is occluded or if the fluid has infiltrated, the medication will not infuse.
- Check the site for redness, swelling, tenderness, and other signs of infiltration or phlebitis.
  Some medications are irritating to the tissue. If the IV fluid has infiltrated the tissue, medication would leak into the tissue and cause injury. IV medications can also irritate the veins and cause phlebitis. Do not infuse a medication into a compromised site.
- Determine the amount of IV solution needed to administer the specific medication.
  Most medications state (on the prescription or on the label) specific dilution to prevent potential harm to the patient.
- Determine the period over which the solution needs to be infused.
  Infusing a medication too slowly may result in an inadequate blood level to achieve therapeutic levels, and infusing a medication too rapidly can cause harm.
- Perform assessments that will provide a basis for evaluating the drug's effectiveness, such as checking blood pressure after administering an antihypertensive agent.

Procedure 26-17A ■ Using a Piggyback Administration Set With a Gravity Infusion

When performing the procedure, always identify your patient according to agency policy, using two identifiers, and be attentive to standard precautions, hand hygiene, patient safety and privacy, body mechanics, and documentation.

Procedure Steps

1. **Obtain the medication.** IV medications usually are premixed and labeled in small bags by the pharmacy. Rarely, you may need to draw up the medication, and inject it into the piggyback solution (see Procedure 26-15). Date and initial the medication bag label. Verify that it has the patient's name, amount of medication, date, and time given.
2. **Obtain and attach** the piggyback tubing to the medication bag. Do not touch the spike.
   Tubing connects the piggyback to the primary line. The piggyback tubing is short. Prevents contamination of tubing and solution.

(continued on next page)

Procedure 26-17 ■ Administering Medication by Intermittent Infusion (continued)

3. **Be sure the slide clamp is closed.** Squeeze the drip chamber, filling it one-third to one-half full.
Clamping prevents excess air coming into the line when you are priming the tubing.

4. **Open the clamp and prime the tubing,** holding the end of the tubing lower than the bag of fluid. Do not let more than one drop of fluid escape from the end of the tubing. Close the clamp.

Alternative: "Backflushing" the Piggyback Line

a. Clamp the piggyback tubing.
b. Scrub all surfaces of the primary "Y" port, and attach the piggyback setup with the needleless connector.
c. Open the clamp on the piggyback tubing, and lower the bag below the primary bag to prime the piggyback line.
d. Once all the air is expelled from the piggyback tubing, clamp the tubing, and finish the procedure.
Priming removes air from the tubing and maintains sterility of the system. Medications are diluted in small amounts of fluid (usually 50 to 100 mL), so you cannot waste any medication. The backflush method ensures you will not do so.

5. **Label the piggyback tubing** with the time, the date, and your initials.
Tubing used for intermittent infusions can be used for 48 to 72 hours, depending on facility policy; labeling allows the nurse to know when it must be changed.

6. **Hang the piggyback container** on the IV pole. Lower the primary IV container to hang below the level of the medication bag.
Gravity causes the higher bag (the piggyback IV setup) to flow instead of the primary IV setup. When the piggyback IV solution has infused, the primary IV line will resume infusing.

7. **Open the clamp** of the piggyback line, and regulate the drip rate with the roller clamp on the primary line. Regulate to the prescribed infusion rate for the medication.
Because the piggyback is the only bag running, the primary roller clamp regulates the speed of the piggyback bag.

8. **When all of the medication is infused,** clamp the piggyback tubing, and move the primary bag back to its original height. Use the roller clamp to reset the primary bag to its correct infusion rate.
This ensures that the primary fluids infuse at their prescribed rate, rather than flowing at the rate the piggyback medication was flowing—which would probably be either faster or slower than the prescribed primary fluid rate.

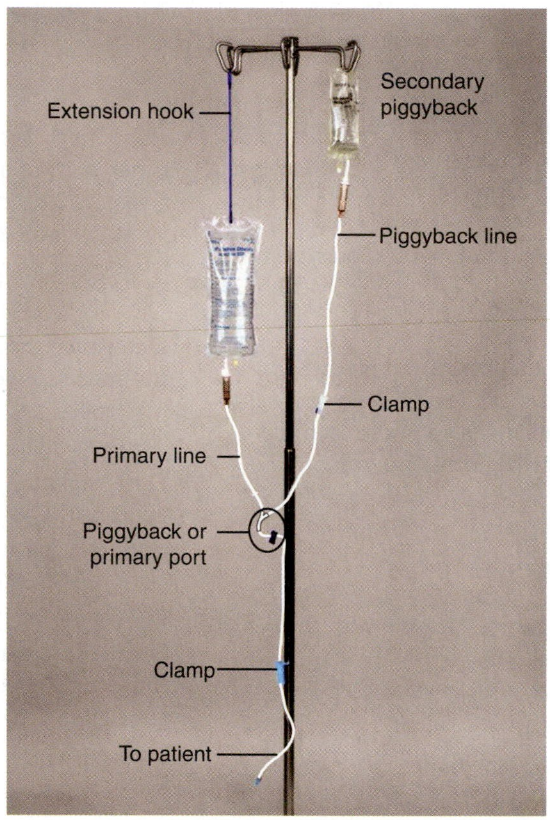

Procedure 26-17B ■ Using a Piggyback Administration Set With an Infusion Pump

➤ For step-by-step instructions in using intermittent infusion devices (pumps), also see Procedure 38-3.

➤ *Note:* This procedure describes the use of a one-piston infusion pump. The steps for using a two-piston pump vary slightly.

➤ When performing the procedure, always identify your patient according to agency policy, using two identifiers, and be attentive to standard precautions, hand hygiene, patient safety and privacy, body mechanics, and documentation.

Procedure Steps

1. **Obtain the medication.** IV medications usually are premixed in small bags and labeled by the pharmacy. If this is not the case, inject the medication into the prescribed piggyback solution (see Procedure 26-15). Date and initial the medication bag label. Verify that it has the patient's name, amount of medication, date, and time given.

2. **Be sure you have the correct secondary infusion tubing.** Hang the piggyback container on the IV pole. Attach the piggyback tubing to the medication bag. Do not touch the spike.

Piggyback tubing is short; tandem tubing is much longer. Secondary tubing connects the piggyback to the primary line. Touching the spike would contaminate the tubing and solution.

3. **Be sure the slide clamp is closed.** Squeeze the drip chamber, filling it one-third to one-half full.
Clamping prevents excess air coming into the line when you are priming the tubing.

4. **Open the clamp and prime the tubing,** holding the end of the tubing lower than the bag of fluid. Do not let more than one drop of fluid escape from the end of the tubing. Close the clamp.

Alternative: "Backflushing" the Piggyback Line

a. With the drip chamber one-third filled, air will be in the secondary tubing.
b. Pause the infusion pump.
c. Scrub all surfaces of the "Y" port on the primary line and attach the piggyback setup with a needleless connector.
d. Open the clamp on the piggyback tubing, and lower the bag below the primary bag to prime the piggyback line. The fluid from the primary line will flow up through the secondary tubing until all air is removed from the tubing. Restart the pump.
e. Once the line is primed, clamp the tubing and finish the procedure.

Priming removes air from the tubing and maintains sterility of the system. Medications are diluted in small amounts of fluid (usually 50 to 100 mL), so you cannot waste any medication. The backflush method ensures you will not do so.

5. **Label the piggyback tubing** with the time, the date, and your initials.
Tubing used for intermittent infusions can be used for 48 to 72 hours, depending on facility policy; labeling allows the nurse to know when it must be changed.

6. **Hang the piggyback container** on the IV pole. Lower the primary IV container to hang below the level of the piggyback medication bag.
The tubing system works such that the higher bag (the piggyback IV setup) flows instead of the primary IV setup.

7. **Program the pump** by selecting the secondary infusion button.
This converts the fluid infusing from the primary line to the secondary line.

8. **Program the rate and total volume** to be infused. (Some pumps allow you to select the medication and dose.)
Ensures accurate infusion amount and restart of primary fluids.

9. **Vigorously scrub the port** of the primary line.
Minimizes the introduction of microorganisms.

10. **Remove the cover** from the secondary tubing, and connect the tubing to the port of the primary line. (This was done at step 4 if the blackflush priming method was used.)

11. **Open the clamp** on the secondary tubing.

12. **Press "start"** on infusion pump.

13. **Check drip chambers** to ensure that the secondary solution is infusing and the primary solution is not.
This ensures that medication is infusing and patient does not receive an overload of fluids.

14. **Check the pump information** again to ensure the correct rate and volume.

15. **At the end of the infusion**, the primary IV line will resume infusing. Once the secondary infusion is complete, the pump programming will reset to the previously programmed primary rate.
This ensures that the primary fluids infuse at their prescribed rate, rather than flowing at the rate the piggyback medication was flowing—which would probably be either faster or slower than the prescribed primary fluid rate.

Procedure 26-17C ■ Using a Volume-Control Administration Set

➤ For step-by-step instructions in using volume-control devices (pumps), see Procedure 38-3. If you have not already done so, affix a label to the secondary bag indicating the name and amount of medication, date and time given, and your name or initials.

➤ When performing the procedure, always identify your patient according to agency policy, using two identifiers, and be attentive to standard precautions, hand hygiene, patient safety and privacy, body mechanics, and documentation.

Procedure Steps

1. **Prepare the volume-control set.**
a. Close both the upper and lower clamps on the tubing, if they are not already closed.
Clamping prevents air bubbles from forming in the tubing.
b. Open the clamp of the air vent on the volume-control chamber.
Venting allows air to escape, which lets the IV solution enter the chamber.
c. Maintaining sterile procedure, attach administration spike of the volume-control set to the primary IV bag.
d. Fill the volume-control chamber with the desired amount of IV solution by opening the clamp between the bag and the volume-control chamber. When the correct amount of solution is in the chamber, close the clamp.
The drip chamber provides solution for priming the tubing and diluting the IV medication.
e. Prime the rest of the tubing by opening the clamp below the chamber and running the IV fluid until all the air has been expelled.
Priming clears the IV tubing of air.

(continued on next page)

Procedure 26-17 ▪ Administering Medication by Intermittent Infusion (continued)

f. Recheck the amount of fluid in the volume control chamber, and add more fluid to the desired amount, if needed.
Priming the tubing alters the volume in the chamber. You must fill to the desired amount.

2. **With an alcohol or CHG-alcohol swab,** gently but thoroughly scrub all surfaces of the injection port closest to the patient.
Thorough cleansing is necessary to remove microorganisms and particles from the IV port, which could potentially enter the patient's bloodstream.

3. **Connect the end of the volume-control IV line** to the patient's IV site (e.g., directly to the IV catheter, to the extension tubing, or to the injection port closest to patient).

4. **Thoroughly scrub the injection port** on the volume-control chamber, attach the medication syringe (preferably with a blunt, needleless device), and inject the medication into the solution in the chamber.

5. **Gently rotate the chamber** to mix the medication in the IV solution.
Distributes the medication within the IV solution.

6. **Open the lower clamp,** and start the infusion at the correct flow rate.
Unclamping allows the infusion of the medication. A correct flow rate infuses the medication over the correct amount of time and prevents a toxic reaction to it.

7. **Label the volume-control chamber** with the date, time, medication and doses added, and your initials, according to agency policy.

8. **When the medication has finished infusing,** add a small amount of the primary IV fluid to the chamber, and flush the tubing. For the flush volume, use twice the volume in the dead space of the tubing; check the tubing package for the amount.
Flushing the line ensures all the medication is given to the patient and does not adhere to the tubing. ➤

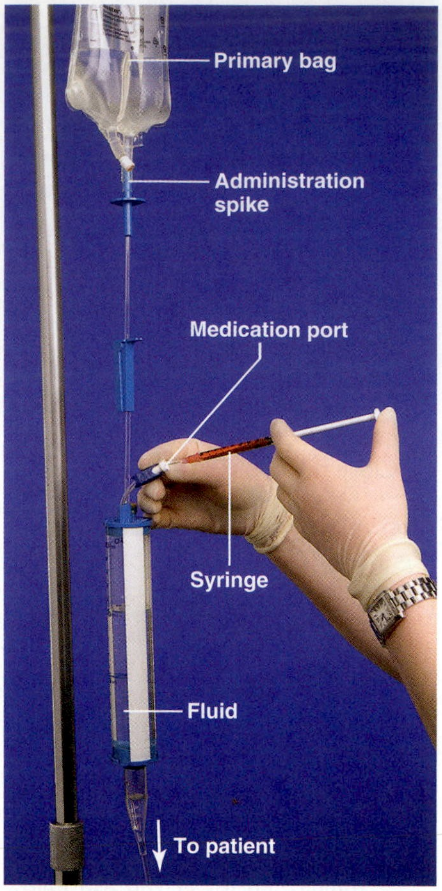

Evaluation

- Assess for pain or discomfort at the site.
- Intermittent infusions via a pump are generally infused over 30 to 60 minutes; therefore, you need to assess the patient as soon as the medication begins infusing and every 15 to 20 minutes until it is absorbed.

Patient Teaching

- Discuss why the medication is being administered intravenously.
- Explain the need to report immediately any reaction to the medication.
- Ask the patient to activate the call device if the infusion pump starts to alarm. Explain common reasons for the alarm to minimize anxiety.

Home Care

- Discuss with the client and/or caregiver how to care for the IV site. Only a nurse should add medications to the IV.
- Explain how to identify problems with the IV site, such as infiltration and phlebitis.
- Assess whether the client has adequate facilities for storing the medication, such as refrigeration, if needed.
- Discuss safety issues, such as keeping medications, needles, and syringes secure and away from children and pets.

Documentation

- Document information according to Medication Guidelines: Steps to Follow for All Medications (Regardless of Type or Route).
- Document related patient assessment findings, such as the appearance of the IV site and patient complaints of pain or discomfort during the administration.

Practice Resources

Gorski L.A., Hadaway L., Hagle M., et al. (2016); Hamilton, S. (2014).

Thinking About the Procedure

The videos **Using a Piggyback Administration Set With a Gravity Infusion, Using a Piggyback Administration Set With an Infusion Pump,** and **Using a Volume-Control Administration Set,** along with questions and suggested responses, are available on the ***Davis's Nursing Skills Videos*** Web site on FADavis.com.

Procedure 26-18 ■ Administering Medication Through a Central Venous Access Device (CVAD)

➤ For steps to follow in *all* procedures, refer to the Universal Steps for All Procedures found on the inside back cover. Also, refer to Medication Guidelines: Steps to Follow for All Medications (Regardless of Type or Route).

Equipment

See Figures 26-36A (Implantable device) and 26-36B (Multilumen catheter with blunt cannula, split septum, needleless access device).

- Syringe appropriate for medication volume (10 mL or larger)

Use of syringes smaller than 10 mL when flushing a CVAD can cause increase pressure and may rupture the CVAD.

- Needleless device or safety syringe with a filter needle for drawing up the medication (You would also need a sterile needle for injection.)
- Two syringes for the flush solution
  - Saline or heparin flush solution, as prescribed. Earlier research recommended flushing with heparin 100 units/mL, rather than with saline solution (Bertolino, Pitassi, Tinelli, et al., 2012); however, more recent research found little evidence to conclude that heparin is more effective than saline flush for CVC maintenance (López-Briz, E., Ruiz, G., Cabello, J., et al., 2018; Zhong, Wang, Xu, et al., 2017)
- Prep pad: CHG-alcohol combination product or appropriate antiseptic solution and gauze pad
- One pair nonsterile procedure gloves

Pre-Procedure Assessment

- Carefully palpate the area around the insertion site through the dressing. If the patient has tenderness, assess further for other signs of infection. Check the surrounding catheter insertion site for intact sutures, redness, swelling, warmth, or drainage.
  This can indicate catheter-related infection.
- Assess the patient's external chest wall for engorged veins at the surface of the skin. If the jugular's site is used, also assess for difficulty moving the neck or jaw, headache, or ear pain.
  This can indicate venous thrombosis.
- PICC line sites should be observed daily for swelling, tenderness, drainage, or streaking. Take site measurements at regular intervals during dressing changes and compare them with the preinsertion arm circumference.
  May indicate problems, such as phlebitis and/or catheter sepsis.
- Conduct a comprehensive pain assessment, looking for unusual pain or discomfort.
  Pain can be associated with the catheter's position in the vein, especially if the line is not in an optimal position.

➤ When performing the procedure, always identify your patient according to agency policy, using two identifiers, and be attentive to standard precautions, hand hygiene, patient safety and privacy, body mechanics, and documentation.

Procedure Steps

1. Prepare the medication.

a. Check compatibility of the medication with the existing IV infusion.

b. Verify that the medication can safely be administered through a central site. Double-check the infusion rate as well.
Some medication might be incompatible with infusion solution or additives. Because dosage may be different for medications given centrally versus peripherally and because the medication enters the heart almost instantly, any error is potentially life threatening.

c. Draw up the medication using a needleless device or a needle with a filter. Then, change to a sterile safety needle or a needleless device for administering the medication.
Filter needles prevent small particles from entering the line.

d. Recap any needles throughout, using a needle-capping device or approved one-handed technique that has a low risk of contaminating the sterile needle (see Procedure 26-10B).
Recapping prevents needlestick injury and, when performed correctly, maintains the sterility of the needle.

e. Dilute the medication, if needed. Fill the medication syringe to the exact volume to be infused; expel excess volume.

f. Label the syringe with the contents, including medication name, dilution, time to be administered, route, and name of person constituting the medication.
Excess volume of medication in the syringe is a risk for inadvertent overdosing.

2. Flush the line.

a. Obtain heparinized or saline solution for flushing the CVAD, following the institution's protocol or the prescription.
The usual concentration for heparin is 10 to 100 units/mL of solution for adults. The recommended volume of flush varies by institution. Most facilities recommend 3 to 5 mL of solution to flush the catheter, although some use 10 mL to flush the line. Some medication might be incompatible with infusion solution or additives.

Dosage for centrally administered drugs is critical because the medication enters the heart almost instantly, so any error is potentially life threatening.

(continued on next page)

Procedure 26-18 ■ Administering Medication Through a Central Venous Access Device (CVAD) (continued)

Using heparin flush in venous access devices is becoming more controversial because of the potential for heparin-induced thrombocytopenia. Be sure to follow the manufacturer's guidelines, prescriber's prescription, and the policy of your institution.

b. Before flushing the CVAD, examine the syringe for bubbles. Remove them by flicking the syringe. Eject the air and bubbles, but be sure you have enough flush solution remaining in the syringe.
Flicking causes the bubbles to rise to the top. Remove bubbles from the syringe before giving medication through the CVAD port to avoid injecting air into the patient's vein and causing an embolus.

c. With clean procedure gloves, using pressure and friction, vigorously scrub all surfaces of the CVAD connectors as well as the luer-locking threads, and the luer-lock, including the extension "tail," with an alcohol wipe, CHG-alcohol combination product, or other antimicrobial product for at least 15 sec. Then, let it dry for 15 sec. Do not touch this connector after cleansing.
Antimicrobial swabs reduce the risk of line-related infection by decreasing colonization of the port and tubing.

d. Insert the flush syringe at a vertical (90°) angle into the port using a needleless system or safety syringe.
A 90° angle reduces stress on the access port, which may cause shearing or mechanical trauma to the material.

e. Open the clamp between the syringe and the patient.
The clamp between the access port and the tubing that goes to the patient must be patent for medication to be injected through the CVAD.

f. Check for blood return, if necessary. Equipment differs regarding the need to aspirate, so follow agency protocols.
In some administration systems, aspiration is one indication that catheter placement is in the vein.

g. Inject saline or heparinized flush solution into the line, per agency protocol or provider's orders and type of catheter. Some catheter types (e.g., Groshong) do not require heparin in the flush solution. Close the clamp.
Saline or heparin flush is used, depending on the type of CVAD, institutional protocol, and manufacturer recommendations.

- *Saline is generally indicated when simple clearing of the line is needed.*
- *If blood is likely to back flow into the line, then heparin might be used in the flush solution to reduce the risk of clot formation.*
- *Most often heparin is used for implanted CVADs to reduce the risk of occlusion from a clot forming on the device.*
- *Different catheters require different volume of flush solutions. Some are more prone to clot formation, depending on whether they are open or closed system devices. The initial flush maintains patency of the line and removes any heparin that was left if the catheter was used previously.*

h. Never force the flush solution into the venous access device if you feel resistance. Look for a closed clamp on the catheter or tubing. Check to see if an inline filter is clogged.
Forcing fluid creates a risk of rupturing the catheter.

i. Disconnect the flush syringe.

CAUTION: Techniques of flushing and clamping may vary, depending on the type of connector you are using. Consult agency protocols and manufacturer's instructions.

If using a needleless connector, in general, do the following:

If Using Negative Fluid Displacement Device

Use a positive-pressure technique:

- For a blunt cannula with split septum, or mechanical valve, withdraw the cannula before the syringe is completely empty, keeping your thumb on the syringe plunger.
- For a mechanical valve device with negative displacement, maintain pressure on the syringe plunger, close the clamp on the IV line between the needleless connector and the patient; and then disconnect the syringe.

If Using a Positive Fluid Displacement Device

Do not use a positive-pressure technique. Flush using a push-pause technique. Wait 10 seconds (or per manufacture guidelines) to allow fluid displacement to occur. Remove syringe, and only then may you clamp the catheter.
The positive-pressure technique would keep the internal mechanism from functioning properly.

For Neutral Fluid Displacement Devices

Any flushing technique can be used. The clamping and disconnecting sequence does not matter.
The clamping sequence is directly dependent upon the needleless connector being used and is critical for the final locking solution.

j. After removing the flush syringe from the port, discard it into a safety disposal container.

3. Administer medication through the CVAD.

a. Scrub all surfaces of the external ports, tubing, and connectors with a CHG-alcohol combination product for at least 15 seconds. Allow the port to dry for 15 more seconds or follow manufacturer's guidelines.
Antimicrobial swabs reduce the risk of line-related infection by decreasing colonization of the port and tubing.

b. Close the clamp to the infusion if a primary IV is running.
The medication could travel back up the line rather than infuse into the patient if the clamp is open.

c. Inject medication into the port, according to the medication prescription (infusion time).
Some medication is infused as a bolus; other medication is given over a period.

4. **After scrubbing all surfaces of the port** again with a CHG-alcohol product or other approved antiseptic, administer the second syringe of flush solution.
The flush prevents incompatible medication or fluid from mixing at later administrations and ensures that all of the medication clears the catheter and enters the bloodstream.

5. **Clamp the tubing** between the syringe and the CVAD port. If there is an infusing primary IV, make sure the tubing is open between the IV fluid and the patient.

What if . . .

- **My patient is a child? How should I secure the line?**

Dress infants and younger children in a one-piece undershirt that fastens between the legs and tape the line to the shirt, leaving a little bit of slack to allow for movement.

- **The line does not flush easily?**
  - Make sure all clamps are unclamped.
  - Check to see if the central line is kinked or twisted.
  - After straightening lines, attempt to flush the central line again. If the flush solution cannot be injected easily from the syringe into the CVAD, do not force the flush.
  Too much flush pressure may dislodge a clot that has formed in the central line.
  - Check to see if an inline filter is clogged.
  - Assess the insertion site to see if the stabilization device or dressing may be causing the occlusion.
  - Try to reposition the patient to lying down and turned to one side.
  - You might also have the patient lift his arms above his head and then attempt to flush the central line.
  - If it is still difficult to flush after repositioning, notify the provider.

- **The central line inadvertently comes out?**

Hold firm, constant pressure on the site to control bleeding. Have a colleague notify the provider immediately.

- **The central line is cracked or leaking?**

Close the clamp between the break or leakage in the line and the patient's line insertion site. Wrap an alcohol wipe and gauze around the broken part of the line. Immediately change the tubing.

- **The clamp on the line is broken?**

Change the tubing. Assure the clamp works properly on the new tubing. This is essential for patient safety.

- **The central line gets caught on or pulled by the patient's clothing?**

Loop the tubing over the dressing and secure with tape.

- **My patient is short of breath or complains of chest pain?**

Notify the provider immediately.
These symptoms could be a sign of fluid overload or other complications, such as a dislodged clot or embolism.

- **My patient feels pain in the neck or ear on the side where an implantable CVAD is located? Or the patient hears swishing noises or has palpitations?**

Notify the provider immediately.
In this case, the implanted device might be dislodged. Placement must be confirmed by x-ray.

Patient Evaluation

- Monitor for signs of catheter complications (e.g., shortness of breath, chest pain, and palpitations).
- Monitor for signs of catheter dislodgement (e.g., neck swelling or pain, bleeding at the site or within the line, palpitations, or gurgling noise).
- Assess for signs of catheter-related infection (e.g., fever, increased WBC count, redness, warmth at the site).
- Observe for leaking or blood backup at the injection ports, tubing connections, and the site.
- Observe for bleeding at the CVAD site.
- Assess for signs of allergic response or adverse effects to medication.

Patient Teaching

- Teach patients, families, and caregivers that the overall goal is to maintain a patent CVAD or PICC line that is free of infection, occlusion, or dislodgement.
- Avoid obtaining blood pressure readings in the arm where a PICC line is inserted.
- If a PICC line is in place, do not immerse the arm in water. The patient may shower if the site is covered by an occlusive dressing.
- Follow prescribed activity restrictions.
- Teach signs of catheter complications including line-related infection, thrombosis, and accidental dislodgement.
- Teach signs of catheter dislodgement to include pain or swelling in the neck or area near the ear of the affected side of the CVAD. Gurgling sounds might also indicate a problem with the placement of the CVAD.

(continued on next page)

Procedure 26-18 ■ Administering Medication Through a Central Venous Access Device (CVAD) (continued)

Home Care

- The goals of home care for clients receiving medication through a CVAD or PICC line are medication safety and maintaining an infection-free line.
- Candidates for home IV therapy through a CVAD or PICC line are those who:
  - Have a family member or other caregiver who can competently provide or assist with care of the line.
  - Have telephone access—either via landline or cell phone.
  - Have access to reliable transportation in case of a line-related emergency.
  - Ideally, caregivers should be able to read instructions for home care.
- Procedures in the home environment are similar to those in the hospital setting, except that clean technique is used instead of sterile technique.
- Home health supplies may be different from the ones used in the hospital.
- After discharge, follow-up care in the home environment is important to ensure safety.

Documentation

- Document any signs of allergic response to or adverse effects of medication.
- Note any signs of catheter complications or dislodgement.
- Document signs of catheter-related infection.
- Document the date and time tubing and port cap are changed.
- Document all medications infused through the CVAD.

Sample Documentation

04/04/2021 1200. PICC line insertion site clean and dry. No redness, swelling, or drainage. Arm circumference 16 inches; same as preinsertion measurement. Pt reports no pain at site. Flushed with 10 mL of NS, no resistance noted. ——— Sue Creas, RN

Practice Resources

Bertolino, G., Pitassi, A., Tinelli, C., et al. (2012); Gorski L.A., Hadaway L., Hagle M., et al. (2016).

Thinking About the Procedure

The videos **Administering Medication Through a Central Venous Access Device,** along with questions and suggested responses, are available on the ***Davis's Nursing Skills Videos*** Web Site on FADavis.com.

CLINICAL INSIGHTS

Clinical Insight 26-1 ➤ Taking Action After a Medication Error

First, check the patient. Take his vital signs, and perform assessments related to the medication that was given.

- If you are unfamiliar with the side effects of the medication, consult a drug reference source.
- Verify that you have made a medication error, and identify the type of error.
- Consult the charge nurse for guidance if this is your first error.
- Notify the prescriber, and follow the prescriptions for intervention.
- Document on the chart that the medication was given, but do not indicate that it was given in error. This alerts anyone reviewing the chart that an error was made.
- Complete an incident report according to the facility's policies. Ask for assistance if you are unfamiliar with the format or requirement of this form. It is important that the information you provide is factual and accurate.
- **Key Point:** *Do not document in the patient's chart that an incident report was filed. This alerts anyone reviewing the chart that an error was made and makes the incident report available for legal review in the event of a lawsuit.*
- When you are calmer and can think clearly, critically reflect on the error. Identify the influences that led to your making the error. Were you rushed? Did you check the prescription? Did you follow the rights of medication? Whatever the reason, use this situation as a learning experience to improve your practice.

Clinical Insight 26-2 ➤ Reusing Needles and Syringes: Home Care

Assess for the Following:

- Is the patient is capable of safely recapping a syringe: adequate vision, manual dexterity, and no obvious tremor?
- Are there contraindications to needle reuse (e.g., poor personal hygiene, an acute illness, open wounds on the hands, or decreased resistance to infection)?

Teach How to Use Needles Safely:

- Consult your healthcare provider before beginning this practice.
- Examine the needle carefully before reusing it. The new 30- and 31-gauge needles can easily be bent at the tip to form a hook, which can lacerate tissue or break off within the skin. Never reuse a needle that is deformed in any way.
- Recap the needle immediately after use if you plan to use it again.
- To recap a needle, hold the syringe in one hand, rest that arm or hand on a solid surface, and with the other, replace the cap with a straight motion of the thumb. Do *not* guide both the needle and cap to meet in midair, because this frequently results in needlestick injury.
- Do not mix insulin types if you reuse needles and syringes. Use one syringe for each insulin type. That means more injections, but certain insulins cannot be mixed without reducing their effectiveness.
- Dispose of needles safely. Do not bend or break a needle; doing so increases the chance of injury. Use a coffee can or other puncture-proof container with a lid to dispose of needles.

Teach Your Patient When to Discard a Needle:

- Discard needles when they become dull. Usually they cannot be used more than 10 times.
- When a needle hurts too much, it's time to discard it. Increased pain means that the silicone coating is wearing off.
- Do not reuse a needle if it has come in contact with anything other than the injection site.

Teach How to Clean and Store Needles:

- Do not use alcohol to cleanse the needle. Alcohol may remove the silicone coating that makes for less painful skin puncture. It is best not to clean the needle after use; just carefully recap it.
- You may store the syringe and needle at room temperature. The potential benefits or risks of refrigerating the syringe are unknown.

Teach How to Recognize and Avoid Infection:

- Be aware that reusing needles and syringes increases the risk of infection, although most insulin preparations have bacteriostatic additives that inhibit growth of bacteria commonly found on the skin.
- Inspect injection sites for redness or swelling. If these signs are present, do not reuse a needle; consult your healthcare provider.
- Never share syringes or needles with another person. This poses a risk of acquiring a bloodborne viral infection (e.g., hepatitis).

Clinical Insight 26-3 ➤ Using Prefilled Unit-Dose Systems

Prefilled systems are commonly used in a variety of healthcare settings and in self-administration.

Technique

1. Check each medication cartridge and dose carefully because all of the cartridges look alike.
2. No medication preparation is necessary.
3. Insert the cartridge into the holder.
4. Swing or twist the plunger into place, depending on the type of syringe you use. Lock it securely at the needle end.
5. Attach the plunger, if necessary. (The system may come with plunger attached.)

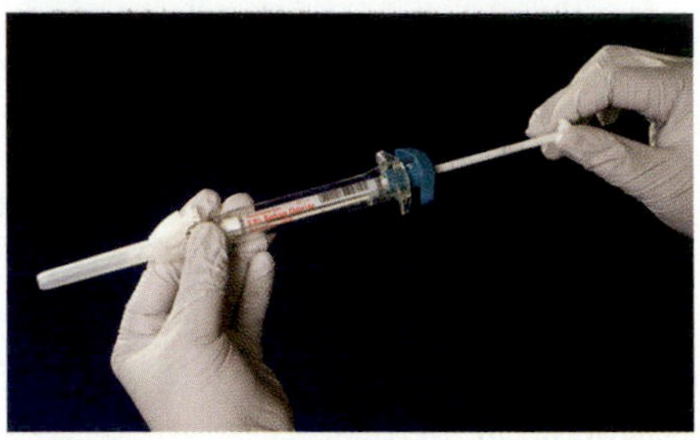

6. Expel air and excess medication.
7. Don gloves.
8. Administer the medication.
9. Dispose of the empty cartridge. Some types can be reused.

Technique Variations

The needle gauge or length is not correct for the patient. You can transfer the medication into a regular, disposable syringe, maintaining sterile technique. There are two ways you can do it.

Cartridge without removable needle:

1. Pull back on the plunger of the regular disposable syringe and keep a capped, sterile needle ready.
2. Insert the cartridge needle through the open tip of the disposable syringe.
3. Eject the medication into the regular syringe.
4. Replace the capped needle onto the regular syringe.
5. Eject the air and check for the correct dosage.

Cartridge with removable needle:
The capped needle can be removed from some prefilled cartridges, allowing the cartridge to be used as a vial. This allows you to safely draw the medications into a different (disposable) syringe, using a vial access device or safety needle. Do not inject air into a cartridge, because the excess pressure may eject the movable bottom.

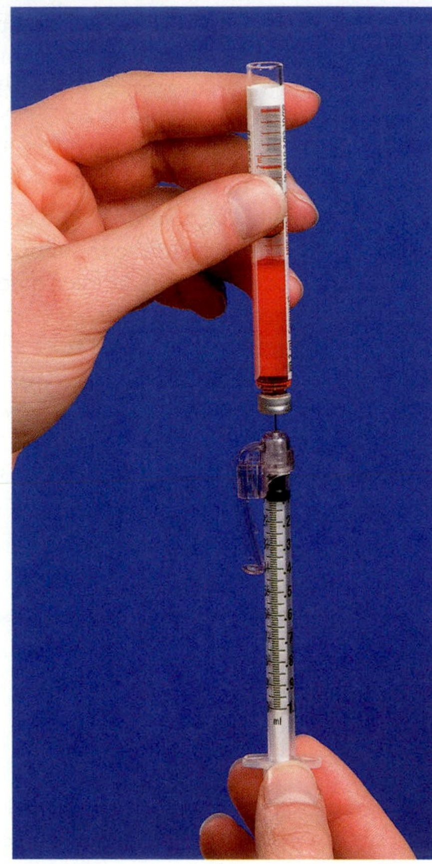

Clinical Insight 26-4 ➤ Reconstituting Medication

1. **Remove the caps of both the medication and diluent vials.**
2. **If a multidose vial is used, scrub the tops of both vials** with alcohol or other antiseptic wipe.
   To clean the cap of dust and reduce the number of microorganisms.
3. **Use a VAD or, if agency policy allows, attach a filter needle to the syringe.**
   To prevent withdrawing glass and rubber particles, which have been found in medications withdrawn from vials and ampules.
4. **Draw up the diluent into the syringe.**
   a. Draw air into the syringe in a volume equal to the amount of diluent you will be withdrawing.
   b. Insert the filter needle (or VAD) carefully through the center of the rubber cap and, keeping the bevel of the needle (or cannula) above the diluent, inject the air.
   The air prevents negative pressure inside the vial when you withdraw the diluent, allowing you to withdraw the diluent easily. Keeping bevel above diluent helps prevent bubbles.
   c. Withdraw the diluent in the specified amount.
5. **Inject diluent into the medication vial** by inserting the VAD carefully through the center of the rubber cap and then injecting the diluent.▼

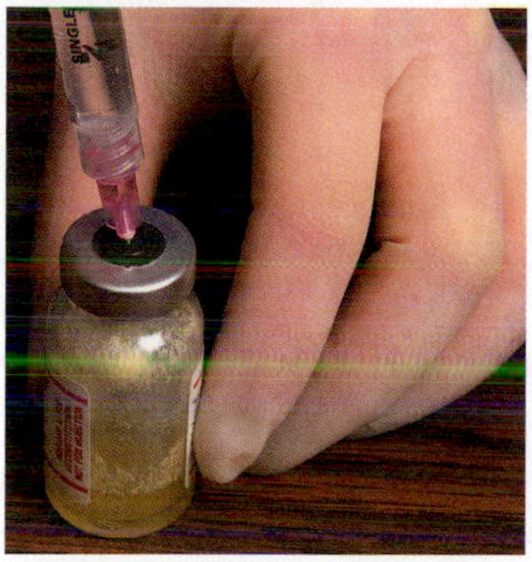

6. **Mix the medication, taking care not to create bubbles** (e.g., roll, do not shake, the vial). If medication does not mix easily, remove the needle or cannula from the vial, and place the syringe and needle on a sterile field (e.g., the wrapper the syringe came in) while you mix more. Alternatively, recap the sterile needle (see Procedure 26-10A).▼

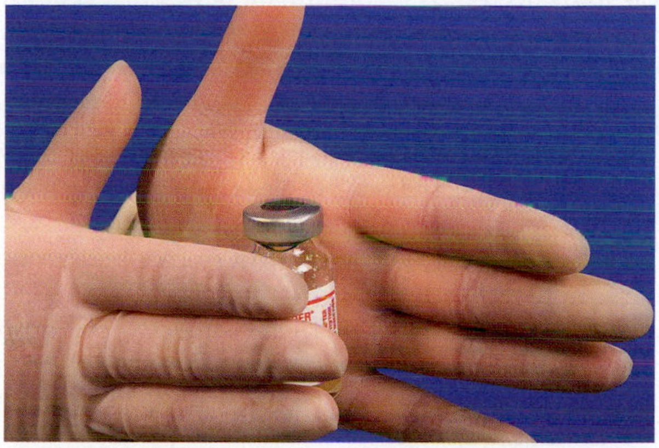

7. **Reinsert filter needle or VAD if it was removed,** and withdraw the reconstituted medication into the syringe.
8. **Remove the filter needle or the cannula from the syringe,** and replace it with a sterile needle before measuring the medication.
   This ensures that the dose is correct and minimizes discomfort. It also prevents tracking of medication through the tissues. Filter needles are usually larger than you need for an injection. In addition, you should not eject fluid through a filter needle.
9. **Hold the syringe vertically, and carefully eject all air** from the syringe, but do not eject the medication. Read the dosage.
10. **If necessary, hold the syringe horizontally to eject unneeded medication** from the syringe to reach the prescribed dose.

Clinical Insight 26-5 ➤ Measuring Dosage When Changing Needles

Note: These are not the old "air lock" techniques.

Using a Nonfilter Needle

When drawing medication from a multidose vial, you may sometimes need to use two regular needles. Alternately, you may use a needleless reconstitution device that is designed with a dispensing spike instead of a needle on one end and a luer-lock port on the other end that attaches to the syringe.

Equipment

One needle (or needless reconstitution device) for drawing up the medication, and one needle for injecting the medication into the patient.

1. **Using needle #1, draw up the prescribed amount of medication.** When using a vial, inject air into the air pocket within the vial. Then, withdraw the correct amount of medication from the vial. Be sure to keep the tip of the needle in the fluid to avoid aspirating air bubbles into the syringe.
2. **Remove bubbles; eject the air.** After drawing up the medication, tap on the barrel of the syringe to remove air bubbles, if necessary. Then eject the air from the syringe (keeping the syringe vertical) while retaining the correct amount of medication in the syringe. Check the volume closely at eye level.
3. **Remove needle #1, and discard it** into a needle-safe container. Put on a fresh needle (needle #2) for injection.
4. **Using needle #2**, pull back on the plunger and draw an extra 0.2 mL of air to account for the air within the needle.
5. **Check the medication dosage.** Your plunger should be 0.2 mL more than the prescribed dose.
6. **Still using needle #2, when you inject the patient**, she will receive the correct dose. The air will drive the medication from the needle into the patient's tissues. This is important when giving irritating medications, such as iron. (This is called an *air lock*.)

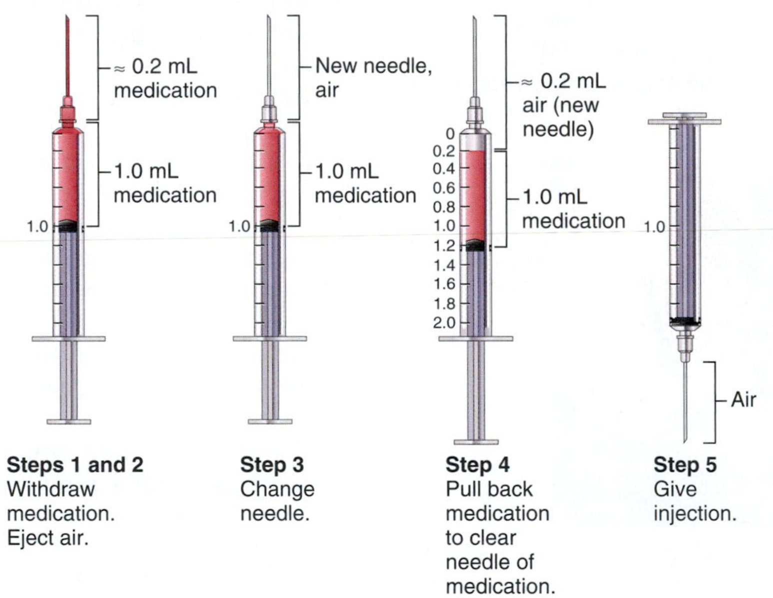

Nonfilter needles

Using a Filter Needle

Always use a filter needle to withdraw medications, if one is available. You must change needles to give the injection because:

- Filter needles are too large. To give the injection, you must use a needle of the correct gauge and length.
- You should not push medication out of the syringe through the filter needle because it can break the filter and release glass (and other) fragments. However, you cannot measure dosage accurately with air in the syringe.

In the following method, pulling air into the syringe allows for exact dosage when the medication is injected. When ejected, the air will clear the needle so that the patient receives all the medication that is in the syringe.

Equipment

One filter needle (or filter cannula) and one regular needle.

1. **With the filter needle (or cannula), withdraw** the exact amount of medication, keeping the syringe vertical as needed to obtain the correct dose. Remember, you must not eject fluid through the filter needle.
2. **Pull back on the plunger to withdraw all the medication from the filter needle (or filter cannula) into the syringe.** Depending on the size of the access cannula, this may be as much as 0.2 mL. It will now appear that you have more than the prescribed dose in the syringe (but you do not; the air is taking up some of the space).

Clinical Insight 26-5 ➤ Measuring Dosage When Changing Needles—cont'd

3. **Change to the needle you are going to use for injection.** Needle #2 has air in it instead of medication.
4. **Hold the syringe vertically, and eject air** until you see a drop of medication at the tip of the needle ("drop to the top").
5. **Measure the medication.** It should be at the correct syringe marking. If it is not, then tip the syringe horizontally, and eject the medication until the dose is correct.
6. **When you inject the patient, she will receive the correct dose,** even though some medication will remain in the needle.
7. **If you are giving an irritating medication** (e.g., iron) draw 0.2 mL of air into the syringe before giving the injection ("air lock").

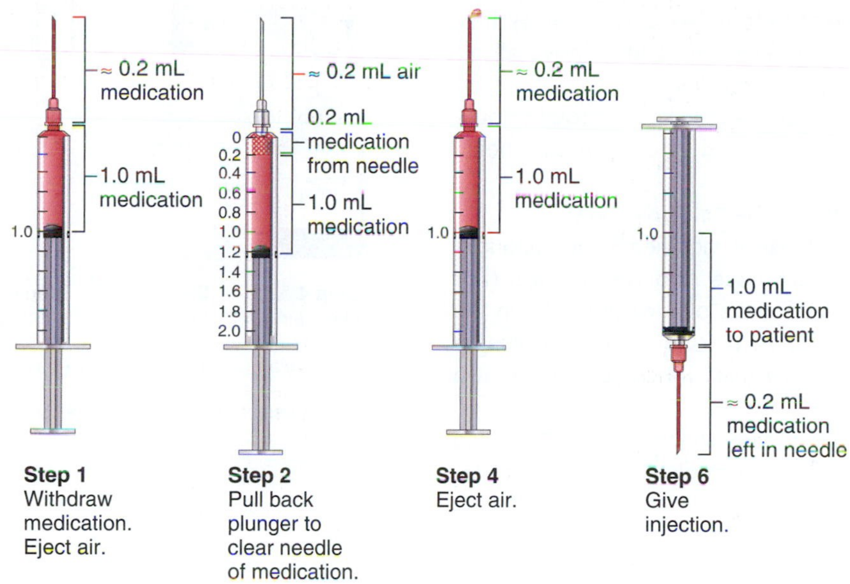

Filter needles

Clinical Insight 26-6 ➤ Mixing Two Kinds of Insulin in One Syringe

What You Should Know

Various combinations of rapid-acting, intermediate-acting, and long-acting insulin may be prescribed. Some can be mixed; some cannot. Insulins may come premixed from pharmacy to minimize the possibility of error. If your agency requires you to mix insulins, carefully follow each step as outlined.

- Lente insulins (Lente and Lantus) can be mixed with each other, but not with neutral protamine Hagedorn (NPH).
- Even though they are compatible, do not mix Lente with regular insulin, except for patients whose diabetes is already controlled on this mixture. Lente will bind with regular insulin, delaying the onset of action.
- A general rule is "clear before cloudy." Regular insulin is clear; all other types are cloudy. Therefore, you would draw up regular insulin into the syringe before Lente or NPH insulin, which are modified. If you draw up a modified type first, the needle may transfer it into the unmodified (regular) vial.

What You Should Do

Follow these steps when drawing up insulin from two vials into one syringe. The procedure assumes you are mixing regular (unmodified) insulin with a modified (e.g., NPH) insulin.

NOTE: If regular insulin is cloudy, do not use it. Return it to pharmacy.

1. **Maintain sterile technique throughout.**
2. **Before preparing the insulin**—rotate the vials between the palms of your hands for at least 1 minute, and invert them to ensure an adequate concentration. Do not shake the vials because this can create bubbles, which take up space and make it difficult to measure the dose precisely.
3. **Scrub vial stoppers** with alcohol or other antiseptic (they are usually multidose vials).

(Continued)

Clinical Insight 26-6 ➤ Mixing Two Kinds of Insulin in One Syringe—cont'd

4. **Inject air into "cloudy" vial**—using an insulin syringe and needle, inject an amount of air equal to the amount of insulin to be withdrawn from the vial of modified insulin (cloudy vial). Do not allow the needle tip to touch the insulin.
5. **Inject air into "clear" vial**—using the same syringe, inject the appropriate amount of air into the vial of regular insulin (clear vial).
6. **Withdraw insulin from "clear" vial**—do not withdraw the needle; withdraw the correct dose of regular insulin.
7. **Measure the dose of "clear"**—remove the syringe from the regular insulin. Eject air, and remove all air bubbles to measure the correct dose.
8. **Calculate combined dose**—calculate the total amount on the syringe that the combined types of insulin should measure.
9. **Withdraw insulin from the "cloudy" vial.**
   a. Return to the (first) vial of modified insulin (cloudy), and draw the correct dose into the syringe. (For example, if you have 5 units of regular insulin in the syringe and you need 10 units of NPH, the plunger should be at the 15-unit mark when you have drawn up the NPH.)
   b. Recall that you have already added air to this vial in a previous step. Draw up the medication slowly and exactly to the total dose, being very careful not to create bubbles and to withdraw only the amount needed. You cannot return any excess to the vial because it is now a mixture of two medications.
10. **Administer the insulin mixture** within 5 minutes after preparation. Even NPH insulin will bind with regular insulin and delay the onset of its action.

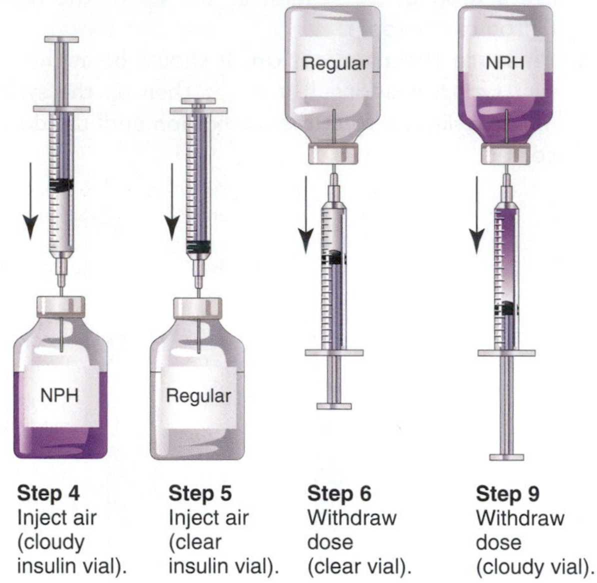

Total dose is mixture of clear and cloudy insulins.

Clinical Insight 26-7 ➤ Administering Anticoagulant Medication Subcutaneously

Because of the anticoagulant properties of heparin and enoxaparin (Lovenox), you should adapt your technique for subcutaneous injections:

- Enoxaparin-prefilled and graduated prefilled syringes are available with a system that shields the needle after injection.
- Use a ⅜-inch, 25- or 26-gauge needle.
- After drawing up the correct dose, add 0.2 mL of air to the syringe.
  To ensure that all of the drug is injected into the subQ tissue and not tracked into the superficial tissue.
- Do not expel the air bubble from the syringe before the injection.
  To avoid the loss of drug when using prefilled syringes.
- With your nondominant hand, pinch or spread the skin; insert the needle at a 90° angle, using your dominant hand.
  - If the patient has very little subQ tissue, use a ⅝-in needle and insert at a 45° angle.
  - Introduce the full length of the needle into a skinfold held between the thumb and forefinger; hold the skinfold throughout the injection.
- Alternate injection sites on the abdomen. Give the injection subQ, deep on the abdomen, at least 2 in from the umbilicus.
- Do not aspirate before injecting.
  This can traumatize tissue and cause bruising.
- Do not massage the site after injecting.
  This can cause bleeding and bruising. It may also cause the heparin to be absorbed more rapidly than desired.
- Keep a record of the sites used. Most agencies have a chart of the body on which to record the sites injected.

Mix-ups between heparin and insulin have been reported. To help avoid this, observe the "3 checks and 6 rights":
1. Do not store heparin and insulin vials beside each other.
2. Have another RN check your preparation before administering IV heparin or insulin.
3. Think critically (e.g., ask yourself if giving heparin or insulin makes sense given the patient's diagnosis) (Mattox, 2012).

TABLES: ABBREVIATIONS

Because abbreviations can be easily misread, you should write out drug names in full. However, some abbreviations are used in medication administration (e.g., mL, mEq), so you should be familiar with them and your facility's approved list of abbreviations. See the table below for a list of medication-related abbreviations you may see when reviewing and documenting medications.

Common Medication-Related Abbreviations

ABBREVIATION	EXPLANATION	ABBREVIATION	EXPLANATION
Ac	before meals: e.g., 0700, 1100, 1700 hours	p.m.	evening
ad lib	as desired	po or PO	by mouth
a.m.	morning	prn	as needed
bid	twice a day: e.g., 0900, 2100 hours	qh, (q1h, q1hr)	every hour
c̄	with	q2h, q2hr	every 2 hours: e.g., 0800, 1000, 1200 hours, etc.
fl oz	fluid ounce	q3h, q3hr	every 3 hours: e.g., 0900, 1200, 1500 hours, etc.
g, gm, or GM	gram	q4h, q4hr	every 4 hours: e.g., 0200, 0600, 1000, 1400, 1800, 2200 hours
gtt	drop	q6h, q6hr	every 6 hours: e.g., 0600, 1200, 1800 hours, 2400.
h, hr	hour	qid or QID	four times a day: e.g., 1000, 1400, 1800, 2200
IM	intramuscular	qs	sufficient quantity
IV	intravenous	s̄	without
IVPB	intravenous piggyback	stat or STAT	at once
Kg or kg	kilogram	sup or supp	suppository
KVO	keep vein open	susp	suspension
L or l	liter	tab	tablet
mEq	milliequivalent	Tbsp	tablespoon
mL or ml	milliliter	tid or TID	three times a day: e.g., 1000, 1400, 1800 hours
OTC	over-the-counter	T or tsp	teaspoon
oz	ounce		
pc	after meals: e.g., 0900, 1300, 1900 hours		

Institute for Safe Medication Practices (ISMP) List of Error-Prone Abbreviations, Symbols, and Dose Designations

ABBREVIATIONS	INTENDED MEANING	MISINTERPRETATION	CORRECTION
µg	Microgram	Mistaken as "mg"	Use "mcg."
AD, AS, AU	Right ear, left ear, each ear	Mistaken as OD, OS, OU (right eye, left eye, each eye)	Use "right ear," "left ear," or "each ear."
OD, OS, OU	Right eye, left eye, each eye	Mistaken as AD, AS, AU (right ear, left ear, each ear)	Use "right eye," "left eye," or "each eye."
BT	Bedtime	Mistaken as "bid" (twice daily)	Use "bedtime."
cc	Cubic centimeters	Mistaken as "u" (units)	Use "mL."
D/C	Discharge or discontinue	Premature discontinuation of medications if D/C (intended to mean: "discharge") has been misinterpreted as "discontinued" when followed by a list of discharge medications	Use "discharge" and "discontinue."
IJ	Injection	Mistaken as "IV" or "intrajugular"	Use "injection."
IN	Intranasal	Mistaken as "IM" or "IV"	Use "intranasal" or "NAS."
HS	Half-strength	Mistaken as bedtime	Use "half-strength."
hs	At bedtime, hours of sleep	Mistaken as half-strength	Use "bedtime."
*IU	International units	Mistaken as IV (intravenous) or 10 (ten)	Use "International units."
o.d. or OD	Once daily	Mistaken as "right eye" (OD-oculus dexter), leading to oral liquid medications administered in the eye	Use "daily."
OJ	Orange juice	Mistaken as OD or OS (right or left eye); drugs meant to be diluted in orange juice may be given in the eye	Use "orange juice."
per os	By mouth, orally	The "os" can be mistaken as "left eye" (OS-oculus sinister)	Use "PO," "by mouth," or "orally."
*q.d. or QD	Every day	Mistaken as q.i.d., especially if the period after the "q" or the tail of the "q" is misunderstood as an "i"	Use "daily."
qhs	Nightly at bedtime	Mistaken as "qhr" or every hour	Use "nightly."
qn	Nightly or at bedtime	Mistaken as "qh" (every hour)	Use "nightly" or "at bedtime."
*q.o.d. or QOD	Every other day	Mistaken as "q.d." (daily) or "q.i.d." (four times daily) if the "o" is poorly written	Use "every other day."
q1d	Daily	Mistaken as qid. (four times daily)	Use "daily."
q6PM, etc.	Every evening at 6 PM	Mistaken as every 6 hours	Use "6 PM nightly" or "6 PM daily."

Institute for Safe Medication Practices (ISMP) List of Error-Prone Abbreviations, Symbols, and Dose Designations—cont'd

ABBREVIATIONS	INTENDED MEANING	MISINTERPRETATION	CORRECTION
SC, SQ, subQ, or subq	Subcutaneous	SC mistaken as SL (sublingual); SQ mistaken as "5 every"; the "q" in "sub q" has been mistaken as "every (e.g., a heparin dose ordered sub q 2 hours before hours before surgery) surgery" misunderstood as every 2	Spell out "subcutaneous."
ss	Sliding scale (insulin)	Mistaken as "55"	Spell out "sliding scale"; use "one-half."
SSRI	Sliding scale regular insulin	Mistaken as "selective-serotonin reuptake inhibitor"	Spell out "sliding scale (insulin)."
SSI	Sliding scale insulin	Mistaken as "strong solution of iodine" (Lugol's)	Spell out "sliding scale (insulin)"
i/d	One daily	Mistaken as "tid"	Use "1 daily."
TIW or tiw	3 times a week	Mistaken as "3 times a day" or "twice in a week"	Use "3 times weekly."
*U or u	Unit	Mistaken as the number 0 or 4, causing a 10-fold overdose or greater (e.g., 4U seen as "40" or 4u seen as "44"); mistaken as "cc" so dose given in volume instead of units (e.g., 4 u seen as 4 cc)	Use "unit."
UD	As directed ("ut dictum")	Mistaken as unit dose (e.g., diltiazem 125 mg IV infusion "UD" misinterpreted as meaning to give the entire infusion as a unit [bolus] dose)	Use "nt"
DOSE DESIGNATIONS OR OTHER INFORMATION	**INTENDED MEANING**	**MISINTERPRETATION**	**CORRECTION**
*Trailing zero after decimal point (e.g., 1.0 mg)	1 mg	Mistaken as 10 mg if the decimal point is not seen expressed in whole numbers	Do not use trailing zeros for doses.
*No leading zero before a decimal dose (e.g., .5 mg)	0.5 mg	Mistaken as 5 mg if the decimal point is not seen	Use zero before a decimal point when the dose is less than a whole unit.
Drug name and drug dose run together (especially problematic for drug names that end in "l" (e.g., Inderal 40 mg)	Inderal 40 mg Tegretol 300 mg	Mistaken as Inderal 140 mg Mistaken as Tegretol 1300 mg	Place adequate space between the drug name, dose, and unit of measurement.
Numeric dose and unit of measurement run together (e.g., 10 mg)	10 mg	The "m" can be mistaken for a zero, leading to a 10-fold dosing error	Place adequate space between the drug name, dose, and unit of measurement.
Abbreviations, such as mg. or mL., with a period following the abbreviation	mg or mL	The period is unnecessary and could be mistaken as the number 1 if written poorly.	Use mg, mL, etc. without a period.

(Continued)

Institute for Safe Medication Practices (ISMP) List of Error-Prone Abbreviations, Symbols, and Dose Designations—cont'd

DOSE DESIGNATIONS OR OTHER INFORMATION	INTENDED MEANING	MISINTERPRETATION	CORRECTION
Large doses without properly placed commas (e.g., 100000 units or 1000000 units)	100,000 or 1,000,000 units	100000 has been mistaken for 10,000 or 1,000,000; 1,000,000 has been mistaken for 100,000.	Use commas for dosing units at or above 1,000 or use such words as 100 "thousand" or 1 "million" to improve readability.

DRUG NAME ABBREVIATIONS	INTENDED MEANING	MISINTERPRETATION	CORRECTION
Note: Pharmacists do not accept prescriptions with abbreviated medication names. To prevent errors, do not abbreviate drug names when communicating medical information.			
APAP	acetaminophen	Not recognized as acetaminophen	Use complete drug name.
ARA A	vidarabine	Mistaken as cytarabine (ARA C)	Use the complete drug name.
AZR	zidovudine (Retrovir)	Mistaken as azathioprine or aztreonam	Use the complete drug name.
CPZ	prochlorperazine (Compazine)	Mistaken as chlorpromazine	Use complete drug name.
DPT	Demerol-Phenergan-Thorazine	Mistaken as diphtheria-pertussis-tetanus	Use complete drug name.
DTO	Diluted tincture of opium, or deodorized tincture of opium (Paregoric)	Mistaken as tincture of opium	Use complete drug name.
HCl	hydrochloric acid or hydrochloride	Mistaken as potassium chloride (The "H" is misinterpreted as "K.")	Use complete drug name unless expressed as a salt of a drug.
HCT	hydrocortisone	Mistaken as hydrochlorothiazide	Use complete drug name.
HCTZ	hydrochlorothiazide	Mistaken as hydrocortisone (seen as HCT 250 mg)	Use complete drug name.
*$MgSO_4$	magnesium sulfate	Mistaken as morphine sulfate	Use complete drug name.
*MS, MSO_4	morphine sulfate	Mistaken as magnesium sulfate	Use complete drug name.
MTX	methotrexate	Mistaken as mitoxantrone	Use complete drug name.
NoAC	Novel/new oral anticoagulant	No anticoagulant	Use complete drug name
PCA	procainamide	Mistaken as patient-controlled analgesia	Use complete drug name.
PTU	propylthiouracil	Mistaken as mercaptopurine	Use complete drug name.
T3	Tylenol with codeine No. 3	Mistaken as liothyronine	Use complete drug name.
TAC	triamcinolone	Mistaken as tetracaine, adrenaline, cocaine	Use complete drug name.
TNK	TNKase	Mistaken as "TPA"	Use complete drug name.

Institute for Safe Medication Practices (ISMP) List of Error-Prone Abbreviations, Symbols, and Dose Designations—cont'd

DRUG NAME ABBREVIATIONS	INTENDED MEANING	MISINTERPRETATION	CORRECTION
TPA or tPA	Tissue plasminogen activator, Activase (alteplase)	Mistaken as TNKase (tenecteplase), or less often as another tissue plasminogen activator, Retavase (retaplase)	Use complete drug name.
$ZnSO_4$	zinc sulfate	Mistaken as morphine sulfate	Use complete drug name.
STEMMED DRUG NAMES	**INTENDED MEANING**	**MISINTERPRETATION**	**CORRECTION**
"nitro drip"	nitroglycerine infusion	Mistaken as sodium nitroprusside infusion	Use complete drug name.
"Norflox"	norfloxacin	Mistaken as Norflex	Use complete drug name.
"IV Vanc"	intravenous vancomycin	Mistaken as Invanz	Use complete drug name.
SYMBOLS	**INTENDED MEANING**	**MISINTERPRETATION**	**CORRECTION**
ʒ	Dram	Symbol for dram mistaken as "3"	Use the metric system.
♏	Minim	Mistaken as "mL"	Use the metric system.
x3d	For 3 days	Mistaken as "3 doses"	Use "for 3 days."
> and <	More than and less than	Mistaken as opposite of intended; mistakenly using incorrect symbols; "<10" mistaken as "40"	Use "more than" or "less than."
/ (slash mark)	Separates two doses or indicates "per"	Mistaken as the number 1 (e.g., "25 units/10 units" misread as "25 units and 110" units)	Use "per" rather than a slash mark to separate doses.
@	At	Mistaken as "2"	Use "at."
&	And	Mistaken as "2"	Use "and."
+	Plus or and	Mistaken as "4"	Use "and"
°	Hour	mistaken as zero (e.g., q2° seen as q 20)	Use "hr", "h", or "hour."
Φ or ⦰	zero, null sign	Mistaken as numerals 4, 6, 8, 9	Use 0 or zero, or describe intent using whole words

Source: Institute for Safe Medication Practices. (2017). *List of Error-Prone Abbreviations, Symbols, and Dose Designations*. Retrieved on November 8, 2018 from, https://www.ismp.org/recommendations/error-prone-abbreviations-list

Report medication errors or near misses to the ISMP Medication Errors Reporting Program (MERP) at 1-800-FAIL-SAF(E) or online at www.ismp.org.

*These abbreviations are included on The Joint Commission's "minimum list" of dangerous abbreviations, acronyms, and symbols that must be included on an organization's "Do Not Use" List, effective January 1, 2004.

MEASURING AND CALCULATING DOSAGE

Medications are not always available in the exact dosage the patient needs. Therefore, you must be proficient in calculating drug dosages to be sure your patients receive the correct amount of medication.

Drugs in solid form (e.g., tablets, powders) are measured by weight (e.g., milligrams [mg], grains). Drugs used for irrigation, infusion, and injection are liquids (usually solutions), measured by volume, generally milliliters (mL).

- A *solution* can be either a solid dissolved in a fluid, or a given volume of one liquid dissolved in a given volume of another liquid.
- Solution concentrations may be expressed as a proportion. A 1⁄100 solution is a solution of 1 gram of solid dissolved in 100 mL of fluid, or 1 mL of fluid mixed with 100 mL of another fluid.
- Think of solutions as a quantity of "solid" drug dissolved in a quantity of "liquid" diluent. The diluent merely carries the medication. When you see a vial marked "50 mg/mL," for example, you will know this means that in each milliliter (mL) of diluent there are 50 mg (in weight) of the solid, active medication.
- Your task is to determine how many milliliters of liquid you need to give the patient to receive the prescribed milligrams of active drug.

Medication Measurement Systems

Medications are usually prescribed and measured using the metric system; however, there are still a few medications that use the apothecary and household systems, so you need to learn how to work with all three systems.

Metric System

The metric system is the preferred system in the healthcare system because it enhances accuracy in the calculation of small drug dosages. It contains the:

- ***Meter,*** the unit for linear measurement is a little longer than a yard.
- ***Liter,*** used for capacity or volume, is a little larger than a quart.
- ***Gram,*** the unit for weight, is a little more than the weight of a steel paper clip. The following are the metric units you will use in preparing medications.

Weights

1 mg (milligram)	=	1,000 mcg or (micrograms)
1 gm (gram)	=	1,000 mg (milligrams)
1 kg (kilogram)	=	1,000 g or gm (grams)

Volume

1,000 mL (milliliters)	=	1 L (liter)
1,000 (cubic centimeters)	=	1 L (liter)

The following are examples of medication prescriptions using the metric system:

- Milk of Magnesia 30 mL orally daily at bedtime
- Cefazolin 1 gm IV q8hr

Apothecary System

The system uses grains, fractions (e.g., gr 1⁄4) instead of decimals (e.g., 0.25 gr), Roman numerals or Arabic numerals. Only a few medications (e.g., aspirin, phenobarbital) are measured using the British apothecary system because it is less precise and less convenient. For example, providers may prescribe aspirin *5 grains,* which might be written as *grains V* or *gr V.* To avoid a dosage error, write out the intended unit of measurement to ensure that *gr* (grains) is not mistaken for *gm* (grams) (The Joint Commission, 2018). **Key Point:** ***Keep in mind the apothecary abbreviations are prone to misinterpretation and error because they are not often used.*** The following are the units used in preparing medications:

Volume

1 minim (m)	=	1 drop (gtt)
1 fluid dram (dr)	=	60 minims
1 fluid ounce (oz)	=	8 fluid drams

Weight

1 dram (dr)	=	27.34 grains (gr)
1 grain	=	60 milligrams (mg)

The following are Roman numerals you will use most often:

M =	1000	X	=	10
D =	500	V	=	5
C =	100	I	=	1
L =	50	II	=	2

The following are examples of medication prescribed using the apothecary system:

Aspirin grains V orally q4hr prn for fever greater than 101°F

Chloramphenicol otic 2 gtts in each ear tid daily

With the exception of drops (gtts), many institutions no longer use the apothecary system of measurement. If used, verify the intended dose with the prescriber and pharmacist.

Household Measurements

This system of measurement is commonly used by the lay person, but is not widely used in healthcare facilities because drug dosages are less precise and can lead to medication dosing errors. The following are household units of measurement with metric conversion:

Volume

1 tsp (t)	=	5 mL		
1 tablespoon (tbsp or T)	=	3 teaspoons (tsp)	=	15 mL

6 tsp or 2 T	=	1 ounce (oz)	=	30 mL
16 T or 8 oz	=	1 cup (c)	=	240 mL
16 T or 8 oz	=	1 glass	=	240 mL
2 C	=	1 pint (pt)	=	480 mL
2 pt	=	1 quart (qt)	=	946.4 mL
4 qt	=	1 gallon (gal)		
Weight				
1 oz	=		=	28.35 gm
16 oz	=	1 pound (lb)	=	0.45 kg
Length				
12 inches (in.)	=	1 foot (ft)	=	30.5 cm
3 feet (ft)	=	1 yard (yd)	=	91.4 cm

The following is an example of a medication prescribed using the household system:

Amoxicillin 250 mg per 5 mL; give 1 tsp PO tid

Special Measurements: Units and Milliequivalent (mEq)

Key Point: ***Note that units and mEq cannot be directly converted to the apothecary, metric, or household system.***

Units Insulin, a drug used by patients with diabetes for control of blood sugar, is measured in ***units.*** The standard strength preparation, is 100 international units (U100). In this strength, 1 mL of the fluid medication contains 100 units of insulin. Heparin (an anticoagulant) and penicillin are also ordered in units.

Be aware that not all units are the same. You must always read the container label to know the number of units per milliliter.

The following are medications prescribed using units:

NPH insulin 14 units subcutaneous every morning
Heparin 4,000 units subcutaneous bid (twice daily)

Milliequivalents (mEq) indicate the strength of the ion concentration in a drug. A milliequivalent is the number of grams of a solid contained in one milliliter of a solution. Electrolytes, such as potassium chloride (KCl), are measured in *mEq.* The following are medications prescribed using *mEq:*

KCl 20 mEq orally bid (twice daily)
D_5W 1,000 mL with KCl 40 mEq q8hr

Calculating Dosages

You should be able to calculate accurately using several different methods and formulas. Inaccurate calculations result in incorrect dosages and could harm the patient. One easy formula to remember is the following:

$$\frac{\text{Dose on hand}}{\text{Quantity (or volume) on hand}} = \frac{\text{Desired dose}}{\text{Quantity (or volume) desired}}$$

Or

$$\frac{DH}{QH} = \frac{DD}{X}$$

Remember: You must pay attention to *both* the milligrams (weight of the drug) marked on the medication container *and* the milliliters (amount of liquid in which the medication is dissolved). For example, the provider prescribes meperidine (Demerol) 25 mg IM now. You have a prefilled syringe containing meperidine (Demerol) 50 mg in 1 mL volume. How much of the liquid (how many mL) would you administer to the patient?

$$\frac{DH}{QH} = \frac{DD}{X} \quad \text{or} \quad \frac{50\ \text{mg}}{1\ \text{mL}} = \frac{25\ \text{mg}}{X}$$

Therefore (recalling your algebra),

50X = 25 mL,
so X = 25 divided by 50,
so X = 0.5 mL

Here is an alternative formula you can use for calculating dosages:

$$\frac{\textbf{Dose desired (DD)}}{\textbf{Dose on hand (DH)}} \times \textbf{quantity on hand (QH) = desired quantity}$$

$$\frac{\text{Dose desired (25 mg)}}{\text{Dose on hand (50 mg)}} \times \text{quantity on hand (1 mL) = desired quantity}$$

ThinkLike a Nurse 26-1A

Mr. Pearson (Meet Your Patients, in Volume 1) has been prescribed nifedipine (Procardia XL) 60 mg orally daily. You have available Procardia XL (extended-release nifedipine) 30-mg tablets. Calculate the number of tablets you will need for one dose. How many tablets per day?

Conversions Within One System

When a drug prescription is written in the same system as the preparation you have on hand, you can easily make conversions. For example, in the metric system, if you want **to convert grams to milligrams,** you simply *multiply* by 1,000 (because 1 g = 1,000 mg). So, if you have 2.5 grams,

2.5 gm × 1,000 = 2,500 mg

To change milligrams to grams, *divide* by 1,000—move the decimal three places to the left. For example, if you wanted to know, in grams, the equivalent of 250 mg:

You know that 1,000 mg = 1 gm
By dividing: 250 mg ÷ 1,000 mg = 0.25 gm
Or by moving the decimal point three places to the left: 250.0 mg = 0.250 gm

Use exactly the same procedures to convert liters (L) and milliliters (mL). For example, if you wanted to know how many milliliters are the equivalent of 0.25 L:

You know that 1 L = 1,000 mL
By multiplying: 0.25 L × 1,000 = 250 mL
By moving the decimal point three places to the right, 0.250 L = 250 mL (Note that you must add a zero to *have* three places to the right.)

Within the apothecary system or the household system, use the equivalents and follow a similar process of multiplying and dividing. ***NOTE: You cannot just move the decimal in these systems.*** For example, suppose you have a dram ii (2-dram) tablet and you need to know how many grains you have (apothecary system). You know that 1 dram = 27.3 grains, so multiply:

2 drams (dr) × 27.3 grains (gr) = 54.6 grain, rounded to 55 grain.

In the household system, suppose you have 4 tbsp of a liquid and you need to know what part of a cup that represents. You know that 1 cup = 16 tablespoons, so substitute the equivalent and divide:

16 tbsp = 1 cup

So,

4 tbsp = 16 ÷ 4 = 1/4 cup

KnowledgeCheck 26-1A

Lanoxin 0.25 mg orally daily is prescribed for a patient with congestive heart failure. The label on the package you have reads "Lanoxin 0.125 mg" How many tablets will you give? Use the "dose on hand (DOH)" formula.

Conversions Between Systems

You will sometimes need to make conversions from one measurement system to another. For example, you may need to convert pounds to kilograms because many medications are prescribed as "milligrams per kilograms" (e.g., "Give 2 mg per kg of body weight"). The following are the basic methods for converting between systems.

- **Metric and Apothecary—Weights**

Grams and grains
(Memorize: 1 gm = 15 gr)
To convert grams to grains—*multiply* the grams by 15
To convert grains to grams—*divide* the grains by 15

Grains and milligrams
(Memorize: 1 gr = 60 mg)
To convert grains to milligrams—*multiply* the grains by 60
To convert milligrams to grains—*divide* the milligrams by 60

- **Metric and Apothecary and Household—Liquid Volume**

Liters and ounces
(Memorize: 1 L = 34.4 oz)
To convert liters to ounces—*multiply* the liters by 34.4
To convert ounces to liters—*divide* the ounces by 34.4

Ounces and milliliters
(Memorize: 1 ounce = 30 mL)
To convert ounces to milliliters—*multiply* the ounces by 30
To convert milliliters to ounces—*divide* the milliliters by 30

Milliliters and drops
(Memorize: 1 mL = 15 drops or 15 minims)
To convert milliliters to minims or drops—*multiply* milliliters by 15
To convert minims and drops to milliliters—*divide* the minims or drops by 15

KnowledgeCheck 26-2A

Work the following conversions:

- How many drops are there in 4 mL?
- How many milliliters are there in 2 oz?
- Convert 16 oz to liters.
- You have 3 gm. How many grains is this?
- You have 10 mg. How many grains is this?

How Should I Calculate Dosage for a Child?

You must be very careful when calculating medication dosages for children and infants.

Confusion between pounds and kilograms is a source of dosing error in pediatrics. Most drug references list normal pediatric ranges, which can serve as additional verification.

Key Point: ***The standard measurement for pediatric patients is kilograms, and prescriptions for pediatric dosages are usually either calculated by the prescriber or stated in terms of "milligrams per kilogram of body weight."***

For example, you might have a prescription for "Erythromycin 30 mg/kg of body weight." You know that 1 kg equals 2.2 lb and that the child weighs 44 lb.

- Convert the weight to kilograms by dividing 44 by 2.2: the child thus weighs 20 kg.
- Multiply the prescribed dose (30 mg) by body weight (20 kg): 30 mg × 20 kg = 600 mg
- 600 mg is the dosage for a 20-kg child.

You should rarely need to calculate a child's dosage on the basis of an adult dose because medication prescriptions should specify the exact dosage for the individual child, and the medication is dispensed using pediatric-specific medication formulations and concentrations. However, if you must calculate a child's dosage, use either the body surface area (BSA) formula by using a nomogram for children, or Clark's Rule for Children, to verify the safety of pediatric orders.

Nomograms To find a child's BSA using a nomogram, you must know the child's height and weight. To use a nomogram, you draw a straight line between the child's height (on the left scale) and weight (on the right scale) and note where the lines cross midline. For an example of a nomogram,

Go to http://www.manuelsweb.com/images/nomogram.png.

Clark's Rule Another formula used in pediatrics to determine safe dosage range is Clark's Rule. This rule is mostly used in children age 2 years and younger. A good example of how to use this rule is with the drug erythromycin, which has a usual adult dose of 250 to 500 mg. To determine the safe dosage range of erythromycin for children 2 years and younger, use Clark's Rule.

1. Using this formula, you assume that an average adult weighs 150 lb (68 kg) (this is the standard for the rule).

$$\textbf{Adult dose} \times \frac{\textbf{Child's weight in pounds}}{\textbf{150}} = \textbf{Child's dose}$$

2. According to Clark's Rule, if the maximum adult dose of erythromycin is 500 mg, then the maximum dose for an infant weighing 15 lb is:

$$500 \times 0.1 = 50 \text{ mg}$$

If you need information about a Web-based dosage calculator,

Go to http://www.manuelsweb.com/nrs_calculators.htm

CLINICALJUDGMENT
Applying the Full-Spectrum Nursing Model

PATIENT SITUATION

Leonard LeMonte is a 57-year-old African American man who has come to his primary care provider because of persistent headaches that have increased in intensity over the course of a day. His overall health has been good, although he is approximately 50 to 60 pounds overweight. His past medical history is significant for borderline primary hypertension and non–insulin-dependent diabetes, type 2 (diet controlled). Mr. LeMonte tells you that he works in a high-stress environment. He shares with you that he fears losing his job and not being able to pay his bills and meet the other financial commitments for his family. He also tells you that he has little time for hobbies or recreational outlets because he works so many hours.

THINKING

1. *Theoretical Knowledge (Facts and Principles):* You see in the medical records that the provider prescribed repaglinide (Prandin) to treat Mr. LeMonte's diabetes. By what route is this medication given?

2. *Critical Thinking (Inquiry):* If you did not know the answer to the first question, specifically how did you get the information? State your source.

DOING

3. *Nursing Process (Assessment):* To evaluate Mr. LeMonte's response to his diabetes medications, what questions do you need to ask him?

4. *Practical Knowledge (Skills):* Mr. LeMonte tells you that he forgot to take his Prandin this morning and also at lunchtime. What should you do?

CARING

5. *Self-Knowledge:* In what areas do you feel compassion for Mr. LeMonte, on which you might build a caring relationship?

6. *Self-Knowledge:* What do you identify as your strength in dealing with Mr. LeMonte's healthcare needs?

7. *Ethical Knowledge:* Mr. LeMonte tells you that he frequently skips doses of his Prandin because he cannot afford the expense. He asks you not to tell his wife about this because he does not want her to worry. What will you do?

Critical Thinking and Clinical Judgment

1. Your patient is prescribed Humulin R insulin 30 units subcutaneously. You have available in a multidose vial Humulin R insulin; the label reads "100 units per mL."
   a. What equipment and supplies do you need to administer this medication? Be specific.
   b. What practical knowledge (psychomotor skills) will you need?
   c. With regard to the psychomotor skills, what are the two aspects that require the most careful attention? Explain your thinking.
   d. What will you do to ensure that you have the correct dosage?
   e. What specific technique steps will you take to decrease the risk for infection?
   f. Suppose that after drawing the insulin into the syringe, you see that instead of the 30 units prescribed, you have only 20 units in the syringe. What will you do?
2. A provider prescribes heparin 4,000 units subcutaneous q12hr for Mr. Dale. You have on hand heparin 10,000 units/mL. How many milliliters should you draw up?

Recall the patients from Chapter 26, Meet Your Patients, in Volume 1. Questions 3 through 6 and 8 below refer to those patients. They are listed here for your convenience.

- Margaret Marks, an 82-year-old woman who has a fractured hip and experiences periods of confusion.
- Cary Pearson, a 70-year-old man with feeding and swallowing difficulties who receives his medications through a gastrostomy tube.
- Cyndi Early, a 32-year-old woman with diabetes who is scheduled for surgery at 1000 today.
- James Bigler, a 44-year-old man who has had a repair of a compound fracture of the right arm and is receiving intravenous fluids and medications.
- Rebecca Jones, an 84-year-old woman with compression fractures of two lumbar vertebrae resulting from a fall.

---

3. It is 0800, and you have begun organizing your medication pass for this shift by verifying the MAR entries against the provider's prescriptions. You notice that Mr. Bigler has been prescribed Toradol 30 mg IM q6hr. His last dose was supposed to have been given at 0600, but there is no documentation that the medication was administered.
   a. What should you do?
   b. Should you assume the night shift nurse administered the medication but forgot to document that she had given it, and give the 0600 dose late? Why, or why not?
   c. When should the next dose be administered?

d. If the night nurse did *not* administer the medication as prescribed, what type of medication error did she make? What factors that could have caused this error?

e. Assuming that the nurse *did* administer the medication as prescribed at 0600, what error did the night nurse make? Which of the "rights of medication" was violated?

4. You receive the laboratory results for Cary Pearson's potassium level and find it to be 3.1 mEq/L. You notify the provider and receive a verbal prescription to add 20 mEq of KCl to his IV of D_5½ NS (5% dextrose in half-strength NS [0.45% saline]) to infuse at 125 mL/hr. The IV infusing is a new 1,000-mL bag that is almost full.

   a. Write the prescription as you would write it on the order sheet.

   b. What information must you put on the additive label for this bag?

   c. Suppose the situation were slightly different. There is only 100 mL of IV fluid left in Mr. Pearson's IV bag when you call the provider, who prescribes, "Add 10 mEq to the IV, and infuse it at 125 mL/hr." Would you ask for clarification of this prescription? Why, or why not?

   d. Change the situation again. You have taken the prescription in this way: "Add 20 mEq of KCl to 1,000 mL of D_5½ NS and infuse at 125 mL/hr." You are preparing this medication and find that Mr. Pearson currently has 500 mL remaining in his IV infusion. Should you add the KCl to the IV that is infusing or wait until you hang a new 1,000-mL bag? If you do add it, how much KCl will you add? What is your rationale for your decision?

   e. You begin preparing the infusion with the 20 mEq of KCl to be added and find you have available a vial containing KCl 40 mEq in a 10-mL vial. How many milliliters of KCl will you add to the bag of fluids?

5. Dr. Xi has prescribed heparin 8,000 units subcutaneous q12hr for Mrs. Marks.

   a. You have vials of heparin containing 10,000 units/mL. How many mL of heparin will you administer?

   b. To prevent tissue trauma and hematoma and to help ensure adequate absorption, what precautions should you take while administering heparin?

   c. What syringe and needle will you select for administration, and why?

6. You are checking Mrs. Early's medical records and find that the provider has prescribed a medication the patient lists as having an allergy. What steps should you take?

7. A patient has been taking warfarin sodium (Coumadin) 3 mg daily for the past 3 years. She has tolerated the medication well, but recently she has noticed more bleeding tendencies, such as nosebleeds and hematuria (blood in the urine). You assess the patient and find that she has gross hematuria today and numerous bruises over her body. To answer the following questions, what theoretical knowledge do you need, and where can you find it? (*Note:* After you get the information you need, answer the following questions.)

   a. What could be causing these bleeding episodes?

   b. What laboratory test is indicated in this situation, and what result do you expect?

   c. What actions should you take in this situation?

8. James Bigler (Meet Your Patients, in Volume 1) has had a postoperative repair of a compound fracture of the right arm and is receiving IV fluids and medications, including opioid analgesics and antibiotics. He also has a herniated intervertebral disk and severe muscle spasms. He received his first dose of an oral muscle relaxant, cyclobenzaprine (Flexeril) 10 mg, at midnight. At 0800, he received another dose. At 0900, he received an IV antibiotic, and while awake, he has been self-administering his opioid analgesic using his patient-controlled analgesia (PCA) IV pump about every 4 hours in a low dose. Consider these facts:
   - The most common side effect of Flexeril is drowsiness. It has a half-life of 24 to 72 hours.
   - Common side effects of opioids are drowsiness, decreased respiratory rate and depth, decreased blood pressure, and constipation (if taken long term).
   - Besides allergies, the most common adverse effect of Mr. Bigler's antibiotic is diarrhea.

   Mr. Bigler's muscle relaxant (Flexeril) is to be administered every 8 hours. When you enter his room to administer his 1600 dose, you find that he is extremely sleepy. He will awaken when you shake him or speak to him, but he falls right back to sleep and is slurring his words. These are new symptoms for him.

   a. Is there anything obvious about his medical diagnosis that might be producing these symptoms? If so, what?

   b. Which of his medications could cause these symptoms, and why?

   c. What would you do? Would you give the 1600 dose of cyclobenzaprine (Flexeril)?

9. Mrs. Thomas lives alone and until a few months ago was able to take care of herself. When her eyesight began to deteriorate, she experienced difficulty self-administering her medications.

   a. Discuss the assessment required to determine whether she is at risk for ineffective management of her medication regimen.

   b. Mrs. Thomas was prescribed lorazepam (Ativan) 1 mg orally. Is this prescription complete? If not, what is missing? What actions should you take?

   c. Mrs. Thomas has a prescription for digoxin (Lanoxin) 1.25 mg orally every morning. You have available Lanoxin 0.25 mg, and you calculate that 5 tablets should be administered. You check a drug guide and find that the usual dose is 0.125 mg to 0.25 mg orally daily. What actions should you take?

10. Calculate dosages for the following medications that you will be administering during your medication pass today. Are there any prescriptions you would question? If so, why?

    a. Cephalexin (Keflex) 500 mg IV q6hr. You have on hand Keflex 1 gram in 1 mL of solution.

    b. Furosemide (Lasix) 280 mg orally daily. You have 40-mg tablets of Lasix available.

    c. Meperidine (Demerol) 10 mg intramuscularly, to a child. You have Demerol 25 mg/mL available in a prefilled syringe. In addition to calculating the dosage, describe the equipment you would use to administer the Demerol to a child.

11. Describe the procedure for giving atropine sulfate 0.4 mg IM along with morphine 10 mg IM using the same syringe. The atropine is in a single-dose vial containing 0.4 mg of atropine in 0.5 mL of fluid. The morphine is in a prefilled 10 mg injectable cartridge containing 10 mg in 1 mL of fluid.

12. You have a prescription to administer injectable phenytoin (Dilantin) and furosemide (Lasix). You would like to administer them in the same syringe. What theoretical and practical knowledge do you need to decide whether you can do this?

13. For each of the following patient problems (1) state what you think might be the cause and (2) state one thing you might have done to prevent the problem.

  a. When you give Mrs. King an intramuscular injection in her ventrogluteal muscle, she complains of pain.

  b. Several weeks after receiving an intramuscular injection in the dorsogluteal site, Mr. Aguilar begins having pain in his left lower back and hip; the pain proceeds down his leg. He is beginning to limp when he walks.

  c. Several days after receiving a subcutaneous injection, Patti Deal's upper arm is red, hot, painful, and swollen. There is pus oozing from the injection site.

  d. Immediately after an intramuscular injection, a patient starts showing severe, unexpected symptoms.

14. For each of the following concepts, use critical thinking to describe how or why it is important to nursing, patient care, or administering medications. Note that these are *not* to be merely definitions.

Pharmacology

Drug classification systems (e.g., according to use or chemical traits)

The United States Pharmacopeia–National Formulary (USP-NF)

Drug excretion

Therapeutic levels

Side effects and adverse reactions

The apothecary system

Household measurements

Units and milliequivalents

Standing prescriptions

"Rights of medication" administration

Ventrogluteal site for intramuscular injection

Medication errors

What Are the Main Points in This Chapter?

- Drugs are classified according to their use, body systems, and chemical or pharmacological traits. Learning the classifications helps you to remember the characteristics of individual drugs.
- The form (preparation) of a drug affects its speed of onset, intensity of action, and route of administration.
- In the United States, the Food and Drug Administration (FDA) regulates the manufacturing, sale, and effectiveness of all medications. Various state and federal agencies and legislation also regulate the administration of medications.
- Controlled substances must be stored, handled, disposed of, and administered according to regulations established by the U.S. Drug Enforcement Agency (DEA).
- In general, intravenous (IV) medications are absorbed most rapidly, followed by intramuscular, subcutaneous, buccal, and oral medications.
- Metabolism is the chemical inactivation of a drug into a form that the body can excrete; drug metabolism takes place mainly in the liver.
- The primary route of drug excretion is from the kidneys; other routes are the liver, gastrointestinal tract, lungs, and exocrine glands.
- The therapeutic level of a drug is the concentration in the blood serum that produces the desired effect without toxicity.
- Medication effects can be primary (therapeutic and intended) or secondary (nontherapeutic and unintended). Secondary effects include side effects, adverse reactions, toxic reactions, allergic reactions, and idiosyncratic reactions.
- The metric system is preferred for medications; however, for a few medications, the apothecary and household systems are still used.

- You are legally responsible for the medications you administer. You must question orders you believe to be incorrect.
- To help prevent medication errors, observe the "three checks" (before and after pouring or drawing up a medication, and at the bedside) and the "six rights of medication" (right drug, right dose, right time, right route, and right patient, as well as right documentation immediately after giving the medication).
- If you make a medication error, it is absolutely necessary that you immediately assess the patient's vital signs and physical status; report findings to the primary care provider; and notify the nurse manager of your unit.
- The oral route is the one most commonly used; it is convenient and safe.
- Buccal and sublingual medications are held in the mouth so that they will be absorbed through the mucous membrane.
- For patients who cannot swallow or who have feeding tubes, you can give oral medications through enteric (e.g., nasogastric [NG] and gastrostomy) tubes. The medications are given one at a time and the tube must be flushed before and after each medication.
- Topical medications may have local and systemic effects; transdermal patches are applied for their systemic effect.
- Nebulization is the production of a fine spray, fog, powder, or mist from a liquid drug.
- Parenteral medications require the use of sterile technique to prevent infection.
- Needle length and gauge are chosen based on the type of medication, the route of administration, and the amount of adipose and muscle tissue the patient has.
- Needleless systems and safety syringes reduce the likelihood of needlestick injury.
- Always dispose of needles in special "sharps" containers. If you must recap a needle, use a one-handed technique.
- The ventrogluteal site is the preferred intramuscular injection site for adults. Other sites are the vastus lateralis and the deltoid. Use the rectus femoris site only if no other sites are available, and never in infants and children. Do not use the dorsogluteal site.
- Experts agree the anterolateral thigh (vastus lateralis) is preferred for infants who are not walking and some recommend using it throughout childhood. Others recommend using the ventrogluteal site when the child starts walking and the gluteal muscle increase in mass. The deltoid can be used for older children if you are certain that the muscle mass is adequate.
- Medications may be given intravenously by adding the medication to a large-volume (primary infusion), by the IV push technique, or by intermittent (piggyback setup) infusion.
- You should report medication errors immediately after they occur; a risk management process for monitoring causative factors should be in place.
- The most common reasons for a patient to have a central venous access device (CVAD) are to:
  - Give long-term IV therapy
  - Provide total parenteral nutrition when the patient cannot eat normally
  - Have blood drawn without the trauma and complications of repeated venipuncture
  - Be used when peripheral IV line placement is difficult

Knowledge Map

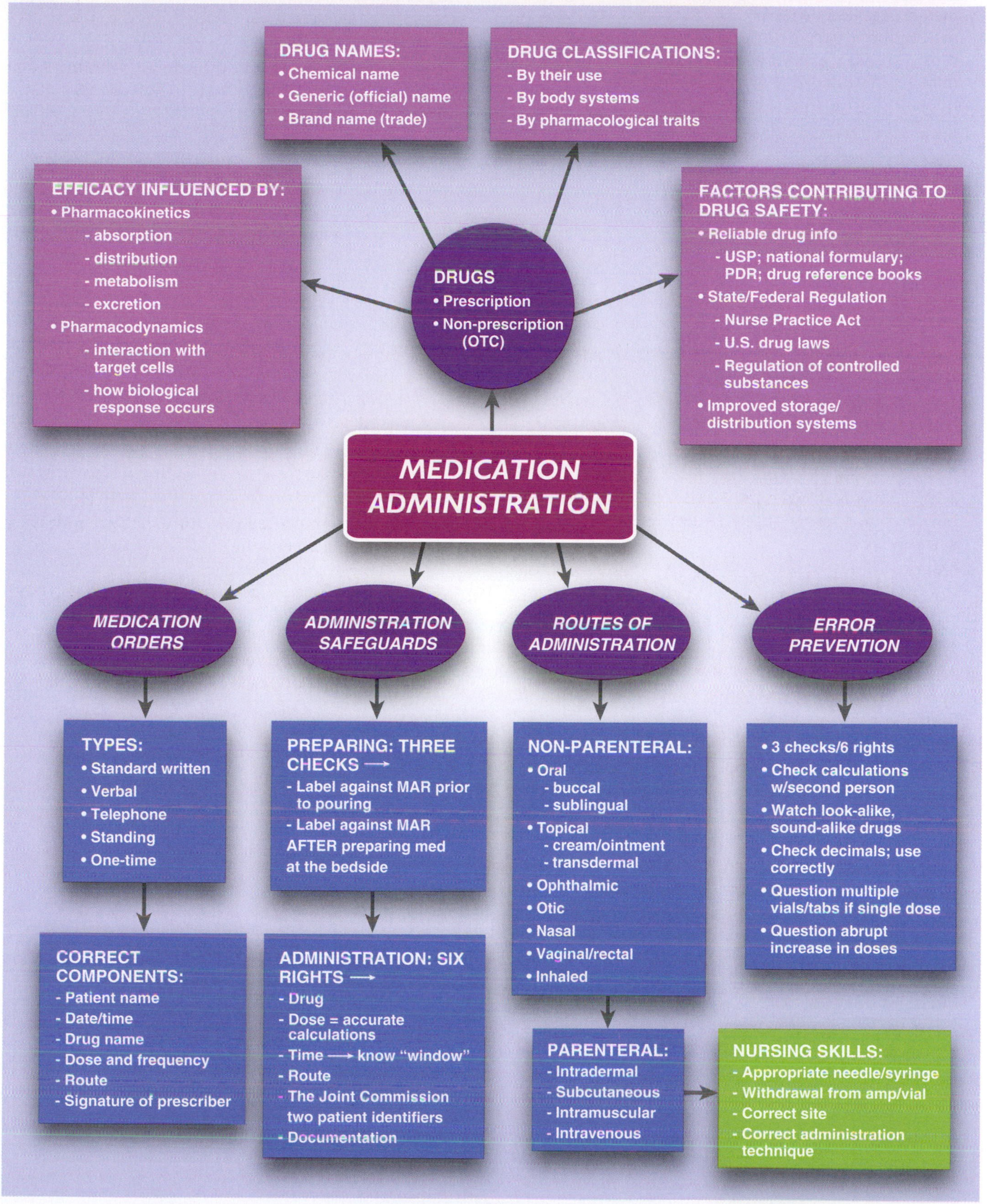

Knowledge Map

UNIT 4

Supporting Physiological Functioning

CHAPTER 27

Nutrition

STUDENT RESOURCES

The questions and exercises in this book allow you to practice the kind of thinking you will use as a full-spectrum nurse. Critical-thinking questions usually have more than one right answer, so we do not provide correct answers for these features. Try to answer these questions yourself. It is more important to develop your nursing judgment than to just cover content. You will learn more by discussing the questions with your peers. If you are still unsure, see the Davis Advantage chapter resources for suggested responses.

To explore learning resources for this chapter,

Go to Davis Advantage and find:

Answers and Suggested Responses for all questions in this chapter

Concept Map

Knowledge Map

References and Bibliography

Lists of NOC Outcomes and NIC Interventions

Key Concepts

Energy

Metabolism

Nutrition

Related Concepts

See the Concept Map on Davis Advantage.

Example Problems

Overweight and Obesity

Undernutrition and Malnutrition

Caring for the Nguyens

Nam Nguyen has been diagnosed with hypertension, type 2 diabetes mellitus, obesity, osteoarthritis, and tobacco abuse. Zach Miller, FNP-BC has advised an 1,800-kcal diabetic diet with no added salt and a daily brisk 30-minute walk. Mr. Nguyen discusses these challenges with his daughter Trinh.

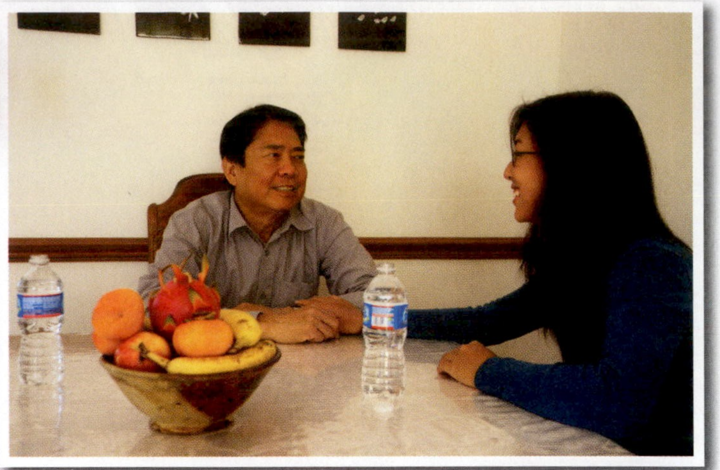

A. Why might Zach have selected this diet plan? Discuss the rationale for each component (i.e., 1,800-kcal, diabetic diet, no added salt).

B. Mr. Nguyen's diet is complex. He tells you he is overwhelmed by the many changes asked of him. How might Zach streamline his instructions about Mr. Nguyen's diet?

C. Nam asks what the best way is for him to monitor his weight loss progress at home and how Zach Miller will monitor his progress. How would you respond?

D. Identify teaching tools that might help Nam understand his diet.

PracticalKnowledge clinical **application**

To apply concepts that support patient nutrition, you will need to master techniques for assessing nutritional status, feeding patients, administering supplemental feedings, and working with nasogastric (NG) and nasoenteric (NE) tubes.

PROCEDURES

Procedure 27-1 ■ Checking Fingerstick (Capillary) Blood Glucose Levels

➤ For steps to follow in all procedures, refer to the Universal Steps for All Procedures found on the inside back cover.

Equipment

- Blood glucose meter
- Test strip
- Sterile lancet (and injector, if available)
- Alcohol (or other antiseptic) pad, if required by policy
- 2 × 2 inch gauze pad or cotton ball
- Procedure gloves

Glucometers, fingerstick devices, and injectors should be assigned to individual patients. If this is not possible, you must clean and disinfect the devices between patients. If they are available, use single-use lancets that permanently retract upon puncture.

Store these supplies on a tray or cart outside patient's room. Do not carry supplies in your pocket. If there are unused supplies, leave them in the room; do not use them for another patient.

These measures help prevent needlestick injury and transmission of bloodborne pathogens (Centers for Disease Control and Prevention [CDC], 2005).

Delegation

Assess the patient first. If the patient's condition allows, you can delegate this procedure to a licensed practical nurse (LPN) or unlicensed assistive personnel (UAP) who has been adequately trained in performing the skill. Most patients perform this procedure independently at home.

Pre-Procedure Assessments

- Assess the patient's comprehension of the procedure.
  Allows you to tailor instructions to the individual patient.

- Assess potential puncture sites for bruising, inflammation, open lesions, poor circulation, or edema.
  Avoid such sites because of risk for infection and inaccurate results.
- Check for factors such as anticoagulant therapy, bleeding disorders, or low platelet count that place the patient at risk for bleeding after skin puncture.

➤ When performing the procedure, always identify your patient according to agency policy, using two identifiers, and be attentive to standard precautions, hand hygiene, patient safety and privacy, body mechanics, and documentation.

➤ *Note:* The steps of this procedure will vary, depending on the type of glucose meter used.

Procedure Steps

1. **Verify the medical prescription** for frequency and timing of testing.
   A prescription is necessary for testing. Timing and frequency of testing are crucial for accurate insulin dosing.

2. **Ask the patient to wash her hands** with soap and warm water, if able, and to dry completely using a clean towel.
   Reduces the risk for infection and dilates capillaries at the puncture site. Also ensures that the testing site is free of any sugar residue.

3. **Turn on the blood glucose meter.** Calibrate it according to the manufacturer's instructions.
   Calibration readies the meter for testing and checks it for accuracy of the machine.

4. **Check that the strip is the correct type** for the monitor. Check the expiration date on the container of reagent strips. If the strips are expired, replace them.
   Expired strips may alter test results. Different brands of monitors use different kinds of reagent strips.

5. **Don procedure gloves.**
   Gloving protects against exposure to blood.

6. **Remove the reagent strip** from the container, and place it into the blood glucose meter. Then, tightly seal the container.
   A tight seal protects reagent strips from exposure to air and light.

7. **Select and clean a fingerstick site.** If the patient is unable to do so, perform hand hygiene for her.
   Helps prevent infection by removing some surface microorganisms.

8. **Use a different site each time** you check the glucose.
   Adult and child—the lateral aspect of a finger (palmar surface, distal phalanx)
   Infant—heel or great toe
   The lateral aspect of the finger contains fewer nerve endings than the central fingertip, so it hurts less. Capillaries in infants are too small to obtain an adequate blood sample.

9. **Position the finger** (or heel or great toe for an infant) in a dependent position, and massage from the base toward the tip of the finger.
   A dependent position promotes blood flow to the site via gravity and pressure, ensuring an adequate specimen. The massaging action increases blood flow to the tip of the finger, which may prevent the need for repuncture.

10. **Prick the finger** (or a different site) with the lancing device.

Semiautomatic Injector

a. Engage the sterile injector, and remove the cover.
b. Place the disposable lancet firmly into the end of the injector.
c. Place the back of the patient's hand on the table, or otherwise secure the finger (e.g., hold the finger and hand firmly).
d. Position the end of the injector firmly against the skin, perpendicular (at a 90° angle) to the chosen puncture site.
e. Push the release switch, allowing the needle to pierce the skin.
   Proper positioning and stabilization of the site ensure that the lancet pierces to the correct depth. This prevents patient injury and allows for adequate blood sampling. Patients tend to pull away as you perform the puncture.

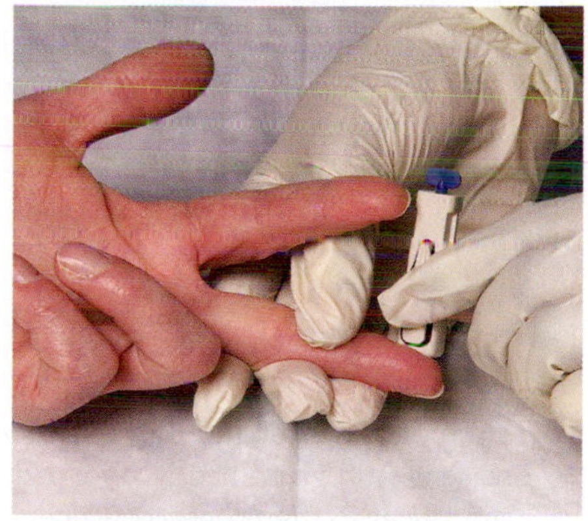

11. **Lightly squeeze the patient's finger** above the puncture site until a drop of blood has collected.
    Squeezing promotes a better blood sample for testing without causing injury to the puncture site.

12. **Place the reagent strip test patch** close to the drop of blood. Allow contact between the drop of blood and the test strip. Do not "smear" the blood over the reagent strip.

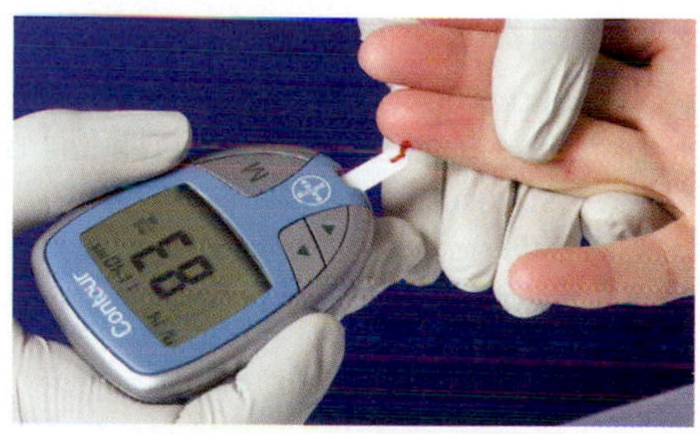

13. **Insert the strip into the meter,** if you have not already done so (follow the manufacturer's instructions); allow the blood sample to remain in contact with the test strip for the amount of time specified.
    For some meters, you insert the test strip before pricking the finger; with others, you put the blood on the reagent strip and then insert the strip into the meter. The blood sample must be on the reagent strip for the specified amount of time to ensure accurate test results.

(continued on next page)

Procedure 27-1 ■ Checking Fingerstick (Capillary) Blood Glucose Levels (continued)

14. **Using a gauze pad, gently apply pressure** to the puncture site.
Pressure stops the bleeding by promoting coagulation.

15. **After the meter signals, read** the blood glucose level indicated on the digital display.

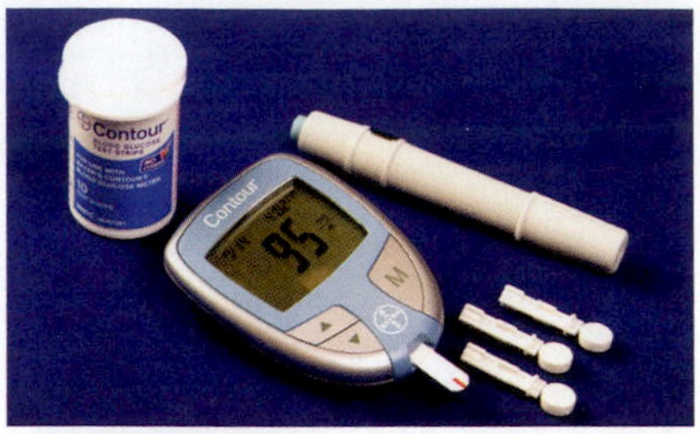

16. **Turn off the meter.** Dispose of the reagent strip, gauze pad, alcohol pad, and lancet in the proper containers (e.g., a sharps container for the lancet).
Proper disposal prevents sharps injury and the spread of infection via bloodborne pathogens.

17. **Remove your gloves,** and dispose of them in the covered trash receptacle or biohazards container. Perform hand hygiene.
Safe disposal reduces the transmission of pathogens.

? What if . . .

- **The patient has poor circulation or is a child or older adult?**

Place a heel warmer or warm cloth on the site for about 10 minutes before obtaining the blood sample. Alternatively, position the patient's hand below the waist for 1 minute.
Capillaries in infants are very small; older adults may have poor peripheral circulation. Warmth dilates the capillaries and may help you obtain an adequate amount of blood; when the extremities are dangled, gravity allows blood to pool in the extremity, making it easier to obtain an ample specimen.

- **The patient is taking an anticoagulant, such as warfarin sodium (Coumadin)?**

After the procedure, hold pressure for 2 min, and then apply a pressure bandage, if needed. Recheck the site after 5 min to make sure bleeding has stopped.

- **The monitor shows an extremely unusual result or an error message?**

Repeat the process using a different finger or site.

- **The patient uses a noninvasive method to measure blood glucose?**

A continuous glucose monitor (CGM) is used to more closely track blood sugar. One type of CGM is worn like a wristwatch. Using an electrical current, it pulls fluid from the skin to give a blood glucose reading. Another style uses a small sensor just below the skin of the abdomen and measures glucose in the interstitial fluid.

  - The CGM will take readings automatically every 5 to 30 minutes and will download data to a computer, tablet, or smartphone.
  - Advise the patient to shave his arm if it is very hairy, or the reading may not be accurate.
  - The patient should wear the device for a 3-hour warm-up before taking a reading and should not bathe or swim during that time.

This does not replace the fingerstick method. Its purpose is to track trends in blood glucose. It also benefits patients whose blood sugar drops dangerously low overnight, which could go undetected.

Evaluation

- Assess the puncture site for bleeding or bruising.
- Evaluate the patient's understanding of the procedure and the test results.
- Promptly notify the primary care provider of abnormal test results, or administer insulin on the basis of test results, if prescribed.

Patient Teaching

- Explain the procedure, test results, and treatment to the patient.
Information allows the patient to participate in his plan of care and typically increases adherence to the therapeutic regimen.
- Discuss the importance of maintaining glycemic control.
- If the patient will be performing fingerstick blood glucose testing at home, teach the patient how to perform the procedure. Ask the patient to perform a return demonstration. Teach the patient to do the following:
  - Read the manufacturer's instructions carefully, and call their toll-free number if you have any questions.
  - Always use the test strips that are recommended for the meter.
  - Take your meter to your healthcare provider's office so that she can make sure you are measuring your blood sugar correctly.
  - Perform quality control checks (read the instructions) to make sure the meter is measuring accurately.
  - Clean the meter according to the manufacturer's directions. Some meters will give you an electronic alert telling you when to clean them.

Home Care

- Assess the client's ability to perform fingerstick blood glucose monitoring independently.
A change in the patient's condition may not allow the patient to perform testing. Certain conditions, such as arthritis and limited vision, may limit dexterity.
- Provide information about purchasing home glucose-monitoring equipment.

- Explain how to dispose of lancets in a labeled, puncture-proof container, such as an empty bleach container.
- Instruct caregivers to wear gloves when obtaining a blood sample for glucose monitoring.
- At home, patients should not cleanse their fingers with an alcohol wipe before puncturing it. However, they should wash their hands with soap and water and dry them well.

Documentation

- Record the fingerstick blood glucose result in the progress notes or special flowsheet, including the date and time the test was performed.
- Note whether the physician was notified, and record any treatment given.
- Document patient teaching.
- If the fingerstick is performed in response to patient symptoms, you may need to write a narrative note.

Sample documentation

8/12/19 1435 Patient reported feeling "cold and shaky." FBBS 62. Alert and able to swallow. Pt ate 5 saltine crackers with peanut butter and drank 3 ounces of orange juice. FSBS 92 at 1430. Will notify physician for further orders. —————————— N. Jones, RN

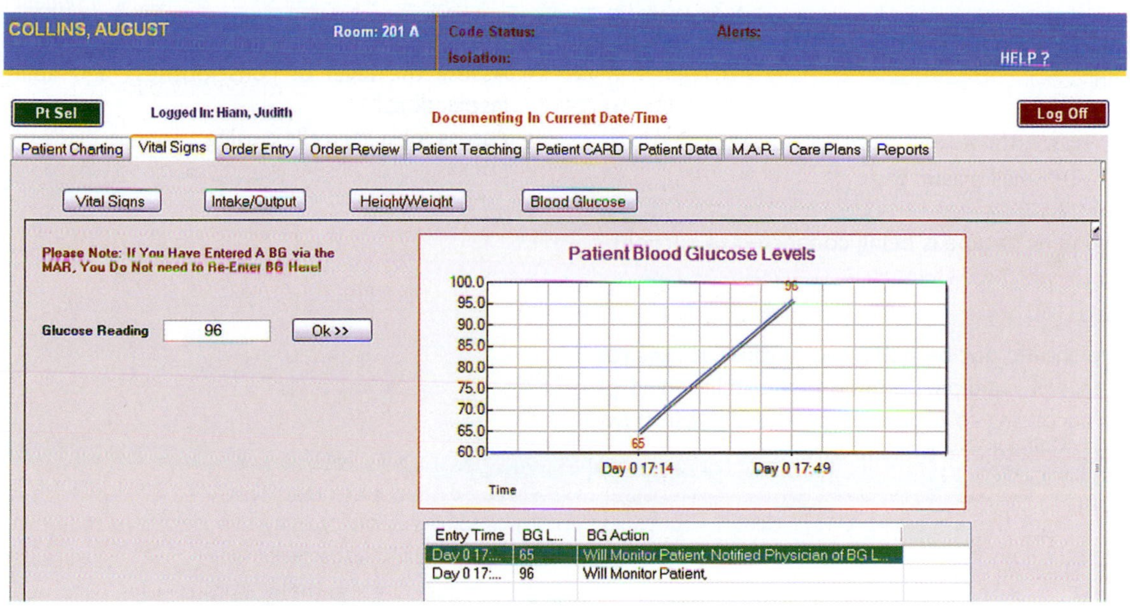

Practice Resources

American Diabetes Association (2018, February 7, last edited); Centers for Disease Control and Prevention (CDC) (2013, February 6, last updated); Hortensius, J., Slingerland, C., Kleefstra, N., et al. (2011); U.S. Food and Drug Administration (FDA) (2018, March 9, updated).

Thinking About the Procedure

The video **Checking Fingerstick (Capillary) Blood Glucose Levels,** along with questions and suggested responses, is available on the ***Davis's Nursing Skills Videos*** Web site on FADavis.com.

Procedure 27-2 ■ Inserting Nasogastric and Nasoenteric Tubes

➤ For steps to follow in all procedures, refer to the Universal Steps for All Procedures found on the inside back cover.

Equipment

- Nasogastric tube (commonly 16- or 18-French (Fr) for adults, but sometimes smaller) or nasoenteric (small bowel) tube (8-Fr, 10-Fr, or 12-Fr)
- Stylet or guidewire (for small-bore tubes), according to agency policy
- Procedure gloves
- Linen-saver pad or towel
- Water-soluble lubricant
- 50- to 60-mL catheter-tip syringe or bulb syringe for Salem sump tubes; 30-mL luer-lock syringe for small-bore feeding tubes
- Hypoallergenic tape (about 2.5 cm [1 in.] wide) or tube fixation device
- Indelible marker
- Skin adhesive
- Stethoscope
- Emesis basin
- Basin with warm water (for plastic tube) or ice (for rubber tube) (Most tubes are plastic.)
- Glass of water with a straw
- Penlight
- Tongue blade
- pH test strip
- Tissues
- Safety pin
- Gauze square or small plastic bag
- Rubber band
- Suction equipment (if tube is being connected to suction)

Delegation

This procedure should not be delegated because it requires knowledge of anatomy and physiology and the ability to adapt the procedure according to patient responses. You can, however, delegate associated oral hygiene care.

Pre-Procedure Assessments

- Verify the medical prescription for type of tube to be placed and whether it is to be attached to suction or drainage.
- Confirm the patient's need for NG or NE intubation (e.g., surgery involving the gastrointestinal (GI) tract, impaired swallowing, or decreased level of consciousness).
  NG or NE intubation decreases the risk for aspiration in these patients. In many institutions, only specially trained nurses are allowed to place small-bowel feeding tubes.
- Assess each naris for patency, deviated septum, and skin breakdown. Ask the patient to close each nostril alternately and breathe. Select the nostril with the greatest air flow. Ask the patient to blow her nose, if not contraindicated.
  A septal defect or facial fracture may cause obstruction, placing the patient at risk for nasal membrane trauma if insertion is attempted through the affected naris.
- Check health history for anticoagulant therapy, coagulopathy, nasal trauma, nasal surgery, epistaxis, or deviated septum, and other conditions that may indicate the need for tube insertion via endoscope or fluoroscope.
  The healthcare provider should be notified if patient history or status places the patient at risk for injury during NG or NE insertion.
- Assess the level of consciousness and ability to follow instructions.
- Assess for a gag reflex, using a tongue blade.
  Diminished or absent gag reflex places the patient at risk for aspiration.

➤ When performing the procedure, always identify your patient according to agency policy, using two identifiers, and be attentive to standard precautions, hand hygiene, patient safety and privacy, body mechanics, and documentation.

Procedure Steps

1. Prepare the tube.

Plastic Tube

Wrap the tube around your index finger, and then unwrap it and proceed, or place in a basin of warm water for 10 minutes and proceed.

Small-Bore Tube

Insert a stylet or guidewire and secure into position, according to agency policy. (Small-bore tubes may come with guidewires in them. If so, flush the tube with tap water to lubricate the wire for easy removal.) Leave the wire in place until the tube is positioned and its placement has been checked on x-ray film. Once the guidewire is removed, do not reinsert it. Agency policy determines which nurses are authorized to place small-bore tubes.

Warm water softens a plastic tube, and ice stiffens the rubber tube to make it easier to insert. (Most tubes are polyurethane or silicone based.) Wrapping a plastic tube around your index finger helps the tube flex into a curve and aids in insertion. A flexible, guidewire facilitates passage of small-bore tube but can cause trauma if not secured in the proper position.

2. Assist the patient into a high-Fowler's position, with a pillow behind the head and shoulders. Raise the bed to a comfortable working level.

This position facilitates tube insertion and prevents aspiration should the patient vomit during tube insertion. Gravity facilitates passage of the tube. Raising the bed reduces strain on the nurse's back.

3. **Measure the tube for placement.**

Nasogastric Tube

Measure the length of the tube to be inserted by measuring from the tip of the nose to the earlobe, and from the earlobe to the end of the sternum at the xiphoid process. Mark the length with tape or indelible ink at the naris.
This measurement indicates how far the tube must be inserted to reach the stomach.

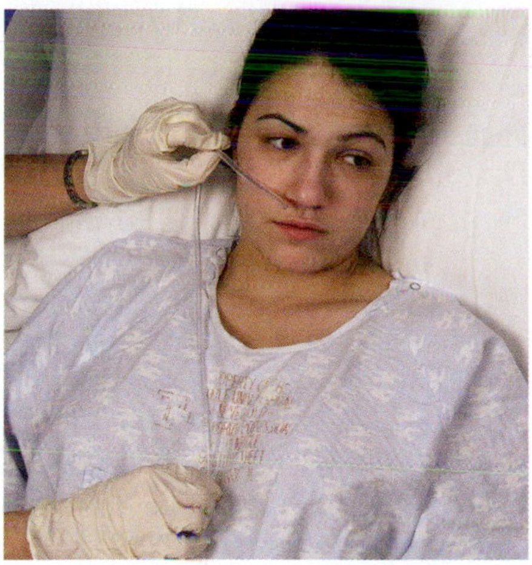

Nasoenteric Tube

Add 8 to 10 cm (3 to 4 in.) to the NG tube measurement, as directed, and mark the tube.

4. **If you are right-handed**, stand on the patient's right side; if you are left-handed, stand on the left side. Drape a linen-saver pad over the patient's chest, and hand her an emesis basin and facial tissues.
Draping protects the patient's gown from becoming soiled during tube insertion.

5. **Prepare the fixation device.** Cut a 10-cm (4-in.) piece of hypoallergenic tape if securing tube with tape; split the bottom end lengthwise 2.5 cm (2 in.). If using a commercial feeding tube attachment device, have it ready at this time.
To secure the tube after insertion.

iCare 6. **Arrange a signal** through which the patient can communicate if she wants to stop (e.g., raising her hand).
Relieves anxiety by giving the patient some control over the procedure.

7. **Don procedure gloves** if you have not already done so.
Reduces the spread of microorganisms.

8. **Wrap 10 to 15 cm (5 to 6 in.)** of the end of the tube tightly around your index finger, then release.
Forms the tube into a curve that helps it conform more easily to the shape of the nasopharynx.

9. **Lubricate the distal 10 cm** (4 in.) of the tube with a water-soluble jelly.
Lubrication eases the passage of the tube and prevents injury to the nasal mucosa. Water-soluble lubricants will dissolve if it is aspirated, whereas oil-based lubricants do not dissolve in the respiratory tract and cause inflammation and blockage of airways if they enter the lungs. Some nurses prefer water as a lubricant because aqueous jelly dries and can block and irritate the nasal passages. Some tubes have a surface lubricant and require only that you dip them in room-temperature water.

10. **Hand the patient a glass of water** with a straw, if she is awake, alert, and able to swallow.
Swallowing during insertion eases passage.

11. **Instruct the patient** to hold her head straight up and extend her neck back against the pillow (slightly hyperextended).
   a. Grasp the end of the tube above the lubricant with the curved end pointing downward.
   b. Carefully insert the tube along the floor of the nasal passage, on the lateral side, aiming toward the ear.
   c. You will feel slight resistance when the tube reaches the nasopharynx; use gentle pressure, but do not force the tube to advance. The patient's eyes may tear; if so, provide tissues.
   d. Continue inserting the tube until just past the nasopharynx by gently rotating the tube toward the client's opposite naris.

Hyperextending the neck straightens the curve where the nasal passage meets the pharynx (nasopharyngeal junction). Gentle insertion prevents trauma to the nasal mucosa. Tears are normal.

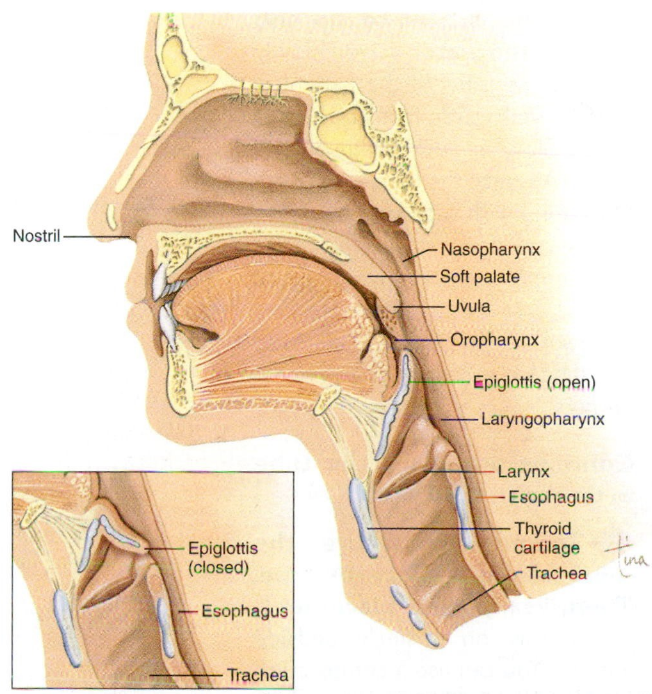

(continued on next page)

Procedure 27-2 ■ Inserting Nasogastric and Nasoenteric Tubes (continued)

12. Pause for a moment to allow the patient to relax and, perhaps, use tissues. Explain that the next step requires her to swallow.
Stopping to relax can give the patient a feeling of control and reduce gagging.

13. Instruct the patient to flex her head toward her chest, take a small sip of water, and swallow.
This maneuver closes the trachea and opens the esophagus.

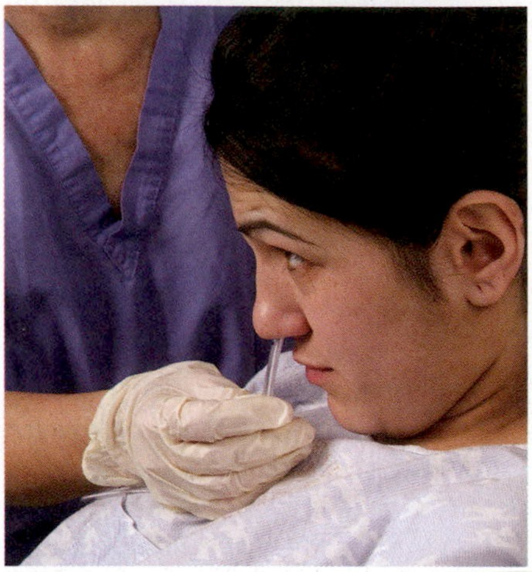

14. Rotate the tube 180°.
Rotation helps redirect the tube so that it will not enter the patient's mouth.

15. Direct the patient to sip and swallow the water as you slowly advance the tube. (If the patient is not allowed water, instruct her to dry-swallow or suck air through a straw.) Advance the tube 5 to 10 cm (2 to 4 in.) with each swallow.
Moving the tube with each swallow uses normal peristaltic movement to help advance the tube into the stomach. Swallowing closes the epiglottis so that the tube cannot advance into the trachea.

16. Continue advancing the tube to the required distance.

17. Temporarily secure the tube with one piece of tape. Then, verify tube placement. Never rely on a single bedside method. You can use a combination of the following methods to verify placement; however, radiographic verification is the only reliable method and should be done before medications or fluids are given through the tube for the first time (AACN, 2016, April; Joanna Briggs Institute, 2012). For detailed steps for verifying placement, see Clinical Insight 27-5, and

Go to Box 27-6: **Comparison of Methods for Checking Nasogastric Tube (NGT) Feeding Tube Placement,** in Volume 1.

If you do not secure the tube temporarily, it may move out of position—especially if you are waiting for placement to be confirmed by x-ray film.

a. Inspect the posterior pharynx for the presence of coiled tube.
Visualization confirms that the tube has gone beyond the oropharynx.

b. Aspirate gently to withdraw stomach contents; measure aspirate pH. Aspirate gently over a period of up to 5 minutes, if necessary, to obtain gastric fluid.
The pH of stomach contents is normally 1 to 5.5; however, many situations commonly alter the pH of gastric contents, so the usefulness of this method is limited. pH testing is helpful only if the fluid is acidic; if it is alkaline, the gastric contents may have been altered (e.g., by enteral feedings or antacids and other medications), or the tube may be in the lung. This procedure does not reliably confirm gastric placement and should be used in combination with other methods. See Box 27-6 in Volume 1.

c. Take note of the amount, color, and consistency of the aspirate.
Gastric aspirates are cloudy tan, off-white, or greenish and may be curdled. Intestinal aspirates will be smaller in quantity, clear, and yellowish because of the presence of bile, and not curdled.

e. Ask the patient to speak.
If she can do so, the tube is probably in the stomach. Use this only to confirm other methods; it is not reliable enough to use as the primary method of verification.

18. After checking for placement, if the tube is not in the stomach, advance it another 2.5 to 5 cm (2 to 4 in.) or as much as directed in the radiologic review. Repeat Steps 17a–e.

19. After you confirm proper placement, clamp the end of the tube or connect it to the drainage bag, feeding, or suction machine.

20. Secure the tube using one of the following methods.

Securing the Tube With 1-Inch (2.5 cm) Tape

a. Apply skin adhesive to the patient's nose; allow it to dry.
A skin adhesive helps the tape to adhere and protects skin from breakdown.

b. Use the 5-cm (2-in.) piece of hypoallergenic tape, split lengthwise to 2.5 cm (1 in.) at one end.
A split tape can be wrapped around the tube in opposite directions to hold the tube in place more securely.

c. Apply the intact end of tape to the patient's nose.

d. Wrap the split strips around the tube where it exits the nose. Fold over the ends if adjustment is needed.

Securing the Tube With Half-Inch Tape

e. Use tape half-inch (1.3-cm) 4 inches (10 cm) long. Apply one end of tape to the patient's nose, and wrap the other end downward around the tube and then back up to secure on the opposite side of the nose (see photo).

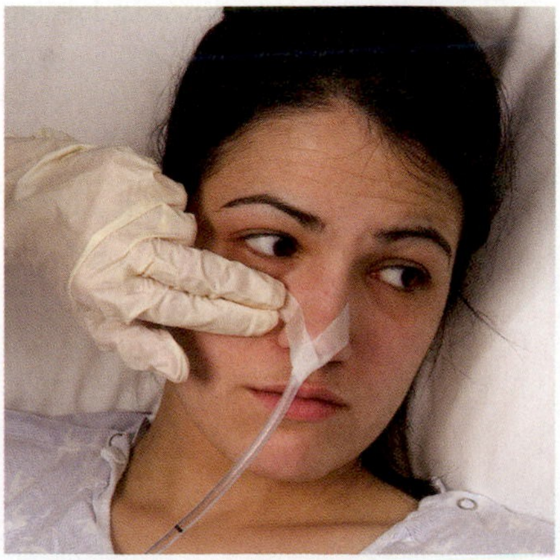

Securing the Tube With a Tube Fixation Device

f. Peel the backing off the pad, and place the wide end of the pad over the bridge of the nose.

g. Position the connector around the NG or NE tube where it exits the nose.

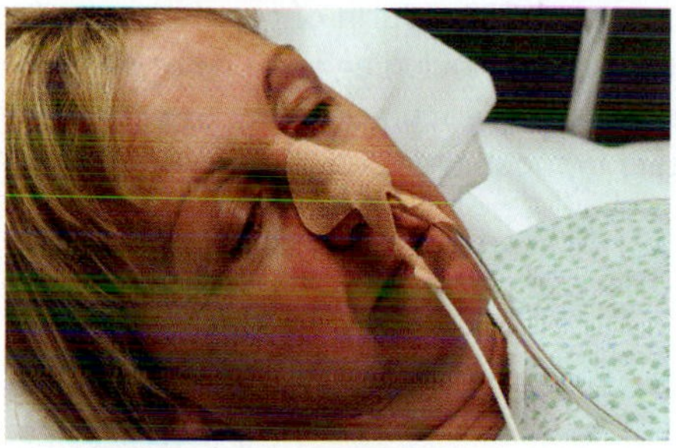

21. Curve and tape the tube to the patient's cheek (not necessary with some commercial tube fixation devices).

Securing the tube to the cheek reduces the tension on the naris.

22. Fasten the tube to the patient's gown: Use a commercial device to secure the tube in place. Or you may tie a slipknot around the tube with a rubber band. Loop a rubber band in a slipknot near the connection. (Alternatively, wrap a short piece of tape around the tube to form a tab.) Then, fasten the rubber band or the tab to the gown with a safety pin (or tape).

Reduces discomfort produced by the weight of the tube and prevents movement that may cause dislocation of the tube and irritation of the nose.

23. Elevate the head of the bed 30° unless contraindicated.

24. Mark the tube with tape where it enters the naris; or measure the length from the naris to the connector.

A marked tube allows you to easily notice whether tube placement has changed.

25. When you finish the procedure, remember the Universal Steps that apply after all procedures. For example, leave the patient in a safe, comfortable position with the call device in easy reach.

? *What if . . .*

- **The patient is confused, combative, or comatose?**

a. If the patient is comatose, place her into a semi-Fowler's position. Have a coworker use a pillow to help position the patient's head forward for insertion.

b. If the patient is confused and combative, ask a coworker to assist you with insertion.

- **The patient gags, coughs, chokes, or vomits [at Steps 11 and 15]?**

a. Stop advancing the tube. Ask the patient to take deep breaths and drink a few sips of water.

Helps suppress the gag reflex.

b. Instruct the patient to breathe easily and take a few sips of water.

c. If coughing continues, pull the tube back slightly.

d. If gagging continues, use a tongue blade and penlight to check the tube position in the back of the throat.

The tube may be coiled in the back of the throat.

e. Continue to advance the tube to the required distance.

f. If the tube is coiled in the back of the throat, the patient coughs excessively during insertion, the tube does not advance with each swallow, or the patient develops respiratory distress (e.g., gasping, coughing, or cyanosis), withdraw the tube completely, and allow the patient to rest before attempting to reinsert.

The tube may be in the patient's trachea.

- **You are unable to obtain an aspirate (at Step 17b) when confirming tube placement?**

a. Use a 50-mL syringe, and aspirate very slowly for at least 5 minutes.

b. Flush the tube with air, then aspirate.

c. Turn the patient to the left side, wait 20 minutes, then aspirate again.

An aspirate might be difficult to obtain with small bore tubes.

- **The prescription states the tube needs to be in the jejunum?**

a. To advance the tube into the jejunum after the tube has been placed in the stomach, position the patient on the right side.

Positioning on the right side allows gravity to assist tube passage through the pyloric sphincter.

b. Advance the tube 5 to 7.5 cm (2 to 3 inches) hourly, over several hours (up to 24 hours) until radiographic study confirms placement.

Weighted tubes will advance by gravity and peristalsis if a loop of the designated length is made at the entrance to the naris. After reading the initial x-ray, the radiologist or primary physician can provide the measurement needed to advance the tube to the required position. Note that specially trained nurses usually place these tubes at the bedside.

- **The procedure is anticipated to cause pain or discomfort?**

iCare Commercial hurricane spray or viscous lidocaine is sometimes used to promote patient comfort. Some practitioners use them for all NG insertions.

a. You may insert 2% viscous lidocaine into the nasal passage using a syringe before tube placement, if prescribed by the primary provider.

b. Alternatively, you can apply an anesthetic spray to the nasal and oropharyngeal mucosae.

- **The patient is a child?**

a. Children usually require a smaller-diameter tube.

iCare b. Encourage parents to comfort infants and children and participate in their care.

c. You may need to apply restraints during insertion to prevent dislodging of the tube.

d. Monitor more frequently for complications.

Small children are not able to communicate about any problems with the tube.

(continued on next page)

Procedure 27-2 ■ Inserting Nasogastric and Nasoenteric Tubes (continued)

Evaluation

- Assess how well the patient tolerated the procedure (e.g., discomfort, gagging, coughing?)
- Note the color, consistency, and pH of NG or NE aspirate.
- Ask the patient whether she feels comfortable.
- Assess and monitor respiratory status.

Patient Teaching

- Explain that the sensation of the tube should decrease with time.
- Explain the importance of immediately reporting tension on the tube or displacement of the tape or fixation device.
- Discuss the need for frequent mouth care while the tube is in place.

Home Care

- Assess the client or caregiver's ability to maintain an NG or NE tube at home.
- Assess the home environment to determine the client's risk for infection.
- Instruct the client or the caregiver about aspirating stomach contents and measuring pH.
- Teach the client or caregiver how to verify tube placement.
- Explain to the client or caregiver how to properly secure the NG or NE tube.
- Reinforce the need for frequent mouth care.

Documentation

- Chart the date and time of insertion, size and type of the NG or NE tube and insertion site (which naris), length of tube from tip of the nose to the end of the tube, tolerance of the procedure, any abnormal findings, and methods for confirming NG or NE tube placement.
- Document the volume and description of gastric contents.
- Document respiratory status, including any sign of distress.
- NG or NE tube insertion is documented in the progress notes and flow sheets in most agencies.

Practice Resources

American Association of Critical-Care Nurses (AACCN) (2016, April); The Joanna Briggs Institute. (2012); Shlamovitz, G. Z., & Shah, N. R. (n.d., updated 2017, May 26); U.S. Food and Drug Administration (USFDA). (n.d.).

Thinking About the Procedure

The video **Inserting Nasogastric and Nasoenteric Feeding Tubes,** along with questions and suggested responses, is available on the ***Davis's Nursing Skills Videos*** Web site on FADavis.com.

Procedure 27-3 ■ Administering Feedings Through Gastric and Enteric Tubes

➤ For steps to follow in all procedures, refer to the Universal Steps for All Procedures found on the inside back cover.

Equipment

- Prescribed feeding formula at room temperature
- Filtered water or prescribed diluent
- Tube feeding administration set with safety adapter that is not compatible with intravenous (IV) tubing, including container for formula
- 60-mL luer-lock or catheter-tip syringe (two needed for syringe feeding)
- Connector to connect administration set to the feeding tube
- Stethoscope
- Enteral feeding infusion pump (if used). Recommended for all continuous feedings.
- IV pole
- Linen-saver pad
- Graduated container
- pH strip
- For gastrostomy and jejunostomy tubes: a small precut gauze dressing

Delegation

You can delegate the procedure to the UAP or the LPN if the patient's condition is stable and the UAP's skills allow. You must verify peristalsis, tube placement, and feeding tube patency before the feeding is started. Remind the UAP to position the patient upright and to report patient discomfort and any difficulty with the infusion.

Pre-Procedure Assessments

- **Verify the feeding tube is in proper placement prior to starting the procedure.**

Go to **Box 27-6** in Volume I for a comparison of bedside methods of verifying tube placement.

Tube placement after insertion must be verified by radiography before the first feeding. For subsequent feedings, use more than one bedside method for verifying correct tube placement. One method is to aspirate and measure gastric residual volume. *(NOTE: For patients with a jejunostomy tube, do not measure the residual volume.)*

- You can also estimate tube placement by checking the length of the exposed tube: (1) Compare the length from the naris with the connector recorded after x-ray confirmation of placement; or (2) observe the mark that was made on it where it entered the nostril after insertion.
  These methods help confirm that the tube has not become displaced since radiography. If there is significant change in length, tube position must again be confirmed by radiography.
- Assess date and time of previous feeding container set change. Containers should be changed every 24 hours or according to unit protocol. Common policies, which can vary by unit, are:
  Sterile feedings may hang for up to 24 hours.
  Nonsterile feedings (i.e., reconstituted powder feedings) may hang for up to 4 hours.
- Assess for fluid volume excess or insufficiency by checking breath sounds, mucous membranes, skin turgor, edema, and intake and output (I&O).
  These signs indicate fluid volume excess or insufficiency.
- Obtain baseline weight and laboratory studies before starting the first feedings.
  Weight change is a sensitive measure reflecting fluid and nutritional status.
- Monitor vital signs before and after feedings.
  Vital signs may vary from baseline because of pain, impaction, or dehydration.
- Auscultate for bowel sounds before each feeding or every 4 to 8 hours for continuous feedings. Also, check for distention, nausea, vomiting, and diarrhea.
  These symptoms may indicate intolerance of tube feedings. If GI motility is impaired, feedings accumulate in the stomach along with gastric secretions, predisposing the patient to reflux and aspiration. Some medications (e.g., opioids) also slow gastric emptying.
- Check patient history for food allergies.
  Helps prevent allergic reaction to ingredients in the feeding formula.
- For gastrostomy and jejunostomy tubes: Assess the exit site at every shift. Report redness or drainage to the primary care provider.
  Leaking of gastric or intestinal contents may cause skin breakdown.

Procedure 27-3A ■ Administering Feedings Through Gastric and Enteric Tubes With an Infusion Pump

➤ When performing the procedure, always identify your patient according to agency policy, using two identifiers, and be attentive to standard precautions, hand hygiene, patient safety and privacy, body mechanics, and documentation.

Procedure Steps

1. **Elevate the head of the bed** (HOB) at least 30° to 45° unless contraindicated. If the patient cannot tolerate a backrest-elevated position, use the reverse Trendelenburg position to elevate the HOB, unless contraindicated. And, place a linen-saver pad under where the connection end of the feeding tube will be.
   A position in which the stomach is higher than the gut reduces the risk for aspiration of gastric contents, a serious risk factor for pneumonia or hypoxia. It also aids in digestion.

2. **Verify the medical prescription** for the type of feeding, rate of infusion, and frequency of feeding.
   A medical prescription is required for enteral feedings. Rate and frequency of feeding are crucial for providing adequate nutrition.

3. **Check the expiration date** of the tube feeding formula and supplies.
   Expired formula should be discarded.

4. **Prepare the formula.**
   a. Inspect the container of feeding solution. If the bag, bottle, or can has been opened or damaged in any way, do not use it.
   b. Shake the feeding formula thoroughly. Examine the solution. It should be uniform in color and consistency.
   c. Keep unopened formula at room temperature. Store opened feeding solutions in the refrigerator in covered and labeled containers. Allow the solution to return to room temperature before giving it to the patient. Discard after 24 hours. Follow the manufacturer's instructions for safe storage.
   Because the formula goes directly into the stomach and is not warmed by the mouth and esophagus, cold formula may cause abdominal cramping and increase the risk for diarrhea.

5. **Prepare the equipment** for administration.
   a. After donning procedure gloves, fill a disposable tube feeding container with a 4- to 6-hr supply of feeding formula. Or use a prefilled bottle with feeding formula. Follow similar procedure for the flush bag if using a two-bag system. Do not transfer sterile feedings into a second container.
   Limit hang-time to help prevent bacterial growth and prevent air from entering the GI tract.
   b. Label the container with the patient's name, room number, date, start time, formula type, feeding rate, and your initials. Write a warning using large, bold letters, for instance, "WARNING! For Enteral Use Only—NOT for IV Use."
   Labeling identifies the formula and prevents misconnection of the feeding tube into an IV line. Labeling also helps avoid administering formula that is past the expiration date.

(continued on next page)

Procedure 27-3 ■ Administering Feedings Through Gastric and Enteric Tubes (continued)

c. Make sure adapters and connectors used in the enteral system are incompatible with female luer-lock rigid connectors used for IV infusion.
Prevents tube feeding misconnection with an IV line.

d. Hang the tube-feeding container on an IV pole with the label facing forward. A prefilled container can safely hang for 24 to 36 hours (some agencies allow for 48 hours).
Closed systems decrease the risk of contamination and prevent air from entering the GI tract.

e. Open the administration set package. Make sure the tubing does not touch the floor. Use sterile equipment and supplies; once you have opened them, handle them as little as possible.

NOTE: Disposable feeding equipment is meant for one-time use. Do not wash and reuse.

f. Close the clamp on the tubing before attaching the set to the container.

g. Remove the cap from the end of safety connector. This adapter must not fit with IV tubing. Do not touch the end of the connector or let it touch another surface.

h. Insert the proximal end of the tubing (with the safety adapter) into the cross-shaped opening of the port on the feeding tube container. Twist the collar in a clockwise direction until it is securely fastened. ▼

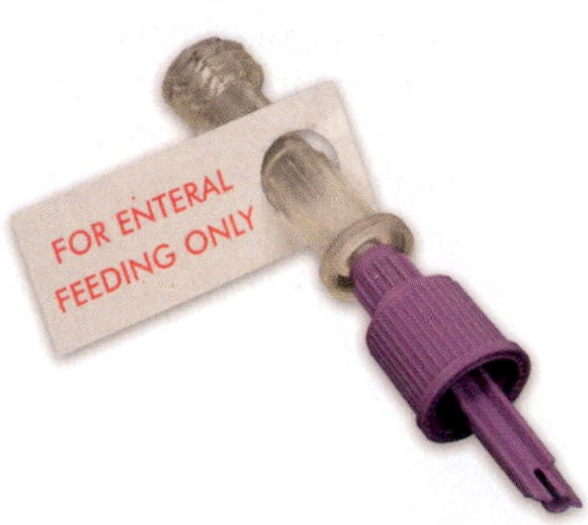

6. **Prime the tubing with the feeding solution.**

7. **Thread the administration set tubing** through the infusion pump, according to the manufacturer's instructions. Be sure to close the roller clamp.
Clamping the tube prevents air from entering the stomach or gastric contents from leaking out. ▼

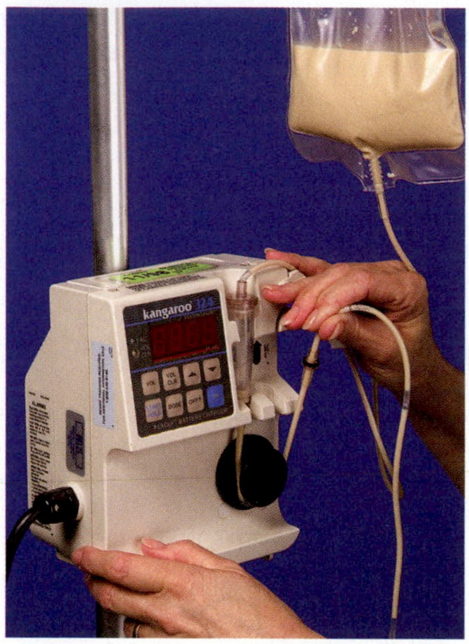

8. **Connect the distal end of the tubing** primed with feeding solution to the connector or directly to the NG or NE tube. Trace the tubing from the container back to the patient before starting the feeding to ensure that you have not inadvertently hooked the feeding bag or bottle to the IV line.

9. **Turn on the infusion pump.** Set the correct infusion rate and volume to be infused. Follow the pump manufacturer's instructions.

10. **Unclamp the tube,** and begin the infusion. Never allow a feeding tube to hang below the height of the patient's stomach.
Follow agency policy regarding how long a solution may be left hanging.

11. **When the feeding volume is complete**, turn off the infusion pump. Close off the end of the feeding tube.

12. **Disconnect the feeding tube** from the administration tubing.

13. **Flush feeding tube** with the prescribed amount of water—typically 50 to 100 mL if there is no fluid restriction. Use sterile water (1) for patients who are immunocompromised, (2) for patients receiving jejunal feeds, or (3) initially after a gastrostomy insertion.

14. **Cap the proximal end** of the feeding tube.
Prevents spillage of gastric contents and stops air from entering the stomach.

15. **Keep the head of the bed elevated** at least 30° to 45° for a minimum of 30 min. after administering the tube feeding.
Facilitates gastric emptying and reduces the risk for aspiration of gastric contents.

16. **Provide or assist with regular oral hygiene,** and encourage frequent gargling.
Oral care reduces oropharyngeal discomfort caused by the tube.

17. **When you finish the procedure**, remember the Universal Steps that apply after all procedures. For example, leave the patient in a safe, comfortable position, with the call device within easy reach.

Procedure 27-3B ■ Administering Feedings Through Gastric and Enteric Tubes Using an Open System: Syringe

Procedure Steps

First, follow Steps 1 through 4, above. Then, proceed as follows:

1. **Prepare the equipment** for administration.
   a. Don procedure gloves.
   b. Label the syringe with the patient's name, room number, date, time, formula type, feeding rate, start time, and your initials.

   Write a warning using large, bold letters, for instance, "WARNING! For Enteral Use Only—NOT for IV Use."
   Labeling identifies the formula and prevents misconnection of the feeding tube into an IV line. Labeling also helps avoid administering formula that is past the expiration date.

2. **Remove the plunger from the syringe.**
3. **Close off** the end of the feeding tube before filling the syringe.
   Prevents air from entering the feeding tube.
4. **Attach the syringe** to the proximal end of the feeding tube.
5. **Fill the syringe** with the prescribed amount of formula.
6. **Unclamp the feeding tube,** and elevate the syringe. Do not elevate the syringe more than 18 inches (45 cm) above the insertion site. Allow the feeding to flow slowly.
   Gravity allows the formula to flow through the feeding tube. Rate of flow is determined by the height of the syringe. Feeding slowly prevents sudden stomach distention, which can lead to diarrhea, cramping, nausea, and vomiting.

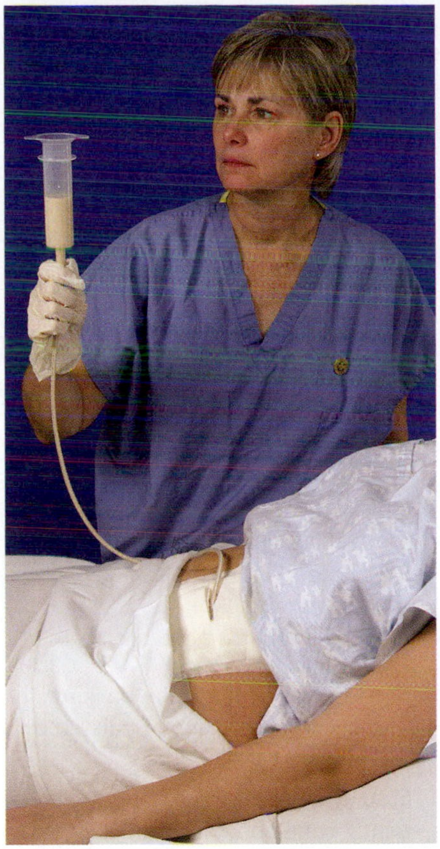

7. **When the syringe is nearly empty**, refill the syringe until the prescribed amount of feeding has been administered.
   If the tubing runs dry, air may enter the stomach and cause discomfort associated with gas.
8. **When the feeding volume is infused, flush the feeding tube** with the prescribed amount of water—typically 50 to 100 mL.
10. **Disconnect the syringe** from the feeding tube.
11. **Cap the proximal end** of the feeding tube, and place the syringe back in the container.
   Prevents spillage of gastric contents and stops air from entering the stomach.
12. **Keep the head of the bed elevated** at least 30° to 45° for a minimum of 30 minutes after administering the tube feeding.
   Elevation facilitates gastric emptying and reduces the risk for aspiration of gastric contents.
13. **Provide or assist with** regular oral hygiene and encourage frequent gargling.
   Oral care helps prevent oropharyngeal discomfort caused by the tube.
14. **When you finish the procedure**, remember the Universal Steps that apply after all procedures. For example, leave the patient in a safe, comfortable position with the call device in easy reach.

? What if . . .

- **When checking for residual, the volume is more than the formula flow rate for 1 hour?**
  - Reinstill the gastric residual volume. Residual gastric contents should be reinfused in the absence of pain or abdominal distension.
  - If the residual is > 250 mL and if there is no abdominal pain or distension, continue the infusion. Recheck in 1 hour. If the residual is still > 250 mL, stop the infusion for 4 hours and recheck. If still > 250 mL, call the healthcare provider (Bankhead, Boullata, Brantley, et al. & the ASPEN Board of Directors, 2009).
  - If residual is < 250 mL, restart the infusion at 50% original rate, and monitor.
  - If the gastric residual volume is ≥ 250 mL after a second gastric residual check, a promotility agent may be considered in adult clients

(continued on next page)

Procedure 27-3 ■ Administering Feedings Through Gastric and Enteric Tubes (continued)

(Bankhead, Boullata, Brantley, et al., & the ASPEN Board of Directors, 2009).
High residual volumes indicate delayed gastric emptying.

- **When checking for residual, none is obtained?**

  Use a large syringe (e.g., 60 mL) and inflate 20 mL of air into the tube, if agency policy permits; this may move the tube away from the gastric wall or clear the tube of any residual formula, medication, or water.

- **When irrigating the feeding tube, resistance is met? Or when instilling the feeding, the fluid does not flow?**
  - Do not force the solution.
  - Do not use any fluid other than water for flushing.
  - Check for kinks in tubing and that the pump is working correctly.
  - Turn the client onto his left side.
  - Remove any enteral feeding solution remaining in the tube. Try instilling 5 mL of warm water into the tube and clamping the tube for 5 min. Then, apply gentle negative pressure to the tube with a syringe.
  - Try flushing with a smaller (e.g., 10 or 20 mL) syringe. If these measures fail, the tube may need to be removed and a new one inserted; contact the primary care provider.

  NOTE: There are other methods, such as the alkalinized enzyme method; these, however, require a medical prescription.

  Forcing the solution may damage the tube. However, you can use a smaller syringe to exert slightly more pressure.

- **The patient has a cuffed tracheostomy tube?**

  Inflate the cuff before administering the feeding, and keep the cuff inflated for at least 15 min. afterward, if the agency permits.
  Cuffing helps prevent aspiration.

- **During the feeding, the patient vomits or complains of nausea or feeling too full?**

  Stop the feeding, and assess the patient's condition. Flush the tube, wait an hour, then measure gastric contents and restart the feeding at a slower rate. You may need to obtain a medical order to decrease the volume of the feedings.

- **The patient has a jejunostomy tube?**
  - Do not instill air into the tube or check for residual before feeding.
    The tube is in the jejunum rather than the stomach. The jejunum is not normally a reservoir; therefore, no residual volume is present in the jejunum. Gastrostomy and jejunostomy tubes are often placed through the upper abdominal wall; these tubes, of course, cannot inadvertently migrate into the airway. Injecting air into the tube is not necessary and introduces air into the GI tract, causing the patient discomfort from gas.
  - Clean the insertion site daily with soap and water. You may apply a small, precut gauze dressing to the site.
    Helps prevent bacterial growth; prevents infection.
  - Be aware that the delivery rate will likely be slower for jejunostomy tubes because of the loss of the stomach as a reservoir.

Evaluation

- Evaluate the patient's tolerance to the tube feeding; did the patient have any abdominal discomfort, nausea, vomiting, or diarrhea?
- Auscultate bowel sounds and vital signs every 4 hours.
- Check gastric residual volume every 4 hours.
- Monitor I&O every 8 hours.
- Weigh patient at least 3 times per week.
- Assess the exit site for signs of skin breakdown.
- Assess characteristics and frequency of bowel movements.
- Check laboratory values to evaluate nutritional status.

Patient Teaching

- Demonstrate the procedure to the patient and caregiver if the patient will be continuing tube feedings at home.
- Explain the importance of flushing the feeding tube with tap water every 4 hours, while the patient is awake, to maintain tube patency and fluid and electrolyte balance.
- Discuss the importance of remaining upright for at least 1 hour after the feeding.

Home Care

- Provide written instructions.
- Be sure the client has a 7-day supply of enteral feedings.
- Identify with the client the person who will be responsible for care of the enteral tube and administration of feedings at home.
- Explain to the client and caregiver how to measure the prescribed amount of tube feeding formula and water for flushes by using household measuring equipment.
- Explain the importance of washing reusable equipment thoroughly with soap and water to prevent the spread of infection.
- Discuss how and where to purchase and store the formula.
- If home feedings are to be delivered by pump:

  Facilitate a home care visit to provide training about the feeding pump.

  Arrange for delivery of the feeding pump before discharge (or refer to the appropriate professional for this).

  Ensure that the client has a 7-day supply of disposable feeding sets and 50- or 60-mL syringes upon discharge.

Documentation

- Chart the type of tube feeding, rate and volume of infusion, amount of gastric residual volume (if any), and tolerance of procedure.
- Tube feeding intake is documented on the I&O portion of the flowsheet in most agencies.
- Record all flushes as intake. Subtract any liquids that you aspirate, and do not reinstill (e.g., when gastric residual is too high).

Practice Resources

American Association of Critical-Care Nurses (AACN). (2016, April); Boullata, J. I., Carrera, A. L., Harvey, L., et al. (2017); Durfee, S. M., Adams, S. C., Arthur, E., et al., and Home and Alternate Site Task Force (2014); The Joint Commission (2014, August 20); McClave, S. A., Taylor, B. E. Martindale, R. G., et al. (2016); Metheny, N., & American Association of Critical-Care Nurses (AACN) (updated 2016); U.S. Food and Drug Administration (USFDA), (n.d.).

Thinking About the Procedure

The videos **Administering Feedings Through Gastric and Enteric Tubes with Infusion Pump** and **Administering Feedings Through Gastric and Enteric Tubes Using an Open-System Syringe,** along with questions and suggested responses, are available on the ***Davis's Nursing Skills Videos*** Web site on FADavis.com.

Procedure 27-4 ■ Removing a Nasogastric or Nasoenteric Tube

➤ For steps to follow in all procedures, refer to the Universal Steps for All Procedures found on the inside back cover.

Equipment

- Linen-saver pad
- 60-mL luer-lock or catheter-tip syringe
- Nonsterile gloves
- Stethoscope
- Disposable plastic bag
- Emesis basin
- Gauze square

Delegation

This procedure should not be delegated to the LPN or the UAP.

Pre-Procedure Assessments

- Auscultate the abdomen for the presence of bowel sounds.
  Bowel sounds and flatus confirm peristalsis, which indicates bowel function is present.
- Assess the patient's ability to consume an oral diet.
  Confirms readiness for discontinuing the NG or NE tube.
- Determine how long it has been since the patient's last enteral feeding.

➤ When performing the procedure, always identify your patient according to agency policy, using two identifiers, and be attentive to standard precautions, hand hygiene, patient safety and privacy, body mechanics, and documentation.

Procedure Steps

1. **Check the patient's health** record to confirm removal of the tube. For feeding tubes, make sure tube feeding has been stopped at least 30 minutes before removal.
2. **Assist the patient to a sitting** position or high-Fowler's position.
   Proper body alignment facilitates tube removal.

iCare 3. **Place the plastic bag and emesis basin** on the bed or within reach. Hand the patient facial tissue. Explain that the procedure may cause some gagging or nasal discomfort but it will be brief.
   Patients often need to blow their nose after this procedure.

4. **Drape a linen-saver pad or towel** across the patient's chest.
   Draping protects the gown and linens from soiling. Maintains universal precautions.
5. **Perform hand hygiene, and don procedure gloves,** if you have not already done so.
6. **If the NG tube is connected to suction,** turn off the suction, and disconnect the tube.
7. **Stand on the patient's right side,** if you are right-handed and on the left side if left-handed.
8. **Attach the syringe** to the proximal end of the NG or NE tube, and flush the tube with 15 mL of water, normal saline, or air.
   Flushing clears the tube of feeding formula or gastric secretions that could cause irritation or be aspirated during tube removal.
9. **Unfasten the tube** from the patient's gown, and then remove the tube from the patient's nose and cheek. Use an adhesive-remover pad to help loosen the tape, as necessary.

(continued on next page)

Procedure 27-4 ■ Removing a Nasogastric or Nasoenteric Tube (continued)

10. **Clamp or pinch the end of the tube** in your hand. Hold gauze up to the patient's nose, and be ready to grab the tube with the towel in the opposite hand upon removal.
Prevents gastric fluids from leaking out the end of the tube onto the nurse or the patient.

11. **Ask the patient to take a deep breath** and hold it.
Breath holding closes the epiglottis and prevents aspiration.

12. **Quickly, steadily, and smoothly withdraw the tube,** and place it in the plastic bag.
Rapid removal in one steady motion avoids causing tissue trauma. The plastic bag acts as a barrier to gastric fluids until the tube can be placed in the trash. Seeing and smelling the tube may cause the patient to become nauseated.

13. **Clean the patient's nares,** and provide mouth care, if the patient cannot do so. Remove the tape residue from her nose with adhesive remover.
Promotes patient comfort and prevents infection.

14. **Measure the drainage, and note the characteristics of the content,** if the NG tube was connected to suction. Dispose of the tube and drainage equipment in a biohazardous waste receptacle, according to facility policy.
For patients receiving enteral feedings or gastric suction, record I&O. Proper equipment disposal prevents the spread of infection.

15. **Remove and dispose of gloves** in the nearest receptacle.

16. **When you finish the procedure,** remember the Universal Steps that apply after all procedures. For example, leave the patient in a safe, comfortable position with the call device in easy reach.

Evaluation

- Assess the nares for signs of skin breakdown or bleeding.
- Monitor the patient for signs of GI dysfunction, such as food intolerance, nausea, vomiting, and abdominal distention. Auscultate for bowel sounds.
GI dysfunction could necessitate reinsertion of the tube.
- Monitor I&O every 8 hours.
- Weigh the patient regularly.
- Check laboratory values to evaluate nutritional status.
- Note any complications following NG or NE tube removal, such as food intolerance, nausea, vomiting, and abdominal distention.

Patient Teaching

- Instruct the patient or caregiver on how to remove the feeding tube.
- Explain the importance of reporting nausea, vomiting, food intolerance, or abdominal distention to the physician.
- Explain the importance of and procedure for drinking fluids, if not contraindicated.

Home Care

The procedure does not require special adaptation for home care, except that you might want to place the tube in a plastic zippered storage bag before discarding it in the trash receptacle.

Documentation

- Chart the date and time of removal as well as the patient's tolerance of the procedure.
- Document the amount of drainage if the tube was connected to suction.

Sample documentation

4/13/19 1010 Explained to pt and wife NG tube was to be removed and procedure for removing NG tube. Pt stated, "I am ready to get this thing out." Untaped NG tube from gown and nose. Removed tube while asking pt to hold his breath. Pt tolerated procedure well without vomiting or bradycardia. Provided mouth care and facial cleansing. ——— A. Hiam, RN

4/13/19 1230 Taking clear liquids since NG tube was removed with no nausea, vomiting, or abdominal distention. Bowel sounds faint but audible in all 4 quadrants. ——— A. Hiam, RN

Practice Resources

National Institutes of Health (NIH) (2016, December 8, reviewed)

Thinking About the Procedure

The video **Removing a Nasogastric or Nasoenteric Tube,** along with questions and suggested responses, is available on the ***Davis's Nursing Skills Videos*** Web site on FADavis.com.

Procedure 27-5 ■ Administering Parenteral Nutrition

➤ For steps to follow in all procedures, refer to the Universal Steps for All Procedures found on the inside back cover.

Equipment

- Parenteral nutrition (PN) solution
  - Keep the PN refrigerated until 60 min before use; do not give the PN cold. Do not hasten warming by placing in a microwave oven or hot water bath.
    Cold solution can cause pain, hypothermia, and venous spasm. Nutrients in PN solution are stable only for this short period. Nutrients could precipitate, causing catheter blockage or emboli.
  - Some pharmacies deliver the solution before infusion. Be sure the PN has not been mixed more than 24 hours beforehand. However, in home care you may find that solutions are mixed and delivered weekly.
- Procedure gloves
- Sterile gloves.

NOTE: If the central line has an injection cap and if IV tubing is connected onto the cap via luer-lock, some agencies do not require gloves.

- IV administration set, extension set, if indicated (free of plasticizers, such as bis(2-ethylhexyl) phthalate [BEHP], when fat emulsion is to be infused)

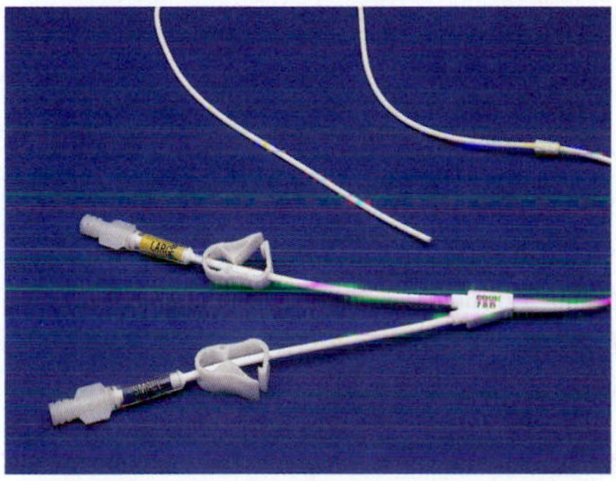

- 0.22-micron filter (1.2-micron filter if solution contains albumin or lipids)
  A 0.22-micron filter will remove most particulates and microorganisms that might have been introduced during mixing, but it is too fine for larger-molecule lipids to infuse properly.
- Time tape
  Even though the PN is delivered by infusion pump, there have been numerous recalls of infusion pumps because of malfunction. This simple tape provides valuable information quickly and is an additional safety measure.
- 70% alcohol pads or chlorhexidine gluconate (CHG)–alcohol (e.g., 2% CHG in 70% isopropyl alcohol)
- Infusion pump
- 10-mL syringe and saline
- Blood glucose testing monitor
- I&O record
- Transparent dressing or sterile gauze and tape (if dressing is to be changed)
- Catheter stabilization device (e.g., StatLock)
  These are recommended for all catheters and must be changed with each dressing change.
- If the dressing is to be changed, you also need a transparent dressing or sterile gauze, tape, and a mask.

Delegation

Do not delegate this skill to the LPN or the UAP because administration of PN requires advanced assessment and critical-thinking skills. The LPN or the UAP can assist by monitoring vital signs, checking blood glucose, and verifying patient identity with you. Instruct her about complications associated with PN, and ask to be informed of any signs or symptoms or change in the patient's condition.

Pre-Procedure Assessments

- Assess nutrition status and nutritional needs (e.g., daily weights, I&O, lab results). Patients requiring PN have complex nutritional needs, and actual nutritional status is assessed by a nurse or dietitian specializing in nutritional support.
- Check the prescriber's orders for type and concentration of additives in each container and for rate of infusion.
  Standardized order forms are recommended by the American Society for Parenteral and Enteral Nutrition (ASPEN).
- Check the patient's record to confirm that proper central venous catheter (CVC) tip placement has been established before the initial PN administration.
- Check agency policy.
  A few may require tubing and filter change with every bottle or bag. The CDC recommends changing the PN set every 72 hours and a fat emulsion set at least every 24 hours.
- Check the blood glucose level.
- Assess for apparent patency of the IV site.
  If PN is being administered continuously by pump and the infusion is running and there is no leakage from the insertion, you can begin the first few steps of the procedure. Actual patency is checked at Step 14.

(continued on next page)

Procedure 27-5 ■ Administering Parenteral Nutrition (continued)

➤ When performing the procedure, always identify your patient according to agency policy, using two identifiers, and be attentive to standard precautions, hand hygiene, patient safety and privacy, body mechanics, and documentation.

Procedure Steps

1. **Gather equipment,** and place at the bedside.
   Promotes efficient use of time.

2. **Identify the patient,** using two identifiers, according to agency policy. Some institutions require, as an extra precaution, that two people identify the patient.
   Multiple patient identifiers help to avoid "wrong patient" errors. PN solutions are mixed to meet individual needs.

3. **Explain to the patient** the procedure and the rationale for it.
   Respects the patient's right to be informed.

4. **Perform hand hygiene.**
   Reduces transmission of infectious microorganisms.

5. **Position the patient supine** in bed.

6. **Obtain and examine the PN container.** Check for leaks, cloudiness, or floating particles. Do not use if any of these are present. Some agencies require that two people examine the solution.

For Solutions Containing Lipids (3-in-1 Admixture)

Do not administer the admixture if it has a brown layer, oil droplets, or oil on the surface. This indicates that the emulsion has "broken," and the large lipid droplets can cause fat emboli, if administered.

Key Point: ***PN solution requires a 1.2-micron filter.***
To reduce the risk of adverse events, such as fat emboli.

7. **Compare the container** to the patient's identification band; check for correct container number, expiration date, and additives and their concentration. Compare with the original prescription. Ask a coworker to verify with you.
   Ensures that the correct solution is administered. Check the expiration date to ensure that the solution will be discarded after that date and time. PN solutions are carefully calculated and prepared using the latest recommendations for sterile compounding of solutions. Therefore, you should not add any medications to the container either before it is hung or while it is infusing.

8. **Connect the IV tubing to the PN solution;** prime the tubing. Priming may be done manually now or later (on the pump after the tubing is loaded into the pump), depending on the design of the pump.
   Be sure to identify the correct port and IV line. Trace the PN tubing from the container to the patient.
   Priming tubing removes air bubbles and prevents air from entering the patient's bloodstream, possibly causing air embolism. If there is PN already infusing, the old tubing must be removed from the pump and the rate regulated manually for the short period it takes to prime the new administration set.

When Using IV Tubing Without an Inline Filter

If the IV tubing does not have an inline filter, attach the filter and the extension tubing before priming. Attach the filter as close to the catheter site as possible.

9. **Place the IV tubing** in the infusion pump. (Prime the tubing if not done in Step 8.) Set the pump to the prescribed rate.
   Administration via pump (preferably volumetric) helps prevent complications associated with too-rapid infusion. PN solutions must be administered by infusion pump with reliable, audible alarms. Catheter tip placement must be confirmed before initial PN administration.

10. **Identify the correct IV catheter** and lumen for the PN. This is usually a peripherally inserted central catheter (PICC) line or a centrally inserted venous line designated solely for PN. Never infuse PN into an IV line that is not central.
    PN must be administered via a CVC (e.g., subclavian catheter, internal jugular, or PICC) whose tip is positioned in the superior vena cava/right atrial juncture.

11. **Clamp the catheter** and the old PN administration set, if still connected, before disconnecting the tubing.
    a. A clamp should be present on the central line catheters with valves built into the catheter itself.
    The central line for the PN should already be clamped if no PN is running. If a previous container is running, always clamp the PN line near the patient before disconnecting. Clamping prevents air from entering the catheter when you open the connection.
    b. As an additional, optional safety measure, instruct the patient to perform the Valsalva maneuver just as you change the tubing.
    c. If Valsalva maneuver is contraindicated for a patient, instruct the patient to exhale at a specific time when the lumen is open.
    The Valsalva maneuver increases intrathoracic pressure and creates positive pressure in the central vessels, also helping prevent air embolism.

12. **Remove and discard gloves.** Perform hand hygiene.
    In Steps 1 through 11, you were observing Universal Precautions. From this step forward, the emphasis is on preventing the introduction of microorganisms into the catheter lumen or the catheter insertion site.

13. **Don clean gloves (or sterile gloves,** if your agency policy requires them). Disconnect the old administration set. Using a CHG-alcohol pad or a 70% alcohol pad, thoroughly cleanse all surfaces of the central line injection cap and extension leg (in a needleless system) or the luer-lock, including threads.
    Because PN solutions are a good medium for growth of pathogens and

because the IV line enters the central circulation, the risk for sepsis is relatively high.

14. Determine patency of the line. Use a 10-mL syringe to aspirate for blood, looking for a brisk return with pulsating pressure; then, flush with saline. The PN running continuously on a pump, absence of occlusion alarms, and dry and intact dressing are also signs—but not proof—of patency.
When PN is running continuously on a pump, the pump creates a constant fluid flow through the lumen to help keep it patent. There is some controversy about this step. Some experts prefer to aspirate for blood only for the first container of a continuous infusion and thereafter to flush without aspirating. As always, follow agency policy.

15. Attach the infusion tubing to the designated PN port, and then turn the luer-lock to secure the connection. "Luer-slip" connections should not be used. Do not use tape. Trace the tubing from the patient back to the PN container to be certain you are using the correct lumen.
Securing the connection with a luer-lock connection prevents separation of the connection and decreases the risk for sepsis or embolism. Tape, even sterile tape, has been found to be a medium for bacterial colonization.

If the Previous Infusion Is Still Connected

Be sure the access line and the line to the "old" infusion container is clamped (Step 11). Quickly disconnect from the central line, thoroughly cleanse the port, and connect the new infusion.

16. Trace the tubing from the patient back to the container. Then, start the infusion. Check again to make sure the catheter tubing connection is secure. Infuse at the rate prescribed (depending on the patient's tolerance, PN is usually started at a rate of 40 to 50 mL/hr and then advanced 25 mL/hr every 6 hours).
PN solutions may contain as much as 70% dextrose. A gradual rate increase allows the patient's pancreatic beta cells time to increase their insulin output to handle the increased glucose load. For lower concentrations of dextrose, you can usually run the same rate for the complete 24-hour volume.

17. Label the tubing with the date and time of change (if it is new tubing or if you have changed the tubing).
Labeling allows other nurses to know when tubing is due to be changed and a new solution must be hung.

18. Remove and discard gloves. Perform hand hygiene.

19. When you finish the procedure, remember the Universal Steps that apply after all procedures. For example, leave the patient in a safe, comfortable position with the call device in easy reach.

? *What if . . .*

- **When you flush the catheter (at Step 14), you meet resistance?**

Examine the insertion site for leaking fluid or inflammation. Aspirate, and try again to flush *gently*. Never forcibly flush against resistance. Remove syringe from luer-lock connection, then reconnect. Reposition the patient and ask him to cough. Roll the patient's shoulder or raise the arm on the same side the catheter is on. If these measures fail, notify the primary healthcare provider.
Occlusion may be caused by a clot; drug precipitation; or catheter migration, kinking, or compression; or may be related to incomplete connection with the luer-lock. Forceful flushing may discharge a clot into circulation. Other measures to clear a catheter require a medical order.

- **The rate falls behind, or the pump gives occlusion alarms?**

First, check to be sure the pump is turned on, the container is not empty, and all clamps are fully open. Change the filter if it is clogged. Perform the steps in the preceding item. If those measures do not work, change the pump, and send it to biomedical engineering to be checked. Do not attempt to catch up by increasing the rate.
A slow rate may indicate a clogged filter or injection cap, a kinked catheter, or a malfunctioning pump. A clogged filter must be changed; you cannot run the PN without a filter.

- **The 24-hour total deviates from the prescribed infusion rate by 10% or more?**

Notify the primary provider or nutrition support team.

- **A PN solution must be discontinued abruptly for any reason?**

Notify the primary provider or nutrition support team. Another solution of 5% or 10% dextrose may be started.
The dextrose solution is started to prevent rebound hypoglycemia. Note that if it is a catheter complication that requires this discontinuation, 10% dextrose is the highest concentration that can be infused through a peripheral vein because infiltrated hyperosmolar fluid causes tissue injury.

- **The patient no longer needs parenteral nutrition?**

You may need to decrease the rate gradually, perhaps over 48 hours, before discontinuing the infusion completely. Be sure the patient either receives enteral nutrition or consumes food during the next few hours after stopping PN.
To prevent rebound hypoglycemia.

(continued on next page)

Procedure 27-5 ■ Administering Parenteral Nutrition (continued)

Evaluation

These are postprocedure evaluations. For ongoing monitoring, see Clinical Insight 27-7.

- Assess vital signs, I&O, and weight.
- Observe that the solution is infusing at the prescribed rate.
- Assess patient's tolerance to the infusion (e.g., observe for pulmonary edema; check lab results).
- Observe for skin rashes, flushing, color changes, or other signs of allergic reactions; notify the primary provider.

  NOTE: These are not common.

- Monitor blood glucose and do not increase the infusion rate until glycemic control is established.

Patient Teaching

- Inform the patient and family of the purpose and duration of the nutritional support.
- Teach them to recognize and report to the nurse symptoms of complications associated with PN.
- Teach the patient that the dressing must remain occlusive and to notify the nurse if it comes loose or gets wet.
- Teach the patient the importance of measures to prevent blood infections.

Home Care

- The home environment must provide dry storage space for supplies, a refrigerator for storing admixtures, a clean low-traffic area for procedure preparation, and electronic outlets for any electronic equipment.
- Teach safe disposal of supplies.
- Provide verbal and written instructions of the procedures; demonstrate and ask for a return demonstration. Role-play "what would you do if . . ." situations with the patient.
- Clients at home often administer their daily 24-hr total over 12 to 16 hr during the night. This allows them to disconnect from the infusion in the morning, flush the central line, and be free to pursue their usual activities during the day.
- Instruct about solution hang time and management of the access device.

  Depending on the anticipated length of therapy, patients may be sent home with a permanent venous access device.

- Provide 24-hr phone numbers for the primary care provider and home care agency.
- Home PN is less expensive than treatment in the hospital and, in many cases, is associated with a lower risk of infection.
- Home nutritional support is usually under the direction of specialized nutrition support teams.

Documentation

- A special form may be used for documenting PN administration:
  - Container number, date and time hung, volume, type of fluid, rate of delivery, additives
  - Date and time of dressing or tubing change (if performed)
  - Patient's tolerance of procedure
  - Pre- and postadministration assessment data, including complications and response to therapy
  - Results of fingerstick blood glucose checks
  - If insulin is required, type, amount, and route/site administered
  - Weight
  - I&O

Practice Resources

American Society for Parenteral and Enteral Nutrition (ASPEN), Board of Directors and Task Force on Parenteral Nutrition Standardization, Kochevar, M., Guenter, P., Holcombe, B., et al. (2007); Ayers, P., Boullata, J., Gervasio, J., et al. (2014); Boitano, M., Bojak, S., McCloskey, S., et al. (2010); Infusion Nurses Society (2016, revised); McClave, S. A., Taylor, B. E., Martindale, R. G., et al. (2016).

Procedure 27-6 ■ Administering Lipids

➤ For steps to follow in all procedures, refer to the Universal Steps for All Procedures found on the inside back cover.

➤ *Note:* If administering through a central line, refer to Procedure 27-5 for precautions associated with central lines.

➤ *Note:* This procedure is for administering fat emulsions. If you are administering an admixture with the parenteral nutrition solution, use Procedure 27-5.

Equipment

- IV lipid solution (not refrigerated)
- Special tubing (infusion set) for lipids (must be without plasticizers [DEHP]. Set should be labeled to that effect)
- Needleless cannula (if using a split septum needleless connector that requires it)
- 70% isopropyl alcohol or CHG-alcohol pads
- Procedure gloves
- Time tape
- Infusion pump
- I&O record
- If a filter is a used, it must be a 1.2-micron filter

  Lipid particles are large and will clog a smaller-size tube.

Delegation

Do not delegate this skill to the LPN or the UAP because administration of lipids requires advanced assessment and critical-thinking skills. The LPN or the UAP can assist by monitoring vital signs and verifying patient identity with you. Instruct him about complications associated with lipids and ask him to inform you of any signs or symptoms or change in the patient's condition.

Pre-Procedure Assessments

- Assess for rash; eczema; dry, scaly skin; poor wound healing; and sparse hair.
  These are signs of essential fatty acid deficits.
- Check the history for anemia; coagulation disorders; and abnormal liver, pancreatic, or respiratory function.
  These factors predispose to fat emboli. Your role as a staff nurse is to be certain the PN prescriber is aware of these factors; they do not necessarily contraindicate PN.
- Check peripheral IV site for erythema, infiltration, and patency. Check the central venous access site for erythema or other signs of infection.
- Take baseline vital signs just before infusing the lipids.
  An immediate reaction can occur upon starting the infusion. Note that not all guidelines require this action.
- Check a baseline blood glucose just before infusing the lipids.
  Infusing lipids can cause an elevation in blood glucose. Note that not all guidelines require this action.

➤ When performing the procedure, always identify your patient according to agency policy, using two identifiers, and be attentive to standard precautions, hand hygiene, patient safety and privacy, body mechanics, and documentation.

Procedure Steps

1. **Review the prescriber's orders,** including lipid concentration and rate of infusion.
   Verifying helps to prevent dosage and "wrong patient" errors. Explaining the procedure respects the patient's right to be informed.

2. **Gather equipment,** and place at bedside. Adjust lighting, as needed.
   Organization promotes efficient use of time.

3. **Perform hand hygiene,** and don procedure gloves.
   Reduces transmission of infectious microorganisms.

4. **Position the patient supine** in bed.

5. **Ensure that lipids are not cold.**
   Cold infusion can cause discomfort.

6. **Examine the container** for a layer of froth or for separation into fat globules or layers.
   Do not use the lipids if these occur.

7. **Label the container** with the patient's name, room number, date, time, rate, and start and stop times. Label the tubing with date and time.

   NOTE: When lipids are infused with parenteral nutrition, the lipid infusion must be completed within 12 hours.

   Labeling helps ensure that the patient receives the correct infusion.

8. **Compare the lipid container** to the patient's wrist band (container number, expiration date); compare with the original prescription. Have a colleague verify.

9. **Determine patency of the IV line.**

10. **Cleanse the stopper on the IV container** with an antiseptic swab; allow to dry.

11. **Connect the special DEHP-free** lipids-infusion tubing to the container, twisting the spike as you insert it. **Key Point:** ***You must use new tubing for each bottle.***
    Twisting the spike helps ensure that particles from the stopper do not fall into the bottle. New tubing reduces the growth of microorganisms (the feeding provides a medium for fungal growth). DEHP is considered a toxin in the bloodstream.

12. **Place the primed tubing** in the pump and attach the tubing to the IV catheter lumen.

    Identify the correct IV line and port for the infusion. Trace the tubing from the container back to the patient.

    a. Thoroughly scrub the catheter injection port or hub and the luer-lock threads with an antiseptic wipe.

    b. If you are infusing lipids simultaneously with PN, attach the primed lipid tubing to the injection port/hub closest to the patient, below the tubing filter, or through a Y-connection at the catheter hub.

    c. Turn the luer-lock to secure the connection.

    d. *NOTE:* If a previous infusion has been running, clamp the catheter lumen and the old administration set tubing before disconnecting and changing the tubing.
    Prevents blood backup in the line.

13. **Begin the infusion.** Ideally, infuse slowly at first: 1.0 mL/min for adults and 0.1 mL/min for children (or as prescribed by the physician). Check again to be sure the catheter-tubing connection is secure.
    Slow infusion allows time to identify adverse reaction to the lipids and to stop the infusion before the patient has received a large volume. Nausea, vomiting, and elevated temperature have been reported when lipids are infused quickly.

14. **Take the vital signs** now, then every 10 minutes for 30 minutes, and according to agency protocol. Observe for side effects (e.g., chills, fever, flushing, dyspnea, nausea, vomiting, headache, back pain).

(continued on next page)

Procedure 27-6 ■ Administering Lipids (continued)

15. **If no reactions occur**, adjust to the prescribed infusion rate, and continue monitoring according to your agency's protocol.
16. **Remove and discard gloves** and perform hand hygiene.
17. **When the infusion is finished**, discard the bottle and IV administration set.

    Formula contains sugars that are a medium for growth of pathogens.
18. **When you finish the procedure**, remember the Universal Steps that apply after all procedures. For example, leave the patient in a safe, comfortable position with the call device in easy reach.

? What if . . .

- **The entire bottle of lipids is not used?**

  Discard partially used bottles to prevent contamination.

Evaluation

- If ordered, monitor serum lipids 4 hours after discontinuing the infusion.
- Monitor the IV site for infection, inflammation, and infiltration.
- Monitor for symptoms of fat emboli.
- Monitor the IV line for patency.
- Monitor for allergic reactions (nausea, vomiting, headache, chest pain, back pain, fever).
- Monitor for lipid intolerance (triglyceride levels, liver function tests, hepatosplenomegaly, decreased coagulation, cyanosis, dyspnea).

Patient Teaching

- Inform the patient and family of the purpose and duration of the nutritional support.
- Teach the patient to recognize and report symptoms of complications associated with lipids infusion.

Home Care

- The home environment must provide dry storage space for supplies, a refrigerator for storing solutions, a clean low-traffic area for procedure preparation, and electronic outlets for any electronic equipment.
- Teach safe disposal of supplies.
- Provide verbal and written instructions for the procedures; demonstrate the steps, and ask for a return demonstration.
- Instruct about solution hang time and management of the access device.
- Provide 24-hour phone numbers for the primary care provider and home care agency.

Documentation

- A special form may be used for documenting lipids and PN administration.
- Lipid container number, date and time hung, volume, type of fluid, and rate of delivery
- Status of dressing, and date and time of dressing or tubing change (if performed)
- Patient's tolerance of the procedure and any problems encountered
- Pre- and postadministration assessment data and blood tests, if any
- Condition of the IV site
- Weight
- I&O

Practice Resources

Infusion Nurses Society (2016, revised); McClave, S. A., Taylor, B. E., Martindale, R. G., et al. (2016).

CLINICAL INSIGHTS

Clinical Insight 27-1 ➤ Skinfold Measurement

- Take measurements directly on the skin, not through clothing.
- Take each reading as soon as the jaws of the caliper come into contact with the skin and the reading has stabilized.
- In each site, take three readings in quick succession, and average the results to the nearest 0.1 mm. *Accuracy of this method varies with the technique.*
- Add the averages of all skinfold sites to arrive at a total skinfold measurement.
- To determine the percentage body fat, compare the final calculated measurement with the values in the appropriate body fat and skinfolds table for the age and gender of the patient.

Measuring Triceps Skinfold

- Locate the midpoint on the posterior side of the dominant upper arm.
- With the client's arm hanging loosely at the side, palpate the measurement site at the midpoint to become familiar with distinguishing muscle from adipose soft tissue.
- From 1 cm above the midpoint, grasp a vertical pinch of skin and only the subcutaneous fat layer between the thumb and index finger. Gently pull the skinfold away from the underlying muscle.
- Place the skinfold caliper at the midpoint, and slowly release the jaw of the caliper while maintaining a grasp of the skinfold (see the figure).

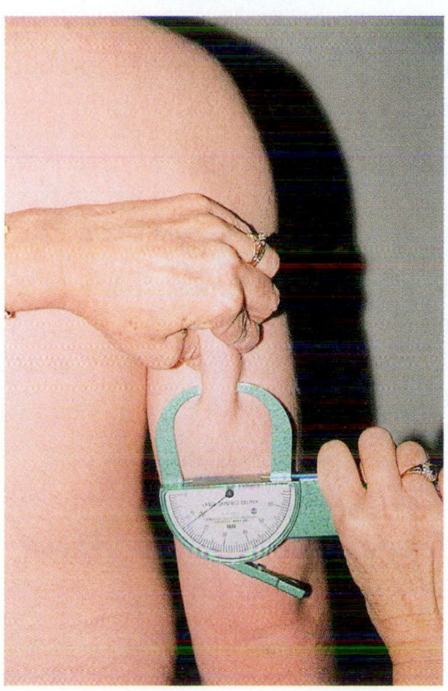

Triceps skinfold.

Measuring Subscapular Skinfold

- Follow the same procedure, except measure on the back, just under the shoulder blade. Grasp below the tip of the inferior angle of the scapula 45° to vertical.

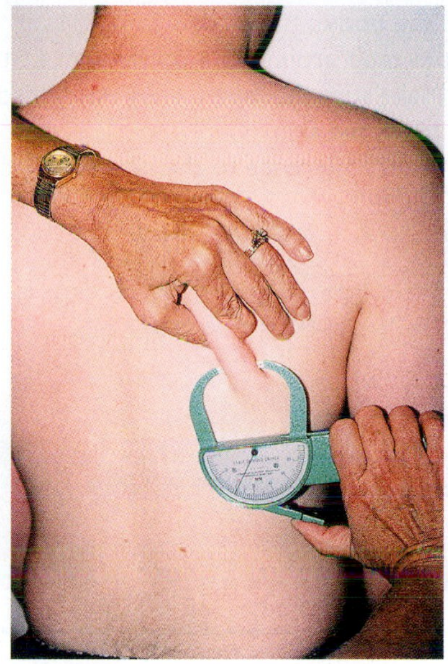

Subscapular skinfold.

Measuring Biceps Skinfold

- Follow the same procedure, except measure the muscle belly of the biceps. With the patient's arm hanging loosely at the side, grasp the skin and subcutaneous fat layer on the front of the upper arm, over the biceps, about level with the nipple.

Measuring Suprailiac Skinfold

- Follow the same procedure, except measure approximately 1 inch above the hipbone, above the iliac crest in the mid-axillary line.

Clinical Insight 27-2 ➤ Measuring Circumferences to Evaluate Body Composition

Measuring Mid-Upper Arm Circumference

- Keeping the client's dominant arm parallel to the body, bend the elbow 90°.
- Using a tape measure, measure the distance between the **acromion** (the bony protrusion of the back of the upper shoulder) and the **olecranon process** (tip of the elbow).
- Mark the midpoint between these two landmarks.
- Ask the client to relax the arm so that it hangs loose and parallel to the body.
- Position the tape around the upper arm at the marked midpoint. Make sure the tape is snug but not so tight as to indent or pinch the skin.
- Record the circumference to the nearest 0.1 cm.

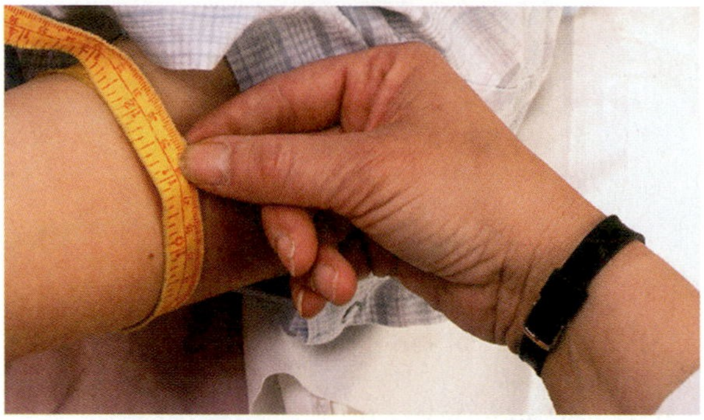

Calculating Waist-to-Hip Ratio (WHR)

WHR > 1.0 in men and > 0.8 in women is considered obese.

- Use a tape measure to measure the circumference of the waist (at the umbilicus with stomach muscles relaxed).
- Use a tape measure to measure the circumference of the hips at their widest point.
- Calculate the WHR using the following formula:

waist circumference (in.) ÷ hip circumference (in.)

NOTE: *Abdominal obesity is defined by World Health Organization (2011) as WHR > 0.85 in women and > 0.9 in men.*

Example: Robert's waist measurement is 32 inches, and his hip measurement is 34 inches. His WHR is 32 ÷ 34 = 0.94.

Clinical Insight 27-3 ➤ Interventions for Patients With Impaired Swallowing

Provide Nutritional Support

Nutritional support includes the following activities from the *Nursing Interventions Classification (NIC): Swallowing Therapy* (Butcher, Bulechek, Dochterman, et al., 2018, p. 370):

- Position the patient in a full upright, 90°, if possible.
- Provide/use assistive devices, as appropriate.
- Avoid use of drinking straws.
- Assist the patient to position head in forward flexion in preparation for swallowing (chin tuck).
- Assist patient to place food at the back of the mouth and on the unaffected side.
- Monitor the patient's tongue movements while she is eating. Frequently cue patient to chew and swallow. Patient may need to double swallow.
- Check mouth for pocketing of food after eating.
- Monitor body weight.
- Monitor body hydration (e.g., intake, output, skin turgor, mucous membranes).

Take Aspiration Precautions

(Butcher, Bulechek, Dochterman, et al., 2018, p. 75):

- Monitor level of consciousness, cough reflex, gag reflex, and swallowing ability.
- Position the patient upright 90° or as far as possible.
- Keep suction setup available.
- Feed in small amounts.
- Avoid liquids.
- Cut food into small pieces.
- Keep HOB elevated for at least 30 to 45 min after feeding.

Clinical Insight 27-4 ➤ Assisting Patients With Meals

Preparation

- Assess for functional deficits that contribute to imbalanced nutrition or difficulty eating independently.
- Monitor intake for nutritional adequacy. Some patients may need liquid oral supplements of protein and calories.
- Collaborate with occupational and physical therapists in planning care.
- Find out about rituals used before meals (blessing of food etc.).
- Provide an opportunity for toileting, oral hygiene, and handwashing before meals.
- Assist the patient to eat and drink only as necessary; encourage independence.
- Provide privacy during meals if the patient is embarrassed; to further maintain dignity, use a napkin, not a bib, over the patient's clothes.
- Check for proper fit of dentures.
- Provide music during the meal if the patient wishes.
- Demonstrate the use of assistive devices and alternative methods for eating and drinking.

Assisting the Patient

- If the patient must eat in bed, place the head of the bed at the highest tolerable level, and adjust the overbed table to be in easy reach.
- If the patient can feed himself, prepare the food on the tray for him (e.g., open food containers, cut the meat, peel an orange, open the milk and butter containers, mash food, if needed).
- If the client is visually impaired, identify the locations of the meal on the tray based on a clock face.
- See that the patient has protein- and energy-enriched meals.
- Provide mid-afternoon snacks.
- Ensure the nutrition prescribed is actually implemented. Assign someone to be responsible for assisting the patient with meals, as necessary. Include this in your instructions to UAPs and other assistive personnel.
- Do not interrupt meals with medications.

iCare Feeding the Patient

- Encourage family members to share mealtimes.
- If the patient's condition allows, encourage her to get out of bed for meals.
- Feed the patient if she is unable to feed herself.
- Sit down while feeding the patient; do not rush.
- Position yourself so you can make eye contact.
- Be sure to provide adequate time for her to chew and swallow.
- If possible, ask the patient what food she would like next.
- Serve one food at a time; serve small amounts.
- Serve finger foods (e.g., fruit, bread) to promote independence.
- Cue older adults, whenever possible, with words or gestures.
- Have casual conversation with the patient while feeding her to make mealtime more pleasant and relaxed.

After the Meal

- Help the patient to wash hands or use the rest room.
- Record the amount of food and fluid the patient consumed.
- Document feeding behaviors.
- Document changes in nutritional status.
- Document staffing and staff education, and availability of a supportive interdisciplinary team.

Assisting Older Adults Who Have Dementia

As do all people, older adults who have dementia differ in their abilities to eat and communicate. The following are general tips, but you should tailor interventions to each person's specific abilities to achieve the best results. In addition to many of the preceding interventions, try some of the following measures:

- Assess the patient's self-feeding abilities.
- Assess the patient's cognitive limitations and communication abilities.
- Assess for and treat pain.
- Minimize distractions: Turn off the TV; discourage people from entering the room.
- Help the patient to a comfortable chair, if possible.
- Assist with oral hygiene and hand hygiene.
- Remove any unnecessary eating utensils; serve only one food at a time.
- Remove items that should not be eaten (e.g., packets of salt or pepper), and hot items that could be spilled.
- Cue the patient verbally to help with self-feeding (e.g., "take a bite," "chew," "swallow").
- Mime eating motions, so the patient can imitate them.
- Place your hand over the patients to begin and guide self-feeding (hand-over-hand).
- When assisting, sit at eye level, and interact socially with the patient.
- Involve family members if they have assisted with feeding at home.
- Train and supervise UAPs in interacting with and feeding patients with dementia.
- Do not assist too soon—give the patient time to eat independently.
- Do not feed too fast. Feed at a rate that is safe and comfortable for the patient.

References

Amella, E. (2008, updated 2012, July); Ebersole, P., Hess, P., Touhy, T., et al. (2016); Joanna Briggs Institute (2011).

Clinical Insight 27-5 ➤ Guidelines for Checking Feeding Tube Placement

Tube placement must be verified by x-ray before the initial feeding is given. Because none of the bedside methods is foolproof, always use pH measurement in combination with one of the other methods for subsequent feedings.

Aspirating Stomach Contents

- Don procedure gloves. This is a clean, not sterile, technique.
- Just before feeding, draw up 10 to 30 mL of air in a 30- to 60-mL syringe, insert the syringe in the distal end of the feeding tube, and inject air.
  To flush out formula, medications, and other substances. This also helps keep a small-bore tube from collapsing when you aspirate.
- With the same syringe, aspirate the air and 20 to 30 mL of stomach or intestinal contents. Use slow, gentle suction—over 3 to 5 min, if necessary.
  It can take a long time to obtain enough fluid, especially from a small-bore tube.
- If you could not aspirate any fluid, inject another 20 mL of air, and use a smaller syringe to aspirate again.
  Using a small (<10 mL) syringe for very small tubes creates less negative pressure and makes it less likely the tube will collapse.
- If you still do not aspirate fluid, repeat the procedure with this variation: Insert air with the large syringe; insert the small syringe into the end of the tubing, and leave it for 15 min to allow fluid to accumulate before aspirating.
- If you are still unsuccessful, reposition the patient and try again after 20 min.
  Repositioning may move the tube into a place where fluid has pooled.

Inspecting the Aspirate

- Aspirate stomach contents, as described above. Gastric contents are normally greenish brown and liquid. If the patient is receiving enteral feedings, gastric contents should be curdled and white or a greenish color; intestinal contents will be a more yellow (bile) color with no curdling.

Intestinal contents are usually yellow-green because of the influence of bile. The colors of gastric and pulmonary secretions are altered by a variety of conditions, so observation of the visual characteristics of feeding tube aspirates is of little value in differentiating between respiratory and GI placement (Joanna Briggs Institute, 2010a, 2010c).

Measuring the Volume and pH of the Aspirate

- Aspirate stomach contents, as described above. Then measure the residual volume of the aspirate.
  Unexpected changes in volume of the aspirate can indicate poor GI motility. Gastric volumes will generally be larger than intestinal or esophageal volumes.
- Measure the pH of the aspirated fluid using nitrazine paper.
  - The lower the pH, the more likely it is that the tube is in the stomach.
    The pH of gastric contents is typically 1 to 5.5. Measuring the pH is useful only if the fluid you aspirate is acidic, indicating gastric placement.
  - Intestinal contents usually have a pH of 6 or greater.
  - The pH of respiratory secretions is ≥ 7; however, respiratory secretions may occasionally have a pH as low as 6.
- Remember that many variables can make the gastric pH results unreliable (e.g., blood in the stomach, antacid medications).
- Measuring bilirubin, trypsin, and pepsin in the aspirate can also be used to diagnose placement of a feeding tube in the respiratory tract (Cirgin Ellet, Cohen, Croffie, et al., 2014; Joanna Briggs Institute, 2010a).

Measuring and Observing the Length of the Tube That Extends From the Body

When the tube was inserted, it should have been marked with indelible marker where it exits the body (e.g., the naris), and the external length recorded. Compare the external length with previous measurements and with the mark made on the tube when it was inserted. If tube placement does not change, the external length should remain the same.

Injecting Air Into the Feeding Tube (not recommended)

This method is no longer recommended, although some professionals still do inject air into the feeding tube. It is the least accurate of the bedside methods and should never be used alone.

- Draw 5 to 30 mL of air into a syringe; place the tip of the syringe in the end of the feeding tube.
- Place a stethoscope over the stomach.
- Listen with the stethoscope as you inject the air through the tube. If you hear a gurgling or whooshing sound in the left upper quadrant, the tube may be in the stomach.
  NOTE: You cannot be sure of this because the lungs and the stomach lie close together, and the sounds created by sending air through the tube can cause you to err in determining placement.

Ongoing Patient Assessments

The following require repeated assessments over time to be useful for confirming other methods of tube placement:

- ***Observe for respiratory distress.*** Note cyanosis or difficulty breathing, coughing, choking.
  - These symptoms are indicators that the tube is in the respiratory tract, but keep in mind that the tube could instead be in the stomach and the symptoms caused by something else.

Clinical Insight 27-5 ➤ Guidelines for Checking Feeding Tube Placement—cont'd

- Absence of symptoms does not necessarily indicate correct placement in the stomach. The tube might be in the airway and not be causing any respiratory symptoms.
- ***Assess whether the patient can speak.*** Keep in mind that some clients can speak even when the tube is in a lung.

Other Bedside Verification Methods

Capnometry measures of carbon dioxide concentration in expired gases. Capnometry and additional tests of gastric juices may also serve as measures to help verify that the tube is correctly placed.

Clinical Insight 27-6 ➤ Monitoring Patients Receiving Enteral Nutrition

Monitor the following:

- **Position of the feeding tube.** Periodically check the placement of the tube. As a rule, check on each shift or at each intermittent feeding. For double-lumen tubes, keep the air vent above the level of the patient's stomach so that it will not act as a siphon and leak stomach contents.
- **NG or NE tube insertion site.** An NG or NE tube is secured by adhesive to the nose. Regularly check the skin, gently cleanse the area (with soap and water, as for normal washing; avoid harsh skin cleansers), and retape the tube, as needed. Report tissue breakdown, epistaxis (nosebleed), or sinusitis.
  These findings may signal a need for insertion of a percutaneous endoscopy gastrostomy (PEG) tube.
- **Gastrostomy tube, PEG/PEJ insertion site.** Inspect the insertion site for erythema or drainage, which are signs of infection. Clean it daily with soap and water.
- **Fluid balance.** Measure all I&O.
- **Weight.** To assess the adequacy of the feeding, regularly weigh the patient. There is usually a medical prescription for frequency of weighing. Frequent weight checks allow for adjustment of the feeding orders to achieve the desired goal.
- **Tube feeding residual volume.** To assess residual volume, aspirate the feeding tube to determine the amount of feeding remaining in the stomach. If the aspirate quantity is equal to or greater than the formula flow rate for 1 hour (alternatively, a total of 150 mL), the patient may be receiving too much fluid or may have delayed gastric emptying. However, you should not automatically stop the feeding; if you obtain a single sample of an increased residual volume, recheck it in 1 hour.
- **Frequency of bowel movements.** Bowel movements should occur regularly.
  Constipation is usually caused by inadequate water or fiber. Some commercial feedings contain fiber. You may add free water and perhaps fiber to other formulas. Diarrhea may indicate intolerance of the formula, excessive feeding, or GI disease.
- **Bowel sounds.** Check before each feeding, or every 4 to 8 hours for continuous feedings. Peristalsis must be present. Flatus is a better indication of complete bowel function than are bowel sounds.
- **Abdominal distention.** Measure abdominal girth daily, at the umbilicus.
- **Serum electrolyte levels.** Monitor regularly (per protocol or prescription).
- **Urine for sugar and acetone.** This is sometimes done as a bedside screen for hyperglycemia. However, treatment is based on blood sugar levels.
- **Skin turgor, hematocrit, and urine specific gravity.** These are indicators of dehydration and overhydration, although skin turgor alone is not a reliable sign.
- **Serum blood urea nitrogen (BUN) and sodium levels.** This is especially important for high-protein formulas. Insufficient fluid intake combined with high protein intake may overload the kidneys so that nitrogenous wastes are not excreted adequately.

Clinical Insight 27-7 ➤ Monitoring and Maintenance for Patients Receiving Parenteral Nutrition

Monitoring

For patients receiving PN, you will need to monitor the following:

Catheter Insertion Site

- Assess catheter insertion site for swelling, redness, drainage, or tenderness (signs of infection and/or phlebitis in PICC lines).
  Hypertonic PN creates a risk for phlebitis.
- Observe for swelling in the extremity on the same side of catheter insertion.
  Sign of infiltration or phlebitis.
- Observe for catheter retraction from the vein; observe the length of the catheter from the insertion site to the hub at insertion and periodically.

Supplies and Equipment

- Monitor tubing connections to see that they are secure.
- Monitor to see that the dressing is secure and dry.
- Check the rate and amount infused at least hourly.
  To ensure the line is patent, the PN is flowing freely, and the pump is functioning properly.

Weight

- Regularly weigh the patient (according to medical order or agency policy, but commonly daily or 3 times per week).
  (1) Frequent weight checks allow for assessing the adequacy of the formula and making adjustments, as needed, to achieve the desired goal. (2) Because of the hypertonicity of the solutions, fluid overload can occur. Rapid weight increase is an indicator.

Glucose

- Check blood glucose every 4 to 6 hours until stable, and then at least daily.
  The high proportion of glucose in the formulas can cause hyperglycemia, the most common complication of PN. You may need to administer regular insulin according to a sliding scale (or the pharmacist may add it directly to the PN solution). The risk for hyperglycemia is less with 3:1 PN solutions.
- You may need to administer regular insulin according to a sliding scale (or the pharmacist may add it directly to the PN solution).

Fluids

Monitor I&O.
Diuresis and dehydration can occur if hypertonic dextrose is infused too rapidly.

Lab Values

Patients receiving PN require regular lab studies (the following are examples and not a comprehensive list). The frequency of the studies depends on the patient's condition.

- Electrolytes, blood sugar, albumin, BUN, and creatinine
  Values are used for formula adjustment and to evaluate electrolyte balance and glucose metabolism.
- Albumin, transferrin, transthyretin (prealbumin), or retinol-binding protein
  May be used to assess visceral protein status.
- 24-hour urine for urine urea nitrogen (weekly)
  To evaluate nitrogen balance.
- Complete blood count (CBC) and differential
  To monitor changes in immune function.
- Liver function studies
- Serum zinc
- Plasma urea
- Plasma and urine osmolality
- Blood gases

Symptoms of Complications

- *Electrolyte imbalances.* Symptoms depend on the electrolytes affected. Monitor lab values.
- *Sepsis.* Temperature greater than 100°F (37.8°C) orally, rapid pulse from baseline, chills, hypothermia, edema or erythema of skin, exudate from catheter insertion site, malaise, leukocytosis (increased white blood cell count), altered level of consciousness.
- *Air embolus.* Cyanosis, tachypnea, hypotension, heart murmur
- *Catheter dislodgement or thrombosis.* Swelling of arm or neck, pain, difficulty flushing catheter, difficulty infusing PN

Nutritional Status

- Calculate the daily calorie intake.
- Perform nutritional assessment at 2-week intervals.
- Possibly measure arm circumference and triceps skinfold thickness.
- Monitor serum albumin levels.
- Most agencies have specialized nutrition teams who will monitor these parameters.

Maintenance

- Change the dressing over the catheter every 24 hr or according to agency policy and when it becomes wet, soiled, or nonocclusive. Use sterile technique.

Clinical Insight 27-7 ➤ Monitoring and Maintenance for Patients Receiving Parenteral Nutrition—cont'd

- Secure connections with luer-lock connectors; do not use tape.
- Change the filter every 24 hr.
- Do not hang PN bottles for more than 12 hr (some guidelines and agency policies specify 24 hr).
  PN solutions are prepared in batches under strict aseptic conditions. Its high nutrient concentration makes PN an excellent feeding alternative; however, it also makes the solution ideal for bacterial growth.
- Use sterile aseptic technique when changing the dressing for a central line, as well as when changing the solution and tubing.
- Do not use the PN infusion line for administering any other medication or solutions.
  Decreases the risk of contamination and infection.
- Infuse PN by pump with a reliable, audible alarm, to protect against "free flow."
- If an infusion falls behind schedule, do not increase the rate in an attempt to catch up.
  This can cause osmotic diuresis and dehydration.
- When PN is discontinued, it may be done gradually (perhaps over as many as 48 hours).
  To prevent a sudden drop in blood sugar.

ASSESSMENT GUIDELINES AND TOOLS

Screening for Nutritional Problems

Clients who have risk factors for nutritional problems should be evaluated using one of the methods in this section: Subjective Global Assessment, Nutrition Screening Initiative (NSI) for Older Adults, and Mini-Nutritional Assessment (MNA).

Focused Assessment

Subjective Global Assessment

Using the subjective global assessment (SGA) method, an experienced clinician examines the general medical history and physical examination to evaluate a client's nutritional status. There are six components pertinent to nutritional status:

1. *Weight history*—over previous 6 months
2. *Dietary history*—including a comparison of usual, recommended, and current intake, as well as changes in eating patterns over the past weeks or months
3. *Gastrointestinal symptoms history*—anorexia, nausea, vomiting, and diarrhea
4. *Energy level*—including activity level and functional abilities
5. *Existing disease*—evaluation of the metabolic demands of any disease states along with acute stressors that may alter those demands
6. *Physical examination data*—regarding loss of fat stores, muscle wasting, and the presence of edema and ascites

As a clinician, you would analyze these components to rate the client's nutritional status as normal, mild, moderate, or severe. The effectiveness of this method depends largely on the experience of the clinician (Detsky, McLaughlin, Baker, et al., 1987).

Focused Assessment

Nutrition Screening Initiative (NSI), for Older Adults: Indications of Impaired Nutritional Status

The NSI requires collection and evaluation of data in four areas: clinical, dietary, body composition, and biochemical. In addition, it identifies indicators of impaired nutritional status.

Major Indicators

- Significant weight loss over time
- Significant high or low weight for height
- Significant change in functional status
- Significant and inappropriate food intake
- Significant reduction in mid-arm circumference
- Significant decrease in skinfold
- Osteoporosis or osteomalacia
- Folate or vitamin B deficiency

Minor Indicators

- Concurrent syndromes
- Alcoholism
- Cognitive impairment
- Chronic renal insufficiency
- Multiple concurrent medications
- Malabsorption syndromes

Symptoms

- Anorexia, nausea, or dysphagia
- Early satiety
- Changed bowel habits
- Fatigue or apathy
- Memory loss

Physical Signs

- Poor oral or dental status
- Dehydration
- Poorly healing wounds
- Loss of subcutaneous fat or muscle mass
- Fluid retention

Lab Values

- Reduced levels of serum albumin, transferrin, or prealbumin
- Folate deficiency
- Iron deficiency
- Zinc deficiency
- Reduced levels of ascorbic acid

Focused Assessment

Mini-Nutritional Assessment

The Mini-Nutritional Assessment (MNA) is a quick and easy method of identifying individuals with nutritional risk or with malnutrition. This tool was developed primarily for use in older clients. It consists of two parts. The first part screens for nutritional risk. The second part is completed only if the individual is identified to be at risk. The final score, which tallies the scores of both parts, is the Malnutrition Indicator Score. Indications of malnutrition require interprofessional follow-up. To see and use the MNA,

Go to the Web site, **www.mna-elderly.com**

References

Guigoz, Y. (2006); Rubenstein, L., Harker, J., Salva, A., et al. (2001); Vellas, B., Villars, H., Abellan, G., et al. (2006)

Focused Nutritional Assessment

If you identify nutritional problems or risks using the screening tools, you should perform a more in-depth nutritional assessment, such as the following. The nutrition component of a focused nutritional assessment includes both subjective (history) and objective (physical examination) data.

Focused Assessment

Focused Nutritional Assessment

Nutritional History

Item	Components
Demographic data	Name, date, age, gender, date of birth, address, occupation, workplace
Chief complaint	Client's subjective statement of health problem, including onset and duration
Present illness and current health	Detailed data about chief complaint as it relates to nutrition status
	Recent diet changes and reasons
	Recent weight loss or gain and over what period
	Usual body weight: 20% above or below desirable weight?
	Change in appetite
	Unusual stress/trauma (surgery, job, family)
	Medications, prescriptions
	Alcohol, nicotine, caffeine consumption
Health history	Previous illnesses, trauma, major dental problems, or issues that could interfere with ability to shop, prepare food, chew, or swallow
	Allergies (i.e., environmental, foods, drugs)
	Eating disorders
	Chronic disease or surgery that affects gastrointestinal (GI) tract
	Substance abuse
	Nutritional programs
	Depression
Family health history	Genetic/familial disorders that could affect nutritional status: cardiovascular or GI disorders, Crohn's disease, diabetes, cancer, sickle cell anemia, allergies, celiac disease, other food intolerances, obesity
Dietary history	Current food intake pattern using one of the following methods: 24-hour–7-day recall, as appropriate; food frequency questionnaire; food record; and comparison to dietary guidelines and Dietary Reference Intakes (DRIs)
	Special dietary considerations, restrictions
	Fad diets
	Vitamin and mineral supplements
	Commercial dietary supplements
	Nonconventional dietary supplements
	Food preferences, dislikes
	Dietary influences from ethnic, cultural, or religious practices
	Counseling needs (based on food knowledge)
Medication history	Recent use of steroids, immunosuppressants, chemotherapy, anticonvulsants, or oral contraceptives
Socioeconomic factors	Adequate food storage, refrigeration, food preparation, payments:
	Supplemental Security Income (SSI), food stamps, Women, Infants, and Children (WIC) program
	Who shops for, prepares, and cooks food?
	Location/availability of retail food/grocery store or availability of transportation
Personal factors	Stress/coping mechanisms, self-concept, social supports
	Daily activity level and exercise regimen

(Continued)

Focused Assessment

Focused Nutritional Assessment—cont'd

Nutrition-Focused Physical Examination

Correlate the following physical examination findings with the dietary history, screening methods, anthropometric measurements, and laboratory results.

I. The General Survey

Assess vital signs, height, weight, and overall impressions.

- ***Overall appearance.*** Does the client look ill? Does he appear adequately nourished? You will want to investigate any hunches as you move through the physical examination.
- ***Temperature.*** An increase in temperature raises the client's metabolic rate and need for fluid, is a sign of infection, and may decrease the client's appetite.
- ***Blood pressure (BP) and heart rate*** are affected by fluid status. An elevated BP may be related to fluid volume excess; a low BP may be a sign of dehydration. Heart rate usually increases when fluid volume is low.
- ***Height and weight.*** Calculate the body mass index (BMI) on the basis of these measures:

  BMI = weight in kilograms ÷ (height in meters)^2

Classification of Body Mass Index Values

Classification	*BMI (kg/m^2)*	*Risk of Comorbidities*
Underweight*	<18.5	Low
Normal weight	18.5–24.9	Average
Pre-obese	25.0–29.9	Mildly increased
Class I obesity	30.0–34.9	Moderate
Class II obesity	35.0–39.9	Severe
Class III obesity	>40.0	Very severe

*NOTE: In adults in long-term care settings or with serious illness, nutritional support should be implemented for those with a BMI less than 21. In this population a BMI of less than 21 is associated with increased mortality (Centers for Disease Control and Prevention, 2016, June 16, last updated).

II. Integumentary System

- ***Skin turgor*** is an indicator of fluid status. Poor skin turgor may result from dehydration. Swelling may result from overhydration.
- ***Skin integrity*** reflects overall nutritional status. Poor wound healing may suggest inadequate intake of protein, vitamin C, or zinc. Patients with uncontrolled diabetes or severely restricted diets often experience slow-healing wounds, especially in the feet and legs.
- ***Areas of warmth or erythema.*** These are signs of inflammation or infection.
- ***Other nutrition-related skin changes*** include red, swollen skin lesions (caused by niacin deficiency); excessive bleeding seen as petechiae or ecchymosis (caused by vitamin K or C deficiency); and xerosis (dry skin).
- ***Abnormal nail findings*** include spoon-shaped, brittle nails (caused by iron deficiency); dull nails with transverse ridge (caused by protein deficiency); pale, poor blanching, or mottled nails (caused by vitamin A or C deficiency); bruising or bleeding beneath nails (caused by protein or caloric deficiency); and splinter hemorrhages (caused by vitamin C deficiency).
- ***Hair*** will grow slowly, thin, or break easily if protein is deficient.

III. The Head and Neck

The condition of the mouth, teeth, and gums has a major effect on a client's choice of food, ability to chew, and ability to swallow.

- ***Facial paralysis or drooping*** of one side of the face may be a result of stroke, injury, or nerve irritation, which also affects the ability to chew and swallow (dysphagia).
- ***Enlarged thyroid gland.*** Look for swelling of the thyroid, which may be related to hypothyroid or hyperthyroid states. Both disorders affect metabolic rate and energy requirements.
- ***Eyes.*** Nutritional deficits may cause the eyes to be red and dry and the conjunctiva pale.
- ***Lips and tongue.*** The lips may be chapped, red, or swollen. The tongue may be bright red, purple, or swollen or may have longitudinal furrows.
- ***Teeth and gums.*** Look for cavities, mottled or missing teeth, and spongy, bleeding, or receding gums.
- ***Lymph nodes.*** Palpate for enlarged or tender lymph nodes under the chin and along the neck. Nodes that are swollen can signal infection, such as a sore throat.

Focused Assessment

Focused Nutritional Assessment—cont'd

IV. Cardiovascular System

You will have gained initial information about the cardiovascular system by taking the vital signs. As you follow up and listen to the heart and check pulses, you should explore any abnormal vital signs.

- ***Bounding pulses*** are associated with fluid overload, fever, and hypertension.
- ***Weak, thready pulse*** may indicate dehydration, shock, or hypotension.
- ***Edema in the extremities*** may be a sign of fluid overload, inadequate protein stores, or electrolyte imbalance.

V. Abdominal Examination

- **A *scaphoid or concave abdomen*** indicates loss of subcutaneous fat, possibly caused by malnutrition.
- **A *round or protuberant abdomen*** points to obesity caused by excess caloric and/or high fat intake.
- **A *generalized enlarged abdomen*** may signify *ascites* (fluid in the abdominal cavity) caused by liver malfunction. Ascites results from three mechanisms: abnormal movement of protein and water into the abdomen; sodium and fluid retention; and decreased albumin production in the liver.
- ***Hyperactive bowel sounds*** are heard with gastrointestinal (GI) infection, laxative use, and malabsorption disorders.
- ***Hypoactive bowel sounds*** suggest sluggish motility in the GI tract.

VI. Musculoskeletal System

- ***Thin extremities with excess skinfolds*** may indicate muscle atrophy and fat loss related to malnutrition, especially protein and calories. This may also occur as a result of prolonged bed rest and inadequate food intake. Skinfold measurement is also useful in assessing muscle and fat stores.
- Look for any obvious ***swelling, deformities, or limitation in range of motion*** of the joints.
- ***Kyphosis*** of the spine may indicate osteoporosis and possible insufficient calcium intake.
- ***Joint pain*** on palpation or with movement is a sign of arthritis or gout. Arthritis may affect ability to shop for groceries, prepare food to eat, and use utensils for eating and drinking. Gout is often induced by diets high in *purines* (food substances that break down into uric acid), obesity, and excess alcohol intake.

VII. Neurological System

The neurological examination will provide insight into the client's ability to perform independent tasks.

- Look for ***altered level of consciousness or signs of behavioral disturbances and dementia*** through general conversation and appropriateness of answers to specific questions.
- Assess ***coordination and reflexes***.
- Assess for ***cognitive deficits or severe psychiatric disorders***. A client with cognitive deficits or severe psychiatric disorders may have difficulty preparing food or judging appropriate nutrient choices.
- Assess for ***motor or sensory deficits***. Clients with motor or sensory deficits may be unable to purchase, prepare, or eat a variety of foods.
- ***Confusion, weakness, diminished reflexes, paresthesia, and sensory loss*** may be cues to vitamin B deficiencies.
- ***Tetany or severe and generalized muscle spasm*** may indicate calcium or magnesium deficits.

VIII. What Are the Signs of Severe Malnutrition?

Malnutrition is a condition of impaired development or function caused by a long-term deficiency, excess, or imbalance in energy and/or nutrient intake.

- Symptoms of undernutrition caused by insufficient food include reduced physical activity, weight loss, and reduced height.
- Children, older adults, and people with chronic illnesses such as cancer, HIV infection, and chronic obstructive pulmonary disease (COPD) are most likely to experience malnutrition. Malnutrition can occur with obesity.
- To assess for malnutrition in children, compare weight, height, and head circumference to the standards (norms) for the child's age.
- Other indicators in children include the presence of iron-deficiency anemia.
- In adolescents, look for a delay of stages of sexual maturation.

DIAGNOSTIC TESTING

Diagnostic Testing

Tests Reflecting Nutritional Status: Norms

NOTE: Norms are for adults (ages 19 to 65 years) unless otherwise noted.

Blood glucose	70 mg/dL to 100 mg/dL. ➤ Capillary blood sugar is frequently assessed at the bedside with a simple fingerstick. ➤ Serum blood glucose levels are assessed by drawing a venous blood sample. The level is measured in the laboratory. The American Diabetes Association (2017) recommends for patients with diabetes a preprandial plasma glucose level of 80 to 130 mg/dL.
Serum albumin	3.4–4.8 g/dL
Prealbumin	12–42 mg/dL (age 6 years–adult)
Globulin	2.3–3.4 g/dL
Blood urea nitrogen (BUN)	5–18 mg/dL (children) 8–21 mg/dL (age 14 years–adult); 10–31 mg/dL (adult older than 90 years)
Creatinine	0.5–1 mg/dL (female) 0.6–1.2 mg/dL (male)
Hemoglobin	13.2–17.3 g/dL (male) 11.7–15.5 g/dL (female) 12.6–17.4 g/dL (male, older adult) 11.7–16.1 g/dL (female, older adult)

CLINICALJUDGMENT
Applying the Full-Spectrum Nursing Model

PATIENT SITUATION

Mrs. Ong is a 75-year-old retired schoolteacher who suffered a stroke 8 months ago. Since leaving the hospital, she has been living in a nursing home. Mrs. Ong has residual weakness on the right side—her dominant side—and has not mastered the use of tableware with her left hand. On admission to the nursing home 7 months ago, she weighed 150 lb. Today, she weighs only 125 lb. Mrs. Ong refuses to go to the dining room for meals. The UAPs report that she eats a few bites of most foods but never eats more than half of anything.

THINKING

1. *Theoretical Knowledge:*

   a. Based on Mrs. Ong's gender, age, and activity level, make a rough estimate of the number of kcal/day she needs.

   b. What are two other, more precise, ways you could determine Mrs. Ong's ideal body weight?

2. *Critical Thinking (Considering Alternatives):* What are some possible explanations for why Mrs. Ong is not eating all her food?

DOING

3. *Practical Knowledge:*

   a. Suppose you have decided to use the general ideal weight guide to determine Mrs. Ong's ideal weight. What, specifically, would you need to do? You do not need to actually calculate; just list the action steps.

b. Suppose you have decided to determine Mrs. Ong's body mass index (BMI). What equipment would you need?

c. What is the formula for calculating BMI from the height and weight?

4. *Nursing Process (Diagnosis):* Write a nursing diagnosis for Mrs. Ong Use just the data provided in the situation. Assume her BMI is 20.

CARING

5. *Self-Knowledge:* What would you be feeling if you were in Mrs. Ong's situation?

6. *Ethical Knowledge:* What are one or two things you would do to help Mrs. Ong feel cared for and cared about?

Critical Thinking and Clinical Judgment

1. Recall the employees (Isaac Schwartz and Sujing Lee) interviewed in the Meet Your Patient scenario in Volume 1. In addition, you now have two more patients, Wakenda Pierre and Luceno Jarin. Their information is provided below.

   - Isaac Schwartz, a 65-year-old accountant, works long hours. He describes a sedentary lifestyle, no tobacco use, infrequent alcohol use, no medical problems, and a nutritional history of skipping meals and daily consumption of restaurant food. You measure his height as 69 in. and weight as 245 lb.

   - Sujing Lee, a 29-year-old project manager, regularly works 65 hours per week. Sujing is 30 weeks pregnant. She does not smoke or drink and has never been hospitalized or had surgery. She has gained a total of 25 lb since becoming pregnant. Her diet consists mainly of traditional Chinese food. She eats three meals a day and always brings lunch from home. Lately, she has been feeling "tired all the time." At the screening, she weighs 126 lb and is 63 in. tall.

   - Wakenda Pierre is a 38-year-old administrative assistant. She exercises at the gym 4 to 5 days per week, smokes an occasional cigarette, has two to three drinks every night before dinner, struggles with keeping her blood pressure under control, and eats fast food for breakfast and lunch every day. She is 72 in. tall and weighs 165 lb.

   - Luceno Jarin is a 65-year-old business executive. He tells you he was diagnosed with type 2 diabetes mellitus 5 years ago. He is struggling to follow his prescribed diet. He drinks alcohol sporadically and walks briskly 30 minutes every day of the week. He is 67 inches tall and weighs 205 lb.

     a. Determine each client's BMI. Based on these results, what conclusions can you make about their weight status?

     b. What are the likely causes of each person's weight status?

     c. What additional work-up would be recommended for each individual?

     d. What indications would lead you to believe that each client has adopted a healthier lifestyle?

2. The following are three clients admitted to the medical–surgical unit of your local hospital. On their admission, the primary nurse collected the following information:

	CLIENT 1	CLIENT 2	CLIENT 3
Weight	175 lb	100 lb	250 lb
Height	70 in.	59 in.	65 in.
Gender/Age	Male/40 years old	Female/18 years old	Male/65 years old
Usual daily caloric intake	2,500 kcal	1,000 kcal	2,500 kcal
Usual activity level	Moderate	High	Light
Serum albumin	Normal	Low	Normal
Serum glucose	Normal	Low	High

a. Identify which client(s) is/are at risk for nutritional imbalance.

b. Which client is at risk for developing malnutrition?

c. What additional information would support this conclusion?

d. What nursing interventions would you initiate at this time?

3. After 3 days, you examine how well each of these clients is doing using the same parameters as admission day.

	CLIENT 1	CLIENT 2	CLIENT 3
Weight	170 lb	103 lb	250 lb
Current daily caloric intake	2,500 kcal	1,500 kcal	1,500 kcal
Intake (mL)	2,000	2,000	1,000
Output (mL)	1,800	1,900	500
Current activity level	Up as tolerated	Up as tolerated	Bedrest
Serum albumin	Normal	Low	Normal
Serum glucose	Normal	Low	High

a. In comparison with the admission data, there are some changes. Which client's health status is a priority now, and why?

b. What is/are the most likely cause(s) of this concern?

c. Which nursing interventions should be initiated for this client while hospitalized? Focus on nutritional needs.

d. Identify appropriate education that should begin during hospitalization for this client.

4. For each of the following concepts, use critical thinking to describe how or why it is important to nursing, patient care, or nutrition. Note that these are *not* to be merely definitions.

Energy balance	Basal metabolic rate
Body mass index	Nutrients
Weight management	Nutritional history
Body weight standards	Enteral feedings
Parenteral nutrition	Special diets
Nutritional screening	

What Are the Main Points in This Chapter?

- Reliable guidelines for designing a nutritious diet include the Dietary Reference Intakes (DRIs), the USDA Dietary Guidelines, and the nutrition facts panel found on packaged foods in the United States.
- ChooseMyPlate is a food guide that illustrates healthful dietary choices. It stresses six concepts for healthy eating: activity, moderation, personalization, proportionality, variety, and gradual improvement.
- Energy nutrients are carbohydrates, proteins, and fats (lipids). Other important nutrients are water and the micronutrients: fat-soluble vitamins, water-soluble vitamins, and minerals.
- Carbohydrates include simple sugars called monosaccharides and disaccharides and complex carbohydrates called *polysaccharides*.
- Glucose, a monosaccharide, is the primary source of energy for the brain, as well as for the body during moderate-to-intense physical activity.
- Proteins are made up of amino acids and are required for cell and tissue growth, maintenance, and repair. They also act as buffers in acid–base balance. Proteins are an energy source.
- Lipids, including fats and oils, are classified as glycerides, sterols, and phospholipids. They are essential components of cells, fuel the body at rest and during light activity, aid in absorption of fat-soluble vitamins, and promote a sense of satiety when eaten. Low-density lipoproteins (LDLs) are the "bad" cholesterol. High-density lipoproteins (HDLs) are the "good" cholesterol.
- Saturated fats and *trans*-fats are less healthful lipid choices than mono- and polyunsaturated fats. Saturated fats and *trans*-fats raise LDL cholesterol levels in the blood.
- The essential fatty acids omega-6 and omega-3 help protect against heart disease when they replace *trans*-fats in the diet. They are found mainly in vegetable oils, nuts, seeds, and fatty fish.
- Nutrients must be consumed at least at a minimal level to meet the body's physiological needs. This level is called Dietary Reference Intake (DRI).
- The fat-soluble vitamins are A, D, E, and K. Water-soluble vitamins are C and B-complex vitamins.
- Minerals (e.g., calcium, iron, magnesium) are important for transmitting nerve impulses, regulating fluid balance, strengthening bones, and producing energy.
- The basal metabolic rate (BMR) is a measure of the energy required by resting tissue to maintain basic function.
- Factors influencing a client's nutritional status include developmental stage, pregnancy and lactation, education, lifestyle choices, vegetarianism, dieting for weight loss, culture, religion, disease processes, functional limitations, economic factors, and modified or special diets.
- Many people must follow a modified diet to assist in managing their illness. In addition, all inpatients must have a diet prescribed by their primary healthcare provider.
- When examining an individual's nutritional balance, it is important to screen for nutritional problems. When risk factors are present, thoroughly assess nutritional history, physical findings, anthropometric measurements, imaging techniques, and biochemical values.
- A food record is the most accurate method of obtaining data about a client's actual food intake.
- The body mass index (BMI), skinfold measurements, and body part circumferences are estimates of body composition.
- Laboratory or biochemical indicators of nutritional status include blood glucose and serum protein levels or indices such as albumin, urea, and hemoglobin.

- Vitamin and mineral supplementation may be appropriate for some people, but they do not replace the need for a balanced diet.
- Government programs provide some assistance for clients who cannot afford to buy food.
- Nutritional requirements of older adults are similar to those for all adults, with a slight reduction in the need for calories, and the more likely need for nutrient supplementation. Nutritional problems are also similar, but the incidence is higher among older adults.
- Nurses can help support nutrition for patients who have deficits in self-care or impairment of swallowing by assisting patients with meals and providing swallowing therapy.
- Nutritional imbalance can range from either inadequate or excessive amounts of a single nutrient relative to overall caloric intake.
- Obesity is a major problem in the United States, both in children and adults.
- Interventions for underweight/undernutrition include measures to improve the patient's appetite, assisting with meals, and providing enteral and parenteral nutrition.
- Nasogastric tubes are inserted to lavage the stomach; collect a specimen of the stomach contents; or prevent nausea, vomiting, and gastric distention. They are also placed to facilitate enteral feeding.
- The most accurate way to check enteral tube placement is by radiographic (x-ray) verification. To check enteral tube placement at the bedside, you could also use a combination of techniques: aspirate stomach contents to observe color and measure the pH (normally 1 to 5.5 for stomach contents); serial observations for respiratory distress, residual volume, length of tube extending outside the body; and capnometry. Do not rely on a single technique.
- Potential complications associated with enteral feedings include aspiration, infection, diarrhea, and electrolyte imbalance.
- Meticulous sterile technique when administering parenteral nutrition is critical because the solution is delivered into a large central vein; if infection occurs, sepsis is almost immediate.

Knowledge Map

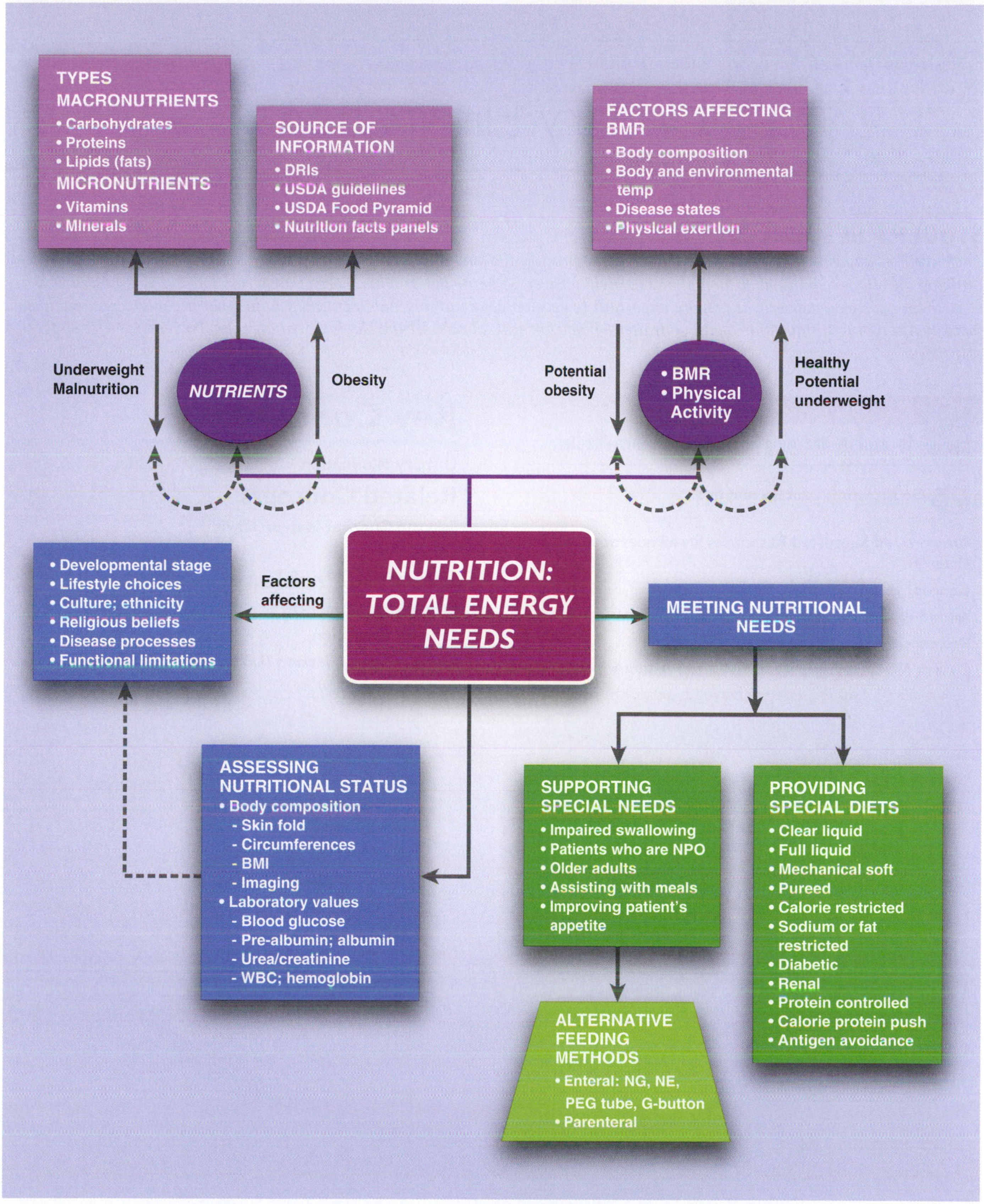

CHAPTER 28

Urinary Elimination

STUDENT RESOURCES

The questions and exercises in this book allow you to practice the kind of thinking you will use as a full-spectrum nurse. Critical-thinking questions usually have more than one right answer, so we do not provide "correct answers" for these features. Try to answer these questions yourself. It is more important to develop your nursing judgment than to just cover content. You will learn more by discussing the questions with your peers. If you are still unsure, see the Davis Advantage chapter resources for suggested responses.

To explore learning resources for this chapter,

Go to Davis Advantage and find:

Answers and Suggested Responses for all questions in this chapter

Concept Map

Knowledge Map

References and Bibliography

Lists of NOC Outcomes and NIC Interventions

Key Concepts

Urinary elimination

Related Concepts

See the Concept Map on Davis Advantage.

Example Problems

Urinary Incontinence

Urinary Retention

Urinary Tract Infection (UTI)

Caring for the Nguyens

At a recent visit to the Family Health Center, Nam and Yen Nguyen confide that Nam's mother Mai Nguyen has had several "accidents." She has denied the problem, but Yen tells you that she helped her mother-in-law with laundry recently and many of the clothes smell of urine. They ask you how to approach Mai about this problem.

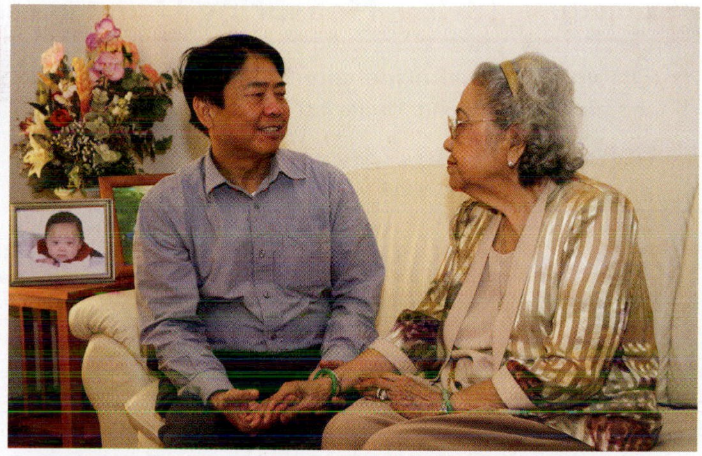

A. How would you respond?

B. What suggestions, if any, could you make to the Nguyens about treatment for Mai?

C. Yen says that she has been told that surgery is the best form of treatment. She asks you whether this is true. How would you answer her question?

PracticalKnowledge clinical application

This section provides procedures and clinical insights you will need to support your patients' urinary function. You will also find assessment guidelines and information about diagnostic tests of urinary function.

PROCEDURES

Procedure 28-1 ■ Measuring Urine

➤ For steps to follow in all procedures, refer to the Universal Steps for All Procedures found on the inside back cover.

Equipment

- Bedpan or urinal
- Clean procedure gloves
- Graduated container
- Toilet paper, as indicated
- Washcloth or towel
- Hand sanitizer for patient's hands

Measuring Post-Void Residual Urine Volume With a Portable Bladder Scanner

- Portable bladder scanning device
- Ultrasound gel
- Clean gloves
- Tissues
- Antiseptic swabs or wipes

Delegation

Measuring urine, including postvoid residual volume (PVR) with the use of a portable bladder scanner, may be delegated to specially trained unlicensed assistive personnel (UAP) in some facilities. However, you must be sure that the UAP knows how to perform the procedure correctly, including proper cleansing of the bedpan/urinal and the graduated container according to the facility's policies. Also, complete the following assessments, and instruct the UAP when to stop the procedure and seek assistance from the nurse and to report the results immediately. In some instances, you may choose to perform the bladder scan to ensure accuracy and expedite any necessary treatment.

Pre-Procedure Assessments

- **Cognitive status.** Determine whether the patient can be instructed to complete this procedure on her own and/or whether she can follow directions.
- **Mobility status.** Determine whether the patient can safely get out of the bed to use the toilet.
- **Urinary status.** Determine the patient's ability to control bladder function.

(continued on next page)

Procedure 28-1 ■ Measuring Urine (continued)

- **Postvoid residual urine volume,** if needed, determine the timing and amount of the last voiding.

  NOTE: A bladder scan should be done as soon as possible after voiding and within no more than 10 to 15 minutes.

- **Palpate the bladder** to assess for distention.

Procedure 28-1A ■ Measuring Urine Output From a Bedpan or Urinal

➤ When performing the procedure, always identify your patient according to agency policy, using two identifiers, and be attentive to standard precautions, hand hygiene, patient safety and privacy, body mechanics, and documentation.

Procedure Steps

1. **Perform hand hygiene,** and don clean procedure gloves.
   Prevents transmission of bacteria.
2. **Place a bedpan or urinal** by positioning the patient in a semi-Fowler's position, with the legs slightly spread.
   a. ***For a male***, place the urinal on the bed between his legs, and insert (or ask him to insert) his penis in the urinal.
   b. ***For a female***, raise the siderails or provide an overhead trapeze so that the patient will have grip holds to maneuver herself onto and off the bedpan.
3. **Remove the bedpan or urinal,** being careful not to spill the urine. Reposition the patient, and transport the urine to the bathroom.
4. **Pour the urine into a graduated** cylinder or calibrated measuring container while still wearing procedure gloves.
   a. Be sure that the measuring device is labeled with the correct patient information (in many institutions, labels are preprinted or barcoded).
   b. Do not use a measuring device for more than one patient.
5. **Place the measuring device on a flat surface** (e.g., shelf, table that is not used for food or personal care products), if available, and read the amount at eye level.
   When looking at fluid level from an angle, the meniscus may appear falsely low or high.
6. **Observe the urine for color,** clarity, and odor.
7. **Discard the urine in the toilet.** If a specimen is required, transfer 30 to 60 mL of urine to the designated container.
8. **Clean the measuring container,** and store in the patient's bathroom.
9. **Remove gloves.** Perform hand hygiene.
10. **Record the time and volume** on the intake and output (I&O) record.

Procedure 28-1B ■ Measuring Urine From an Indwelling Catheter

➤ When performing the procedure, always identify your patient according to agency policy, using two identifiers, and be attentive to standard precautions, hand hygiene, patient safety and privacy, body mechanics, and documentation.

Procedure Steps

1. **Wearing clean gloves**, place the drainage spout for the collection bag inside a calibrated measuring container. Avoid touching the spout to the inside of the container.
   Prevents transmission of bacteria.
2. **Unclamp the drainage spout**, and direct the flow of urine into the measuring device, still keeping the spout away from the sides of the container.
   Prevents contaminating the drainage spout.▼

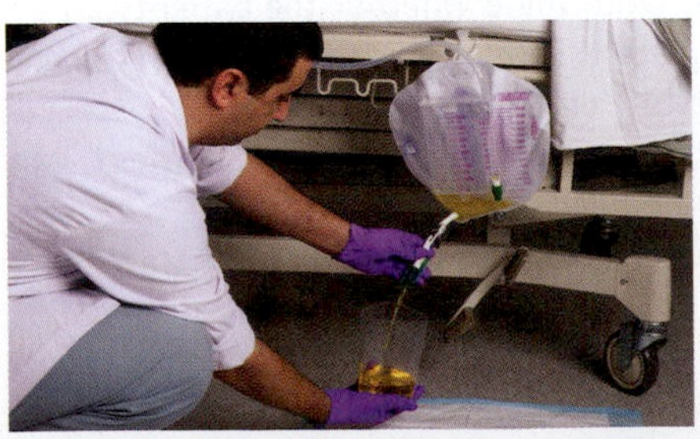

3. **Reclamp the spout** when the collection bag is empty.
4. **Wipe the drainage spout** with an alcohol pad or disinfecting wipe, then replace the spout into the slot on the collection bag.
   A clean spout reduces transmission of bacteria when the nurse touches it.
5. **Measure urine output** from the indwelling catheter at the end of each shift, or if the urine bag is getting full.▼

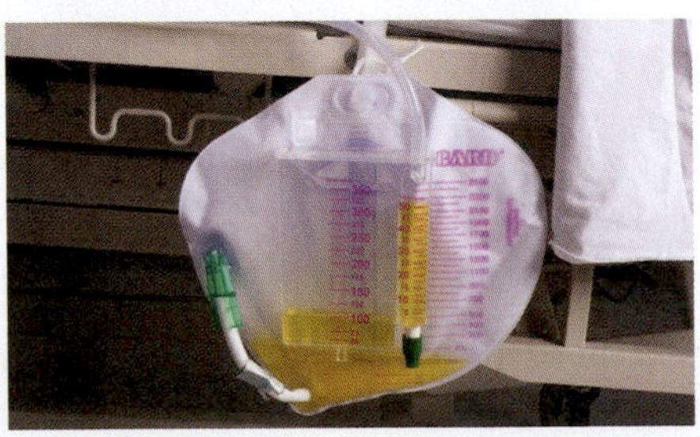

6. **Discard the urine in the toilet.**
7. **Remove gloves, and perform hand hygiene**.
8. **Record the time and amount** on the I&O record; record urine color, clarity, and odor.

Procedure 28-1C ■ Measuring Postvoid Residual Urine Volume With a Portable Bladder Scanner

➤ When performing the procedure, always identify your patient according to agency policy, using two identifiers, and be attentive to standard precautions, hand hygiene, patient safety and privacy, body mechanics, and documentation.

Procedure Steps

1. **Perform hand hygiene,** and don clean gloves.
   Prevents transmission of bacteria.

2. **Assist the patient to a supine** position. Uncover only the patient's lower abdomen and suprapubic area.

3. **Clean the scanner head** with antiseptic wipes.
   Prevents transmission of microorganisms between patients.

4. **Turn the device on.**

5. **Select the patient's gender.** If a woman has had a hysterectomy, follow manufacturer's directions for gender selection. In some cases, you will select the MALE icon for a woman who has undergone hysterectomy.
   The device is calibrated to adjust for uterus and bladder anatomy.

6. **Palpate the symphysis pubis,** and then apply an ample quantity of warmed ultrasound gel midline on the abdomen, approximately 2.5 to 4 cm (1 to 1.5 in.) above the symphysis pubis.
   The gel ensures proper transmission of the ultrasound. Warm gel is more comfortable for the patient.

7. **Position the scanner head** in the gel, and aim it toward the bladder, pointing slightly downward toward the patient's coccyx.
   Proper placement allows for an accurate reading.

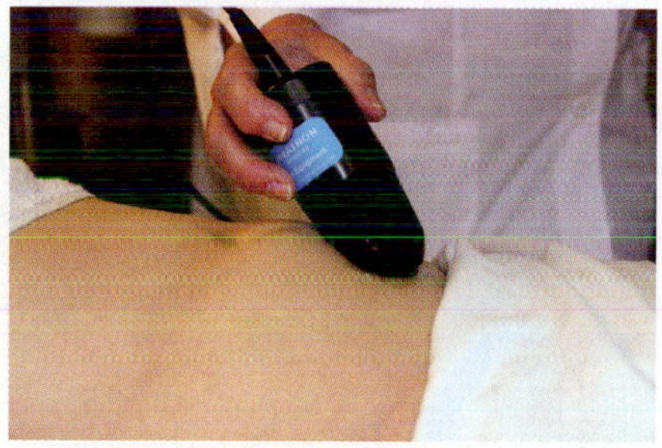

8. **Press and release the SCAN** button. Hold the scanner head steady until the scan is finished.
   An audible tone indicates the scan is complete.

9. **Read the bladder volume measurement.** Repeat the scan several times to ensure accuracy. NOTE: Some scanners will also display an image of the bladder. The bladder image should be centered on the crossbars. If it is not, reposition the scanner head, and repeat the scan.

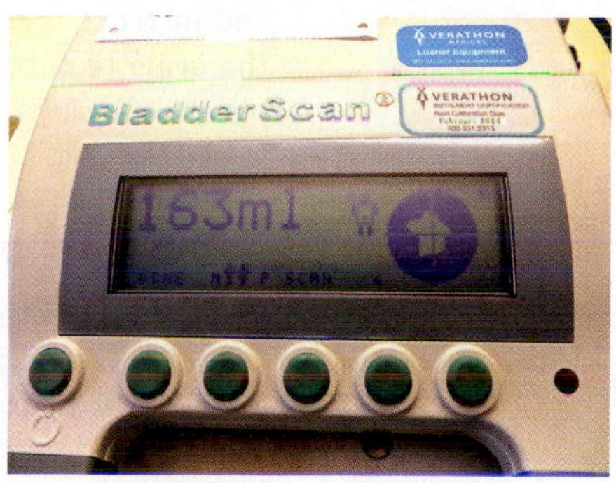

   Taking several readings ensures maximum accuracy.

10. **Press DONE when finished.** Print the results by pressing PRINT.
    A printout provides for accurate documentation and may, in some facilities, be added to the patient record.

11. **Wipe the gel from** the patient's skin with tissue, cover the patient, and return the patient to a comfortable position.

12. **Clean the scanner head** with antiseptic. Remove gloves and perform hand hygiene.

? What if . . .

- **The provider orders hourly monitoring of the patient's urine output?**

  Obtain a special collection bag with a small measuring chamber; document urine output on the I&O record every hour. Be sure that the cylinder does not overflow in the hour. Check the collection bag more frequently if the input is increased or if the patient has diuretic.

Evaluation

- Note any unusual characteristics of the urine (e.g., color, odor, presence of sediment or mucus).
- Note any difficulties with urination (e.g., pain, dribbling, difficulty beginning urination).
- Continue to monitor that urine is flowing freely from the indwelling catheter and that the drainage bag is below the level of the bladder.
- Assess for bladder distention.
  Bladder distention indicates poor bladder emptying.

NOTE: If the facility has a bladder-scanning device, scan to determine whether there is residual urine. A normal post-void residual volume is less than 150 mL.

Patient Teaching

Instruct the patient and/or primary caregiver to document fluid intake and urine output on the I&O record.

Home Care

Teach the client and/or the primary caregiver how to collect and measure urine and how to document fluid intake and urine output on the I&O record.

Documentation

- Record urine volume and record the time and date the specimen was collected, per agency policy (e.g., in the

(continued on next page)

Procedure 28-1 ■ Measuring Urine (continued)

nurse's notes or a patient graphic flow sheet, depending on the agency).

- Document the characteristics of the urine, including color, odor, particulate matter, blood, and clarity.
- Document any difficulty with voiding, including pain or burning with urination, frequency, or difficulty starting the urine flow.
- For PVR, document the time and amount of the last void prior to the scan and the amount of residual urine. Follow agency policy related to attaching a printout of the bladder scan to the patient record.

Sample documentation

12/15/20 1500 Voided 75 mL of clear, yellow urine with no odor, blood, or mucus. Pt states that he still feels full. Bladder palpated just above level of symphysis pubis. Bladder scan performed—350 mL of residual urine in bladder. Dr. Roy contacted and straight catheterization prescribed. ——————————— S. Tran, RN

Practice Resources

Appendix C. Sample Bladder Scan Policy.(2017, December, last reviewed); Boyer, D. R., Steltzer, N., & Larrabee, J. H. (2009); Jones, J., Sibai, J., & Fakih, M. J. (2016, February); Siegel, J. D., Rhinehart, E., Jackson, M., et al. (2007).

Thinking About the Procedures

The videos **Measuring Urine Output From a Bedpan or Urinal, Measuring Urine From an Indwelling Catheter,** and **Measuring Postvoid Residual Urine Volume With a Portable Bladder Scanner,** along with questions and suggested responses, are available on the ***Davis's Nursing Skills Videos*** Web site on FADavis.com.

Procedure 28-2 ■ Obtaining a Urine Specimen for Testing

➤ For steps to follow in all procedures, refer to the Universal Steps for All Procedures found on the inside back cover.

Equipment

Collecting a Clean-Catch Urine Specimen

- Prepackaged collection kit
- If no kit is available:
  - Sterile specimen container
  - Antiseptic solution
  - Sterile cotton balls or 2 × 2 inch gauze pads
- Washcloth and towel, or perineal wipes
- Perineal wash solution
- Two pairs of clean procedure gloves
- Patient identification labels
- Bedpan or bedside commode for an immobile patient

Obtaining a Sterile Urine Specimen From a Catheter

- Clean gloves
- Antiseptic swab or wipe
- Sterile specimen container with a lid
- Patient identification label
- Sterile 5- to 10-mL syringe with a sterile 21- to 25-gauge needleless access device

Collecting a 24-Hour Urine Specimen

NOTE: Some tests require using a double-storage container. Be sure to find out if you need a double-storage container and preservative, and if there are special instructions for collection of the sample.

- Basin and ice, possibly. Check with the laboratory to determine whether the specimen needs to be kept on ice during the 24-hour collection.
- Large collection container

Delegation

You may delegate this procedure to the UAP, but you must be sure that she knows how to perform the procedure correctly, including proper cleansing and maintaining sterility of the container. You must complete the following assessments and instruct the UAP to report any abnormalities seen in the urine (e.g., blood, foul odor, mucus) or any patient complaints of dysuria. The UAP should bring the specimen to you for inspection.

Pre-Procedure Assessments

- **Cognitive status**: Determine whether the patient can follow directions and complete this procedure on her own.
- **Mobility status**: Assess the patient's ability to ambulate to the bathroom or bedside commode.
  To determine where the specimen will be collected.
- **Urinary status**: Assess the patient's ability to control urinary flow.
  To plan how to best collect a urine specimen.

Procedure 28-2A ■ Collecting a Clean-Catch Urine Specimen

➤ When performing the procedure, always identify your patient according to agency policy, using two identifiers, and be attentive to standard precautions, hand hygiene, patient safety and privacy, body mechanics, and documentation.

Procedure Steps

1. **Don procedure gloves.** Wash the perineal area with periwash solution. Remove soiled gloves, perform hand hygiene, and apply new gloves.
2. **Cleanse, or instruct the patient to cleanse,** around the urinary meatus. Allow the area to dry.
Cleansing prevents contamination of the specimen with surface bacteria.
3. **Remove soiled gloves**, perform hand hygiene, and don clean procedure gloves.
4. **Open the prepackaged kit** (if available), and remove the contents.
   - Open the sterile specimen cup, being careful not to touch the inside of the lid or container, and place within easy reach.
   - Make sure to place the lid with the inside surface facing upward.
5. **Cleanse the perineum and urethra.**

For Women:

a. Open the antiseptic towelette provided in the prepackaged kit. If there is no towelette, pour the antiseptic solution over the cotton balls.

b. To cleanse the perineum, spread the labia, and wipe down one side of the meatus using one pad and discard it. Then wipe the other side with a second pad. Wipe down the center over the urinary meatus with the third pad and discard. Clean the perineal area at least twice; use each towelette or cotton ball only once.
Following the "clean to dirty" principle decreases the likelihood of contamination of the specimen and the urethra with feces. ▼

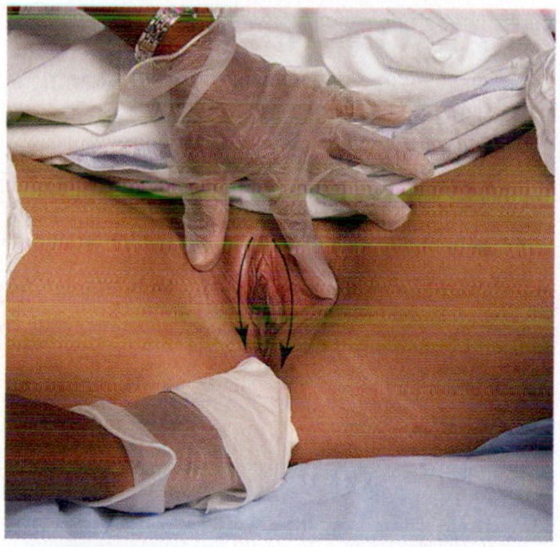

For Men:

c. If the penis is uncircumcised, retract the foreskin back from the end of the penis.
Allows for better access when cleansing the area around the meatus.

d. Use the towelette provided in the prepackaged kit, or pour antiseptic solution over cotton balls. You might also use 2 × 2 in. gauze pad soaked with povidone–iodine to cleanse the periurethral area.

> Before using an iodine-based solution, be sure to check the patient's health history for allergy to iodine.

e. With one hand, grasp the penis gently. With the other hand, cleanse the meatus in a circular motion from the meatus outward away from the urethral opening. Cleanse down the shaft of the penis. Repeat this cleansing two more times, using each towelette or cotton ball only once.
Cleansing the site in this manner helps prevent contaminating the specimen with bacteria.

f. Keep one hand in place to retract the foreskin (if uncircumcised); or to hold the penis (for a patient who is unable to assist).

6. **Pick up the sterile specimen container,** and hold it near the meatus. Instruct the patient to begin voiding.

For Men:

a. Keep the foreskin retracted during voiding, if uncircumcised. If the patient is unable to assist, it will be necessary to hold the penis.

For Women:

b. Separate and hold the labia apart; or have the patient do so.
To help keep bacteria from the labia from contaminating the urine specimen.

7. **Allow a small stream of urine to pass**; then, without stopping the urine stream, place the specimen container into the stream, collecting approximately 30 to 60 mL. Check with the agency lab to determine how much urine to collect.
Midstream urine collection prevents specimen contamination.
8. **Remove the container from the stream,** and allow the patient to finish emptying the bladder.

NOTE: For men, if the penis is uncircumcised, replace the foreskin over the glans when the procedure is finished.

9. **Carefully replace the container lid**, touching only the outside of the cap and container. Avoid touching the rim of the cup to the genital area. Do not get toilet paper, feces, pubic hair, menstrual blood, or anything else in the urine sample.
Maintains sterility of specimen and prevents cross-contamination.

(continued on next page)

Procedure 28-2 ■ Obtaining a Urine Specimen for Testing (continued)

10. **Remove your gloves, and perform hand hygiene.** If the specimen has been obtained from a patient on a bedpan, leave your gloves on until you have removed, emptied, and stored the bedpan properly.
Hand hygiene and gloving prevent transmission of bacteria.

11. **Label the container** with the correct patient information (in many institutions, labels are preprinted or barcoded). Place the container in a facility-specific carrier (usually a plastic bag) for transport to the lab.

12. **Assist the patient back to bed,** or remove the bedpan or urinal, if applicable. (See Procedure 29-2 for instructions on removing a bedpan.) Raise the siderails, and place the call bell in a convenient location.

13. **Transport the specimen** to the lab in a timely manner.
Delayed testing can cause inaccurate results (e.g., casts in the urine will break up if urine is allowed to sit for an extended period).

Procedure 28-2B ■ Obtaining a Sterile Urine Specimen From a Catheter

➤ When performing the procedure, always identify your patient according to agency policy, using two identifiers, and be attentive to standard precautions, hand hygiene, patient safety and privacy, body mechanics, and documentation.

Procedure Steps

1. **Don procedure gloves,** and empty the drainage tube of urine.

2. **Clamp the drainage tube** below the level of the specimen port for 15 to 30 minutes to allow a fresh sample to collect. If the client's urine is flowing briskly, you may not need to clamp the catheter.

3. **Remove your contaminated gloves, and perform hand hygiene. Then don** a sterile pair before scrubbing the specimen port with an antiseptic swab or wipe.
Aseptic technique is used to obtain a catheter sample of urine (Loveday, Pratt, Wilson, et al., 2014).

4. **Insert the needleless access device** with a 10-mL syringe into the specimen port, and aspirate to withdraw the amount of urine you need.

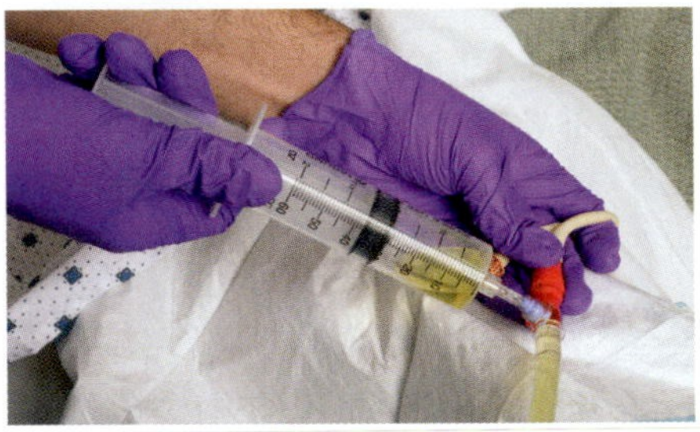

5. **Once you have the sample,** transfer the specimen into a sterile specimen container.

6. **Discard the needleless access device** and syringe in a safe container.

7. **Tightly cap** the specimen container.

8. **Remove the clamp** from the catheter. Remove gloves and perform hand hygiene.

Be sure to unclamp the tubing of the urinary collection bag after you obtain the sample.

Urine backflow can cause bladder distention and lead to stasis-induced urinary tract infection (UTI).

9. **Label and package the specimen** with the correct patient identification, according to agency policy.
To avoid a "wrong patient" error.

10. **Transport the specimen to the lab.** If immediate transport is not possible, refrigerate the sample, per agency policy.

Never disconnect the catheter from the drainage tube to obtain a sample. Interrupting the system creates a portal of entry for pathogens, thereby increasing the risk of contamination.

Procedure 28-2C ■ Collecting a 24-Hour Urine Specimen

➤ When performing the procedure, always identify your patient according to agency policy, using two identifiers, and be attentive to standard precautions, hand hygiene, patient safety and privacy, body mechanics, and documentation.

Procedure Steps

1. **Use a large collection container** (usually supplied by the lab), and collect all urine voided in the 24-hour period. If you need to use more than one container during the 24-hour period, use one container at a time. When it is full, collect the urine in the next container. Label it with the patient's name, date and time of first voiding (labels may be preprinted or bar coded).

2. **To begin collection,** have the patient void, and record the time.
NOTE: Discard this first voiding.
This urine was produced before the start of the collection period and should not be part of the specimen collection.

3. **Collect all urine voided** during the next 24 hours. (e.g., if the first voiding was at 9:00 a.m. on Monday, collect all urine voided until 9:00 a.m.

on Tuesday). Just before the collection period ends, ask the patient to void again, and add this last specimen to the collection container. Store the collection container in a designated refrigerator or surrounded by ice.
If the lab does not receive the entire collection, the results will be inaccurate.

4. **Inform the patient and all staff** about the collection.
Communication can help prevent accidental discarding of urine.

5. **Post signs in prominent** locations, such as the patient's bathroom or entry door, to remind staff of the ongoing collection.
Key Point: ***It is essential that none of the urine voided during the 24-hour period is accidentally discarded.***

6. **Check to be sure the container is properly labeled** with the correct patient information (name, date, and time the test ended). Place the container in a facility-specific carrier (usually a plastic bag), and transport it to the lab in a timely manner, following agency protocol.

? What if . . .

- **A urine culture is ordered on the specimen?**

Be sure to list current antibiotic therapy on the laboratory request form.
This information is important to accurately determine sensitivity of the microorganisms.

- **A clean-catch urine sample is needed for an immobile patient?**

For the patient using a bedpan, raise the head of the bed to a semi-Fowler's position.
Facilitates correct direction of urine flow down into the specimen container you are holding. In addition, this is the anatomical position for voiding.

- **You need to collect a urine sample from an infant?**

1. Remove the paper covering adhesive patches on the back side of the specimen bag before applying it to the clean and dry perineal area. Start at the narrow area between the anus and the vaginal or scrotal area. Press the adhesive sides firmly against the skin while avoiding wrinkles in the skin against the patch.
2. It is easier to apply the lower portion of the bag first. The area must also be dry for the adhesive to stick to the skin. Because infants urinate frequently, it is best to work quickly to catch the specimen. Work upward to secure the bag around the entire genital area.
3. After the specimen bag is has been applied, put a diaper on the infant/child. Remember to check the collection bag every 15 to 30 minutes to see if there is a specimen. If the infant has not urinated in 2 to 3 hours, discard the bag, recleanse the area, and apply a new bag.
It is possible there was a leak in the seal between the skin and the adhesive sides of the specimen collection bag.
4. Once a specimen is obtained in the bag, remove it gently, and pour the urine into a sterile specimen cup. Label it with the patient-identifying information.

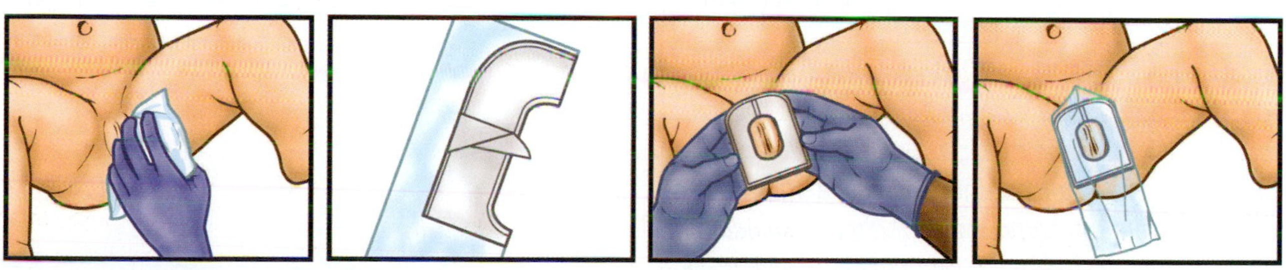

Evaluation

- Note any unusual characteristics of the urine (e.g., color, odor, clarity, crystals, blood, mucus).
- Note any difficulties with urination (e.g., pain, burning, dribbling, difficulty beginning).

Patient Teaching

- ***For a clean catch specimen***, teach the patient how to collect the specimen, focusing on how to maintain sterility of the specimen.
- ***For the 24-hour urine specimen***, emphasize the need to collect all urine during the 24-hour period. If the procedure is to be completed at home, tell the patient to refrigerate the urine specimen for up to 24 hours until it can be transported to the lab. Instruct the patient to place the specimen in a plastic bag, separate it from food items, and label it appropriately.
- ***For clean-catch and 24-hour urine specimens***, instruct a menstruating woman that perineal cleansing is especially important. The woman may use a tampon to prevent leakage during specimen collection. Instruct her to notify the lab that she is menstruating.
- Explain that prepackaged antiseptic wipes cannot be flushed down the toilet.

(continued on next page)

Procedure 28-2 ■ Obtaining a Urine Specimen for Testing (continued)

Documentation

- Urine volume in the patient record, per agency protocol, and the time and date that the specimen was collected. Some facilities use a Kardex or flow sheet; others require documentation in nursing notes or electronic health records.
- Characteristics of the urine—color, odor, particulate matter, blood, clarity, or other qualities.
- Any difficulty with voiding, including pain or burning with urination, frequency, or difficulty starting the urine flow.

Sample documentation

mm/dd/yyyy 0800 Order noted for clean-catch urine specimen. Explained to client the procedure for cleaning and obtaining urine specimen. Client stated "I must clean my bottom from front to back using the toilet in here. Then begin to void and stop voiding. Then void directly into this container." Assisted client to bedside commode. 100 mL of clear yellow urine without foul odor, blood, or particles collected. Pt. denies difficulty voiding, pain, and burning. Urine container labeled per protocol and sent to laboratory. ——— L. Schaaf, RN

mm/dd/yyyy 1000 Order noted for sterile urine specimen. Foley catheter clamped for 15 minutes. Port on Foley cleansed with antiseptic agent. 30 mL of pink tinged-urine without foul odor or sediment removed. Specimen labeled per protocol and sent to laboratory. ——— L. Schaaf, RN

mm/dd/yyyy 1200 Order noted for 24-hour urine collection. Explained procedure to client. Client stated, "I will call you when I void. This first void will be flushed and the test will begin. During the test, I will void in the white hat that is in the commode. Then every time that I void, I will call you to empty the urine into the big container. The big container for the urine must be kept cold with ice." ——— L. Schaaf, RN

Practice Resources

Dolan, V. J., & Cornish, N. E. (2013); Loveday, H. P., Pratt, R. J., Wilson, R.A. et al. (2014); Van Leeuwen, A. M., & Bladh, M. L. (2019).

Thinking About the Procedure

The video **Obtaining a Sterile Urine Specimen From a Catheter,** along with questions and suggested responses, is available on the ***Davis's Nursing Skills Videos*** Web site on FADavis.com.

Procedure 28-3 ■ Testing Urine at the Bedside

➤ For steps to follow in all procedures, refer to the Universal Steps for All Procedures found on the inside back cover.

Equipment

Dipstick Testing

- Procedure gloves
- Dipstick testing kit

Refractometer Testing

- Refractometer
- Procedure gloves
- Distilled water
- Dropper
- Small urine sample

Delegation

You may delegate bedside urine testing to the UAP if you know that he has the knowledge and skill to perform the procedure. Ask the UAP to report the test results to you and to save the urine sample in case you need to repeat the test.

Pre-Procedure Assessments

- Mobility status—determine where the specimen will be collected (e.g., toilet, bedside commode, bedpan).
- Urinary status—determine whether or not the patient has an indwelling catheter.

Procedure 28-3A ■ Dipstick Testing of Urine

➤ When performing the procedure, always identify your patient according to agency policy, using two identifiers, and be attentive to standard precautions, hand hygiene, patient safety and privacy, body mechanics, and documentation.

Procedure Steps

1. **Read the instructions,** and check the expiration date on the diagnostic kit.
2. **Perform hand hygiene,** and don procedure gloves.
3. **Have the patient void** into the collection container or obtain urine from the indwelling urinary catheter. See Procedures 28-1A and 28-1B for measuring urine.
4. **Obtain a test strip from the kit,** dip it into the urine, and begin timing. Follow the manufacturer's directions regarding the time needed for the reagent to develop.
5. **Compare the results to the color** chart at the specified time. Be sure there is good lighting to accurately evaluate the results.
6. **Document the test results.**

Procedure 28-3B ■ Measuring Specific Gravity of Urine

➤ When performing the procedure, always identify your patient according to agency policy, using two identifiers, and be attentive to standard precautions, hand hygiene, patient safety and privacy, body mechanics, and documentation.

Procedure Steps

1. **Clean the equipment lens** with distilled water, and dry with a soft, nonabrasive cloth.
   To ensure accurate results.
2. **Calibrate the refractometer** before use, following the manufacturer's instructions. When calibrated, the refractometer should read 1.000.
3. **Perform hand hygiene,** and don clean procedure gloves.
4. **Use fresh urine**; if you cannot perform the test within 1 hour, refrigerate the specimen.
5. **Wearing procedure gloves,** use the dropper to place one or two drops of urine on the prism surface (at the notched bottom of the cover).
6. **Hold the refractometer** horizontally, and turn toward the light. Rotate the eyepiece until the scale is in focus.
7. **Read the scale** at the point where the dividing line between bright and dark fields crosses the scale. The scale reads from 1.000 to 1.035 in increments of 0.001.
8. **Record the results.**
9. **When you are finished,** add a drop of distilled water to cleanse the prism. Dry the equipment with a soft, nonabrasive cloth.

? What if . . .

- **The diagnostic kit for dipstick testing is outdated?**

  Contact the pharmacy, and/or work with the patient's caregiver to obtain a kit that is not expired.

Evaluation

- Characteristics of urine output (e.g., volume of output, color, clots, mucus).
- Abnormally concentrated or dilute urine

Patient Teaching

- Explain the test procedure to the patient and the patient's caregiver and family members, as indicated.

Home Care

- Teach the client or the caregiver the steps of the procedure.
- Tell the client or the caregiver that the urine specimen must be tested within an hour or refrigerate the specimen to test later.
- Instruct the client or the caregiver that the specimen should be tested, as ordered by the healthcare provider.
- Teach the client or the caregiver to record the results on the flow sheet, per agency protocol.

Documentation

- Document urine volume and the time and date that the specimen was collected, per agency protocol (e.g., on a Kardex card, a checklist, or the nursing notes).
- Document the urine specific gravity and pH, and note the presence of hemoglobin, glucose, ketones, protein, white blood cells (WBCs), bilirubin, casts, crystal, and nitrites.
- Chart other characteristics of the urine—color, odor, clarity, particulate matter, gross blood, mucus shreds, or other qualities.
- Record any difficulty with voiding, including pain or burning with urination, frequency, or difficulty starting the urine flow.

(continued on next page)

Procedure 28-3 ■ Testing Urine at the Bedside (continued)

Sample documentation

3/4/20 1515 Pt voided in bedside commode. Urine is straw-colored with sediment. No unusual odor, blood, or mucus evident. No hemoglobin, glucose, ketones, protein, WBCs, bilirubin, casts, or crystal nitrates noted on urine dipstick. Specific gravity 1.015, pH 6.6, and 3+ protein noted. ——————————— M. Clary, RN

Practice Resources

Ban, K. M., & Easter, J. S. (2017); Chernecky, C. C., & Berger, B. J. (2013).

Procedure 28-4 ■ Inserting an Intermittent Urinary Catheter (Straight Catheter)

➤ For steps to follow in all procedures, refer to the Universal Steps for All Procedures found on the inside back cover.

Equipment

- Washcloth and towel
- Periwash solution
- Procedure gloves, at least two pairs
- Catheter insertion kit containing:
  - Sterile gloves
  - Urinary catheter
  - Antiseptic cleansing agent, forceps, and cotton balls or a packet of sterile antiseptic swabs or wipes
  - Sterile waterproof drapes
  - Sterile lubricant
  - Urine receptacle
  - Specimen container
- Extra pair of sterile gloves and extra sterile catheter
  Obtaining extra supplies prevents the need to leave the bedside to obtain additional supplies should the gloves or catheter become contaminated.
- Bath blanket
- Procedure lamp or flashlight
- Topical anesthetic gel (e.g., 2% lidocaine, [Xylocaine]), according to agency policy and patient need ▼

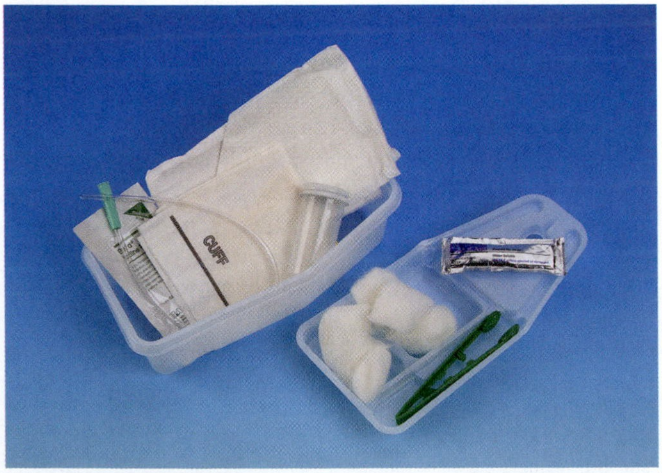

Straight catheter kit

Delegation

In some institutions, UAPs receive special training to learn this skill. In such instances, you may delegate this task to the UAP. However, you must complete the following assessments and instruct the UAP when to stop the procedure and what abnormal findings to report. You must, from time to time, supervise to ensure that the procedure is being performed correctly.

Pre-Procedure Assessments

- Assess the patient's cognitive level.
  To determine whether the patient will be able to follow instructions.
- Assess for the presence of conditions that may impair the patient's ability to assume the necessary position.
  To determine whether you will need assistance to help the patient maintain the correct position.
- Assess the presence and degree of bladder distention.
  To establish a baseline against which to evaluate future data.
- Determine time of last voiding or last catheterization.
  To interpret the significance of the amount of urine obtained in this catheterization.
- Assess the general body size of the patient and size of the urinary meatus.
  To determine whether you need to choose a different-sized catheter.
- ✚ Determine whether the patient is allergic to iodine (if that is the antiseptic solution in the kit). If so, use a different solution or sterile, normal saline.
- Determine whether the patient is allergic to latex.
  Many catheters are made of latex.
- Note any signs and symptoms of bladder infection (e.g., elevated temperature, urinary frequency, dysuria).
- Note any conditions (e.g., enlarged prostate in men) that may make it difficult to pass the catheter.
- Assess the need for additional lighting.
  It is sometimes difficult to visualize a woman's urinary meatus. Supplemental, direct lighting helps.

➤ When performing the procedure, always identify your patient according to agency policy, using two identifiers, and be attentive to standard precautions, hand hygiene, patient safety and privacy, body mechanics, and documentation.

➤ *Note: Before starting the procedure, gather the appropriate supplies and prepare the patient. Explain to the patient the reason for the catheter insertion, the expected length of time the catheter will be needed, and the sensations she is likely to have.*

Procedure Steps

NOTE: The following steps are described for a female patient. If your patient is a male, refer to the procedure variation for Intermittent Urinary Catheterization (Straight Catheter) for a Male Patient, immediately following the Procedure Steps for females.

1. **If you are right-handed,** stand and work at the patient's right side; if you are left-handed, stand and work on the patient's left side.

2. **Place the patient supine** (dorsal recumbent), to allow you to see the urinary meatus:
   a. Flex the patient's knees; and place her feet flat on the bed.
   b. Instruct the patient to relax her thighs and allow them to rotate externally. Obtain help if the patient is confused, unable to cooperate or follow directions, or unable to hold her legs in position.
   The urinary meatus is sometimes difficult to visualize on women because it may resemble skinfolds or other anatomical landmarks in the area.

3. **Don clean procedure gloves.**

iCare 4. **Drape the patient.** Fold the blanket in a diamond shape, wrapping the corners around the patient's legs and folding the upper corner down over the perineum. (To review draping, see Procedure 25-4: Providing Perineal Care.)
Providing privacy promotes comfort.

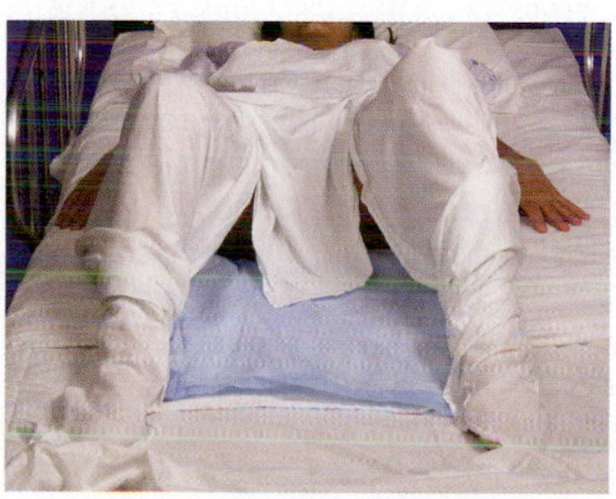

5. **Lift the corner of the privacy drape** to expose the perineum; position the procedure light to allow optimal visualization of the perineum, and then locate the urinary meatus.
Locating the meatus during this step helps prevent delays at subsequent steps when it is important to maintain sterile technique.

6. **Cleanse the perineal area** with periwash solution; let dry.
Cleansing the perineum before inserting the catheter reduces the number of skin bacteria, thereby helping to prevent transmission of microorganisms into the bladder.

7. **Remove and discard gloves.** Perform hand hygiene.
To prevent the transmission of microbes.

8. **Organize your work area.**
   a. Arrange the bedside table or overbed table within your reach.
   b. Open the sterile catheter kit, according to manufacturer's instructions, and place it on the bedside or overbed table.
   c. Position a biohazard bag or other trash receptacle so that you will not have to reach across the sterile field (between the patient's legs) to dispose of soiled cotton (e.g., a trashcan on the floor beside the bed; a trash bag on the bed near, but not between, the patient's feet; or the outer wrapping of the catheter kit).
   Carrying contaminated objects above a sterile field can contaminate the field.
   d. Position a procedure light in a location that will illuminate the perineum.

9. **Place the sterile underpad and drape.**

   NOTE: This step assumes the waterproof drape is packed as the top item in the kit. If your kit is different, see the What if … section.

   The drapes provide sterile work surfaces and help prevent contamination of your gloves and sterile supplies.
   a. Remove the underpad from the kit carefully, allowing it to fall open as you remove it. Do not touch other kit items. Place it flat on the bed, shiny side down, and tuck the top edge under the buttocks, taking care to touch only the corners of the drape.
   b. Remove the sterile glove package, and don sterile gloves (see Procedure 23-7: Sterile Gloves [Open Method]). *NOTE: Once you are wearing the sterile gloves, you may touch items inside the catheter kit, arranging the supplies as needed.*
   c. Place the fenestrated drape. This has a hole in the center. Pick up the drape, allowing it to unfold as you remove it, without touching any other objects from the kit. Place the drape over the perineum with the hole over the labia. See the photos below and in Step 11.

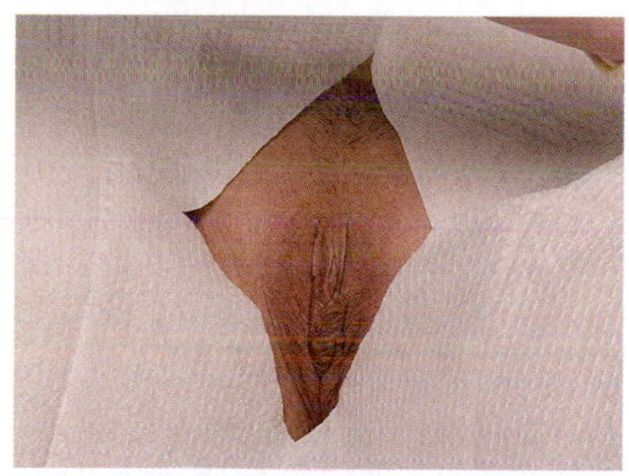

10. **Organize kit supplies on the sterile field**, and prepare the supplies in the kit.
    a. Open the antiseptic package, and pour solution over the cotton balls; or use sterile, normal saline to moisten cotton balls.

    NOTE: Some kits contain a packet of sterile antiseptic swabs or wipes. Open the end of the packet where you feel the "sticks," leaving the swabs covered by the packet.

(continued on next page)

Procedure 28-4 ■ Inserting an Intermittent Urinary Catheter (Straight Catheter) (continued)

NOTE: Newest guidelines indicate there is no advantage in using antiseptic solutions for cleansing the urethral meatus prior to catheter insertion. Nevertheless, follow agency policy.

b. Place the forceps near the cotton balls. Omit this step if using swabs.
c. Open the specimen container if you need to collect a specimen.
d. Remove any unneeded supplies, such as the urine specimen container, from the urine collection basin.
e. Remove the plastic wrapper from the catheter, if it is covered.
f. Open the packet or uncap the syringe filled with sterile lubricant.
g. Squeeze sterile lubricant into the kit tray; roll the catheter slowly in the lubricant to generously lubricate the first 2.5 to 5 cm (1 to 2 in.). Leave the catheter tip in the lubricant or on the sterile field until ready to use.
Lubrication allows for ease of insertion of the catheter. Prevents trauma to the mucosa.
h. Touching only the box or sterile side of the wrapping, place the sterile catheter kit down onto the sterile field between the woman's legs or at bedside.
This approach allows you to reach supplies during catheter insertion. It also extends the sterile field created by the sterile underpad.

11. Cleanse the urinary meatus.

a. Place your nondominant hand above the labia majora, and with your thumb and forefinger, spread the patient's labia, pulling up (or anteriorly) at the same time, to expose the urinary meatus. Hold this position throughout the procedure—firm pressure is necessary. If the labia slip back over the urinary meatus, it is considered contaminated, and you will need to change gloves and repeat the cleansing procedure.
When a woman is supine, gravity may cause tissues above the meatus to fall downward and obscure the meatus from sight. Once placed on the patient's perineal area, your hand is considered contaminated.
b. With your dominant hand, pick up a moistened cotton ball with the forceps (or swab), and cleanse the perineal area, taking care not to contaminate your sterile glove.
   - Use one stroke and a new cotton ball or swab for each area.
   - Wipe from front to back (clitoris to anus).
   - ***If there are five cotton balls or swabs:*** Wipe in this order: far labium majora, near labium majora, inside far labium, inside near labium, and directly down the center over the urinary meatus.
   - ***If there are only three cotton balls or swabs:*** Cleanse only the inside far labium minora, inside near labium minora, and down the center of the urethral meatus.
   - Discard the used cotton balls or swabs as you use them. Be careful not to move them across the open and sterile kit.

Because the urethra is close to the anus in female patients, thorough cleansing of the perineum is very important to reduce contamination of the catheter and prevent bacteria from being introduced into the urethra. Following the "clean to dirty" principle prevents recontamination of the cleansed area.

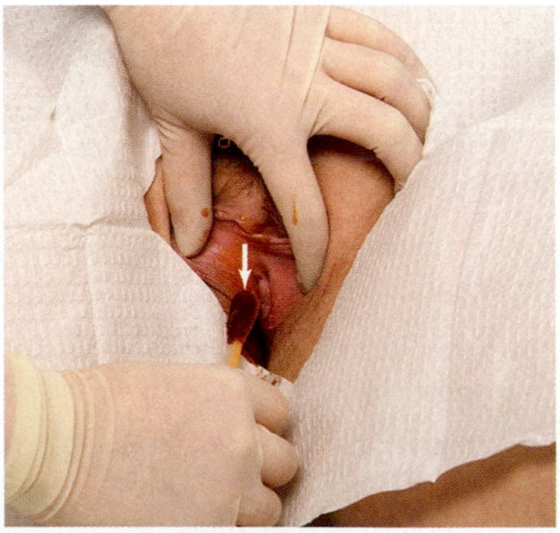

12. Prepare the urine receptacle. Place it 10 cm (4 in.) from the meatus (for women).
The end of the catheter will need to reach into the container to catch the draining urine.

13. Insert the catheter.

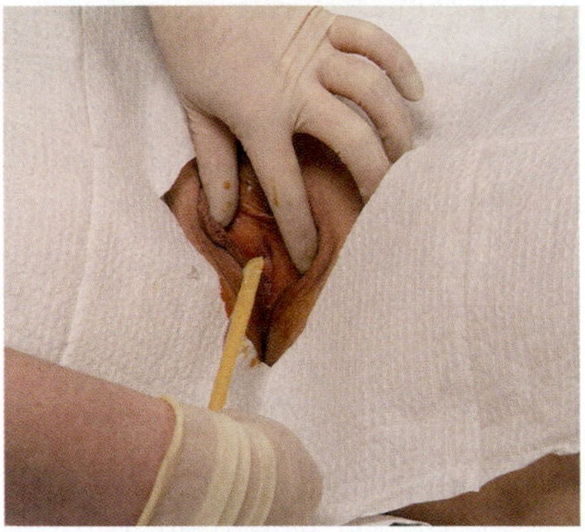

a. Grasp the catheter with your dominant hand, no more than 5 to 7.5 cm (2 to 3 in.) from the tip. Keep the rest of the catheter coiled in the palm of your hand. Slowly insert the end of the catheter into the meatus. Ask the patient to take slow, deep breaths until the initial discomfort has passed.
Bearing down helps relax the external sphincter and makes insertion easier and more comfortable. Holding the catheter close to the distal end will help to keep the tip stable and prevent it from being inserted into the vaginal opening. Deep breathing by the patient helps relax the sphincters. Coiling the catheter in your hand keeps you from contaminating the catheter.
b. Ask the woman to bear down as though she is trying to void.
c. Continue inserting the catheter gently until urine flows, for a distance of 5 to 7.5 cm (2 to 3 in.). After you see urine, insert the catheter another 2.5 to 5 cm (1 to 2 in.).

d. If you feel slight resistance as the catheter goes through the sphincters, twist the catheter slightly, or apply gentle pressure, but do not force the catheter while inserting it. You might need to remove it and cautiously attempt the insertion action again using a new catheter.
Forcing may damage mucosa. Insert the catheter more deeply after urine flow to be sure the catheter is well into the bladder so that the bladder can empty completely. The catheter might not advance while being inserted when it is misplaced in the vagina or if there is a stricture within the urethra or sphincter spasm.

e. If the catheter touches the labia or unsterile linens or if you inadvertently place it in the vagina, it is contaminated; and you must insert a new, sterile catheter. Leave the contaminated catheter in the vagina while you are inserting the new one into the meatus.
Leaving the catheter in the incorrect location serves as a visual landmark and helps avoid making the same mistake again.

14. Manage the catheter and/or urine collection device.

a. Continue to hold the catheter securely with your nondominant hand while the urine drains from the bladder.
Holding the catheter like this prevents the catheter from being expelled by the bladder or urethral contractions.

b. If you are to collect a urine specimen, use your dominant hand to take the specimen container, and put it into the flow of urine until you obtain the correct amount of urine. Cap the container, maintaining sterile technique. See Procedure 28-2B.

c. When the flow of urine stops and the bladder has been emptied, pinch the catheter, and slowly withdraw it from the meatus. Discard the catheter in an appropriate receptacle.
Withdrawing slowly promotes adequate urinary drainage, preventing urinary stasis. Pinching prevents urine from dribbling out of the end of the catheter.

d. Remove the urine-filled receptacle; set it aside outside the patient care area to be emptied when the procedure is finished.
Keeps the urine from spilling on the bed.

15. Cleanse the patient's perineal area, as needed; dry.
This removes residual antiseptic solution from the area, an especially important step if you used povidone–iodine (Betadine). Betadine left on intact healthy skin can cause irritation.

16. Remove and discard disposable supplies (e.g., drapes).

17. Remove your gloves, and perform hand hygiene.
Prevents transmission of bacteria.

18. Return the patient to a comfortable position, with the call device within reach.

Intermittent Urinary Catheterization (Straight Catheter) for a Male Patient

Procedure Steps	Nursing Action
1. Position the patient.	Position the patient supine, legs straight and slightly apart.
2. Drape the patient.	Cover the patient's upper body with a blanket; fold bed sheets down to expose the penis.
3. Don procedure gloves, and cleanse the perineum.	After donning procedure gloves, wash the penis and perineal area with perineal wash solution; dry. If you are using a topical anesthetic gel (e.g., Xylocaine), use a syringe (no needle) to insert it into the urethra now. ▪ Remove and discard gloves. ▪ Perform hand hygiene.
4. Organize the work area.	▪ Open the sterile catheter kit and place on overhead table without contaminating the inside of the wrap. ▪ Position a trash receptacle nearby.
5. Place the sterile underpad and sterile drape.	▪ Remove underpad from the kit before donning sterile gloves. ▪ Place the drape shiny side down between or across the patient's thighs.
6. Don sterile gloves.	Remove the sterile glove package, and don sterile gloves (see Procedure 23-7: Sterile Gloves [Open Method]).
	NOTE: Once you are wearing the sterile gloves, you may touch items inside the catheter kit, arranging the supplies as needed.
7. Place the fenestrated drape.	Allow the fenestrated drape to fall open while removing it from the kit and without touching other kit items. Place the drape with the center hole over the penis.
8. Organize kit supplies on the sterile drape.	▪ Open the antiseptic package and pour over cotton balls or use antiseptic swabs or wipes. Sterile, normal saline is also acceptable for cleansing the urethral opening (follow agency guidelines). ▪ Open the sterile specimen container.

(continued on next page)

Procedure 28-4 ■ Inserting an Intermittent Urinary Catheter (Straight Catheter) (continued)

Procedure Steps	Nursing Action
	■ Remove any unneeded supplies. ■ Remove the wrapper from the catheter. ■ Touching only the kit or inside of the wrapping, place the sterile catheter kit down onto the sterile field between the patient's legs.
9. Lubricate the catheter.	■ Do not lubricate the catheter if you have already inserted a lubricant (lidocaine-based product) directly into the urethra. ■ If the lubricant comes in a packet, squeeze it into the kit tray, and roll the catheter slowly in it to generously lubricate 12.5 to 17.5 cm (5 to 7 in.) of the catheter. Leave the catheter tip in sterile lubricant or on the sterile field until ready to use. ■ If your kit contains a prefilled syringe of lubricant, gently insert the tip of the syringe into the urethra, and instill the lubricant.
10. Expose the urinary meatus.	■ With your nondominant hand, grasp the penis, taking care not to contaminate the surrounding drape. This glove is no longer sterile. ■ Hold the penis gently, but firmly, at a 90° angle to the body, exerting gentle traction. ■ If the penis is uncircumcised, retract the foreskin to fully expose the meatus. If the foreskin accidentally falls over meatus and does not remain retracted, or if you release the penis during cleansing, you must change gloves and repeat the cleansing procedure.
11. Cleanse the urinary meatus.	■ Continuing to hold the penis with your nondominant hand, hold the forceps in your dominant hand and pick up a cotton ball. Cleanse the glans in a series of circular motions, starting at the meatus and working partially down the shaft of the penis. ■ Repeat with at least two more cotton balls or swabs. Discard the cotton balls or swabs as they are used. Do not move them across the open sterile kit and field.
12. Prepare the urine receptacle.	■ Maintaining sterile technique, with your dominant hand place the plastic urine receptacle between the patient's thighs, close enough to the urinary meatus for the end of the catheter to rest inside the container as the urine drains. ■ With the dominant hand, hold the catheter 5 to 7.5 cm (2 to 3 in.) from the tip with remainder coiled in the palm of the hand and the distal end of the catheter is in the plastic container.
13. Insert the catheter into the urinary meatus.	■ Ask the patient to bear down as though trying to void; slowly insert the end of the catheter into the meatus. Instruct the patient to take slow, deep breaths until the initial discomfort has passed. If you feel resistance, withdraw the catheter. Do not force against resistance. ■ Continue inserting the catheter to about 17.5 to 22.5 cm (7 to 9 in.) or until urine flows. After you see urine, insert the catheter another 2.5 to 5 cm (1 to 2 in.).
14. Collect a specimen, if needed.	If a urine specimen is to be collected, continue to grasp the penis, and use your dominant hand to place the specimen container into the flow of urine; cap container using sterile technique.
15. Manage the catheter.	■ When the flow of urine stops and the bladder has been emptied, pinch the catheter, and slowly withdraw it from the meatus. ■ Replace the foreskin, if uncircumcised. ■ Discard the catheter in a biohazardous waste receptacle.
16. Finish the procedure.	Remove gloves and perform hand hygiene. Return patient to a comfortable position with the call device within reach.

? *What if . . .*

- **The sterile gloves are packed as the top item in the catheter kit?**
- **A woman is unable to maintain a dorsal recumbent position?**
- **The patient is having a menstrual period?**
- **A man has an erection during the procedure?**

You will find instructions for all of these situations at the end of Procedure 28-5.

Evaluation

- Note any difficulty with catheter insertion.
  This can indicate structural problems, especially in an older male patient with an enlarged prostate gland.
- Note the characteristics of the urine obtained (e.g., amount, color, odor, presence of sediment or mucus).
- Assess and palpate for absence of bladder distention.

  NOTE: Some facilities have a portable bladder-scanning device that will allow you to determine whether residual urine remains.

  Palpating the bladder helps you to determine whether it has been emptied.

Documentation

- Document the reason for the catheter and/or clinical indication for continuing catheterization.
- Document the time and date of the procedure.
- Document the size of catheter used.
- Record the amount of urine obtained on the I&O portion of the graphics sheet. Record the color of urine, odor, presence of mucus, blood, and so on, in the nursing notes.
- Record the patient's subjective statements.
- If you collected a specimen, document it, and note the time it was sent to the lab.
- Some facilities require that you record the amount of saline used to inflate the balloon.

Practice Resources

Foley catheter care and maintenance guide: Patient education guide. (2013); Gould, C.V., Umscheid, C. A., Agarwal, R. K., et al. (2009);); Loveday, H. P., Pratt, R. J., Wilson, R.A. et al. (2014); Newman, D. K., Cumbee, R. P., & Rovner, E. S. (2017); Vahr, S., Cobussen-Boekhorst, H., Eikenboom, J., et al. (2013, March); Wound, Ostomy, and Continence Nurses Society (WOCN). (2016).

Thinking About the Procedure

The video **Intermittent Urinary Catheterization,** along with questions and suggested responses, is available on the ***Davis's Nursing Skills Videos*** Web site on FADavis.com.

Procedure 28-5 ■ Inserting an Indwelling Urinary Catheter

➤ For steps to follow in *all* procedures, refer to the Universal Steps for All Procedures found on the inside back cover.

Equipment

- Washcloth and towel
- Periwash solution
- Procedure gloves, at least two pairs
- Catheter insertion kit containing:
  - Sterile gloves
  - A double-lumen or triple-lumen catheter with a balloon tip for inflation
  - Antiseptic cleansing agent or sterile, normal saline
  - Forceps
  - Cotton balls
  - Sterile waterproof drapes
  - Sterile lubricant
  - Prefilled syringe with sterile water (to inflate the catheter balloon)
  - Urine collection bag with drainage tubing (often the tubing is preconnected to the catheter)
  - Specimen container
- Extra pair of sterile gloves and extra sterile catheter
  Obtaining extra supplies prevents the need to leave the bedside to obtain additional supplies should the gloves or catheter become contaminated.
- Bath blanket
- Procedure lamp or flashlight
- Topical anesthetic gel (e.g., 2% lidocaine [Xylocaine]), according to agency policy and patient need
- Commercial securement device (e.g., Velcro leg strap). If not available, use hypoallergenic tape.
- Safety pin and elastic band (if needed to secure tubing to the bed; you can usually use the clamp that is on the drainage tubing.)

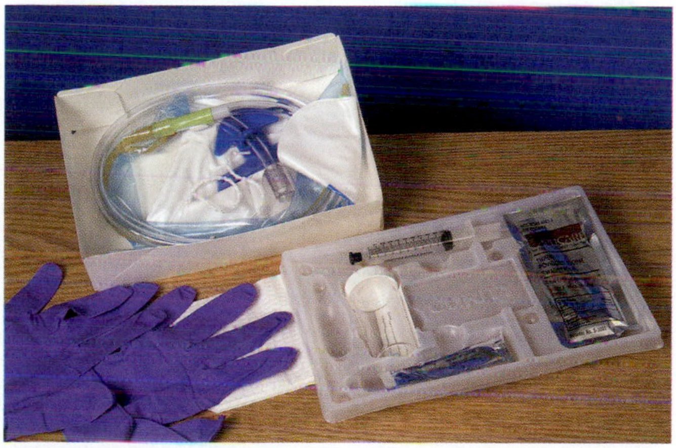

Indwelling catheter kit

Delegation

In some institutions, UAPs undergo special training to learn this skill. In such instances, you may delegate this task to the UAP. However, you must complete the following assessments and instruct the UAP when to stop the procedure and what abnormal findings to report. You must from time to time supervise to ensure that the procedure is being performed correctly.

(continued on next page)

Procedure 28-5 ■ Inserting an Indwelling Urinary Catheter (continued)

Pre-Procedure Assessments

- Assess the patient's cognitive level.
  To determine whether the patient will be able to follow instructions.
- Assess for conditions that may impair the patient's ability to assume the necessary position.
  To determine whether you will need assistance to help the patient maintain the correct position for catheter insertion.
- Assess the presence and degree of bladder distension.
  To establish a baseline against which to evaluate future data.
- Determine time of last voiding or last catheterization.
  To interpret the significance of the amount of urine obtained in this catheterization.
- Assess the general body size of the patient and size of the urinary meatus.
  To determine whether you need to choose a different-sized catheter.
- Determine whether the patient is allergic to iodine (if that is the antiseptic solution in the kit). If so, use a different solution or sterile, normal saline.
- Determine whether the patient is allergic to latex.
  Many catheters are made of latex.
- Note signs and symptoms of bladder infection (e.g., elevated temperature, urinary frequency, dysuria).
- Note any conditions (e.g., enlarged prostate in men) that may make it difficult to pass the catheter.
- Assess the need for extra lighting.
  It is sometimes difficult to visualize a woman's urinary meatus. Supplemental, direct lighting helps.

➤ When performing the procedure, always identify your patient according to agency policy, using two identifiers, and be attentive to standard precautions, hand hygiene, patient safety and privacy, body mechanics, and documentation.

➤ *Note:* **The following steps are described for a male patient.** If your patient is a female, refer to the Procedure Variations for Women, immediately following the procedure steps.

Procedure Steps

1. **Place the patient supine,** with legs straight and slightly apart. If the patient is confused, unable to follow directions, or unable to hold his legs in correct position, obtain help with the procedure.
2. **If you are right-handed,** stand and work at the patient's right side; if you are left-handed, stand and work on the patient's left side.
3. iCare **Drape the patient.** Cover the patient's upper body with a blanket; fold the bedsheets down to expose the penis.
   Covering the patient preserves modesty and enhances a feeling of security, while ensuring that you can visualize the urinary meatus.
4. **Don clean procedure gloves.** Cleanse the penis and perineal area with antiseptic solution; allow to dry.
   Cleansing the area of skin bacteria reduces the risk of transmitting microbes into the bladder.
5. **If you are using topical anesthetic** gel, use a syringe (no needle) to insert it into the urethra.
   This is frequently used for men to provide local anesthesia. You insert it now because it takes 5 minutes for the gel to take effect at the time you are ready to insert the catheter.
6. **Remove and discard gloves.** Perform hand hygiene.
   To prevent the transmission of microbes.
7. **Organize your work area:**
   a. Arrange the bedside table or overbed table within your reach.
   b. Open the sterile catheter kit, according to the manufacturer's instructions, and place it on the bedside or overbed table.
   c. Position a plastic bag or other trash receptacle so that you will not have to reach across the sterile field to dispose of soiled cotton balls and so forth (e.g., a trash can on the floor beside the bed; a trash bag or the kit outer wrapper on the bed near, but not between, the patient's feet).
   Carrying contaminated objects above a sterile field can contaminate the field.
8. **Place the sterile underpad** and drape.

   NOTE: This step assumes the waterproof drape is packed as the top item in the kit. If your kit is different, see the What If … section.

   These drapes provide sterile work surfaces and help prevent contaminating your gloves and sterile supplies.
   a. Remove the underpad from the kit carefully. Drop the underpad shiny side down between or across the patient's thighs, touching only the corners.
   b. Remove the sterile glove package and don sterile gloves (see Procedure 23-7: Sterile Glove [Open Method]).

   NOTE: Once you are wearing the sterile gloves, you may touch any items inside the catheter kit, arranging the supplies as needed.

   c. Place the fenestrated drape. This has a hole in the center. Pick up the drape, allowing it to unfold as you remove it, without touching any other objects. Place it with the center hole over the penis.
9. **Organize the kit supplies** on the sterile field; and prepare the supplies in the kit.
   a. Pour antiseptic solution or sterile, normal saline over the cotton balls.

   NOTE: Some kits contain a packet of sterile antiseptic swabs or wipes. Open the end of the packet where you can feel the "sticks," leaving the swabs covered by the remainder of the packet.

b. Lay the forceps near the cotton balls.

c. Open the specimen container, if you are to collect a specimen.

d. Remove any unneeded supplies, such as the specimen container, from the kit. Remove the plastic wrapper from the catheter, if it is covered.

e. Do not lubricate the catheter if you have already inserted a lubricant (xylocaine gel) directly into the urethra.

Variation: Lubricant in a Syringe

If the sterile lubricant in the kit is packaged in a syringe, you will insert the lubricant into the urethra at Step 11.

Variation: Lubricant in a Packet

If the lubricant comes in a packet, squeeze the lubricant into the kit tray and roll the catheter slowly in the lubricant. Generously lubricate 12.5 to 17.5 cm (5 to 7 in.) of the catheter. Leave the catheter tip in sterile lubricant or on the sterile field until ready to use.

f. Attach the sterile water-filled syringe to the balloon port of the catheter.

g. Touching only the box or sterile side of the wrapping, place the sterile catheter kit down onto the sterile field on top of the man's thighs. You may, alternatively, set up the sterile field between his legs.
Placement of supplies in this manner allows you to reach supplies during catheter insertion.

h. If the bedside bag is preconnected to the catheter itself, leave the bag on or near the sterile field until after the catheter is inserted.

10. Cleanse the urinary meatus.▼

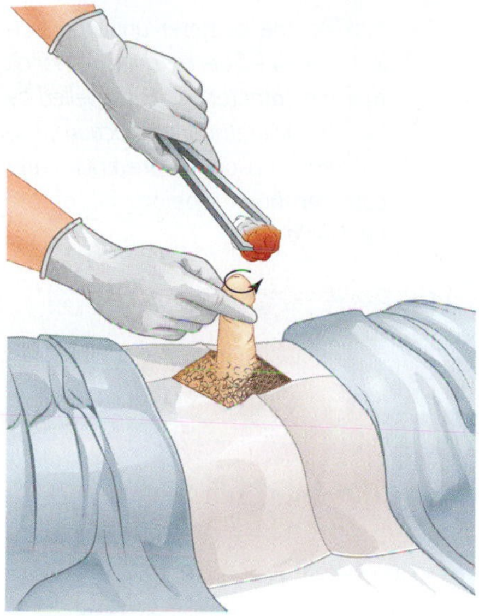

a. With your nondominant hand, reach through the opening in the fenestrated drape and grasp the penis, taking care not to contaminate the surrounding drape. This glove is no longer sterile.

b. Hold the penis gently, but firmly, at a 90° angle to the body, exerting gentle traction.
Supporting the shaft with the fingers straightens the urethra, easing insertion of the catheter.

c. If the penis is uncircumcised, retract the foreskin to fully expose the meatus. If the foreskin accidentally falls over the meatus or if you drop the penis during cleansing, you must change gloves and repeat the cleansing procedure.
Retracting the foreskin allows for full cleansing of the area.

d. Continuing to hold the penis with your nondominant hand, hold the forceps in your dominant hand and pick up a cotton ball. Cleanse the glans in a series of circular motions, starting at the meatus and working partially down the shaft of the penis.

e. Repeat with at least two more cotton balls or swabs. Discard the cotton balls or swabs as you use them. Do not move them across the open sterile kit and field.
Following the "clean to dirty" principle prevents recontamination of the cleansed area.

f. Continue to grasp the penis with your nondominant hand during the next steps. This glove is no longer sterile.

11. Instill lubricant (if not done previously).

Variation: Lubricant Packaged in a Syringe

Before beginning the procedure, you should have made sure that the catheter kit contains a prefilled syringe of lubricant rather than a packet. Gently insert the tip of the prefilled syringe into the urethra, and instill the lubricant (unless you have already inserted Xylocaine gel).

Variation: Lubricant in a Packet

If the kit contains a single packet of lubricant, make sure you have already generously lubricated 12.5 to 17.5 cm (5 to 7 in.) of the catheter. This is not the technique of choice.

12. Insert the catheter.▼

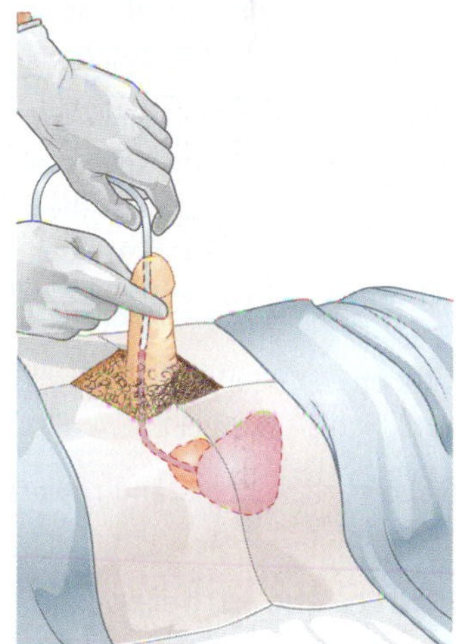

a. With your dominant hand, stabilize the catheter before inserting it by holding the catheter approximately 5 to 7.5 cm (2 to 3 in.) from the tip. Keep the rest of the catheter coiled in the palm of your hand if the catheter is not already preconnected to the drainage tube.
Coiling the catheter in your hand keeps you from contaminating the catheter. When you preconnect the drainage bag before you insert the catheter, you keep the urine from draining onto the bed. Frequently, the catheter and drainage bag are connected by the manufacturer.

(continued on next page)

Procedure 28-5 ■ Inserting an Indwelling Urinary Catheter (continued)

b. With your nondominant hand, continue to hold the penis gently, but firmly, at a 90° angle to the body, exerting gentle traction.
Supporting the shaft with the fingers straightens the urethra, easing insertion of the catheter.

c. Ask the patient to bear down as though trying to void; slowly insert the end of the catheter into the meatus. Ask the patient to take slow deep breaths until the initial discomfort has passed.
These strategies help the patient to relax the external sphincter and make insertion easier and more comfortable.

d. Continue inserting the catheter to about 17.5 to 22.5 cm (7 to 9 in.) or until urine flows. You will feel slight resistance at the level of the internal sphincter. Continue to advance almost to the bifurcation (Y-connector).

You will commonly feel resistance at the prostatic sphincter. Hold the catheter firmly against the sphincter until the resistance eases. Then advance the catheter, but do not force it.
This prevents compromised circulation and painful swelling.

e. Lower the penis, and replace the foreskin.

13. Manage the catheter.

a. Continue to hold the catheter securely with your nondominant hand to stabilize the catheter's position in the urethra. Use your other hand to pick up the water-filled syringe and inflate the catheter balloon.
Holding the catheter until the balloon is inflated decreases the chance that the catheter will be expelled by bladder or urethral contractions. The inflated balloon prevents the catheter from slipping out of the bladder.

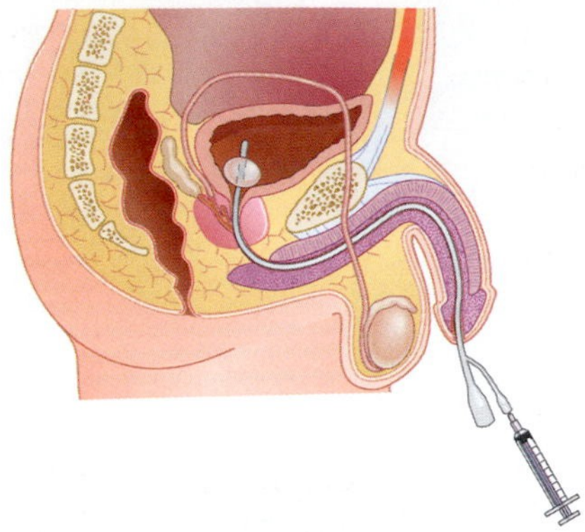

A Catheter placement, male.

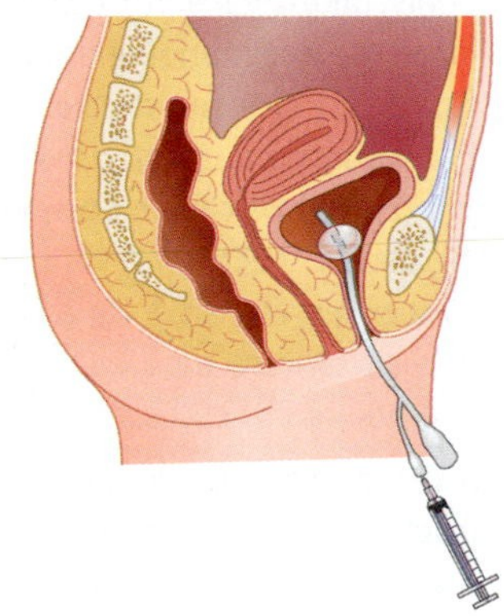

B Catheter placement, female.

b. If the patient complains of pain on inflation of the balloon, withdraw the water from the balloon, and reposition the catheter by advancing it 2.5 cm (1 in.).
Pain usually indicates that the balloon was in the urethra instead of in the bladder.

c. After the balloon is inflated, pull back gently on the catheter until you feel resistance. Lower the penis, and replace the foreskin.
This indicates that the balloon is correctly positioned at the neck of the bladder.

14. Connect the drainage bag to the end of the catheter if it is not already preconnected. Hang the drainage bag on the side of the bed, below the level of the bladder.
Hanging the drainage bag below the bladder promotes adequate urinary drainage by gravity, preventing urinary stasis.

15. Using a commercial catheter securement device (e.g., a catheter tube holder or Velcro leg strap), secure the catheter to the thigh or the abdomen. If you must use tape, use hypoallergenic tape.
Securing the catheter prevents urethral irritation related to tugging or pulling of the catheter. Commercial catheter securement devices are preferable to tape for catheter securement.

16. Cleanse the patient's perineal area, as needed; dry. Cover the patient.
Removes residual antiseptic solution from the area, an especially important step if you used povidone–iodine (Betadine). Betadine left on intact healthy skin can cause irritation.

17. Remove and discard disposable supplies (e.g., drapes).

18. Remove gloves, and discard them into biohazard receptacle. Perform hand hygiene.

19. Return the patient to a comfortable position, with the call device within reach.

Procedure Variation: Indwelling Catheter Insertion for a Female Patient

Procedure Steps	Nursing Action
1. Position the patient.	Flex the patient's knees; and place her feet flat on the bed (dorsal recumbent position). Instruct the patient to relax her thighs and allow them to rotate externally. *NOTE: Obtain help if the patient is confused, unable to follow directions, or unable to hold her legs in the correct position.*
2. Drape the patient.	Fold the blanket in a diamond shape, wrapping the corners around the patient's legs and folding the upper corner down over the perineum. See Procedure 28-4, Step 4.
3. Cleanse the perineal area.	■ Don clean procedure gloves. ■ Lift the corner of the privacy drape to expose the perineum. ■ Position the procedure light to allow optimal visualization of the perineum, and then locate the urinary meatus. ■ Cleanse the perineal area with antiseptic solution or sterile normal saline (per agency policy); dry. ■ Remove and discard gloves. Perform hand hygiene.
4. Organize the work area.	■ Arrange the bedside table or overbed table within your reach. ■ Open the sterile catheter kit, according to the directions; and place it on the table. ■ Position a plastic bag or other trash receptacle so that you will not have to reach across the sterile field to dispose of soiled cotton balls and other items.
5. Apply the sterile underpad and fenestrated drape.	■ Remove the sterile underpad from the kit before donning sterile gloves. Be sure not touch other kit items with bare hands. Touching only the corners, place the drape shiny side down under the patient's buttocks. ■ Carefully remove the sterile glove package from the kit, and don sterile gloves. ■ Pick up the fenestrated drape; allow it to unfold without touching other objects; place over the perineum with the hole over the labia.
6. Organize the kit supplies on the sterile field.	■ Open the antiseptic packet and pour solution over the cotton balls, and position forceps nearby. Or if the kit comes with antiseptic swabs, open the packet so the sticks are convenient to grasp. You may also use sterile, normal saline for cleansing the urethral opening (follow agency policy) ■ Open the specimen container if a specimen is to be collected. Remove any unneeded supplies. ■ Remove the plastic wrapper from the catheter, if it is covered. Squeeze the sterile lubricant into the kit tray. Roll the catheter slowly in the lubricant, being sure to generously lubricate the first 2.5 to 5 cm (1 to 2 in.) of the catheter. Leave the catheter tip in the sterile lubricant or on the sterile field until ready to use. ■ Attach the sterile water-filled syringe to the balloon port of the catheter. Leave the syringe attached to the catheter. ■ Touching only the box or sterile side of the wrapping, place the sterile catheter kit down onto the sterile field. You may, as an alternative, set up the sterile field between her legs.
7. Spread the labia, and cleanse the urinary meatus.	■ Place your nondominant hand above the labia majora and, with thumb and forefinger, spread the patient's labia, pulling up at the same time to expose the urinary meatus. Use firm pressure to hold this position throughout the procedure. If the labia accidentally slip back over the meatus during cleansing, change your gloves, and repeat this step. ■ Wipe from the clitoris to the anus, wiping in the order of: far labium majora, near labium majora, inside far labium, inside near labium, and directly down the center over the urinary meatus. ■ Discard cotton balls or swabs as they are used; do not move them across the open, sterile kit and field. Use only one stroke and a new cotton ball or swab for each area.
8. Insert the catheter.	■ Ask the woman to bear down as though she is trying to void. ■ Grasp the catheter with your dominant hand, no more than 5 to 7.5 cm (2 to 3 in.) from the tip. Slowly insert the end of the catheter into the meatus. ■ Ask the patient to take slow, deep breaths until the initial discomfort has passed.

(continued on next page)

Procedure 28-5 ■ Inserting an Indwelling Urinary Catheter (continued)

Procedure Steps	Nursing Action
9. Manage the catheter.	■ If the catheter touches the labia or unsterile linens, or if you inadvertently place it in the vagina, it is contaminated; and you must insert a new, sterile catheter. Leave the contaminated catheter in the vagina while you are inserting the new one into the meatus; this keeps you from making the same mistake again. ■ Continue inserting the catheter gently until urine flows, for a distance of 5 to 7.5 cm (2 to 3 in.). After you see urine, insert the catheter another 2.5 to 5 cm (1 to 2 in.). ■ After urine flows, stabilize the catheter in the urethra with your nondominant hand; use the dominant hand to pick up the sterile water-filled syringe and inflate the catheter balloon. If the patient complains of pain when inflating the balloon, withdraw the water out of the balloon. Then reposition the catheter by advancing it 2.5 cm (1 in.).
10. Secure the catheter.	■ Hang the drainage bag on the side of the bed below the level of the bladder. ■ Using a commercial catheter securement device, if available, secure the catheter to the thigh.
11. Finish up.	■ Remove and discard disposable supplies in a biohazard receptacle. ■ Remove and discard gloves. Perform hand hygiene. ■ Return the patient to a comfortable position, with the call device within reach.

? What if . . .

- **The sterile gloves are packed as the top item in the catheter kit?**
  - Grasp the corner and remove the sterile glove package, taking care not to touch anything else in the package. Don the sterile gloves. Once you have donned the sterile gloves, you may touch any item inside the catheter kit, arranging the supplies as needed.
  - Place the sterile underpad: Grasp the edges of the sterile drape. Fold the entire edge down 5 to 7.5 cm (2 to 3 in.) and toward you, making a "cuff" to protect your gloves. Be careful not to touch unsterile objects with your gloves or the drape.

    For women: Carefully slide the drape under the patient's buttocks without contaminating your gloves. Ask the patient to raise her hips slightly if she can.

    For men: Drop the sterile underpad across thighs.
  - Continue with the fenestrated drape, as described in the standard procedures.

- **The patient is having a menstrual period?**

  Note on the lab form that the patient is having a menstrual period before sending a specimen for diagnostic testing.

  Blood in the urine from a menstrual period might lead to misinterpretation of the result.

- **A woman is unable to maintain a dorsal recumbent position?**

  Use Sims' position (side-lying with the upper leg flexed at the hip). Cover the rectal area.

  Prevents contamination from the rectal area to the urethra.

- **A man has an erection during the procedure?**

  Treat the situation professionally. Take a break until the erection goes away. Never force the catheter.

  Forcing the catheter can cause urethral trauma.

Evaluation

- Note any difficulty with catheter insertion.

  This can indicate structural problems, especially in an older male patient with an enlarged prostate gland.
- Note the characteristics of the urine obtained (e.g., amount, color, odor, presence of sediment or mucus).
- Assess and palpate for absence of bladder distention.

NOTE: Some facilities have a portable bladder-scanning device that will allow you to determine whether residual urine remains.

Palpating the bladder helps you to determine if it has been emptied. A portable bladder scanner may also be used to help you determine whether residual urine remains.

- For indwelling catheters, continue to monitor that drainage is not obstructed and that the drainage bag is below the level of the bladder.

Home Care

For inserting indwelling catheters in the home, teach clients:

- When to change the catheter
  Changing indwelling catheters at routine, fixed intervals is generally not recommended (Gould, Umscheid, Agarwal, et al., 2009). Clients should be taught to change catheters based on clinical indications, such as impaired urine drainage or encrustation.
- How to prevent catheter blockage (e.g., increase fluid intake)
  Fluids increase the urine volume, helping to reduce the deposit of sediment or other particles in the tubing.
- To empty the drainage bag frequently and to keep the bag below the level of the bladder
- How to prevent UTIs (e.g., maintain a closed system, handwashing prior to handling catheter equipment, prevent blockage of urine outflow, adequate fluid intake, taking a shower rather than a bath.)
- How to prevent discomfort at the urethra
- Use of a leg bag
- To eat foods that help acidify urine: meat, eggs, cheese, prunes, cranberries, and whole grains
- How to obtain additional supplies suitable for individual needs

Documentation

- Document the reason for indwelling urinary catheterization.
- Time and date of the procedure.
- The size of catheter used.
- Amount of urine obtained (on the I&O portion of the graphics sheet).
- Color of urine, odor, presence of mucus, blood, and so on, (in the nursing notes).
- The patient's subjective statements.
- Any specimen collected; note the time it was sent to the lab.
- For an indwelling catheter: In addition, some facilities require that you record the amount of sterile water used to inflate the balloon.
- Include a date for removal or review for continued need.

Sample documentation

3/4/20 1010 Order noted for insertion of indwelling catheter. Explained the procedure to pt and reason for insertion. Pt verbalized understanding of the procedure and need for catheter. Placed pt in a dorsal recumbent position with blankets to keep pt warm and provide privacy. Perineal care completed. 14 Fr. Foley catheter inserted using sterile technique per protocol. Foley draining dark yellow urine with sediment and foul odor. No mucus or blood noted in urine. Bladder is not distended. Client returned to semi-Fowler's position. No needs noted at this time. Reminded pt to call nurse if there is any discomfort associated with urinary catheterization. Call light placed in pt's dominant hand.——— C. Chin, RN

Practice Resources

Clayton, J. L. (2017, April); Gould, C.V., Umscheid, C. A., Agarwal, R. K., et al. (2009); Foley catheter care and maintenance guide: Patient education guide. (2013); Loveday, H. P., Pratt, R. J., Wilson, R.A. et al. (2014); Newman, D. K., Cumbee, R. P., & Rovner, E. S. (2017); Vahr, S., Cobussen-Boekhorst, H., Eikenboom, J., et al. (2013, March); Wound, Ostomy, and Continence Nurses Society (2009).

Thinking About the Procedure

The video **Indwelling Urinary Catheterization,** along with questions and suggested responses, is available on the ***Davis's Nursing Skills Videos*** Web site on FADavis.com.

Procedure 28-6 ■ Applying an External (Condom) Catheter

➤ For steps to follow in all procedures, refer to the Universal Steps for All Procedures found on the inside back cover.

Equipment

- Condom catheter
- Two pairs of clean procedure gloves
- Washcloth and towel
- Disposable basin of soap and purified water or antiseptic wash or sterile, normal saline
- Bath blanket, if available
- Urine collection bag (e.g., bedside drainage bag or leg bag)
- Disposable tape measure
- Skin prep (per agency policy)
- Scissors
- Commercial leg strap

Delegation

You may delegate the application of a condom catheter to the UAP once you have assessed the UAP's skill level and completed the pre-procedure assessments. Instruct the UAP to report any alterations in the skin integrity along the shaft of the penis.

Pre-Procedure Assessments

- Assess the patient's cognitive status.
  Knowing whether the patient can follow directions helps determine how to approach the procedure and also to know if the patient may be prone to pulling on the catheter.
- Assess pattern of voiding (e.g., degree and time of incontinence).
  Helps you to determine when the condom catheter should be applied.
- Assess the skin along the shaft of the penis, the glans, and the meatus (for swelling or excoriation).
  The condom catheter cannot be used on excoriated, irritated skin or over areas of impaired skin integrity.

(continued on next page)

Procedure 28-6 ■ Applying an External (Condom) Catheter (continued)

- Note whether and how much the penis is retracted toward the body.
  There is an increased risk of nonadherence and leakage of urine in a patient with a retracted penis.
- Assess for the presence of neuropathy.
  Patients with neuropathies that affect sensation in the penis may not feel skin irritation from the condom catheter and will need to be assessed more frequently.

➤ When performing the procedure, always identify your patient according to agency policy, using two identifiers, and be attentive to standard precautions, hand hygiene, patient safety and privacy, body mechanics, and documentation.

Procedure Steps

1. **Determine appropriate size** of the external catheter by measuring the circumference of the penis using a disposable paper tape. Obtain a correctly sized catheter.
   A catheter that is too small impairs circulation. A catheter that is too large allows leakage of urine.
2. **Perform hand hygiene,** and don clean procedure gloves.
   Hand hygiene and gloving prevent the transmission of bacteria.
3. **Organize supplies,** and prepare the leg bag or bedside drainage bag for attachment to the condom catheter by removing it from the packaging and placing the end of the connecting tubing near the perineal area.
4. **Position the patient supine.** If the patient has difficulty breathing, raise the head of the bed to 30°.
5. **Fold down the bedcovers** to expose the penis, and drape the patient using the bath blanket.
   Covering the patient reduces patient embarrassment.
6. **Gently cleanse the penis** with soap and filtered water or antiseptic perineal wipes. Rinse and dry it thoroughly. If the patient is uncircumcised, retract the foreskin, cleanse the glans, and replace the foreskin. Excess hair along the shaft of the penis may be carefully clipped off with the scissors.
   Cleansing the penis not only helps to prevent infection but it also helps the condom catheter to adhere better to the shaft.
7. **Perform hand hygiene,** and change procedure gloves.
8. **Apply skin prep** (if used by your agency), and allow it to dry.
   NOTE: Some external condom catheters require the placement of the special adhesive strip onto the penis before the application of the condom. Follow the manufacturer's directions.
9. **Hold the penis** in your nondominant hand. With your dominant hand, place the condom catheter at the end of the penis, and slowly unroll it along the shaft toward the patient's body. Leave 2.5 to 5 cm (1 to 2 in.) between the end of the penis and the drainage tube on the catheter.
   Careful unrolling in this manner helps prevent irritation of the glans caused by rubbing and allows for expansion of the penis if an erection were to occur.

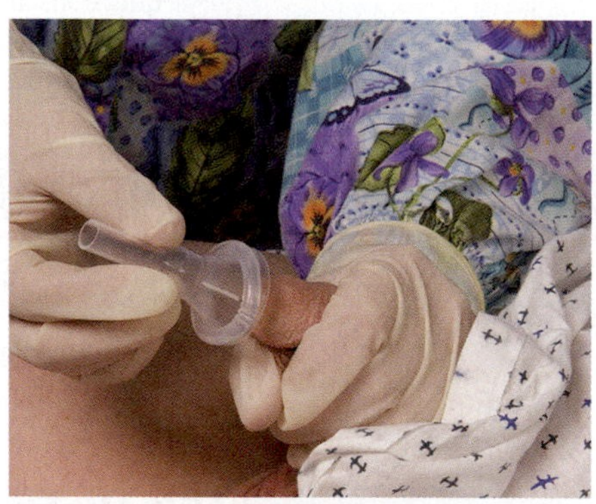

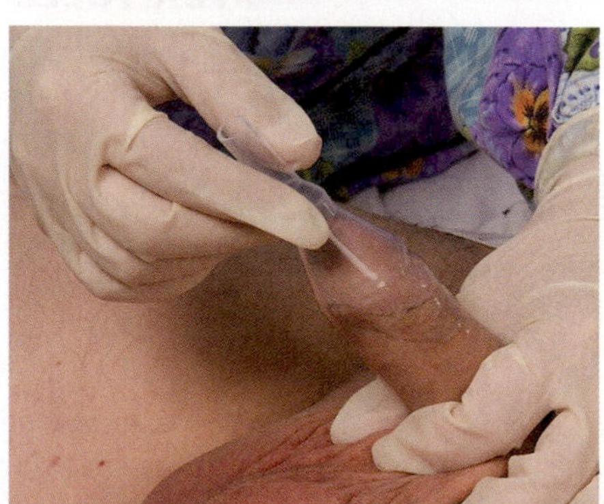

10. **Secure the condom catheter** in place on the penis.
    a. Ensure that the condom is not twisted.
    Twisting can obstruct urine flow.
    b. Do not use regular bandage or surgical dressing tape to hold an external condom catheter in place.
    Regular tape does not expand and could lead to decreased blood flow to the penis.

Variation: Catheter With Internal Adhesive

    c. Gently grasp the penis and compress so that the entire shaft comes in contact with the condom.

Variation: Catheter With External Adhesive Strip

    d. Wrap the strip around the outside of the condom in a spiral direction, taking care not to overlap the ends.
    Prevents constriction of blood flow to the penis.

11. **Assess the proximal end** of the condom catheter. If a large portion of the condom is still rolled above the adhesive strip, you may need to clip the roll.
    Clipping the roll prevents constriction of blood flow.
12. **Attach the tube end** of the condom catheter to a drainage system (e.g., a leg bag). Make sure there are no kinks in the tubing.
    Kinks impede the flow of urine. Urine that does not drain away from the meatus can cause irritation and skin breakdown and possibly cause the condom catheter to fall off.

13. Secure the catheter tubing to the patient's thigh using a commercial leg strap. (Hypoallergenic tape may be used if a commercial leg strap is unavailable. Follow agency protocol.)

A leg strap controls movement of the tubing and accidental pulling on the condom catheter.

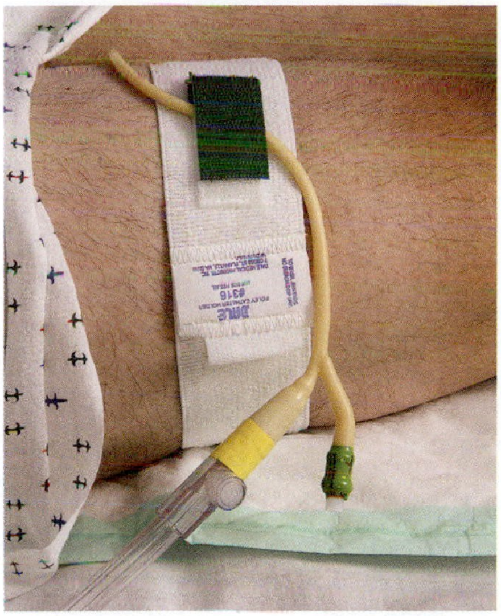

14. Cover the patient, and return him to a comfortable position, with the call bell within reach. Raise the siderails, and lower the bed.

15. Remove your gloves, and perform hand hygiene.

16. Change the condom daily or more often, if needed.

This helps to prevent urinary tract infection and allows for inspection of the skin.

? What if . . .

- **The urine flow becomes obstructed?**

  Check the catheter and collecting tube for kinking; readjust, if needed, and make certain that the tubing is secured properly to the patient's thigh. Replace the catheter and tubing, if necessary.

Evaluation

Within 30 minutes of condom application, assess for:

- Urine flow (should not be obstructed)
- Swelling or discoloration of the penis

  Swelling or discoloration might indicate that the condom is too tight.

Monitor:

- Penis for circulatory changes
- Position and patency of the drainage tubing
- Characteristics of the urine (e.g., amount, color, odor, bleeding)
- Patient comfort
- Leakage of urine

Home Care

- Clients and caregivers should wash their hands before and after any manipulation of the penis or apparatus.
- Daily bag decontamination with a diluted (1:10) bleach solution has been found effective in reducing bacteria.
- Teach the client and the caregiver to recognize the signs and symptoms of skin irritation and excoriation, as well as the symptoms of UTI.
- Teach the client and the caregiver to notify the care provider and discontinue use of the condom catheter if skin irritation or swelling occurs; if urine becomes thick and cloudy, pink or red; if urine has mucus in it; or if no urine has drained from the catheter in 6 to 8 hours.
- Change the external condom catheter every 24 hours.
- Keep the collecting bag below the level of the bladder.
- Regularly empty the collection bag before it becomes completely full.
- Never allow the draining spigot to come in contact with the nonsterile collecting container.
- Disinfect the catheter–tubing junction before disconnecting them (if they must be disconnected).
- Avoid disconnecting the catheter and drainage tube unless the catheter must be irrigated.

Documentation

- Document the date and time of application of the external catheter in the nursing notes.
- Note any unusual findings related to the condition of the skin on the penis.
- Document characteristics of urine (e.g., color, odor, consistency, blood).

Practice Resources

Newman, D. K., & Wein, A. J. (2018); Wound, Ostomy, and Continence Nurses Society (n.d.).

Thinking About the Procedure

The video **Applying an External Condom Catheter,** along with questions and suggested responses, is available on the ***Davis's Nursing Skills Videos*** Web site on FADavis.com.

Procedure 28-7 ■ Removing an Indwelling Catheter

➤ For steps to follow in all procedures, refer to the Universal Steps for All Procedures found on the inside back cover.

Equipment

- Syringe (5 to 30 mL, depending on balloon size)
- Clean procedure gloves
- Towel or drape
- Receptacle for the catheter, such as an emesis basin)
- Hygiene supplies (washcloth, warm filtered water or perineal wash solution, towel)

Delegation

In some institutions, unlicensed UAPs undergo special training to learn this skill. In such instances, you may delegate this task to the UAP. However, you must complete the following assessments and instruct the UAP about what abnormal findings to report.

Pre-Procedure Assessments

- Assess the patient's cognitive level.
  Knowing whether the patient can follow directions or not helps you to determine how to approach the procedure and also to know if the patient may be prone to pulling on the catheter or your hands when you are removing the catheter.
- Assess the condition of bladder (e.g., distention), perineum, and meatus (e.g., color, swelling, crusting, drainage, lesions).
  This information helps you to establish a baseline for later assessment.

➤ When performing the procedure, always identify your patient according to agency policy, using two identifiers, and be attentive to standard precautions, hand hygiene, patient safety and privacy, body mechanics, and documentation.

Procedure Steps

1. **Gather the necessary supplies.**
2. **Tell the patient what you are about to do,** what she will feel, and that you will need to monitor her urination after removal.
3. **Perform hand hygiene** before and after removing the catheter.
4. **Wear clean procedure gloves** during the removal.
   Gloving prevents transmission of bacteria.
5. iCare **Explain that this procedure** is nearly always pain-free, but patients may feel a little pressure as the balloon deflates and catheter is removed.
6. **Instruct** the patient to assume a supine position.
7. **Place the catheter receptacle** near the patient (e.g., on the bed).
8. **Place a waterproof drape** or towel.

Variation: Female: Place the drape between the patient's legs and up by the urethral meatus.

Variation: Male: Place the drape on his thighs.

These methods preserve modesty and a feeling of security; and prevent soiling of the bed.

9. **Obtain a sterile specimen** (see Procedure 28-2B), if needed. Some agencies require a culture and sensitivity test of the urine when an indwelling catheter is removed.
10. **Wash the perineum** with soapy water or periwash prior to removal of the catheter.
    The perineum and surface of the colonized with bacteria. Cleansing this area reduces the risk for urinary catheter-associated infection.
11. **Remove the device securing** the catheter to the patient.
12. **Deflate the balloon completely** by inserting a syringe into the balloon valve and allowing the balloon to self-deflate. Allow at least 30 seconds for the balloon to deflate.

    NOTE: Follow the manufacturer's directions for balloon deflation. If the direction is to attempt aspiration, it should be done slowly and gently.

    Aspiration of the balloon may collapse the lumen and cause the formation of creases and ridges that may make removal of the catheter difficult.
13. **Verify that the total fluid** volume has been removed by checking the balloon size written on the balloon port.
    If water remains in the balloon, removal of the catheter may cause urethral trauma.
14. **Ask the patient to relax** and take a few deep breaths as you slowly withdraw the catheter from the urethra. Pinch the catheter while removing it.
    Deep breathing helps the patient to relax the sphincters.
15. **Wrap the catheter in the towel** or drape or place in the catheter receptacle.
16. **Again, cleanse the perineal area** with warm filtered water or perineal wash solution on gauze pads or perineal disposable wipes. A mild soap may also be used.
    Cleansing the perineum prevents transmission of bacteria.
17. **Measure the urine,** and then empty it in the toilet; discard the catheter, drainage tube, and collection bag in the biohazard waste.

18. **Explain to the patient** the need to monitor the first few voidings after catheter removal. If the patient toilets independently, place a receptacle in the toilet or use a bedside commode. Ask the patient to notify the nurse when she voids and to save the urine.

19. **Remove and discard gloves**; perform hand hygiene.

20. **Record the procedure** (see Documentation, below).

21. **Return the patient to** a position of comfort with the call device within reach.

? What if . . .

- **The balloon does not empty completely when you aspirate?**

  Do not pull on the catheter. Report to the charge nurse or the primary healthcare provider before continuing the procedure.

  Pulling on the catheter could cause injury to the urethra.

Evaluation

- Observe for signs and symptoms of infection.
  Signs of a catheter-associated urinary tract infection include the presence of significant bacteriuria in a patient with signs or symptoms of UTI, such as fever, malaise, flank pain, dysuria, altered mental status, or hematuria.
- Observe the condition of the meatus.
- Monitor the next few voidings. Place a collection container in the commode if the patient is ambulatory.
- Assess the characteristics of the urine at the time the catheter is removed. Then note the time of the first voiding and the amount voided, and observe the urine for color, amount, odor, and presence of blood.
- Compare voidings over the next 8 to 10 hours to the patient's intake.
- Monitor for bladder distention. A portable bladder-scanning device may be used to quantify any residual urine.

Patient Teaching

- Explain to the patient that you need to monitor the first few voidings after catheter removal to ensure that he does not have difficulty re-establishing bladder control.
- Teach the patient to notify you when he voids and to save the urine (if the patient toilets independently).

Home Care

For clients who will have catheters at home, teach the client and family the following:

- Steps for removing the catheter that you learned in this procedure
- To notify a healthcare provider if the client is unable to urinate within 8 hours after catheter removal, or if his abdomen becomes distended and painful
- The signs and symptoms of UTI
  Signs and symptoms of UTI develop rapidly and can include a strong, persistent urge to urinate; a burning sensation when urinating; passing frequent, small amounts of urine; blood in the urine (hematuria); fever; flank pain; or an alteration in mental status.
- Increase fluid intake if not contraindicated by other health conditions.
- The client should never remove a catheter unless trained by a healthcare provider. Remove the catheter only when prescribed by the provider.

Documentation

- Date and time the catheter was removed
- Amount of urine (on the I&O portion of the graphics sheet)
- Characteristics of urine (e.g., color, odor, cloudiness, turbidity, or blood)
- Time the specimen was sent to the lab
- Amount of fluid returned from balloon by self-deflation, amount of urine in drainage bag, and notification of first void
- Any unusual findings in your assessment of the perineum
- How the patient tolerated the procedure
- Patient teaching

Sample documentation

3/4/20 1010 Order noted for removal of indwelling catheter. Explained the procedure to patient. Pt stated, "I'm finally getting this thing out." Placed Pt in a dorsal recumbent position with blanket to provide privacy. Perineal care completed. Allowed retention balloon to self-deflate, obtaining 10 mL of liquid. Removed catheter, using gentle pulling motion. Pt expressed no discomfort during removal. Perineal care again given. 250 mL of clear, yellow, strong-smelling urine noted in drainage bag. Instructed client to increase fluid intake, especially water, and to notify a nurse when she voids for the first time.————————— D. Drumpf, RN

Practice Resources

Clayton, J. L. (2017); Foley catheter care and maintenance guide: Patient education guide. (2013); Griffiths, R., & Fernandez, R. (2009); Hooton, T. M., Bradley, S. F., Cardenas, D. D., et al. (2010); Jones, J., Sibai, J., & Fakih, M. J. (2016, February); Newman, D. K., Cumbee, R. P., & Rovner, E. S. (2017): Wound, Ostomy, and Continence Nurses Society (2016);

Thinking About the Procedure

The video **Removing an Indwelling Urinary Catheter,** along with questions and suggested responses, is available on the ***Davis's Nursing Skills Videos*** Web site on FADavis.com.

Procedure 28-8 ■ Irrigating the Bladder or Catheter

➤ For steps to follow in all procedures, refer to the Universal Steps for All Procedures found on the inside back cover.

Equipment

Intermittent Irrigation Through a Three-Way Catheter

- Bag of sterile irrigation solution
- Connecting tubing (to connect the bag to the irrigation port)
- IV pole
- Antiseptic swabs or wipes
- Bath blanket

Intermittent Irrigation via the Specimen Port Using a Syringe

- Sterile container
- Sterile 60-mL syringe with large-gauge needleless access device
- Sterile irrigation solution
- Two pairs of clean procedure gloves
- Antiseptic swabs or wipes

Continuous Bladder Irrigation

- Three-way (or triple-lumen) indwelling catheter in place
- Sterile irrigation solution at room temperature
- Connecting tubing
- Antiseptic swabs or wipes
- IV pole
- Bath blanket
- Measuring container
- Pair of clean procedure gloves

Delegation

Irrigation of an indwelling catheter requires nursing assessment and clinical decision-making. Because of the high potential for urinary tract infection, you should not delegate this procedure to the UAP. Bladder/catheter irrigation may be delegated with supervision to qualified LPNs who are trained in the procedure.

Pre-Procedure Assessments

- Note the characteristics of the urine (e.g., amount, color, odor, presence of clots or mucus).
- Assess for the presence and degree of bladder distension.
  This information helps you to establish a baseline for assessment.
- Note patient complaints of discomfort.
- Assess the patient's cognitive status.
  To determine whether the patient can remain still during the procedure.
- Check the chart for the amount and type of sterile solution to use.
- Determine whether the irrigant is to remain in the bladder for any length of time.

Procedure 28-8A ■ Intermittent Bladder or Catheter Irrigation

➤ When performing the procedure, always identify your patient according to agency policy, using two identifiers, and be attentive to standard precautions, hand hygiene, patient safety and privacy, body mechanics, and documentation.

➤ *Note:* This is the procedure for the closed methods of irrigation. The "open" method is no longer recommended. Because of the risk for infection, you should never disconnect the drainage tubing from the catheter.

Procedure Steps

Procedure Variation: Three-Way (Triple-Lumen) Indwelling Catheter

1. **Before starting irrigation**, prepare the connection tubing and irrigation solution warmed to room temperature.
   a. Close the clamp on the connection tubing.
   b. Spike the tubing into the appropriate portal on the irrigation solution bag, using aseptic technique.
   c. Invert the solution and hang it on an IV pole.
   d. Remove the protective cap from the distal end of the connection tubing. Hold the end of the tubing over the sink or trash receptacle. Open the roller clamp; and allow the solution to fill the tubing. Be sure to keep the end sterile.
   e. Reclamp the roller on the tubing to stop the flow of irrigation solution.
   f. Recap the tubing.
2. **Perform hand hygiene,** and don procedure gloves.
   To reduce the transmission of microbes.
3. **Position the patient in the supine.**
4. iCare **Drape the patient** so only the connection port on the indwelling catheter is visible.
   Protects patient privacy.
5. **Before beginning the flow** of irrigation solution, empty any urine that is in the drainage bag, and perform hand hygiene. Then document the volume on the I&O record.
   Starting the procedure with an empty drainage bag gives you a baseline for correct calculation of true urine output during irrigation.
6. **Scrub the catheter port** with antiseptic swabs or wipe or sterile, normal saline.
   To remove microorganisms and help prevent UTI.
7. **Connect the irrigation tubing** to the catheter port.
8. **Slowly open the roller clamp** on the irrigation tubing to the desired flow rate.
   Slow instillation prevents patient discomfort.

9. **Instill or irrigate** with the prescribed amount of irrigant. If the irrigant is to remain in the bladder for a certain period, clamp the drainage tubing for that time.

10. **When the correct amount** of irrigant has been used and/or the goals of the irrigation have been met, close the roller clamp on the irrigation tubing, leaving the tubing connected to the catheter for use during the next irrigation.
You can assess whether the goals of irrigation have been met by inspecting the color of the urine and assessing for presence of clots, mucus, or blood. Clamping the drainage tubing prevents immediate outflow.

11. **Remove gloves,** perform hand hygiene, and return the patient to a position of comfort.

Procedure Variation: Two-Way Indwelling Catheter

12. **Don clean procedure gloves.** Empty any urine currently found in the bedside drainage bag.
Emptying the bag will ensure accurate output results.

13. **Perform hand hygiene,** and then apply clean gloves.
Gloving prevents the transmission of microorganisms.

iCare 14. **Drape the patient** so that only the specimen removal port on the drainage tubing is exposed. Place a waterproof drape beneath the exposed port.
Draping ensures patient privacy and prevents soiling of the bed linens.

15. **Open the sterile irrigation** supplies. Pour approximately 100 mL of the irrigating solution, warmed to room temperature, into the sterile container, using aseptic technique.
Warm solution is more comfortable to the patient.

16. **Scrub all surfaces** of the specimen removal port with an antiseptic swab or wipe.
Cleaning the port reduces the risk of transmission of pathogens into the bladder.

17. **Draw up irrigation solution** into the syringe. Connect the syringe to the specimen port. For catheter irrigation, use a total of 30 to 40 mL; for bladder irrigation the amount is usually 100 to 200 mL, unless irrigation is prescribed postoperatively (in which case more irrigation might be needed).

18. **Clamp or pinch the drainage** tubing distal to the specimen port.
Clamping prevents irrigant from going down into the drainage bag instead of into the catheter and/or bladder.

19. **Inject the solution into the port.** Hold the specimen port slightly above the level of the bladder. If you meet resistance, have the patient turn slightly, and attempt a second time. If resistance continues, stop the procedure, and notify the primary care provider.
Holding the port above the level of the bladder enhances gravitational flow of irrigant into the bladder.

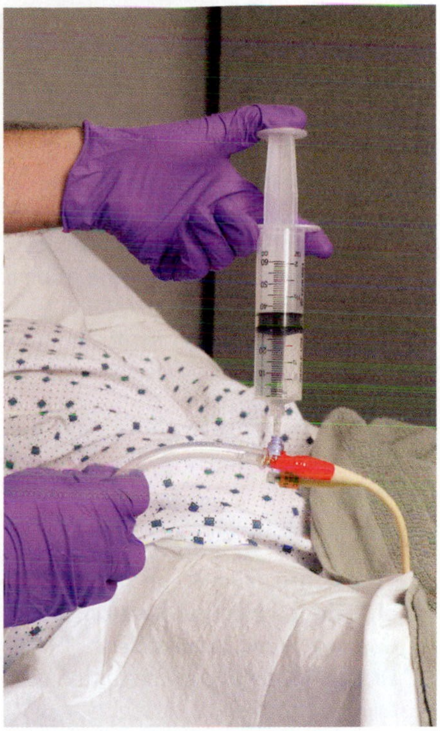

20. **When the irrigant has been injected,** remove the syringe. Refill the syringe, if necessary.

21. **Unclamp or release** the drainage tubing, and allow the irrigant and urine to flow into the bedside drainage bag by gravity. (If the solution is to remain in the bladder for a prescribed time, leave the tubing clamped for that period.)

22. **Repeat the procedure, as necessary,** until the prescribed amount has been instilled or until the goal of the irrigation is met (e.g., removal of clots and mucus, free flowing of urine).

23. **Remove gloves,** perform hand hygiene, and return the patient to a position of comfort with the call device within reach.

Procedure 28-8B ■ Continuous Bladder Irrigation

➤ When performing the procedure, always identify your patient according to agency policy, using two identifiers, and be attentive to standard precautions, hand hygiene, patient safety and privacy, body mechanics, and documentation.

Procedure Steps

1. **If one is not already present,** insert a three-way (triple-lumen) indwelling catheter.
A triple-lumen catheter provides an access for the irrigation solution without disrupting the sterile drainage unit.

2. **Prepare the irrigation fluid** and tubing by warming it to room temperature:
   a. Close the clamp on the connecting tubing.
   b. Spike the tubing into the portal on the irrigation solution container, using aseptic technique.
   This prevents the introduction of microorganisms into the solution.
   c. Invert the container and hang it on the IV pole.
   The elevated bag allows the solution to flow by gravity.

(continued on next page)

Procedure 28-8 ■ Irrigating the Bladder or Catheter (continued)

d. Remove the protective cap from the distal end of the connecting tubing. Hold the end of the tubing over a sink or other receptacle. Open the roll clamp slowly; and allow the solution to fill the tubing completely. Reclamp the tubing. Recap the tubing.
Priming the tubing flushes air from tubing, preventing bladder distension.

3. **Perform hand hygiene,** and don clean procedure gloves.
To prevent the spread of microorganisms.

iCare 4. **Place the patient supine,** and drape him so that only the connection port on the indwelling catheter is visible.
Draping prevents exposure of the genital area and protects patient privacy.

5. **Place a waterproof barrier** drape under the irrigation port. Scrub the irrigation port with antiseptic swabs or wipes. Pinching the tubing and using aseptic technique, connect the end of the irrigation infusion tubing to the irrigation port of the catheter.

6. **Before beginning the flow** of irrigation solution, empty any urine that may be in the bedside drainage bag, and document the volume on the I&O record.
Starting the procedure with an empty bag gives you a baseline for correct calculation of true urine output during irrigation. The I&O record provides data for evaluating urinary status.

7. **Remove your gloves,** and perform hand hygiene.
Gloving and hand hygiene prevent the transmission of microorganisms.

8. **Cover the patient**; and return him to a position of comfort, with the call device within reach.

9. **Open the roller clamp** on the tubing; and regulate the flow of the irrigation solution to meet the desired outcome for the irrigation.
The goal of continuous bladder irrigation for patients who have had transurethral resection of the prostate is to keep urine light pink to clear.

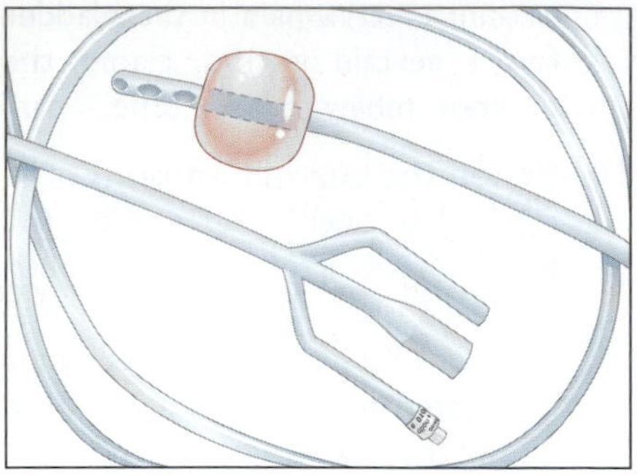

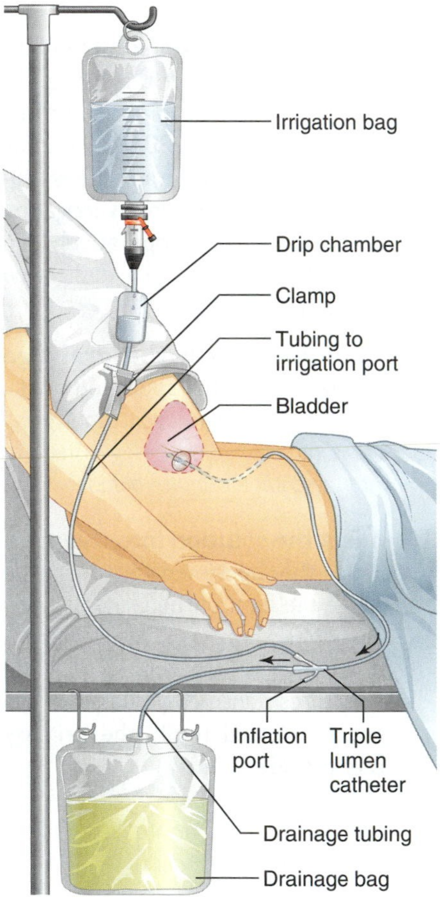

10. **Monitor the flow rate** for 1 to 2 minutes to ensure accuracy.
Monitoring the irrigation fluid for a minute or two prevents rapid introduction of solution into the bladder, which would cause patient discomfort.

What if . . .

- **The draining irrigant solution and/or urine looks like it has red blood cells (RBCs) in it?**

  Stop the irrigation and report to the primary care provider.
  Increased RBCs in urine may indicate bladder irritation and possible trauma to the inner mucosal lining of the bladder.

- **You meet resistance when irrigating?**

  Ask the patient to turn slightly; and attempt a second time. If resistance continues, stop the procedure, and notify the primary care provider.

Evaluation

- Note the flow rate of irrigant and/or inability to instill irrigant into the catheter.
- Note the characteristics of urine output (e.g., presence of output, color, amount, clots, mucus).
- Note patient report of discomfort (e.g., pain, spasms).
- Assess for development of bladder distention accompanied by lack of urine outflow. A portable bladder scanner may be used to quantify the amount of fluid retained in the bladder.

Home Care

For clients who will have continuous bladder irrigation at home, you will need to teach the family the necessary steps of the procedure. Also teach them to:

- Empty the urine collection device before beginning the procedure.
- Use strict aseptic technique when irrigating the bladder or catheter.

- Irrigate the catheter using the closed method, which carries the least risk for introducing bacteria into the bladder. The catheter and drainage tubing should never be disconnected.
- Identify signs and symptoms of urinary retention and UTI.
- Wash their hands before and after any manipulation of the catheter site or apparatus.
- Be certain to maintain unobstructed flow.
- For the syringe method, the client will need access to syringes and needleless access devices and a process to dispose of them properly.

Documentation

- Date and time of procedure, the type of irrigant, and the total volume infused
- Characteristics of the urine (e.g., color, odor, clarity, sediment, presence of clots or mucus)
- Evidence of catheter patency (e.g., flow of urine, absence of distention)

Sample documentation

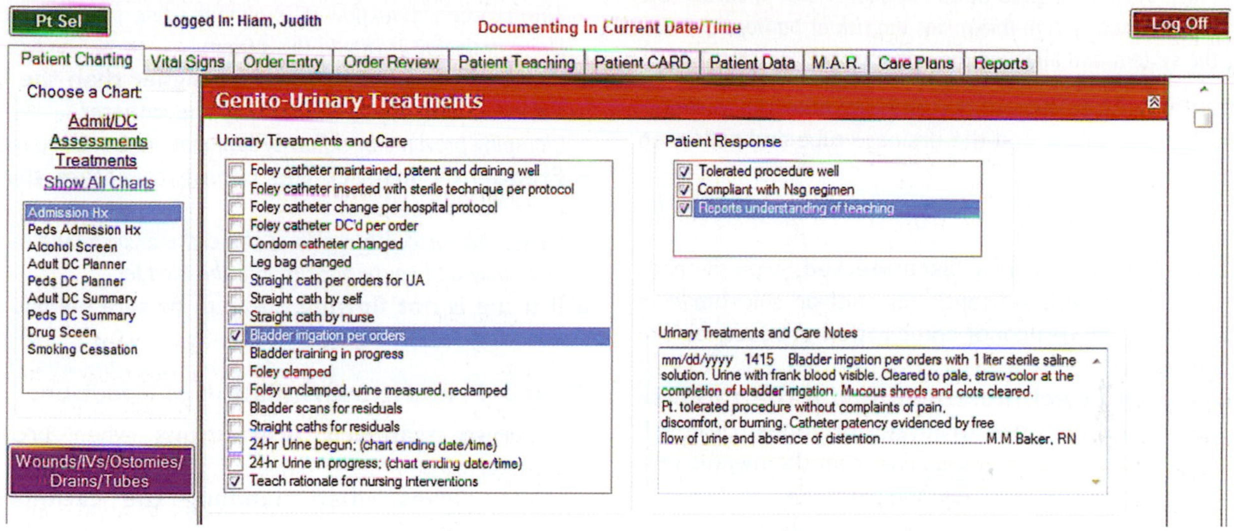

Practice Resources

Appendix C. Sample Bladder Scan Policy (2017); Hooton, T. M., Bradley, S. F., Cardenas, D. D., et al. (2010); Shepherd, A. J., Mackay, W. G., & Hagan, S. (2017, March 6); Weber, J., Purvis, S., VanDenBergh, S., et al. (2017).

Thinking About the Procedure

The videos **Intermittent Bladder Irrigation: Three-Way (Triple-Lumen) Indwelling Catheter; Intermittent Bladder Irrigation: Two-Way Indwelling Catheter;** and **Continuous Bladder Irrigation,** along with questions and suggested responses, are available on the ***Davis's Nursing Skills Videos*** Web site on FADavis.com.

CLINICAL INSIGHTS

Clinical Insight 28-1 ➤ Caring for a Patient With an Indwelling Catheter

An indwelling catheter is connected to a drainage tube and collection bag, which constitute a closed system.

Goal 1: Prevent urinary tract infection.

- **Do not disconnect the tubing** or open the drainage system (e.g., to obtain specimens or measure the urine). *A closed system minimizes the risk of pathogens entering the system and infecting the urinary tract.*
- **Regularly check connections** between the catheter and drainage tubing and the drainage tube and collection bag.
  Loose connections cause leaks and serve as entry points for pathogens.
- **If the system becomes disconnected,** wipe the ends of both tubes with antiseptic (alcohol or chlorhexidine gluconate [CHG]–alcohol combination product) before reconnecting them.
- **After each bowel movement and if the catheter becomes soiled from drainage or feces,** cleanse it with mild soap and water, cleaning from the meatus outward. Rinse the catheter well, and pat it dry.
  This removes the medium for growth of microorganisms.
- **Empty the collection bag** at least every 8 hours and more frequently if urine output is high.
  This prevents stagnation of urine.
- **Do not touch the spout to any surfaces** when emptying the collection bag. If the spout is accidentally contaminated, cleanse it with an antiseptic (alcohol or CHG–alcohol combination product).
- **Keep collection bag below the level of the bladder, but do not let it touch the floor** (see Goal 2).
  The floor is considered contaminated.
- **Teach the patient to report signs of UTI;** observe for cloudy, strong-smelling urine, chills, or fever.
- **Change the indwelling catheter only when necessary** (e.g., when sediment collects in the tubing or catheter or the urine does not drain well), **and discontinue it as soon it is no longer necessary**.
  Some agency policies specify that catheters be changed at specific intervals (e.g., monthly). However, this is not advisable because the more often a catheter is changed, the more likely an infection will develop.
- **Routine hygiene is all that is necessary for meatal cleansing.**
  Antiseptic solutions are no more effective than sterile, normal saline for cleansing; they may irritate or dry the skin at the urinary meatus.

Goal 2: Maintain free flow of urine.

Maintaining free flow of urine prevents backflow of urine into the bladder, which can cause bladder distension and injury. Stasis of urine also provides a medium for growth of microorganisms.

Note that some of the interventions in this section are the same as those for preventing infection (Goal 1).

- **Keep the tubing and bag below bladder level.** Never place the bag on the floor or the bed.
  This prevents backflow of stagnant urine into the bladder. Urine drains by gravity in this system.
- **If the collecting bag must be higher than the bladder** at any time, you must clamp the catheter.
  Clamping prevents backflow of stagnant urine into the bladder.
- **Frequently inspect the tubing** to ensure that the urine flows freely.
  Kinks, coils, or compression of the catheter or tubing may impede flow and cause backup into the bladder.
- **If urine is not flowing**, check to be sure the patient is not lying on the tubing.

Goal 3: Prevent transmission of infection.

- **Observe standard precautions** when providing catheter care.
- **Wear gloves when handling the catheter** or drainage system.
  Gloving prevents possible exposure to body fluids.
- **Always perform hand hygiene before and after providing care** to any patient, including one with an indwelling catheter.

Goal 4: Promote normal urine production.

Adequate urine production flushes pathogens out of the bladder, provides natural irrigation of the tubing, and prevents stasis of urine.

- **Encourage oral intake of at least 8 to 10 glasses** (approximately 2,000 to 2,500 mL) of fluid per day, unless contraindicated by other health problems (Frellick, 2017; Turner & Dickens, 2011; Wound, Ostomy, and Continence Nurses Society, 2009). For patients who are unable to take oral liquid, provide an equivalent amount of parenteral or enteral fluids.
- **Monitor I&O at least every 8 hours** (more frequently if the patient is experiencing fluid and electrolyte imbalance).
- **For accurate determination of output,** empty the urine into a calibrated container. Volume markings on the urine collection bag are only approximate.
- **Observe the urine output for color and other characteristics**. Report evidence of blood, sediment, or infection to the primary care provider.
- **Encourage the patient to be active and out of bed** as much as possible.
  This promotes blood flow to the kidneys for better urinary function.

Clinical Insight 28-1 ➤ Caring for a Patient With an Indwelling Catheter—cont'd

Goal 5: Maintain skin and mucosal integrity.

Perineal skin and mucosa can be irritated by feces and by movement or encrustation of the catheter.

- **Secure the tubing to the patient's thigh** by applying a commercial catheter securement device, such as a catheter tube holder or a Velcro strap (or hypoallergenic tape if a securement device is unavailable).
  Failure to secure the tubing may cause significant injury to the bladder neck and urethra. Although the inflated balloon holds the catheter in the bladder, you must secure the tubing to prevent traction on the bladder and urethral meatus.
- **Assist with routine hygiene care, as needed.** Cleanse the area around the meatus with mild soap and filtered tap water or perineal wash solution daily, after each bowel movement, and more often if there is drainage or excessive sweating. Rinse well and pat dry.
  Routine hygiene care normally provides adequate cleanliness. Rinsing helps to avoid skin irritation by soap residue.
- **Avoid using powders or lotions in the perineal area.**
  Topical products can be irritating to the skin.
- **Monitor the urethral meatus and upper drainage tube.**
  Encrustation, as evidenced by sandy particles at the meatus, irritates the mucosa and signals the need to change the catheter.

Clinical Insight 28-2 ➤ Teaching Clients About Clean, Intermittent Self-Catheterization

You will need to teach self-catheterization to clients who have compromised ability to spontaneously empty their bladders. In the home setting, this is a clean procedure rather than a sterile one. It is referred to as clean, intermittent self-catheterization (CISC).

Goals of Intermittent Self-Catheterization

1. Completely empty the bladder
2. Prevent urinary tract infections

Teaching Considerations

- In teaching the steps of the procedure, consider the client's physical ability to manipulate the catheter equipment and reach the urethra (e.g., range of motion, fine motor skills, degree of sensation).
- Encourage the client to drink 8 to 10 eight-ounce glasses of fluid without caffeine each day to ensure a quantity of urine adequate to flush the bladder.
- Teach the client to report the signs and symptoms of urinary tract infection: burning, frequency, urgency, dull abdominal ache, fever, or malaise; or urine that contains sediment or becomes cloudy.

Older adults may experience confusion before the other signs and symptoms occur.

- Advise the client to contact a healthcare provider if there is bleeding, pain, or difficulty inserting the catheter.
- Some CISC catheters can be reused; some are disposable.
- Instruct the patient to wash her hands thoroughly before handling the equipment or performing the catheterization.
- Tell the client to catheterize as often as needed. Most patients will need to catheterize 4 to 6 times daily.
- Instruct the client to discard a reusable catheter when it becomes difficult to clean or difficult to insert. A CISC catheter may be reused for up to 7 days.
- Recommendations for cleaning a reusable catheter include washing with soap and water, boiling or microwave sterilization, or soaking in an antiseptic solution. Running tap water forcefully through the catheter may remove encrustation or mucus deposits. The client should follow the specific cleaning recommendations from the catheter manufacturer.

Procedure for Men

1. **Try to void before catheterization.** If you are unable to void or if the amount is less than 3 ounces (or the amount specified by your healthcare provider), then insert the catheter.
2. **Assemble the catheter, lubricant, and drainage receptacle.**
3. **Thoroughly wash** your hands with soap and water; cleanse the penis and the urethral opening.
4. **Lubricate** the catheter to 15 cm (6 in.).
5. **Stand over the toilet,** or assume a comfortable position (e.g., sitting on the toilet).
6. **Hold the penis** perpendicular (at a right angle) to your body.
7. **Gently insert** and advance the catheter.
8. **When you meet resistance**, at the level of the prostate, take deep breaths to try to relax, and advance the catheter.
9. **When the urine flow starts,** advance the catheter 2.5 cm (1 in.) more; return the penis to its natural position; hold the catheter in place until the urine flow stops and the bladder is empty.
10. **Withdraw the catheter** slowly in small increments to be sure the entire bladder empties.
11. **Wash the catheter** with soap and water, if it is reusable (or follow the manufacturer's instructions for cleaning). Rinse and dry it well. If it is disposable, discard it immediately.

(Continued)

Clinical Insight 28-2 ➤ Teaching Clients About Clean, Intermittent Self-Catheterization—cont'd

12. **Store catheters** in a clean, dry, secure place.
13. **Record the amount** of urine obtained.

Procedure for Women

1. **Try to void before catheterization.** If you are unable to void or if the urine amount is less than 3 ounces (or less than the amount specified by your healthcare provider), then insert the catheter.
2. **Assemble the catheter, lubricant, and drainage receptacle;** a good light is important for women.
3. **Thoroughly wash your hands** with soap and water.
4. **Cleanse your labia and urethra** with soap and water or with a moist towelette; rinse well. Cleanse and rinse from front to back.
5. **Lubricate the catheter** to about 2.5 cm (1 in.).
6. **Assume a comfortable position** for urinating. Some women perform CISC standing up with one foot on the toilet.
7. **Use a hand mirror** to locate the urethral opening, which is between the clitoris and the vagina.
8. **Spread your labia** with the second and fourth fingers; use the middle finger to feel for the urethral opening.
9. **Gently insert the catheter** into the opening, guiding it upward toward your umbilicus (belly button) until urine flows. This is usually 5 to 8 cm (2 to 3 in.) past the urethral opening.
10. **When urine flows,** advance the catheter another 2.5 cm (1 in.). Hold it in place until the urine flow stops and your bladder is empty.
11. **Withdraw the catheter slowly** in small increments, to be sure the entire bladder empties.
12. **If the catheter is reusable,** wash it with soap and water; rinse and dry it well (or follow the manufacturer's instructions for cleaning). If it is disposable, discard it immediately.
13. **Store catheters** in a clean, dry, secure place.
14. **Record the amount** of urine obtained.

Practice Resources

Adams, J., Watts, R., Yearwood, M., et. al. (2011); Newman, D., & Willson, M. M. (2011); Zhang, L., Thompson, D., Arya, L. A., et al. (2018).

Clinical Insight 28-3 ➤ Guidelines for Bladder Training and Pelvic Floor Exercises

Most cases of urinary incontinence (UI) are managed with skin care and behavioural interventions, but UI is sometimes treated with medications and other collaborative interventions.

Bladder Training

The goal of bladder training is to enable the patient to hold increasingly greater volumes of urine in the bladder and to increase the interval between voidings.

- Teach the mechanisms of urination.
- Teach distraction and relaxation strategies to help inhibit the urge to void. For example:
  - The patient can perform serial subtractions or engage in an activity that requires concentration (e.g., a crossword puzzle) when she feels the urge to void.
  - Alternatively, the patient might perform several rapid pelvic floor muscle contractions to quiet the sensations from the bladder.
  - Other techniques include deep breathing and guided imagery.
- **Scheduled voiding** is a form of bladder training involving timed voiding and habit retraining. The patient must be mentally and physically capable of self-toileting.
  - Assist the patient to the toilet, commode, or bedpan on a timed schedule. Initially, this may be every 2 hours or even more often.
  - As a pattern develops and the person gains greater control, the length of time between voiding may be increased.
  - Scheduled voiding is usually combined with other techniques, including lifestyle adjustments and pelvic muscle exercises.
  - Ask the patient to keep a daily record of her adherence to the schedule and of the number of incontinence episodes.
  - When the patient can adhere to the schedule comfortably, the voiding interval can be increased by 15 to 30 min.

Pelvic Floor Muscle Rehabilitation

Theoretical Knowledge: Pelvic floor muscle exercises (PFMEs), also known as *Kegel exercises,* are a mainstay of UI treatment for women.

- PFMEs strengthen perineal muscles and help prevent and treat stress, urge, and mixed UI.
- PFMEs are the most commonly used method for preventing and reversing incontinence in women for the first year after giving birth.
- PFMEs may also prevent or reduce urinary incontinence in older women and in men undergoing prostate surgery.
- **Key Point:** *To be successful, the patient must do the exercises correctly and practice them daily.*

Clinical Insight 28-3 ➤ Guidelines for Bladder Training and Pelvic Floor Exercises—cont'd

Kegel Routine

Teach patients the following routine to strengthen pelvic floor muscles:

- A period of 2 to 3 months may be required before treatment is effective.
- Imagine that you are urinating and wish to stop the flow; also tighten your rectum as though you are trying to keep from passing gas. The muscles you contract to interrupt flow are the pelvic floor muscles.

NOTE: Caution the patient against doing PFMEs while actually urinating because this may cause backflow of urine.

- You should feel your rectum tighten. Women may also feel the vagina tighten. Your abdomen should not tighten—check by placing your hand lightly on your abdomen. Do not contract the thigh and gluteal muscles.
- Hold each contraction for 5 to 10 sec and then rest for 5 to 10 sec. Some people may be able to hold for only 3 seconds at first. Count, "one-and-two-and-three …." Keep contraction and relaxation times equal. That is, if you hold a contraction for 5 sec, rest 5 sec before the next contraction.
- A recommended daily exercise routine is to perform 10 to 15 PFMEs three times a day. Do not do all 30 to 45 exercises at one time; spread them out through the day.
- One way to remember to perform your exercises it to associate them with an activity. For example, do PFMEs at every stoplight or stop sign when you are in the car. Or do some of these exercises every time you go to the bathroom—but not while you are urinating.

Practice Resources

Angelini, K. (2017); Dumoulin, C., Cacciari, L. P., Hay-Smith, E. J. C. (2018); Hay-Smith, E. J., Herderschee, R., Dumoulin, C., et al. (2011); Nahon, I., Martin, M., & Adams, R. (2014).

Clinical Insight 28-4 ➤ Caring for Patients With Urinary Diversion

A patient with a urinary diversion requires physical and psychological care. Initially, you will care for the ostomy. However, the long-term goals are for the patient to become comfortable with his changed body and to assume self-care.

- **Perform a thorough assessment.** A healthy stoma ranges in color from deep pink to brick red, regardless of skin color, and is shiny and moist at all times. A pale, dusky, or black stoma often indicates inadequate blood supply. Immediately document and report such findings to the surgeon.
- **Assess the skin surrounding the stoma for signs of irritation,** such as redness, tenderness, and skin breakdown. **Key Point:** *Skin care is critical. When the normally acidic urine remains in contact with the skin, it becomes alkaline. Encrustations collect on the skin, and the skin becomes macerated and excoriated. Skin breakdown may lead to infection, pain, and leakage.*
- **Be certain that the collection device fits** snugly against the skin. A moisture-proof skin barrier is usually placed around the stoma.
  Moisture on the skin can lead to irritation and maceration.
- **Barrier creams** may be prescribed for irritated skin; if fungal infection develops, nystatin may be prescribed.
- **Monitor the amount and type of drainage** from the stoma.
- **Empty the device frequently** during the day; connect it to a larger collection bag during the night when the patient is sleeping.

iCare ■ **Be available to discuss the patient's reaction** to the stoma. Be careful that your facial expressions do not convey disgust or disapproval when working with the patient and his stoma.

- **Provide ample time** to explain stoma care and use of ostomy appliances.

For most patients this is a life-long task; therefore, patient teaching is essential.

Continent Urinary Reservoir

These patients will also need instruction about catheterizing their reservoir to drain the urine. Once healed, the reservoir will need to be catheterized four or five times a day. See Clinical Insight 28-2.

Neobladder

- These patients will not have a stoma but will require bladder training once the postoperative retention catheter has been removed.
- Instruct the patient to perform pelvic floor muscle exercises three times a day and empty the bladder on a schedule, as often as every 2 hours initially. Once bladder capacity builds, the interval between voidings may be increased.
- Teach the patient to relax the pelvic muscles and bear down to release urine from the bladder. He may also need to use **Credé's maneuver**—applying manual pressure over the bladder to promote emptying.
- If the patient is unable to fully empty the bladder with these techniques, he may need to perform intermittent self-catheterization.

ASSESSMENT GUIDELINES AND TOOLS

Focused Assessment

Urinary Elimination History Questions

Usual Urination Pattern

- How often do you urinate?
- Do you get up in the middle of the night to urinate?
- Do you have difficulty getting to the bathroom in time to urinate?
- Do you ever leak urine when you cough, laugh, or exercise?
- Do you ever leak urine on the way to the bathroom?
- Do you need to use pads or tissue in your underwear to catch urine?
- Do you have any difficulty starting to void?

Appearance of Urine

- How would you describe your urine?
- Have you noticed unusual odor with urination?

Changes in Urination Habits or Urine Appearance

- Have you experienced any changes in your voiding pattern recently?
- Have you experienced any changes in the appearance or odor of your urine?

History of Urination Problems

- Have you experienced any problems with urinary tract infections or kidney and bladder problems?
- Have you ever lost control of your urination?
- Have you ever had urinary tract surgery or diagnostic procedures?

Use of Urination Aids

- What aids, if any, do you use to help you urinate?
- What is your usual fluid intake over the course of a day?
- What medications are you taking? Have they had any effect on your urination pattern?

Lifestyle Questions

- Where is your bathroom located? Can you get to it easily?
- Can you manage your clothing when you go to the bathroom?
- How much fluid do you drink each day?
- How many caffeinated beverages do you drink?
- Do you smoke?
- Are you bothered with constipation?
- Do you do high-impact exercise (e.g., jogging)?

Presence of Urinary Diversions

- Have you ever had urinary tract surgery?
- If so, what and when?
- Gather data on the client's usual care of the stoma, use of appliances, and adjustment to the ostomy.

For Infants and Young Children

- Has the child been toilet-trained?
- What elimination routines have been established?

Focused Assessment

Guidelines for Physical Assessment for Urinary Elimination

Physical assessment for urinary elimination includes examination of the kidneys, bladder, urethra, and skin surrounding the genitals, as appropriate. For a complete discussion of physical examination of the genitourinary system, see Chapter 22, Procedures 22-17 and 22-18, in this volume.

Technique	*Rationale*
The Kidneys	
The **costovertebral (CV) angle** is formed by the junction of the 12th rib and the spine on both sides of the back. Place one palm flat on the CV angle and lightly strike it with the closed fist of the other hand (see the accompanying figure).	You cannot usually palpate the kidneys. Instead, examine them by assessing for costovertebral angle tenderness (CVAT). If kidney inflammation is present, percussion of this angle produces pain.

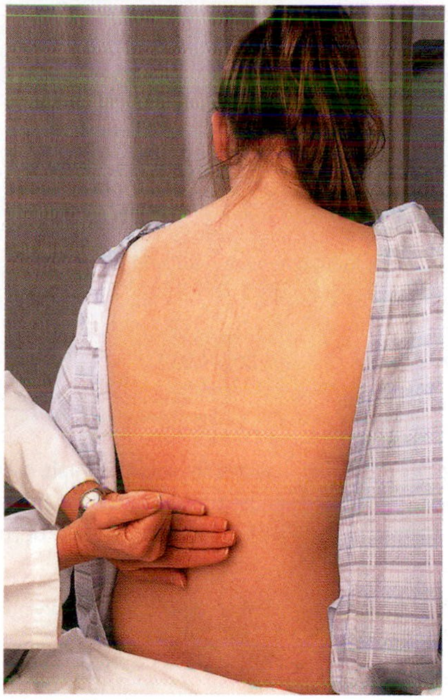

The Bladder

Inspect, palpate, and percuss the lower abdomen. Correlate your findings with data about the client's fluid intake and voiding.

➤ Inspect the lower abdomen.	➤ An empty bladder, or one with limited urine, is small and sits below the symphysis pubis. ➤ In contrast, a distended bladder rises above the symphysis pubis. If it is very distended, you may be able to see a rounded swelling above the symphysis pubis.
➤ Lightly palpate the lower abdomen to define the bladder margin. Observe the patient's response to palpation, noting signs of tenderness or discomfort.	An empty bladder, or one with limited urine, will not be palpable.
➤ Percuss the area.	A distended bladder produces a dull sound as opposed to the normal tympanic sound of intestinal air.
The Urethra	
➤ Inspect the urethral orifice. Look for erythema, discharge, swelling, or odor.	These are all signs of infection, trauma, or inflammation.
The Perineal Area	
➤ Frequently inspect skin color, condition, texture, turgor, and presence of urine or stool.	Clients who have urine leakage or a urinary catheter are at risk for perineal skin problems. Ammonia in urine may cause skin excoriation, skin breakdown, and subsequent infection. If both urine and stool are present on the skin, the likelihood of skin breakdown increases.

DIAGNOSTIC TESTING

Diagnostic Testing

Urinalysis

Characteristic Findings	Expected	Variations
Color	A freshly voided sample is pale yellow to deep amber.	➤ Color is lighter, or even clear, if fluid intake is high or urine output is excessive. ➤ Color is darker as it becomes more concentrated (e.g., with decreased fluid intake or excessive fluid loss. ➤ Color is also affected by certain foods (e. g., beets, carrots, asparagus) and medications (e.g., antacids, phenazopyridine). ➤ Dark, tea-colored urine can indicate liver disease or vasculitis. ➤ Color is also affected by some medications.
pH	5.0–9.0	➤ Indicates the kidneys' ability to help maintain balanced hydrogen ion concentration (acid–base balance) in the blood. ➤ The pH increases (more alkaline) if the client eats dairy products or citrus fruits or has a vegetarian diet. ➤ The pH decreases (more acidic) if the client eats a high-protein diet or consumes cranberry juice.
Specific gravity	1.002–1.030	➤ Reflects the kidneys' ability to concentrate urine. ➤ Rises with dehydration or kidney disease. ➤ Decreases as fluid intake increases.
Clarity	A freshly voided sample should be translucent. If the urine sits for some time, it will become cloudy.	➤ Cloudiness in a freshly voided sample indicates the presence of other constituents in the urine (e.g., bacteria, RBCs, WBCs, sperm, prostatic fluid, or vaginal discharge).
Odor	Fresh urine is mildly odorous.	➤ Certain foods, such as garlic, onions, and asparagus, may give urine a distinctive odor. ➤ Vitamins (e.g., B_6) and medication can change the odor of urine. ➤ Bacteria with a bladder or kidney infection give urine an ammonia-like odor. ➤ A sweet odor may indicate an inborn metabolic disorder (maple syrup urine disease). ➤ Diabetes and liver failure can cause a different odor.
Protein	<20 mg/dL	➤ Most common indicator of renal disease (e.g., diabetic nephropathy, glomerulonephritis, nephrosis, or toxemia of pregnancy). ➤ May be increased in benign proteinuria secondary to stress or physical exercise. ➤ Foamy urine can mean there is more protein than normal.
Glucose	Negative	➤ Indicates elevated blood sugar (as in diabetes).
Ketones	Negative	➤ Indicates impaired carbohydrate metabolism. ➤ May be detected with diabetes, fever, fasting, high-protein or low-carbohydrate diet, vomiting, and during the postanesthesia period.
Hemoglobin	➤ Negative on dipstick ➤ If RBCs are assessed via microscopic exam: <5 per high-power field	➤ Detected with UTI, bladder or kidney disease or cancer, enlarged prostate, trauma, lupus, or sickle cell anemia. It also may be present in samples from women during menstruation.
Bilirubin	Negative	➤ Increased bilirubin occurs with liver disease, cancer, gallstones, or hepatitis.
Urobilinogen	Up to 1 mg/dL	➤ Increased in cirrhosis, heart failure, liver disease, infectious mononucleosis, malaria, and pernicious anemia.
Nitrite	Negative	➤ Increased in bacteriuria, presence of nitrite-forming bacteria, such as *Escherichia coli*.

Diagnostic Testing

Urinalysis—cont'd

Characteristic Findings	Expected	Variations
Leukocyte esterase	➤ Negative ➤ If WBCs are assessed via microscopic exam: <5 per high-power field	➤ Increased in bacterial infection, calculus formation, fungal or parasitic infection, glomerulonephritis, interstitial nephritis, or tumor.
Renal cells	None seen	➤ Indicates damage to the tubular network. (Renal cells come from the lining of the collecting ducts.)
Transitional cells	None seen	➤ Occurs with infection, trauma, and malignancy. (Transitional cells line the renal pelvis, ureter, bladder, and proximal urethra.)
Squamous cells	Rare	➤ Typically insignificant. (Squamous cells line the vagina and distal portion of the urethra.)
Casts	Rare hyaline; otherwise negative	➤ Large numbers of *hyaline casts* are seen in renal disease, hypertension, with diuretic use, and in fever. ➤ *Granular casts* occur in renal disease, viral infection, or lead intoxication.
Crystals	Absent in freshly voided sample	➤ May indicate an old sample, stone formation in the urinary tract, gout, high dietary intake of oxalates, liver disease, or side effect of chemotherapy.
Bacteria, yeast, parasites	None seen	➤ Microbes in urine indicate urinary tract infection (UTI).

Source: Adapted from Van Leeuwen, A. M., Poelhuis-Leth, D. J., & Bladh, M. L. (2019). *Davis's comprehensive manual of laboratory and diagnostic tests with nursing implications,* (8th ed.). Philadelphia, PA: F. A. Davis.

Diagnostic Testing

Blood Studies: BUN and Creatinine

Normal Ranges		Levels May Be Increased in:	Levels May Be Decreased in:
Blood urea nitrogen (BUN)	8–21 mg/dL	➤ Renal failure	➤ Inadequate protein intake
Creatinine	0.5–1.2 mg/dL	➤ Impaired renal perfusion	➤ Malabsorption syndromes
		➤ Kidney inflammation	➤ Liver disease
		➤ Kidney obstruction	
		➤ Dehydration	
		➤ Excessive protein intake	
		➤ Use of total parenteral nutrition (TPN)	

Source: Adapted from Van Leeuwen, A. M., Poelhuis-Leth, D. J., & Bladh, M. L. (2019). *Davis's comprehensive manual of laboratory and diagnostic tests with nursing implications,* (8th ed.). Philadelphia, PA: F. A. Davis.

Diagnostic Testing

Studies of the Urinary System

Direct Visualization Studies

Cystoscopy

Direct visualization of the urethra, bladder, and ureteral orifices by insertion of a scope. May be used to obtain biopsies and treat any pathology of visualized areas.

PREPARATION

- Instruct the patient that the procedure is performed under anesthesia. This anesthesia may be general, spinal, or local.
- Ensure that a signed consent form is included with the chart.
- Restrict food and fluids for 8 hours if the patient is receiving general anesthesia. For local anesthesia, allow intake of only clear liquids for 8 hours before the procedure.

POSTPROCEDURE CARE

- Monitor vital signs and intake and output (I&O).
- Observe the characteristics of urine after the procedure.
- Encourage increased fluid intake.
- Report suprapubic or flank pain, chills, or difficulty urinating.

Cystometry

Done to determine whether a muscle or nerve problem is causing problems with how well the bladder holds or releases urine. A catheter is inserted into the bladder and a pressure probe into the rectum. Warm fluid is injected and connected to the *cystometer*, which measures how much the bladder can hold and the pressure in the bladder. A gas or contrast material is sometimes used.

PREPARATION

- Ensure a signed consent form is included with the chart.
- Explain that patient cooperation with positioning and activity is crucial during the test.
- There are no food or fluid restrictions before the test.

POSTPROCEDURE CARE

- Monitor vital signs and I&O.
- Encourage increased fluid intake.
- Report suprapubic or flank pain, chills, or difficulty urinating.

Indirect Visualization Studies

Intravenous Pyelography (IVP) and Retrograde Pyelography

IVP uses IV radiopaque contrast medium to visualize the kidneys, ureters, bladder, and renal pelvis. It evaluates renal function by analyzing flow of contrast over time.

Retrograde pyelography uses radiopaque contrast medium to visualize the renal collecting system. Contrast media is injected via a ureteral catheter inserted through a cystoscope.

PREPARATION

- Assess for history of allergies. Radiopaque dyes can be highly allergenic for some patients; therefore, this test is contraindicated for patients with allergies to shellfish or iodinated dye.
- Ensure baseline BUN and creatinine results are available. This test is contraindicated for patients experiencing renal failure.
- Ensure that a signed consent form is included with the chart.
- Restrict food and fluids for 8 hours prior to the procedure. Check agency protocols for specific guidelines, especially related to fluid intake.
- Some patients may require a laxative the evening before the surgery to clear the gastrointestinal tract and improve visualization.
- Check to be sure diabetic patients who take insulin make an adjustment to the insulin dose when fasting for this examination.
- Determine the patient is not pregnant, breastfeeding, or with an intrauterine device (IUD) in place.
- Ask whether the patient has had an x-ray test using barium contrast material (e.g., barium enema) or have taken a medication containing bismuth (e. g., Pepto-Bismol) in the 4 days prior to the test. These can affect the test results.
- Check for a history of bleeding disorders or if the patient is taking any anticoagulant, aspirin, or other medications that affect blood clotting. It may be necessary to hold these medications prior to the procedure.

POSTPROCEDURE CARE

- Encourage increased fluid intake.
- Monitor vital signs and I&O.
- Observe for reactions to the contrast media: rash, nausea, hives.

Ultrasonography

Ultrasound (US) uses high-frequency sound waves to assess the size, shape, and location of the kidneys within the surrounding structures. Using a transducer on the skin, a picture is created with sound waves that reflect from the organs at different speeds, depending on the density of the tissue.

PREPARATION

- Ensure a signed consent form is included with the chart.
- There are no food or fluid restrictions with renal ultrasonography. A patient undergoing bladder ultrasonography may be required to drink five to six glasses of fluid 90 minutes before the procedure to ensure a full bladder.

POSTPROCEDURE CARE

- No special care is required.

Computed Tomography

Using contrast media, CT examines body sections from different angles by using a narrow x-ray beam to produce a three-dimensional image of the area of the body being scanned.

PREPARATION

- Obtain history of allergies. This test is contraindicated in patients with allergies to shellfish or iodinated dye.
- Ensure a signed consent form is included with the chart.
- For renal CT, food and fluids are usually restricted for 2 to 4 hours prior to the procedure.
- Remove all metal objects from the patient's body (e.g., eyeglasses, rings, safety pins).

Diagnostic Testing

Studies of the Urinary System—cont'd

POSTPROCEDURE CARE
- Monitor vital signs and I&O.
- Observe for reactions to the contrast media: rash, nausea, hives.

Renal Biopsy
Removal of a piece of kidney tissue for microscopic evaluation, usually done with ultrasound guidance.
PREPARATION
- Ensure baseline coagulation studies and hemoglobin results are available.
- Ensure a signed consent form is on the chart.
- Nothing by mouth (NPO) 6 to 8 hours prior to an open biopsy procedure and at least 4 hours prior to a needle biopsy procedure. Protocols may vary among facilities.
- Instruct the patient that sedation and/or pain medication may be given.

POSTPROCEDURE CARE
- Monitor vital signs and I&O.
- The patient will be on bedrest for 6 to 24 hours, as ordered.
- Monitor biopsy site for bleeding.
- Monitor urine for presence of blood.

Source: Adapted from Van Leeuwen, A. M., Poelhuis-Leth, D. J., & Bladh, M. L. (2019). *Davis's comprehensive manual of laboratory and diagnostic tests with nursing implications*, (8th ed.). Philadelphia, PA: F.A. Davis.

CLINICALJUDGMENT
Applying the Full-Spectrum Nursing Model

PATIENT SITUATION

An older adult woman, Mrs. Patel, has several health concerns, including diabetes and obesity. She seeks healthcare because she is experiencing burning with urination, frequency, and urgency. You explain to her these are signs of a urinary tract infection (UTI). You discover while taking the nursing history that she also is experiencing urinary incontinence (UI). When asked about toileting habits, she tells you she often doesn't "make it to the bathroom" even at home. This has been going on for about 3 years now. She has trouble getting up and walking upstairs to the bathroom because of a foot ulcer that isn't healing well. Mrs. Patel's affect is flat, with little expression. During your time with her, she seems to have little interest in talking about her health concerns. When you ask her about what she does to get out or socialize, she is hesitant to go far because she is afraid of wetting without knowing it and carrying an odor that would be embarrassing to her.

THINKING

1. *Theoretical Knowledge (Recall of Facts and Principles):*
   a. What kind(s) of UI is this patient likely to have?

   b. What are this patient's risk factors for UI?

2. *Critical Thinking (Contextual Awareness):*
   a. What aspects of this situation have you experienced or observed before in your role as a caregiver?

   b. How might those past experiences affect your perception in this situation?

DOING

3. *Practical Knowledge (Patient Teaching):*
   a. How could you encourage this woman to seek healthcare for managing her urinary incontinence?

   b. What might you ask your patient to do in order to get a better idea of her bladder history and toileting habits?

   c. By looking at Mrs. Patel's bladder diary, you see a pattern suggestive of UI. What other behavioral strategies might you suggest for improving her ability to have control of her bladder?

CARING

4. *Self-Knowledge:*

   a. Have you ever personally experienced urinary urgency, when you had trouble getting to the bathroom in time? Reflect on this experience, and examine how you might feel if you were incontinent much of the time.

   b. In what way(s) can you show compassion for the patient who has urinary incontinence?

Critical Thinking and Clinical Judgment

1. You receive a report from the UAP that a patient with no history of urinary elimination problems has had 150 mL of oral liquids in 6 hours and has voided 100 mL of clear, dark amber urine. His vital signs at the start of the shift were as follows: blood pressure 108/76 mm Hg; pulse 72 beats/min; respirations 18 breaths/min; temperature 98.6°F (37.0°C). The most recent check revealed blood pressure 112/80 mm Hg; pulse 88 beats/min; respirations 22 breaths/min; and temperature, 100.4°F (38.0°C).

   a. What conclusion might you draw about what has caused these symptoms?

   b. What actions should you take?

2. As you make patient rounds, you discover a collection bag for an indwelling catheter placed on the bed above the level of the patient's bladder.

   a. What should you do first? What assessments should you make?

   b. What teaching would be important in this situation?

3. Unlicensed assistive personnel (UAP) complain that Mr. Jones, a patient with dementia, keeps urinating in his trashcan and in the hallway.

   a. What special measures could be taken to assist Mr. Jones in finding the bathroom?

   b. What data could be helpful in developing a plan for Mr. Jones?

4. For each of the following concepts, use critical thinking to describe how or why it is important to nursing, patient care, or urinary elimination. Note that these are *not* to be merely definitions.

   Blood pressure

   Hydration

   Kidney tubules

   Specific gravity

   Developmental stage

   Urinary incontinence

   Privacy

What Are the Main Points in This Chapter?

- The urinary system consists of two kidneys, two ureters, the urinary bladder, and the urethra.
- The kidneys filter nitrogen and other metabolic wastes, toxins, excess ions, and water from the bloodstream and excrete them as urine.
- The bladder has a normal average storage capacity of 500 mL (1 pint), but it may distend, when needed, to a capacity twice that amount.
- Voiding occurs when contraction of the detrusor muscle pushes stored urine through the relaxed internal urethral sphincter into the urethra.
- The kidneys produce urine at a rate of approximately 60 mL per hour, or 1,500 mL per day. Most people urinate about five to six times per day.
- Voiding and control of urination require normal functioning of the bladder and the urethra, as well as an intact brain, spinal cord, and nerves supplying the bladder and the urethra.
- As adults age, the number of functional nephrons gradually decreases, along with the ability to dilute and concentrate urine. The potential volume of the bladder also decreases as the bladder wall loses elasticity; thus, older adults need to urinate more frequently.
- Substances that contain caffeine act as diuretics and increase urine production.
- A diet high in salt causes water retention and decreases urine production.
- Medications with anticholinergic effects inhibit the free flow of urine and may contribute to urinary retention.
- An adequately hydrated adult produces clear yellow urine. Concentrated urine is darker in color, but dilute urine can appear colorless.
- A clean-catch urine specimen is preferred for many diagnostic tests. To collect this specimen, the client must cleanse the genitalia before voiding and collect the sample in midstream.
- Sterile urine specimens may be obtained by inserting a catheter into the bladder or withdrawing a sample from an indwelling catheter.
- Twenty-four-hour urine collection requires collection of all urine voided in that period. The start time of the 24-hour collection begins when the first-voided urine is discarded.
- A routine urinalysis is one of the most commonly ordered laboratory tests. It is used as an overall screening test as well as an aid to diagnose renal, hepatic, and other diseases.
- Normal urine is free of bacteria, viruses, and fungi. Urinary tract infections are often caused by the introduction of *Escherichia coli*, which normally live in the colon, into the urethra and bladder.
- Urinary retention is an inability to empty the bladder. It may occur because of obstruction, neurological problems, infection, surgery, medications, or anxiety.
- Urinary catheterization is the introduction of a pliable tube (catheter) into the bladder to allow drainage of urine.
- Urinary incontinence (UI) is a lack of voluntary control over urination. Nurses can independently perform the primary interventions to manage UI.
- A urinary diversion is required when the bladder must be removed or bypassed. There are three options: a conventional urostomy or ileal conduit, a continent urinary reservoir, or a neobladder.
- A patient with a urinary diversion requires physical and psychological care. The goal is to have the patient become comfortable with his changed body and assume self-care.

Knowledge Map

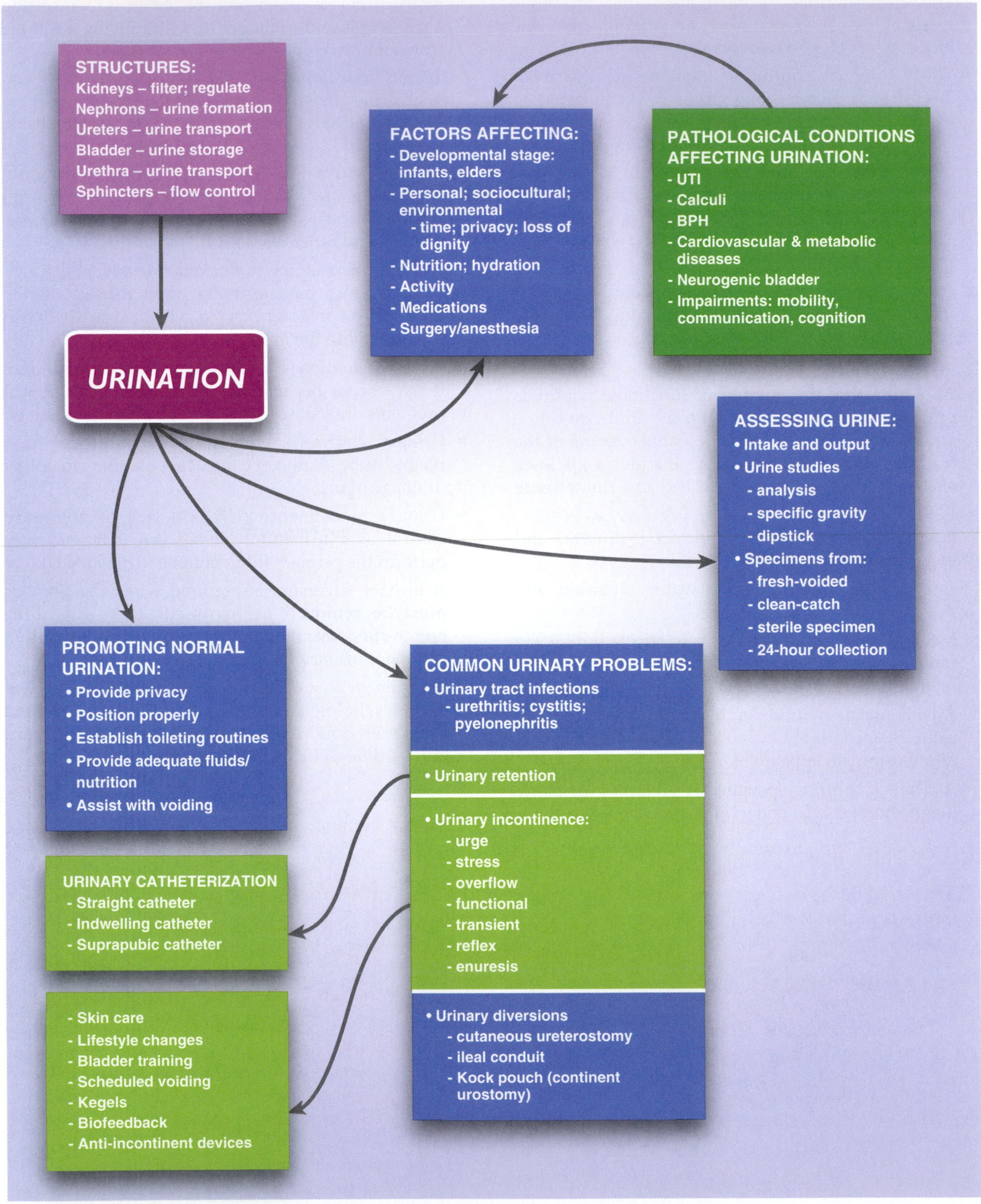

CHAPTER 29

Bowel Elimination

STUDENT RESOURCES

The questions and exercises in this book allow you to practice the kind of thinking you will use as a full-spectrum nurse. Critical-thinking questions usually have more than one right answer, so we do not provide "correct answers" for these features. Try to answer these questions yourself. It is more important to develop your nursing judgment than to just cover content. You will learn more by discussing the questions with your peers. If you are still unsure, see the Davis Advantage chapter resources for suggested responses.

To explore learning resources for this chapter,

Go to Davis Advantage and find:

Answers and Suggested Responses for all questions in this chapter
Concept Map
Knowledge Map
References and Bibliography
Lists of NOC Outcomes and NIC Interventions

Key Concepts

Bowel elimination
Motility

Related Concepts

See the Concept Map on Davis Advantage.

Example Problems

Bowel incontinence
Constipation and impaction
Diarrhea

Caring for the Nguyens

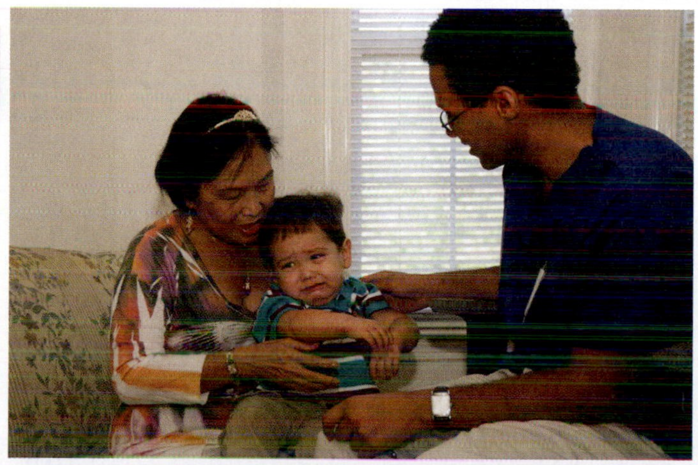

Yen Nguyen arrives at the family health center for a scheduled appointment, accompanied by her grandson Kim Phan. Recently, Yen has been constipated and has had several episodes of bleeding with bowel movements (BMs). She has read that a change in bowel habits is a sign of colon cancer and is worried about that. She brought her grandson along because he is also having bowel problems. Kim's bowel habits are erratic. At times he has a soft BM daily. However, he has also had bouts of constipation and diarrhea. Yen would like advice on her grandson's elimination status. As a critical thinker, you will begin by obtaining accurate, credible information.

(Continued)

Caring for the Nguyens (continued)

A. What history questions would be appropriate to ask Yen regarding her bowel concerns? What data do you need? How can you get the data? Are the data accurate? What information is important; what is not? Write some specific questions, just as you would ask them in an interview.

B. What physical assessments would you conduct for Yen to add to, and possibly to validate, your subjective data?

C. Now you must consider the context. What factors must you consider when gathering a history on Kim?

D. The family nurse practitioner (FNP) examines Yen and determines that she has external hemorrhoids that have been bleeding because of recent straining at stool. The FNP prescribes rectal suppositories to decrease the swelling of the hemorrhoids and asks you to teach Yen about necessary lifestyle changes. What additional information will you need to gather to provide this teaching? Recall that you have already obtained a significant amount of information from the history questions. Again, think about context: Whatever the content of your teaching, Yen will be using that information to care for herself and her grandson in her home.

E. The FNP examines Kim and tells you that the examination is normal. Use your theoretical knowledge of bowel elimination and Kim's developmental stage to think of possible reasons for his erratic bowel pattern.

PracticalKnowledge clinical application

To help you promote normal bowel elimination and support patients who have bowel elimination problems, this section applies concepts from Volume 1 to provide practical knowledge of procedures and clinical insights. You will also find assessment guidelines for assisting patients who are having diagnostic studies of the gastrointestinal (GI) system.

PROCEDURES

The procedures in this chapter will help you provide care to patients who have problems with bowel elimination.

Procedure 29-1 ■ Testing Stool for Occult Blood

➤ For steps to follow in *all* procedures, refer to the Universal Steps for All Procedures found on the inside back cover.

Equipment

- Clean gloves
- Tongue blade or other wooden applicator
- Clean, dry collection container to place in the commode, or a clean, dry bedpan
- Facility-specific fecal occult blood test (FOBT) slide or test paper
- Developing solution

Delegation

You can delegate the collection and testing of a stool sample for occult blood to the unlicensed assistive personnel (UAP) if the UAP has the necessary skills and the patient's condition is stable. Inform the UAP of any special considerations (e.g., the need to assist the patient with ambulation or the need for a bedpan). Instruct the UAP to inform you if there is visible blood in the stool and to show you the FOBT slide for evaluation of results when the test is complete.

Pre-Procedure Assessments

- Assess the patient's mobility status.
  Determines the patient's ability to participate in stool collection, the need for a bedpan or commode, and so forth.
- Assess the patient's dietary history for the past 24 to 48 hours.
  Some foods, such as red meat, chicken, fish, horseradish, turnips, or raw vegetables, may lead to a false-positive reading. Vitamin C in excess of 250 mg per day can produce a false-negative result (MEDLINE Plus, 2018).

- Assess medication history.
  If the patient is taking medications, such as salicylates, nonsteroidal antiinflammatory drugs (NSAIDs), iron, oxidizing drugs (e.g., iodine salts, boric acid), reserpine, corticosteroids, anticoagulants, colchicines, consult with a physician. These medications may cause a false-positive reading. If possible, they will be discontinued for 7 days before the test. If the patient must have them, then the results must be interpreted taking use of these medications into consideration.
- Assess for the presence of hemorrhoids.
  Any source of blood may cause a false-positive result for intestinal bleeding.
- If the patient is female, ask whether she is menstruating.
- Check the expiration date on the developing solution for the FOBT test slide.
- Assess the patient's or family's understanding of the need for the stool test.
  Provides a baseline for health teaching.

➤ When performing the procedure, always identify your patient according to agency policy, using two identifiers, and be attentive to standard precautions, hand hygiene, patient safety and privacy, body mechanics, and documentation.

Procedure Steps

1. **Determine whether the test will be done by the nurse** at the point of care (e.g., in the home or at the bedside) or by lab personnel.
   Because of the regulatory and billing practices in some settings, this test may be completed by lab personnel.
2. **Gather the necessary testing supplies**. Be sure you understand the directions for the testing kit you are using.
   This procedure gives instructions for using the FOBT slide method.
3. **Ask the patient to void** before collecting the stool specimen.
   Helps prevent contaminating the stool with urine.
4. **Perform hand hygiene, and don procedure gloves.**
5. **Place a clean, dry container** for the stool specimen into the toilet or bedside commode in such a manner that any urine falls into the toilet and the fecal specimen falls into the container. Obtain a clean, dry bedpan for a patient who is immobile.
   Using a sample of stool that comes in contact with either urine or water may produce an inaccurate test result.
6. **Instruct the patient to defecate** into the container, or place the patient on the bedpan. Do not contaminate the specimen with toilet tissue.
7. **Once the specimen has been obtained** and the bedpan removed or the patient assisted to bed, as necessary, perform hand hygiene, and don clean procedure gloves.
   Prevents the spread of intestinal bacteria.
8. **Explain the purpose of the test.** Explain to the patient that serial specimens may be needed.
   Testing serial specimens decreases the chances of a false-negative finding.
9. **Open the specimen side** of the FOBT slide. With a tongue depressor or other applicator, collect a small sample of stool and spread it thinly onto one "window" of the FOBT slide.
10. **With a different applicator** or the opposite end of the tongue blade, collect a second small sample of stool from a different location in the large sample. Spread the second sample thinly onto the second "window" of the slide.
    Reduces the possibility of a false-negative result.

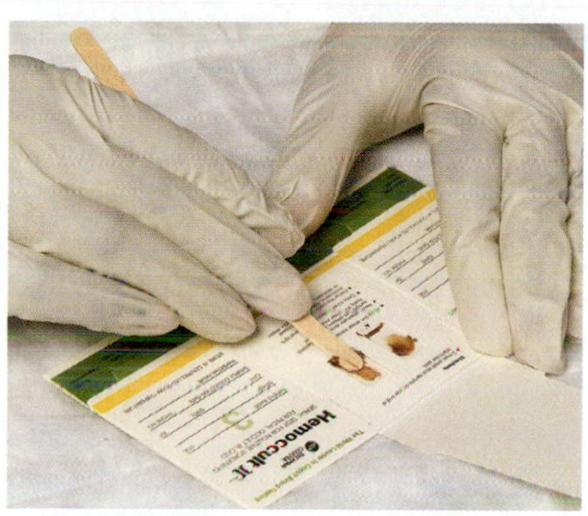

11. **Wrap the tongue depressor** in tissue and a paper towel; place it in a waste receptacle. Do not flush it.
    Prevents transfer of microorganisms. Flushing would likely clog the plumbing.
12. **Close the FOBT slide.**
    Prevents the transfer of microorganisms from the specimen smears on the slide.
13. **If the test is to be done by laboratory personnel**, transfer the specimen to a clean dry container, being careful not to contaminate the outside of the container with feces. Label the specimen in the presence of the patient according to agency policy, and place it into the proper receptacle for transportation to the lab.
14. **If you are to perform the test**, turn the slide over, and open the opposite side of the FOBT slide. Follow the directions on the package regarding the number of drops of the developing solution.
    Ensures an accurate reading.

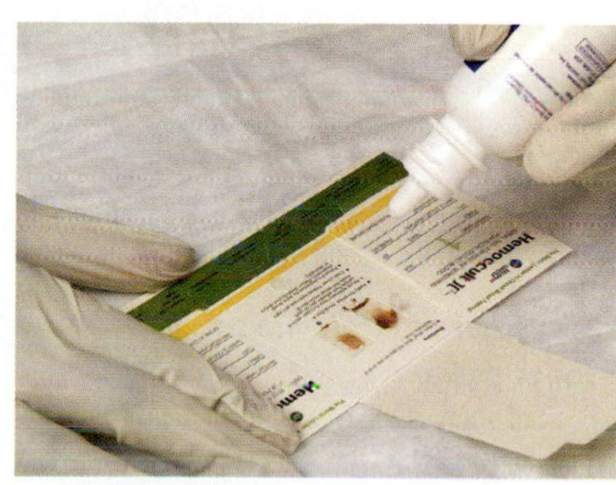

15. **Remove gloves,** and perform hand hygiene.

(continued on next page)

Procedure 29-1 ■ Testing Stool for Occult Blood (continued)

Evaluation

- Observe the color of the paper inside the FOBT slide windows for 30 to 60 sec.
- If the paper turns blue, consider the test for occult blood to be positive.

Patient Teaching

- Inform the patient of the reasons for performing the test.
- Explain the possible implications of a positive occult blood test, if one is obtained.

Home Care

- Determine the client's level of cognition and manual dexterity to assess his ability to follow instructions and physically perform the test.
- Explain necessary dietary and medication restrictions (see the Pre-Procedure Assessments section of this procedure).
- Instruct the client to collect the specimen in a clean, dry container. If an appropriate container is not available, the client may use the toilet.
- If the client is going to defecate in the toilet, the toilet should be flushed immediately prior to obtaining the sample. If commercial toilet bowl cleaners are in use, remove them from the tank, and flush twice before the client defecates. Then, lay rice paper (from the kit) directly on the water; it is okay to get it wet. When using the probe to take the stool sample, take the sample from any area of stool that is above the water line.
- Protect the slide from heat, light, and household chemicals.
- Home collection slides come in a kit, connected together as a set of three. Instruct the client not to tear them apart.
- Emphasize to the client that each sample should be from separate bowel movements on separate days.
- After all three specimens have been collected over the course of at least 3 days, store the slide in a paper envelope to air dry.
- The client must place the slides in the special mailing pouch that comes with the slides, if they are to be sent back to the lab. The slides should be returned to the care provider or the lab no later than 14 days after the first sample was collected. For additional instructions,

Go to the **Hemoccult Web site** at https://www.beckmancoulter.com/download/wsr-118305

Documentation

- Document the date and time of the specimen collection, both in the patient record and on the specimen container or FOBT kit.
- Note the appearance of the stool (e.g., color, odor) and the presence of blood, mucus, or other abnormal constituents.
- Note any rectal bleeding or discomfort during and after defecation.
- Document the test results on the appropriate agency form.
- Notify the appropriate care provider of the results.

Sample documentation

06/14/20 0915 Specimen taken from 2 separate sections of yellowish-brown soft stool containing mucus. No rectal bleeding or discomfort with defecation. Specimen sent to lab; test results pending. ——— S. Hoeszle, RN

Practice Resources

American Cancer Society (2016a); Bibbins-Domingo, K., Grossman, D. C., Curry, S. J., et al., (2016); Gomella L., & Haist, S. (2006); Leggett, B. A., & Hewett, D. G. (2015); Siegel, J., Rhinehart, E., Jackson, M., et al. (2007); The Joint Commission Accreditation Program (2018).

Procedure 29-2 ■ Placing and Removing a Bedpan

➤ For steps to follow in *all* procedures, refer to the Universal Steps for All Procedures found on the inside back cover.

Equipment

- Bedpan
- Two pairs of clean gloves
- Toilet tissue
- Prepackaged disposable wipes
- Waterproof pad
- Bedpan cover
- Linen-saver pad

Delegation

You may delegate the placement and removal of a bedpan to the UAP after ensuring that the UAP has the necessary skills and that the patient's condition is stable. Complete the pre-procedure assessments, and inform the UAP of any special considerations (e.g., medical or surgical conditions that will necessitate the use of a fracture pan and extra care with turning or required positioning based on medical condition).

Pre-Procedure Assessments

- Assess the patient's level of consciousness, ability to follow directions, mobility status, and physical status.
  Helps determine whether one or two persons are needed to complete the procedure.

- Determine the patient's comfort level—note the presence of rectal or abdominal pain, hemorrhoids, or perianal irritation.
Pain can cause difficulty with positioning and bearing down during defecation. Any unexplained pain should be evaluated by the primary care provider.
- Identify factors that will necessitate the use of a fracture pan. (Examples include a fractured pelvis; total hip replacement; lower back surgery; presence of casts, splints, or braces on lower limbs; or obesity.)
- Auscultate bowel sounds, and palpate for distention, if indicated.
The colon when full with fecal matter is a rounded, firm mass. A smooth, round mass above the symphysis pubis is a distended bladder.
- Review the patient's chart to determine the need to obtain a stool specimen.
Promotes efficiency by allowing you to obtain a specimen container before placing the patient on the bedpan.

Procedure 29-2A ■ Placing a Bedpan

➤ When performing the procedure, always identify your patient according to agency policy, using two identifiers, and be attentive to standard precautions, hand hygiene, patient safety and privacy, body mechanics, and documentation.

Procedure Steps

1. **Obtain the necessary supplies,** and take them to the patient's room. Warm prepackaged disposable wipes, and leave at the bedside for use during bedpan removal.
The patient will need to wash her hands after using the bedpan.

2. **If the bedpan is metal,** place it under warm, running water for a few seconds. Then, dry it, making sure bedpan is not too hot.
A warm bedpan allows the patient to be more comfortable and helps relax the anal sphincter. Most bedpans now are made of disposable plastic.

3. **Raise the siderail** on the opposite side from where you are working.
Prevents patient from falling out of bed and gives the patient something to hold onto while moving around in bed.

4. **Raise the bed** to a comfortable working height.
Allows you to use good body mechanics and prevents muscle strain.

5. **Prepare the patient** by folding down the covers to a point that will allow for placement of the bedpan, yet exposing only as much of her body as necessary.
Privacy facilitates elimination by promoting relaxation.

6. **Perform hand hygiene,** and don clean procedure gloves.
Prevents the spread of microorganisms via contact with urine or feces.

7. **Observe for the presence of** dressings, drains, intravenous (IV) fluids, and traction, and be sure there is a linen-saver pad in place.
These appliances may hinder the patient from assisting with the procedure and may create the need for assistance from another caregiver.

Procedure Variation: For the Patient Able to Move/Turn Independently in Bed

8. **Position the patient.**

Variation: Supine Position

a. Lower the head of the bed, placing the patient in a supine position.
b. Ask the patient to lift her hips. The patient may need to raise her knees to a flexed position, place her feet flat on the bed, and push up. You can also assist the patient to raise her hips by sliding a hand under the small of her back.

Variation: Semi-Fowler's Position

c. Place the bed in a semi-Fowler's position.
d. Ask the patient to raise the hips by pushing up on raised siderails or by using an overhead trapeze.

9. **Place the bedpan.**

Variation: Regular Bedpan

a. Place the bedpan under the patient's buttocks so that the wide, rounded end is toward the back.
Sliding the pan against the patient's skin may cause damage to skin.

Variation: Fracture Pan

b. Place the wide, rounded end of the pan toward the front.

10. **Instruct or assist the patient** to lower her hips onto the bedpan. Move to Step 16.

Procedure Variation: For the Patient Unable to Move/Turn Independently

11. **Ask for help** from another healthcare worker if the patient's condition warrants.

12. **With the patient in a supine position,** lower the head of the bed.

13. **Assist the patient** to a side-lying position. Use a turn sheet, if necessary.

14. **Place the bedpan.**

Variation: Regular Bedpan

a. Place the bedpan under the patient's buttocks so that the wide, rounded end is toward the back. Do not push the pan under the patient's buttocks. ▼

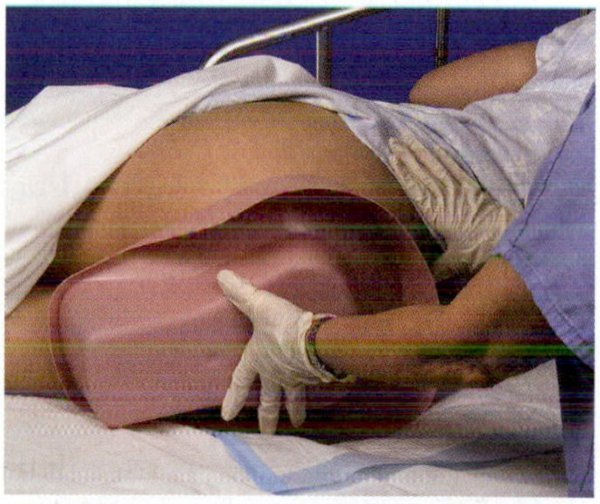

(continued on next page)

Procedure 29-2 ■ Placing and Removing a Bedpan (continued)

Variation: Fracture Pan

b. Place the wide, rounded end toward the front.

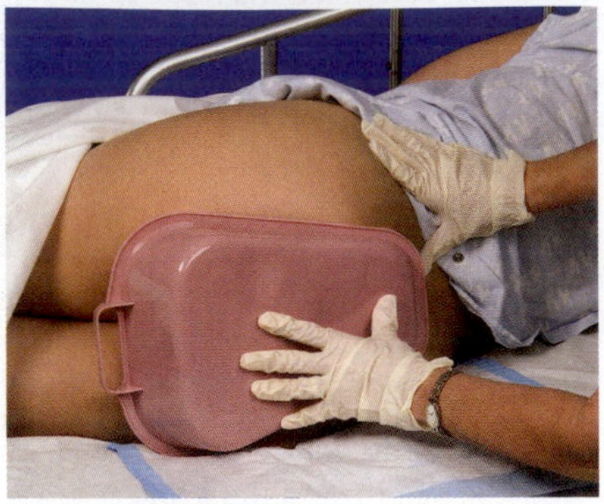

15. Holding the bedpan in place, slowly roll the patient back and onto the bedpan.

16. Replace the covers; raise the head of the bed to a position of comfort for the patient. Place a rolled towel, blanket, or small pillow under the sacrum (lumbar curve of the back).

17. Place the call light and toilet tissue within the patient's reach. Return the bed to its lowest position if not already done, and raise the upper siderails.
Provides privacy, comfort, and safety.

18. Remove your gloves, and perform hand hygiene.
Prevents the transmission of intestinal bacteria.

Procedure 29-2B ■ Removing a Bedpan

➤ When performing the procedure, always identify your patient according to agency policy, using two identifiers, and be attentive to standard precautions, hand hygiene, patient safety and privacy, body mechanics, and documentation.

Procedure Steps

1. Don clean procedure gloves. Open the prepackaged disposable wipes, and place them near the work area.

2. If the patient is immobile, lower the head of the patient's bed. Pull down the covers only as far as needed to remove the bedpan.
Lowering the head of the bed is necessary only if the patient is immobile.

3. Offer the patient toilet paper. Assist patients who are unable to complete this task independently.

4. Ask the mobile patient to raise her hips. Stabilize and remove the bedpan. If the patient is unable to raise her hips, stabilize the bedpan and assist her to a side-lying position.
Stabilizing the bedpan prevents spillage of contents.

5. Cleanse the buttocks with a warm, prepackaged disposable wipe. Allow to air dry.
Provides comfort and hygiene and decreases the risk of skin irritation and breakdown.

6. Replace covers, and position the patient for comfort. Offer the patient the second wipe to cleanse her hands.
Encourages independence with personal hygiene and decreases transmission of bacteria.

7. Empty the bedpan into the patient's toilet. Measure the output if that is part of the treatment plan. Clean the bedpan, following facility-specific guidelines.
If there is no toilet in the patient's room, cover the bedpan and carry it to the nearest toilet or soiled utility room for emptying.

8. Remove the soiled gloves, and perform hand hygiene.
Prevents transmission of infectious microorganisms.

? What if . . .

■ **Your patient is an older adult?**

Offer a bedpan at set intervals, perhaps in conjunction with a turning schedule. For elderly clients with limited mobility, you may wish to keep the bedpan readily available.
To minimize episodes of incontinence and/or falls. Trying to get out of bed to use the toilet is a common cause of falls.

Evaluation

- Assess the amount and characteristics of any urine and/or stool.
- Observe the skin on the perineum and buttocks for redness and skin breakdown.
- Note the presence of any unusual characteristics of either stool or urine, and include a description in the nursing notes. If there are no unusual characteristics, document the passage of stool or urine in the graphic records.

Home Care

Teach the patient's family the steps of this procedure.

Documentation

- Document the amount of urine voided if intake and output (I&O) are being recorded.

Practice Resources

Ayello, E., & Sibbald, R. (2016); Balas, M., Casey, C., & Happ, M. (2016); Gray-Micelli, D. (2016); Siegel, J., Rhinehart, E., Jackson, M., et al. (2007).

Thinking About the Procedure

The video, **Placing a Bedpan and Removing a Bedpan,** along with questions and suggested responses, is available on the ***Davis's Nursing Skills Videos*** Web site on FADavis.com.

Procedure 29-3 ■ Administering an Enema

➤ For steps to follow in *all* procedures, refer to the Universal Steps for All Procedures found on the inside back cover.

Equipment

- Enema administration container, correct enema solution, or prepackaged enema—depends on the type of enema ordered.
  - *Enema kit:* This may be a grouping of supplies that includes a small plastic bucket or a 1-liter plastic bag with attached tubing, disposable toweling, lubricant, and castile soap.
  - *Prepackaged enema solution:* If a prepackaged enema (e.g., Fleets) is ordered, you may need to obtain the preparation from the pharmacy or central supply department.
- Prepackaged disposable wipes and/or toilet tissue
- Bath blanket
- Waterproof pad
- Bedpan with cover or bedside commode, if needed
- Water-soluble lubricant
- Clean procedure gloves
- IV pole

Delegation

You may delegate this procedure to the UAP if the UAP is trained and the patient is stable. Complete the pre-procedure assessments, and instruct the UAP about conditions under which the procedure should be stopped (e.g., severe abdominal pain occurs, bleeding is seen, or the patient is unable to retain the solution). Instruct the UAP to report the results of the enema and show you any stool that appears to be abnormal (e.g., containing blood or pus).

Pre-Procedure Assessments

- Assess for history of bowel disorders (e.g., diverticulitis, ulcerative colitis, recent bowel surgery, abdominal pain, abdominal distention, hemorrhoids).
  Some disorders put the patient at risk for complications, such as mucosal irritation or perforation. Abdominal pain along with hypoactive bowel sounds and distention could indicate a bowel obstruction.
- Inspect the abdomen for the presence of distention.
  Establishes baseline for effectiveness of the enema.
- ✚ Review the patient's chart for the presence of increased intracranial pressure, glaucoma, or recent rectal or prostate surgery.
  An enema may cause the patient to strain, increasing the pressure on the brain or surgical incisions.
- Review lab results, paying particular attention to blood urea nitrogen (BUN), creatinine, and electrolytes.
  Hypertonic and hypotonic enemas have been linked to fluid and electrolyte changes. Phosphate enemas (Fleets) have been associated with hyperphosphatemia and hypocalcemia.
- Note the date and time of the patient's last bowel movement, recent bowel movement pattern, and bowel sounds.
  Establishes baseline for evaluating bowel function.
- Assess the patient's cognitive level and mobility.
  Determines the patient's ability to follow instructions and the need for placing him on a bedpan for the enema.
- Assess the patient's rectal sphincter control.
  Will determine whether you need to administer the enema with the patient on the bedpan. Also influences the amount of solution to instill.
- Assess for fecal impaction.
  May necessitate the need to obtain a prescription for a different type of enema.

Procedure 29-3A ■ Administering a Cleansing Enema

➤ When performing the procedure, always identify your patient according to agency policy, using two identifiers, and be attentive to standard precautions, hand hygiene, patient safety and privacy, body mechanics, and documentation.

Procedure Steps

1. **Before administering** a prescribed enema, explain the purpose of the enema and what the patient can expect (e.g., the patient will probably experience some cramping with a large-volume enema). Reassure the patient that you will be immediately available to help him to the restroom or bedpan.
2. **Place the bedpan nearby** or the commode near the bed.
   So you can reach the bedpan during the procedure or the patient can easily get to the commode.
3. **Open the enema supplies or kit.** Attach the tubing to the enema pail, if you are using a pail.
   The 1-liter enema bag comes with preconnected tubing.
4. **Close the clamp on the tubing,** and fill the container with 500 to 1,000 mL of warm solution. The water temperature should be lukewarm—105°F to 110°F (40°C to 43°C).
   ✚ Check the temperature with a bath thermometer. Never warm the enema solution in a microwave oven.
   a. For infants—use 50 to 150 mL of solution.
   b. For toddlers—use 250 to 350 mL of solution.
   c. For school-age children—use 300 to 500 mL of solution.
   Cold solution causes intestinal cramping. Very hot solution can damage the intestinal mucosa. Use the correct amount of solution to decrease the necessity of repeating the procedure.

(continued on next page)

Procedure 29-3 ■ Administering an Enema (continued)

5. **Add castile soap** (or the soap solution used by your facility) to the fluid at this time if a soapsuds enema has been prescribed.
Soap causes mucosal irritation, which stimulates peristalsis and defecation.

6. **Hang the container** on the IV pole. Holding the end of the tubing over a sink or waste can, open the clamp and slowly allow the tubing to prime (fill) with solution. Reclamp the tubing when the tubing is filled.
Expresses air from the tubing. Air introduced into the bowel may cause intestinal distention and discomfort.

7. **Don clean procedure gloves.**
Prevents the transmission of intestinal bacteria.

8. **Position the patient:** Ask or assist the patient to turn to a left side-lying position with the right knee flexed.
Allows the enema solution to fill the rectum and lower intestine following the natural flow of gravity.
   a. If the patient has shortness of breath associated with a respiratory condition, elevate the head of the bed very slightly. Avoid the semi-Fowler's position.
   The semi-Fowler's position increases the likelihood that gravity will cause the solution to leak out.
   b. Do not administer the enema with the patient on the toilet. The curved rectal tubing can scrape the rectal wall.
   c. If the patient has poor sphincter control, position him on the bedpan in a comfortable dorsal recumbent position.
   He will not be able to retain all of the enema solution.

9. **Place the waterproof pad** under the patient's buttocks or hips.
Prevents soiling of bed linens.

iCare 10. **Drape the patient** with the bath blanket, exposing only the buttocks and rectum. See Procedure 25-4 to review the procedure for draping.
Promotes patient privacy.

11. **Depending on the patient's** mobility status, place the bedpan flat on the bed, directly beneath the rectum, up against the patient's buttocks.

12. **Lubricate the tip of the enema** tubing generously.
Allows for ease of insertion, decreases patient discomfort, and helps prevent mucosal irritation.

13. **If necessary, lift the superior buttock** to expose the anus. Slowly and gently insert the tip of the tubing approximately 7 to 10 cm (3 to 4 in.) into the rectum. Have the patient take slow, deep breaths as you complete this step. If the tube does not pass with ease, do not force it. Allow a small amount of fluid to infuse, and then try again, inserting the tube slowly.
Helps the patient to relax, provides additional lubrication, and decreases reflex tightening of the anal sphincter.

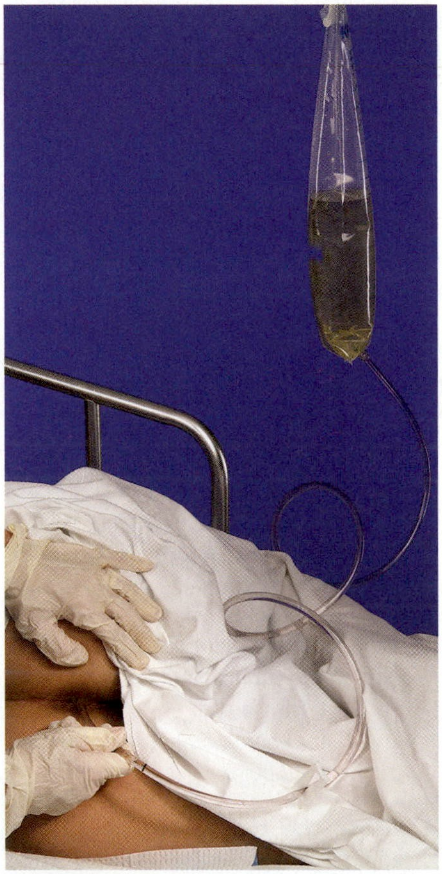

14. **Remove the container from the IV pole**, and hold it at the level of the patient's hips. Unclamp to begin instilling the solution.
Lowering the container slows the force of the instillation, decreasing pressure, cramping, discomfort, and reflex expulsion of the solution.

15. **Slowly raise the level** of the container, so that it is 30 to 45 cm (12 to 18 in.) above the level of the hips. Adjust the pole, and rehang the container. Continue a slow, steady instillation of the enema solution.
The height of the container determines the speed of the flow. A slow, steady rate of infusion decreases cramping and increases the patient's ability to retain the solution.

16. **Continuously monitor the patient** for pain or discomfort and ability to retain the solution. If the patient has difficulty with retaining the solution, lower the container, stop the flow for 15 to 30 seconds, and then resume the procedure.

If the patient feels pain or you meet with resistance at any time during the procedure, stop and consult with the primary care provider.

17. **When the correct amount** of solution has been instilled, clamp the tubing, and remove it slowly from the rectum. If there is stool on the tubing, wrap the end of the tubing in a disposable wipe or toilet tissue until it can be rinsed or disposed of.
Prevents transmission of pathogens.

18. **Clean the rectal area**, cover the patient, and instruct him to hold the enema solution for approximately 5 to 15 minutes. Be certain the call device is within reach.
- Retention of the enema solution will distend the bowel and increase the stimulus to defecate.
- Leaving the solution in the bowel too long may result in fluid and electrolyte complications.
- Retaining hypertonic solutions may result in dehydration related to large amounts of fluids moving from the capillary bed into the bowel. Excessive retention of hypotonic solutions may cause fluid overload.

19. **Dispose of the enema supplies** or, if they are reusable, clean and store them in an appropriate location in the patient's room.
Maintains a pleasant environment and helps prevent transfer of pathogens.

20. **Remove your gloves, and perform hand hygiene.**
Prevents transmission of intestinal pathogens.

21. **Depending on the patient's mobility**, assist him onto the bedpan, to the bedside commode, or to the toilet when he feels the need to defecate. Perform hand hygiene and use clean procedure gloves as necessary.

22. **After the patient has defecated**, remove the bedpan or assist the patient to bed; inspect the stool for color, consistency, and quantity.

Procedure 29-3B ■ Administering a Prepackaged Enema

➤ When performing the procedure, always identify your patient according to agency policy, using two identifiers, and be attentive to standard precautions, hand hygiene, patient safety and privacy, body mechanics, and documentation.

Procedure Steps

1. **Open the prepackaged enema.** Remove the plastic cap from the container. Clip the tip of the container if it does not have a hole in it. The tip of the enema container comes prelubricated. However, you may need to add extra lubricant.
Extra lubricant decreases discomfort and eases insertion of the tube into the rectum.

2. **Follow Steps 7 through 13 of Procedure 29-3A** (regarding gloving, positioning, draping, and inserting the enema tip).

3. **Tilt the container slightly,** and roll and squeeze the container slowly until all of the solution is instilled.
Ensures that the container empties completely and that an adequate amount of solution is instilled.

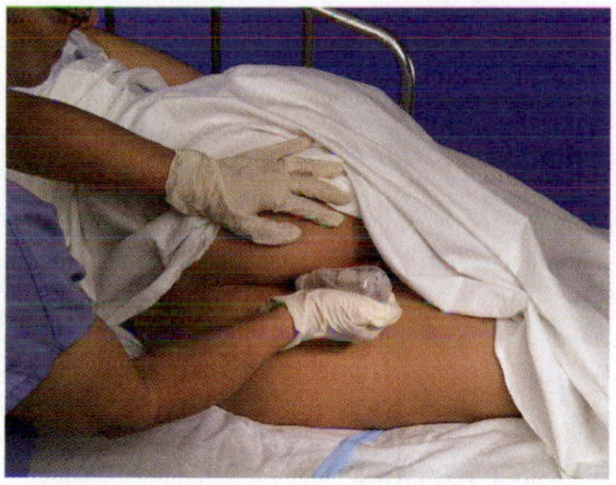

4. **Withdraw the container tip** from the rectum. Wipe the area with a disposable wipe or toilet tissue.
Prevents transmission of pathogens.

5. **Cover the patient, and instruct** him to hold the enema solution for approximately 5 to 10 minutes. Be certain the call light within reach.
Retention of the enema solution will distend the bowel and increase the stimulus to defecate. Retaining the solution for longer than the prescribed time has been associated with dehydration and electrolyte imbalances.

6. **Dispose of the empty container.**
Maintains a pleasant environment.

7. **Follow Steps 19 through 22 of Procedure 29-3A** (regarding equipment disposal, assisting the patient, and observations of stool).

Procedure 29-3C ■ Administering an Oil-Retention Enema

➤ When performing the procedure, always identify your patient according to agency policy, using two identifiers, and be attentive to standard precautions, hand hygiene, patient safety and privacy, body mechanics, and documentation.

➤ *Note:* An oil-retention enema may be administered to help a client pass hard stool; it also may be administered before digital removal of stool; or it may be given at least 1 hour before a cleansing enema. See Procedure 29-4 for digital removal of stool.

Procedure Steps

1. **Obtain a commercial oil-retention enema kit;** these kits include a small rectal tube. If a commercial kit is not available, use a small tube and about 90 to 120 mL of the prescribed solution.
A small tube allows for slower infusion, which minimizes cramping and thereby promotes retention.

2. **Warm the oil** to body temperature by running warm tap water over the container. Test a drop on your arm.
If the oil is too cold, it will cause cramping and expulsion of the oil. If it is too warm, it may injure the patient.

3. **Follow Steps 7 through 13 of Procedure 29-3A** (regarding gloving, positioning, draping, and inserting the enema tip).

4. **Instill the oil into the rectum.**
Softens stool and lubricates the rectum for easier passage of stool.

5. **Withdraw the container tip** from the rectum. Wipe the area with a disposable wipe or toilet tissue.

6. **Cover the patient, and instruct** the patient to retain the oil for at least 30 minutes.

7. **Follow Steps 19 through 22 of Procedure 29-3A** (regarding equipment disposal, assisting the patient, and observations of stool).

(continued on next page)

Procedure 29-3 ■ Administering an Enema (continued)

Procedure 29-3D ■ Administering a Return-Flow Enema

➤ When performing the procedure, always identify your patient according to agency policy, using two identifiers, and be attentive to standard precautions, hand hygiene, patient safety and privacy, body mechanics, and documentation.

➤ *Note: A return-flow enema (Harris flush) may be ordered to help a patient expel flatus and relieve abdominal distention.*

Procedure Steps

1. **Obtain a rectal tube and solution** container (e.g., bag or pail).
2. **Prepare 100 to 200 mL** (for adults) of tap water or saline, the temperature should be lukewarm—105°F to 110°F (40°C to 43°C).
3. **Follow Steps 7 through 13 of Procedure 29-3A** (regarding gloving, positioning, draping, and inserting the enema tip).
4. **Instill all the solution** into the patient's rectum.
5. **Lower the tube and container** below the level of the rectum, and allow the solution to flow back into the container.
6. **Repeat this process several times** or until the distention is relieved.
7. **Follow Steps 19 through 22 of Procedure 29-3A** (regarding equipment disposal, assisting the patient, and observations of stool).

? What if . . .

- **The solution for a return-flow enema becomes thick with fecal matter?**

  Discard it, and begin again with new solution.

Evaluation

- Observe the amount, color, and consistency of the stool.
- Evaluate the patient's tolerance of the procedure (e.g., amount of cramping, discomfort).
- Determine whether the prescriber's orders require subsequent enema administration.
- Some bowel exams require repeated enemas or enemas administered until the returns are "clear." For the latter, you will need to examine the return and determine whether stool particles are still present. "Clear" does not mean absence of color but, rather, absence of stool particles and transparency of the liquid.

Patient Teaching

- Teach the patient that dependence on enemas can disrupt the normal process that stimulates defecation.
- Teach dietary and lifestyle changes that promote regular elimination (e.g., increased fluid intake, diet high in fiber, increased exercise).

Home Care

- Show the patient the box for a prepackaged enema, and instruct him that he may purchase this type of enema at a local grocery or pharmacy.
- Assess the patient's ability to administer his own enema. If you determine that he will be unable to do so, encourage him to seek assistance and instruct the caregiver in the task.
- Teach the patient or the caregiver proper handwashing. Encourage them to purchase nonsterile procedure gloves.
  Patients and caregivers may not be aware of the serious infections that can be caused by gram-negative intestinal bacteria.
- If the patient will be attempting to self-administer a cleansing enema, help him determine how and where to hang the container so that it is at the proper height.
- If a soapsuds enema is to be administered in the home setting, teach the patient which household soaps may be substituted for castile soap.
  Some soaps used in the home may be too harsh and irritating to the intestinal mucosa.

Documentation

- Document on the nursing notes type of enema given and, if applicable, the amount of the solution instilled; patient's tolerance of the procedure; characteristics and amount of stool.
- If the prescription is to administer enemas until the returns are clear, document the color of the return solution and the amount of stool seen.
- For prepackaged enemas, some facilities require documentation on the medication administration record (MAR) of the time given and the nurse's initials.

Sample documentation

06/04/2020 0825 Fleets enema administered (see MAR). Patient had no cramping; retained enema for 5 minutes. Passed moderate amount of solid, formed, brown stool with no mucus, but with streaks of bright red blood on the surface. ——— R. Cline, RN

Thinking About the Procedure

The video, **Administering a Cleansing Enema**, along with questions and suggested responses, is available on the ***Davis's Nursing Skills Videos*** Web site on FADavis.com.

Procedure 29-4 ■ Removing Stool Digitally

➤ For steps to follow in *all* procedures, refer to the Universal Steps for All Procedures found on the inside back cover.

Equipment

- Two pairs of clean procedure gloves
- Water-soluble lubricant (containing lidocaine, if agency policy permits)
- Bedpan and cover
- Prepackaged disposable wipes (or moistened towelettes)
- Bath blanket
- Waterproof pad

Delegation

This procedure should not be delegated to a UAP. Ongoing assessment of the patient by the professional nurse is required when stool is manually removed from the rectum. The nurse must monitor the patient for complications, such as bleeding and vagal nerve stimulation. Nursing judgment is necessary in determining the need to halt the procedure.

Pre-Procedure Assessments

- Assess the patient's baseline vital signs and history of heart disease. Be sure to monitor the patient's pulse before and during the procedure.
  Digital removal of stool can stimulate the vagus nerve, causing bradycardia. Patients who have a history of heart disease or dysrhythmia are at greater risk. You should check the physician's order before performing this procedure.
- Assess the patient's white blood cell (WBC) count.
  If the patient has a compromised immune status, evidenced by a low WBC count, you should discuss this procedure with the primary care provider to evaluate the risks and benefits of the procedure.
- Assess the patient's cognitive level and mobility.
  Determines the patient's ability to follow directions and turn in bed.
- Determine the time of the patient's last bowel movement.
  The longer stool remains in the lower bowel, the more water can be absorbed and the more likely it is that hard stool may form in the rectum.
- Assess the patient for history of fecal impaction.
  Can be a recurrent problem for immobile, disabled, or institutionalized patients.
- Assess stool consistency.
  Patients who are immobilized may become incontinent of watery stool. They may be able to pass small sections of hard stool or small quantities of watery stool. The latter, which may be intermittent or continuous, is a symptom of high colon impaction.
- Ask whether the patient has pain on defecation.
  Pain can cause the patient to suppress defecation.
- Assess the patient's pattern of bowel movements, diet, exercise, mobility, and medications (e.g., iron supplements or opioid analgesics).
  Determine whether any of these factors contribute to the problem, and add this information to the nursing care plan to help prevent recurrence.
- Assess bowel sounds and any abdominal distention.
  Peristalsis may be present without GI patency. This creates abdominal distention, which can aggravate constipation.

Guidelines

- Prevention of fecal impaction is the best treatment, but if impaction has occurred, the stool must be removed. The procedure is both painful and embarrassing to your patient.
- An order from the healthcare practitioner may be necessary to perform digital disimpaction. Check your facility policy.
- Some practitioners may prescribe an oil-retention enema before the procedure to soften and moisten the stool, making removal easier.
- Many also advise that you follow digital removal of stool with either an oil-retention enema or a tap water enema to ensure evacuation of stool that may not have been reached by digital removal.
- Trim and file your fingernails if they extend past the end of your fingertips.
- **CAUTION:** Some resources suggest that this procedure should be done in small steps (no more than four finger insertions in one session), giving a series of suppositories between stool removal episodes. This is thought to prevent patient fatigue and pain, reduce the risk of injury to the rectal tissue, and minimize vagal stimulation.

➤ When performing the procedure, always identify your patient according to agency policy, using two identifiers, and be attentive to standard precautions, hand hygiene, patient safety and privacy, body mechanics, and documentation.

Procedure Steps

1. **Determine whether lubricant containing lidocaine is to be used,** and obtain the correct lubricant.
   May decrease rectal discomfort for the patient.
2. **Drape the patient** with the bath blanket. Go to Procedure 25-4 to review the procedure for draping. Assist him to turn on his left side, with his right knee flexed toward his head. Place the waterproof pad halfway beneath his left hip.
   Provides privacy and exposes the anus for visualization. The pad protects the bed from becoming soiled.

(continued on next page)

Procedure 29-4 ■ Removing Stool Digitally (continued)

3. **Don clean procedure gloves.** Some sources recommend double-gloving.
Prevents the transmission of intestinal bacteria.

4. **Expose the buttocks.** Place a clean, dry bedpan on the waterproof pad next to the buttocks in line with the rectum.

5. **Open the packet of prepackaged disposable** wipes, or have toilet tissue ready to cleanse the rectal area when you complete the procedure.

6. **Generously lubricate** either the gloved forefinger or the middle finger of your dominant hand.
Helps prevent discomfort, pain, and mucosal injury.

7. **Slowly slide one lubricated finger** into the rectum. Observe for perianal irritation.
The patient may need skin care to reduce pain during additional bowel evacuation.

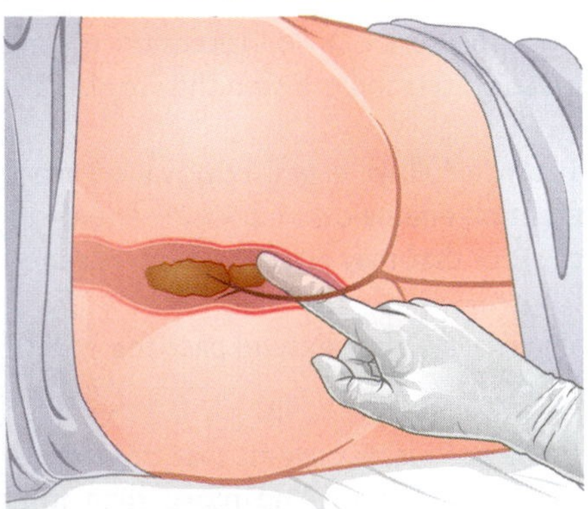

8. **Gently rotate your finger** around the mass and/or into the mass.
Assists in determining the amount and texture of the fecal bulk.

9. **Begin to break the stool** into smaller pieces. At this point, you may insert a second finger and gently "slice" apart the stool, using a scissoring motion. Remove pieces of stool via the rectum as it becomes separated, and place the pieces in the bedpan.

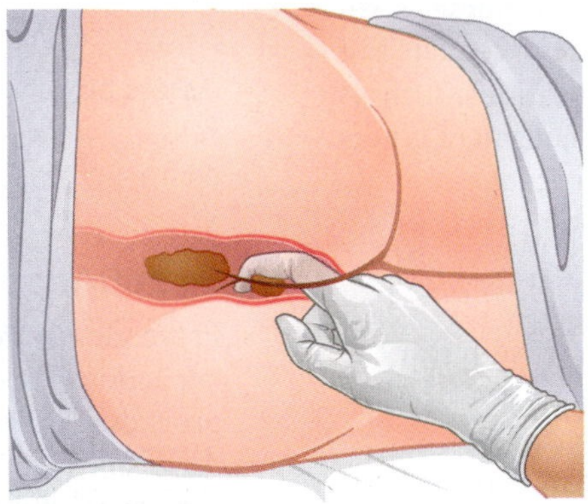

10. **As you proceed, instruct the patient** to take slow, deep breaths.
Helps the patient to relax his anal sphincter.

11. **Continue to manipulate** and remove pieces of stool, allowing the patient to rest at intervals. Reapply lubricant (containing lidocaine, if permitted) each time you reinsert your fingers.
Rest periods allow for assessment of and attention to the patient's comfort level and tolerance for the procedure.

12. **Assess the patient's heart rate** at regular intervals.
Bradycardia is a sign of vagal stimulation. Stop the procedure if the patient's heart rate falls or the rhythm changes from your initial assessment.

13. **When removal of stool** is complete, cover the bedpan, and set it aside. Use a prepackaged disposable wipe and/or toilet tissue to cleanse the rectal area.
Provides personal hygiene and decreases transmission of pathogens.

14. **Assist the patient to return to a position of comfort.** Note the color, amount, and consistency of the stool, and dispose of it properly.

15. **Remove your gloves,** and perform hand hygiene.
Prevents transmission of intestinal pathogens.

? What if . . .

- **The patient is an infant?**

When treating infants with fecal impactions, avoid enemas and mineral oils. Glycerin suppositories may be used to soften the stool before removal.

Evaluation

- Determine whether evacuation of the retained stool was complete. Perform a rectal exam to assess for presence of stool.
- Reassess vital signs, and compare the results to the initial assessment. Continue to monitor for 1 hour for bradycardia.
- Assess bowel sounds.
- Palpate the abdomen for tenderness and firmness.
- Ask the patient whether he feels relief from rectal pressure or abdominal discomfort.

Patient Teaching

Retained stool is most often the result of poor dietary habits, lack of fluid intake, lack of exercise, inattentiveness to the urge to defecate, and laxative abuse. Focus patient teaching on lifestyle changes that will facilitate a regular bowel elimination pattern.

Home Care

Home care should focus on preventing constipation that would require the digital removal of stool. Teach clients about high-fiber foods, adequate water intake, and the importance of exercise. Digital removal of stool may be necessary for some clients as part of a bowel-training program, (e.g., patients who are paraplegic or quadriplegic). You can teach this procedure to the caregiver in the home.

Documentation

- Document the bowel movement on the graphic record.
- Document the procedure and the patient's tolerance for the procedure in the nursing notes.
- Record the patient's pulse rate on the vital signs record.
- Document any unusual characteristics of the stool (e.g., black or green color, blood, or mucus).

Sample documentation

07/11/20 1815 Impacted stool removed digitally. No perianal irritation noted. Removed moderate amount (approximately 6 oz [170 g]) dry, hard, gray-colored stool. Pulse 78 before removal; 84 after. Encouraged 8 oz of fluid every hour. ——— C. Bryan, RNC

Practice Resources

Collins, B. R., & O'Brien, L. (2015); McKay, S. L., Fravel, M., & Scanlon, C. (2012); Siegel, J., Rhinehart, E., Jackson, M., et al. (2007).

Procedure 29-5 ■ Inserting a Rectal Tube

➤ For steps to follow in *all* procedures, refer to the Universal Steps for All Procedures found on the inside back cover.

Equipment

- 22- to 34-French (Fr) rectal tube for adults (Choose the size according to the size of the client. For children or petite adults, a smaller size tube [12- to 18-Fr] may be required.)
- Water-soluble lubricant
- Procedure gloves
- Toilet paper
- Skin care items (e.g., soap, skin cleanser, disposable wipes)
- Collecting device (waterproof pad, graduated cylinder partially filled with water, a urine collection bag nicked at the top to vent)
- Paper tape
- Stool specimen container, if needed

Pre-Procedure Assessments

- Obtain baseline vital signs.
- Auscultate bowel sounds; percuss for tympany.
- Observe and palpate the degree of abdominal distention.
- Ask whether the patient is passing any flatus.
- Assess for discomfort caused by flatulence.
- Assess the condition of the perianal tissues.
- Assess for any history of cardiac disease.
  Insertion of a rectal tube can stimulate the vagus nerve, causing bradycardia.

➤ When performing the procedure, always identify your patient according to agency policy, using two identifiers, and be attentive to standard precautions, hand hygiene, patient safety and privacy, body mechanics, and documentation.

Procedure Steps

1. **Wear procedure gloves.**
   Follows standard precautions.

2. **Ask the patient to lift his hips** or roll from side to side to place a waterproof pad.
   Protects against soiling of linens.

3. **Attach a collecting device** to the end of the rectal tube: Tape a plastic bag or urine collection bag around the distal end of the rectal tube, and vent the upper side of the bag. Alternatively, use one of these variations:

   Variations: Use One of These Alternatives:

   - Insert the tube into the specimen container.
   - Place the end of the tube in a graduated container partially filled with water.
     Collects small pieces of stool expelled with flatus. Venting the plastic bag prevents overinflation and bursting the bag. An advantage of using water in the container is that gas generates bubbles, and you will be able to assess the effectiveness of the rectal tube based on the amount of bubbling in the container.

4. **Place patient in a left side-lying position.** Drape for privacy.
   Allows the tube to follow the normal curve of the rectum and sigmoid colon when inserted.

5. **Lubricate the tip** of the rectal tube.
   Prevents trauma to the rectal mucosa.

6. **Separate the buttocks,** and ask the patient to take a deep breath. Gently insert the tube into the rectum.
   Adults—10 to 12.5 cm (4 to 5 in.)
   Children—5 to 10 cm (2 to 4 in.).
   Deep breaths relax the anal sphincter and ease tube insertion.

(continued on next page)

Procedure 29-5 ■ Inserting a Rectal Tube (continued)

7. **For adults, tape the tube** in place; for children, hold it manually.

8. **Leave the rectal tube in place** for 15 to 20 minutes. If distention persists, you may reinsert the tube every 2 to 3 hours.
Leaving the tube in place for more than 20 minutes may cause pressure necrosis of the mucosa; prolonged stimulation of the anal sphincter may result in loss of the neuromuscular response.

9. **Assist the patient to move** about in bed to promote gas expulsion. A knee–chest position is ideal.
Because gas is lighter than fluid or solid, the position promotes passage of flatus. Unfortunately, many patients cannot tolerate this position.

10. **Remove the tube**, wipe the patient's buttocks with tissue, and assist to clean the rectal area, as needed.
Prevents transmission of microorganisms from feces; promotes patient comfort and skin integrity.

11. **Dispose of used equipment**; or clean it if it is to be reused. Follow agency procedures for cleaning.

Evaluation

- Evaluate the patient's response to the procedure (e.g., vital signs, fatigue).
- Assess for abdominal distention and abdominal discomfort.

Patient Teaching

- Teach the patient that chewing gum, sucking on hard candy, using a straw, smoking, and drinking carbonated beverages increase air swallowing and abdominal distention.
- Teach factors that promote normal elimination (e.g., exercise, increased fluid intake, adequate dietary fiber).

Documentation

Record the following:
- Date and time tube was inserted
- Size of tube and characteristics of feces collected
- Abdominal distention before and after the procedure
- Pulse and respiratory rates before and after the procedure
- Tolerance of procedure and any complications
- Patient and family teaching

Procedure 29-6 ■ Changing an Ostomy Appliance

➤ For steps to follow in *all* procedures, refer to the Universal Steps for All Procedures found on the inside back cover.

➤ *Note: Some pouches come with the wafer attached and some without. These instructions assume that the wafer is attached.*

➤ *Note:* Also see Clinical Insight 29-2: Guidelines for Ostomy Care.

Equipment

- Ostomy pouch
  - One-piece pouch with the wafer attached or a two-piece system with a separate wafer and pouch
  - Clamp for pouches with an opening at the bottom (a new clamp is not used each time; usually one clamp is packaged with each box of pouches)
- Skin care items per agency protocol or recommended by the enterostomal therapist (e.g., pH-balanced skin cleanser, skin prep, skin barrier wipe, adhesive remover, adhesive paste, and stoma paste, if needed, to fill and smooth skin surface)
- Stoma measuring guide (or precut template)
- Scissors
- Pen or pencil
- Two pairs of clean procedure gloves
- Prepackaged disposable wipes
- Toilet tissue
- 4 × 4 inch gauze pad
- Bedpan or container for *effluent* (fecal material)
- Plastic bag (for disposal of used pouch)
- Plastic bag for disposal of other contaminated articles
- Waterproof pad
- Ostomy deodorant
- Hypoallergenic paper tape (optional) or ostomy belt
- Bath blanket

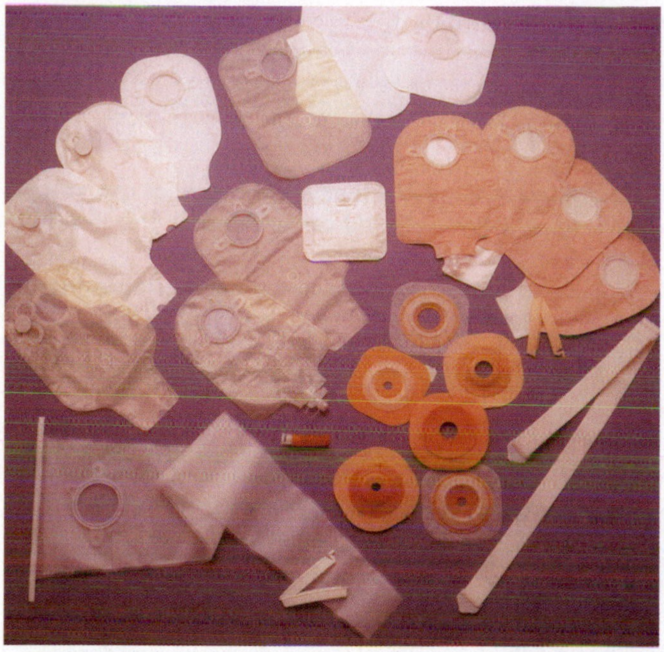

Delegation

During the immediate postoperative period, the professional nurse must assess the newly created stoma and peristomal skin area and use clinical judgment when changing a pouch. You may delegate to a UAP if it is a preexisting, stable stoma and if you are sure the UAP is qualified to perform the task. If you do delegate this task, instruct the UAP to report any changes or unusual findings (e.g., changes in stoma color, swelling, peristomal redness, excoriation, deviations from expected amount) and color and consistency of drainage from the stoma.

Pre-Procedure Assessments

- Assess the type of stoma (e.g., ileostomy, colostomy, urostomy), number of stomas, and location on the abdomen (e.g., is the stoma near structures that will impact care?).
  Determines the type of pouch or system to use.
- Assess stoma color, shape, size, and/or length of protrusion or retraction; stoma construction (end, loop, double barrel); direction of stoma lumen; and discharge. Does the stoma lie flat, or does it protrude?
  The stoma should be moist and red or pink. Alterations in stoma color (purple, black, or blue) may indicate poor circulation and possible necrosis and should be reported to the primary care provider. Protruding or retracted stomas will need special adjustments in wafer measurement and placement. It is normal for a new stoma to have yellow or blood-tinged mucus or dried blood on it.
- Assess peristomal skin for redness, rash, irritation, or excoriation. Observe the existing skin barrier and pouch for leakage and length of time in place. You may have to remove the pouch to observe the stoma fully, depending on the type of pouch (i.e., if the pouch is opaque). Notify the healthcare provider or an ostomy specialist immediately if you note peristomal skin abnormalities.
  Preserving peristomal skin is critical because skin excoriation may cause an ineffective seal between the wafer and the skin and leakage of effluent. This, in turn, causes more skin and tissue damage. Leakage may indicate the need for a different type of pouch system or sealant.
- Determine the changing schedule for the pouch.
  Pouches are usually changed every 3 to 5 days, preferably before leakage occurs. Frequency also depends on the type of stoma, the equipment used (e.g., one- or two-piece pouch), the effluent, the patient's preference, and the climate (i.e., pouches are changed more frequently during the summer). To decrease skin irritation, avoid changing the entire system. In a one-piece or two-piece pouching system, change the skin barrier only every 3 to 7 days, never daily.
- Observe abdominal shape and incision, if present.
  Abdominal shape determines the proper placement of the pouch. Because of stomal and abdominal characteristics, some patients may need convexity in their ostomy pouching system to avoid leakage.
- Assess the patient's willingness to look at the stoma, touch the appliance, and discuss or participate in the task.
  May indicate a readiness or desire to learn.
- Assess the patient's condition and self-care ability. Consider vision, dexterity or mobility, and cognitive ability.
  Helps determine best type of appliance to use.
- Auscultate for bowel sounds.
  Determines the presence of peristalsis.
- Observe for effluent from the stoma, and document your findings.
  Change the skin barrier pouch at times of lower effluent output. Avoid changing after meals, when the gastrocolic reflux increases chance of fecal effluent output. Mucus secretion is normal.
- Assess whether a new clamp will be needed or the one on the pouch can be used again.
- Consult a peristomal nurse or the primary care provider to determine whether an ostomy should be irrigated.
  Many patients with left-end colostomies may be safely irrigated as a method of continence management. An ileostomy, however, drains liquid containing high concentrations of sodium, chloride, potassium, magnesium, and bicarbonate.

Ileostomies should never be irrigated, except in cases of food blockage near the stomal outlet. Only a qualified person, such as an enterostomal therapy nurse, may perform a gentle lavage.

(continued on next page)

Procedure 29-6 ■ Changing an Ostomy Appliance (continued)

➤ When performing the procedure, always identify your patient according to agency policy, using two identifiers, and be attentive to standard precautions, hand hygiene, patient safety and privacy, body mechanics, and documentation.

Procedure Steps

1. **Perform hand hygiene,** and don clean procedure gloves.
Prevents transmission of pathogens.

2. **Fold down the bed covers** to expose the ostomy site. Place a clean towel across the patient's abdomen under the existing pouch.
Helps prevent spilling effluent onto the patient.

3. **Position the patient** so that no skinfolds occur along the line of the stoma.
Ensures an adequate seal between the wafer and the skin, preventing leakage.

4. **If the present ostomy pouch** is drainable, empty it into the bedpan.
Pouches should be drained when they are one-third to one-half full because the weight of the contents may dislodge the skin seal; ostomy drainage is irritating to the skin. The pouch also collects flatus, which needs to be expelled because it can disrupt the skin seal.
   a. To calculate the amount of output in milliliters for an ostomy with a liquid effluent (e.g., ileostomy or urostomy), use a graduated measuring container.
   b. For pouches that you open by unrolling them at the bottom, you must remove a clamp to empty the pouch. Save this clamp for reuse.

NOTE: Some pouches cannot be drained.

5. **Remove the appliance** by applying a silicone-based (hexamethyldisiloxane) adhesive remover, with one hand as you press the skin away from the wafer barrier with your other hand. Avoid pulling the appliance straight off. Begin at the top and work downward.
Silicone-based adhesive removers are preferred over alcohol- or oil-based products. Pulling the appliance from the skin tends to strip the loosely bound epidermal skin layers, making the skin more susceptible to moisture loss and irritation from effluent. Silicone-based products reduce the bind strength, whereas alcohol dissolves the adhesives; thus alcohol may cause dryness and irritation. It also causes pain if the skin is not intact. If you use an oil-based solvent, the new pouch will not adhere to the oily skin.▼

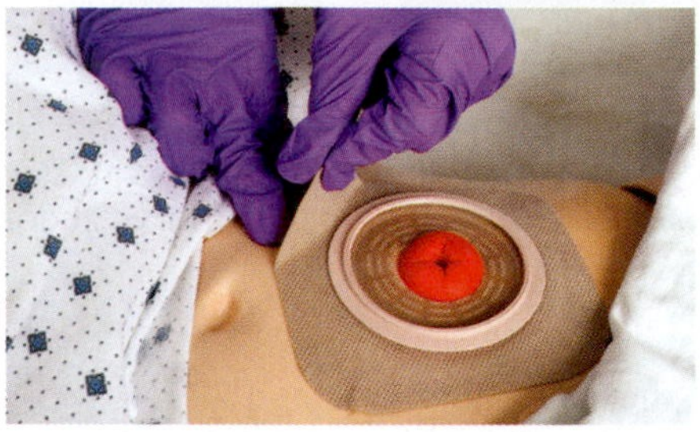

6. **Place the old pouch and wafer** in the plastic bag for disposal. If the pouch is not a drainable one, dispose of it according to agency protocol.
Prevents transmission of infections caused by fecal bacteria.

7. **Inspect the stoma** and peristomal skin area for redness, rash, irritation, or excoriation (see Pre-Procedure Assessments).

8. **Remove your gloves, and perform hand hygiene.**
Decreases the spread of intestinal bacteria.

9. **Don clean procedure gloves.**

10. **Cleanse the stoma** and surrounding skin using a skin cleansing agent with a pH of 5.5 that is designed to both cleanse and moisturize the skin.
Removes old adhesive and any effluent that has leaked. Helps prevent skin irritation and/or breakdown and maintain skin moisture. Select cleansing agents that protect the stratum corneum lipids and proteins.

11. **Remove gloves and perform hand hygiene.**

12. **Measure the size of the stoma.** You can accomplish this in several ways.
   a. Place a standard stoma measuring guide over the stoma.
   b. Reuse a previously cut template.
   c. Measure the stoma from side to side (approximating the circumference).
   The stoma may need to be remeasured frequently during the initial postoperative period because the size of the stoma may change as edema subsides.▼

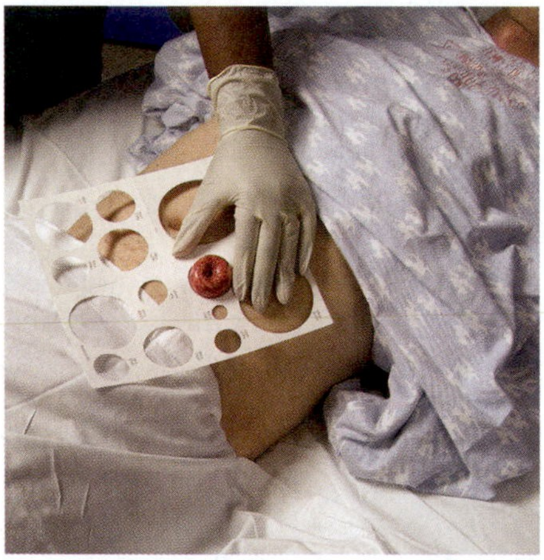

13. **Place a clean 4 × 4 in. gauze pad** over the stoma.
Gauze will absorb any leaking effluent, keeping the skin clean and dry during application of the new pouch.

14. **Trace the size of the opening** (obtained in Step 12) onto the paper on the back of the new wafer. Cut the opening. The opening in the wafer should be approximately 1/16 to 1/8 in. (1.5 to 3 mm) larger than the circumference of the stoma. Holding the wafer between the palms of your hand to warm the adhesive ring.
Allows for skin movement with activity and prevents impaired circulation to the stoma. Warming the adhesive ring enhances the integrity of the seal by making the ring more "sticky" so that it will bond better with the skin.

15. **Don clean procedure gloves.**

16. **Apply ostomy skin care products** at this time, using your clinical judgment, hospital protocol, or the recommendations of the enterostomal therapist (e.g., wipe around stoma with skin prep, apply skin barrier powder or paste, or apply extra adhesive paste).
These products prevent or treat excoriated skin and/or ensure a tight seal between the wafer and the skin.

17. **Remove the gauze** from the stoma. Center the wafer opening around the stoma, and gently press it down. Make sure the bag is pointed toward the patient's feet. Press your hand firmly against the newly applied wafer and hold for 30 to 60 seconds.

18. **Peel the paper off the wafer.** Center the wafer opening around the stoma, and gently press it down. Make sure the bag is pointed toward the patient's feet. Press your hand firmly against the newly applied wafer, and hold for 30 to 60 seconds.
Heat from the hand activates the adhesive ring, making it adhere better, thus, promoting optimal wear time. Some sources also suggest taping down the edges of the wafer.

19. **Remove your gloves,** and perform hand hygiene.

20. **Return the patient** to a comfortable position.

21. **Dispose of the used ostomy** pouch following your facility's policy for biohazardous waste.

? *What if . . .*

- **My patient has a two-piece pouch?**
After applying the wafer around the stoma with a good seal (Step 16), attach the bag following manufacturer's instructions.
- **My patient's ostomy uses an open-ended pouch?**
After applying the wafer securely around the stoma, fold the end of the pouch over the clamp, and close the clamp, listening for a "click" to ensure that it is secure.
- **When cleansing the stoma (Step 10), you notice that the stoma is bleeding?**
Slight bleeding of the stoma is normal; report excessive bleeding to the primary care provider.

Evaluation

Make the following observations:

- Characteristics of stoma: color, size, presence of edema, and shape
- Presence of blisters, redness, or excoriation on peristomal skin
- Amount and characteristics of effluent: color, odor, consistency
- Whether the patient expressed a desire to participate in the task
- Whether the patient demonstrated nonverbal cues that she is ready to learn about the task (e.g., looking at the stoma)

Patient Teaching

Patient teaching is aimed at preparing the patient to complete this skill at home. She (or a caregiver) will need to be instructed in how to complete all the steps of the procedure.

Home Care

- Assess the patient's self-care ability and assist the client to establish a routine for changing the stoma wafer/pouch (see Clinical Insight 29-2). The client may need to stand in front of a mirror or sit to change her ostomy appliance if she is unable to view the stoma easily.
- Teach the client that slight bleeding is normal when the stoma is washed.
- The client should not use soaps and lotions containing oils. They decrease the adhesiveness of the wafer.
- The appliance and the wafer cannot be flushed down the toilet.
- Teach the client to report changes in the color or size of the stoma and/or the presence of peristomal irritation or skin breakdown to the primary care provider.
- Provide information about ostomy supply vendors and community support groups, such as Ostomates (https://www.ostomy.org/support-group-finder/).

Documentation

Document the following:

- Your assessment of the stoma and peristomal skin area
- Patient's tolerance of the procedure
- Type of appliance used, including the manufacturer and part number
- Use of any special ostomy skin care products
- Amount of liquid effluent (on the I&O portion of the graphics record)
- Patient teaching and the degree to which the patient participated in the procedure

(continued on next page)

Procedure 29-6 ■ Changing an Ostomy Appliance (continued)

Sample EHR documentation

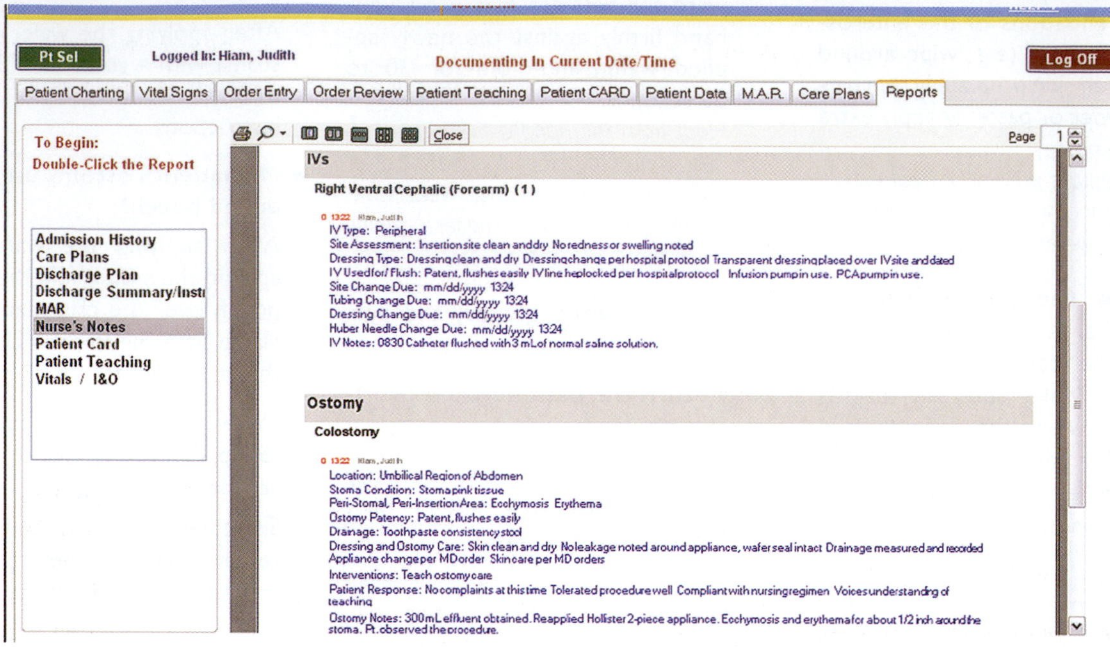

Practice Resources

Burch, J. (2014); Gray, M., Colwell, J. C., Doughty, et al. (2013); Siegel, J., Rhinehart, E., Jackson, M., et al. (2007); Tam, K. W., Lai, J. H., Chen, H. C., et al. (2014).

Thinking About the Procedure

The video, **Changing an Ostomy Appliance**, along with questions and suggested responses, is available on the ***Davis's Nursing Skills Videos*** Web site on FADavis.com.

Procedure 29-7 ■ Irrigating a Colostomy

➤ For steps to follow in *all* procedures, refer to the Universal Steps for All Procedures found on the inside back cover.

Equipment

- Irrigation equipment
  - One-piece system with a fluid container connected to tubing with cone or two-piece system with a container separate from tubing with cone
  - Irrigation sleeve (A sleeve without adhesive backing requires a belt to hold it in place.)
  - Clamp for a sleeve with an opening at the top
  - Prescribed irrigating solution—usually 500 to 1,000 mL warm tap water, 100°F to 105°F (40°C to 43°C)
- IV pole or other equipment to hang the irrigation container
- Chair
- Water-soluble lubricant
- Silicone-based adhesive remover
- Skin cleansers and barriers as recommended by your agency
- Toilet tissue
- Prepackaged disposable wipes
- Waterproof pad
- Two pairs of clean procedure gloves
- Toilet facilities that include a flushable toilet and a hook or some other device to hold the irrigation container; or bedpan or bedside commode (for patients with impaired mobility)
- New ostomy appliance and skin barrier or stoma cap cover
- Ostomy deodorant (optional)
- Plastic bag for disposal of the used pouch

Delegation

The initial irrigation of a newly created colostomy requires nursing judgment and clinical decision making. Initially, this procedure should not be delegated to the UAP, although in some situations it may be delegated to an LPN, depending on agency policy.

Pre-Procedure Assessments

- Evaluate the defecation pattern (or absence) nature of stool, placement of stoma, abdominal distention, and nutritional pattern.
  Findings may indicate the need to irrigate to stimulate elimination function; consistency of stool varies along the length of the GI tract.

- **Identify the type of ostomy.**
  Many patients with left-end colostomies may be safely irrigated as a method of continence management. However, do not irrigate an ileostomy.
- **Assess the patient's usual bowel pattern.**
  The purpose for irrigating a colostomy is to promote a regular pattern of bowel elimination.
- **Assess for abdominal distention.**
  Report distention to the primary care provider, as it may indicate excess gas or inflammation.
- **Assess hydration.**
  The colon may absorb some of the irrigation fluid if the patient is very dehydrated.
- **Assess cognitive level and mobility.**
  Determines the necessity for a bedpan or bedside commode. Also determines whether patient teaching will be effective.
- **Assess the patient's ability to maintain a sitting position.**

➤ When performing the procedure, always identify your patient according to agency policy, using two identifiers, and be attentive to standard precautions, hand hygiene, patient safety and privacy, body mechanics, and documentation.

Procedure Steps

1. **Place an IV pole near** the location of the procedure (e.g., in the bathroom, next to the bedside commode, or next to the bed).
   Allows you to work efficiently.

2. **Assist the patient to the bathroom** or commode, if possible. Ask the patient whether she prefers to sit directly on the toilet or on a chair in front of it. If the patient must remain in bed, elevate the head of the bed.
   Patients with impaired mobility can sit directly on or in front of the bedside commode or may remain in bed in a side-lying position.

3. **Prepare the irrigation container.**
   a. For two-piece systems, connect the tubing to the container. Clamp the tubing. Fill the container with 500 to 1,000 mL of warm tap water.

   Water that is too cold will cause cramping, nausea, and discomfort. Water that is too hot will damage the intestinal mucosa.

   NOTE: Some ostomy resources suggest that using 1,000 mL of water will promote a more effective irrigation of the entire colon and decrease the necessity to irrigate more than once a day.

4. **Hang the solution container** on the IV pole. Adjust the pole so that it reaches the height of the patient's shoulder (approximately 45 cm [18 in.] above the stoma).
   The height of the container regulates the force of the flow.

5. **Unclamp the tubing to prime it,** and allow it to fill.
   Removes air from the tubing, preventing gas pains.

6. **Perform hand hygiene,** and don clean procedure gloves.
   Prevents the transmission of pathogens.

7. **Remove the existing colostomy appliance** (if the patient is wearing one) following the steps in Procedure 29-6.
   Use of ostomy skin care preparations may be needed when you replace the pouch.

8. **Dispose of the used colostomy** appliance properly. Empty the contents into the bedpan or toilet, and discard the pouch in a moisture-proof (e.g., plastic) bag.
   Prevents transmission of intestinal bacteria.

9. **Assess the characteristics** of the stoma and the surrounding skin (see Clinical Insight 29-2).

10. **Apply the colostomy irrigation sleeve,** following the manufacturer's directions.
    - ***If your patient is sitting on a toilet*** or bedside commode, then the end of the sleeve should hang down past the patient's pubic area, but not down into the water. Place a waterproof pad under the sleeve over the patient's thighs.
    - ***If your patient is in bed,*** place the end of the sleeve into the bedpan.
    Prevents leakage and spilling of irrigation fluid and effluent.

11. **Generously lubricate the cone** at the end of the irrigation tubing with water-soluble lubricant.
    Prevents irritation and damage to the stoma and intestinal lumen.

12. **Open the top of the irrigation sleeve;** insert the cone gently into the colostomy stoma, and hold it solidly in place.
    Gentle insertion prevents damage to the mucosa.

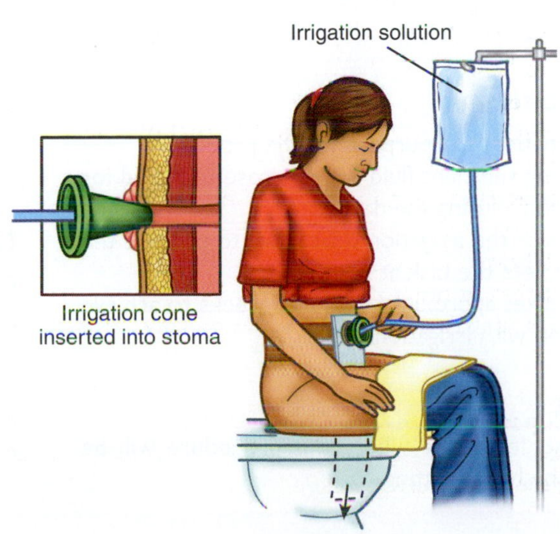

(continued on next page)

Procedure 29-7 ■ Irrigating a Colostomy (continued)

13. **Open the clamp on the tubing,** and slowly begin the flow of water. The fluid should flow for about 10 to 15 minutes or as the patient can tolerate.
Proceeding slowly allows the patient to adjust to the distention of the bowel.

14. **If the patient complains** of discomfort, stop the flow for 15 to 30 seconds, and ask the patient take deep breaths.
Allows the patient to rest and adjust to the pressure of solution. Cramping may indicate that the bowel is ready to empty, the water is too cold, the flow is too fast, or the tube contains air.

15. **When the correct amount of solution** has instilled, clamp the tubing, and remove the cone from the stoma.

16. **Wrap the end of the cone** in tissue or paper towel until you can clean or dispose of it properly.
Prevents transmission of intestinal bacteria.

17. **Close the top of the irrigation sleeve** with a clamp.
Prevents spillage of irrigation fluid and feces.

18. **Wait for evacuation to occur:**
    - ***If the patient is sitting***, ask her to remain sitting until most of the irrigation fluid and bowel contents have evacuated. Alternatively, you can clamp the end of the sleeve and ask the patient to ambulate to stimulate complete evacuation of stool.
    - ***If the patient is in bed***, massaging the abdomen may also help stimulate return.

    This should take about 30 minutes on average. You might wait for about an hour to be certain all the fecal material has been returned.

19. **When evacuation is complete,** open the top clamp, and rinse and remove the irrigation sleeve. Set it aside.
The irrigation sleeve is reusable, but it should be rinsed promptly to make thorough cleansing easier in the following steps.

20. **Change gloves.**

21. **Cleanse the stoma** and peristomal skin area with a warm prepackaged disposable wipe. Prep the skin and apply a new colostomy appliance, if the patient is wearing one, following the steps in Procedure 29-6. Otherwise, cover the stoma with a small gauze bandage.

22. **Clean the irrigation sleeve** with mild soap and water. Allow it to dry. Place the irrigation supplies in the proper place (e.g., in a plastic container or plastic bag).
The irrigation sleeve must be cleaned well to avoid odors and transmission of pathogens.

23. **Remove your gloves** and perform hand hygiene.
Prevents healthcare-associated infections.

24. **Assist the patient back to** a position of comfort.

? What if . . .

- **Your patient has a colostomy sleeve without an adhesive backing?**
Place the belt around the patient's waist, and attach the ends to the pouch flange on either side.

Evaluation

Observe the following:

- Characteristics of the stool: color, amount, consistency
- Signs of bleeding from stoma or bowel
- Presence or absence of abdominal distention
- Patient's tolerance of procedure (e.g., cramps, fatigue)
- Patient's ability to participate in the irrigation

Patient Teaching

- Explain to the patient the purpose for the procedure.
- Explain that using sufficient fluid will decrease the need for multiple irrigations during the day.
- Teach the steps of the irrigation procedure to prepare the patient to complete the task at home.
- Explain that it takes approximately 6 to 8 weeks to achieve bowel regulation with irrigations.

Home Care

- Help the client determine where this procedure will be completed in the home setting.
- Make sure the client has resources for purchasing the supplies for the irrigation. Provide contact information.
- Help the client locate a place to hang the irrigation container. For instance, there may be a hook on the bathroom wall.
- If the irrigating solution does not flow well, the client should:
  Check the tubing for kinks
  Change the position of the cone
  Put the container at a slightly higher level
- Explain and demonstrate how to care for the irrigation supplies (e.g., how to rinse and clean the sleeve and/or belt, if used).

Documentation

Document:

- Your assessment of the stoma and peristomal area
- The amount of irrigation solution used
- The date and time that you performed the irrigation
- Characteristics of the stool returned in the irrigation fluid
- Patient teaching

Sample documentation

06/14/20 0830 AM Ostomy irrigated with 750 mL warm tap water. Small amount of loose, formed, flakey stool returned in the fluid, with some undigested food apparent. No blood; very small amount of mucus. Stoma pink, peristomal area without redness. Explained procedure steps to patient as it was performed. Patient stated he will do some of the steps tomorrow. ——————— C. Hiam, RNC

Practice Resources

Avent, Y. (2012); Bauer, C., Arnold-Long, M., & Kent, D. J. (2016); Cobb, M. D., Grant, M., Tallman, N. J., et al. (2015); Kent, D. J., Arnold- Long, M., & Bauer, C. (2015); Siegel, J., Rhinehart, E., Jackson, M., et al. and the Healthcare Infection Control Practices Advisory Committee (2007).

Thinking About the Procedure

The video, **Irrigating a Colostomy,** along with questions and suggested responses, is available on the ***Davis's Nursing Skills Videos*** Web site on FADavis.com.

Procedure 29-8 ■ Placing Fecal Drainage Devices

➤ For steps to follow in *all* procedures, refer to the Universal Steps for All Procedures found on the inside back cover.

Equipment

External Fecal Collection Device

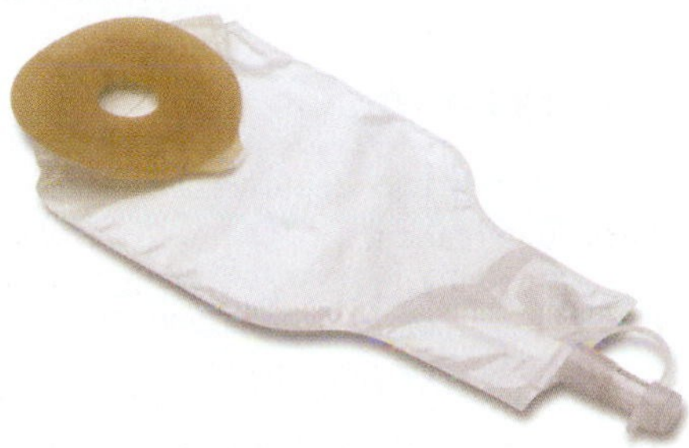

- pH-balanced soap and water or recommended skin cleanser
- Skin protection wipes (e.g., peristomal wipes to protect skin and improve adherence)
- Self-adhesive fecal containment device
- Procedure gloves
- Linen-saver pad
- Scissors

Internal Fecal Collection System

- Fecal device kit: Contains soft silicone catheter tube assembly, a syringe, and a collection bag.
- Water-soluble lubricant
- Approximately 100-mL container of tap water or saline (Follow the manufacturer's directions for amount and type of solution.)
- 500 mL of lukewarm irrigant (water or saline)
- 60-mL luer-tip syringe and a catheter tip syringe (if not contained in the kit)
- Protective skin-care dressing (e.g., Stomahesive, DuoDerm)
- Tape
- Procedure gloves, mask, and goggles
- pH-balanced soap and water or recommended skin cleanser
- Scissors
- Linen-saver pad

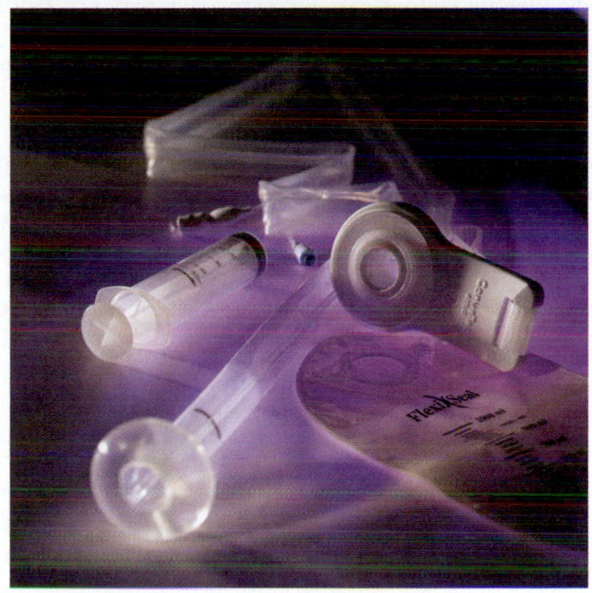

Delegation

Application of an external fecal collection system may be delegated to the UAP. Insertion of an internal fecal collection device is usually performed by a professional nurse, but may be delegated to an LPN, depending on agency policy.

Pre-Procedure Assessments

- Assess the patient's bowel patterns.
  Fecal diversion is indicated when the patient is incontinent of liquid or semi-liquid stools (flowing).
- Assess for allergies to silicone. If the patient is sensitive or allergic to any of the materials in the device, it cannot be used.
- Inspect perirectal skin.
  External devices should not be used in patients with impaired skin integrity.

(continued on next page)

Procedure 29-8 ■ Placing Fecal Drainage Devices (continued)

For Indwelling Devices, in Addition:

- Assess whether the patient has had a recent bowel movement.
  Patients who have not had a bowel movement for 2 or more days should be considered as having firm stool and will likely be given a bowel prep or enema before insertion of the indwelling device.
- Check for the presence of any indwelling anal or rectal device (e.g., thermometer for continuous temperature monitoring).
  The treatment plan may need to be changed. If suppositories or enemas are a part of the current treatment plan, collaborate with the prescriber, as these medication delivery mechanisms will need to be changed.
- Identify factors that increase your patient's risk for bleeding, including medications (anticoagulant and/or antiplatelet therapy) and lab results (prothrombin time [PT], partial thromboplastin time [PTT], platelets).
  Patients with an increased risk of bleeding should be monitored carefully.
- Check the chart for contraindications to an indwelling fecal management system (e.g., proctitis, lacerations, rectal surgery in the past year, large or painful hemorrhoids).
  If your patient has a history of any of these problems, contact the primary care provider immediately. You may elect to use an external device, but an internal fecal catheter is contraindicated.
- Internal fecal catheters should not be used for children.

Procedure 29-8A ■ Applying an External Fecal Collection System

➤ When performing the procedure, always identify your patient according to agency policy, using two identifiers, and be attentive to standard precautions, hand hygiene, patient safety and privacy, body mechanics, and documentation.

Procedure Steps

1. **Recruit another nurse** or nursing assistant to help you. Assist the patient to a side-lying position, and drape to expose the buttocks.
   For successful application (without leakage) it is best to have one caregiver position the patient and a second person apply the device.
2. **Don procedure gloves.**
   Observes standard precautions.
3. **Cleanse the perineal area,** and dry well. If perianal hair is present, trim it away.
4. **Wipe the area** with skin protectant wipes.
   To obtain a leak-proof seal, the device should be attached to clean, dry skin. The wipes protect the skin and improve adherence.
5. **Spread the buttocks apart** to expose the anus.
6. **Remove the backing from the adhesive** on the fecal bag, then apply it, being careful to place the opening in the bag over the anus and to avoid gaps and creases.
   Careful application helps to obtain a leak-proof seal.
7. **Release the buttocks.** Connect the fecal incontinence pouch to a drainage bag.
8. **Hang drainage bag below the patient.**
   To collect and promote gravity drainage of fecal material.

Procedure 29-8B ■ Inserting an Indwelling Fecal Drainage Device

➤ When performing the procedure, always identify your patient according to agency policy, using two identifiers, and be attentive to standard precautions, hand hygiene, patient safety and privacy, body mechanics, and documentation.

➤ *Note: Because devices differ markedly, it is best to follow the manufacturer's instructions for placing the device. The following are generic instructions.*

➤ *Note:* Also see Clinical Insight 29-1: Caring for a Patient With an Indwelling Fecal Drainage Device.

Procedure Steps

1. **Ensure that a primary care provider has performed a digital rectal exam.**
To assess for contraindications and to check sphincter tone. When sphincter tone is compromised, the patient may not be able to retain the device.

2. **Don procedure gloves, mask, and goggles.**
To protect from splatters when irrigating or disconnecting the device. Usually, the devices are used for incontinence of loose, if not liquid, stool.

3. **Position the patient** in a left side-lying position.
Allows access to the rectum.

4. **Remove any indwelling device.**
The presence of a foreign body between the inflated balloon and rectum may damage rectal mucosa, and a seal cannot be maintained.

5. **Depending on the type** of device, verify proper inflation and deflation of the intraluminal balloon. Attach the syringe, inflate with the recommended amount of air, deflate, and remove the syringe.

6. **Again depending on the device,** fill the retention cuff with 35 to 40 mL of water; disconnect syringe and check for leaks. After verifying function, slowly and completely aspirate all fluid from cuff and balloon, and disconnect the syringe.

7. **Connect the indwelling tube** to the collection bag. Clamp and hang the bag lower than the level of the patient.

8. **Some systems have an** "introducer," which you must inflate with about 25 mL of air through a connector on the tube. Disconnect the syringe. ▼

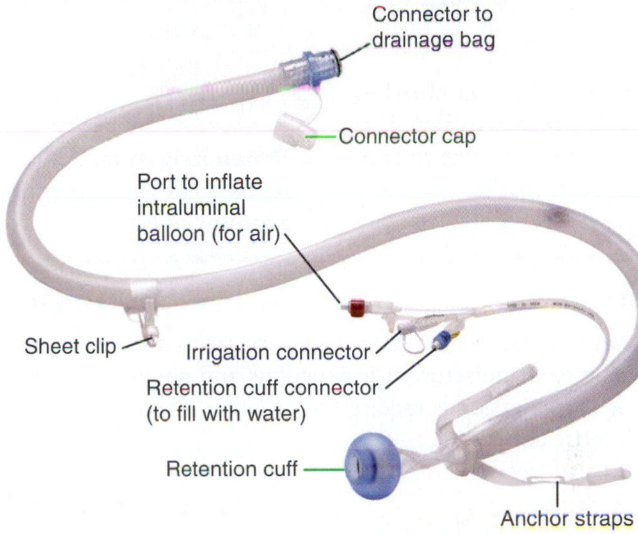

9. **Insert your lubricated, gloved index finger** into the balloon cuff finger pocket (located above the position indicator line), and coat the balloon generously with lubricant.
This allows for digital guidance during insertion.

10. **Gently insert the balloon end** of the catheter through the anal sphincter until the balloon is beyond the anus and well inside the rectal vault.
This helps prevent accidental expulsion of the device.

11. **Inflate the retention cuff** with water or saline, per the manufacturer's guidelines. Do not overfill. If the catheter will not accept the recommended amount of fluid, see the What If . . . ? section at the end of this procedure. ➤

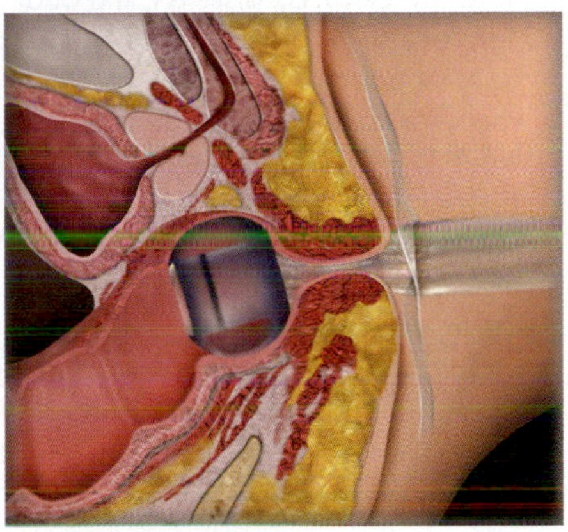

12. **Remove the syringe** from the inflation port and put gentle traction on the catheter.
To determine whether the balloon is securely in the rectum and appropriately positioned against the rectal floor.

(continued on next page)

Procedure 29-8 ■ Placing Fecal Drainage Devices (continued)

13. If you inflated an intraluminal balloon or introducer in Step 8, you must now completely aspirate the air from it.

Do not leave an air-inflated intraluminal balloon inflated in an unattended patient.

An inflated balloon can cause tissue necrosis after some time.

14. If the device has anchoring straps, apply protective skin care dressing, and tape one strap to each of the patient's buttocks.

Prevents internal migration of the tube and occlusion by twisting of the tube.

15. Position the tubing along the patient's leg, avoiding kinks and obstruction, and position the collection bag lower than the patient.

Promotes flow of stool from the rectum to the collection bag.

? What if . . .

- **When irrigating, the catheter will not accept the recommended amount of fluid?**

  Deflate the balloon and reposition the catheter.

  The catheter is probably not positioned correctly. Do not use more than the recommended amount of fluid as this would result in excessive pressure on the rectal vault and may cause mucosal or sphincter damage.

- **Rectal bleeding occurs with an internal fecal management device?**

  Discontinue the device, and notify the physician.

  Bleeding may indicate pressure necrosis from the device.

Evaluation

- Confirm catheter/bowel lumen patency by irrigating the bowel, according to manufacturer's instructions and physician order. Regular irrigation is required to facilitate evacuation through most devices.

  Stool needs to be of loose consistency to pass through the indwelling tube.
- Assess how well the patient tolerated the procedure.
- Note the color, consistency, and odor of stool.
- Monitor the amount of stool in the collection bag. Change the fecal pouch at least every 72 hours (per protocol) and whenever there is evidence of leakage.
- When the collection bag is approximately two-thirds full, change it.
- Monitor for abdominal distention and pain.
- Regularly assess that connections are secure and that the device is not leaking.
- In addition, for indwelling devices monitor:
  - Length of time the device is in place

    Not intended for use longer than 29 days.
  - Rectal bleeding

    May indicate tissue necrosis, bowel perforation, or fistula formation; device must be removed.

Documentation

- Date, time, and type of collection device used
- Your assessment of the perineal skin
- Patient's tolerance of the procedure
- Characteristics and amount of stool in the collection bag (output)
- Patient/family teaching

Sample documentation

09/15/20 1435 After prepping skin, an external fecal collection device was applied. Patient tolerated procedure well. Rationale for device was explained. Pt and family verbalized they will report leaking, pain, or discomfort. Device is draining large amounts of brown liquid stool, with no visible mucus or blood.——— J. Smiley, RN

Practice Resources

Ayello, E., & Sibbald, R. (2016); Lukacz, E. S., Segall, M. M., & Wexner, S. D. (2015); Neilson, J., Avital, L., Willock, J., et al. (2014); Pittman, J., Beeson, T., Carter, B., et al. (2015); Siegel, J., Rhinehart, E., Jackson, M., et al. (2007); Wound, Ostomy and Continence Nurses Society (2017).

Thinking About the Procedure

The video, **Applying an External Fecal Collection System,** along with questions and suggested responses, is available on the ***Davis's Nursing Skills Videos*** Web site on FADavis.com.

CLINICAL INSIGHTS

Clinical Insight 29-1 ➤ Caring for a Patient With an Indwelling Fecal Drainage Device

With an indwelling fecal drainage device, a catheter is present in the rectum and connected to a drainage tube and collection bag.

Nursing Goal 1: Prevent Injury to Rectal Sphincter and/or Rectal Mucosa.

- Do not add air or fluid to the balloon port of the catheter.
- Check the catheter frequently for kinks or obstructions.
- Monitor for signs of complications, and notify the health-care provider immediately if the patient experiences rectal pain, rectal bleeding, abdominal distention, or abdominal pain.
- Monitor stool for change in consistency (solid or soft-formed stool cannot pass through the catheter and will cause an obstruction).
- How to discontinue the catheter:
  1. Attach a 60-mL syringe to the balloon inflation port, and deflate the retention balloon by pulling back on the plunger.
  2. Grasp the catheter as close to the patient as possible, and slowly slide it out of the anus.
  3. Dispose of the device, according to the agency policy for disposal of medical waste.

Nursing Goal 2: Maintain Free Flow of Liquid Stool.

- Monitor the patient for changes in stool consistency. If the stool is no longer liquid and flowing, the device must be discontinued.
- Make sure the tubing and bag remain below the level of the patient.
- Irrigate the tube as often as necessary to maintain patency:
  1. Fill a 60-mL syringe with room-temperature tap water.
  2. Attach it to the irrigation port of the catheter and flush by depressing the plunger.
     Be sure you are using the irrigation port, *not* the balloon inflation port.
  3. Be sure to subtract the irrigation fluid from the stool volume to maintain an accurate record of intake and output.
- Change the collection bag when it is three-fourths full.
  1. Remove the collection bag from the tubing. Snap the cap onto the used bag and dispose of it, according to agency policy for medical waste.
  2. Snap new collection bag securely onto the device.

Nursing Goal 3: Prevent Transmission of Pathogens to Others.

- Follow the agency protocol for hand hygiene. Always wear clean procedure gloves when handling the fecal management device.
- Monitor stool cultures and implement isolation protocols, as indicated. If a stool sample is ordered, you may obtain it from the collection bag:
  1. If the collection bag is more than 24 hours, old place a new collection bag before obtaining a sample.
  2. Cut the collection bag at the bottom, and transfer stool to an appropriate container for transport to the lab.
  3. Apply a new collection bag to the connector at the end of the catheter.

Nursing Goal 4: Maintain Perineal Skin Integrity or Prevent Wounds from Being Contaminated by Stool.

- Monitor insertion site for leakage and signs of infection.
- If perineal wounds are present, keep clean and dry; notify the primary provider if signs of infection are present.
- Perform perineal care, according to agency policy.

Clinical Insight 29-2 ➤ Guidelines for Ostomy Care

Assess Stoma Appearance.

- The stoma should be moist and red or pink.
- Immediately report to the surgeon a stoma that is pale, dusky, or black in color; dry; or with sloughing tissues. These are signs of inadequate blood supply to, and possible necrosis of, the portion of intestine that has been externalized.
- Protruding or retracted stomas will need special adjustments in wafer measurement and placement. It is normal for a new stoma to have yellow or blood-tinged mucus or dried blood on it.

Preserve Peristomal Skin.

- Preserving peristomal skin is critical because skin excoriation may cause an ineffective seal between the wafer and the skin and leakage of effluent. This, in turn, causes more skin and tissue damage. Leakage may indicate the need for a different type of pouch system or sealant.
- Use recommended moisture-proof barrier creams and skin care products.

Plan for and Change the Pouch as Scheduled.

- Change the skin barrier pouch at times of lower effluent.
- Avoid changing after meals, when the gastrocolic reflux increases chance of fecal effluent. Mucus secretion is normal.
- Pouches are usually changed every 3 to 5 days, preferably before leakage occurs. Frequency also depends on the type of stoma, the type of equipment used (e.g., one- or two-piece pouch), the effluent, the patient's preference, and the climate (e.g., pouches are changed more frequently during the summer).
- To decrease skin irritation, avoid changing the entire system. In a one-piece or two-piece pouching system, change the skin barrier only every 3 to 7 days, never daily.

Assess the Patient's Self-Care Ability.

- Patients with poor vision may need to use magnification mirrors and yellow-tinted sunglasses to help reduce glare and improve contrast when they perform stoma care.
- Patients with immobility or spinal cord injury may need equipment that has a longer pouch that the patient can empty independently when sitting.
- Impaired dexterity or vision may warrant the use of a one-piece system or precut pouch and skin barrier, whereas a two-piece system may be better for patients who need to keep the skin barrier in place for several days and change just the pouch.
- Patients who are blind can be taught to change the equipment by themselves.

Determine Whether the Ostomy Should be Irrigated.

- Consult a peristomal nurse or the primary care provider to determine whether an ostomy should be irrigated.
- Many patients with left-end colostomies may be safely irrigated as a method of continence management. An ileostomy, however, drains liquid containing high concentrations of sodium, chloride, potassium, magnesium, and bicarbonate.
- Ileostomies should never be irrigated, except in cases of food blockage near the stomal outlet. Only a qualified person, such as an enterostomal therapy nurse, may perform a gentle lavage. For lavage, normal saline is preferred because excessive lavage could lead to a serious fluid and electrolyte imbalance.

Promote Psychological Adaptation.

- Be available to discuss the patient's reaction to the stoma. Your attitude and willingness to discuss the patient's body changes will help your patient begin adapting.
- Show acceptance when working with the patient and the stoma.
- Provide adequate ventilation and odor control when assessing the stoma or ostomy appliance.
- Provide ample time to explain stoma care and use of ostomy appliances. For most patients, this is a lifelong task; therefore, patient teaching is essential.
- Teach the client about diet modifications.
- Encourage patients to return to their usual activities as much as possible.
- Encourage patients to discuss intimacy issues associated with the ostomy. Use the PLISSIT model (in Chapter 33) if necessary, and convey to them that sexual functioning is an appropriate topic to discuss. You may wish to use The United Ostomy Associations of America's *Intimacy After Ostomy Surgery Guide*, or give it to the patient (Schuler, 2013).
- Refer the patient to the local ostomy association, if one is available. Most of the counselors are skillful because, they, too, have ostomies. They are able to share practical and personal information based on their own experience with similar challenges. To find the local chapter consult your phone book, or

Go to the **United Ostomy Associations of America** Web site at https://www.ostomy.org/

ASSESSMENT GUIDELINES AND TOOLS

Focused Assessment

Bowel Elimination

Nursing History

Ask the following questions such as:

1. **Normal bowel pattern**
   - How often do you have a bowel movement (BM)?
   - What time of day do you usually have a BM?
   - Do you follow any routines to help you have a BM?
2. **Appearance of stool**
   - How would you describe your stool?
   - What color is your stool?
   - How would you describe the texture of your stool—hard, soft, or watery?
   - What shape is the stool?
   - Have you noticed unusual odor with your stool?
3. **Changes in bowel habits or stool appearance**
   - Have you had any changes in your bowel pattern recently?
   - Have you noticed any changes in the appearance, texture, or odor of your stool?
4. **For clients with a bowel diversion**, also gather data on the client's usual care of the stoma, use of appliances, and adjustment to the ostomy.
5. **History of elimination problems**
   - What has been your experience with bowel elimination problems?
   - Have you had any problems with constipation, diarrhea, or severe bloating or gas?
   - Have you ever lost control of your bowels?
   - Have you ever had bowel surgery or diagnostic procedures of the digestive tract?
6. **Use of bowel elimination aids**, including diet, exercise, medications, and remedies
   - What aids, if any, do you use to help you have a BM?
   - What foods help you maintain your bowel pattern?
   - What foods do you avoid? What effect do these foods have on you?
   - What is your usual fluid intake over the course of a day?
   - What is your usual exercise pattern?
   - What medications are you taking? Have they had any effect on your bowel elimination pattern?
   - What is your current stress level? What effect does stress have on your bowel elimination pattern?

Physical Assessment

Examine the abdomen, rectum, and anus.

- Recall that in abdominal assessment, the order of the exam is inspection, auscultation, percussion, and palpation.
- Observe the size, shape, and contour of the abdomen.
- Percuss and palpate the abdomen for tenderness, presence of air or solid, and presence of masses.
- Inspect the anus for signs of hemorrhoids.
- Depending on the policies of your institution as well as your skill with assessment, you might also palpate the anus and rectum for the presence of stool or masses.
- When listening to bowel sounds, note the presence and timing of the sounds and the presence of any bruits. Note whether the sounds are normal, hyperactive, hypoactive, or absent. (If you need to review, see Focused Nursing History in Volume 1.)
- If, after listening for 3 to 5 minutes, you hear no bowel sounds, you should listen in several areas before describing them as absent.

For a complete discussion of physical examination of the abdomen, rectum, and anus,

Go to Chapter 22, **Procedure 22-14: Assessing the Abdomen,** and **Procedure 22-19: Assessing the Anus and Rectum,** in Volume 2.

DIAGNOSTIC TESTING

Diagnostic Testing

Direct Visualization Studies of the Gastrointestinal Tract

- These studies are invasive procedures; ensure that the patient has signed an informed consent.
- All of the procedures require some degree of advance preparation, such as fasting. Check agency policy, as preparation may vary.
- Preparing the patient includes telling him what he will experience and feel during the procedure.
- When the patient is sedated (e.g., with midazolam or diazepam), a crash cart must be in the room during the procedure and the patient monitored with pulse oximetry.
- All of the procedures require teaching for aftercare.
- For all tests, explain that rectal bleeding is normal for a few days if polyps were removed or a biopsy was taken.

Esophagogastroduodenoscopy (EGD)

A *fiberoptic endoscope*, a long, flexible tube with a light and lens, is introduced through the mouth and advanced for visualization of the esophagus, stomach, and duodenum. The physician may also perform tissue biopsies or coagulate bleeding sites through the endoscope.

Preparation

- Instruct the patient to fast for 6 to 12 hours before the test (instructions usually are "NPO [nothing by mouth] after midnight").
- Remove dentures and eyewear prior to the test.
- Because the tube is introduced through the mouth, patients often require sedation to limit gagging.

During the Test

- The patient will be sedated but awake.
- A local anesthetic will be sprayed into his mouth and throat to lessen the gag reflex.

Post-Test Care

- Check vital signs and gag reflex (per agency protocol).
- Keep the patient NPO until the gag reflex returns; then instruct him to have light meals during the next 12 to 24 hours.
- Instruct the patient to resume normal activity, medications, and diet in 24 hours.
- Observe and teach the patient to observe for Potential Complication: esophageal or bowel perforation—cyanosis, substernal or abdominal pain, vomiting blood, continuing difficulty swallowing, or black, tarry stools.
- Explain to the patient that he will have a sore throat and hoarseness for a few days. Suggest gargling with saltwater and using throat lozenges.
- Caution the patient to notify the physician immediately if he experiences severe pain, fever, difficulty breathing, or expectoration of blood.
- Inform the patient that belching, bloating, or flatulence is a result of introducing air into the intestine and will be temporary.

Sigmoidoscopy

A rigid metal scope or a flexible fiberoptic scope is used to visualize the anal canal, rectum, and sigmoid colon. The patient is usually not sedated. During the exam, the physician may perform a biopsy, remove polyps (small growths), or coagulate sources of bleeding in the area. This procedure is also used as a screen for colon cancer.

Preparation

- A light meal before the test may be allowed. For flexible sigmoidoscopy, the patient may be asked to follow a clear liquid diet for a day before the exam.
- Administer two commercially prepared, small-volume enemas before the test.
- For a flexible sigmoidoscopy, a strong laxative solution may also be prescribed.
- Have the patient void before the procedure.

During the Test

- Drape the patient for modesty.
- The patient may feel pressure, cramping, or the urge to defecate; encourage slow, deep breathing through the mouth to help alleviate the feeling.

Post-Test Care

- Observe for Potential Complication: bowel perforation (see discussion of EGD).
- The patient may resume normal activity.
- Explain that air was introduced into the intestines to distend them for better visibility and that this may cause gas pains or flatulence for a few hours.
- A small amount of blood in the first bowel movement is normal. Notify the physician of significant bleeding.

Fiberoptic Colonoscopy

Provides direct visualization of the rectum, colon, entire large intestine, and distal small bowel. A flexible scope is inserted through the rectum and advanced to the cecum. Colonoscopy is useful in detecting lower GI disease. It is also often used instead of a sigmoidoscopy for cancer screening because colonoscopy provides greater visualization of the colon. This is the preferred test for clients with suspected problems above the level of the sigmoid colon.

Preparation

- The colon and rectum must be empty and clean so the physician can view the linings during the exam. Practitioners have different colon-cleansing routines to achieve this, such as the following:
  - Instruct the patient to take strong cathartic and laxative (e.g., Dulcolax) tablets the day before the test and an enema on day of the test, until returns are clear.

Diagnostic Testing

Direct Visualization Studies of the Gastrointestinal Tract—cont'd

- Instruct the patient to consume a clear liquid diet for 24 to 48 hours before the test (nothing red or purple) and to remain NPO after midnight the night before the exam.
- The patient will be sedated before the test, so she may need a ride home from someone.

During the Test
- Position the patient on her side with knees flexed. Drape for modesty.
- Monitor vital signs.
- The patient may feel pressure, cramping, or the urge to defecate; encourage slow, deep breathing through the mouth to help alleviate the feeling.

Post-Test Care
- Monitor vital signs (per agency protocol).
- Observe for Potential Complication: Bowel perforation (see discussion of EGD).
- Explain that air was introduced into the intestines to distend them for better visibility and that, as a result, the patient may experience gas pains or flatulence for a few hours.
- Instruct the patient to resume a normal diet when she has recovered from sedation.

Source: American Cancer Society. (2018). Colorectal cancer. Retrieved August 9, 2018, from https://www.cancer.org/cancer/colon-rectal-cancer.html; Van Leeuwen, A. M., Poelhuis-Leth, D. J., & Bladh, M. L. (2019). *Davis's comprehensive handbook of laboratory and diagnostic tests with nursing implications,* (8th ed.). Philadelphia, PA: F.A. Davis.

Diagnostic Testing

Indirect Visualization Studies of the Gastrointestinal Tract

Abdominal Flat Plate

An anterior-to-posterior (AP) x-ray view of the abdomen is used to detect gallstones, fecal impaction, and distended bowel. This test requires no preparation and no special post-test care.

Barium Enema (BE)

Radiological examination of the rectum, colon, and distal small bowel. A rectal tube is inserted into the rectum or an existing ostomy. Barium (a contrast medium) is instilled. The patient must retain the barium through several position changes while air is instilled and radiographs are obtained. The test is especially useful for visualizing polyps, diverticula, and tumors. In addition, it may be used to reduce certain obstructions. As a rule, patients are not sedated.

Preparation
- The test is invasive, so a signed informed consent is necessary.
- Patient instructions: Low-residue diet for several days prior to the procedure; consume only clear liquids the evening before the procedure; NPO for 8 hours before the test; possibly avoid dairy products that day.
- Administer a laxative, suppository, or cleansing enema the day before the test and cleansing enemas on the morning of the procedure (check agency policy). Enema administration is discussed in this chapter. For complete instructions for inserting a suppository, see Chapter 26, Procedure 26-6: Inserting a Rectal Suppository.

Post-Test Care
- The patient may have bloating and cramping after the test and will probably feel the need to empty her bowels as soon as the test is done.
- Instruct the client to resume food, fluids, and medications withheld before the procedure.
- Instruct the client to take a mild laxative and increase fluid intake (four glasses) to aid in elimination of barium (unless contraindicated). Barium can cause constipation for a few days.
- Explain that stools will be white or light colored for 2 to 3 days; if patient is unable to eliminate the barium, she should call the physician.

Ultrasonography

Detects tissue abnormalities, such as masses, cysts, edema, or stones. An ultrasound probe, called a *transducer,* is moved over the skin surface of the abdomen. The probe emits a sound wave that abdominal tissue and organs reflect back based on their density. The sound waves may be transformed into images visible on a computer screen.

Computed Tomography (CT)

Useful in diagnosis of many abdominal disorders. Examines body sections from different angles using a narrow x-ray beam and produces a three-dimensional image of the area of the body being scanned. The patient needs to lie very still during the procedure. A CT scan may be enhanced by injecting contrast dye that allows for improved visualization of circulatory function.

Preparation

If contrast dye is to be used:
- Determine that the patient is not allergic to contrast medium, iodine, or shellfish.
- Check blood urea nitrogen and creatinine levels to ensure adequate kidney function.

(Continued)

Diagnostic Testing

Indirect Visualization Studies of the Gastrointestinal Tract—cont'd

- Patients taking metformin (Glucophage) should discontinue it on the day of the test and withhold it for 48 hours after to prevent lactic acidosis.
- Restrict food and fluids for 6 to 8 hours if contrast medium is to be given.
- Sometimes the patient is asked to drink about 450 mL of a dilute barium solution 1 hour before the CT scan to distinguish the GI tract from other abdominal organs.

During the Test

- Explain that the patient may feel nausea or warmth or experience a metallic taste or a transient headache after injection of contrast medium. Instruct the patient to take slow, deep breaths if this occurs.

Post-Test Care

- The patient may resume normal diet, activity, and medication.
- Renal function should be assessed before metformin (Glucophage) is restarted.
- The patient should increase fluid intake to help eliminate contrast medium.
- Diarrhea may occur after ingestion of oral contrast medium.
- Observe for delayed allergic reactions (e.g., hives, headache, nausea, vomiting) if contrast medium was used.

Magnetic Resonance Imaging (MRI)

Produces cross-sectional images of the body. MRI utilizes a strong magnetic field and radio waves. This type of diagnostic test does not use ionizing radiation, so it is free of the hazards of x-rays. MRI is very sensitive and may be used to detect edema, hemorrhage, blood flow, infarcts, tumors, and infections in organ structures. When used, the contrast medium is noniodinated, and it is administered intravenously to enhance contrast between normal and abnormal tissues. The patient must lie still in a narrow tube, sometimes for up to an hour.

Preparation

- Determine the presence of metal in the body, such as shrapnel or flecks of ferrous metal in the eye.
- Instruct the patient to remove all external metallic objects before entering the scanning room (e.g., jewelry, body piercing rings, eyeglasses, hairpins, credit cards).
- Food and fluids are not always restricted. The patient may be instructed to be NPO for 4 to 6 hours before the exam.
- Have the patient void before the procedure.

Post-Test Care

- The patient can resume normal activity, medication, and diet.
- If a contrast medium was used, observe for delayed allergic reactions.

Source: Van Leeuwen, A. M., Poelhuis-Leth, D. J., & Bladh, M. L. (2019). *Davis's comprehensive handbook of laboratory and diagnostic tests with nursing implications,* (8th ed.). Philadelphia, PA: F.A. Davis.

STANDARDIZED NURSING LANGUAGE

Nursing Diagnoses Associated with Bowel Elimination

LABEL, DEFINITION, DISCUSSION	DEFINING CHARACTERISTICS/ RISK FACTORS	ETIOLOGIES/RELATED FACTORS
Bowel Incontinence. Change in normal bowel pattern characterized by involuntary defecation.	*Subjective*: Urgency, inability to recognize the urge to defecate or inability to feel rectal fullness *Objective*: Leakage of soft stool, red perianal skin, fecal odor, fecal soiling of clothing or bedding, and inability to delay defecation	High abdominal or intestinal pressure, chronic diarrhea, colorectal lesions, dietary habits, medications, decline in muscle tone, immobility (inability to get to the bathroom), inaccessibility of bathroom facilities, impaction, stress, Toileting Self-care Deficit, Impaired Cognition, laxative abuse, loss of rectal sphincter control, and motor nerve damage.

Nursing Diagnoses Associated with Bowel Elimination—cont'd

LABEL, DEFINITION, DISCUSSION	DEFINING CHARACTERISTICS/ RISK FACTORS	ETIOLOGIES/RELATED FACTORS
Constipation. Because frequency of bowel elimination varies, constipation is usually defined as infrequent bowel movements or difficult passage of hard, dry feces. Constipation can be a temporary problem with symptoms resolving in a short time. Most people experience constipation at some point. Unrelieved constipation may eventually result in a fecal impaction, in which dry, hard stools lodged in the rectum cannot be passed.	*Subjective:* Abdominal pain, a feeling of rectal fullness, straining or pain with defecation, and some rectal bleeding. The person may report needing to perform manual maneuvers to pass stool (e.g., pressing on the anus or pressing on the posterior vaginal wall).	Abdominal muscle weakness, ignoring the urge to defecate, insufficient physical activity, depression, emotional stress, medications, changes in eating patterns, and insufficient fiber or fluid intake. Habitual laxative use may also cause constipation as the colon becomes responsive only to the stimulating effect of the laxative.
Constipation Risk. At risk for a decrease in normal frequency of defecation accompanied by infrequent or difficult passage of hard, dry feces.	*Risk factors:* Abdominal muscle weakness, habitually ignoring the urge to defecate, insufficient intake of fluid and fiber, dehydration, and certain medications (e.g., opioids, anticholinergics, calcium channel blockers), surgery. Constipation is more common among women than men, and increases with age. It is associated with depression, lower socioeconomic status, and lower education levels.	Not applicable.
Perceived Constipation is an appropriate diagnosis for a client who has an impression of infrequent or difficult passage of hard, dry feces without cause.	*Subjective:* Expectation of a daily bowel movement, or at the same time every day; overuse of laxatives, enemas, or suppositories.	Cultural and family health beliefs and impaired thought processes.
Diarrhea is the abnormal increased frequency and fluidity of feces (loose, watery stools). Persistent diarrhea threatens fluid and electrolyte balance, especially in young children and older adults.	*Subjective:* Abdominal pain, cramping, and urgency. *Objective:* At least three loose, liquid stools per day; and hyperactive bowel sounds. The patient may also experience bloating, fever, and blood in the stools, depending on the cause of the diarrhea.	Anxiety, high stress levels, radiation, toxins, travel, tube feedings, medication side effects, alcohol abuse, contaminants, laxative abuse, infections, inflammation, irritation, malabsorption, parasite. The most common cause is GI infection; however, diarrhea may occur with a chronic disease, such as celiac disease or irritable bowel syndrome.
Gastrointestinal Motility Alteration is the change in or modification of peristaltic activity within the GI system. If you use this label, you need to specify whether the GI motility is increased, decreased, and so on (e.g., dysfunctional GI motility: increased).	Because the diagnosis is defined so broadly, defining characteristics include symptoms of both diarrhea and constipation, as well as nausea, regurgitation, vomiting, increased gastric residual, bile-colored gastric residual, and accelerated gastric emptying.	Aging, anxiety, tube feedings, food intolerance (e.g., lactose intolerance), immobility, contaminates (e.g., in food), malnutrition, medications, anesthesia, surgery prematurity, sedentary lifestyle.
Risk for Gastrointestinal Motility Alteration is the risk for change in or modification of peristaltic activity within the GI system.	***Risk Factors:*** Abdominal surgery, aging, anxiety, change in food or eating habits, decreased GI circulation, diabetes mellitus, food intolerance, gastroesophageal reflux disease (GERD), immobility, infection, medications, prematurity, sedentary lifestyle, stress, or unsanitary food preparation.	Not applicable.

(Continued)

Nursing Diagnoses Associated with Bowel Elimination—cont'd

LABEL, DEFINITION, DISCUSSION	DEFINING CHARACTERISTICS/ RISK FACTORS	ETIOLOGIES/RELATED FACTORS
Toileting Deficit is impaired ability to urinate or defecate for oneself. Strictly speaking, this is not a bowel problem. Bowel function may be normal, but the person simply cannot manage toileting.	Use this diagnosis for patients who cannot manipulate their clothing for toileting, perform adequate toilet hygiene, flush the toilet, get to the toilet or commode, or sit on or rise from the toilet or commode.	Impaired cognitive ability, lack of motivation, fatigue, impaired mobility, musculoskeletal or neuromuscular impairment, pain, impaired ability to respond to stimuli, severe anxiety, weakness, environmental factors.

Selected Standardized Outcomes and Interventions for Bowel Elimination Diagnoses

NURSING DIAGNOSIS	NURSING OUTCOMES CLASSIFICATION (NOC) OUTCOMES AND SCALE*	NOC OUTCOME INDICATORS	NURSING INTERVENTIONS CLASSIFICATION (NIC) INTERVENTIONS AND ACTIVITIES
Bowel Incontinence	Bowel Continence (m and t) Tissue Integrity: Skin and Mucous Membranes (a and n)	Recognizes urge to defecate Maintains control of stool passage Responds to urge in timely manner Control of bowel movements Elimination pattern Diarrhea Mucus in stool Skin integrity Erythema Skin lesions	***Bowel Incontinence Care: Encopresis*** Determine … cause of fecal incontinence. Keep bed and clothing clean. Place on incontinent pads, as needed. ***Bowel Management*** Teach patient/family members to record color, volume, frequency, and consistency of stools. ***Bowel Training*** Initiate an uninterrupted, consistent time for defecation. Teach patient/family the principles of bowel training.
Constipation	Bowel Elimination (a and n) Ostomy Self-care (a and n)	Stool soft and formed Ease of stool passage Pain with passage of stool Passage of stool without aids Maintains ostomy for elimination	***Bowel Management*** Monitor BMs, including frequency, consistency, shape, volume, and color, as appropriate. Instruct the patient on foods high in fiber, as appropriate. Insert rectal suppository, as needed. ***Constipation/Impaction Management*** Monitor for impaction. Institute a toileting schedule, as appropriate. Teach patient/family on the relationship of diet, exercise, and fluid intake to constipation/impaction. Bowel management: Ostomy care. Teach patient/family on the relationship of diet and fluid intake as a means of preventing constipation. Teach patient psychomotor skills needed to maintain ostomy.

Selected Standardized Outcomes and Interventions for Bowel Elimination Diagnoses—cont'd

NURSING DIAGNOSIS	NURSING OUTCOMES CLASSIFICATION (NOC) OUTCOMES AND SCALE*	NOC OUTCOME INDICATORS	NURSING INTERVENTIONS CLASSIFICATION (NIC) INTERVENTIONS AND ACTIVITIES
Constipation, Perceived	Health Beliefs (n) Bowel Elimination (a and n)	Perceived importance of taking action Perceived threat from inaction Perceived benefits of action Abuse of elimination aids Passage of stool without aids Elimination pattern	***Teaching: Individual*** Determine patient's learning needs. Determine ability to learn specific information (i.e., developmental level, pain, fatigue, emotional state. Reinforce behavior, as appropriate. ***Behavior Modification*** Encourage the patient to list values that guide behavior in various settings and types of situations. Encourage consideration of the issues and consequences of behavior.
Diarrhea	Bowel Elimination (a and n) Bowel Continence (a and n) Symptom Severity (n)	Elimination pattern Fat in stool Blood in stool Mucus in stool Diarrhea Symptom intensity Impaired life enjoyment	***Bowel Management*** Monitor BMs, including frequency, consistency, shape, volume, and color, as appropriate. ***Diarrhea Management*** Evaluate medication profile for gastrointestinal side effects. Encourage frequent, small feedings, adding bulk gradually. Suggest trial elimination of foods containing lactose. Instruct the patient to notify the staff of each episode of diarrhea. Monitor the skin in the perianal area for irritation and ulceration. Measure diarrhea/bowel output.
Gastrointestinal Motility Alteration	Bowel Elimination (a and n) Gastrointestinal Function (a and n)	Bowel sounds Elimination pattern Abdominal distention Increase in visible peristalsis Regurgitation Frequency of stools Gastric aspirates: amount of residuals Frequency of nausea Frequency of vomiting Fecal odor of emesis Excessive secretion of saliva	***Bowel Management*** Monitor bowel sounds. Monitor BMs. Note preexisting bowel problems, bowel routine, and use of laxatives. Evaluate medication profile for gastrointestinal (GI) side effects. Nutrition management and diet teaching Monitor for signs and symptoms of diarrhea, constipation, and impaction. ***Vomiting Management*** Measure or estimate emesis volume. Use oral hygiene to clean mouth and nose. Control environmental factors that may evoke vomiting (e.g., smells).
Toileting Deficit	Refer to Chapter 25.		

Sources: Butcher, H., Bulechek, G., Dochterman, J., et al. (Eds.). (2018). *Nursing interventions classification (NIC)* (7th ed.). St. Louis, MO: Elsevier; Moorhead, S., Swanson, E., Johnson, M., et al. (Eds.). (2018). *Nursing outcomes classification (NOC)* (6th ed.). St. Louis, MO: Elsevier; NANDA International. (2017). *NANDA nursing diagnoses: Definitions and classification 2018–2020. Thieme.* Used with permission.
*For a list of NOC measurement scales, see Chapter 5.

CLINICALJUDGMENT

Applying the Full-Spectrum Nursing Model

PATIENT SITUATION

Lucy Franklin is a frail, elderly woman, a long-time resident in a long-term care facility. She can no longer communicate and lies in whatever position the UAPs place her in bed, seldom moving. She is very thin, does not eat or drink, and is being fed entirely through a gastrostomy tube. She is incontinent of both stool and urine and has recently started having copious diarrhea, probably from the tube feedings, but that has not been established definitively. The skin on Lucy's back, buttocks, and perineum is still intact, but it is quite red now. The healthcare team is considering various measures for controlling the diarrhea, but until that can be achieved, nurses want to protect her skin integrity.

THINKING

1. *Theoretical Knowledge:*

   a. Other than tube feedings, what else could be causing Lucy's diarrhea?

   b. In addition to Skin Integrity Impairment, what are some other risks associated with diarrhea?

   c. Why is fecal incontinence, especially with diarrhea, a risk factor for Skin Integrity Impairment?

2. *Critical Thinking:*

   a. *(Contextual Awareness):* What other factors in Lucy's situation do you think might make her even more vulnerable to Skin Integrity Impairment? If you do not yet have the theoretical knowledge you need, draw on your own experiences—and think carefully about everything you know about Lucy.

   b. *(Considering Alternatives):* A fecal incontinence pouch is being discussed as an intervention to preserve Lucy's skin integrity. Do you think it should be an external system or an internal system? Why?

DOING

3. *Practical Knowledge:*

   It has been decided that an external fecal collection system will be used. Describe the steps you will take to apply this system after you have made the necessary assessments.

4. *Nursing Process (Assessments):*

   What ongoing assessments will you need to make after the fecal collection system is applied?

CARING

5. *Self-Knowledge:*

   How comfortable would you be applying Lucy's fecal collection system? What aspects of the situation make you most uncomfortable?

Critical Thinking and Clinical Judgment

1. Your neighbor is aware that you are a nursing student and calls you for advice. She has a 12-year-old daughter with diarrhea. "Everything runs through her," states the mother. There are also two other children in the house, ages 6 years and 18 months. Both have had watery stools this morning. Your neighbor explains that her husband has an ileostomy and has been hospitalized since yesterday. Your neighbor has no symptoms but is very worried. She asks, "Do we all need to go to the hospital?"
   a. Consider alternatives. What are the most likely explanations for the diarrhea?
   b. Based on your theoretical knowledge, how would you explain why her husband was hospitalized, while the rest of the family members, who have the same symptoms, remain at home?
   c. After reassuring her, what advice should you offer your neighbor about self-care for her and the children's elimination problem?

2. Consider the following patients:
   - A 54-year-old man diagnosed with colon cancer who now has a new sigmoid colostomy
   - A 21-year-old woman with Crohn's disease (an inflammatory bowel disorder) who has just had an ileostomy
   - A 36-year-old trauma victim who has a new double-barreled transverse colostomy

   a. How are these patients similar?
   b. With regard to their surgery, what nursing care priorities do these patients share?
   c. How do the major concerns for these patients differ? (Consider the context. How are their surgical and self-care situations different?)

3. For each of the following concepts, use critical thinking to describe how or why it is important to nursing, patient care, or bowel elimination. Note that these are *not* to be merely definitions.

   Digestion (in the mouth, esophagus, stomach, and small intestine)

   Large intestine (colon)

   Rectum and anus

   Fluid intake

   Location of a bowel diversion

   Bowel sounds

   Providing privacy

   Diarrhea

What Are the Main Points in This Chapter?

- Bowel elimination is a normal process by which waste products are eliminated from the body.
- Feces are a mixture of insoluble fiber and other indigestible material, bacteria, and water.
- During defecation, the internal and external anal sphincters relax; the rectum contracts; and peristalsis increases in the sigmoid colon, propelling feces through the anus.
- The frequency of bowel movements (BMs) varies. As long as stools are passed without excessive urgency, with minimal effort and no straining, and without the use of laxatives, bowel function is regarded as normal.
- The bowel pattern set in childhood normally continues into adulthood. Adequate fiber, fluid, and exercise are required to maintain this pattern.
- Factors affecting bowel function include developmental stage, personal and sociocultural factors, nutrition, hydration, activity level, stress, anesthesia, medications, pregnancy, surgery and other procedures, and pathological conditions.
- To promote regular defecation, provide privacy for the patient, and allow time to use the toilet.
- Constipation is a decrease in frequency of BMs and the passage of dry, hard stool that requires more effort to pass.
- Bulking agents are the preferred medication for treating constipation.
- Habitual use of laxatives, with the exception of bulking agents, may cause reliance on medication for bowel elimination.
- Fecal impaction is detected by digital examination of the rectum. To treat a fecal impaction, enemas or digital removal of stool is required.
- Enema is the introduction of solution into the rectum to soften feces, distend the colon, and stimulate peristalsis and evacuation of feces.
- Monitor patients with diarrhea for intake and output, body weight, and vital signs to assess for fluid losses; provide hygiene measures to protect the skin.
- Bowel incontinence may be managed by providing assistance to the bathroom at regular intervals and at the times BMs are most likely to occur, and by beginning a bowel training program.
- External or internal fecal collection devices can be used to protect perianal skin or to collect large stool samples. They minimize odor, allow for accurate measurement of output, and improve patient comfort.
- A bowel diversion is a surgically created opening for elimination of digestive waste products.
- The *effluent* (fecal matter) of an ostomy ranges from liquid to solid, depending on the part of the bowel that is being diverted.
- A healthy stoma ranges in color from deep pink to brick red and is shiny and moist at all times.
- A client with a bowel diversion must adapt to the stoma for elimination and learn to care for the stoma.

Knowledge Map

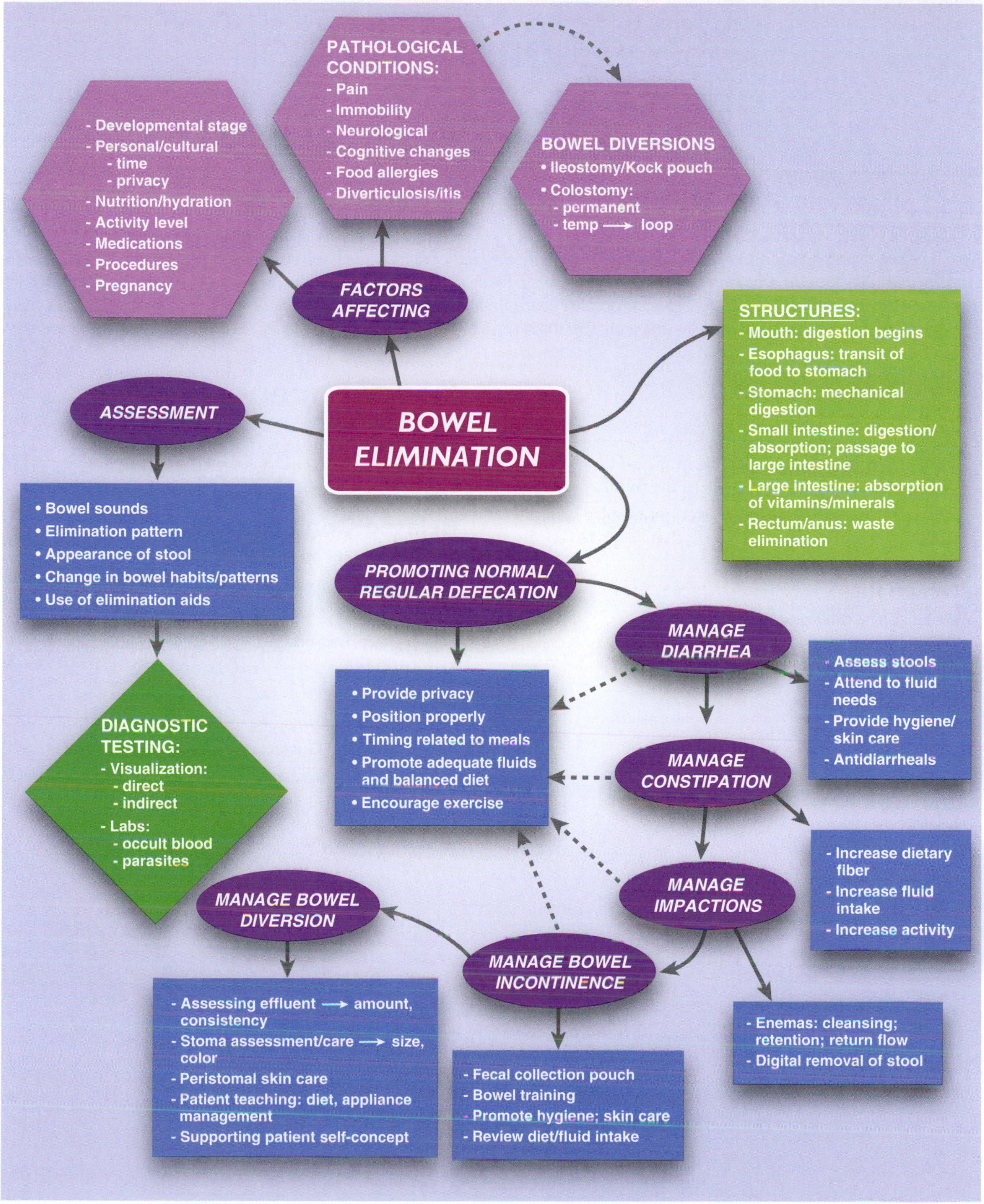

CHAPTER 30

Sensation, Perception, & Response

STUDENT RESOURCES

The questions and exercises in this book allow you to practice the kind of thinking you will use as a full-spectrum nurse. Critical-thinking questions usually have more than one right answer, so we do not provide "correct answers" for these features. Try to answer these questions yourself. It is more important to develop your nursing judgment than to just cover content. You will learn more by discussing the questions with your peers. If you are still unsure, see the Davis Advantage chapter resources for suggested responses.

To explore learning resources for this chapter,

Go to Davis Advantage and find:

Answers and Suggested Responses for all questions in this chapter
Concept Map
Knowledge Map
References and Bibliography
Lists of NOC Outcomes and NIC Interventions

Key Concepts

Perception
Reception
Sensation

Related Concepts

See the Concept Map on Davis Advantage.

Example Problems

Sensory Deprivation
Sensory Overload
Sensory Deficits
- **Visual and Hearing**
- **Olfactory and Gustatory**
- **Tactile and Kinesthetic**

Seizures

Caring for the Nguyens

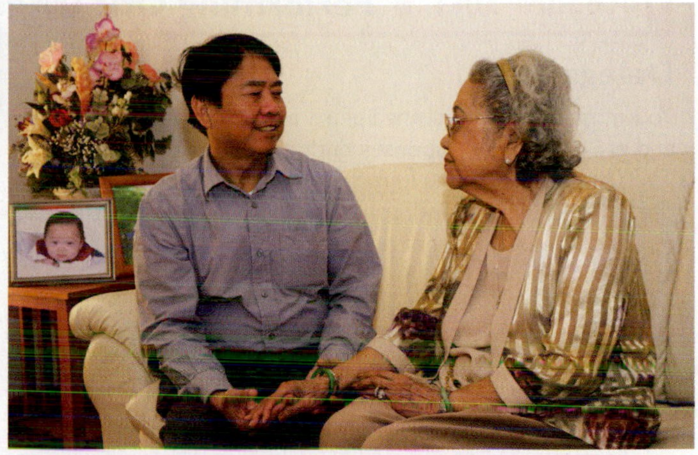

Mai Nguyen, Nam Nguyen's mother, has been experiencing blurred vision. At a recent ophthalmology appointment, she was told she has bilateral cataracts that will require surgical removal. She reports to the primary care clinic today, accompanied by Nam. Mai tells you, "I don't know what happened. I was pulling into a parking space at the grocery store, and the next thing you know, I hear this loud boom. I don't know how I did it, but I hit the car next to me. I just didn't see it."

Nam is very concerned and questions whether his mother should be allowed to drive. Mai is visibly upset. "I don't want to hurt anyone, but I don't want to lose all my freedom." Nam insisted on this appointment to discuss his concerns.

A. What data will you need to gather from Mai and Nam?

B. What assessments will you need to perform?

C. How will cataract surgery most likely affect Mai? You will need to learn about the surgery and recovery to answer this question.

D. What information would you offer to Mai and Nam?

PracticalKnowledge clinical **application**

To provide support for patients with sensorineural alterations, you will need practical knowledge about assessing and diagnosing sensorineural functions. You will find those in Assessment Guidelines and Tools.

Nursing interventions involve caring for patients who have vision and hearing deficits. This section includes a procedure for otic irrigations, which may be used to correct hearing loss resulting from a cerumen blocked ear canal. Some procedures to support sensory function, such as instilling medications and irrigating the eye, are presented in the procedures in Chapter 26 of this volume. For other interventions, see Volume 1 of this chapter.

PROCEDURES

Procedure 30-1 ■ Performing Otic Irrigation

➤ For steps to follow in *all* procedures, refer to the Universal Steps for All Procedures found on the inside back cover.

Equipment

- An ear irrigation system, such as the Welch Allyn ear wash system or an electronic jet ear irrigator

Using a metal syringe is no longer recommended and is considered dangerous. An ear irrigation system is also preferred over an Asepto or bulb syringe because of the better ability to control pressure and remove cerumen (Harkin, n.d.).

- Asepto syringe, or rubber bulb syringe (if an ear irrigation system is not available)
- Irrigating solution (usually normal saline solution or sterile water, but may be an antiseptic solution), warmed to body temperature
- Bath towel and moisture-resistant towel
- A headlight, if one is available
- Emesis basin
- Otoscope
- Cotton balls
- Procedure gloves

(continued on next page)

Procedure 30-1 ■ Performing Otic Irrigation (continued)

Delegation

You must assess the client before performing this procedure and evaluate client responses during and after the procedure. The procedure requires knowledge of anatomy and physiology, use of an otoscope, and, sometimes, use of sterile technique. Therefore, you should not delegate otic irrigation to unlicensed assistive personnel (UAP).

Pre-Procedure Assessments

- Determine whether there are contraindications for ear irrigation.
  Contraindications include ruptured tympanic membrane, present or recent middle ear infection, prior surgery on the ear, cleft palate, or acute inflammation of the ear canal.
- Assess the external ear for drainage.
  Do not irrigate the ears if drainage is present. Drainage from the ear may be a sign of rupture of the tympanic membrane.
- Assess the external ear for cerumen.
  Impacted cerumen is the most common reason for the need to perform ear irrigation.
- Assess the external ear canal for redness, swelling, or foreign objects; visualize the tympanic membrane. If a foreign object is present, attempt to remove it before irrigation.
  Establishes the baseline. If you irrigate with a foreign object in the ear, it may cause the object to swell and become more difficult to remove. Also, if you cannot visualize the tympanic membrane, it may be perforated; if so, otic irrigation is contraindicated.
- Assess for pain or hearing loss.
  Establishes the baseline. Cerumen blockage in the ear canal may result in conductive hearing loss.

➤ When performing the procedure, always identify your patient according to agency policy, using two identifiers, and be attentive to standard precautions, hand hygiene, patient safety and privacy, documentation, and body mechanics.

Procedure Steps

1. **Warm the irrigating solution** to body temperature; fill the reservoir of the irrigator.
   Placing cool solutions in the ear can cause dizziness.
2. **Assemble the irrigator,** if necessary; place a clean disposable tip on it.
3. **Assist the client** into a sitting or lying position, with the head tilted slightly toward the affected ear. Explain what you are going to do.
   Positioning facilitates administering the solution and allows fluid to run along the roof of the ear canal. Knowing what to expect may decrease patient anxiety and improve his ability to cooperate during the procedure.
4. **Don gloves;** put on the headlight.
   The gloves are needed because of the risk of exposure to body fluids. The headlight facilitates direct vision.
5. **Drape the client** with a plastic drape; place a towel on the client's shoulder on the side being irrigated. Ask the client to hold an emesis basin under his ear to collect the irrigating fluid that drains out of the ear.
   NOTE: An emesis basin is not necessary if a comprehensive ear wash system is used. The drape and the towel protect the client's clothing.
6. **Set the irrigator pressure** to the minimum level. Let it run for 20 to 30 sec to prime the tubing or nozzle before irrigation. (If you must use an Asepto or rubber bulb syringe, fill the syringe with about 50 mL of the irrigating solution, and expel any remaining air.)
7. **Straighten the ear canal.**
   a. For a child younger than 3 years old, pull the pinna down and back.
   b. For older children and adults, pull the pinna upward and outward.
   Straightens the ear canal so that the solution can flow through the length of the canal.
8. **Instruct the client to notify you** if he experiences any pain or dizziness during the irrigation. Explain to the client that he may feel warmth, fullness, or pressure when the fluid reaches the tympanic membrane.
   Pain or dizziness may indicate a contraindication to the procedure.
9. **Place the tip of the nozzle** (or syringe) about 1 cm (½ in.) above the entrance of the ear canal; direct the stream of irrigating solution gently along the top of the ear canal toward the back of the client's head.
   a. Do not occlude the ear canal with the nozzle.
   b. Instill the solution slowly.
   c. Allow the solution to flow out as it is instilled.
   d. Repeat these steps for 5 minutes or until you can see cerumen in the return solution.
   Directing the flow directly onto the tympanic membrane could injure the membrane. Strong pressure can cause discomfort and may even damage the tympanic membrane. ▼

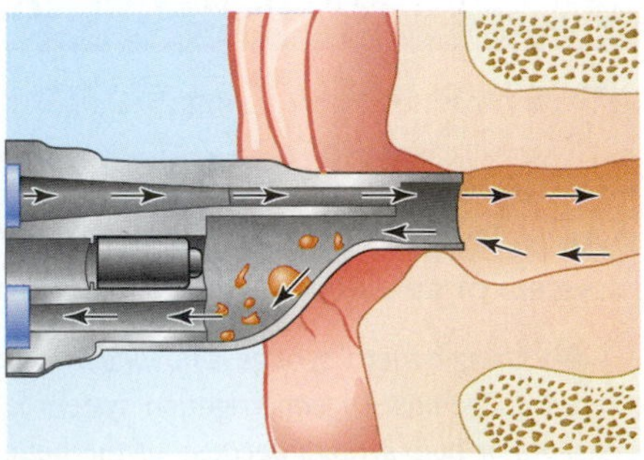

10. **Inspect the ear** with an otoscope to evaluate cerumen removal. See Procedure 22-7: Assessing the Ears and Hearing if you need to review otoscopic examination.
Allows visualization of the canal.

11. **Continue irrigating** until the examination indicates the canal is cleaned of cerumen and debris.
The irrigating solution will soften the cerumen, easing removal. Blocking the canal prevents the outward flow of the solution.

12. **Place a cotton ball loosely** in the ear canal; ask the client to lie on the side of the affected ear.
The cotton ball will absorb excess fluid that drains by gravity.

13. **Clean and disinfect the irrigator**, according to the manufacturer's instructions or agency protocols. Dispose of the disposable tips.

? What if . . .

- **The cerumen is very hard or you have difficulty removing it?**
  The irrigating solution will help soften it, so you may attempt again after 15 minutes.
- **Your patient is an infant or young child?**
  Ask another caregiver to hold the child still during the irrigation.

Evaluation

- Observe the quantity and quality of ear cerumen you removed.
- Observe the appearance of the ear canal.
- Assess for complaints of pain or dizziness.
- Assess for improvement in hearing acuity.
- Reassess for drainage on the cotton ball.

Patient Teaching

- Avoid use of cotton-tipped swabs.
  They simply push cerumen deeper into the ear.
- Keep the ear dry for a few days. Use cotton balls coated with petroleum jelly when bathing.
  Exposure to a wet environment, such as a swimming pool, may increase the risk of bacterial or fungal infection. Petroleum jelly serves as a barrier to keep water from entering the ear.
- Clean ears daily with washcloth, soap, and water. If wax buildup is a problem, over-the-counter preparations (oils) can be used.
- Notify the primary care provider if you experience ear pain, vertigo, or "ringing in the ears."
  Ear irrigation is an invasive procedure and may result in otitis media, trauma to the external meatus, vertigo, tinnitus, and perforation of the tympanic membrane, although this is not common.

Home Care

- Provide the caregiver with instructions on ear care as stated above.
- Teach parents to avoid irrigation in young children unless absolutely necessary. Oil- or water-based ear drops may be used to treat a wax problem in a child, applying the oil when the child is asleep.

- Teach clients that ear candling is a not advisable. Candling consists of putting a hollow cone soaked in beeswax or paraffin in the ear and lighting the other end. The heat is supposed to draw out wax, but there is no evidence that it is effective. People using ear candles have burned themselves, blocked their ear canals with candle wax, and punctured their tympanic membranes (eardrums).

Documentation

- Document the ear solution used, the quantity, character, and odor of cerumen or drainage.
- Chart the condition of the ear canal and tympanic membrane after the irrigation.

Sample documentation

mm/dd/yyyy 1400 *Pt c/o bilateral decreased hearing acuity. External ear canals occluded with dried cerumen. Irrigated with warm water using electronic jet ear irrigation system. Large amount of dry, brown cerumen removed with irrigation. External canals and tympanic membrane intact to otoscopic inspection after irrigation. —N. Ephrain, RN*

Practice Resources

Chau, J., Lee, D., & Lo, S. (2012); Harkin, H. (n.d.); Schwartz, S. R., Magit, A. E., Rosenfeld, R. M., et al. (2017).

CLINICAL INSIGHTS

Clinical Insight 30-1 ➤ Communicating With Visually Impaired Clients

iCare
- Introduce yourself when you enter the room.
- Call the client by name so that she can be certain you are addressing her.
- When you enter a room with a client who is visually impaired, describe the room, the room's layout, and the activities that are occurring.
- Explain unfamiliar sounds, such as the paging system and the monitor and pump alarms.
- If the client has limited vision, be sure to position yourself in the client's field of vision.
- Speak to the visually impaired person before you touch her so that she is prepared for your touch.
- Do not speak loudly unless the client has a hearing impairment.
- Let the client know when you are leaving the room.
- Use the words "see" and "look" as you would with a sighted person.
- Avoid expressions, such as "over there" or "right here." Guide the client to the location or place her hand on the object.

Clinical Insight 30-2 ➤ Communicating With Hearing-Impaired Clients

iCare Difficulty communicating can be anxiety provoking for patients and frustrating for both patients and caregivers, especially in a healthcare setting. A caring nurse will:

Assess the Patient's Method of Receiving Speech.

- If the patient wears a hearing aid, check to see that it is turned on.
- If not, does the patient read lips or use sign language? (Only about ⅓ of spoken words can be understood by speech reading.)
- If possible, arrange a hearing evaluation for the client and construction of any required hearing aids.

Position Yourself and Minimize Noise.

- Do not chew gum or eat while talking. Many clients use lip reading to interpret speech.
- Make sure you are clearly visible to the client before you start speaking.
- Face the client directly; keep your hands away from your mouth.
- If the hearing deficit is predominantly in one ear, move closer to the less affected ear.
- Minimize environmental noise (e.g., turn off the television).

Send the Message.

- Speak slowly and articulate clearly, in a natural way. Do not shout. Shouting distorts your words.
- Do not drop your voice at the end of a sentence.
- Use simple, plain language, but longer phrases (e.g., "Would you like me to get you a drink of water?" instead of "Do you want a drink?")
- Use gestures to provide visual cues (e.g., act out what you want the patient to do).
- Use paper, pencil, or computer communication, when necessary. Consider the client's literacy skills.

Interpret the Client's Responses.

- Observe the client's verbal responses, facial expressions, and body language for clues to understanding. An inappropriate response is a sign of misunderstanding.
- Be aware the person may nod agreement or say "yes" even when she does not understand what is being said.
- Confirm that the client understood you by asking her to repeat what you said, especially if you are giving specific information, such as a time or place. Many numbers and words sound alike (e.g., "fifteen" and "fifty"; or "Prozac" and "Prograf").
- If the person does not understand what you have said, rephrase your statement. Do not repeat the same words.

- **For older adults:** Use a low-pitched voice. The ability to hear high-pitched tones is lost first with aging.

ASSESSMENT GUIDELINES AND TOOLS

Always consider your client's sensory–perceptual status. Sensory deficits, deprivation, and overload have a significant influence on quality of life and may be especially troublesome for institutionalized clients.

Hearing Screening in Older Adults

Nurses may administer the ***Hearing Handicap Inventory for the Elderly Screening Version (HHIE-S)*** to assess the emotional and social effects of hearing impairment in older adults (Ventry & Weinstein, 1983). The HHIE-S is a simple to administer, 10-question, highly reliable tool that has been used worldwide since the 1980s. It is designed for older adults in clinical and community settings. This tool does not determine the extent of hearing loss as audiometric testing in a sound-protected environment does; rather, it assesses the effect on the hearing impairment on everyday life. The goal of the HHIE-S is to identify individuals who would likely benefit from intervention. To see a copy of the HHIE-S,

Go to the U. S. Preventive Services Task Force at https://www.uspreventiveservicestaskforce.org/Home/GetFileByID/231

Other Sensory Assessment Tools

Focused Assessment

Nursing History: Overall Sensory Perceptual Status

Usual Sensory Function

Ask the following questions such as:

- How would you rate your vision?
- How would you evaluate your ability to see objects up close or at a distance?
- Do you have any difficulty hearing conversations or listening to the radio or television?
- Have you experienced any difficulty locating sounds?
- Do you experience ringing or buzzing in your ears?
- Do you enjoy the taste of food?
- Do you notice any difficulty with your ability to smell?
- Are you experiencing any pain or discomfort?
- Do you have any areas of numbness or tingling on your body?
- Do you have any difficulty with sensing hot or cold?
- Describe your level of coordination.
- What medications are you taking? Have they had any effect on your vision, hearing, sense of taste, smell, touch, or balance?
- What is your current stress level?
- What is your usual activity level?
- What is your preferred activity level?

Assess for Risk Factors for Impaired Sensory Function

- Developmental level (e.g., older adults)
- Health status (usual and current state of health, current health concerns (e.g., Ménière's disease), history of hospitalizations and surgeries)
- Medications (i.e., look up side effects to determine what, if any, effect the medications have on sensory function)
- Stress (current and usual stress level, major sources of stressors, usual coping mechanisms)
- Lifestyle (normal activity, noise, interaction levels, hobbies, and usual lifestyle)

History of Sensory Problems

Ask about the following:

- Have you experienced any problems with blurred vision, double vision, sensitivity to light, blind spots, objects moving in front of your eyes, or eye pain?
- Have you ever felt unable to follow a conversation because of difficulty hearing?
- Have you ever had problems with your ability to taste or smell?
- Have you ever had areas of numbness or tingling?
- Has anyone in your family ever been diagnosed with a stroke or circulation problem?
- Have you ever had episodes of confusion or disorientation?

Use of Sensory Aids, Including Diet, Exercise, Medications, and Remedies

- Does the client wear glasses or contact lenses at any time? If so, determine the following:

  When was the client's last eye exam?

  Are the glasses clean and in good repair? Are the glasses within easy reach?

  Are contact lenses in good condition? Is the client able to care for them?

- Does the client wear a hearing aid? If so, determine the following:

  Can the client hear adequately with the hearing aid in place?

(Continued)

Focused Assessment

Nursing History: Overall Sensory Perceptual Status—cont'd

Are the batteries working?

Is the hearing aid clean?

How much help does the client need to place the hearing aid in his ear?

- Does the client use a cane or walker? If so:

Has the cane or walker been properly fitted to the client?

How often does the client use the device when walking?

- What factors determine when the device will be used?

Assess Mental Status

- Assess behavior, appearance, response to stimuli, speech, memory, and judgment. If you need more specific instructions, see Procedure 22-16, Steps 1–10 and Questions for Evaluating Cognitive Status, at the end of the procedure.

- **For older adults**, a tool called the Mini-Cog is especially useful (Borson, Scanlan, Brush, et al., 2000). It consists of 3 memory questions and instructions to draw a clock face. To use this tool,

Go to https://consultgeri.org/try-this/general-assessment/issue-3.1

- Assess level of orientation: Have the client tell you his name, the date, and his current location. If he person can answer these questions correctly, describe him as "awake, alert, and oriented to person, place, and time" (AA&O (3).

Assess Level of Consciousness

Alert	Is the patient awake and aware of the environment and himself, speaking clearly, making eye contact?
Confused	Are actions and speech inappropriate?
Lethargic	Is speech slow or sluggish? Are mental processes and movements sluggish?
Obtunded	This is a low level of awareness and response to environment. Document it if it occurs.
Stuporous	This occurs when the patient can be aroused by vigorous stimulation but seems confused during periods of arousal.
Comatose	In this state, there is no spontaneous movement, no verbalization, and only nonpurposeful movement with stimulation. (Huntley, 2008)

- Also see Chapter 22, Procedure 22-16: Assessing the Sensory–Neurological System, Glasgow Coma Scale, and Full Outline of UnResponsiveness Scale.

Assess Support Network for Clients With Sensory Deficit

- Are there support persons to help the client by assuming chores he can no longer perform?
- Are there people who provide comfort to ease the client's distress about sensory losses?
- Who can provide sensory stimulation?
- Who can help reorient and calm the client?
- Does the client need help with transportation to maintain social contact?

Focused Assessment

Bedside Assessment of Sensory Function

Sense	Assessment Process
Vision	Use the Snellen chart, or have the client read a newspaper.
	Observe for squinting.
Hearing	Perform the whisper test.
	Inspect the ear canals for hardened cerumen.
	Observe client conversations. Are there frequent requests for repeating information or misunderstandings?
	How loud is the client's radio or television?
	To screen hearing in older adults, you will find a useful tool if you
	Go to http://consultgerirn.org/uploads/File/trythis/try_this_12.pdf
Smell	Ask the client to close his eyes and identify common smells (e.g., coffee, vanilla, cloves, tobacco).
Taste	Ask the client to close his eyes and identify common tastes (e.g., salt, lemon, and sugar). Give water between tastes.
Tactile	With his eyes closed, touch the client with a wisp of cotton. Have him identify when you have touched him. Repeat this process with a sharp object, such as a needle.
	With his eyes closed, ask the client to identify where you are touching his body.
Kinesthesia	Have the client perform the Romberg test. See Procedure 22-7.
	Have the client perform alternating rapid motions, such as tapping heels or clapping.
	Observe the client's gait and movement.

CLINICALJUDGMENT

Applying the Full-Spectrum Nursing Model

PATIENT SITUATION

Clint Gossage is an 85-year-old man who lives at home alone. His wife moved to a nursing home a year ago. Although Mr. Gossage has many self-care deficits, he is still able to live at home, with regular visits from a home health nurse and community services to help with some meals and bathing. When you visit him, you notice that he shouts when talking to you, looks at you intently when you speak, and constantly asks you to repeat what you say. You examine his external ear canal and note that there is some hardened cerumen in the canal. He is not wearing a hearing aid. The patient record reveals tympanic membrane scarring and a diagnosis of conductive hearing loss.

THINKING

1. *Theoretical Knowledge:* Describe the pathophysiology of conductive hearing loss.

2. *Critical Thinking (Considering Alternatives):* Based on your knowledge of conductive hearing loss and your assessment of Mr. Gossage, what is the first follow-up question you would ask him about his hearing?

DOING

3. *Practical Knowledge:* At a subsequent visit, you discover that Mr. Gossage has impacted cerumen in his left ear. After obtaining a medical order, you prepare to perform an otic irrigation.
   a. To what temperature would you warm the solution?
   b. What position would you use for Mr. Gossage?
   c. Describe how you would place the tip of the syringe (or ear wash system) for irrigating.
   d. After the ear is cleared of cerumen and you have finished irrigating, what should you do next? And what position would you have Mr. Gossage assume when you do it?

4. *Nursing Process (Diagnosis):*
   a. Write a nursing diagnosis that focuses on Mr. Gossage's safety and that relates to hearing.
   b. Based on your nursing diagnosis, what safety measures would you recommend for Mr. Gossage's home? (Do not address the hearing aid issue here.)

CARING

5. *Ethical Knowledge:* Now, think back to the first visit with Mr. Gossage. What are some reasons that he might not have been wearing a hearing aid? Consider physical changes associated with aging.

Critical Thinking and Clinical Judgment

1. Review the following client scenarios.
   - Margaret is 84 years old. She is a retired schoolteacher, who loves to read, work in her garden, and volunteer at the local children's hospital. She is a light-eyed, older adult with a long history of smoking. She lived in the southern region most of her life, reporting that she rarely used sunglasses most of her life. She has developed macular degeneration and is progressively losing her sight.
   - Rocky is 55 years old. He is a former guitar player in a heavy metal band. He now works in music production. He has significant hearing loss related to chronic exposure to loud music. Most recently, he has developed tinnitus, which has exacerbated his hearing loss.
   - Abdul is 31 years old. He is a chef at a local four-star restaurant. He suffered a head injury in a motor vehicle accident. A few days after his injury, he notices that he has difficulty smelling and tasting food and a change in his appetite. In addition to tiring easily and failure to remember the events after his injury, Abdul also experiences sensitivity to light and noise. He acts cranky and isolates himself from others.
   - Vitoria is 35 years old. She is a licensed architect working for a firm in the downtown area. She has been taking birth control pills for 5 years. Recently, she has been under a lot of stress. She began drinking lots of coffee, smoking cigarettes, and working long hours. She was admitted to the hospital with right-sided weakness and slurred speech. She is being evaluated for a cerebrovascular accident.

   a. For each client, write a nursing diagnosis to reflect his or her sensory perception problem. Write one other nursing diagnosis that might result from the sensory perception problem. Explain your thinking.

   b. Each of the clients is experiencing a sensory deficit. What interventions would be most appropriate to address each client's concerns?

   c. Which client(s) is/are most likely to have difficulty adapting to the sensory deficit? How would you determine how each client is adapting?

   d. Which client, if any, is most likely to be experiencing sensory overload?

2. Examine the clinical unit that you are visiting for your current clinical rotation. What unit factors contribute to the development of sensory overload?

3. What factors in the clinical unit contribute to the development of sensory deprivation?

4. For each of the following concepts, use critical thinking to describe how or why it is important to nursing, patient care, or sensory perception. Note that these are *not* to be merely definitions.

   Sensory stimulation　　Sensory deficits

   Sensory overload　　Sensory aids

   Sensory deprivation

What Are the Main Points in This Chapter?

- The purpose of sensation is to allow the body to respond to changing situations and maintain homeostasis.
- A sensory experience involves four components: stimulus, reception, perception, and an arousal mechanism.
- Reception is the process of receiving stimuli from nerve endings in the skin and body.
- Perception is the ability to interpret the impulses transmitted from the receptors and give meaning to the stimuli.
- Humans respond to sensations when they are alert and receptive to stimulation. The response to a stimulus is based on intensity, contrast, adaptation, previous experience, illness, or injury.
- Sensory deprivation is caused by a deficiency of meaningful stimuli.
- Sensory deprivation can be caused by environmental conditions or to interference with the reception or perception of stimuli.
- Sensory overload develops when either environmental or internal stimuli—or a combination of both—exceed a level that the client's sensory system can effectively process. It can also occur in clients with neurological or psychiatric disorders unable to adapt to continuing, nonmeaningful stimuli.
- Impaired vision and hearing are the sensory deficits most commonly encountered in nursing practice.
- The client with impaired vision, hearing, tactile sensation, olfactory sensation, or kinesthesia is at risk for injury.
- Visual and hearing changes may diminish the ability to communicate and may hamper social interaction.
- Developmental issues, culture, health status, medications, stress level, and individual preferences affect sensory perception.
- To assess sensory perceptual function, assess factors affecting sensory perception, mental status, recent changes in sensory stimulation, use of sensory aids, the client's environment, and the support network.
- Nursing strategies to address impaired sensory perception include activities to promote sensory function, prevent and treat sensory overload and deprivation, assist clients with sensory deficits, and communicate with clients with altered mental status.

Knowledge Map

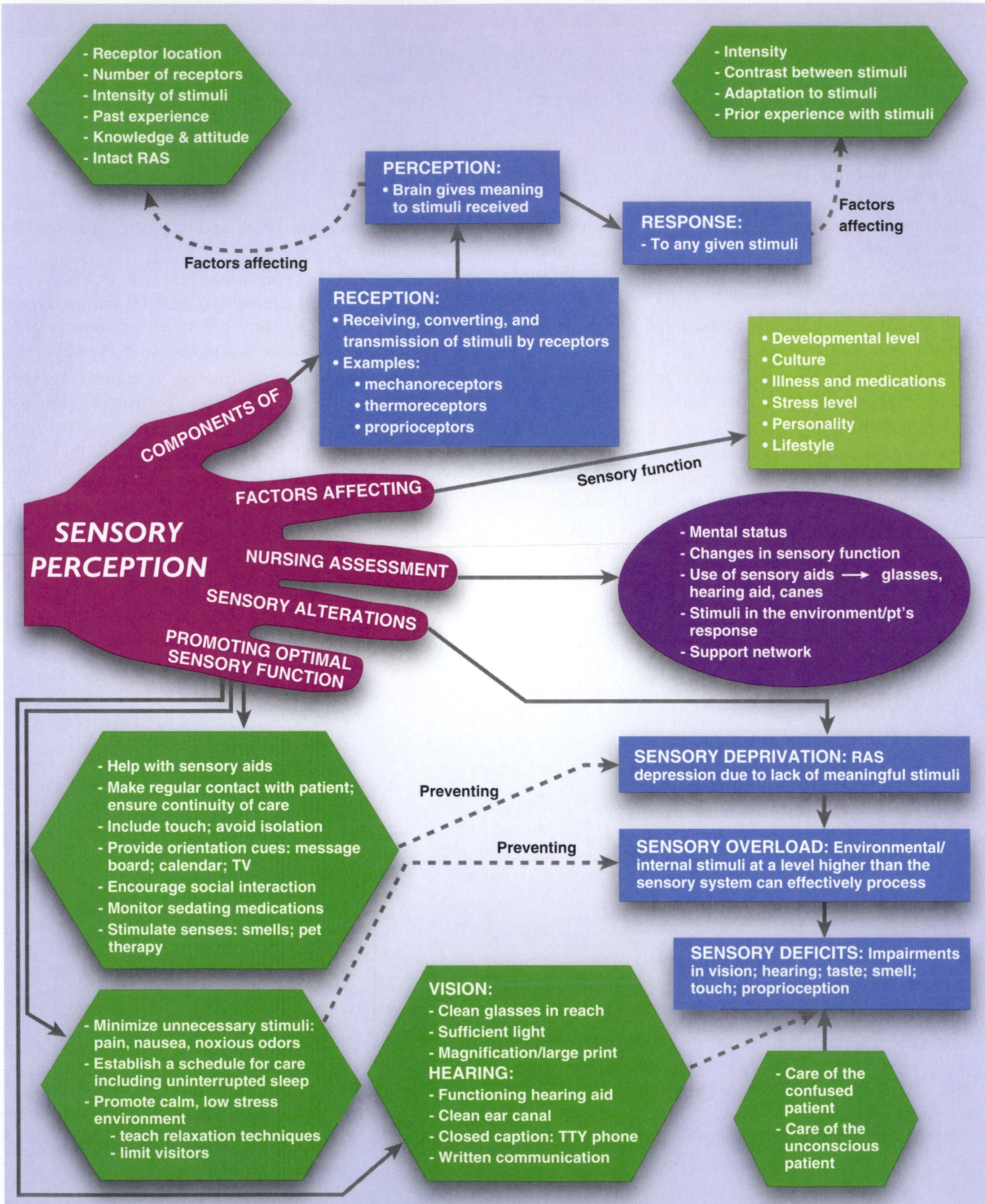

CHAPTER 31

Pain

STUDENT RESOURCES

The questions and exercises in this book allow you to practice the kind of thinking you will use as a full-spectrum nurse. Critical-thinking questions usually have more than one right answer, so we do not provide "correct answers" for these features. Try to answer these questions yourself. It is more important to develop your nursing judgment than to just cover content. You will learn more by discussing the questions with your peers. If you are still unsure, see the Davis Advantage chapter resources for suggested responses.

To explore learning resources for this chapter,

Go to Davis Advantage and find:

Answers and Suggested Responses for all questions in this chapter

Concept Map

Knowledge Map

References and Bibliography

Lists of NOC Outcomes and NIC Interventions

Key Concepts

Pain

Pain management

Related Concepts

See the Concept Map on Davis Advantage.

Caring for the Nguyens

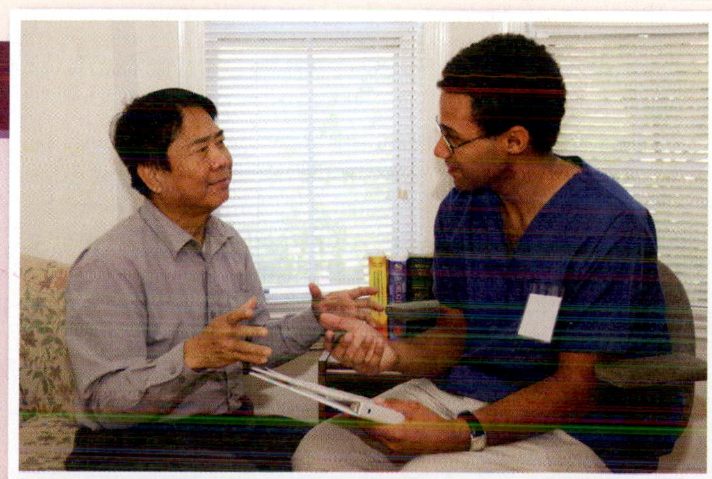

Review the introduction to the Nguyens at the front of this volume. Nam Nguyen has bilateral knee pain secondary to osteoarthritis.

(Continued)

Caring for the Nguyens (continued)

A. To develop a pain management plan, what patient data do you need to know?

B. How will you get the data you need? What sources should you use?

C. What types of nursing knowledge (theoretical, practical, ethical, or self-knowledge) are needed to develop a pain management plan?

PracticalKnowledge knowing **how**

When caring for patients with pain, you will need to be skilled in medication administration, including use of patient-controlled analgesia (PCA) pumps and caring for patients who have an epidural catheter.

PROCEDURES

Procedure 31-1 ■ Setting Up and Managing Patient-Controlled Analgesia by Pump

➤ For steps to follow in *all* procedures, refer to the Universal Steps for All Procedures found on the page facing the inside back cover.

Equipment

- PCA pump (infuser and central unit)
- Manufacturer's instructions for the pump
- Cartridge, syringe, or other type of sealed unit containing the medication
- Connecting tubing (to connect the PCA device to the patient's intravenous [IV] line)
- Maintenance IV supplies, as needed
- IV pole
- Antiseptic swab
- Flowsheet (electronic or paper)
- One pair of clean procedure gloves (if venipuncture is necessary)

Delegation

Because an opioid medication is delivered intravenously to the patient, this procedure is outside the scope of the practice of unlicensed assistive personnel (UAP) and should never be delegated. Furthermore, the UAP should not administer a dose for the patient, even if he asks her to do so. You can inform the UAP of expected side effects and ask her to report her observations to you.

Pre-Procedure Assessment

- Assess physical conditions that can affect respirations.
  Respiratory diseases (e.g., chronic obstructive pulmonary disease [COPD] and asthma) and conditions such as head injury and sleep apnea increase the risk for respiratory depression with opioid use (American Pain Society, 2016).
- Assess level of consciousness and cognitive level.
  Determines whether the patient will be able to follow directions for self-dosing.
- Review lab values reflecting liver and kidney function, such as blood urea nitrogen (BUN), creatinine, and liver enzymes.
  Opioid analgesics are typically metabolized through the liver or kidneys.
- Assess the baseline respiratory rate, pulse, blood pressure, and oxygen saturation.
  A change in vital signs (e.g., hypotension, respiratory rate less than 8) may indicate adverse responses to opioid administration.
- Be aware of the patient's age and weight.
  Age is a factor when you are verifying the dose. Older patients and very young children are at increased risk for respiratory suppression and so may require lower doses. Pediatric doses are based on the child's weight.
- Assess the patient's baseline pain level using a standardized pain assessment tool or numeric scale ranging from 0 to 10.
  A quantified self-report is one of the most accurate measures of pain.
- Assess the patient's manual dexterity.
  Patients with impaired fine motor control or upper extremity injury may not be able to operate the self-dosing mechanism.
- Review medications currently in use.
  The risk of respiratory depression increases when a PCA pump is used in conjunction with other central nervous system depressants, such as diazepam (Valium).
- Assess the extent of family involvement. Identify any family anxiety over the patient's pain. Reinforce that only the patient should use the PCA button.
  Only the patient should administer the medication. "PCA by proxy" (someone other than the patient pushing the dosing button) is a major factor contributing to adverse patient outcomes (Wuhrman, Cooney, Dunwoody, et al., 2007).

➤ When performing the procedure, always identify your patient according to agency policy, using two identifiers, and be attentive to standard precautions, hand hygiene, patient safety and privacy, body mechanics, and documentation.

Procedure Steps

1. **Don clean procedure gloves;** initiate IV therapy if the patient does not currently have an IV solution infusing. Refer to Procedure 38-1 as needed.

2. **Obtain the medication and double-check it** with the original prescription before starting the infusion or wasting medication. You may need to remove air from the vial by pushing the injector into the vial.
Some vials may not be completely filled with medication. Ejecting the air makes it faster to prime the connecting tubing.

3. **Double-check your dose calculation with another nurse** before starting the infusion or wasting medication.
To prevent errors in dosing.

4. **Connect the PCA tubing to the vial or cartridge.** Then:
   a. Prime the tubing.
   b. Clamp the tubing above the connector.
   Priming prevents air from entering the pump and causing malfunction. Clamping prevents an accidental bolus of medication getting to the patient.

5. **Insert the cartridge or vial** into the pump; lock the pump. Follow the manufacturer's instruction manual (e.g., some pumps can be set only if the door is closed and locked).
Depending on the pump, it may be a syringe, a cartridge, or other sealed container that can be "locked" into the pump. Locking the pump prevents unauthorized access to the opioid and dosing features.

6. **Turn the pump on; set** the desired pump settings according to the prescription and calculation verifying the dose.
PCA settings for preventing unintended dosing include:
   a. **"On-demand" dose**—the amount of drug to be delivered with each push of the button).
   b. **The "lockout" interval**—the number of minutes allowed between each administration of an on-demand dose (e.g., every 10 minutes). Even if the patient pushes the button more frequently, the PCA pump will not administer a dose until the preset time between doses has been met.
   c. **Basal rate or continuous infusion**—the amount of medication to be delivered automatically by the pump over 1 hour should be used with caution. Giving the medication continuously without the patient having to push a button takes away some of the inherent safety of a PCA.
   d. **One-time "bolus"**—*loading* dose that you administer after setting up the pump.
   e. **The 1-hour or 4-hour lockout interval**—the maximum dose allowed in that time frame. For example, if the patient has a 4-mg on-demand dose with a 10-minute lockout interval, the patient can receive a maximum of six 4-mg doses per hour for a total of 24 mg/hr and a maximum dose of 96 mg in 4 hours.

   NOTE: PCA prescriptions are usually written in milligrams; however, pump settings may be in milliliters. In such cases, you must verify the concentration (milligrams per milliliter) to set the pump correctly.

7. **Scrub the port on the IV** tubing closest to the patient, using alcohol or a chlorhexidine gluconate (CHG)–alcohol product; then connect the PCA pump tubing.
Removes gross contamination and discourages growth of pathogens.

8. **Open the clamp and administer the bolus** (loading) dose if prescribed. Remain with the patient as the dose is delivered.
A loading dose is usually larger than the basal and on-demand doses because pain is likely to be more severe before the pump is initiated. Remaining with the patient allows you to observe for adverse effects.

9. **Close the pump door and lock the settings.**

10. **Check for flashing lights** or alarms that may indicate the need to correct settings or check the infusion site.

11. **Be sure to release tubing clamps** if you previously clamped the tubing; press the start button to begin pump operation.

12. **Ensure that the battery life** is sufficient or, preferably, that the pump is plugged in to an appropriate electrical outlet.
To avoid battery failure.

13. **Place the control button** for on-demand doses within the patient's reach. Be sure the PCA cord is placed away from the call device.
To avoid error in self-dosing with PCA.

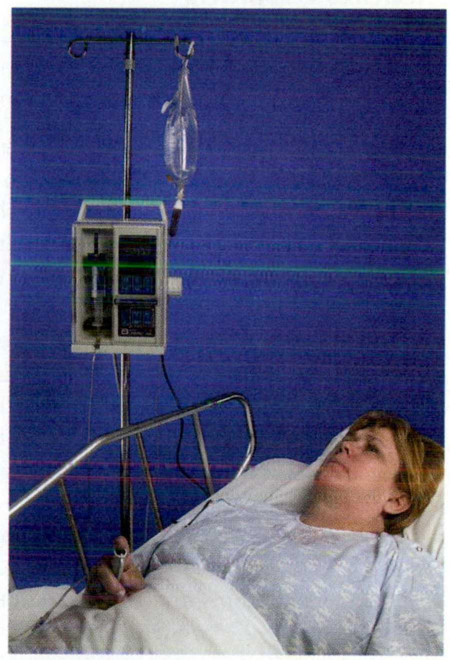

14. **Leave the patient in a safe, comfortable position** with the call device within reach.

? What if . . .

- **The patient cannot verbally communicate pain status?**

Use an alternate standardized pain tool, such as the FACES pain scale or

(continued on next page)

Procedure 31-1 ■ Setting Up and Managing Patient-Controlled Analgesia by Pump (continued)

a behavioral measure, to determine pain level.

Pain assessment in patients who are uncommunicative may include behavioral or physiological indicators to assess and monitor the effectiveness of pain medication.

- **The infusion infiltrates?**

  Discontinue the IV and establish another IV site. Follow facility policy for application of cold or warm compresses to the infiltrated area. Assess pain level. You may need to contact the prescriber for a bolus dose if the IV has been interrupted for an extended period or the patient has insufficient pain relief.

Evaluation

- Monitor the patient's pain level, sedation level, and respiratory rate at least every hour for the first 24 hours or according to facility policy after initiating PCA.

  Promotes the early detection of respiratory depression, oversedation, or inadequate pain control.
- Perform routine assessment of number and frequency of doses and pump settings per facility protocol.
- Check the IV site for redness, infiltration, or phlebitis.
- Check the IV tubing for patency (e.g., for kinks) to be sure the medication is infusing.

Patient Teaching

Patients who are candidates for use of PCA should be trained before surgery rather than in the immediate postoperative period, when the effects of anesthesia impair learning. Reinforce or teach the patient and family the following:

- Safe and correct use of the PCA pump
- Benefits of PCA for controlling pain
- The pump will deliver only the amount of medication prescribed. Pushing the button too many times will not result in overdosing.
- The patient cannot accidentally roll over on the button and unintentionally give additional medication.
- If pain is not being relieved, the patient should tell the nurse, so adjustments can be made to the PCA.
- The pump will alarm when nearly empty, alerting nurses to change the syringe.
- The PCA button is to relieve pain—not to help the patient sleep.
- Signs and symptoms of allergic reaction and which ones to report
- How to rate pain using a standard pain scale
- The patient is the only one who may push the pain-dosing button. Explain why family members should not give "doses by proxy."

Documentation

You will usually document PCA initiation on a specialized checklist or flowsheet. Items charted include:

- Time the infusion was begun, including the drug, the patient demand dose, the loading dose, the basal dose if applicable, lockout interval, and hourly limit
- Patient's baseline pain level and evaluation of subsequent pain level performed at intervals determined by facility policy
- Baseline respiratory rate, pulse, blood pressure, and oxygen saturation; routine evaluation of subsequent vital signs performed at intervals determined by facility policy
- Sedation level
- Continuous monitoring of vital signs, level of consciousness, and pain status, as well as the number and frequency of doses
- Unusual occurrences (e.g., oversedation, IV infiltration) in the electronic health record (EHR)

Practice Resources

Portenoy, R. K., & McCafferty, M. (2011).

Thinking About the Procedure

The video **Setting up and Managing Patient-Controlled Analgesia by Pump,** along with questions and suggested responses, is available on the ***Davis's Nursing Skills Videos*** Web site on FADavis.com.

CLINICAL INSIGHTS

Clinical Insight 31-1 ➤ Caring for the Patient With an Epidural Catheter

Nursing care of the patient with epidural analgesia focuses on the following:
- Safely administering analgesia
- Assessing pain while achieving maximum pain control
- Preventing or identifying adverse reactions

Contraindications

Epidural analgesia is contraindicated in patients who have the following:
- Increased risk for bleeding: anticoagulant therapy; other bleeding problems
- Infection at the insertion site or in the bloodstream
- Increased intracranial pressure
- Allergy to local anesthetic or opioid
- As a general rule, those who have spinal defects, previous spinal surgery, or certain neurological conditions (e.g., multiple sclerosis)

Monitoring

- **Monitor vital signs,** especially for respiratory depression and hypotension (every hour for the first 24 hours, then every 4 hours if the patient is stable).
- **Assess pain intensity** using a pain rating scale (per institution's protocol) and degree of motor and sensory block.
- **Monitor the site** for leaking or drainage.
- **Check connections for leaks.** This can be fixed by carefully retightening connections. If the filter is cracked, replace with a new one using sterile technique.
- **Assess for urine retention.** Keep careful intake and output (I&O) records.
  Urinary retention is one side effect of epidural opioids.
- **Observe for verbal and nonverbal signs of headache** as a result of dural puncture. Treatment consists of bedrest, analgesics, and liberal hydration. Caffeine is also helpful and may be administered IV. If unresolved after 72 hours, patient might receive an epidural blood patch.
  An epidural blood patch is an injection of the patient's own blood into the epidural space to prevent headache.
- **Observe for signs of catheter migration:** nausea, a decrease in blood pressure, and a loss of motor function without a recognizable cause.
- **Observe for signs of local anesthesia toxicity** occurring when anesthesia is injected directly into the bloodstream instead of the epidural space. The patient might report numbness or tingling around the mouth or ringing in the ears (tinnitus); or you may assess irritability, tremors, seizures, or cardiac arrhythmias (Portenoy & McCaffery, 2011; Sawheney, 2012).

Prevention

- **Clearly label solutions with "For epidural use only"** using large font. Store IV and epidural medication in separate locations.
  Prevents errors in medication administration.
- **Mark all lines *clearly*:** Most epidural tubing is marked with a yellow stripe.
  Epidural lines must not be confused with IV solution for an arterial or venous catheter.
- **Ensure the tape is secure on the tubing** connected to the patient.
  To prevent catheter migration.
- **Use strict aseptic technique** when changing tubing, including mask and sterile gloves for access and maintenance procedures.

Discontinuing the Catheter

- **If you are specially trained to remove an epidural catheter**:
  1. Loosen the tape securing the catheter.
  2. While wearing clean gloves, apply slow, steady pressure to withdraw the catheter.
  3. Inspect the catheter on removal. You must be able to see the tip of the catheter. If not, a portion of the catheter may still be lodged in the patient's epidural space. Notify the anesthesia team immediately of this finding.
- If the catheter cannot be withdrawn with minimal force, try repositioning the patient to the same position for removal as the patient was in during insertion of the catheter.
- Cleanse the insertion site, and cover with a dry sterile dressing.

ASSESSMENT GUIDELINES AND TOOLS

Focused Assessment

Pain Assessment

Taking a Pain History

Taking a pain history is the most effective way to perform an assessment. Each agency has a different assessment form for this history, but the questions typically will include the following:

- Do you have pain now?
- When did the pain begin?
- Where is the pain located?
- How do you rate your pain? (Use a pain scale.)
- How would you describe your pain? Sharp? Dull? Achy? Burning?
- How often do you have pain? Is it constant or intermittent?
- Is there a rhythm or pattern to your pain? Is there anything you do that triggers the pain?
- What makes the pain better? What makes it worse?
- How many days this past week has pain interfered in your ability to do what you would like to do?
- Does pain interfere with your ability to take care of yourself?
- Does pain wake you up at night?
- Does pain interrupt your concentration and reduce your ability to think clearly?
- Does pain prevent you from participating in pleasurable activities, hobbies, and socializing with friends?
- Have you experienced this type of pain in the past?
- Do you have any other symptoms (such as nausea and vomiting) when you are experiencing pain?
- Have you used any medications to treat the pain? If so, were they effective? How often do you need to take pain relievers?
- What, if any, alternative treatments have you used for pain?
- What past experiences or cultural factors, if any, influence the pain?

Observing for Nonverbal Indicators of Pain

Physiological (Involuntary) Responses

SYMPATHETIC RESPONSES (ACUTE PAIN)

- Increased systolic blood pressure
- Increased heart rate and force of contraction
- Increased respiratory rate
- Increased alertness (resulting from dilated blood vessels to the brain)
- Dilated pupils
- Rapid speech

PARASYMPATHETIC RESPONSES (DEEP OR PROLONGED PAIN)

- Decreased systolic blood pressure, possible syncope
- Decreased pulse rate
- Changeable breathing patterns
- Withdrawal
- Constricted pupils
- Slow, monotonous speech

BEHAVIORAL RESPONSES (VOLUNTARY)

- Withdrawing from painful stimuli
- Moaning
- Facial grimacing
- Crying
- Agitation
- Guarding the painful area

Psychological (Affective) Responses

- Anxiety
- Depression
- Anger
- Fear
- Exhaustion
- Hopelessness
- Irritability

Using Pain Scales

The most commonly used pain scales are the Visual Analog Scale, the Numeric Rating Scale, the Simple Descriptor Scale, and the Wong-Baker FACES rating scale.

The Visual Analog Scale

The Visual Analog Scale (VAS) is a 10-cm horizontal line in which "No pain" is written on the left side and "Worst pain imaginable" is written on the right. Patients point to a location on the line that reflects their current pain. Although this rating system is simple and quick, some patients have problems with the abstract nature of the scale.

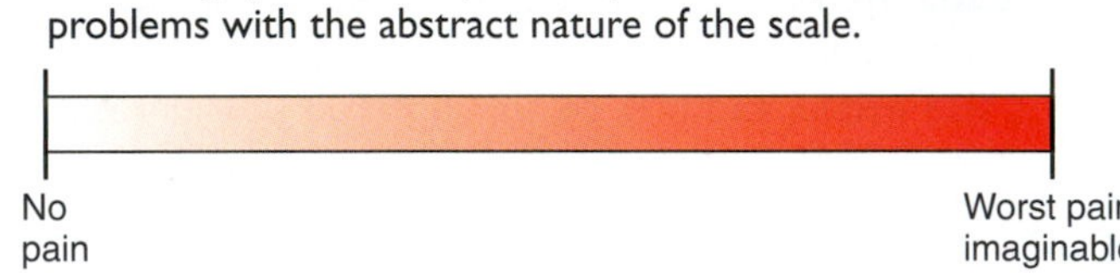

The Numeric Rating Scale

The Numeric Rating Scale (NRS) is a line numbered from 0 to 10. Zero indicates no pain at all, whereas a 10 indicates the worst possible pain. Patients choose a number from 0 to 10 to denote their level of pain. To use this scale, the patient must be able to count to 10. A scale of 0 to 5 may be more helpful for cognitively impaired patients.

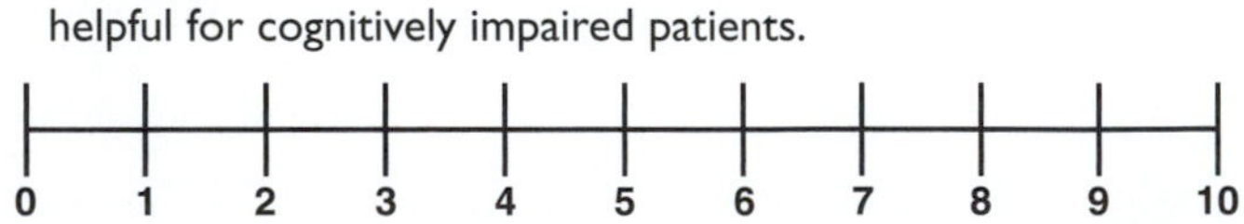

Focused Assessment

Pain Assessment—cont'd

The Simple Descriptor Scale

The Simple Descriptor Scale (SDS) is a list of adjectives that describe different levels of pain intensity. The simplest version of this scale uses the words *mild, moderate,* and *severe*. An SDS with many words is not recommended; it is time consuming to describe and may not be understood by many patients.

The Wong-Baker FACES Pain Rating Scale

The FACES Scale uses simple illustrations of faces to depict various levels of pain. It requires no numerical or reading skill. Initially developed for use with children older than the age of 3, the scale has proved to be extremely useful for adults with communication and cognitive impairments as well.

Wong-Baker FACES Pain Rating Scale

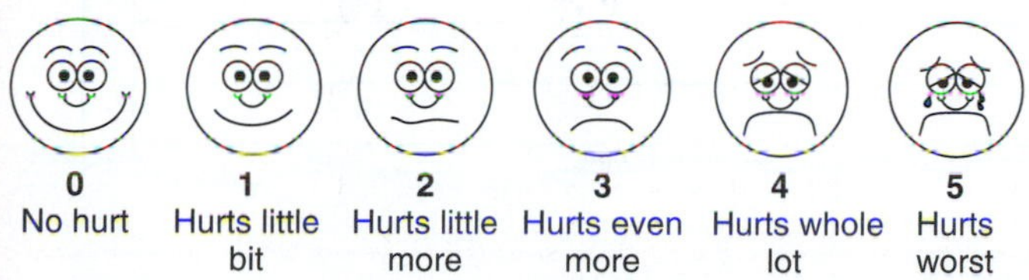

Explain to the person that each face is for a person who feels happy because he has no pain (hurt) or sad because he has some or a lot of pain. Face 0 is very happy because he doesn't hurt at all. Face 2 hurts a little more. Face 3 hurts even more. Face 4 hurts a whole lot. Face 5 hurts as much as you can imagine, although you do not have to be crying to feel this bad. Ask the person to choose the face that best describes how he is feeling. Rating scale is recommended for persons age 3 and older.

From Wong-Baker FACES Foundation (2018). Wong-Baker FACES® Pain Rating Scale. Retrieved February 7, 2019 with permission from http://www.WongBakerFACES.org. Originally published in *Whaley & Wong's Nursing Care of Infants and Children*. © Elsevier Inc.

Revised Faces Pain Scales

The Faces Pain Scale—Revised (FPS-R) is a self-reported measure of pain intensity developed for children. It was adapted from the FACES Pain Scale to make it possible to score pain levels using the widely accepted 0-to-10 metric. The use of grimacing can reflect the experience of pain more accurately than rating faces with smiles and tears.

Give direction for patients to score the chosen face 0, 2, 4, 6, 8, or 10, where 0 means *no pain* and 10 means *very much pain*. This scale is intended to measure how they feel inside, not how their face looks.

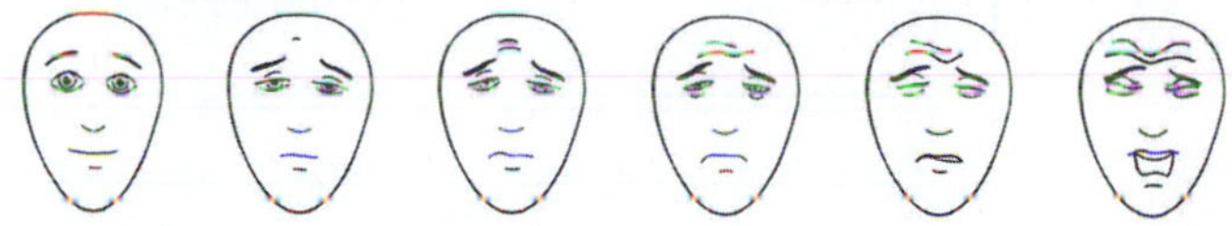

From Hicks, C. L., von Baeyer, C. L., Spafford, P. van Korlaar, I., Goodenough, B. (2001). The Faces Pain Scale—Revised: Toward a common metric in pediatric pain measurement. *Pain, 93,* 173–183; Bieri, D., Reeve, R., Champion, G. D., Addicoat, L., & Ziegler, J. (1990). The Faces Pain Scale for the self-assessment of the severity of pain experienced by children: Development, initial validation and preliminary investigation for ratio scale properties. *Pain, 41,* 139–150.

To see FACES scales using photos of children of various ethnicities,

Go to the **OUCHER! Web site** at www.oucher.org

Focused Assessment

Pain Relief Diary

Client Pain Relief Diary

For pain relief I am using:

Medications ______________________

Alternative therapy (relaxation, distraction, etc.) ______________________

I will call my physician if ______________________ (filled in by nurse before discharge)

My goals are a pain rating of ______________________

Date	Time	Number of pills	Pain scale 0 1 2 3 4 5 6 7 8 9 10	Goal met? Yes No	Activity

Focused Assessment

Richmond Agitation-Sedation Scale

Score	Term	Description
+4	Combative	Overtly combative or violent; immediate danger to staff
+3	Very agitated	Pulls on or removes tube(s) or catheter(s) or has aggressive behavior toward staff
+2	Agitated	Frequent nonpurposeful movement or patient–ventilator dyssynchrony
+1	Restless	Anxious or apprehensive but movements not aggressive or vigorous
0	Alert and calm	
–1	Drowsy	Not fully alert but has sustained (more than 10 seconds) awakening, with eye contact, to voice
–2	Light sedation	Briefly (less than 10 seconds) awakens with eye contact to voice
–3	Moderate sedation	Any movement (but no eye contact) to voice
–4	Deep sedation	No response to voice, but any movement to physical stimulation
–5	Unarousable	No response to voice or physical stimulation

Sessler, C. N., Gosnell, M.S., Grap, M. J., et al. (2002). The Richmond Agitation–Sedation Scale: Validity and reliability in adult intensive care unit patients. *American Journal of Respiratory Critical Care Medicine, 166*, 1338–1344.

CLINICALJUDGMENT

Applying the Full-Spectrum Nursing Model

PATIENT SITUATION

Dieter Schmidt is a 48-year-old man with a 2-year history of cervical spine injury that began after a motor vehicle accident. Presenting symptoms were neck pain when turning his head, biceps weakness, and pain down the arm with tingling into the fingertips. He is unable to sit for extended periods or walk distances. Initially he received treatment with medication, transcutaneous electrical nerve stimulation (TENS) to the site, physical therapy, and cervical fusion. Despite trying all treatments available to him, including surgery, Dieter continues to suffer chronic pain and fatigue. After prolonged suffering with no relief, he develops a cynical attitude toward healthcare. He begins missing more and more scheduled appointments for physical therapy. He describes the stress he feels from the economic downturn impacting his land development business and fears bankruptcy. As a result, he has given up previous hobbies and most social activities. His relationships with his family and friends are increasingly strained as the pain persists over time.

THINKING

1. *Theoretical Knowledge:*
   What is the mechanism that explains how pain is transmitted in the spine?

2. *Critical Thinking (Considering Alternatives, Deciding What to Do):*
   a. When planning care for Dieter, what approach would you take in helping him to set goals for his rehabilitation?
   b. Why do you think Dieter displays a negative attitude and reduced compliance toward rehabilitative therapies?

DOING

3. *Practical Knowledge:*
   a. *(Nursing Process: Assessment)*: What questions would you ask Dieter to assess the impact of pain on his daily living and quality of life?
   b. *(Nursing Process: Interventions)*: In addition to drug therapy, what other measures might you teach Dieter to do to control his pain and increase his comfort?

CARING

4. *Self-Knowledge:*
   Have you ever experienced chronic pain, such as back pain, fibromyalgia, arthritis, migraines, sports injuries, or other types? If so, how has it affected your daily life? Has your pain impacted your relationships? Has it interfered with your job or recreational activities? In what other ways would you say chronic pain has reduced the quality of your life?

Critical Thinking and Clinical Judgment

1. Mrs. J is a 29-year-old woman with terminal metastatic breast cancer. She knows she is dying. She has a devoted husband and two children, ages 2 and 4. Her husband has been taking care of her at home, but she is currently hospitalized for intractable pain. She does not want to be heavily sedated because she wants to spend as much time with her family as she can. She has no pain management plan.
   a. What is it about the patient's situation that may intensify her pain?
   b. Would you suggest using alternative therapies? Why or why not?

2. Mr. L is a 39-year-old construction worker who fell from a roof at a construction site 8 months ago and is still having back pain from the accident. To manage pain, he is prescribed an oral opioid every 4 hours on an as-needed (prn) basis. He is still out of work and has great difficulty walking, so he spends most of the day in a recliner watching TV and drinking beer. Mr. L also sleeps most nights in the recliner. He states that the alcohol is the only thing that helps his pain. How would you alter his pain management plan to get better relief? What is your rationale for these changes?
3. If you were delegating vital signs to UAP, what instructions would you give?
4. For each of the following concepts, use critical thinking to describe how or why it is important to nursing, patient care, or pain management. Note that these are *not* to be merely definitions.

Nociceptive pain	Opioid pain medications
Neuropathic pain	Adjuvant therapies
Unrelieved pain	Fear of addiction
Pain scales	Nonpharmacological pain management
Pain flowsheets	Nonopioid pain medications

What Are the Main Points in This Chapter?

- Pain is whatever the person says it is and exists whenever the person says it does.
- Pain has a protective function, warning us of potential or actual tissue damage and prompting us to act.
- Pain can be classified by its origin, cause, duration, and quality.
- Nociceptive pain results from injury to body tissues. Pain begins when mechanical, thermal, or chemical stimuli activate nociceptors, which send pain impulses to the spinal cord.
- Neuropathic pain occurs when there is injury to one or more nerves. A pain signal is transmitted even in the absence of painful stimuli.
- Fast pain impulses are carried on large-diameter A-delta fibers, whereas slow pain impulses are carried on thinner C fibers.
- Perception of pain occurs in the frontal cortex of the brain.
- Pain can be modulated by the endogenous analgesic system or by the gate control mechanism.
- Some of the factors that influence pain are emotional factors, life span variations, past pain experiences, sociocultural factors, inability to communicate, and cognitive impairment.
- Serious physiological, emotional, and psychological problems can result from unrelieved pain.
- Nonpharmacological pain relief measures include cutaneous stimulation, immobilization, and cognitive–behavioral intervention.
- Pharmacological measures include nonopioid analgesics, opioid analgesics, and adjuvant analgesics.
- Local and regional anesthesia, nerve blocks, and ablation therapy can relieve short- and long-term pain.
- Surgical interruption of pain conduction pathways is an option for intractable pain. Options depend on the type and location of pain.
- Opioid addiction among individuals being treated for pain is rare.
- The nurse assesses the patient for pain thoroughly and often (e.g., when the patient is admitted to a healthcare facility and whenever checking vital signs, before and after an intervention, change in clinical condition, and when the patient reports pain).
- The patient's self-report is the most reliable indicator of pain, especially for those suffering chronic pain.
- Misconceptions about pain can interfere in pain management.
- Older adults are at risk for undertreatment of pain.
- Planning for the patient's pain management program includes discovering the patient's own goals, educating the patient and family, and developing a nursing plan of care.
- It is important to assess continually the effectiveness of pain management strategies.

Knowledge Map

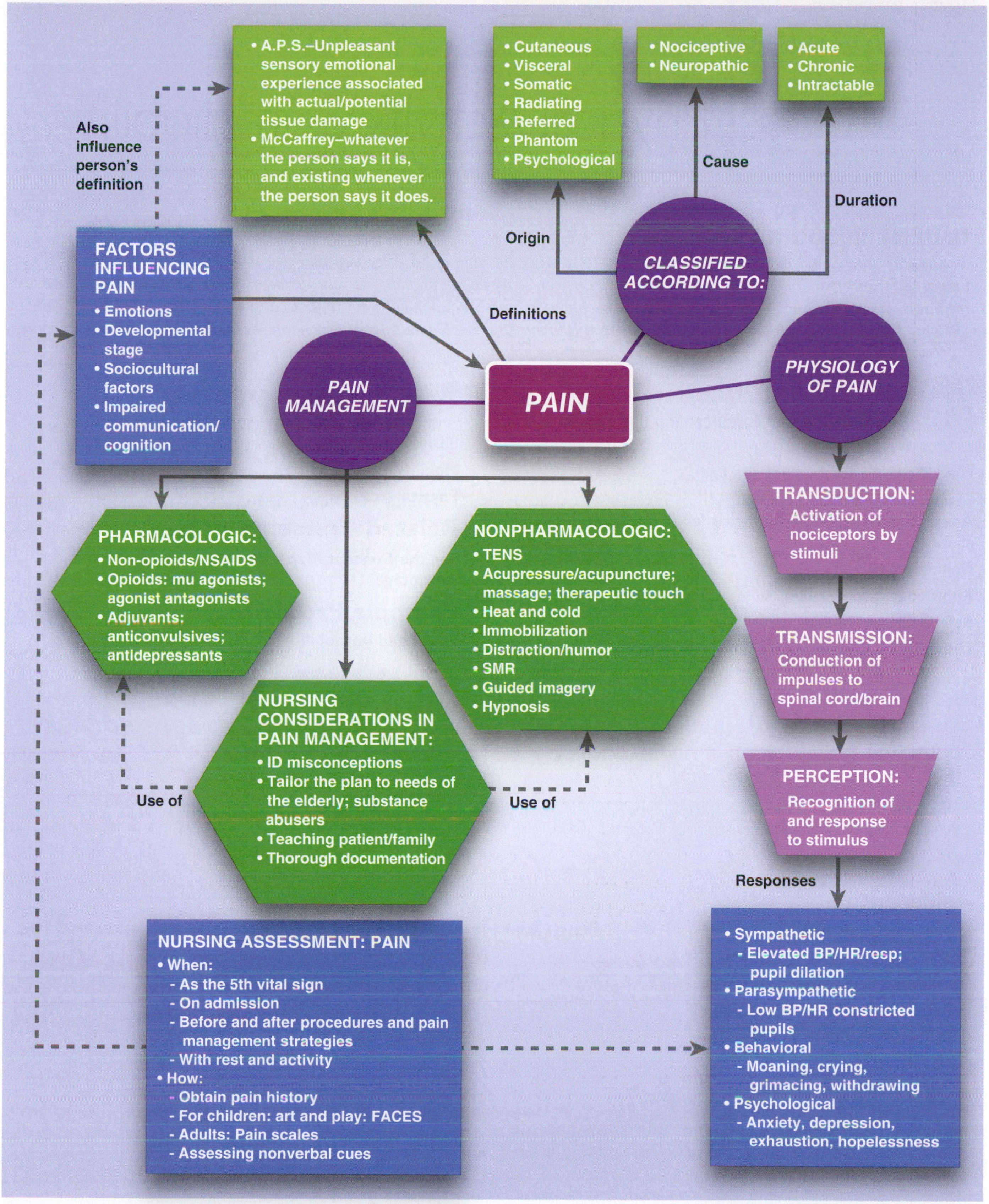

CHAPTER 32

Physical Activity & Immobility

STUDENT RESOURCES

The questions and exercises in this book allow you to practice the kind of thinking you will use as a full-spectrum nurse. Critical-thinking questions usually have more than one right answer, so we do not provide "correct answers" for these features. Try to answer these questions yourself. It is more important to develop your nursing judgment than to just cover content. You will learn more by discussing the questions with your peers. If you are still unsure, see the Davis Advantage chapter resources for suggested responses.

To explore learning resources for this chapter,

Go to Davis Advantage and find:

Answers and Suggested Responses for all questions in this chapter

Concept Map

Knowledge Map

References and Bibliography

Lists of NOC Outcomes and NIC Interventions

Key Concepts

Fitness

Mobility

Physical Activity

Related Concepts

See the Concept Map on Davis Advantage

Example Problem

Prolonged Immobility

Caring for the Nguyens

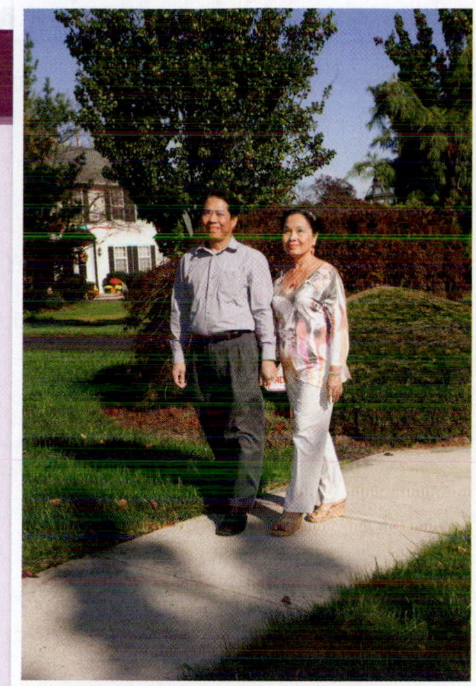

As you may recall, Nam Nguyen has been advised to diet and exercise as part of the treatment plan for hypertension, type 2 diabetes mellitus, obesity, and osteoarthritis. Zach Miller's exam has revealed no other cardiovascular problems.

A. Design a fitness program for Nam. Describe the program in detail. Recall that Nam has been relatively sedentary.

B. Compare the type of program you would recommend for Nam with the type of program appropriate for his grandson, Kim.

C. What type of fitness program would be most appropriate for Mai Nguyen, Nam's mother? What additional information do you need to know to answer this question?

PracticalKnowledge clinical **application**

In the next sections you will learn about procedures and techniques for positioning, moving, turning, transferring, and ambulating patients safely. Although the American Nurses Association (ANA, 2013) recommends that you use assistive equipment for all patient lifting and transferring, you may encounter situations in which equipment is not available or you do not have time to get it (e.g., in an emergency). In such situations, using good body mechanics may help you decrease the risk of injury to you and the patient.

PROCEDURES

Procedure 32-1 ■ Moving and Turning Patients in Bed

➤ For steps to follow in *all* procedures, refer to the Universal Steps for All Procedures found on the page facing the inside back cover.

Equipment

- Nonlatex gloves, if you may be exposed to body fluids
- Friction-reducing device, such as a transfer roller sheet or scoot sheet
- Pull or lift (draw) sheet
- Pillows, as needed

Delegation

You may ask unlicensed assistive personnel (UAP) to assist with moving a patient up in bed, turning a patient, or logrolling a patient after ensuring that the UAP has the necessary skills and that the patient's condition is stable. Complete the assessment; inform the UAP of any special considerations when moving the patient.

(continued on next page)

Procedure 32-1 ■ Moving and Turning Patients in Bed (continued)

Pre-Procedure Assessment

Assess the following:

- Level of comfort
  If the patient is uncomfortable, you may need to administer an analgesic before moving.
- Level of consciousness, ability to follow directions, and ability to assist with the move
- Any restrictions in movement or position (ask the patient and check the provider's orders
- Physical size of the patient and the assistive devices available
- The patient's health status. Identify problems that may affect positioning (e.g., respiratory or cardiac problems, pain).
- Presence of equipment such as intravenous (IV) setups, pumps, or casts and know what must be moved with the patient
  The preceding assessments all help determine how many assistants and what equipment you need, the patient's ability to assist in the procedure, and how to proceed with the move safely.

Procedure 32-1A ■ Moving a Patient Up in Bed

➤ When performing the procedure, always identify your patient according to agency policy, using two identifiers, and be attentive to standard precautions, hand hygiene, patient safety and privacy, body mechanics, and documentation.

Procedure Steps

Key Point: ***Medicate the patient for pain, if needed, before moving the patient in bed.***

1. **Lock the bed wheels.** Lower the head of the bed; place the patient in a supine position. Position one nurse on each side of the bed. Lower the siderails on the "working" side of the bed. Raise the height of the bed to waist level.
   These actions allow you to work with gravity and move the patient more easily while maintaining good body mechanics.
2. **Ensure that a friction-reducing** device, such as a transfer roller sheet, is in place under the drawsheet. If it is not in place, turn the patient from side to side to place the device under the drawsheet. You can improvise this device by placing a clean, unused plastic bag or plastic film under the drawsheet.
   A transfer roller sheet facilitates movement by reducing friction. This also helps to reduce back injury to the nurse.

   NOTE: This procedure uses a transfer roller sheet. This device is inexpensive and readily available. Scoot sheets further reduce the risk of back and musculoskeletal injury; however, their availability varies. Having a second person to help move a patient up in bed is the safest approach for staff and patients. Also follow the guidelines in Clinical Insight 32-1.
3. **Remove the pillow** from under the patient's head. Place it at the head of the bed.
   A pillow prevents patient from hitting his head on the headboard.
4. **Instruct the patient to fold** his arms across his chest. If an overhead trapeze is in place, ask the patient to hold the trapeze with both hands if able. Have the patient bend his knees with feet flat on the bed.
   This position facilitates the patient's assistance with the move.
5. **Instruct the patient to flex** his neck.
   Protects the neck while moving.
6. **With a nurse positioned** on either side of the patient, grasp and roll the drawsheet close to the patient.
7. **Stand as close as possible** to the client without twisting your back.
8. **Position your feet with a wide** base of support. Point your feet toward the direction of the move. Flex your knees and hips.
   Allows you to maintain proper body mechanics and prevents injury while moving the patient.

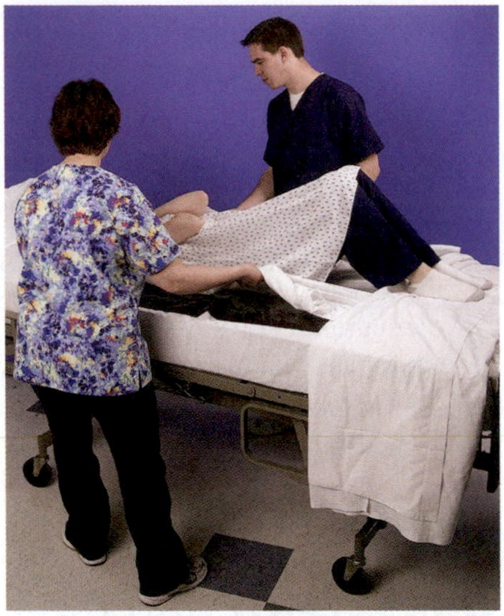

9. **Instruct the patient,** on the count of 3, to lift his trunk and push off with his heels toward the head of the bed. **With your weight on your foot** nearest to the foot of the bed, lean forward toward the head of the bed. Move along the patient's side instead of reaching. Use gentle rocking motions to reduce exertion.
   Shifting your weight allows you to use your momentum to move the patient, which helps protect your back from injury.
10. **Repeat until the patient** is positioned near the head of the bed. If you used a plastic sheet to reduce friction, remove it now.
    Plastic is water impermeable, so it allows moisture to pool under the patient and creates a risk for Impaired Skin Integrity.

11. Straighten the drawsheet; tuck it in tightly at the sides of the bed.
A wrinkle-free sheet prevents uneven pressure, discomfort, and skin irritation.

12. Place a pillow under the patient's head; assist him to a comfortable position.
Provides comfort and good body alignment.

13. Place the bed in low position; raise the siderail.
Helps prevent falls.

14. Place the call light in a position where the patient can easily reach it.
Allows patient to call for help, if needed.

Procedure Variation: Use of an Approved Mechanical Lifting Device

15. Lock the bed wheels. Lower the head of the bed; place the patient in a supine position. Position at least one nurse on each side of the bed. Lower the siderails. Raise the height of the bed to waist level.

16. Using the drawsheet, turn the patient to one side of the bed. Position the midline of the full body sling at the patient's back. Tightly roll the remaining half of the sling; tuck the fabric under the drawsheet.

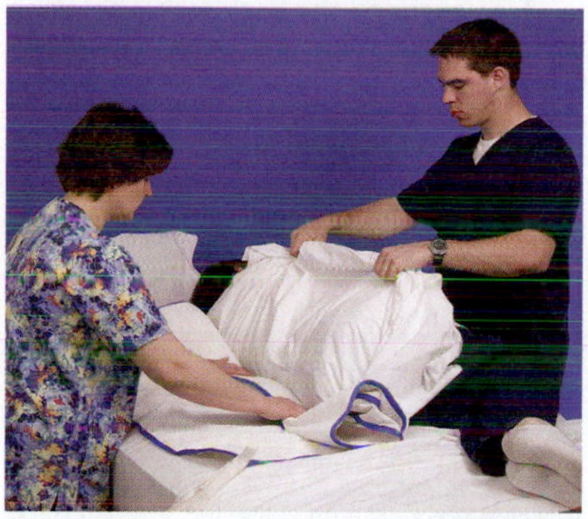

17. With a second nurse positioned on either side of the patient, use the drawsheet to turn the patient to the opposite side of the bed. Unroll the full body sling; reposition the patient supine.

18. Attach the sling to the overbed lifting device or mechanical lift. Be sure the fasteners are securely attached to the lifting device.

19. Engage the lift to raise the patient completely off the bed. Advance the lift toward the head of the bed until the patient is at the desired level.

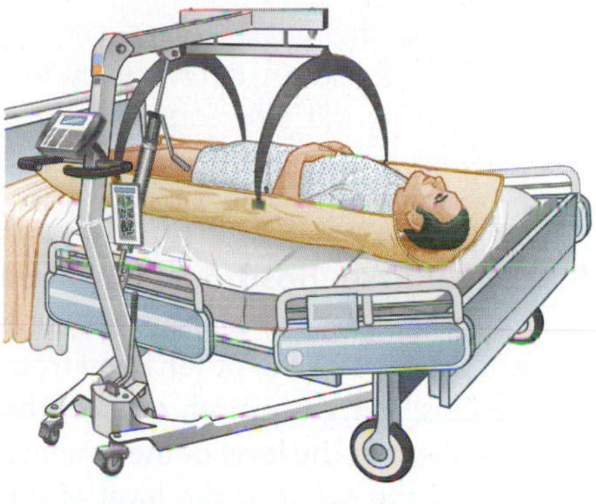

20. Lower the lift; turn the patient to the desired position. You may leave the sling in place for future movement, or you may remove it by turning the patient from side to side.

NOTE: If a full body sling is not available, use a friction-reducing device, such as a transfer roller sheet, and at least three staff members.

Procedure 32-1B ■ Turning a Patient in Bed

➤ When performing the procedure, always identify your patient according to agency policy, using two identifiers, and be attentive to standard precautions, hand hygiene, patient safety and privacy, body mechanics, and documentation.

➤ *Note:* This procedure describes the use of a transfer roller sheet. This device is inexpensive and readily available.

➤ *Note:* This procedure describes turning the patient by two nurses. With one nurse, some details differ.

Procedure Steps

1. Lock the bed wheels. Lower the head of the bed; place the patient in a supine position. Position one nurse on each side of the bed. Lower the siderail. Raise the height of the bed to waist level.
Lowering the siderails and raising the bed allow you to move the patient while maintaining good body mechanics and working with gravity to prevent injury.

2. Position the patient for turning.
a. Remove the pillow from under the patient's head and place it at the head of the bed.
b. Stand as close as possible to the patient without twisting your back.
c. Roll the patient side to side and place a friction-reducing device under the drawsheet. Smooth any wrinkles as needed. Tuck the friction-reducing device snugly under the mattress. *Note:* You can improvise this device by placing a large, clean plastic bag or plastic film under the drawsheet.
d. Move the patient to the side of the bed you are turning him away from by rolling up the drawsheet close to the patient's body and pulling it.
e. Align the patient's legs and head with the trunk.
This allows you to position the patient in the center of the bed after turning. ➤

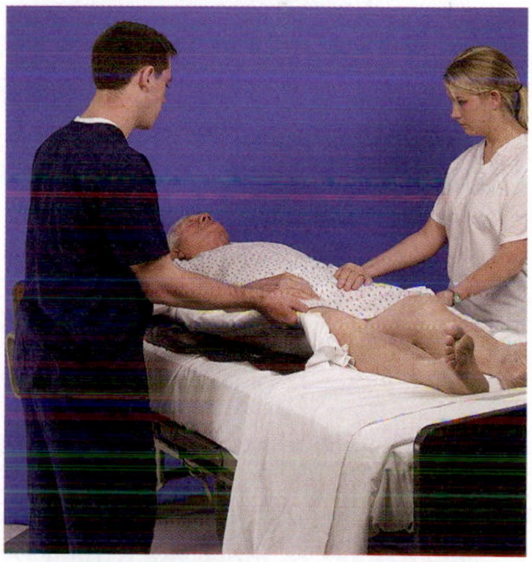

3. Place the patient's near leg and foot across the far leg (e.g., when turning the patient to his right, place his left leg over his right leg).

(continued on next page)

Procedure 32-1 ■ Moving and Turning Patients in Bed (continued)

4. **Place the patient's near arm** (e.g., left when turning right) across his chest. And, position the patient's underneath arm up and away from his body.
Positioning the patient's legs and his near arm facilitates turning. Abducting and rotating the other arm prevent it from being caught under the patient during the turn.

5. **Each nurse positions her feet** with a wide base of support with one foot forward of the other. Bend from the hips, and grasp both ends of the drawsheet at the level of the patient's hip and the other at the level of the shoulder.
A wide base of support allows you to maintain good body mechanics while performing the move.

6. **Instruct the patient** that the turn will occur on the count of three.
Counting coordinates and facilitates patient cooperation with the move.

7. **On the count of three, flex** your knees and hips and shift your weight. The nurse positioned on the side toward which the patient will turn shifts his weight to the back foot. The nurse on the opposite side shifts her weight forward. Move along the patient's side instead of reaching. Use gentle rocking motions to reduce exertion.
Provides the best leverage to turn the patient.

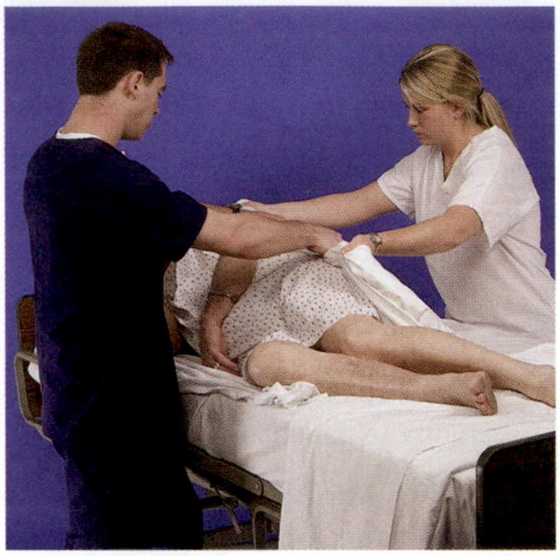

8. **If a plastic film is used,** remove it after you turn the patient.

9. **Position the dependent shoulder** forward. Place pillows behind the patient's back and between legs to maintain the patient in the lateral position. Replace the pillow under the patient's head.
Positioning ensures that the patient is not putting excess pressure on the inferior shoulder. Pillows help maintain good body alignment.

Go to Chapter 32, **Table 32-2: Positioning a Bed-Bound Patient,** in Volume 1.

10. **Place the bed in low position**; raise the siderail.
Helps ensure patient safety.

11. **Place the call device** in a position where the patient can easily reach it.
Allows patient to call for help, if needed.

Procedure 32-1C ■ Logrolling a Patient

➤ When performing the procedure, always identify your patient according to agency policy, using two identifiers, and be attentive to standard precautions, hand hygiene, patient safety and privacy, body mechanics, and documentation.

Procedure Steps

1. **Lock the bed wheels.** Lower the head of the bed with the patient supine. Lower the siderail on the side where you are standing but keep the opposite rail in the up position. Raise the height of the bed to waist level.
Lowering the siderail and raising the bed allows you to move the patient while maintaining good body mechanics and working with gravity to prevent back injury.

2. **You should already have** a drawsheet with an underlying friction-reducing device, such as a transfer roller sheet, to move the patient to the side of the bed on which you are standing. (You can improvise this device by placing a clean, unused plastic bag or plastic film under the drawsheet.)

3. **Position one staff member** at the patient's head and shoulders; she is responsible for moving the head and neck as a unit. Position the other person at the patient's hips. If you need three staff members, position one at the shoulders, one at the waist, and the third at thigh level. One staff member must maintain the patient's head and neck in alignment. The other members assist with moving the rest of the body in alignment.

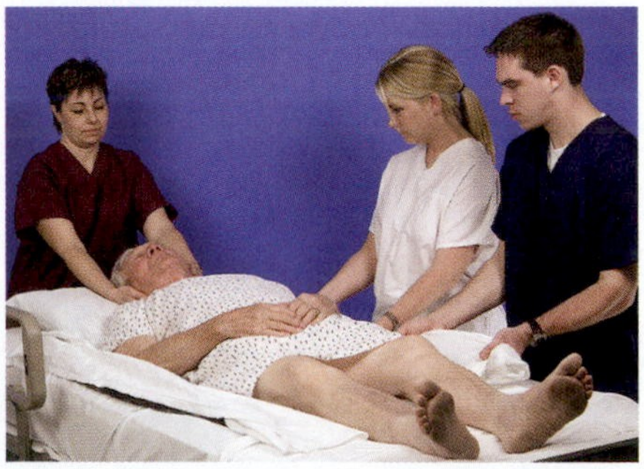

4. **Each nurse should position her** feet with a wide base of support with one foot slightly more forward than the other.
Facilitates proper body mechanics and minimizes risk of injury to staff members.

5. **Use the drawsheet** or transfer sheet to move the patient to the side of the bed on which the nurses are standing. The move must be smooth so that the patient's head and hips are kept in alignment. Position the patient's head with a pillow.
A transfer sheet maintains straight alignment of the spine.

6. **Instruct the patient to fold** his arms across his chest.

7. **Place a pillow** between the patient's knees.
A pillow prevents internal rotation of the hip and spine with movement. Maintains straight alignment of the spine.

8. Raise the siderail; move to opposite side of the bed.
Siderails keep the patient from falling out of bed.

9. Lower the siderail on the "new" side of the bed; face the patient. All nurses should position their feet with a wide base of support, with one foot forward of the other. Place your weight on the forward foot. Bend from the hips; position your hands evenly along the length of the drawsheet.
Provides the best leverage to turn the patient while maintaining spine alignment.

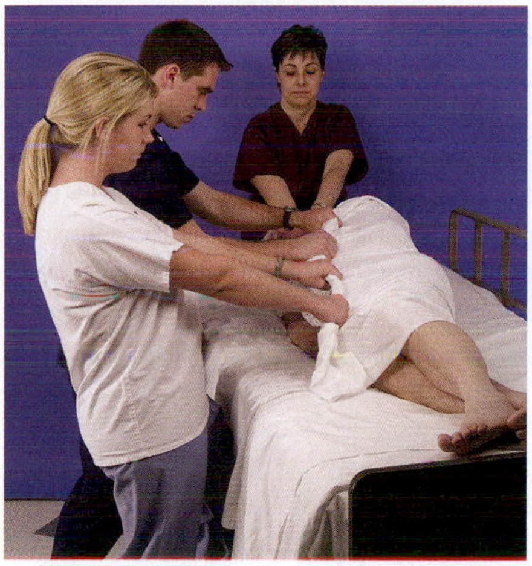

10. All nurses flex their knees and hips and shift their weight to the back foot on the count of 3. Be sure to support the head as the patient is rolled to his side.
Allows you to maintain straight alignment and body mechanics while performing the move.

11. Place pillows to maintain the patient in the lateral position.

Go to Chapter 32, **Table 32-2: Positioning a Bed-Bound Patient,** in Volume 1.

A pillow provides support and maintains proper alignment.

12. Place the bed in low position; raise the siderail.

13. Place the call device in a position where the patient can easily reach it.
Allows patient to call for help, if needed.

? What if . . .

- **Your facility has instituted a no-lift policy and you have to pull the patient up in bed?**
  Use assistive equipment, such as friction-reducing devices, mechanical lifts, air-powered mattresses, and/or lateral transfer devices to help prevent work-related injuries.
- **Your patient is obese or unable to assist (totally dependent) and you need to lift him?**
  Minimize manual lifting in all cases and eliminate it where feasible. Therefore, follow facility recommendations/protocols and use approved devices. You should be familiar with the lift devices in your facility.
- **Your patient has had a total hip replacement and you have to turn or logroll your patient?**
  Maintain the affected leg in abduction, by using a pillow or abduction wedge between the legs.
  To ensure the hip will not become dislocated during turning.
- **Your patient has a cast or is in traction and you have to turn or logroll your patient?**
  Designate a person to assist in the turning by guiding the affected extremity.
- **Your patient has an external fixation device and you have to turn or logroll your patient?**
  Secure the device in place to keep it from moving when lifting or moving the limb as needed.
  By holding onto the device to secure it and keep it from moving, there is less movement of the healing bone, and therefore less trauma and pain.

Evaluation

- Assess the patient's comfort level after the position change.
- Assess body position and alignment after position change.
- Assess skin for pressure areas.

Patient Teaching

- Explain to the patient the importance of maintaining spine alignment.
- Explain to the patient the importance of frequent position changes.
- Instruct the patient to ask the nurse when she needs to be turned sooner than scheduled.
- Teach the patient how she can assist with moving and turning.

Home Care

- Instruct the family member or caregiver in the techniques for moving, turning, or logrolling the client.
- Discuss the shearing effects on the skin from sliding down in bed (see Chapter 35).
- Provide instruction on importance of changing position and maintaining proper body alignment.

Documentation

Repositioning and turning patients are considered routine aspects of care and are not usually charted every time they are done. However, document in the nursing notes any problems with positioning the patient or any areas of skin breakdown. You might also chart turning as an intervention when charting

(continued on next page)

Procedure 32-1 ■ Moving and Turning Patients in Bed (continued)

to a specific problem. For example, if the patient has Impaired Skin Integrity, you might describe the skin and chart, "Position changed hourly." Some facilities have flowsheets on which you indicate by a checkmark each time a patient is repositioned.

Practice Resources

Centers for Disease Control and Prevention (2012, updated 2016); Collins, J. W., Nelson, A., & Sublet, V. (2006); National Institute for Occupational Safety and Health (NIOSH). (2018, August 28, updated); Nelson, A., & Baptiste, A. S. (2004); Occupational Safety and Health Administration, U.S. Department of Labor (2014); Waters, T. R. (2007); Waters, T. R., Nelson, A. N., Hughes, N., et al. (2009).

Thinking About the Procedure

The videos **Moving a Patient Up in Bed, Moving a Patient Up in Bed Using a Mechanical Lifting Device, Turning a Patient in Bed,** and **Logrolling a Patient,** along with questions and suggested responses, are available on the ***Davis's Nursing Skills Videos*** Web site on FADavis.com.

Procedure 32-2 ■ Transferring Patients

➤ For steps to follow in *all* procedures, refer to the Universal Steps for All Procedures found on the page facing the inside back cover.

Equipment

- Nonlatex gloves, if you may be exposed to body fluids
- Transfer board (for transferring from bed to stretcher, and sometimes bed to chair)
- Pull or lift (draw) sheet (for transfers)
- Gait transfer belt (for dangling and transferring from bed to chair)

Delegation

You may ask unlicensed assistive personnel (UAP) to dangle, transfer a patient from bed to stretcher, or transfer a patient from bed to chair. Ensure that the UAP has the necessary skills and that the patient's condition is stable. Inform the UAP of any special considerations when dangling or transferring the patient and evaluate the patient after transfer.

Pre-Procedure Assessment

- Assess for any restrictions in movement or position by asking the patient and checking the provider's orders.
- Observe for the presence of equipment such as IV lines, drains, or catheters.
- Assess possible side effects of medications (e.g., dizziness and sedation). Assess the patient's level of consciousness, ability to follow directions, and ability to assist with the move.
- Assess the physical size of the patient and your own strength and ability to move the patient.
- Before transferring a patient to a chair, assess the patient's tolerance of dangling.
  The preceding assessments inform you about activity tolerance, readiness to get out of bed, and ability to participate in the transfer. They help you determine how many assistants you need, the appropriate transfer device, and how to proceed with the move while preventing injury and dislodging of equipment.
- Assess vital signs; monitor for postural hypotension (lightheadedness when sitting or standing up quickly from a recumbent position).
  If the patient is at risk for postural hypotension, you may need to allow additional time for the patient to change position.
- Assess the patient's level of comfort using a standardized pain scale.
  If the patient is experiencing pain, you may need to administer an analgesic before moving.

Procedure 32-2A ■ Transferring a Patient From Bed to Stretcher

➤ When performing the procedure, always identify your patient according to agency policy, using two identifiers, and be attentive to standard precautions, hand hygiene, patient safety and privacy, body mechanics, and documentation.

Procedure Steps

1. **Lock the wheels on the bed.** Position the bed so that it is flat (if the patient can tolerate being supine) and at the height of the stretcher.
   Locking the wheels ensures client safety during the transfer. Having the bed flat helps prevent injury to staff, because the patient is easier to move.
2. **Lower the siderails** and position at least one nurse on each side of the bed. Move the patient to the side of the bed where the stretcher will be placed by rolling up the drawsheet close to the patient's body and pulling it toward the designated side. Align the patient's legs and head with her trunk.
   Positions patient to enable nurses to move her to the stretcher.
3. **Position the stretcher** next to the bed. Lock the stretcher wheels.
   Locking the wheels keeps the stretcher from moving during the transfer and prevents falls.
4. **Place the transfer board** against the patient's back.
   a. Place a friction-reducing device, such as a transfer roller sheet, over the transfer board. (You can improvise this device by placing a

clean, unused plastic bag or plastic film under the drawsheet.)

b. The nurse on the side opposite the stretcher uses the drawsheet to turn the patient away from the stretcher, while the other nurse places the transfer board against the patient's back halfway between bed and stretcher. Turn the patient to her back and onto the transfer board.
Safely positions the transfer board under the patient, without friction. ▼

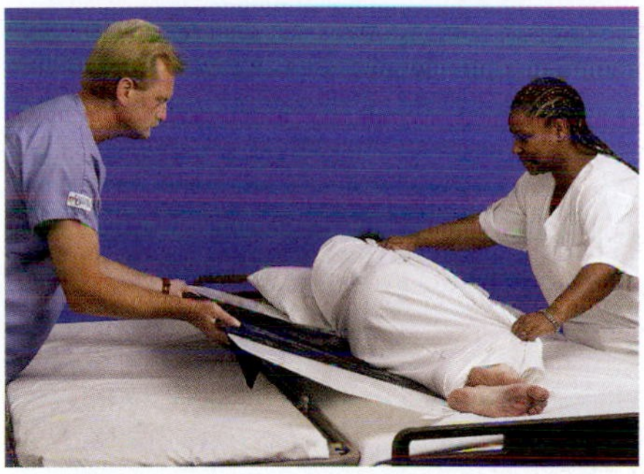

5. **Ensure the patient's feet** and shoulder are over the edge of the transfer board.
To prevent injury to the patient from the edge of the board.

6. **Ask the patient to raise her head** if able. Use the drawsheet to slide her across the transfer board onto the stretcher.
Facilitates the move to the stretcher; prevents friction on patient's skin. ▼

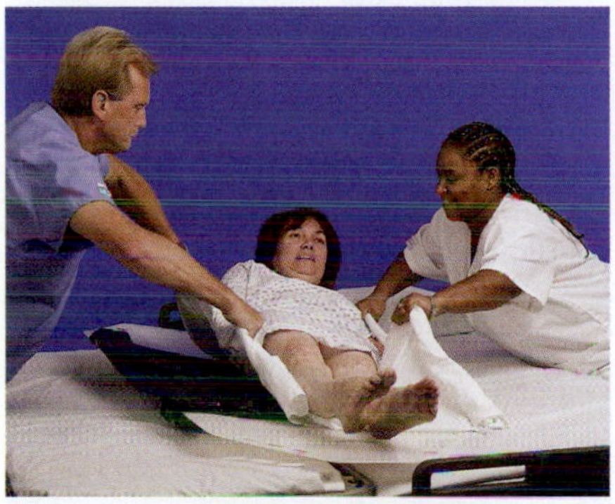

Procedure Variation: If Transferring a Patient From Bed to Stretcher With a Slipsheet

A slipsheet may be used instead of a transfer board. A slipsheet is a large, low-friction fabric that facilitates transfer.

7. **With the drawsheet, turn** the patient away from the bed; remove the board and roller sheet.

8. **Position the midline of the slipsheet** under the patient. Roll the remaining half tightly and tuck it under the patient.

9. **Turn the patient back over to the** side near to the stretcher; and pull the slipsheet through from under the patient.

10. **Place the patient supine**; lower the siderail on the side where the stretcher will be placed.

11. **Move the stretcher** next to the bed and lock the wheels on the stretcher.

12. **Position at least two nurses** on the far side of the stretcher. Using the slipsheet, pull the patient onto the stretcher. ▼

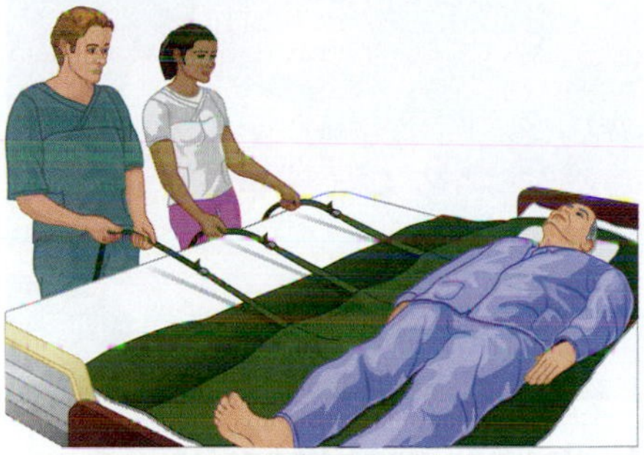

13. **Be sure the stretcher** wheels are locked and the siderails raised for patient safety.

14. **Place the call device in reach** of the patient or position the patient where she can be seen by staff members at all times.

Procedure 32-2B ■ Dangling a Patient at the Side of the Bed

➤ When performing the procedure, always identify your patient according to agency policy, using two identifiers, and be attentive to standard precautions, hand hygiene, patient safety and privacy, body mechanics, and documentation.

Procedure Steps

1. **Lock the bed wheels.** Place the patient in a supine position; raise the head of the bed to 90°. Keep the siderail elevated on the side opposite where you are standing.
Locking the wheels prevents the bed from moving as you move the patient. Raising the head of the bed prepares the patient to be dangled and requires less effort from you to help the patient sit erect.

2. **Apply a gait transfer belt** to the patient at waist level. Be sure the belt is snug but not uncomfortable.

3. **Place the bed in the low position.**
Ensures patient safety and proper body mechanics.

4. **Instruct the patient to bend** his knees and turn the patient onto his side, if possible, keeping knees flexed.
Prepares the patient to be able to dangle his legs over side of bed.

5. **Stand at the side of the bed,** facing the patient and using a wide base of support. Place your foot closest to the head of the bed forward of the other foot. Lean forward, bending at the hips, with your knees flexed. Instruct the patient to use his arm to push off the bed.

(continued on next page)

Procedure 32-2 ■ Transferring Patients (continued)

Allows you to maintain proper body mechanics and prevents injury.

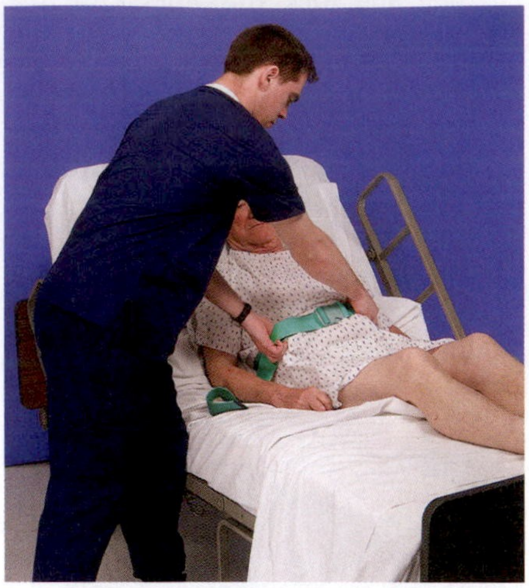

6. **Position your hands** on each side of the gait transfer belt.
7. **Rock onto your back foot** as you assist the patient toward you with the gait transfer belt, thereby moving the patient into a sitting position at the side of the bed.

Uses your body weight as leverage to reposition the patient, preventing injury to your back.

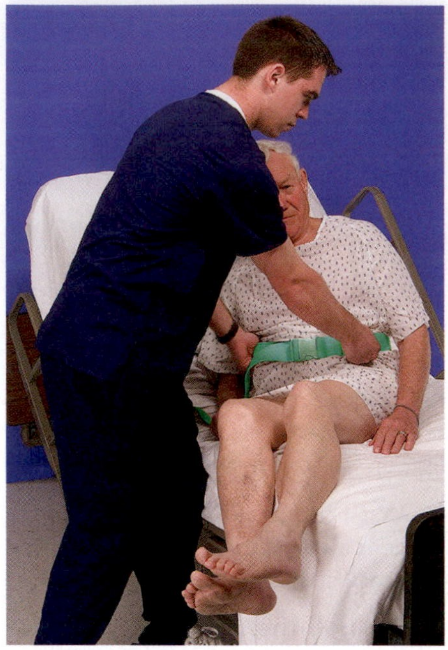

8. **Stay with the patient** as he dangles. Reassess comfort level and for dizziness.
Helps prevent falls.

Procedure 32-2C ■ Transferring a Patient From Bed to Chair

➤ When performing the procedure, always identify your patient according to agency policy, using two identifiers, and be attentive to standard precautions, hand hygiene, patient safety and privacy, body mechanics, and documentation.

Procedure Steps

1. **Position the chair** next to the bed. If possible, lock the chair.
Prevents the chair from moving during transfer. Ensures patient safety.
2. **Put nonskid footwear** on the patient.
Prevents the patient from slipping during transfer.
3. **Place the bed in a low position**; lock the bed wheels.
Prevents the bed from moving during the transfer. Low position allows patient to place feet firmly on the floor.
4. **Apply a transfer belt.**
Facilitates transfer of the patient to the chair and helps prevent back injury to the nurse.
5. **Assist the patient to dangle** at the side of the bed (see Procedure 32-2B). Be sure the patient doesn't need support before releasing him.
6. **Stand toward the bed,** facing the patient. Brace your feet and knees against the patient's legs. Pay particular attention to any known weakness. Bend your hips and knees, and, keeping your back straight, hold on to the transfer belt on both sides. If two nurses are available to assist with the transfer, one nurse should be on each side of the patient.
Bracing provides stability. Bending the hips and knees allows you to use the major muscle groups and limit the risk of injury. Lifting the patient at waist level prevents injury to the arm or shoulder. ➤

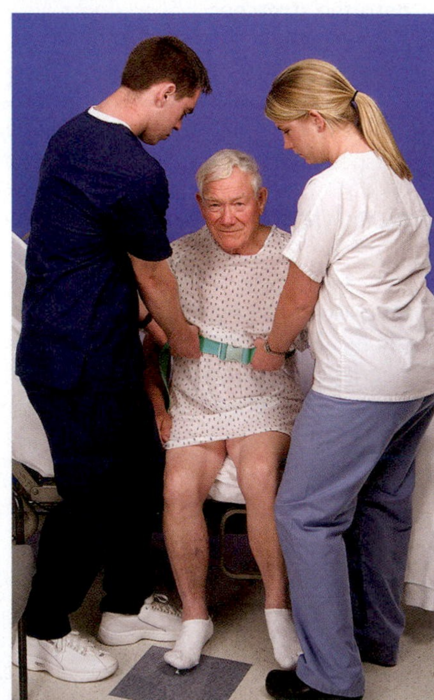

7. **Instruct the patient** to place his hands by his sides and help to push off of the bed.
Having the patient help to push off of the bed reduces the risk for injury to your back or neck.

8. **Ask the patient to stand** as you move to an upright position by straightening your legs and hips.
Straightening your thighs and hips uses your large muscle groups and prevents injury to your back.

9. **Allow the patient to steady** himself for a moment. Ask whether he is feeling light-headed.
Provides the patient an opportunity to rest before further movement. Allows you to evaluate his tolerance to activity and ability to maintain an upright posture before continuing.

10. **Instruct the patient to pivot** and turn with you toward the chair.
Pivoting helps prevent twisting and straining the patient's back muscles.

11. **Assist the patient to position** himself in front of the chair. Have the patient flex his hips and knees, and as he lowers himself to the chair, reach for arms of the chair. Guide his motion while maintaining a firm hold on him and keeping your back straight.
Maintains good body mechanics and balance and ensures patient safety.

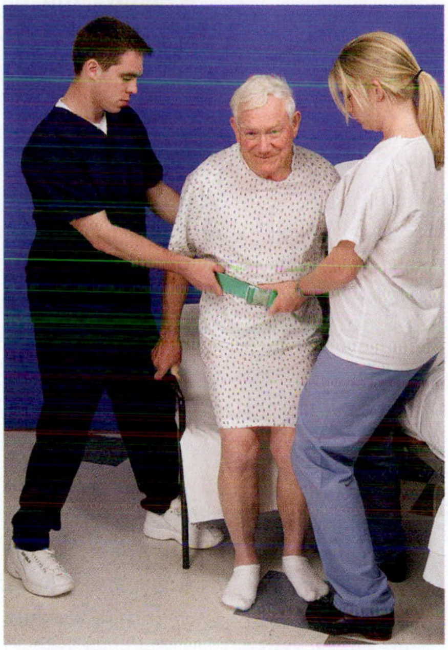

12. **Assist the patient** to a comfortable position in the chair.

13. **Provide a blanket** if needed for warmth or privacy.

14. **Place the call device in reach** of the patient or position the patient where he can be seen by staff members at all times.

? What if . . .

- **Your patient is obese?**
If your patient is obese or unable to assist, use a full body sling that allows the patient to assume a seated position. You may also use a powered standing assist lift, if one is available.

- **Your patient has had hip surgery (replacement or fracture repair).**
When assisting the patient out of bed, raise the bed to a position that is high enough to allow the patient to exit the bed without acute hip flexion.
To avoid hip injury or dislocation.

- **Your patient becomes dizzy during the transfer?**
Return the patient to sitting or recumbent position and assess his vital signs.

- **Your patient has a weaker side, for example, from a cerebrovascular accident (CVA) or surgical procedure?**
Instruct the patient to exit the bed from his unaffected side. Stand on the patient's weaker side.
The stronger side should lead a transfer.

Evaluation

- Assess the level of patient participation in the transfer.
- Assess the patient's comfort level during the transfer and in the new position.
- Assess proper body position and alignment after his position change.
- Assess the patient's vital signs for postural hypotension after dangling or transferring to a chair.

Patient Teaching

- Explain the importance of frequent position changes and getting out of bed to avoid complications of immobility.

Home Care

- Instruct the family member or caregiver in the proper technique for assisting the client to dangle at the bedside or transfer to a chair.
- Provide instruction in the importance of changing position and maintaining proper body alignment.

Documentation

Patients are usually moved to a stretcher for transport to a test or procedure. The movement is a routine aspect of care and is not documented. When dangling or transferring a patient to a chair, document in the nursing notes how much assistance was required, the use of assistive devices, any problems with positioning the patient, how long the patient was out of bed, and how the patient tolerated the activity.

Practice Resources

Centers for Disease Control and Prevention (CDC) (2012, updated 2016); Collins, J. W., Nelson, A., & Sublet, V. (2006); National Institute for Occupational Safety and Health (NIOSH). (2018); Occupational Safety and Health Administration, U.S. Department of Labor (2014); Waters, T. R. (2007); Waters, T. R., Nelson, A. N., Hughes, N., et al. (2009).

Thinking About the Procedure

The videos **Transferring a Patient From Bed to Stretcher, Dangling a Patient at the Side of the Bed,** and **Transferring a Patient From Bed to Chair,** along with questions and suggested responses, are available on the ***Davis's Nursing Skills Videos*** Web site on FADavis.com.

Procedure 32-3 ■ Assisting With Ambulation

➤ For steps to follow in *all* procedures, refer to the Universal Steps for All Procedures found on the page facing the inside back cover.

Equipment

- Nonlatex gloves, if you may be exposed to body fluids
- Transfer belt
- Nonskid footwear

Delegation

You may ask unlicensed assistive personnel (UAP) to assist with ambulation. Ensure that the UAP has the necessary skills and that the patient's condition is stable. Inform the UAP of any special considerations when assisting a patient with ambulation and evaluate the patient after the activity.

Pre-Procedure Assessment

- Assess for any restrictions in movement or position by asking the patient and checking the provider's orders.
- Observe for the presence of equipment such as IV lines, drains, or catheters.
- Assess possible side effects of medications (e.g., dizziness and sedation).
- Assess the patient's level of consciousness, ability to follow directions, and ability to assist with the move.
- Assess the physical size of the patient and your own strength and ability to move the patient.
- Assess the patient's tolerance when dangling before beginning to ambulate.
  The preceding assessments inform you about activity tolerance, readiness to get out of bed, and ability to participate in the transfer. They help you determine how many assistants you need, the appropriate transfer device, and how to proceed with the move while preventing injury and dislodging of equipment.
- Assess vital signs; monitor for postural hypotension.
  If the patient is at risk for postural hypotension, you may need to allow additional time for the patient to change position and plan for adequate help.
- Assess the patient's level of comfort using a standardized pain scale.
  If the patient is uncomfortable, you may need to administer an analgesic before moving.
- Assess for factors that may increase the risk of falls (elderly, muscle weakness, chronic disease, gait disturbance).
  Identifies patients at risk.

Procedure 32-3A ■ Assisting With Ambulation (One Nurse)

➤ When performing the procedure, always identify your patient according to agency policy, using two identifiers, and be attentive to standard precautions, hand hygiene, patient safety and privacy, body mechanics, and documentation.

Procedure Steps

1. **Put nonskid footwear** on the patient.
   Prevents the patient from slipping while transferring and ambulating.
2. **Apply the transfer belt.**
   Allows you to safely support the patient during the transfer and ambulation.
3. **Place the bed in a low position**; lock the bed.
   Prevents the bed from moving during transfer. Makes it easier for the patient's feet to reach the floor.
4. **Assist the patient to dangle** at the side of the bed (see Procedure 32-2B, if you need to review).
5. **Face the patient.** Brace your feet and knees against the patient's feet and knees. Pay particular attention to any known weakness. Bend your hips and knees, and hold on to the transfer belt.
   Bracing provides stability of the patient's legs. Bending the hips and knees allows you to use the major muscle groups and limit injury. Lifting at the patient's waist level prevents injury to his arm or shoulder.
6. **Instruct the patient** to place his arms around you between the shoulders and waist (the location depends on your height and the height of the patient). Ask the patient to stand as you move to an upright position by straightening your legs and hips.
   Having the patient hold you on your trunk prevents injury to your neck. Straightening your thighs and hips uses your large muscle groups and promotes good body mechanics.
7. **Allow the patient to steady** himself for a moment.
   Allows the patient an opportunity to rest before further movement and to regain equilibrium before walking.
8. **Stand at the patient's side,** placing both hands on the transfer belt. If the patient is weak on one side, position yourself on the weaker side.
   By standing on the weaker side, the patient is freer to reach with the stronger arm and grip wall or bed rails with his strong-side hand and use the stronger side for strength and balance. This position also keeps you clear of a cane or other assistive device, which would be used on the strong side, and allows you

to support the weaker side to prevent the patient from falling.

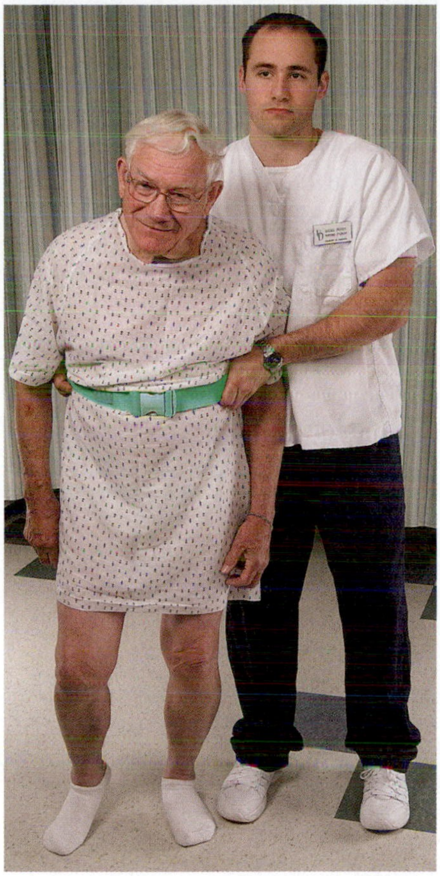

9. **Slowly guide the patient** forward. Observe for signs of fatigue or dizziness.
Helps prevent falls.

10. **If the patient has an IV pole**, ask him to hold on to the pole on the side where you are standing. Assist the patient to advance the pole as you ambulate. Be sure the patient does not rely on the pole for support.
Provides a grip for the patient and positions the IV pole near you so that you can assist the patient to move the pole.

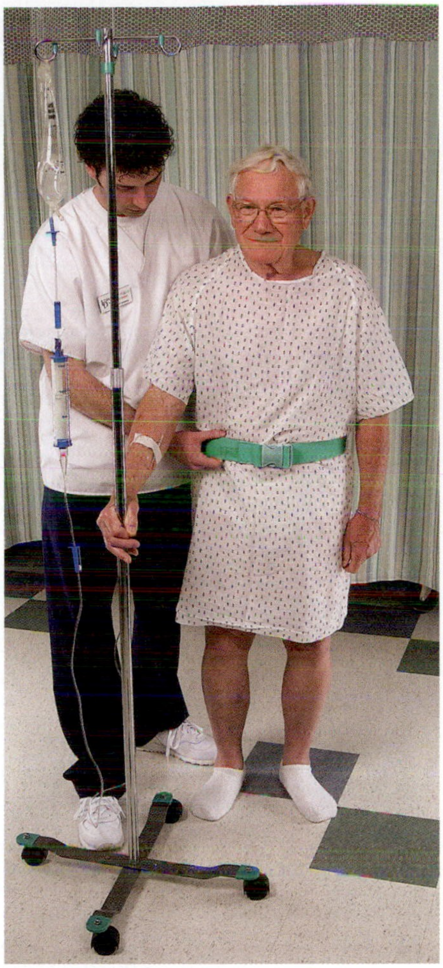

Procedure 32-3B ■ Assisting With Ambulation (Two Nurses)

When performing the procedure, always identify your patient according to agency policy, using two identifiers, and be attentive to standard precautions, hand hygiene, patient safety and privacy, body mechanics, and documentation.

Procedure Steps

1. **Put nonskid footwear** on the patient.
Prevents the patient from slipping during the transfer and ambulation.

2. **Apply the transfer belt.**
Allows you to support client during transfer and ambulation.

3. **Place the bed in low position**; lock the bed.
Prevents the bed from moving during transfer and prevents the patient from falling.

4. **Assist the patient to dangle** at the side of the bed (see Procedure 32-2B, as needed).

5. **Each nurse should stand facing** the patient on opposite sides of the patient. Brace your feet and knees against the patient, paying particular attention to any known weakness. Bend from the hips and knees and hold onto the transfer belt.
Bracing provides stability. Bending the hips and knees allows you to use the major muscle groups and limit injury. Lifting at the patient's waist level prevents injury to his arm or shoulder.

6. **Instruct the patient to place** his arms around each of you between the shoulders and waist (the location depends on your height and the height of the patient). Ask the patient to stand as each of you move to an upright position by straightening your legs and hips.

7. **Allow the patient to steady** himself for a moment.
Allows the patient an opportunity to rest before further movement and to regain equilibrium. Allows you to evaluate the patient's tolerance to activity and ability to maintain an upright posture before ambulating.

(continued on next page)

Procedure 32-3 ■ Assisting With Ambulation (continued)

8. **Both nurses stand at** the patient's sides, grasping hold of the transfer belt. If no belt is available, the nurses grasp each other's arms at the patient's waist.
   Helps patient maintain an erect posture.

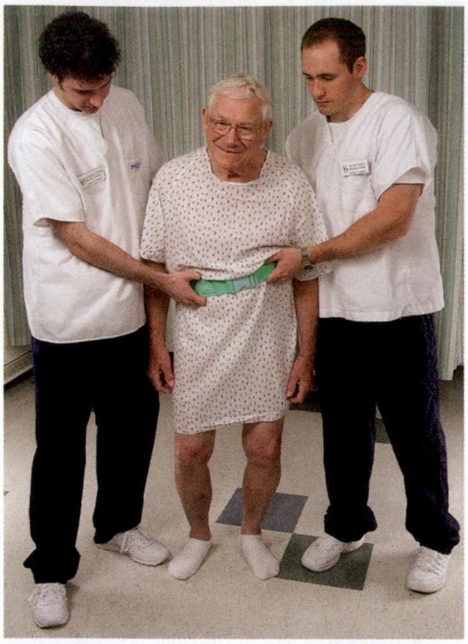

9. **Slowly guide the patient forward.** Observe for signs of fatigue or dizziness.
   Ensures client safety.

10. **If the patient has an IV pole,** one nurse advances the IV pole along the side of the patient by holding the pole with the outside hand.
    Remind the patient not to use the IV pole for support.
    Positions the IV pole out of the path of the patient. Because the IV pole is on rollers, it will not support the patient if he starts to fall.

? What if . . .

- **Your patient has a weaker side (e.g., from a stroke or musculoskeletal injury)?**

  If the patient has weakness on one side, provide additional support but allow him to use that side as he is able.
  This will require him to use his weaker side.

Evaluation

- Assess the level of patient participation in the transfer.
- Assess patient comfort with ambulation.
- Assess posture and base of support.
- Assess vital signs for postural hypotension.

Patient Teaching

- Instruct the patient to inform you if he feels dizzy or weak.
- Explain the importance of ambulation to prevent complications of immobility.

Home Care

- Teach family members or caregivers how to assist the client with ambulation.
- Provide instruction on importance of ambulation.

Documentation

Document in the nursing notes how much assistance was required, any problems with ambulation, and the distance walked.

Sample Documentation

11/11/20 0630 Pt assisted to ambulate to doorway in room. Required minimal assistance from one nurse. Placed in chair for 30 min and then assisted back to bed. Required maximum assist from two nurses to return to bed. ———————— B. Bowen, RN

Practice Resources

Centers for Disease Control and Prevention (2012, updated 2016); National Institute for Occupational Safety and Health (NIOSH) (2018); Occupational Safety and Health Administration (2009); Waters, T. R., Nelson, A. N., Hughes, N., et al. (2009).

Thinking About the Procedure

The videos **Assisting With Ambulation (One Nurse),** and **Assisting With Ambulation (Two Nurses),** along with questions and suggested responses, are available on the ***Davis's Nursing Skills Videos*** Web site on FADavis.com.

CLINICAL INSIGHTS

Clinical Insight 32-1 ➤ Applying Principles of Body Mechanics

Principles of body mechanics are the rules that enable you to move your body without causing injury. Use the following guidelines to decrease the risk of back and other injuries. Teach them to your patients as well.

The American Nurses Association (2013) states you should use mechanical equipment (e.g., lift, transfer board) or get assistance for lifting and transferring whenever possible. Do not rely on body mechanics alone to prevent injury.

Account for Patient Factors

- **Assess patient dependency levels** and select equipment after determining the patient's ability to assist in the transfer. You will also want to be aware of the patient's strength and ability to bear weight. Height and weight of the patient factor into how you transfer the patient safely.

Transferring Patients According to Dependency Level

PATIENT LEVEL OF DEPENDENCE	ASSISTIVE DEVICE
Complete dependence (immobile; no assistance)	Mechanical lift with full sling
Extensive dependence (holds on to device but with minimal strength)	Mechanical lift with full sling or stand/assist lift
Moderate dependence (no patient assist for lifting from floor)	Mechanical lift with full sling, or if transfer is manual, more than one helper might be needed
Patient assists with limited mobility	Transfer belt or gait belt
Limited dependence	Stand/assist lift or friction-reducing device

Source: Adapted from American Nurses Association (ANA) (2013). *Safe patient handling and mobility: Interprofessional national standards.* Silver Springs, MD: Author.

Make Use of Inanimate Objects and Get Help When Possible

- **Raise the height of the bed and overbed table to waist level** when you are working with a patient.
- **Get help to move a heavy object** or patient. Assess the object or patient you are going to lift. If you have any doubt that you can do it by yourself, get help from a coworker.
- **Use assistive devices at all times** to limit the risk of back and musculoskeletal injury.
- **Maintain competency** in using all assistive and transfer devices.

Use Your Body Correctly

- **Use a wide base of support** (feet spread apart).
- **Minimize bending and twisting.** These movements increase the stress on the back. Instead, face the object or person, and bend at the hips or squat.
- **Squat to lift heavy objects** from the floor. (Squatting lowers your center of gravity.) Push against the strong hip and thigh muscles to raise yourself to a standing position. Avoid bending at the waist.
- **Use the muscles in your legs** as the power for lifting. Bend your knees, keep your back straight, and lift smoothly. Repeat the same movements for setting the object down.
- **Keep objects close to your body** when you lift, move, or carry them. The closer an object is to the center of gravity, the greater the stability and the less strain on the back.
- **Use both hands and arms** when you lift, move, or carry heavy objects.
- **Do not stand on tiptoes to reach** an object. If you must use a ladder or stepstool to reach for an object, make sure it is stable and adequate to position your body close to the object.
- **Push, slide, or pull heavy objects** whenever possible rather than lifting.
- **Maintain a good grip** on the patient or object you are moving before attempting to move it.
- **When possible, keep your elbows bent** when you carry an object.
- **Work with smooth and even movements.** Avoid sudden or jerky motions.

Clinical Insight 32-2 ➤ Using Common Positioning Devices

Applying a Trochanter Roll

Trochanter rolls prevent external hip rotation when the patient is in a supine position.

- Fold a towel or bath blanket lengthwise.
- Roll the towel or bath blanket tightly.
- Invert the roll. Turning the patient to one side, place the bath blanket or towel under the patient's hip and thigh. Repeat on the other side if needed.
- Roll the sheet or towel under until it is snug against the patient's hip and thigh.
  The patient's weight should keep the roll from moving and help to prevent external (outward) rotation of the hips.
- Make sure the roll does not extend as far as the knee.
  To avoid nerve compression and palsy that can lead to footdrop.

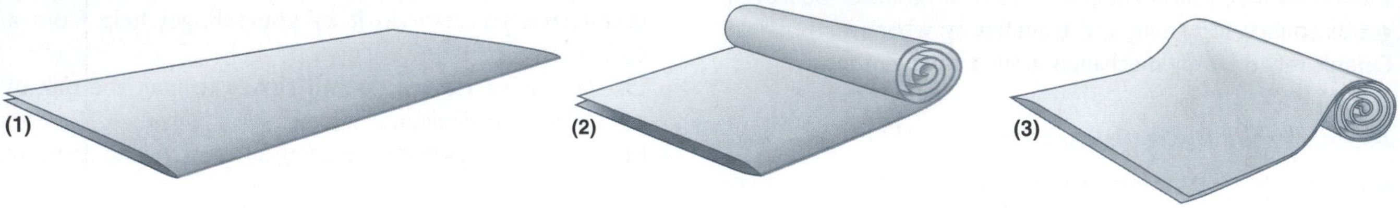

- Alternately, you can place the patient on a sheet that has been folded so that the top edge is at the top of the hips, and the lower edge is about one-third the way down the thighs. Then place the rolled towels under the sheet and roll the sheet under tightly.

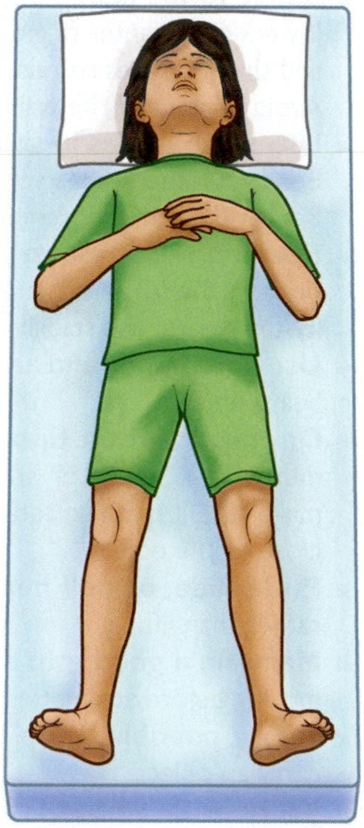

External rotation can occur without a trochanter roll.

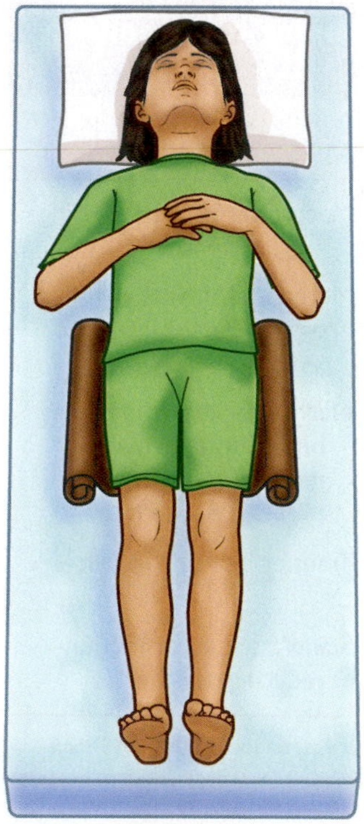

Proper alignment using a trochanter roll.

Clinical Insight 32-2 ➤ Using Common Positioning Devices—cont'd

Applying Hand Rolls

Hand rolls help prevent hand contractures.

- Place a commercial hand roll or even a rolled washcloth in the patient's palm to maintain a neutral position. For an illustration,

Go to **Figure 32-6** in Volume 1.

- Secure the strap, if present.
- Roll soft gauze around the hand and secure with nonallergenic, adhesive tape to keep it from falling out of the patient's hand.
- Place another roll in the patient's other hand, if needed.

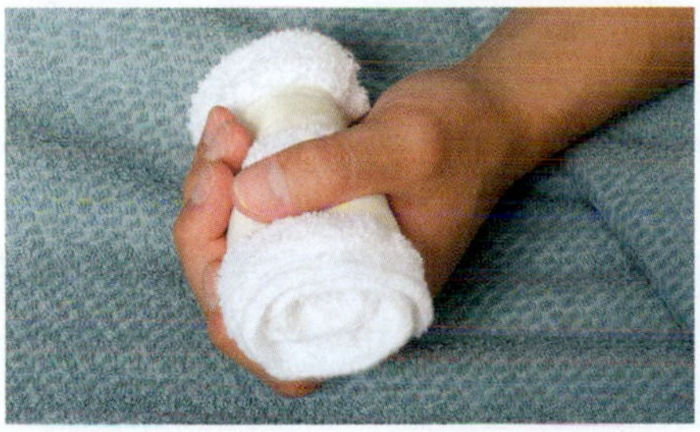

Applying Cradle Boots

Cradle boots prevent footdrop, hip rotation, and pressure on bony prominences, which lead to skin breakdown.

- Open the slit on the top surface of the boot.
- Place the patient's heel in the round cutout for the heel. If the patient is positioned on her side, you may put the boot on the bottom foot.
- Support the flexed top foot with a pillow.
- Apply the boot to the other foot, as needed.
- Position the patient's legs in neutral alignment with slight flexion.
  Neutral positioning prevents strain on hip ligaments.

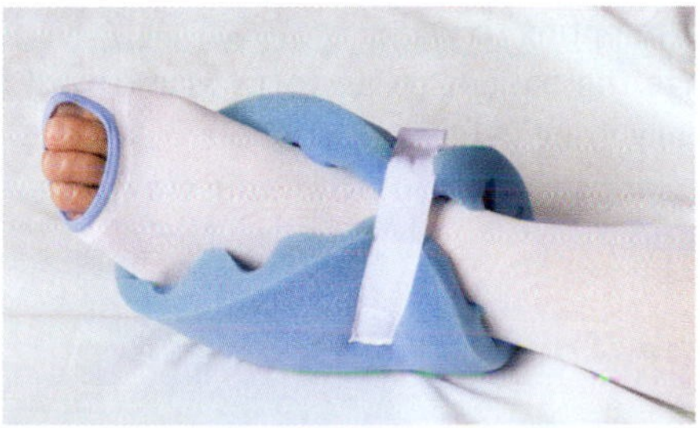

Applying Hip Abduction Pillow

Hip abduction pillows prevent internal hip rotation and hip adduction when the patient is in a supine position.

- Place the wedge-shaped, spongy pillow between the patient's legs when she is lying on her back.
- Slide it toward the groin so it touches the legs all along the inside of the thigh.
- Place both upper legs in the pillow's lateral indentations.
- Secure the straps to prevent the pillow from slipping down the mattress.

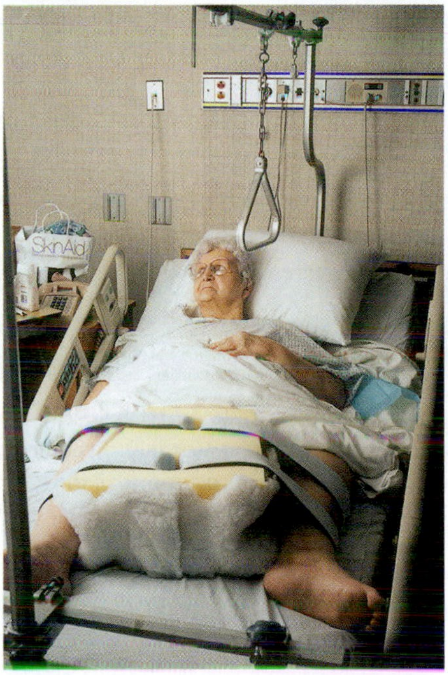

Clinical Insight 32-3 ➤ Performing Passive Range-of-Motion Exercises

Passive range of motion (PROM) is the movement of the joints through their full range of motion by another person. Nurses often perform PROM to maintain joint mobility. Refer to the Range of Motion at the Joints table after Assessment Guidelines and Tools.

- **Explain the purpose of PROM.** You may also wish to teach family members and caregivers about the importance of ROM exercises and enlist their help in exercising the patient when they visit.
- **Observe the patient as you perform PROM.** You may need to perform the exercises in several short segments if the patient tires easily or experiences discomfort.
- **Support the patient's limb** above and below the joint that is to be exercised.
- **Move the joint in a slow, smooth, rhythmic manner.** Avoid fast movements; they may cause muscle spasm.
- **Never force a joint.** Some patients may have limited ROM. Move each joint to the point of resistance. This should not be painful.
- **Perform PROM** at least twice daily. Move each joint through ROM three to five times with each session. Consider incorporating PROM into care activities, for example, while bathing or turning the patient.
- **Return the joint to a neutral position** when exercise is complete.
- **Encourage active exercise** whenever possible.

Thinking About the Procedure

The video **Performing Passive Range-of-Motion Exercises,** along with questions and suggested responses, is available on the ***Davis's Nursing Skills Videos*** Web site on FADavis.com.

Clinical Insight 32-4 ➤ Assisting With Physical Conditioning Exercises to Prepare for Ambulation

Patients who have been confined to bed for more than a week or who have sustained major injury require conditioning before they are able to resume walking. Conditioning exercises include the following.

Quadriceps and Gluteal Drills

- Ask the patient to tighten her thigh muscles by pushing downward with her knees and flexing her feet. Each leg may be done separately if moving both is contraindicated.
- Ask the patient to hold the position for a count of 5 and then relax.
- Repeat this process two to three times per hour during the waking hours.
- To exercise the gluteal muscles, ask the patient to pinch her buttocks together.
- Do this exercise when the patient exercises her quadriceps muscles.
- Instruct the patient not to hold her breath as she exercises.

Arm Exercises

- Install a trapeze bar on the patient's bed. Ask the patient to do pull-ups on the bar from a lying position. This exercises the biceps muscles.
- To exercise the triceps muscles, ask the patient to lift his upper body off the mattress by firmly pressing down with the palms.
- The patient can also do pushups from a seated position at the side of the bed or from a stationary chair or wheelchair.

Dangling

- Dangling is a seated position at the side of the bed, feet resting on the floor.
- Provide a footstool if the patient's feet do not reach the floor.
- Assess for light-headedness or postural hypotension.
- Do not progress to ambulation until the patient is comfortable and stable in the dangling position.

Daily Activities

- Encourage your patient to be active in bed by repositioning and turning herself.
- Encourage the patient to get out of bed and into a chair before attempting to walk.
- Encourage the patient to perform as much of her activities of daily living (ADLs) as possible.
- ADLs exercise many of the muscle groups used in ambulation.

Thinking About the Procedure

The video **Physical Conditioning Exercises: Quadriceps, Gluteal, Arm, and Dangling,** along with questions and suggested responses, is available on the ***Davis's Nursing Skills Videos*** Web site on FADavis.com.

Clinical Insight 32-5 ➤ Sizing Walking Aids

Sizing Canes

- Ask the patient to stand erect; place the cane tip 20 cm (4 in.) to the side of the foot.
- The top of the cane should reach the top of the hip joint so that the patient can hold the cane with her elbow flexed 30°.

Sizing Walkers

- Ask the patient to stand erect, holding onto the walker.
- The walker should extend from the floor to the hip joint so that the patient can comfortably hold the walker with 30° flexion of the elbow.

Sizing Crutches

To measure a patient for an axillary crutch, follow these guidelines:

- Ask the patient to lie down wearing the nonskid shoes that she will use when walking.
- Measure the distance between the heel and the anterior fold of the axilla, then add 2.5 cm (1 in.).
- Select a crutch that can be adjusted to this height.
- Have the patient stand; position the crutch tip 10 to 15 cm (4 to 6 in.) to the side of the heel. Adjust the axillary crutch pad three fingerbreadths below the axilla.
- Adjust the handgrips so that the patient can comfortably grasp the bar while the elbow is slightly flexed. The patient's axilla should not rest on the crutchpad.

Clinical Insight 32-6 ➤ Teaching Patients to Use Canes, Walkers, and Crutches

Canes

After ensuring the cane is the proper size (refer to Clinical Insight 32-5), instruct the patient to do the following:

- Hold the cane on the stronger side.
- Distribute weight evenly between the feet and cane.
- Advance the cane and weaker leg simultaneously, then bring the stronger leg through.
- Avoid leaning over or on the cane.
- Maintain the integrity of the rubber tip for traction.

Walkers

After ensuring the walker is the proper size (refer to Clinical Insight 32-5), provide the following instructions:

- Stand between the back legs of the walker. Do not stand too far behind the walker.
- Pick up the walker and advance it as you step ahead. Do not advance it so far as to lose balance.
- If one leg is weaker, move it forward as the walker moves forward.
- Do not slide the walker (unless it has wheels).

Crutches

After ensuring the crutches are the proper size (refer to Clinical Insight 32-5), do the following:

- When first teaching crutch walking, instruct the patient to stand near a wall with a chair behind him. Help the patient to stand and grip the crutches. Ask the patient to sway from side to side on the crutches to become accustomed to weight bearing by the arms.
- *Tripod position* is the basic crutch gait standing position. Place crutches 15 cm (6 in.) in front of the feet, with the crutch point 15 cm from the patient's center. In this position, a triangle is formed by the crutches and the body.
- Five crutch gaits exist (see accompanying chart): 2-point gait, 3-point gait, 4-point gait, swing-to gait, and swing-through gait.

To teach the patient how to go up and down stairs, instruct him to lead with the unaffected leg when going up the stairs and to lead with the affected leg coming down the stairs.

Navigating stairs with crutches can be dangerous. When possible, have the patient practice this technique before discharge. When having a patient practice, the nurse should always stand below the patient on the stairs to prevent falling.

(Continued)

Clinical Insight 32-6 ➤ Teaching Patients to Use Canes, Walkers, and Crutches—cont'd

***NOTE:* Read this table from bottom to top.**

2-Point gait	3-Point gait	4-Point gait	Swing to	Swing through
• Partial weight bearing, both feet; faster, but less support than a 4-point gait	• Non-weight bearing; faster than a 4-point gait; can use with walker	• Partial weight bearing, both feet; patient must shift weight constantly	• Weight bearing, both feet; can use with walker	• Weight bearing; requires the most coordination and balance
4. Advance right foot and left crutch	4. Advance right foot	4. Advance right foot	4. Lift both feet; swing them forward, landing feet next to the crutches	4. Lift both feet; swing them forward, landing feet in front of the crutches
3. Advance left foot and right crutch	3. Advance left foot and both crutches	3. Advance left crutch	3. Advance both crutches	3. Advance both crutches
2. Advance right foot and left crutch	2. Advance right foot	2. Advance left foot	2. Lift both feet; swing them forward, landing feet next to the crutches	2. Lift both feet; swing them forward, landing feet in front of the crutches
1. Advance left foot and right crutch	1. Advance left foot and both crutches	1. Advance right crutch	1. Advance both crutches	1. Advance both crutches
Tripod position	Tripod position	Tripod position	Tripod position	Tripod position

Crutch gaits. The shaded area represents weight-bearing. The arrow shows movement.

ASSESSMENT GUIDELINES AND TOOLS

Focused Assessment

Assessing Activity and Exercise

Suggested History Questions

Usual Activity

Describe your typical daily activity level.

If the patient has very restricted activity, ask the following questions:

- Are you able to care for yourself in regard to hygiene, dressing, toileting, and getting out of bed?
- If the patient has ADL limitations: Who helps you with these daily activities?

If the patient does not indicate restricted activity, ask the following questions:

- What is your usual form of exercise?
- How often do you exercise?
- How long are your exercise sessions?
- How long have you been engaged in this type of activity?
- What types of exercise or sports have you participated in the past?
- Describe your activity level over the last 10 years.
- Are you exercising more or less than in the past?
- What factors have changed your activity level?

Fitness Goals

What aspects of exercise do you enjoy? What aspects of exercise do you dislike?

What do you think are the benefits of exercise?

How do you schedule your exercise?

What motivates you to exercise?

What are your current fitness goals?

Mobility Concerns

Do you have any pain or discomfort with activity?

Do you avoid any activities because of pain, discomfort, shortness of breath, or chest pain?

If the patient answered *yes* to either question, describe the following:

- Type of problem
- Onset of concern
- Frequency of problem
- Activities that trigger and relieve
- Severity and type of symptoms
- Effect of problem on day-to-day activities
- Treatments used to alleviate and how they worked

Underlying Health Concerns

Do you have any healthcare problem that affects your ability to engage in activity or exercise?

If so, describe the problem and the effect.

What medications do you take?

Have you ever been told you have a bone problem? If so, what was the nature of the problem?

Have you ever experienced a fracture, strain, or sprain? If so, where was the problem? When did it occur? How did it occur?

Have you ever had weakness of the muscles or problems coordinating movement?

Do you have any cardiac or respiratory problems that affect your ability to perform activities?

Have you ever experienced anxiety or depression that affected your ability to participate in activities?

Lifestyle

What kind of work do you do?

Describe your typical work activities.

How many hours per week do you work?

What other commitments do you have (school, family, other obligations)?

External Factors

Are there any restrictions in your home that limit your ability to be active?

Do you feel you need an assistive device?

Are you comfortable exercising outside your home or in your neighborhood?

Focused Physical Assessments for Activity and Body Alignment

With the patient standing, observe from the anterior, posterior, and lateral views. Check for the following:

Shoulders and hips are level.

Toes are pointed forward.

The spine is straight, with no abnormal curvatures noted.

The posture is not slumped.

Ask the patient to sit down; observe as he does so.

Does he have difficulty lowering his torso?

Can he control the movement?

Is he able to get into this position with ease?

When he sits, does he slump?

If the patient cannot stand or sit, assess his alignment in bed. Look for ability to move in bed, as well as the posture the patient maintains.

(Continued)

Focused Assessment

Assessing Activity and Exercise—cont'd

Joint Function

Assessing joint function includes inspection and palpation of the joints and assessment of range of motion.

Begin your assessment at the neck and systematically work your way through each of the joints.

At each joint observe for swelling, erythema, asymmetry, or obvious deformity.

Compare the size of the muscles above and below the joint and on each side of the body.

Palpate the joint for temperature and crepitus. Warmth over a joint indicates inflammation or infection. Be sure to compare body temperature over several joints and right to left. **Crepitus** is a grating sensation when the joint is moved. It can often be heard as well as felt. Crepitus is associated with degenerative joint disease or arthritic changes in the joint.

As you palpate the joint, move it through its range of motion.

Muscle Strength

Assess muscle strength by having the patient push and then pull against your hands.

Start at the neck; test the strength of all major joints' range of motion.

To see a nurse using a performing passive range-of-motion exercise,

Go to the video **Performing Passive Range-of-Motion Exercises**, along with questions and suggested responses, is available on the ***Davis's Nursing Skills Videos*** Web site on FADavis.com.

Gait

Gait is divided into two phases: stance and swing.

Stance—In the stance phase, the heel of one foot strikes the ground while the opposite foot pushes off and leaves the ground.

Swing—In the swing phase, the leg from behind moves in front of the body. When the right leg is in stance mode, the left leg is in swing mode.

You must observe the patient walking. Normal gait includes the following features:

- Head is erect, gaze forward.
- Heel strikes the ground before the toe.
- Opposite arm moves forward at the same time.
- Feet are dorsiflexed in the swing phase.
- Gait is coordinated and rhythmic.
- Weight is evenly distributed, with minimal swing from side to side.
- Movement starts and stops with ease.
- Movement is at a moderate pace.

If the patient uses an assistive device, such as a cane, crutch, or walker, pay attention to how he uses it. Ask the patient to ambulate a short distance with and without the device to determine if the device is actually providing stability.

Activity Tolerance

Assess and record vital signs before having the patient engage in 3 minutes of activity.

Select an activity appropriate for the patient. For example, if the patient uses a walker, ask the patient to walk down the hallway. For a patient without obvious health limitations, consider asking her to run in place for 3 minutes.

Observe the patient throughout the exercise. If she shows any signs of distress, stop the exercise, immediately take a set of vital signs, and repeat the vital signs every minute until they have returned to baseline.

If the patient can exercise continuously for 3 minutes, assess the patient at the end of the 3-minute period and at 1-minute intervals. Note the change in heart rate, blood pressure, and respiratory rate.

This type of approach is not appropriate for patients who easily become short of breath, develop chest pain, or are very unsteady on their feet. Instead, for example, limit your assessment to determining the amount of assistance the patient needs to turn in bed or get out of bed.

Muscle Mass and Strength

As you observe the patient, compare muscle mass on the right and left sides. If you notice an obvious discrepancy in size, measure the circumference of the limbs and compare.

To assess strength, ask the patient to push against your hand with the hands and feet. Once again, compare both sides.

For guidelines for assessing mobility in the home,

Go to Chapter 32, **Home Care: Home Assessment for a Patient With Mobility Concerns,** in Volume 1.

TABLES

Range of Motion at the Joints	
JOINT	**ILLUSTRATION**
Neck (Pivot Joint) The joint is formed by a ring-like object that turns on a pivot. Motion is limited to rotation.	
Flexion—Move the head from upright midline position to the chin, resting the head on the chest. *Normal Range:* 45° from midline ***Extension***—Move the head from flexed to upright midline position. *Normal Range:* 45° from midline ***Hyperextension***—Move the head from upright midline position to as far back as possible. *Normal Range:* 10°	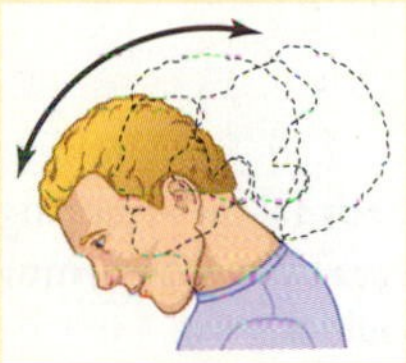
Lateral flexion—Tilt the head laterally from midline position toward the shoulder. *Normal Range:* 40° from midline	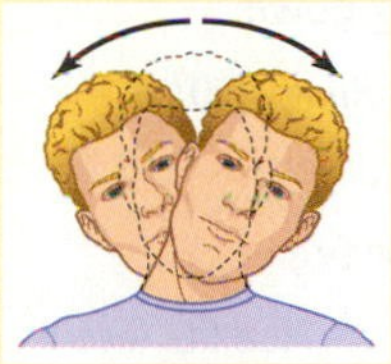
Rotation—Rotate the head in a circular motion from upright midline position to as far right or left as possible. *Normal Range:* 180°	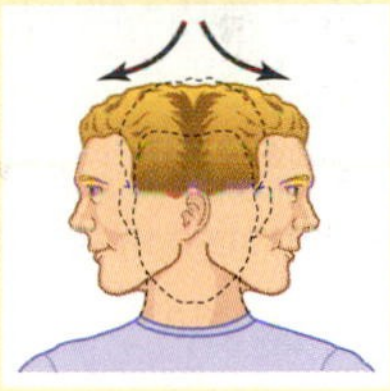
Shoulder (Ball-and-Socket Joint) A rounded head (ball) fits into a cup-like structure (socket) to allow movement in all planes in addition to rotation.	
Flexion—Raise the arm from a neutral position at the side to alongside the head. *Normal Range:* 180° ***Extension***—Move the arm from flexed to a neutral position at the side of the body. *Normal Range:* 180° ***Hyperextension***—Move the arm, keeping the elbow straight, from a neutral position at the side of the bed to behind the body. *Normal Range:* 45°–60°	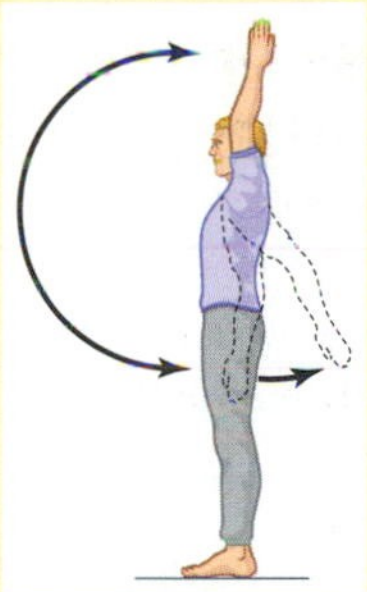
Abduction—Raise the arm laterally from a neutral position at the side of the body to a position at the side of the head, palm facing outward. *Normal Range:* 180° ***Adduction***—Move the arm downward from a position beside the head to across the front of the body as far as possible. *Normal Range:* 230°–320°	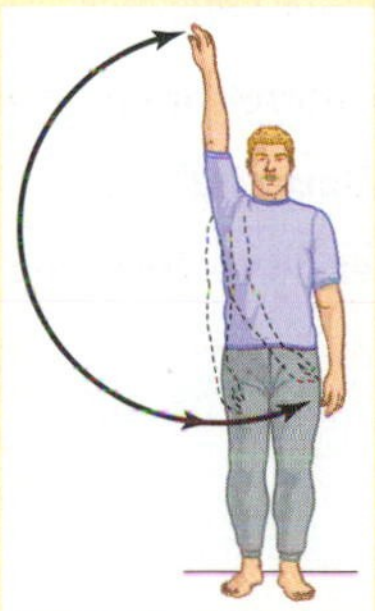

(Continued)

Range of Motion at the Joints—cont'd

JOINT	ILLUSTRATION
Circumduction—Circle the arm from the shoulder. *Normal Range:* 360°	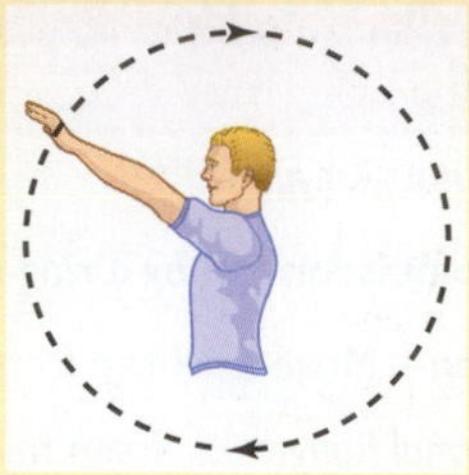
External rotation—Keeping arm held out to the side at shoulder level and bent to a right angle, fingers pointing down, move the arm upward so that the fingers point upward and are above the shoulder. *Normal Range:* 90° ***Internal rotation***—Move the arm forward and down to return to the starting position, fingers pointing down. *Normal Range:* 90°	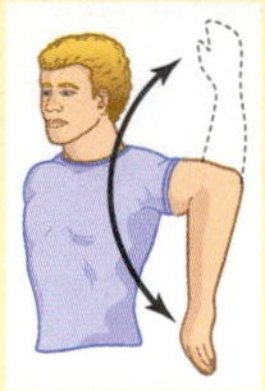
Elbow (Hinge Joint) A convex surface fits into a cavity, allowing flexion and extension.	
Flexion—Bend at the elbow to move the forearm from a straightened position up toward the shoulder. *Normal Range:* 150° ***Extension***—Straighten the arm by bringing the lower arm forward and down. *Normal Range:* 150°	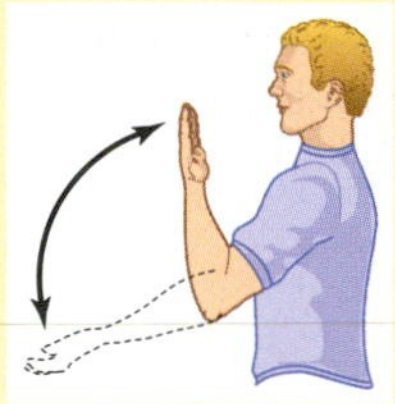
Rotation (for supination)—With the arm at the side, elbow bent, move the hand and forearm so that the palm is facing upward. *Normal Range:* 70°–90° ***Rotation (for pronation)***—With the arm at the side, elbow bent, move the hand and forearm so that the palm is facing downward. *Normal Range:* 70°–90°	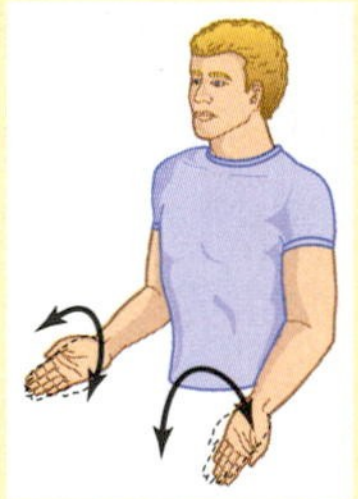
Wrist (Condyloid Joint) An oval-shaped bone fits into an elliptical cavity to allow movement in two planes at right angles to each other.	
Flexion—Bend the fingers of the hand toward the inner aspect of the forearm. *Normal Range:* 80°–90° ***Extension***—Straighten the wrist so that it is on the same plane as the forearm. *Normal Range:* 80°–90° ***Hyperextension***—Bend the wrist as far back as possible toward the outer aspect of the forearm. *Normal Range:* 70°–90°	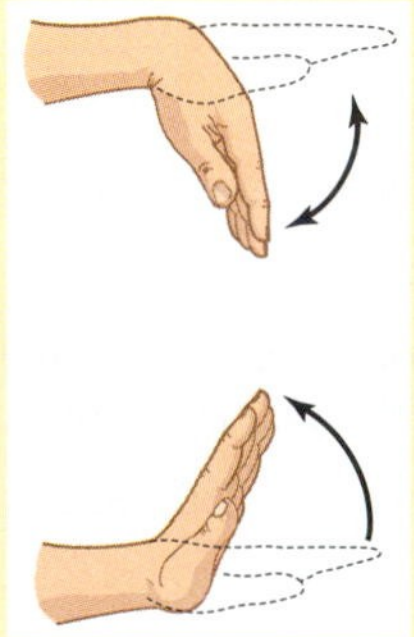

Range of Motion at the Joints—cont'd

JOINT	ILLUSTRATION
Abduction (radial flexion)—With the hand supinated, bend each wrist laterally toward the thumb side. *Normal Range:* 0°–20° ***Adduction (ulnar flexion)***—With the hand supinated, bend each wrist laterally toward the fifth finger side. *Normal Range:* 30°–50°	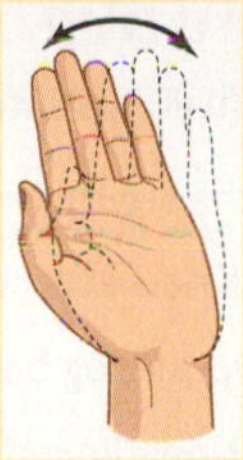
Hands and Fingers (Condyloid Joints: Interphalangeal Joints Are Hinges)	
Flexion—Bend the fingers into a fist. *Normal Range:* 90° ***Extension***—Straighten the fingers. *Normal Range:* 90° ***Hyperextension***—Bend the fingers back. *Normal Range:* 30°	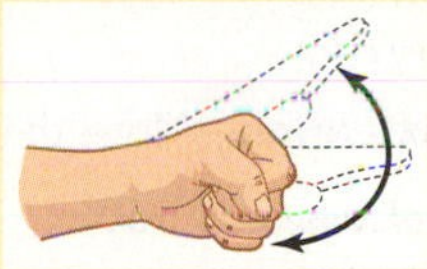
Abduction—Spread the fingers apart. *Normal Range:* 20° ***Adduction***—Bring the fingers together. *Normal Range:* 20°	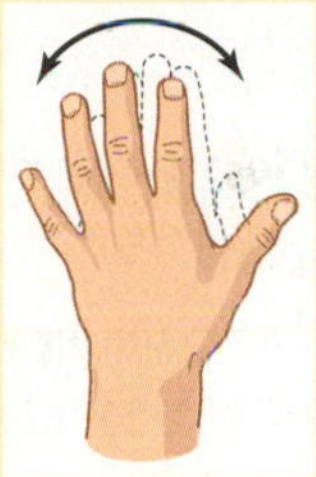
Thumb (Saddle Joint) One bone surface is concave in one direction and convex in the other. The other surface has the opposite construction so that the bones fit together. Movement occurs in two planes at right angles to each other.	
Flexion—Move the thumb across the palm of the hand toward the fifth finger. *Normal Range:* 90° ***Extension***—Move the thumb laterally away from the fingers. *Normal Range:* 90°	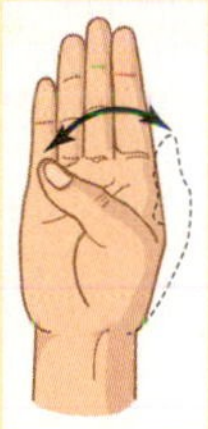
Opposition—Touch the thumb to the top of each finger of the same hand. *Normal Range:* NA	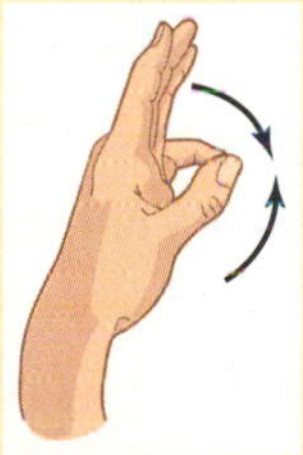

(Continued)

Range of Motion at the Joints—cont'd

JOINT	ILLUSTRATION
Hip (Ball-and-Socket Joint) A rounded head (ball) fits into a cup-like structure (socket) to allow movement in all planes in addition to rotation.	
Flexion—Move the leg forward and up. *Normal Range:* Knee extended 90° ***Extension***—Move the leg back down beside the other. *Normal Range:* Knee flexed 120°	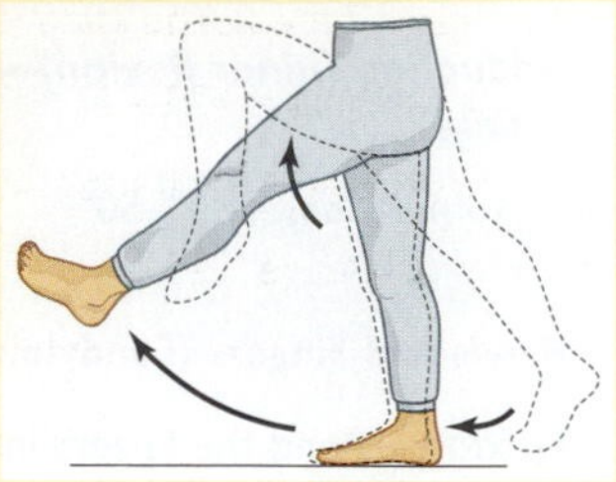
Hyperextension—Move the leg back behind the body. *Normal Range:* 30°–50°	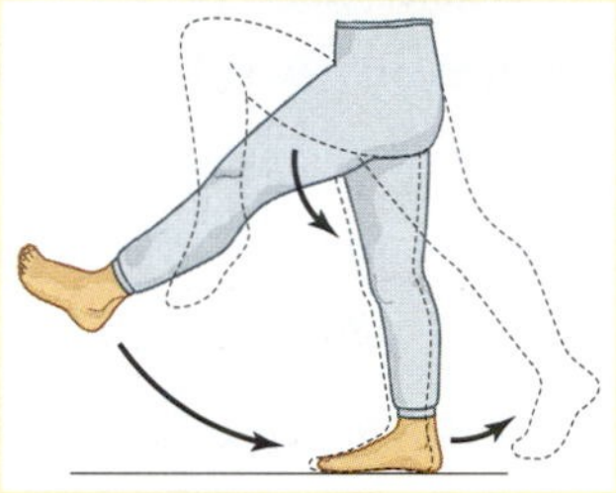
Abduction—Move the leg laterally. *Normal Range:* 45°–50° ***Adduction***—Sweep the leg inward across the midline. *Normal Range:* 20°–30° beyond the other leg	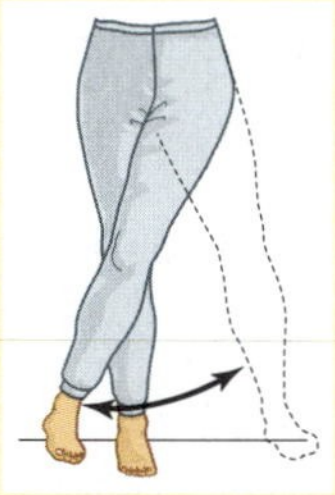
Circumduction—Circle the leg, keeping the knee straight. *Normal Range:* 360°	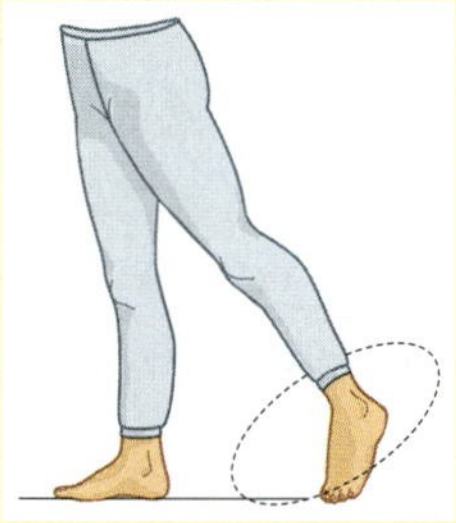
Internal rotation—Turn the foot and leg inward toward the other leg. *Normal Range:* 90° ***External rotation***—Turn the foot and leg outward, pointing the toes as far as possible away from the other leg. *Normal Range:* 90°	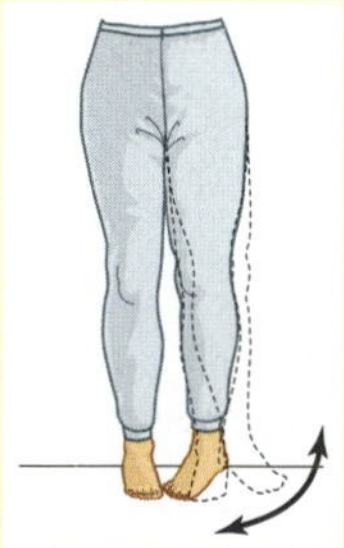

Range of Motion at the Joints—cont'd

JOINT	ILLUSTRATION
Knee (Hinge Joint) A convex surface fits into a cavity, allowing flexion and extension.	
Flexion—Bend at the knee, bringing the heel back toward the buttocks. *Normal Range:* 120°–130° ***Extension***—Straighten the knee, returning the leg to its original position. *Normal Range:* 120°–130°	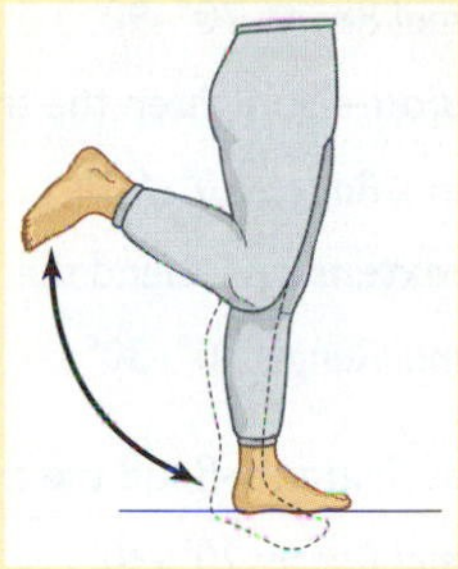
Ankle (Hinge Joint) A convex surface fits into a cavity, allowing flexion and extension.	
Extension (plantar flexion)—Point the toes and foot downward. *Normal Range:* 45°–50° ***Flexion (dorsiflexion)***—Pull the toes and foot upward. *Normal Range:* 20°	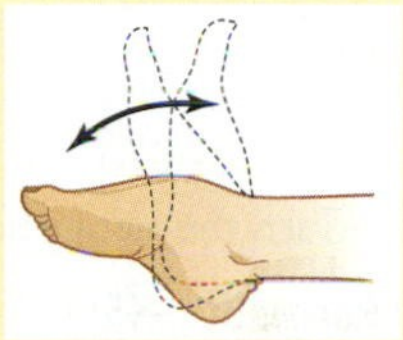
Foot (Gliding Joint) Two flat plane surfaces move past each other.	
Eversion—Turn the sole of the foot laterally. *Normal Range:* 5° ***Inversion***—Turn the sole of the foot medially. *Normal Range:* 5°	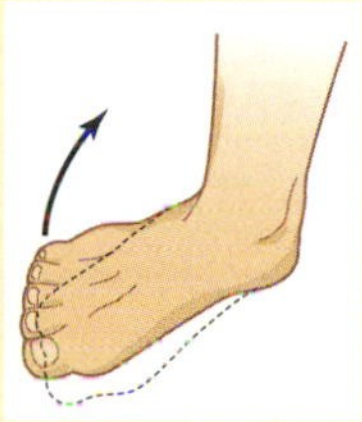
Toes (Hinge Joint except intertarsal joints, which are Gliding Joints) A convex surface fits into a cavity, allowing flexion and extension.	
Flexion—Curl the toes downward. *Normal Range:* 35°–60° ***Extension***—Straighten the toes. *Normal Range:* 35°–60°	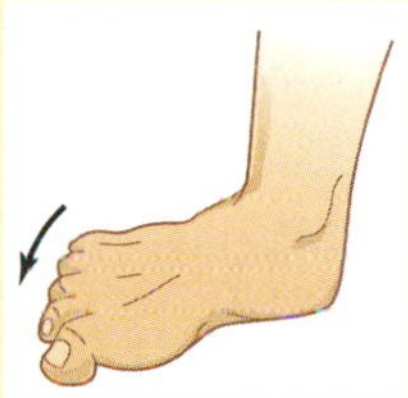
Abduction—Spread the toes apart. *Normal Range:* 0°–15° ***Adduction***—Bring the toes together. *Normal Range:* 0°–15°	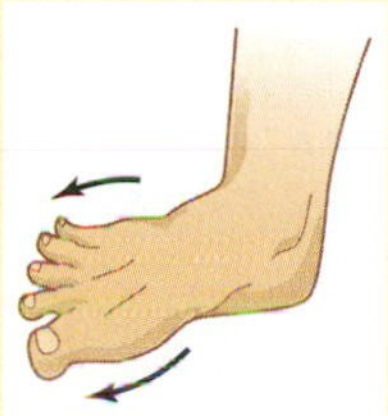

(Continued)

Range of Motion at the Joints—cont'd

JOINT	ILLUSTRATION
Trunk	
Flexion—At the waist, bend forward toward the toes. *Normal Range:* 70°–90° ***Extension***—Straighten the trunk from the flexed position. *Normal Range:* 70°–90° ***Hyperextension***—Bend the trunk backward. *Normal Range:* 20°–30°	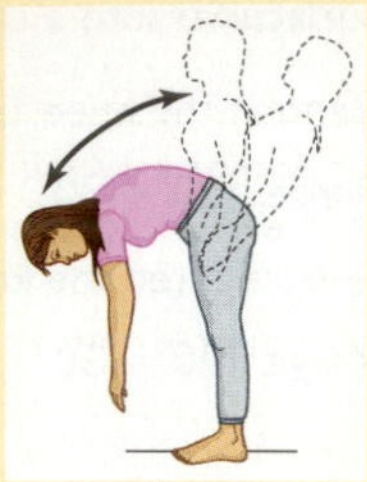
Lateral flexion—Bend the trunk to the side. *Normal Range:* 20°–40°	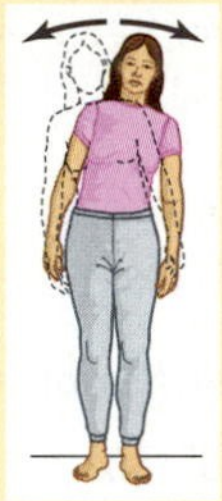
Rotation—Turn the upper body from side to side (twist at the waist). *Normal Range:* 30°–45°	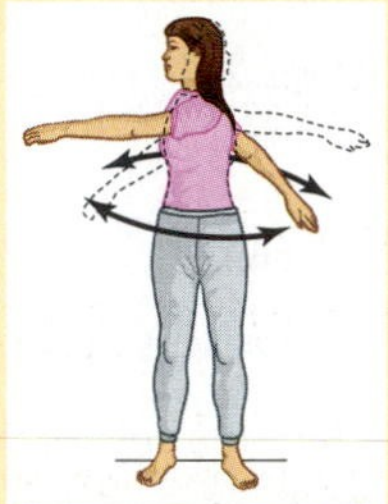

NA, not applicable.

STANDARDIZED LANGUAGE

Standardized Language

Diagnoses for Activity and Exercise Problems

Nursing Diagnosis	Defining Characteristics	Etiologies
Activity Intolerance—insufficient physiological or psychological energy to endure or complete required or desired daily activities (NANDA International, 2018)	*Subjective:* fatigue, weakness, discomfort on exertion, dyspnea, and verbalization of no interest in activity *Objective:* changes in heart rate, blood pressure disproportionate to activity, dysrhythmias or evidence of ischemia on electrocardiogram (ECG), and pallor or cyanosis with activity	Conditions that affect tissue oxygenation (e.g., chronic obstructive pulmonary disease or cardiac disease) Conditions that produce fatigue, such as depression, prolonged immobility, bed rest, and sedentary lifestyle
Impaired Physical Mobility—Limitation of independent purposeful movement of the body or of one or more extremities (NANDA International, 2018) (specify level of independence using a standardized functional scale)	*Subjective:* pain or discomfort with movement, exertional dyspnea *Objective:* limited ROM, limitations in fine or gross motor movement, poor coordination with movement, difficulty turning, unstable gait, decreased reaction time, postural instability, slowed movement, and difficulty performing ADLs	Neuromuscular, sensoriperceptual, or musculoskeletal impairment; reduced one mass; malnutrition; obesity; deconditioning due to sedentary lifestyle; lack of knowledge about the importance of activity and exercise for maintenance of health; anxiety; cognitive impairment or developmental delay; discomfort; limited cardiovascular endurance; medications; pain; prescribed movement restrictions

Note: *Impaired Physical Mobility* is a broad, general diagnosis. Use the following, more descriptive diagnoses when the patient has specific deficits:

Impaired Bed Mobility	Impaired Walking	Sedentary Lifestyle
Impaired Wheelchair Mobility	Impaired Transfer Ability	

Mobility Problems as Etiologies of Other Diagnoses

Note: Mobility problems may also be the etiology of other diagnoses. The following are examples:

- *Risk for Ineffective Peripheral Tissue Perfusion* (specify) r/t blood flow compromised by reduced mobility
- *Risk for Disuse Syndrome* occurs when there is a risk for deterioration of body systems due to musculoskeletal inactivity. Risk factors include prescribed bed rest, severe pain, altered level of consciousness, mechanical immobilization (traction), and paralysis.
- *Acute Pain* r/t musculoskeletal injury
- *Ineffective Health Maintenance* r/t prescribed bed rest
- *Risk for Injury* r/t unsteady gait
- *Self-Care Deficit* (or more specific deficits: *Bathing/Hygiene Deficit, Feeding Deficit, Dressing/Grooming Deficit, Toileting Deficit)* (Saba, 2017) r/t Impaired Physical Mobility

Sources: NANDA International (2017). *Nursing diagnoses: Definitions & classification 2018–2020* (11th ed.), Herdman, T. H. & Kamitsuru, S. (eds.). New York, NY: Thieme; and Saba, V. K. (2017). *Clinical care classification (CCC) system, version 2.5: User's guide.* Retrieved from https://sabacare.com/Custom/Tables/Diagnoses.php?SF=DiagCode&SO=Asc

Standardized Language

Selected NIC Interventions for Mobility Diagnoses

Class: Activity and Exercise Management	Class: Immobility Management
Body Mechanics Promotion	Bed Rest Care
Energy Management	Cast Care: Maintenance
Exercise Promotion	Cast Care: Wet
Exercise Promotion: Strength Training	Physical Restraint
Exercise Promotion: Stretching	Positioning
Exercise Therapy: Ambulation	Positioning: Wheelchair
Exercise Therapy: Balance	Self-Care Assistance: Transfer
Exercise Therapy: Joint Mobility	Splinting
Exercise Therapy: Muscle Control	Traction/Immobilization Care
Teaching: Prescribed Activity/Exercise	Transfer

Source: Butcher, H., Bulechek, G., Dochterman, J., et al. (eds.). (2018). *Nursing interventions classification (NIC)* (7th ed.). St. Louis, MO: Elsevier. Used with permission.

CLINICALJUDGMENT
Applying the Full-Spectrum Nursing Model

PATIENT SITUATION

Mr. Ronald Ornduff is a 72-year-old retired man who lives with his wife in a one-story home. He has excellent general health with no significant health problems. Ronald typically walks with a moderate to vigorous pace in his neighborhood or at the mall in the winter. He belongs to a health club and works out two or three times a week, walking on the treadmill, using the weight machines, or taking a basic conditioning class. Ronald considers himself fit and of an acceptable weight for his age. When going outdoors to pick up the morning paper, he slipped on a patch of ice and fell. You are now caring for him 2 days after hip surgery. He is experiencing pain and seems fearful his injury could be the beginning of a decline in his health.

THINKING

1. *Theoretical Knowledge:*
   a. Based on Mr. Ornduff's age, physical condition, and activity level, make a rough estimate of the number of minutes per week of physical activity he should have after he recovers from surgery and resumes full mobility. What are the benefits of this physical activity?

   b. As a nurse planning the care for a patient after hip surgery, what complications of immobility should you assess for?

2. *Critical Thinking (Considering Alternatives):* What are some possible barriers for an older adult's participating in physical activity? What might you teach your patient to do to overcome those barriers?

DOING

3. *Practical Knowledge:*
   a. How might you position your patient after hip surgery?

   b. What equipment would you need to position your patient after surgery? Is there anything you can set up that will help your patient move around in bed when he can tolerate it?

   c. What type of physical activity would you recommend Mr. Ornduff incorporate into his exercise plan after he experiences full recovery from his surgery? What benefit will these exercises provide?

4. *Nursing Process (Diagnosis):* Write at least two nursing diagnoses for Mr. Ornduff. Use just the data provided in the situation. Assume he is 2 days postoperative.

CARING

5. *Self-Knowledge:* What would you be feeling if you were in Mr. Ornduff's situation of being physically fit one day and suffering pain and immobility the next?

6. *Ethical Knowledge:* What are one or two things you would do to help Mr. Ornduff feel cared for and cared about?

Critical Thinking and Clinical Judgment

1. In Volume 1, you were introduced (Meet Your Patient) to Helen Jillian, a 72-year-old woman with hypertension, high cholesterol levels, and chest pain. She is 61 inches tall and weighs 290 pounds. Ms. Jillian is admitted to the hospital for another episode of chest pain. You are assigned to care for her. Her provider has ordered her to be out of bed in the chair at least twice daily and to ambulate every day. How will you safely move this patient from bed to chair and assist her with ambulation? Work through that decision by answering the following questions.
   a. What aspects of this situation require the most careful attention (what are the risks; what could go wrong)?
   b. What steps can you take to prevent those difficulties?

2. Ms. Jillian is refusing to get out of bed. "I'm sick," she tells you. "If you make me get out of bed, I'll probably have chest pain." How would you respond to this statement?

3. Vince Fulk is an 85-year-old man who sustained a massive cerebrovascular accident (stroke). He is unresponsive and immobile. What activity or mobility interventions should you incorporate into his plan of care? What is your rationale for these interventions?

4. For each of the following concepts, use critical thinking to describe how or why it is important to nursing, patient care, or activity and exercise. Note that these are *not* to be merely definitions.

   Body mechanics

   Exercise

   Immobility

   Activity tolerance

   Assistive devices

What Are the Main Points in This Chapter?

- The skeletal system includes bones, cartilage, ligaments, and tendons. The skeleton forms the framework of the body and protects the internal organs.
- Movement depends on the interaction between the skeleton and the muscles. The ligaments, tendons, and cartilage serve as the interface between these two systems.
- Contraction of skeletal muscles causes the muscles to shorten, thus causing the bones to move at the joints.
- There are four natural curves to the spine. Proper posture maintains these natural curves in good alignment.
- In the human body, the center of gravity is below the umbilicus at the top of the pelvis. The feet provide the base of support.
- Range of motion (ROM) is the degree of maximum movement at a joint. Active range of motion (AROM) is when the patient independently moves his joints through flexion, extension, abduction, adduction, and circular rotation. Passive range of motion (PROM) is performed by another person when the patient is unable to do so for himself.
- Principles of body mechanics are the rules that allow you to move your body with proper alignment, strength, and balance without causing injury.

- The U.S. Department of Health and Human Services recommends a minimum of 150 minutes per week of moderate-intensity or 75 minutes per week of vigorous-intensity aerobic physical activity, or an equivalent combination of moderate- and vigorous-intensity aerobic physical activity.
- A well-rounded exercise program focuses on flexibility and balance, resistance training, and aerobic conditioning.
- Regular physical activity each week, sustained for months and years, can produce long-term health benefits. Strong evidence links regular physical activity with a lower risk for early death, heart disease, stroke, type 2 diabetes, hypertension, colon and breast cancers, and depression.
- Together with a healthy diet, regular physical activity aids in weight management, better heart and lung function and muscular fitness, fall prevention, and improved memory and mental clarity in older adults.
- People who are physically active tend to feel better and have more energy. Sleep quality is improved. And, overall, for many people, physical activity promotes a sense of optimism and positive self-esteem.
- Factors that influence activity and exercise level include developmental stage, health concerns, nutrition, lifestyle, attitudes, and external factors.
- Severe illness associated with prolonged immobilization causes physiological changes in almost every body system.
- A nursing history focused on activity and exercise assesses usual activity, commitment to fitness goals, mobility concerns, underlying health concerns and injuries, lifestyle, attitude of hardiness and persistence, and external factors.
- Physical assessment that is focused on activity and exercise examines the musculoskeletal system and activity tolerance. Important data include vital signs, height, weight, body mass index, body alignment, joint function, gait, and activity tolerance.
- Patients require a change of position at least every 2 hours to prevent pressure injury, muscle discomfort, damage to superficial nerves and blood vessels, or contractures.
- Range-of-motion exercises maintain joint mobility and limit the complications of immobility.
- Patients who have been confined to bed for more than a week or who have sustained major injury require ROM and muscle strength conditioning before they are able to resume walking.
- Canes, braces, walkers, and crutches promote stability for patients to walk independently and more safely.

Knowledge Map

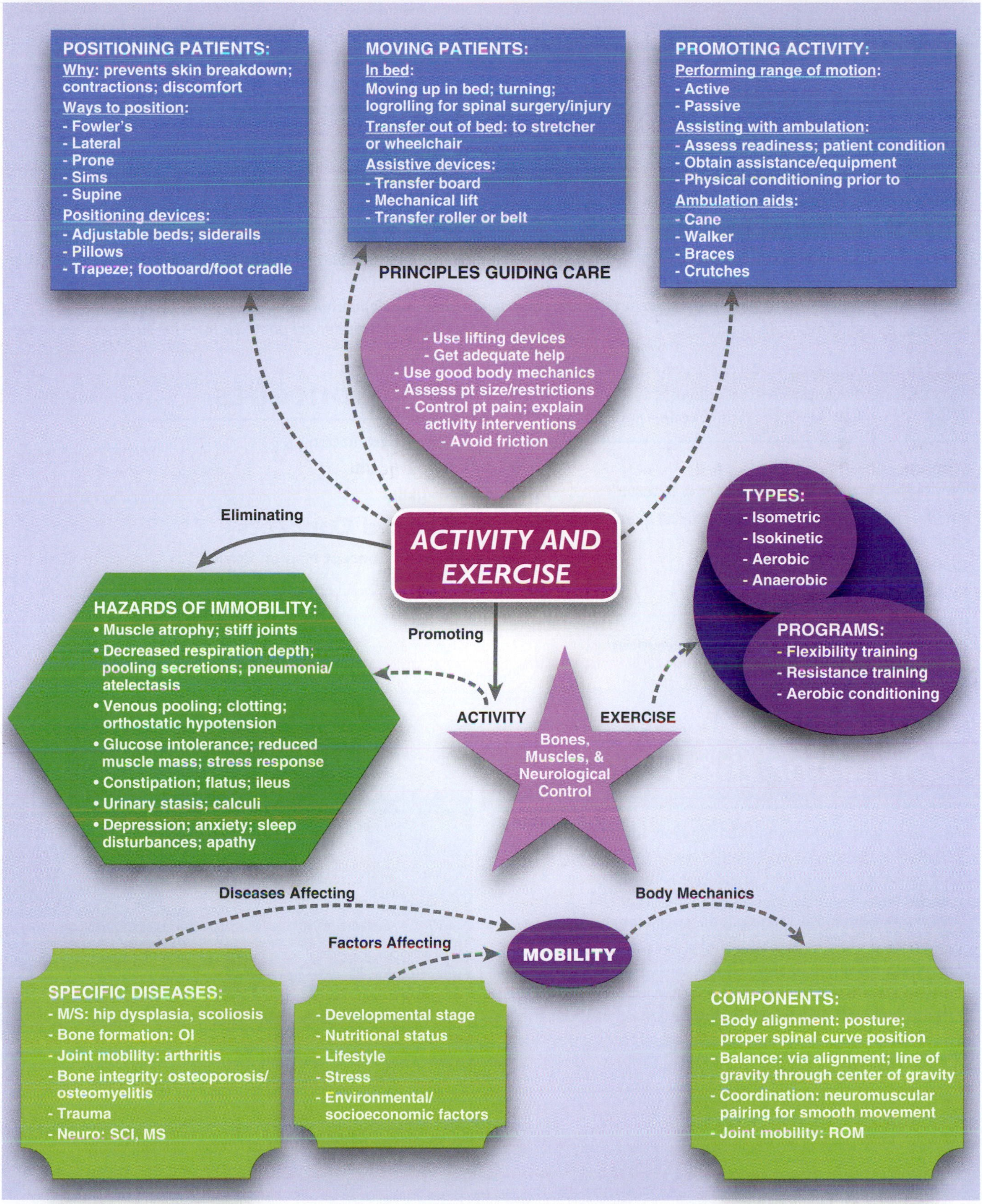

CHAPTER 33

Sexual Health

STUDENT RESOURCES

The questions and exercises in Volume 2 allow you to practice the kind of thinking you will use as a full-spectrum nurse. Critical-thinking questions usually have more than one correct answer, so we do not provide "correct answers" for these features. Try to answer these questions yourself. It is more important to develop your nursing judgment than to just cover content. You will learn by discussing the questions with your peers. If you are still unsure, see the Davis Advantage chapter resources for suggested responses.

To explore learning resources for this chapter,

Go to Davis Advantage and find:

Answers and Suggested Responses for all questions in this chapter
Concept Map
Knowledge Map
References and Bibliography
Lists of NOC Outcomes and NIC Interventions

Key Concepts

Sexual dysfunction
Sexual health
Sexuality

Related Concepts

See the Concept Map on Davis Advantage

Caring for the Nguyens

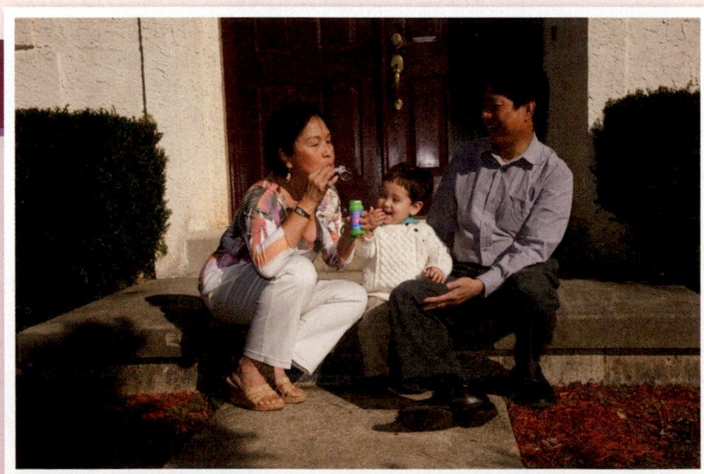

As you may recall, Nam and Yen Nguyen are raising their 3-year-old grandson, Kim. Kim has made friends with Dinh, another little boy at preschool. Kim has asked whether they can play together. Yen works at the preschool and knows Dinh and his family. She is unsure whether she should allow her grandson to play with Dinh because Yen is uncomfortable with the boy's family. Dinh was conceived via artificial insemination and is being raised by a lesbian couple. His parents are open about the relationship and shared the conception information with Yen voluntarily.

Caring for the Nguyens (continued)

A. Yen calls the clinic to speak with you. She explains the situation and asks you whether you think it would be a problem to allow the children to play together. She is concerned that being around this family may be a bad influence on Kim. How would you respond?

B. Yen remains concerned and presses you for more information. She is concerned that Kim's interest in Dinh may indicate that Kim has homosexual tendencies. How would you address her concerns?

C. Yen admits that Nam does not agree with her. "He told me that sexual orientation is genetic." How would you react to this statement?

Practical Knowledge clinical application

In this section you will find guidelines to assist you in assessing and planning care related to patients' sexual health.

CLINICAL INSIGHTS

Clinical Insight 33-1 ➤ Providing Care After Sexual Assault

- **Carefully collect information about the incident** and document findings in a fact-based manner, following your institution's protocol.
- **Be sensitive to the victim's fear, anxiety, and guilt** related to the event.
  Open discussion without communicating judgment or disapproval helps with fact finding for better care.
- **Assess the victim's emotional status,** including sexual identity, stress disorder, and risks for suicide and self-harm. Also discuss the potential for sexual and physical violence, including violence within relationships.
- **When collecting a nursing history for people with disabilities, be sure to screen for sexual violence.**
- **Administer prophylactic treatment** to patients who have been assaulted (vaginally, anally, or orally) to prevent sexually transmitted infections (STIs), such as chlamydia and gonorrhea. If there is a significant risk for HIV, prophylaxis may be prescribed within 72 hours of exposure.
- **Administer vaccines to prevent hepatitis B and human papillomavirus (HPV),** as prescribed and according to your agency's policy.
- **Administer emergency pregnancy prevention** (e.g., the "morning after" pill) to patients who have been vaginally assaulted even if penetration is uncertain, according to your agency's policy.
- **Document pregnancy status** with a urine or blood sample.
- **Teach follow-up care.** The victim should receive follow-up care within 1 week after the event to assess for healing of injuries and presence of STIs. Advise a female victim who has had vaginal penetration to obtain pregnancy testing again 2 weeks after the event.
- **Follow the current reporting requirements** for sexual assault in your state. Some states require reporting assault of children and adolescents, even if they do not consent to the reporting.
- **Know support services** available in your community for victims of abuse. Refer the victim to a sexual assault center for support, counseling, and additional information. Because of the long-term psychological and emotional consequences of sexual assault, most victims benefit from counseling.

Clinical Insight 33-2 ➤ Guidelines for Taking a Sexual History

iCare 1. **Provide privacy.**
- Usually it is not enough merely to pull the curtains around the bed. Ask others who may be able to overhear private conversation behind the curtain to leave the room.
- Talk to the client alone.
- In some situations, it is also beneficial to talk to the partners as a unit, with the consent of both of course.

2. **Protect confidentiality.** Assure your client that information will not be shared with others, unless directly related to planning or delivering healthcare.
3. **Be relaxed in your approach**, and allow the client time to fully answer your questions. Your manner and attitude are critical in putting the client at ease.
4. **Make eye contact.** Do not act embarrassed or allow your body language to show your discomfort.
5. **Avoid communication stoppers**, such as the following:
   - "I'm only asking you these questions because I have to."
   - "I know that you probably won't want to tell me but..."
   - "You're not having any sexual problems, are you?"
6. **Consider a more inviting opening:**
   - "Many people are embarrassed when asked questions about their sexuality, but whatever you tell me will remain confidential."
   - "Many people hesitate to talk about sexual problems. However, your sexual health is important to your overall health, and I would like to ask you a few questions about that."
7. **Be aware of verbal and nonverbal cues** that indicate concerns. Many people will cloak their concerns in comments such as, "I suppose that I won't need to worry about sexy lingerie any longer," or "Sex is for the young. I just have to accept that I'm sick and older now." Be careful that your response to such statements does not either negate or validate your patient's identity as a sexual being. Follow up with comments that encourage the client to provide more details (see Chapter 21 if you would like to review communication techniques).
8. **Realize the client may be embarrassed.** If the client is uncomfortable discussing topics about his own sexual health, reassure him by letting him know that some information, because of its private nature, may be difficult to discuss but is important.
9. **Encourage your client to use terminology that he is comfortable with.**
10. **Help the client feel comfortable.** Consider statements such as the following:
    - "Most people wonder how this surgery [or illness] may affect their sexual functioning."
    - "Whenever these medications are suggested, there are questions about sexual side effects."
    - "Have you thought about the kinds of adaptations you may have to make in your sex life after this surgery/treatment/illness?"
11. **Begin with a less sensitive topic** such as "When was your last menstrual period?" or "How is your relationship with your partner [spouse]?" Then you can move into more sensitive areas: "Many older women have some vaginal dryness that creates discomfort during intercourse. Do you have any concerns about this?"

Clinical Insight 33-3 ➤ Teaching Your Patient to Use a Condom

Using Male Condoms

The male condom is a sheath that covers the penis during sexual activity.

- Put the condom on before the penis touches the vagina, mouth, or anus.
- Inspect the package to ensure that the condom has not been damaged.
- Open the package without tearing the condom.
- Squeeze out the air at the tip of the condom, and unroll it over the erect penis, leaving some space at the tip to collect the ejaculate.
- After sex, to avoid breaking the condom, hold the condom at the rim as the penis is withdrawn. Discard the condom. Wash your hands.
- Use a new condom if you want to have sex again.

Using Female Condoms

The female condom is a plastic pouch that fits inside the vagina so that all vaginal tissue is protected from contact with the penis. The condom is inserted with the inner ring placed high in the vagina near the cervix and the outer ring on the labia.

- Insert the condom before the penis touches the vagina.
- Inspect the package to ensure that the condom has not been damaged.
- Open the package without tearing the condom.
- Put the inner ring and pouch inside the vagina.
- Push the inner ring as far into the vagina as it will go.
- Ensure that the outer ring stays outside the vagina.
- If needed, add lubricant to the inside of the condom.
- After sex, gently pull out the condom and discard.

Do

- Use latex condoms unless you or your partner are allergic to latex, or use polyurethane condoms.
- Treat condoms gently, and keep them out of the sun.
- Use only water-based lubricants to reduce friction and prevent tearing.
- Check the expiration date of the condom and packaging. Old condoms may be brittle and more likely to break.

Don't

- Don't store condoms in your wallet or other place where body heat can break down the latex.
- Don't use fingernails or teeth to open the condom wrapper; doing so can tear the condom.
- Don't reuse a condom.
- Don't use lotions or oils with condoms; these may cause breakage.

TABLES

Methods of Contraception

CONTRACEPTION METHOD	ADVANTAGES	DISADVANTAGES
Abstinence—No sexual intercourse	100% effective Cost free	Lack of sexual expression May create stress in relationship
Fertility awareness (natural family planning, rhythm method)—Intercourse only when a woman is thought to be in the infertile phase of her menstrual cycle	Cost free May be consistent with religious teachings No physical side effect	Requires cooperation of both partners Menstrual cycle must be regular Relatively high failure rate: Pregnancy may result The woman must be motivated and capable of carefully tracking her menstrual cycle. No protection against STIs
Withdrawal (coitus interruptus)—Removal of the penis from the vagina before ejaculation	Cost free	Requires discipline and mutual cooperation Pre-ejaculatory fluid may contain sperm Relatively high failure rate; pregnancy may result No protection against STIs
Male and female condoms	Obtained without a prescription Relatively inexpensive Protects against STIs	Must be put on before penetration; therefore, may diminish spontaneity of intercourse May decrease sensation for both partners Cannot use certain types of condoms if either partner has latex allergy
Spermicides—Jelly, creams, or foams placed in the vagina	Obtained without a prescription More effective when used with a barrier (condom)	Significant pregnancy rate when used without a barrier (condom) No protection against STIs
Contraceptive sponge	May offer some protection against STIs Can be inserted into the vagina up to 24 hours before intercourse Inexpensive	Not fully effective against pregnancy
Vaginal ring	Highly effective in preventing pregnancy Does not have to be inserted before each act of intercourse—can be left in place for weeks to months, depending on the type	Requires a prescription because it is a hormonal method Similar risks as oral contraceptives Costs similar to or greater than those oral contraceptives Correct insertion is key factor in effectiveness of the method
Oral contraceptives (birth control pills)	Highly effective Do not interfere with intercourse Regulate menstrual flow Decrease menstrual cramps	Require a healthcare visit and prescription Significant cost Must be taken as prescribed to be effective Drug interactions No protection against STIs

Methods of Contraception—cont'd

CONTRACEPTION METHOD	ADVANTAGES	DISADVANTAGES
		Carry some undesirable side effects Contraindicated for some women (e.g., those who smoke, who have significant varicose veins)
Depo-Provera injections	Last 3 months Highly effective Do not interfere with intercourse	Require a healthcare provider visit Amenorrhea (may be seen as an advantage) No protection against STIs
Intrauterine device (IUD)—A small piece of plastic that also may contain metal or a hormone: placed through the cervix into the uterus by a healthcare provider	Highly effective May remain in place for years Does not interfere with intercourse	Increased risk of pelvic inflammatory disease (PID) Must be inserted by a healthcare provider Increased menstrual flow and cramping No protection against STIs
Diaphragm—Latex dome-shaped cup with a flexible rim that is inserted in the vagina and fits over the cervix Note: Cervical (silicone) cups provide a better fit for women who have not been pregnant or had vaginal deliveries.	Few side effects Quite effective if used properly with spermicide	Must be inserted before intercourse, thereby compromising spontaneity Must be removed about 6 hours after intercourse Must be used with a spermicide Increased risk of urinary tract infection (UTI) No protection against STIs
Hormonal implant—Small rod(s) containing hormones that are inserted under the skin, usually in the back of upper arm	One of the safest and most effective forms of birth control available (World Health Organization, 2006, updated 2018) Users do not have to think about their birth control every day or for every sexual intercourse Menstrual periods are fewer and lighter for most women Effective for 3 years Can be removed at any time Does not contain estrogen	No protection against STIs May be able to see the rod if the woman is very thin A small number of women have longer and heavier periods with breakthrough bleeding May be limited availability More expensive than some other birth control methods Surgical procedure
Female sterilization (tubal ligation)	Effective Long-term cost-effectiveness May be reversible	May be reversible in some cases, but usually is not No protection against STIs
Male sterilization (vasectomy)	Effective Long-term cost-effectiveness Does not interfere with sexual performance May be reversible in some cases	Psychological effects No protection against STIs

ASSESSMENT GUIDELINES AND TOOLS

Focused Assessment

Guidelines and Questions for Taking a Sexual History

Topics to Include in a Sexual History

The topics to include in the sexual history depend on the nature of the patient's concern. The following topics are most commonly included:

- Reproductive history
- Sexual self-concept
- History of sexually transmitted infections
- History of sexual dysfunction
- Present sexual functioning
- Other factors that affect sexuality, such as medications and diseases
- Signs or symptoms of sexual abuse (see Procedure 9-1: Assessing for Abuse)
- Knowledge level about sex, reproduction, and contraception

Tailor your assessment to meet the client's needs. For example, Frank Thanee (Meet Your Patients, in Volume 1) is concerned about his family's reaction to his lifestyle and sexual orientation. In his situation, you would focus your assessment on his sexual self-concept, family relationships, present sexual functioning, and specific concerns about his heart and the impending family visit.

Questions to Ask Women

Menstrual Cycle

- How old were you when you started your menstrual periods?
- When was your last menstrual period?
- How often are your periods? How would you describe the flow? How long does your period last?
- Do you have any problems with your periods, such as cramping, breast pain, or heavy flow?
- Does your menstrual period ever prevent you from going to work or school or participating in the activities you enjoy?
- What products do you use during your period, such as tampons and pads? Do you ever use douches, either during your period or at other times?

Cancer Screening

- When was your last Pap smear?
- Have you ever had an abnormal Pap smear? If so, how was it treated?
- Have you received a vaccine for HPV?
- Do you examine your breasts? If so, how often?
- Have you noticed asymmetry, lumps, or masses in your breasts? If so, describe them and show me where they are.
- When was your last mammogram? What were the results?
- Is there any history of breast cancer in your family?

Childbearing History

- How many living children do you have?
- How many times have you been pregnant?
- Have you ever had a miscarriage? An abortion?
- How many of your births were preterm (before 38 weeks)? Term?

Sexual Activity

- How often do you typically have sexual intercourse per month?
- Are you satisfied with the frequency or quality of sexual activity?
- Is there anything in your life that prevents you from sexual activity?
- Do you have any difficulty achieving orgasm?
- Is sexual intercourse ever painful for you?
- Are you sexually attracted to women? Have you had oral or genital sexual intercourse with women?

Questions to Ask Men

Sexual Activity

- How many times a month do you typically have sexual intercourse?
- Do you have any difficulty achieving or maintaining an erection or orgasm?
- Are you satisfied with the firmness of your erection?
- Do you experience premature ejaculation or have difficulty achieving sexual orgasm?
- Are you sexually attracted to men? Have you had oral or anal intercourse with men?

Cancer Screening

- Have you been taught to examine your testicles? Do you practice testicular self-exam?
- Is there a history of testicular cancer in your family?

Questions to Ask Both Men and Women

Illnesses and Medications

- What types of illnesses have you been treated for in the past?
- Have you ever been hospitalized? Have you ever had surgery?
- What medications, herbal remedies, or over-the-counter medicines do you take?
- Has any medical treatment, surgery, or medication affected your sexual functioning?

Focused Assessment

Guidelines and Questions for Taking a Sexual History—cont'd

Family Responsibilities

- Do you have children? If so, how many? How many are still at home? Dependent on you?
- Are you responsible for other children or adults? (This question may reveal whether the person continues to care for an adult, disabled child, or grandchildren.)

Genitalia

- Have you noticed any redness, swelling, discharge, itching, or odor in your genital area?
- Have you noticed asymmetry, lumps, or masses in the genitals? If so, describe them and show me where they are.
- Have you ever been told you have a hernia?
- Have you ever had trauma to your genitals?
- Are you having any problems urinating?

Sexual Patterns

- Are you sexually active? If not, have you ever been?
- Do you have sex with men, women, or both?
- What types of sexual activity do you engage in? Oral, anal, or genital?
- How many partners do you currently have? How many partners have you had in the past 6 months?
- How would you describe your satisfaction with your current sexual relationship?
- What are your thoughts about how this procedure/illness may affect your sexual relationship?
- Have you experienced any recent changes in your sexual function—in your level of desire, your sexual activity, participation, or satisfaction?
- Do you have any concerns about your sexual function, including your level of desire, activity, participation, or satisfaction?

Contraception (as appropriate)

- Do you use birth control? If so, what type and how often?
- How satisfied are you with your method of contraception?

Sexually Transmitted Infections

- Have you ever been treated for an STI? If so, what type?
- Are you concerned about STIs or HIV?
- What precautions do you take to avoid STIs?

Abuse

- Have you ever been forced to have sex against your will?
- Have you ever been threatened or abused by a partner?
- Do you ever feel threatened by your partner?

For guidelines for your approach to taking a sexual history, see Clinical Insight 33-2.

STANDARDIZED LANGUAGE

Standardized Language

Examples of Nursing Interventions Classifications (NICs) for Sexuality Problems

For Ineffective Sexuality Pattern:

Body Image Enhancement
Coping Enhancement
Family Planning: Contraception
Role Enhancement
Self-Esteem Enhancement
Sexual Counseling
Teaching: Safe Sex

For Sexual Dysfunction:

Abuse Protection Support
Behavior Management: Sexual
Infection Protection
Risk Identification
Sexual Counseling
Teaching: Sexuality

Source: Adapted from Butcher, H., Bulechek, G., Dochterman, J., et al. (Eds.). (2018). *Nursing interventions classification (NIC)* (7th ed.). St. Louis, MO: Elsevier. Used with permission.

CLINICAL JUDGMENT
Applying the Full-Spectrum Nursing Model

PATIENT SITUATION

Debra is perimenopausal at age 52, and her husband Roberto is 59. She has been feeling tired in the afternoon and moody at times. At her annual women's health visit, Debra tells you that she feels a lower level of sexual desire than she used to. Debra says, "I chalk it up to being very busy at work and yet still having so many demands on my time and energy with care of our three kids and housework." Debra is physically active, exercising four times a week, and is in good general health. She takes no medication and is within 15 pounds of her normal weight. Debra still has her period, but the flow is very heavy and cramping is more uncomfortable than it ever had been.

Recently, Debra has noticed that Roberto has been taking longer to achieve an erection, and his erection is not as firm as it used to be. He is in general good health except for high blood pressure and high blood cholesterol levels. He takes medication for both conditions.

THINKING

1. *Theoretical Knowledge (Factual Information):*
   a. What are the common physical and emotional manifestations occurring with perimenopause?

2. *Critical Thinking (Analyzing Alternatives, Deciding What to Do):*
   a. How would you respond to Debra when she asks for information and support regarding her husband's erectile dysfunction?

   b. Debra asks you whether her desire for sexual intimacy will continue to decline after she goes through "the change of life." Describe in detail what you would tell her.

DOING

3. *Practical Knowledge:*
   a. What general topics would you explore with Debra to assess her sexual history?

   b. What questions would you ask Roberto to assess his sexual history?

CARING

4. *Self-Knowledge:* What might you be feeling if you were in Debra's situation?

5. *Ethical Knowledge:* What are one or two things you would do to help Debra and Roberto feel cared for and cared about?

Critical Thinking and Clinical Judgment

1. A 34-year-old married woman was hospitalized yesterday following an alleged rape. You are assigned to provide her nursing care. She will remain hospitalized for several days because of a head injury she suffered during the rape.
   a. How can you best approach this woman to establish a positive rapport?

   b. What fears is this patient likely to express?

   c. The patient's spouse is coming to visit. What concerns do you think that he may have?

   d. You begin to feel overwhelmed by this couple's emotions and questions. What can you do to help provide this couple with optimal care?

2. You are assigned a 26-year-old male patient who recently had a spinal cord injury. The doctors have talked to him about the possibility of regaining motor function and perhaps being able to walk again after intense therapy. He now seems most concerned about his relationship with his 25-year-old fiancée.
   a. What aspects of their relationship do you think he is concerned about?
   b. Do you have enough theoretical and patient information regarding his injury to answer all of his concerns?
   c. As you consider some of the changes in sexual functioning that may follow a spinal cord injury, what suggestions might you share with him?
   d. What clues would indicate that talking to the fiancée may be appropriate?
3. You are seeing Jessica, a 14-year-old girl, at the clinic. Her throat culture is positive for gonorrhea. The girl's mother has gone down to the coffee shop. The doctor has left a prescription for antibiotics. You are left to take care of the discharge from the clinic.
   a. How would you explain the culture results to Jessica?
   b. Jessica tells you that she cannot possibly have a sexually transmitted infection (STI) because she has not had sexual intercourse. How would you respond?
   c. Jessica tells you that she has had oral sex with her boyfriend, but no one else. What education regarding STIs and antibiotics would be appropriate?
   d. What information would you give the mother when she returns?
4. A 45-year-old married man with young children has just been informed that he is HIV positive. He is shocked by the news. He admits he had an extramarital relationship with a man 7 years ago.
   a. What concerns is he likely to have? As his nurse, what biases will you have to put aside to help him?
   b. What theoretical knowledge would you need at a later time to help him deal with questions about sexual activity?
   c. What patient information would you need to help him deal with questions about sexual activity?
5. Review the following scenarios from Meet Your Patients in Volume 1.
   - **Jocelyn Carter.** Two days after undergoing a fine-needle aspiration to evaluate a small breast mass, Jocelyn Carter's surgeon informed her that the mass was malignant. He recommended a mastectomy (removal of the breast). Today, she arrives alone at the surgery registration area. You ask how she is feeling, and she tells you that the past week has been a whirlwind of activity. "I had to arrange child care, cancel a business trip, and organize the house so that I could take a few days off to have the surgery. My husband is working overseas this fall, so he couldn't be here to help me. Honestly, I don't know how I'm feeling. I haven't had time to think about it." A few minutes later, as she waits in the surgery holding area, she begins to cry. You hold her hand and ask whether she would like to talk. She asks you, "Do you think my husband will still want me? I'm afraid he will be turned off when he looks at me."
   - **Gabriel Thomas.** This patient comes to the outpatient clinic complaining of a throbbing headache for the past 3 days. He explains that he has tried several over-the-counter medicines and has had no relief. You check his blood pressure, and measure the reading at 240/130 mm Hg. When you ask whether he has ever been treated for high blood pressure, he replies, "Are you another one of these people trying to get me to take drugs that will ruin my sex life?"
   - **Frank Thanee.** Frank has heart disease, had a mitral valve replacement 3 days ago. He has been transferred to the cardiology floor for an additional day of hospitalization. His partner, Greg, has spent the last 3 days at the hospital and has just left to check on the apartment and feed their cat. Frank confides that he is worried about his parents' expected visit. "I've never been able to tell them about Greg. They wouldn't be able to understand our relationship, much less approve of it. I don't know how to handle this. What do you think I should do?"

a. Write etiologies for each of the patients. The nursing diagnosis label is provided for you in each case.

Jocelyn Carter—Ineffective Sexuality Patterns

Gabriel Thomas—Ineffective Sexuality Patterns

Frank Thanee—Sexual Dysfunction

b. For each of the patients, instead of the sexuality diagnosis, identify another nursing diagnosis label that you should explore to see whether it fits the situation better. Consult a nursing diagnosis handbook, as needed.

Jocelyn Carter:

Gabriel Thomas:

Frank Thanee:

6. For each of the following concepts, use critical thinking to describe how or why it is important to nursing, patient care, or sexual health. Note that these are *not* to be merely definitions.

Sexual health	Sexual expression
Gender	Sexually transmitted infections
Sexual orientation	Fertility control

7. An infant is born with ambiguous sex organs. The provider has informed the parents that they will need to make a decision regarding which gender they want to assign to the child. They also have the option of waiting and letting the child decide at a later date.

a. What do you think the parents need to consider in making this decision?

b. What emotional factors may be involved in this decision?

What Are the Main Points in This Chapter?

- Sexuality is a broad and complex aspect of the self, with physical, emotional, social, and spiritual dimensions.
- Sexuality involves how we feel about ourselves as individuals and how we interact with others and our environment.
- Gender, gender roles, gender identity, and sexual orientation contribute to expression of our sexuality throughout the life cycle.
- There are both typical and atypical forms of sexual expression.
- Culture, religion, lifestyle, sexual knowledge, and physical health all influence our attitudes toward sexuality, sexual behaviors, and intimate relationships.
- Sexual victimization is a societal and healthcare concern.
- Physical and psychological health status affects sexuality and sexual functioning.
- Sexual health is challenged by high-risk sexual behaviors, STIs, negative interpersonal relationships, and sexual dysfunctions.
- Four phases of the sexual response cycle are excitement, plateau, orgasm, and resolution.
- A sexual history is a component of the nursing assessment.
- There are strategies you can use to help you gain comfort and competence in collecting sexual data.
- The PLISSIT model was developed as a guideline for counseling for sexual problems: Permission, Limited Information, Specific Suggestions, and Intensive Therapy.
- Sexual well-being may be enhanced through nursing interventions such as counseling for sexual problems; dealing with inappropriate sexual behavior; and teaching about body function and reproduction, self-care, contraception, and prevention of STIs.

Knowledge Map: Sexuality

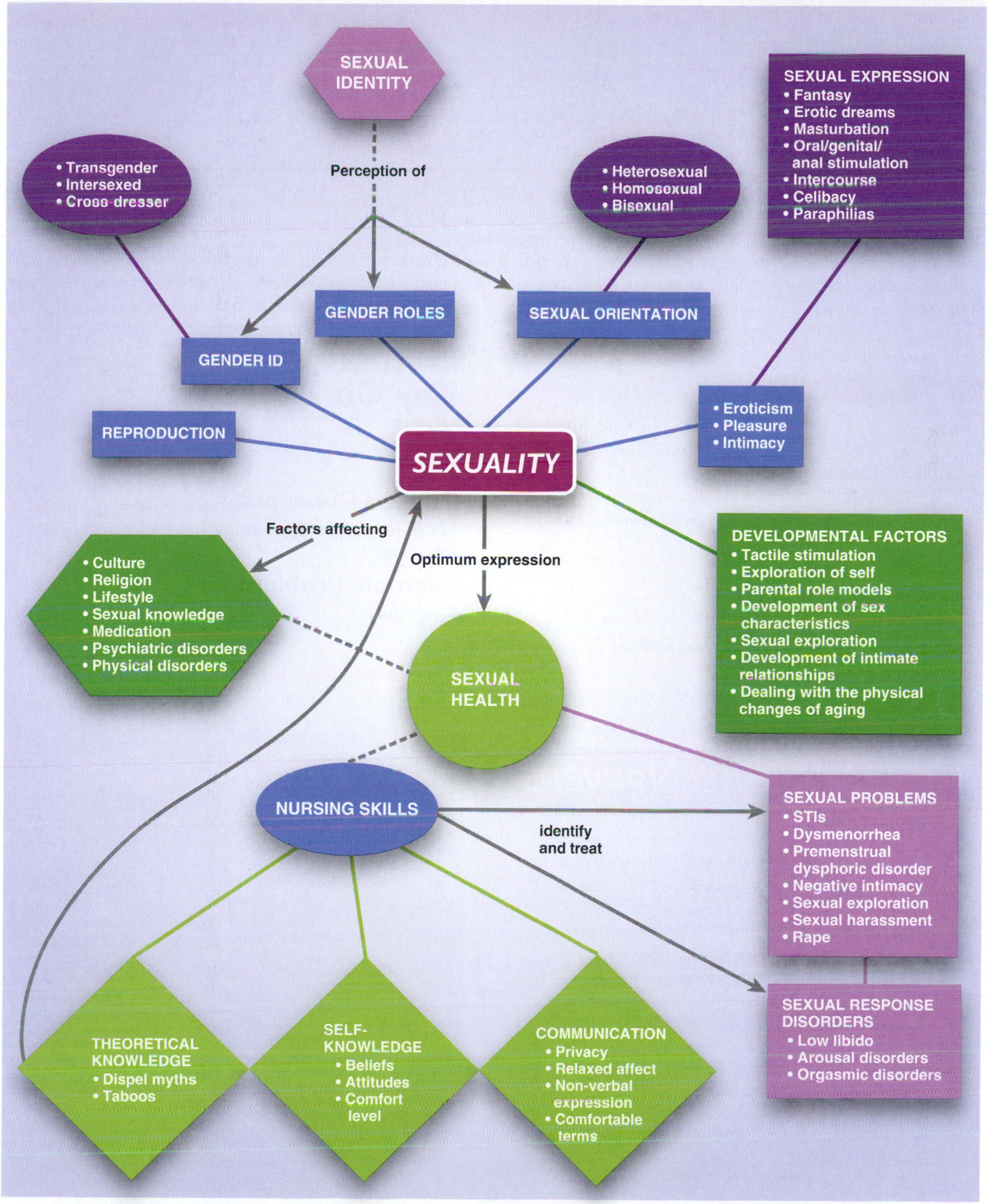

CHAPTER 34

Sleep & Rest

STUDENT RESOURCES

The questions and exercises in this book allow you to practice the kind of thinking you will use as a full-spectrum nurse. Critical-thinking questions usually have more than one right answer, so we do not provide "correct answers" for these features. Try to answer these questions yourself. It is more important to develop your nursing judgment than to just cover content. You will learn more by discussing the questions with your peers. If you are still unsure, see the Davis Advantage chapter resources for suggested responses.

To explore learning resources for this chapter,

Go to Davis Advantage and find:

Answers and Suggested Responses for all questions in this chapter
Concept Map
Knowledge Map
References and Bibliography
Lists of NOC Outcomes and NIC Interventions

Key Concepts

Rest
Sleep

Related Concepts

See the Concept Map on Davis Advantage

Example Problem

Sleep Apnea

Caring for the Nguyens

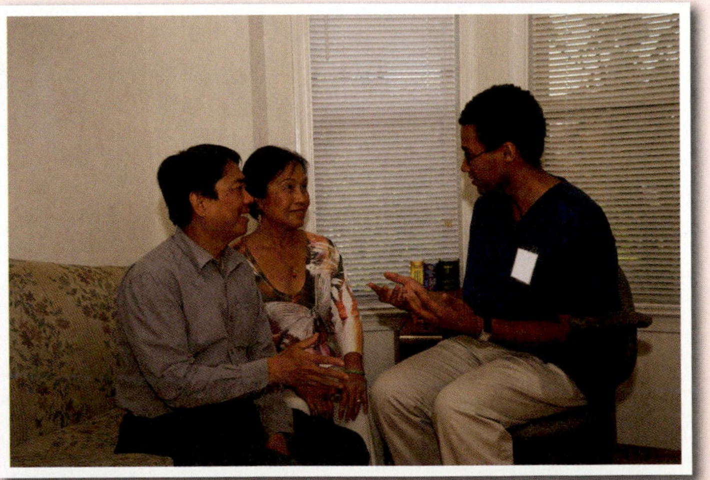

Yen Nguyen arrives at the clinic accompanied by her husband, Nam. She appears very tired. Nam tells you that she has been sleeping poorly. "She worries so much. She worries about Kim, our grandchild. She worries about our kids. Now she's worried about my mother. When we were going through that mammogram scare, she was even worse!"

Mrs. Nguyen shrugs her shoulders. "I can't help it. I'm like that. I've always been a worrier. But it's gotten worse lately. Now I worry and get so emotional. I lie in bed thinking about all this stuff and end up in tears. Then, when I finally get to sleep, I wake up covered with sweat. I've tried extra soy for hot flashes, melatonin from the health food store, herbal tea, and even Benadryl—but nothing seems to work. I'm so tired. But when I get up, I have to deal with all these little kids at work. They're bouncing all over the place and noisy. I just get so short-tempered with them. That's not like me. I can't take this anymore."

Caring for the Nguyens (continued)

A. *Patient data:* Clearly Mrs. Nguyen has a sleep problem. Underline the data that are defining characteristics (symptoms) of a sleep problem.

B. *Patient data:* Which data suggest ideas about the etiologies (causes) of Mrs. Nguyen's sleep problem?

C. *Nursing diagnosis:* Two NANDA-I sleep-related nursing diagnoses are Sleep Deprivation and Disturbed Sleep Pattern. You have already identified the patient's defining characteristics. Now, what *knowledge* do you need to decide which of these NANDA-I labels to use?

D. How could you obtain this knowledge?

E. Sleep Deprivation is defined as "prolonged periods of time without sleep" and Disturbed Sleep Pattern is defined as "time-limited disruption of sleep." Can you make the diagnoses on the basis of this knowledge? Why or why not?

F. In the next column are some of the defining characteristics for these two nursing diagnoses. Certainly there is some overlap between the two sets of symptoms. Nevertheless, which set seems to be a better fit for Mrs. Nguyen? Why?

Disturbed Sleep Pattern

- Verbal complaints of not feeling well rested
- Dissatisfaction with sleep
- Change in normal sleep pattern
- Decreased ability to function
- Reports being awakened
- Reports no difficulty falling asleep

Sleep Deprivation

- Daytime drowsiness
- Apathy
- Decreased ability to function
- Agitation
- Irritability
- Hallucinations
- Anxiety
- Inability to concentrate
- Slowed reactions
- Combativeness
- Fatigue
- Fleeting nystagmus
- Hand tremors
- Heightened sensitivity to pain
- Lethargy, listlessness, malaise
- Perceptual disorders (e.g., disturbed body sensation, delusions, feeling afloat)
- Restlessness
- Transient paranoia

G. Write a nursing diagnosis for Mrs. Nguyen.

PracticalKnowledge clinical application

This section will help you learn to give a back massage, assist you in obtaining a sleep history, and provide standardized language to use in planning care for clients with sleep problems.

PROCEDURES

In the not-so-distant past, a relaxing back massage was a part of the evening care routine for every hospitalized patient. In this era of cost containment, this sleep enhancer has become a "nice but not essential" procedure in most agencies. Massage has therapeutic benefits, however. It promotes circulation, physical and emotional comfort, and sleep. Furthermore, it is an independent nursing activity for which you do not need a medical prescription (except in very rare circumstances). Try to offer a back rub whenever you can; and teach and encourage unlicensed assistive personnel (UAP) to do so as well. Refer to the following procedure.

Procedure 34-1 ■ Giving a Back Massage

➤ For steps to follow in *all* procedures, refer to the Universal Steps for All Procedures found on the page facing the inside back cover.

Equipment

Skin care lotion

Pre-Procedure Assessment

Check the skin for reddened areas or skin breakdown.

Delegation

You can delegate back massage to the UAP if the patient's condition and the UAP's skills allow. However, giving the back rub yourself provides an excellent opportunity to assess the patient, develop rapport, and provide emotional support.

➤ When performing the procedure, always identify your patient according to agency policy, using two identifiers, and be attentive to standard precautions, hand hygiene, patient safety and privacy, body mechanics, and documentation.

Procedure Steps

1. **Warm the lotion** by placing the bottle in warm water.
   Cold lotion can cause muscle contraction; warming the lotion helps relax the muscles.
2. **Raise the bed to working height.**
   Prevents back strain of the nurse.
3. **Position the patient comfortably** on her side or prone.
   a. Untie the patient's gown; expose her back.
   b. Raise the siderail on the opposite side of the bed.
   Siderails prevent the patient from falling off the bed when you turn her toward the side of the bed away from you.
   c. Don procedure gloves.
   d. Wash the patient's back with warm water, if needed.
   Warm water will help relax the muscles while removing any sweat and soiling.
4. **Place lotion on your hands.**
   Placing the lotion directly on the back may cause the patient's muscles to tighten.
5. **Place your hands on either side** of the spine at the base of the neck. Using gentle, continuous pressure, rub down the length and then up the sides of the back.
   a. Repeat this motion several times.
   b. Never rub directly over the spine.
   The spine is a vulnerable area.

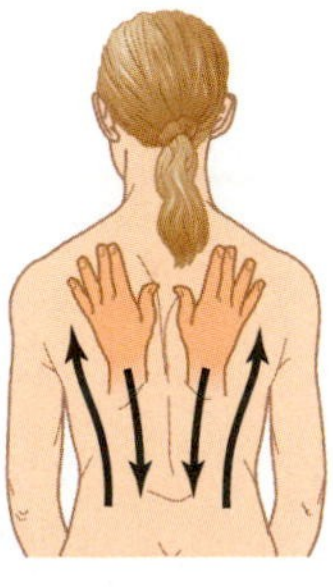

6. **Apply gentle thumb pressure** (using the fleshy part of your thumbs) on either side of the spine at the midback, pushing outward for about 2.5 cm (1 in.).
   a. Repeat from the midback to the base of the neck in a series of small, outward strokes.
   Strokes should be along the muscle length and not across the muscle to help stretch and relax it.
   b. Ask the patient whether the amount of pressure is comfortable. Be careful not to cause the patient discomfort, which might cause further muscle tightness.
   c. Always apply pressure away from the spine, not toward it.
   This gently stretches the muscles and helps prevent placing pressure on the spine.

d. If you are unable to massage both sides at the same time, work on one side and then the other.
Work as symmetrically as possible to increase muscle relaxation.▼

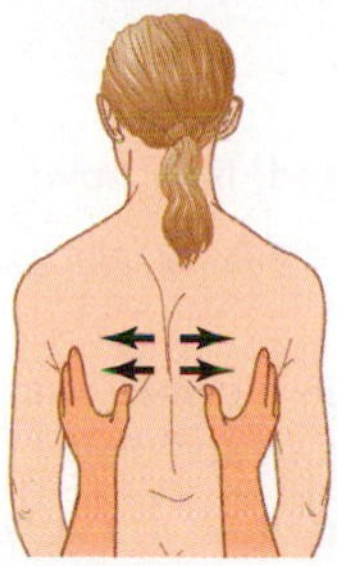

7. **Now go to the spots that felt** the tightest or that the patient states are tight. Work in small circles, using gentle thumb pressure.
Small circular movements can help release muscle "knots" and relax tightened muscles.▼

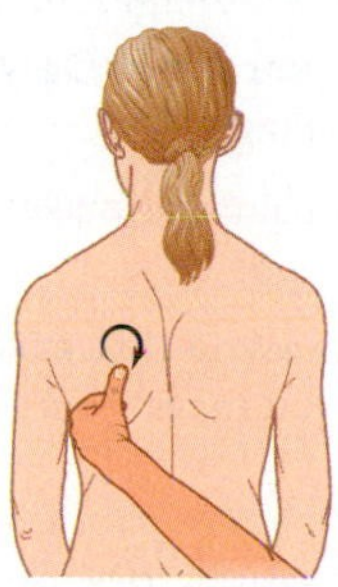

8. **Gently shake the scapulae.** Place your palm on one scapula, and gently shake it by quickly moving your palm back and forth. Repeat on the other side.
Movement of the scapula decreases when muscles tighten; gently vibrating the scapula helps loosen the muscles.▼

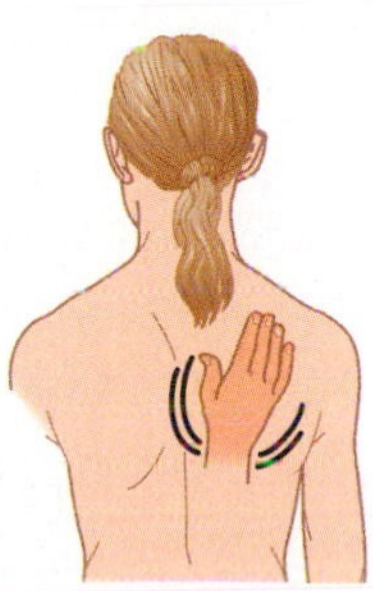

9. **Apply horizontal strokes** across the scapula, using your thumb. Using horizontal strokes from near the spine across the bottom of the scapula, push out all the way across the scapula from the spine. Move up and repeat until you have covered the entire scapula and top of the shoulder. Repeat on the other side.
This movement helps loosen the trapezius muscle.▼

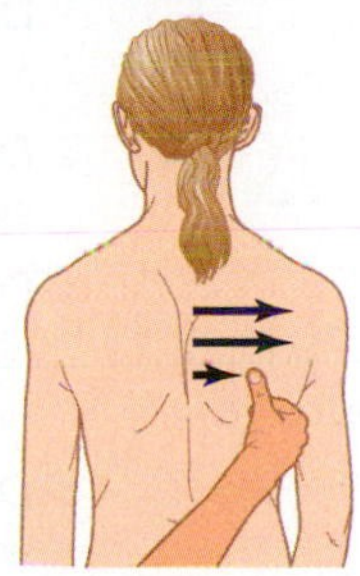

10. **If you find tender spots,** use the fleshy parts of your fingers in a small circular motion.

11. **Apply pressure in circles** using the heels of your hands down both sides of the spine. Beginning at the upper shoulder and working down to the lower back, apply pressure in medium-sized circles down the sides of the spine with the heels of your hands. Be cautious not to apply too much pressure. Assess patient for comfort.
The circular motion helps relax tightened areas in the paraspinal muscles.▼

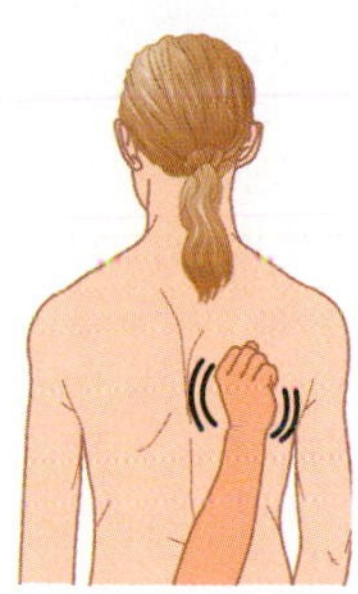

12. **Apply horizontal strokes** using the heels of your hands across the latissimus dorsi muscle. Using horizontal strokes from near the spine below the scapula, push out from the spine across to the ribs, and work down across the lower back with the heels of your hands.
This movement helps relax the latissimus dorsi muscle.

13. **Gently rub your hands up either side** of the spine from the base of the back to the base of the neck and then down the sides of the back. Repeat several times.
Long strokes help increase circulation and promote relaxation of the back muscles.

NOTE: If you are unable to do a complete back massage, ask the patient where she is most uncomfortable, and massage those areas. If the patient has general tightness, use the long strokes down each side of the spine and back up the sides.

Evaluation

Assess the patient's report of comfort, relaxation, and how soon she falls asleep.

Documentation

This is a routine aspect of care and is usually documented on a flowsheet.

Practice Resources

Dosey, B., & Keegan. L. (2016); Fritz, S. (2019).

ASSESSMENT GUIDELINES AND TOOLS

This section will assist you in screening for sleep problems.

Focused Assessment

Questions for a Sleep History

A brief assessment for all patients should include questions about the following:

Usual Sleeping Pattern

- When do you go to sleep and wake up?
- How many hours do you sleep?
- Do you have a regular sleep schedule?
- How would you rate the quality of your sleep on a scale of 1 to 10, with 10 meaning "great"?
- Do you take a nap? If you do, for how long?
- How often do you waken during sleep, for example, to go to the bathroom?
- Do you feel adequately rested when you wake up?

Sleeping Environment

- Would you like a night-light?
- What room temperature do you prefer?
- What noise level do you prefer (for example, radio, television, absolute quiet)?

Bedtime Routines/Rituals

- What do you typically do in the hour before bedtime?
- What do you do to help you fall asleep?

Sleep Aids

- Do you need a special pillow or positioning aid?
- Do you take any sleep medications or other drugs, natural sleep aids, or homeopathic remedies that may affect sleep?

Sleep Changes or Problems

- Have your sleep patterns changed? If so, how?
- How often do you experience difficulty falling asleep? Staying asleep?
- Do you currently, or have you in the past, ever experienced a sleep disorder (e.g., narcolepsy, insomnia)?
- Do you remember your dreams after you wake? Do you ever have night terrors? Do you sleepwalk?
- Do you ever experience an unpleasant creeping feeling, crawling, or tingling, relieved only by moving the legs at night?
- Do you snore? Does your own snoring or grunting ever wake you or anyone in the room?
- Do you wear a cap at night? Do you require oxygen at night? Or any other medical aid or therapy while you sleep?
- Do you grind your teeth while you sleep? Do you wear a dental appliance to prevent grinding?
- Do you experience any kind of pain that makes it difficult for you to fall asleep or stay asleep?
- Is there anything that I have not asked that might help you sleep while you are in the hospital (having surgery, receiving home care)?

If the client reports experiencing satisfactory sleep, that is an adequate assessment, and you merely need to support her usual sleep patterns and rituals. When you suspect a sleep problem, you will perform a more in-depth assessment, such as a detailed sleep history or sleep diary.

Focused Assessment

Sleep Log

A sleep log provides specific information on the patient's sleep–wakefulness patterns over a long period. The log is usually kept for 14 days and may include the following.

Note: If you work a night shift, adjust the time for sleep and waking in these questions accordingly.

Completed in the Morning

1. Time you went to bed: ________
2. Approximate time you fell asleep: ________
3. Times you woke during the night: ________
4. Times you fell back to sleep: ________
5. Time you woke up in the morning: ________
6. Did you feel refreshed upon wakening? ________
7. What did you eat or drink just before bedtime? ________
8. What mental and physical activities did you engage in the 2 to 3 hours before bedtime? ________
9. Were you worried or anxious about anything when you went to bed? ________
10. Sleep medications you have taken: ________ Any repeated doses? ________ Times: ________

Completed in the Evening

1. How sleepy did you feel during the day?
   - ______ Sleepy; struggled to stay awake during the day
   - ______ Somewhat tired
   - ______ Fairly alert
   - ______ Wide awake
2. Any naps during the day? ________ If so, for how long? ________
3. Frequency of pain medication taken and times ________
4. Exercise during the day? ________ If so, for how long? ________ What time of the day? ________
5. Number of alcoholic drinks ________ What time: ________
6. Number of caffeinated drinks ________ What time: ________
7. Number of tobacco products ________ What time: ________

CLINICAL JUDGMENT

Applying the Full-Spectrum Nursing Model

PATIENT SITUATION

A 43-year-old healthy woman, Maria Lupe, is being seen for her annual women's health visit. She tells you she lies awake in bed for hours before falling asleep at night. Sometimes she falls asleep without problems but will wake up and then have trouble going back to sleep. After feeling as though she had been awake nearly all night, Maria wakes in the morning feeling exhausted. She tells you she feels tired all the time and can't seem to get things done during her time off because of her fatigue. Maria admits to feeling irritable with her coworkers and children. Because of her lack of rest, she doesn't have the desire to do things socially anymore.

THINKING

1. *Theoretical Knowledge:* The NANDA-I definition and defining characteristics of Insomnia differ slightly from the medical diagnosis of insomnia.
   a. What is insomnia, as defined medically (e.g., by the National Sleep Foundation)?
   b. What other health conditions might a medical diagnosis of insomnia be confused with?
   c. What factors either lead to or aggravate insomnia, as described medically?
2. *Critical Thinking (Contextual Awareness):*
   a. Obviously Maria has trouble sleeping. Based on the data you have, do you consider her difficulty sleeping significant enough to require consultation with her primary healthcare provider? Explain your thinking.

(continued)

(continued)

DOING

3. *Nursing Process (Assessments):*

   a. When conducting a sleep history for Maria, what questions would you ask her in order to (1) describe more fully her sleeping problem and (2) identify the cause of her sleeping problem?

   b. What would you suggest Maria do to help you gain more information about her sleeping problem?

4. *Nursing Process (Nursing Diagnosis):* Based on the data in the Patient Situation, would you use a nursing diagnosis of Sleep Deprivation or Insomnia for Maria? Explain your thinking. Use a nursing diagnosis handbook, as needed, to compare the defining characteristics of the two diagnoses.

5. *Nursing Process (Interventions):* How might you help your patient manage her Insomnia other than using prescription medication? What might you suggest?

CARING

6. *Self-Knowledge:*

   a. Have you ever had trouble falling or staying asleep? How did you feel at the time and in the morning? Describe your experience.

   b. How might you provide better emotional care and support to your patient after recalling your own episodes of sleeping difficulty?

Critical Thinking and Clinical Judgment

1. You are a nurse working on a psychiatric unit. You are assigned to the care of Sheryl, a 23-year-old woman with the diagnosis of anorexia nervosa (a potentially life-threatening eating disorder characterized by an intense fear of weight gain and extremely restrictive food intake). Sheryl attends therapy each day, seems to be taking her medications, and is eating the required amount of food at each meal. But she continues to lose weight. The nurse working the night shift reports that Sheryl is unable to sleep at night; seems frightened, almost panicky; paces the hall; and cries. Sheryl is unwilling to talk about her inability to sleep, but you read in her chart that she was sexually abused during the night while she was in a foster home. As you are straightening up in her room, you find several of Sheryl's sleeping pills. Sheryl walks into the room and begs you to be her friend and not to tell anyone. She promises to take her pills that night.

   a. What do you think may be contributing to Sheryl's inability to sleep? Explain your reasoning.

   b. How do you *feel* about keeping Sheryl's secret? Why might you want to tell other caregivers about the sleeping pills? What reasons can you think of for *not* telling?

   c. For you to deal effectively with Sheryl's sleep problem, what theoretical knowledge would you need?

   d. Now assess your current theoretical knowledge. Do you need more knowledge about certain topics to help Sheryl? If so, where can you find out what you need to know?

2. Imagine that you are a registered nurse at a local nursing home. Gwen, a 74-year-old woman, has captured your heart. Gwen has severe rheumatoid arthritis with pain and joint deformities, so she cannot ambulate or perform activities of daily living independently. Gwen's family visits every weekend, and they always bring cookies or candy, usually chocolate. Gwen likes to eat these treats just before bedtime, right after her bedtime medications. She receives a stool softener, a sleeping pill, and a pain pill for her arthritis. Lately she has been awakening at least twice each night, seeming quite confused. She tells the day shift nurse that she needs another sleeping pill at bedtime because "I'm not sleeping as well as I used to, because I have to get up so many times to go to the bathroom." She also seems more sluggish than usual during the day. You will need to integrate all available information. Don't worry if you do not know much about arthritis or if there

are other things you have not yet studied. Just try to reason out the questions based on the knowledge you *do* have.

a. If you have not yet studied arthritis and urinary elimination, you may lack some theoretical knowledge you need to answer the following questions. What information do you need? Where would you go to get it?

b. What are some reasons that Gwen might be awakening?

c. What might be causing her confusion at night?

d. Should you address the problem of having chocolate before bed? Why or why not?

e. List as many different interventions as you can that you might use to address the problem of eating sweets before bed.

f. Consider the consequences. How might her family react if you suggest that they bring something besides sweets?

g. What teaching might you do with the family?

3. You are a home health nurse. One of your patients is a 55-year-old man named Grant. He is homebound because of complications of diabetes. He states that he sleeps during the day, taking several naps. His chief complaint today is a pain in his left foot. There are books about alternative medicine and bottles of vitamins and minerals all over the house. He believes he can cure his diabetes with herbs. He refuses to take any medications that are prescribed for him by his physician.

a. Do you have enough information to conclude that Grant has a sleep problem? Explain your answer.

b. Examine the patient situation (context). What factors lead you to suspect that Grant may not be sleeping enough at night?

c. What would you do to find out whether Grant is getting enough sleep?

d. Imagine how you would feel about Grant's decision to forgo his medication and use herbal treatments.

e. What personal values and biases do you have that will affect the way you respond to Grant?

4. For each of the following concepts, use critical thinking to describe how or why it is important to nursing, patient care, or sleep and rest. Note that these are *not* to be merely definitions.

Sleep

Rest

Theoretical knowledge about the physiology of sleep

Circadian rhythm

Stages of sleep (e.g., REM sleep)

Sleep apnea

Sedatives

Sleep log

What Are the Main Points in This Chapter?

- Sleep is a basic physiological need.
- Sleep and rest promote physical, mental, and spiritual well-being by restoring energy and reducing body demands while the body repairs itself.
- Illness can interfere with the ability to sleep and rest; conversely, people who suffer from sleep disorders have an increased susceptibility to illnesses.
- The hypothalamus and various neurotransmitters are involved in the physiology of sleep.
- Circadian rhythm is a biorhythm that is influenced by both internal and external stimuli, especially the light–dark patterns of day and night.
- The brain waves produced during REM sleep are similar to those of alert wakefulness. REM is characterized by rapid eye movements and dreaming.
- Duration of sleep varies according to age.
- Factors affecting sleep include developmental needs and stressors, work, exercise, foods, other lifestyle factors, use of medications, illness, pain, and the environment.
- Common sleep disorders include insomnia, sleep apnea, and narcolepsy.
- It is important to obtain information about the patient's usual sleep patterns and rituals; this may require use of a sleep diary.
- Nursing interventions to promote sleep include scheduling nursing care, creating a restful environment, promoting comfort, and supporting bedtime rituals and routines.
- Pain is one of the main deterrents to sleep. Hormonal fluctuations and stress also contribute to sleep difficulties.
- Sleep medications, as a rule, should be used only as a temporary measure.
- Teaching patients and their families about the importance of rest and sleep is an important health promotion intervention.

Knowledge Map

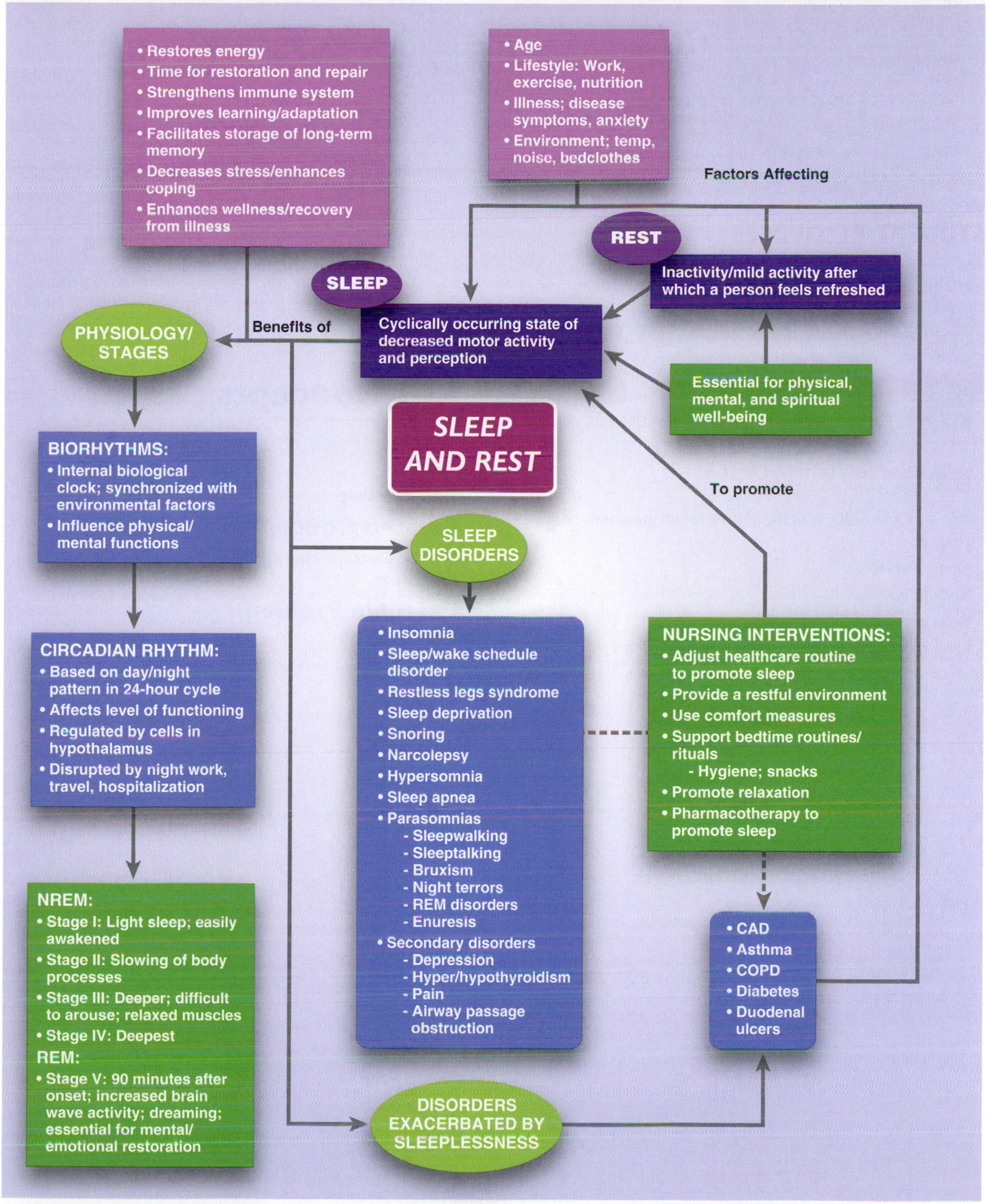

CHAPTER 35

Skin Integrity & Wound Healing

STUDENT RESOURCES

The questions and exercises in this book allow you to practice the kind of thinking you will use as a full-spectrum nurse. Critical-thinking questions usually have more than one right answer, so we do not provide "correct answers" for these features. Try to answer these questions yourself. It is more important to develop your nursing judgment than to just cover content. You will learn more by discussing the questions with your peers. If you are still unsure, see the Davis Advantage chapter resources for suggested responses.

To explore learning resources for this chapter,

Go to Davis Advantage and find:

Answers and Suggested Responses for all questions in this chapter
Concept Map
Knowledge Map
References and Bibliography
Lists of NOC Outcomes and NIC Interventions

Key Concepts

Skin integrity
Wound
Wound healing

Related Concepts

See the Concept Map on Davis Advantage

Example Problem

Pressure Injury

Caring for the Nguyens

Kim Phan, Nam and Yen Nguyen's 3-year-old grandchild, fell at the neighborhood playground. He has abrasions on his knees, a deep puncture wound on his left hand, and a laceration on his scalp. Mr. and Mrs. Nguyen bring him to the clinic for assessment. He is crying loudly and moving all extremities. No treatment has been given.

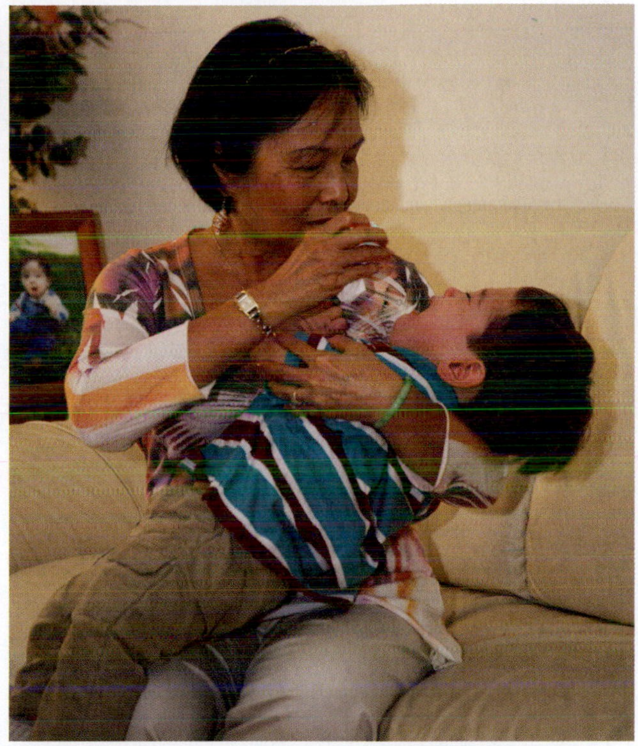

A. What should be your first course of action?

B. What kind of care will Kim need at the clinic?

C. You determine that the scalp laceration will need to be sutured. What actions should you take to prepare Kim for the suturing?

D. One week later, Kim arrives at the clinic with his grandmother to have the sutures removed. The scalp laceration is dried and healed. When you inspect his other wounds, you notice that his left knee is erythematous, warm, and painful to touch and that there is a moderate amount of purulent drainage. What assessment questions should you ask?

E. Yen Nguyen tells you that Kim would not allow her to clean or dress the abraded knees. You cleanse the knee and remove several small pieces of gravel from the wound bed. The wound is yellow and malodorous. What kind of care will Yen need to provide to Kim to heal the left knee?

PracticalKnowledge clinical **application**

As a nurse, you will care for many patients who have wounds or who are at risk for impaired skin integrity. In order to apply your theoretical knowledge of wound assessment and wound care, you will need practical knowledge found in the Procedures and Clinical Insights following.

PROCEDURES

All wounds require a focused assessment. Assessment frequency depends on the condition of the wound, the patient care setting, the patient's overall condition and underlying disease process, the type of wound, and the type of treatment used for the wound. If you are providing wound care, you will assess the wound with every treatment.

Specific nursing interventions directed at maintaining skin integrity or healing wounds make use of procedures for obtaining wound cultures, cleansing wounds, and dressing wounds; for placing and removing wound closures, caring for wound drains, and applying binders and bandages; and Clinical Insights for applying local heat and cold therapy.

Procedure 35-1 ■ Obtaining a Wound Culture by Swab

➤ For steps to follow in *all* procedures, refer to the Universal Steps for All Procedures found on the page facing the inside back cover.

➤ *Note:* This procedure uses modified sterile technique because wound care is now usually performed using a clean approach rather than strict sterile technique.

Equipment

- Three pairs of clean nonsterile gloves
- Aerobic culturette tube with sterile calcium alginate or rayon swab
- Sterile 4 in. × 4 in. gauze in an impermeable tray or separate 4 × 4 packs and an impermeable barrier
- Sterile 0.9% (normal) saline solution for irrigation, warmed to body temperature when possible
  Cold solution lowers the temperature of the wound bed and slows the healing process.
- 20-mL syringe
- 19-gauge angiocatheter
- Gown and face shield
- Emesis basin
- Water-resistant disposable drapes

Delegation

This procedure requires knowledge of wound healing. It needs to be performed by a registered nurse. Do not delegate this skill to unlicensed assistive personnel (UAP).

Pre-Procedure Assessments

NOTE: If the wound is covered when you begin, you will make these assessments once you remove the soiled dressing *and* after cleansing the wound.

- Assess for pain.
  Wounds may be very painful, and wound irrigation may increase pain. Provide prescribed pain medication 30 minutes before performing the procedure, if indicated.
- Determine whether the wound requires sterile, modified sterile, or clean technique.
  Sterile technique is used for acute surgical wounds and for wounds that have undergone recent sharp débridement, or when the healthcare provider prescribes it. Chronic wounds are colonized with bacteria and may be cared for using clean technique, as in this procedure. To perform sterile wound irrigation, see Procedure 35-2.
- Assess the amount and type of tissue present in the wound bed.
  Granulating tissue is beefy red with a velvety appearance. It appears with the growth of new blood vessels and connective tissue. Pale pink tissue may indicate compromised blood supply to the wound bed. Necrotic tissue, which is black, brown, or yellow in appearance, is nonviable, and inhibits healing. Only red granulating tissue should be swabbed for a culture.
- Assess the type and amount of exudate.
  Exudate may be a sign of infection.
- Assess the wound for odor.
  A foul odor may indicate infection. Cleanse wounds before you assess for odor because some dressings interact with wound drainage to produce an odor.
- Assess the tissue surrounding the wound edge.
  Surrounding tissue that is red, warm, and/or edematous may indicate infection.

➤ When performing the procedure, always identify your patient according to agency policy, using two identifiers, and be attentive to standard precautions, hand hygiene, patient safety and privacy, body mechanics, and documentation.

Procedure Steps

NOTE: Steps are for aerobic culture.

1. **Place the patient** in a comfortable position that provides easy access to the wound and will allow the irrigation solution to flow freely from the wound, with the assistance of gravity. Position a water-resistant disposable drape between the patient and the bed to protect the bedding from any possible runoff.
2. **After performing hand hygiene,** don gown, face shield, and clean nonsterile gloves.
3. **Remove the soiled dressing.** Dispose of gloves and soiled dressing in a biohazard bag.
4. **Again perform hand hygiene; then don clean, nonsterile gloves.**
5. **Place an emesis basin** at the bottom of the wound to collect irrigation runoff. Avoid touching the wound with the basin.
   Prevents contamination of wound from the emesis basin; protects linens from runoff.
6. **Using a 19-gauge angiocatheter,** remove the metal stylet needle and dispose into a sharps container. Attach the angiocatheter to a 35-mL syringe and fill with normal saline irrigation solution. Commercial irrigation kits containing a piston tip syringe may also be used. Their use is discussed in Procedure 35-2.
   Prevents contamination and needlestick injury. A 19-gauge angiocatheter with a 35-mL syringe provides 8 psi (pounds per square inch) of pressure and is effective for removing bacteria, necrotic tissue, exudate, and/or metabolic wastes.

7. **Holding the angiocatheter** tip 2 cm from the wound bed, gently irrigate the wound with a back-and-forth motion, moving from the superior aspect to the inferior aspect (or from clean to dirty).
Irrigating from top to bottom prevents flow of contaminated solution over the cleansed area.

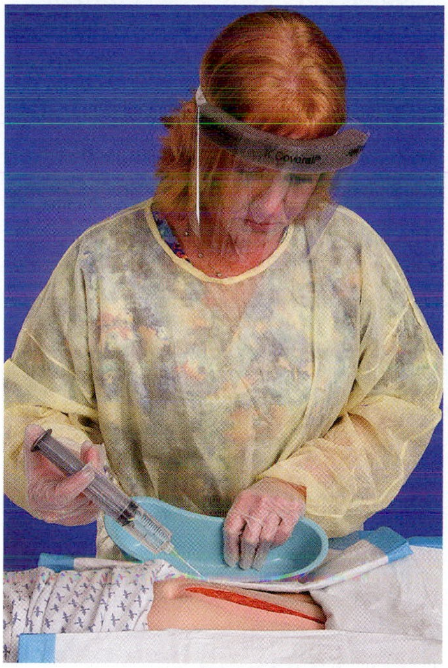

8. **Dispose of the syringe** and angiocatheter in the sharp disposal container, and gloves in the biohazardous waste receptacle.
Prevents contamination and needle-stick injury.

9. **Obtain an aerobic culturette tube** with calcium alginate or rayon swab (not cotton tip); twist the top of the tube to loosen the swab.
Swab specimens are not suitable for anaerobic culture. Culture for anaerobic organisms may be obtained in tissue biopsy or needle aspiration specimens only.

10. **Don clean nonsterile gloves**, and locate an area of red, granulating tissue in the wound bed.

Using Levine Technique

a. Withdraw the swab from the culturette tube. Press the swab against the granulating area with sufficient pressure to express fluid from the wound tissue, and rotate the swab using a rolling motion.
Fluid from deeper within the wound bed is more indicative of the microbial colonization than culturing surface of a wound.

Using Z-Stroke Technique

b. Swab the wound from margin to margin in a 10-point zigzag pattern, avoiding contact with the wound edge.
Provides a sampling in different areas of the wound bed.

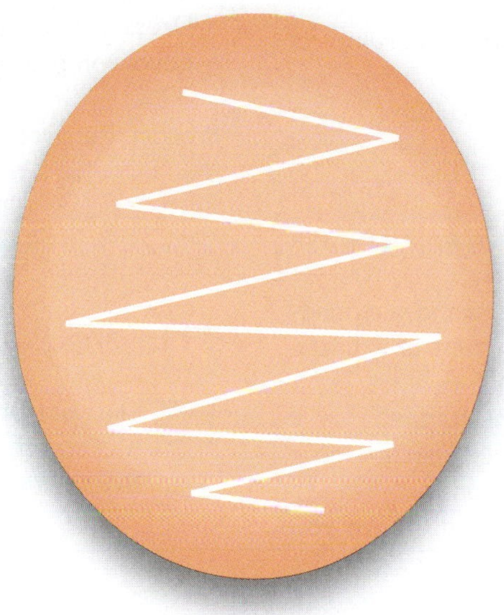

For Both Technique Variations

c. Do not allow the swab to touch anything other than the granulating area of the wound. Avoid wound edges.

d. Do not swab culture areas where slough or eschar is present.
These are areas of avascular or necrotic tissue and are contaminated with bacteria. Swab cultures detect only surface bacteria and are not a reliable means for diagnosing wound infection.

e. Do not roll the swab around in a pool of exudative material.
Pus is a collection of white blood cells that have already done their work; includes the microorganisms that have already died. Obtaining a culture from this material would not produce reliable culture result. The culture specimen must be of "tissue" or "tissue fluid," not surface fluid or exudate.

f. Do not swab multiple sites with the same culturette. Use more than one culturette if several areas need to be cultured.

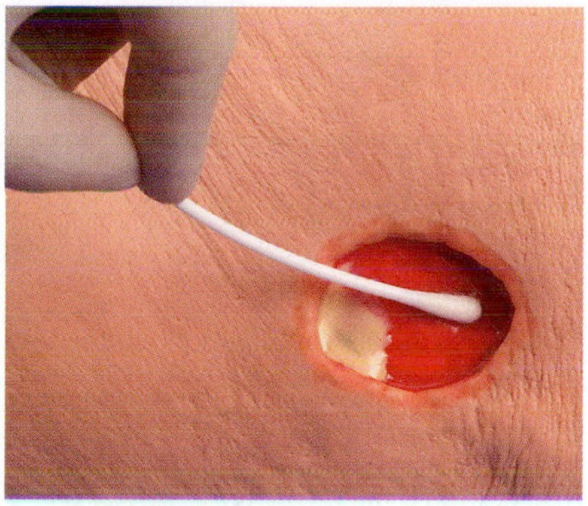

11. **Carefully insert the swab** back into the aerobic culturette tube, making sure it does not make contact with the opening of the tube on reinsertion. Twist the cap to secure the tube.
Decreases risk of contamination; ensures that any microorganisms that grow in the culture are from the wound and were not introduced from the environment.

12. **Crush the ampule** of culture medium at the bottom of the tube. (*NOTE: Inspect the culture tube to determine whether this step is required. In some systems it is not.*)
The ampule contains medium for growth of microorganisms.

13. **Label the culturette tube** with the patient's name, patient identifier, birthdate, source of specimen, and date and time of collection.
Labeling ensures obtaining the results for the correct patient.

(continued on next page)

Procedure 35-1 ■ Obtaining a Wound Culture by Swab (continued)

14. Apply a clean dressing to the wound, as needed.

15. Arrange for transport of the specimen for culture to the lab immediately. Do not refrigerate the specimen.

? What if . . .

- **You determined this wound requires sterile technique?**

  After removal of soiled dressing, apply sterile gloves for irrigating, obtaining culture, and applying new sterile dressing.

  Sterile technique is used for acute surgical wounds and for wounds that have undergone recent, sharp débridement, or when the healthcare provider prescribes it.

- **The culture tube is not sent to the lab within 72 hours?**

  If the culture swab is not sent to the lab within 48 to 72 hours, it must be discarded. Be sure to check the policy within your institution.

  The swab culture needs to be exposed to ideal laboratory conditions to allow microbial growth. If the culture sits on the unit too long, the culture medium might not produce reliable results. Most swab transport systems are validated for 48 to 72 hours after collection. However, if bacteria are suspected, the quicker the specimen is sent to the lab, the better.

- **The wound care and culture supplies are kept on a common treatment cart?**

  Common treatment carts should be left in the hall and not taken into individual rooms.

  When a mobile cart is rolled into a room, it is a source for possible cross-contamination.

Evaluation

- Assess the patient's pain level. Medicate according to prescriptions.
- Monitor lab reports for results of the swab culture.

Documentation

Document the following information (some agencies use a wound/skin flowsheet):

- Appearance, size, and location of the wound and surrounding tissue. Note type, consistency, and amount of exudate, as well as odor, if present, after irrigation.
- Patient's pain level before you obtained the culture
- If the patient was medicated for pain, document the drug and dose used, time given, and patient response.
- Method by which the wound was cleansed before you obtained the swab culture
- Description of the area where the culture was obtained
- Dressing reapplied to wound, if applicable
- Education provided to the patient

Practice Resources

Association for the Advancement of Wound Care (AAWC) (2014); Baranoski, S., & Ayello, E. (2015); Benbow, M. (2010); Bonham, P.A. (2012); Levine, N. S., Lindberg, R. B., Mason, A. D., et al. (1976); McCulloch, J. M., & Kloth, L. C. (2010); Non, L. R., (2012, updated); Rushing, J. (2007).

Thinking About the Procedure

The video **Obtaining a Wound Culture by Swab,** along with questions and suggested responses, is available on the ***Davis's Nursing Skills Videos*** Web site on FADavis.com.

Procedure 35-2 ■ Performing a Sterile Wound Irrigation

➤ For steps to follow in *all* procedures, refer to the Universal Steps for All Procedures found on the page facing the inside back cover.

Equipment

- Nonsterile gloves
- Sterile gloves
- Gown and face shield
- Water-resistant, disposable drapes
- Tepid (body temperature) irrigation solution

  Cold solution lowers temperature of wound bed and slows the healing process.
- Sterile gauze
- Dressing supplies
- Biohazardous waste container
- Sterile impermeable barrier
- Sterile bowl

When Using an Angiocatheter (Step 10A)

- Sterile emesis basin
- 35-mL syringe
- 19-gauge angiocatheter (needle removed)
- Skin protectant

When Using a Piston-Tip Syringe (Step 10B)

- Sterile commercial irrigation kit containing a sterile basin and piston-tip syringe

Delegation

This is an invasive, sterile procedure that requires nursing assessment, judgment, evaluation, and teaching during the procedure. It requires knowledge of wound healing and should be performed by a registered nurse. Do not delegate this skill to UAP.

Pre-Procedure Assessments

NOTE: If the wound is covered when you begin, you will make these assessments when you remove the soiled dressing and after cleansing the wound.

- Assess the amount and type of tissue present in the wound bed.
  Granulating tissue is beefy red with a velvety appearance. It appears with the growth of new blood vessels and connective tissue. Pale pink tissue may indicate a delay in wound healing due to compromised blood supply to the wound bed or lack of proper nutrition. Necrotic tissue, which is black, brown, or yellow in appearance, is nonviable and inhibits healing and is a source of bacterial growth.
- Determine whether the wound requires sterile, modified sterile, or clean technique for irrigation.
  Irrigation helps wounds to heal because it removes bacteria, old drainage, and necrotic tissue from the wound bed. Sterile technique is used for acute surgical wounds, for wounds that have undergone recent sharp débridement, or when the healthcare provider has ordered it. Chronic wounds are colonized with bacteria and may be irrigated with clean technique. Irrigation using clean technique is presented in Steps 1 through 8 of Procedure 35-1.
- Identify any allergies to irrigation solutions or medications.
- Assess the wound for signs of infection (erythema, induration, amount and type of drainage).
  Exudate may be a sign of infection. Infected wounds require higher flow pressures for irrigation.
- Assess the wound for odor.
  A foul odor may indicate infection. Cleanse wounds before you assess for odor, because some dressings interact with wound drainage to produce an odor.
- Assess the tissue surrounding the wound edge.
  Surrounding tissue that is red, warm, and/or edematous may indicate infection. Tissue that is macerated (white and moist) indicates too much fluid is being held against the skin, usually from saturated dressings.
- Assess for pain and the need to premedicate.
  Wound irrigation may be very painful.

➤ When performing the procedure, always identify your patient according to agency policy, using two identifiers, and be attentive to standard precautions, hand hygiene, patient safety and privacy, body mechanics, and documentation.

Procedure Steps

1. **Administer pain medication** 30 minutes before the treatment, if necessary.

2. **Place the patient in a** comfortable position that provides easy access to the wound and will allow the irrigation solution to flow freely from the wound, with the assistance of gravity. Position a water-resistant disposable drape to protect the bedding from any possible runoff.

3. **After performing hand hygiene,** apply a gown, face shield, and clean, nonsterile gloves.
   Personal protective equipment (PPE) provides a barrier against splattering that commonly occurs during wound irrigation.

4. **Remove the soiled dressing.** Dispose of gloves and soiled dressing in a biohazard bag.
   Soiled dressings contain body fluids and other contaminants and should be treated as biohazardous waste.

5. **Set up a sterile field** on a clean, dry surface. Add the following supplies to the field:
   Sterile gauze
   Sterile bowl
   Dressing supplies
   A sterile commercial irrigation kit, *or* a 19-gauge angiocatheter, 35-mL syringe, and sterile emesis basin
   Setting up a sterile field at bedside provides easy access to equipment for irrigation and reduces the risk for contamination when retrieving supplies after getting started.

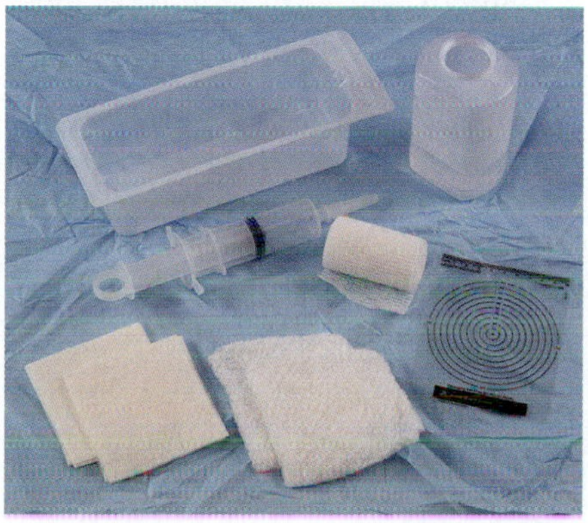

6. **Select irrigation solution** based on the wound assessment and goals of therapy. Sterile saline or sterile water is the solution of choice for irrigation, although commercial cleansers may be used for irrigation for wounds with debris or in dirty, necrotic wounds.

   Do not use povidone-iodine (Betadine) if the patient has an iodine allergy.
   Cleansers contain surfactant (soap-like substance) that removes bacteria and cellular debris with less force and slow growth of bacteria, molds, and fungi. However, some antiseptic solutions can be harmful to healing tissues (e.g., hydrogen peroxide, acetic acid, povidone-iodine, bleach solutions, and sodium hypochlorite solutions [Dakin's solution]).

7. **Pour the tepid (room temperature) irrigation solution** into the sterile bowl.
   Local cooling of wound tissues impairs healing. This can occur if you irrigate with refrigerated solutions and change dressings frequently.

(continued on next page)

Procedure 35-2 ■ Performing a Sterile Wound Irrigation (continued)

8. **Don sterile gloves.**
Gloving maintains sterile technique.

9. **Place the sterile basin** at the bottom of the wound to collect irrigation runoff.

10. **Fill the irrigation syringe.**

If Using an Angiocatheter

a. Attach the 19-gauge angiocatheter (with needle removed) to the 35-mL syringe; fill with the irrigation solution.
A 19-gauge angiocatheter (with needle removed) and 35-mL syringe provide 8 psi of pressure and are effective for removing bacteria, necrotic tissue, exudate, and/or metabolic wastes.

If Using a Piston-Tip Syringe

b. Fill a piston-tip syringe with irrigation solution.

11. **Gently irrigate the wound.** Hold the angiocatheter tip or syringe tip 2 cm above the wound bed and use a back-and-forth motion, moving from the clean to dirty areas of the wound.
Irrigating from clean to dirty prevents flow of contaminated solution over cleansed area. Irrigating a clean, noninfected wound with gentle low pressure (8 psi) reduces disruption of the healthy, healing tissue. Irrigating an infected wound with higher flow (but <15 psi) selectively débrides necrotic tissue while protecting healthy tissue.

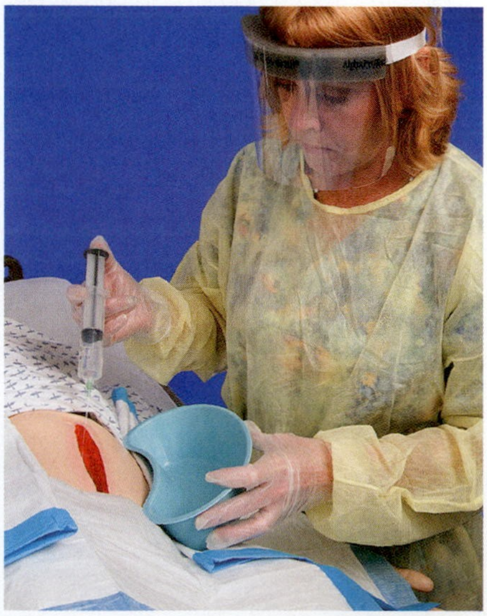

a. Ensure any undermining or tunneling is irrigated as well.
b. Repeat the irrigation until the solution returns clear.
Flushing removes exudate, debris, and some surface bacteria.

12. **Remove the basin** or sterile container from the base of the wound.

13. **Gently pat the skin surrounding** the wound dry with sterile gauze, beginning at the top of the wound and working downward.
Moisture on the surrounding tissue may lead to maceration and further breakdown of the wound margins.

14. **Dress the wound as prescribed.**

15. **Consider applying a** waterproof skin protectant around the wound if drainage is heavy.
Wound drainage contains irritating chemicals that can damage healthy tissues, especially at the wound edge and surrounding skin. Solutions used to keep the wound bed moist can also macerate or damage healthy skin if allowed to remain on intact skin.

16. **Dispose of the contaminated** irrigation fluid in a biohazardous waste receptacle.
Contaminated fluid is biohazardous waste.

17. **Remove soiled drapes** from the patient area.

18. **Remove your gloves, face shield,** and gown. Dispose of these items appropriately.
Contaminants from the irrigation may be present on these items, and they should also be considered biohazardous.

19. **Reposition the patient** to a comfortable position. Change any linen that may have become wet during the procedure.

20. **Perform hand hygiene.**
Hand hygiene prevents cross-contamination.

? What if . . .

- **Your client has a wound covering a large area of the body?**
A general rule is that the larger the wound, the more solution needed to clean it.
The purpose of cleansing a wound is to remove bacteria and debris by flushing the wound.

- **Peroxide or another antiseptic solution is prescribed?**
First, identify the reason that the solution was ordered for the wound type. Then identify the length of time it is to be used. Weigh the benefit of using the solution with the potential risks to healing tissues. Finally, discuss any concerns with the healthcare provider.
Peroxide is indicated more for acute, traumatic wounds to remove dirt and other debris. Peroxide and other commercial antiseptics can damage fibroblasts and cause air embolism if used to forcefully irrigate or pack a tunneling wound. Fibroblasts produce collagen, the major structural protein of skin and healing tissues.

Evaluation

- Determine whether the patient remains comfortable. If not, medicate according to prescriptions.
- Reassess the wound at regular intervals.

Patient Teaching

- Answer any questions the patient may have.
- Teach the patient about the expected healing process.
- Inform the patient and caregiver about signs and symptoms of infection and the need to report these findings.

Home Care

- Wound irrigation is commonly done in the home. In most cases, clean technique is used in the home setting.
- Irrigation solutions, such as saline, can be made and stored up to 7 days if refrigerated.
- Review with the family proper disposal of contaminated supplies.

Documentation

Document the following information (many agencies use a wound/skin flowsheet):

- Method by which the wound was cleansed, including amount and type of irrigant
- Appearance and location of the wound, size, tissue in wound base, periwound tissue, type and amount of exudate, and odor, if present, after irrigation. A photograph is an accurate method for documenting the condition of a wound.
- The patient's pain level. If the patient was medicated for pain, document the drug and dose used, time given, and patient response.
- Dressing reapplied to the wound, if applicable
- Education provided to the patient

Sample documentation

04/22/2021 0800 Dressing change to sacral wound using modified sterile technique due to saturation of old dressing with serious drainage. Patient premedicated with Lortab 5 mg PO 30 minutes prior to dressing change. Wound irrigated with normal saline using 19-gauge needleless angiocatheter and 35-cc syringe. Wound repacked with saline-moistened fluffed gauze and ABD to cover. Healing stage 4 pressure injury with 100% granulation tissue to the wound bed; 4 × 3.5 cm, with 1 cm of undermining at 6:00; copious serous drainage though no odor was noted. Periwound is slightly macerated; therefore, zinc-based barrier cream applied for protection. Patient reported no pain with procedure. Will continue to monitor and change dressing as needed. ———————————— L. Syzmanski, RN

Practice Resources

Fernandez, R., & Griffiths, R. (2008, updated 2012); ICSI (2012); Gabriel & Schraga, 2017; Myers, B. A. (2011); Wilkins, R. G., & Unverdorben, M. (2013); Wound, Ostomy and Continence Nurses Society (WOCNS) (2010, revised 2016).

Procedure 35-3 ■ Taping a Dressing

➤ For steps to follow in *all* procedures, refer to the Universal Steps for All Procedures found on the page facing the inside back cover.

Equipment

- Nonsterile gloves
- Tape (cloth, plastic, foam, silk-like, etc.)

Delegation

As a nurse, you are responsible for assessing the wound and evaluating interventions. However, this procedure may be delegated to UAP.

Pre-Procedure Assessments

- Assess the degree of importance of the dressing.
  The more critical the dressing, the more adhesion required.
- Assess the characteristics of the dressing material, weight and conformability, and the device or tubing to be held.
  Heavier dressings require higher adhesion. Bulky dressings may need high conformability or greater adhesion.
- Assess the skin surface (i.e., dry, damp, diaphoretic, oily, hairy, edematous, fragile, or impaired skin integrity).
  Fragile skin may require less adhesion while damp or oily skin may require higher adhesion.
- Assess the anticipated wear time.
  Tape adhesion gets stronger over time. Breathable tapes can be used longer. Occlusive plastic tapes build up moisture and are used when adhesion is intended for a shorter period.
- Assess the patient's history and current medical conditions.
  Review allergies or sensitivities to tapes. Review medical conditions that may be affected by adhesives.
- Assess for activity level of the patient and the anticipated length of time the dressing will be needed.
  The more active the patient is, the more adhesion will be required.

(continued on next page)

Procedure 35-3 ■ Taping a Dressing (continued)

➤ When performing the procedure, always identify your patient according to agency policy, using two identifiers, and be attentive to standard precautions, hand hygiene, patient safety and privacy, body mechanics, and documentation.

Procedure Steps

1. **Perform hand hygiene. Don gloves.**
2. **Choose the type of tape** based on wound size, location, amount of drainage or edema, frequency of dressing changes, patient's activity level, and type of dressings used.
   Tapes come in many different adhesive types and backings. Select the tape based on individual characteristics.
   a. Choose tape of the width that is appropriate for the dressing. The larger the dressing, the wider the tape needed for securing.
   For example, a large abdominal dressing may require 3-inch tape, whereas a small incision on an extremity may need only ½-inch tape.
   b. Choose a tape that stretches if the area is at risk for distention, edema, hematoma formation, or movement.
   Skin distention under tape may cause blistering or skin tears.
3. **Tear strips that extend** ½ to 1½ inches beyond the dressing, depending on the size of the dressing.
   To anchor the dressing to the skin.
4. **Place the tape perpendicular** to the incision.
   Fewer skin tension injuries occur with perpendicular taping.
   a. When taping over joints, apply the tape at a right angle to the direction of joint movement, or at a right angle to a body crease. For example, tape a shoulder or knee horizontally, not lengthwise.
   b. Apply tape with an even amount tension on both sides, being careful not to pull at the edges.
   Reduces the risk of skin damage.
5. **Smooth tape in place** with your fingertips.
   To maximize the tape's adhesion to the skin surface.
6. **Replace tape if site becomes** edematous, or the skin is not intact. ▼

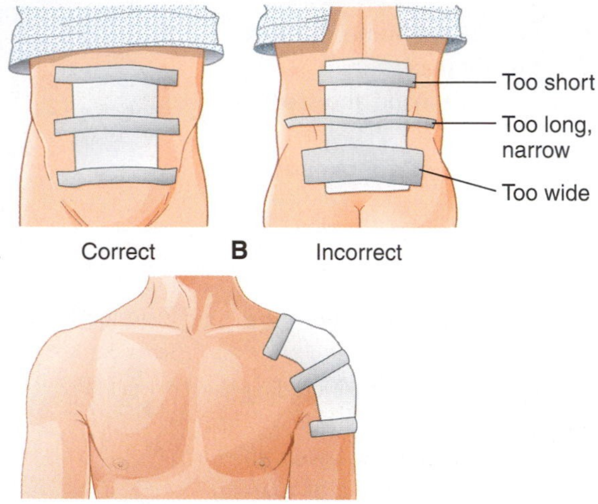

A Correct B Incorrect

C Correct

? What if . . .

■ **The tape will not adhere to the patient's skin because of excess hair?**

Remove the hair with clippers or scissors. Do not shave the site with a razor.
Shaving can cause nicks or abrasions to the skin that could become a portal of entry for bacteria.

■ **Your patient's skin is diaphoretic or excessively oily?**

Cleanse the skin with soap and water before the dressing change. Allow the skin to dry before applying the dressing and tape. You may also use polymer skin barriers to place a seal over the skin and allow the tape adhesive to adhere.

■ **Your patient has fragile skin (e.g., is an older adult)?**

Use skin sealant preparations under adhesives. Use the least adhesive product possible.
The junction between the epidermis and dermis on the older adult is not as strong as it is in a younger person.

■ **Your patient is allergic to tape adhesives?**

Use hypoallergenic products.
Circular wraps, ace bandages, or other such products may be used to secure dressings.

Evaluation

- Verify type of tape that is appropriate for the patient and dressing.
- Note whether the tape adheres comfortably to the skin.
- Ensure that the patient verbalized understanding of the treatment.
- Inspect the dressing daily for intactness, edema, or hematoma.

Patient Teaching

- Teach the patient about the expected healing process.
- Educate the patient about the purpose of the procedure.
- Instruct the patient to keep the dressing dry.

Documentation

Document the following information (many agencies use a wound/skin flowsheet):

- Type of dressing and tape applied
- Location and characteristics of wound
- Education given to patient

Sample documentation

2/16/21 0800 Dressing applied to left hip incision using conformable cloth tape. Wound edges are well approximated with no drainage noted. Periwound skin is dry and intact without erythema, induration, or odor. Wound cleaned with normal saline using sterile technique. Educated patient about the purpose of the dressing and expected course for wound healing. Will continue to monitor ——————— B. Hopkins, RN

Procedure 35-4 ■ Removing and Applying Dry Dressings

➤ For steps to follow in *all* procedures, refer to the Universal Steps for All Procedures found on the page facing the inside back cover.

➤ *Note:* This procedure uses clean technique because wound care is now usually performed using clean rather than sterile technique.

Equipment

- Three pairs of clean nonsterile gloves
- Normal saline solution for irrigation, warmed to body temperature when possible
  Cold solution lowers the temperature of wound bed and slows the healing process.
- Tray of sterile 4 in. × 4 in. gauze.
- Sterile gauze for dressings
- Tape
- Adhesive removal pads

Delegation

This procedure requires knowledge of wound healing. It should be performed by a registered nurse. Do not delegate this skill.

Pre-Procedure Assessments

NOTE: When you begin, the wound will likely be covered with a dressing. You will make these assessments when you remove the soiled dressing and after cleansing the wound.

- Assess for pain at least 30 minutes before performing the procedure.
  Wounds may be very painful. Provide pain medication 30 minutes before performing the procedure if needed, to allow the medication time to be distributed in target tissues. Changes in the quality or severity of pain are some symptoms linked with infection.
- Assess the type and amount of exudate.
  Exudate may be a sign of infection.
- Assess the wound for odor.
  A foul odor may indicate infection. Clean wounds before you assess for odor, because some dressings interact with wound drainage to produce an odor.
- Assess the tissue surrounding the wound edge.
  Surrounding tissue that is red, warm, and/or edematous may indicate infection.
- Determine the type of dressing needed.
  The type of dressing depends on the characteristics of the wound and the goal of treatment. Dry dressings are appropriate when there is no need to keep the wound bed moist, such as a wound healing by primary intention or a wound covered by eschar. Removing a dry dressing can also interfere with wound healing by disrupting granulation tissue and can cause pain to the patient.

➤ When performing the procedure, always identify your patient according to agency policy, using two identifiers, and be attentive to standard precautions, hand hygiene, patient safety and privacy, body mechanics, and documentation.

(continued on next page)

Procedure 35-4 ■ Removing and Applying Dry Dressings (continued)

Procedure Steps for Removing the Dressing

1. **Place the patient in a** comfortable position that provides easy access to the wound.
   Provides for patient comfort and proper nurse body mechanics during dressing change.

2. **Perform hand hygiene,** and don nonsterile gloves.
   Handwashing is one of the most important measures for preventing infection transmission.

3. **Gently loosen the edges of the tape** of the old dressing at an angle parallel to the skin.
   a. Hold that edge with one hand and gently raise the edge until it is taut but not pulling on the skin.
   b. Using your other hand, push down on the exposed skin at the point where the tape and skin meet. Push the skin off of the tape. Adhesive remover pads are advised to help prevent tearing of fragile skin.
   The pull–push method will help prevent skin stripping from the adhesive and reduce discomfort and skin trauma as you remove the tape.

4. **Beginning at the edges** of the dressing, lift the dressing toward the center of the wound. If the dressing sticks, moisten it with normal saline before removing it completely.
   Moistening the dressing decreases the risk of bleeding and/or removal of granulating tissue.

5. **Assess the type and amount** of drainage on the soiled dressing.
   Allows for evaluation of wound healing. Purulent drainage is an indication of infection.

6. **Dispose of the soiled** dressing and gloves in a biohazard receptacle.
   Soiled dressings contain bodily fluids and other contaminants and should be disposed of as biohazardous waste.

7. **Remove the cover of a tray** of sterile 4 in. × 4 in. gauze. Moisten the gauze with sterile saline.
   The sterile container tray is impermeable and allows you to moisten the gauze while maintaining sterility. Gauze will not shed fibers into the wound (as do cotton balls). Fibers and any other foreign bodies in a wound promote inflammation and delay healing.

8. **Don clean nonsterile gloves.**

9. **Gather a gauze pad** by pulling the four corners up toward the middle. Use the center ball of the gauze to cleanse the wound.
   Forming a ball with the gauze pads prevents contamination of gloved hands during cleansing.

10. **Gently cleanse the wound** with the saline-moistened gauze by lightly wiping a section of the wound from the center toward the wound edge (work from clean to dirty). Discard the gauze in a biohazard receptacle; repeat in the next section using a new piece of gauze with each wiping pass.
    Removes surface bacteria and exudate.

11. **Discard the gloves** and soiled gauze into a biohazard bag.

12. **Reassess wound** for size, color of tissue present, amount and type of exudate, and odor.

Procedure Steps for Applying Dry Dressing

13. **Perform hand hygiene**; use an antiseptic hand rub at the bedside.

14. **Open sterile gauze packages** on a clean, dry surface.
    Maintains sterility of gauze.

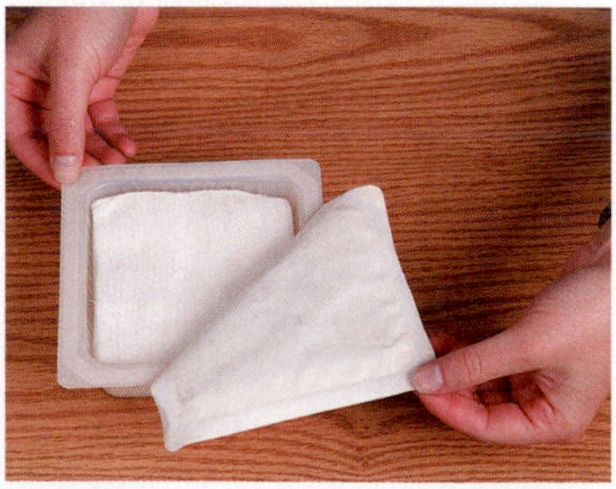

15. **Don clean nonsterile gloves.**

16. **Apply a layer of dry dressings** over the wound. If drainage is expected, use an additional layer of dressings.
    The first layer serves as a wick for drainage. A second layer is needed if increased absorption is required.

17. **Place strips of tape at the ends** of the dressing and evenly spaced over the remainder of the dressing. Use strips that are sufficiently long to secure the dressing in place. Tape the dressing around all edges, "windowpaning," if appropriate.
    Edges remain taped down and dressing stays intact.

18. **Remove gloves**; discard them in a biohazard receptacle.

19. **Assist the patient** to a comfortable position.

? What if . . .

- **Signs of infection are noted with wound assessment?**
  Notify the healthcare provider. Cultures, wound care interventions, and potentially even antibiotics may be required.
- **The wound is not approximated?**
  Place the patient in a supine position, apply adhesive skin closures, and cover with sterile saline dressings. Notify primary healthcare provider.
  This could indicate wound dehiscence.
- **The skin surrounding the incision is not intact?**
  Clean the area with sterile saline, dry thoroughly, and apply protective moisture barrier dressing. Consider using Montgomery straps.
  Montgomery straps are useful when dressings must be changed frequently because they do not cause trauma to the skin.
- **A drain or drainage tube is present?**
  Always clean the drain site after cleaning the primary incision site.
  Reduces the risk of cross-contamination.

Evaluation

- Determine whether the dressing is clean, dry, and intact.
- Verify that the patient experienced minimal discomfort during the procedure.

Patient Teaching

- Teach the patient about the expected healing process.
- Inform the patient and caregiver about the signs and symptoms of infection and the need to report these findings.

Home Care

- Help the client to store dressings appropriately to keep them clean, for example, in a plastic container with a lid.
- Teach the client or caregivers to dispose of contaminated dressings and gloves by double-bagging them in moisture-proof bags (e.g., plastic grocery bags).
- Advise the client and family whether they can get the wound wet (e.g., during bathing). If it must be kept dry, demonstrate how to cover it with a waterproof barrier (e.g., a plastic bag).

Documentation

Document the following information (many agencies use a wound/skin flowsheet):

- Appearance, size, and location of the wound, type and amount of exudate, and odor, if present, after cleansing
- The patient's pain level before the procedure. If the patient was medicated for pain, document the drug and dose used, time given, and patient response.
- Method of cleansing the wound
- Type of dressing applied to the wound
- Education provided to the patient

Sample documentation

10/22/22 1420 Pt with no report of pain. Gauze dressing removed from lateral aspect of right forearm without difficulty. No drainage noted on gauze. Surrounding skin intact. Abrasion on right, lateral forearm cleansed with normal saline. Sterile gauze dressing reapplied to wound and anchored with cloth tape. Pt instructed to report any change at wound site, such as bleeding, drainage, or increase in pain ——— D. Enferma, RN

Practice Resources

Armstrong, D. G., & Meyer, A. J. (2013, updated 2018, August 20).

Thinking About the Procedure

The video **Removing and Applying Dry Dressings,** along with questions and suggested responses, is available on the ***Davis's Nursing Skills Videos*** Web site on FADavis.com.

Procedure 35-5 ■ Removing and Applying Wet-to-Damp Dressings

➤ For steps to follow in *all* procedures, refer to the Universal Steps for All Procedures found on the page facing the inside back cover.

➤ *Note:* This procedure uses clean technique because wound care is now usually done using a clean or modified sterile approach rather than sterile technique. However, sterile technique is recommended for wounds that have recently had sharp débridement, have a drain, or are fresh surgical wounds. Sterile technique might also be used for patients with immunodeficiency.

Equipment

- Three pairs of clean nonsterile gloves
- Sterile or clean solution, typically saline or distilled water (in the hospital setting), warmed to body temperature when possible.
  Cold solution reduces the temperature of the wound bed and slows the healing process.
- Water-resistant disposable drapes
- Sterile fine-mesh gauze in a tray for dressing
- Surgipad
- Tape or Montgomery straps
- Adhesive removal pads

Delegation

This is an invasive procedure that requires knowledge of wound healing. It should be performed by a registered nurse. Do not delegate this skill to UAP.

Pre-Procedure Assessments

NOTE: When you begin, the wound will likely be covered with a dressing. You will make these assessments when you remove the soiled dressing and after cleansing the wound.

- Assess the amount and type of tissue present in the wound bed.

(continued on next page)

Procedure 35-5 ■ Removing and Applying Wet-to-Damp Dressings (continued)

Granulating tissue is beefy red with a velvety appearance. It appears with the growth of new blood vessels and connective tissue. Pale pink tissue may indicate compromised blood supply to the wound bed. Necrotic tissue, which is black, brown, or yellow in appearance, is nonviable and inhibits healing.

- Assess the type and amount of exudate.
  Exudate may be a sign of infection.
- Assess the wound for odor.
  A foul odor may indicate infection. Clean wounds before you assess for odor, because some dressings interact with wound drainage to produce an odor.
- Assess the tissue surrounding the wound edge.
  Surrounding tissue that is red, warm, and/or edematous may indicate infection.
- Assess for pain.
  Wounds may be very painful. Assess for pain and provide prescribed pain medication 30 minutes before performing procedure, if needed. A change in the quality or intensity of pain may be a sign of infection.

➤ When performing the procedure, always identify your patient according to agency policy, using two identifiers, and be attentive to standard precautions, hand hygiene, patient safety and privacy, body mechanics, and documentation.

Procedure Steps for Removing the Wet-to-Damp Dressing

1. **Place the patient** in a comfortable position that provides easy access to the wound.
   Provides for patient comfort during dressing change.
2. **Perform hand hygiene,** and don clean nonsterile gloves.
   Handwashing complies with standard precautions, helping to prevent transfer of pathogens.
3. **Gently loosen the edges** of the tape of the old dressing. Hold that edge with one hand and gently raise the edge until it is taut but not pulling on the skin. Using your other hand, push down on the exposed skin at the point where the tape and skin meet. Push the skin off of the tape. Use adhesive remover pads to avoid tearing fragile skin.
   The pull–push method will help prevent skin stripping from the adhesive and reduce discomfort and skin trauma as you remove the tape.
4. **Beginning with the top layer,** lift the dressing from the corner toward the center of the wound. If the dressing sticks, moisten it with normal saline or bacteriostatic water before completely removing it. Remove first from one side of the wound, first toward the wound, and then from the other side. Continue to remove layers until you have removed the entire dressing.
   Moistening the dressing decreases the risk of bleeding and/or removal of granulating tissue. ▼

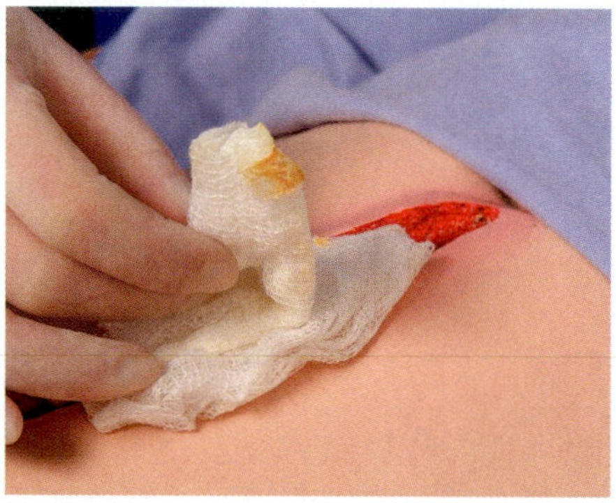

5. **Assess the type and amount** of drainage present on the soiled dressing.
   Type of drainage is an indication of the stage of healing. Purulent drainage is an indication of infection.
6. **Dispose of the soiled dressing** and gloves in a biohazard container. Wash your hands.
   Soiled dressings contain body fluid contaminants and should be disposed of as biohazardous waste.
7. **Remove the cover of a tray** of sterile 4 in. × 4 in. gauze. Moisten the gauze with sterile saline or water.
   The sterile container tray is impermeable and allows you to moisten the gauze while maintaining sterility. Gauze will not shed fibers into the wound (as do cotton balls). Fibers and any other foreign bodies in a wound promote inflammation and delay healing.
8. **Don clean procedure gloves.**
   Avoids introducing microorganisms into the wound.
9. **Gather a gauze pad** by pulling the four corners up toward the middle. Use the center of the gauze to cleanse the wound.
   Prevents contamination of your gloves during wound cleansing.
10. **Using gauze moistened** with saline or potable water, gently wipe a section of the wound from the center toward the wound edge. Discard the gauze in a biohazard receptacle; repeat in the next section using a new piece of gauze with each wiping pass.
    Removes surface bacteria and exudate. Prevents transfer of microorganisms from the skin to the wound.
11. **Reassess the wound** for location, amount of tissue present, exudate, and odor.
    Allows for determination of most effective treatment and type of dressing.
12. **Discard the gloves** and soiled gauze into a biohazard bag. Perform hand hygiene.
    Soiled gauze contains contaminants and should be disposed of as biohazardous waste.

Procedure Steps for Applying a Wet-to-Damp Dressing

13. **After establishing a sterile** field using a sterile impermeable barrier, open a sterile gauze pack tray and a surgipad. The amount of gauze you use depends on the size of the wound.
    Maintains sterile field and supplies.

14. **Moisten sterile gauze** with saline solution or potable water for irrigation.

15. **Don clean nonsterile** gloves.

16. **Squeeze out excess moisture** from the gauze.
    a. Apply a single layer of moist, fine-mesh gauze to the wound.
    b. Be sure to place gauze in all depressions or crevices of the wound. You may need to use forceps or a cotton applicator to ensure that you fill deep depressions or sinus tracts with gauze.
    c. "Fluff" the mesh gauze before placing in the wound so as it dries it acts as a wick for any drainage.
    Maintains a moist environment for the wound bed.

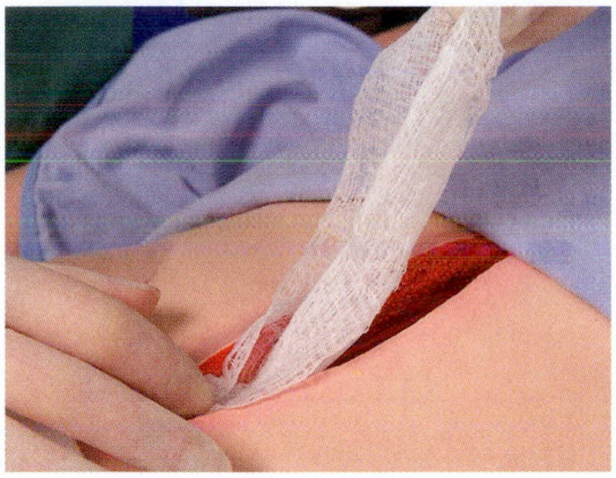

17. **Apply a secondary moist layer** over the first layer. Repeat this process until the wound is completely filled with moistened sterile gauze—but do not tightly *pack* the gauze into the wound. Do not extend the moist dressing onto the surrounding skin.
    Packing the gauze tightly can restrict blood flow to the area. Moist dressings on the surrounding skin can cause maceration.

18. **Cover the moistened gauze** with a surgipad.
    Protects the wound from external contaminants.

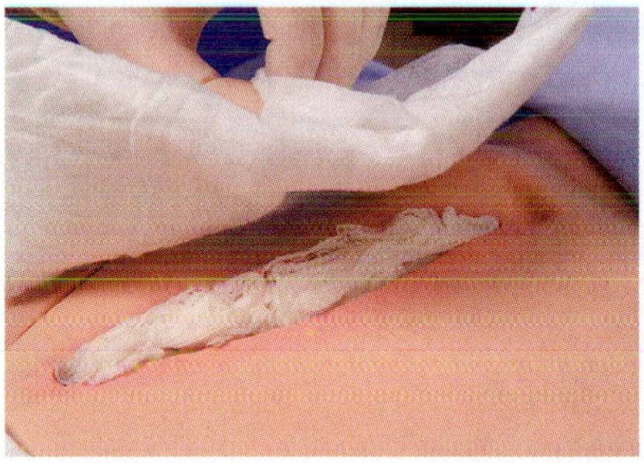

19. **Secure the dressing** with tape or Montgomery straps.
    Montgomery straps are useful when dressings must be frequently changed because they do not cause trauma to the skin.

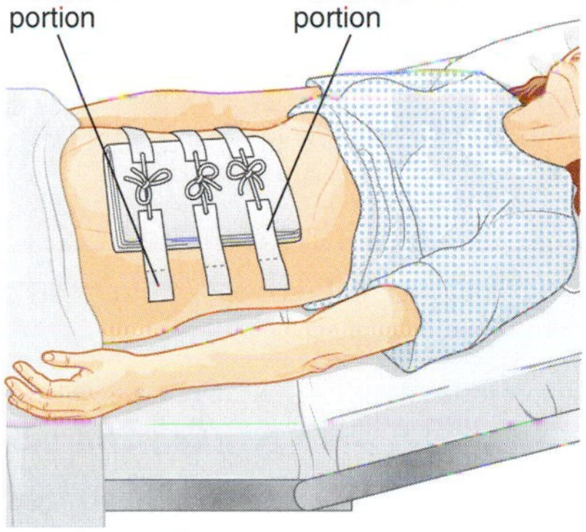

Montgomery straps

20. **Dispose of gloves** and materials in the biohazard waste receptacle. Perform hand hygiene and date and time the dressing.

21. **Assist the patient** to a comfortable position.

? What if . . .

- **Gauze becomes dry between dressing changes?**
  Moisten dressings with sterile saline before removing them; change dressing more frequently; consider using a semiocclusive dressing.
  A moistened dressing prevents débridement of granulating tissue, maintains a moist environment, and prevents tissue injury. Dressings that become too dry will injure healthy tissue and impair healing.
- **Your patient has multiple wounds?**
  The most infected wound should be treated last. Remember to always change your gloves in between wound dressing changes.
  The risk of cross-contamination is reduced when moving from clean to dirty and with fresh gloves.

Evaluation

- Evaluate whether the patient experiences pain with the procedure and afterward.
- Note whether the patient verbalizes understanding of the procedure.

Patient Teaching

- Teach the patient about the expected healing process.
- Inform the patient and caregiver about signs and symptoms of infection and the need to report these findings.

Home Care

- Help the client store dressings appropriately to keep them clean, for example, in a plastic container with a lid.
- Teach the client or caregivers to dispose of contaminated dressings and gloves by double-bagging them in moisture-proof bags (e.g., plastic grocery bags).
- Advise the client and family whether they can get the wound wet (e.g., during bathing). If it must be kept dry, demonstrate how to cover it with a waterproof barrier (e.g., a plastic bag).

(continued on next page)

Procedure 35-5 ■ Removing and Applying Wet-to-Damp Dressings (continued)

Documentation

Document the following information (many agencies use a wound/skin flowsheet):

- Appearance, size, color and location of the wound, type and amount of exudate, and odor, if present after cleansing
- The patient's pain level before and after the procedure
- Pain medication given including the dose, time, your name, and the patient's response
- Method of cleansing the wound
- Type of dressing applied to the wound
- Education provided to the patient

Sample documentation

09/20/22 2120 Red granulating tissue noted throughout the wound bed of a stage 4 pressure injury on sacrum. No tunneling or undermining observed. Minimal amount of serosanguineous drainage on old dressing. Wound cleansed with normal saline prior to application of new dressing. Wet-to-damp dressing applied. Pt tolerated procedure well with no verbalization of pain throughout procedure. Pt placed on 2-hr turn schedule and educated about pressure relief measures. Pt reports understanding. ———————— W. Earl, RN

Practice Resources

Bhimji, S. (2017, updated); Wound, Ostomy and Continence Nurses Society (WOCN), Doughty, D. B., & McNichol, L. L. (2016).

Thinking About the Procedure

The video **Removing and Applying Wet-to-Damp Dressings**, along with questions and suggested responses, is available on the ***Davis's Nursing Skills Videos*** Web site on FADavis.com.

Procedure 35-6 ■ Applying a Negative Pressure Wound Therapy (NPWT) Device

➤ For steps to follow in *all* procedures, refer to the Universal Steps for All Procedures found on the page facing the inside back cover.

Equipment

- Suction unit (pump)
- Collection canister with connecting tubing
- Open-pore reticulated polyurethane foam dressing
- Semipermeable transparent adhesive dressing
- Skin preparation product or sealant (skin prep)
- Sterile 4 in. × 4 in. gauze
- Clean nonsterile gloves
- Two pairs of sterile gloves (if using sterile technique)
- Sterile scissors (if using sterile technique)
- Waterproof pad
- Bath blanket
- Goggles or safety glasses, mask, and protective gown
- 10- to 20-mL irrigation syringe
- Normal saline for irrigation
- Emesis basis
- Biohazard bag for contaminated materials

Procedure 35-6A Open-Pore Reticulated Polyurethane Foam Therapy

- GranuFoam (black), white, or silver foam dressing
- Therapeutic regulated accurate care (TRAC) pad

Procedure 35-6B Gauze Dressing Application (i.e., Chariker–Jeter Dressing Method)

- Fenestrated drain
- Ostomy paste

Delegation

As a nurse, you are responsible for assessing the wound and evaluating interventions. You should not delegate application of a negative pressure wound therapy device to UAP. However, you may ask the UAP to report to you any changes in the wound dressing, pressure in the unit, or alarms.

Pre-Procedure Assessments

- Assess the type of wound to be treated with negative pressure.
  Negative pressure wound therapy is used to promote wound healing by secondary or tertiary intention in acute, chronic, traumatic, and dehisced wounds; partial-thickness burns; or flaps and grafts. NPWT will prepare the wound bed for closure, reduce edema, promote granulation formation, and remove exudate and infective material.

- Determine if there is any contraindication to use of a NPWT: nonenteric or unexplored fistulas; necrotic tissue with eschar; untreated osteomyelitis; malignancy in the wound or in exposed blood vessels, anastomosis sites, organs, or nerves.
- Assess patients for active or prolonged bleeding; patients who are on anticoagulant therapy or platelet aggregation inhibitors; or patients with infected, damaged, irradiated, or sutured blood vessels.
  Patients who are at increased risk for bleeding should be closely monitored. These conditions could be fatal if negative pressure is applied and bleeding is uncontrolled (exsanguination could occur). Notify the healthcare provider of these conditions.
- Assess the wound for bone fragments or sharp edges.
  When NPWT is activated, mechanical stress is placed upon the wound. Sharp edges or bone may puncture protective barriers, vessels, or organs, causing injury, and bleeding, if uncontrolled, could be fatal.
- Assess the wound for infection.
  Monitor infected wounds closely because they may require more frequent dressing changes than noninfected wounds.
- Assess the wound for size (length, width, and depth in centimeters); location and depth of undermining or tunneling; amount, character, and odor of drainage; type and percentage of tissue present in wound bed (granulation, slough, fibrin, necrotic); and periwound condition (i.e., intact, denuded, erythema, induration, or maceration).
  If no response or improvement in the wound condition occurs in 2 weeks, use of NPWT should be reevaluated.
- Assess the patient's nutritional status.
  Adequate protein stores are needed for wounds to heal. Evaluate the patient's albumin or prealbumin level before initiating therapy because NPWT may deplete these levels and prevent healing.
- Assess for pain.
  Wound care is very painful. Poorly controlled wound pain can lead to wound bed hypoxia. This impairs wound healing and increases infection rates. Wound pain also negatively affects the patient's quality of life.

➤ When performing the procedure, always identify your patient according to agency policy, using two identifiers, and be attentive to standard precautions, hand hygiene, patient safety and privacy, body mechanics, and documentation.

➤ *Note:* The success of NPWT partially depends on the training and expertise of the clinician. Allow adequate time for this procedure. Experienced nurses need at least 15 to 30 minutes. You will need more time if problems arise, and even more if you are a novice.

➤ *Note:* This procedure assumes you are performing the initial application of vacuum-assisted closure (VAC) therapy. If you are changing the dressing, first read the What If … section near the end of this procedure.

Procedure Steps

1. **Consider administering pain medication before initiating negative pressure wound therapy.**
   Allow sufficient time for the medication to take effect.

2. **Select the appropriate dressing** (per NPWT system used) to fill the entire wound cavity.
   Dressings should be placed directly against the wound surface to allow for equal suction/pressure throughout the wound bed.

3. **Obtain suction pump** unit as prescribed.
   Negative pressure wound therapy is provided by several different manufacturers. Use the unit and dressing method that is approved by your facility.
   a. Place the suction unit upright on a level surface.
   b. Remove the canister from the sterile package and insert it into the pump.
   c. Connect the tubing to the canister.
   d. Ensure the opposite end of the tubing remains clean before connecting with the tubing from the dressing.
   e. You may place the suction unit at the end of the bed or hang it on an intravenous (IV) pole.
   f. Do not place the unit on the floor. Ensure the unit is not knocked over because drainage from the canister can back up and contaminate the pump's filter, blocking suction.

4. **Place the waterproof bag** or trash receptacle so you can reach it easily during the procedure.
   Convenient placement facilitates access to safe disposal of the dressing into a trash receptacle for biohazardous waste.

5. **Assist the patient** to a comfortable position that allows for easy access to the wound and a position that allows gravity to direct the flow of the irrigant from the clean end toward the dirty end of the wound.
   Facilitates access to the wound site with less contamination and promotes good body mechanics for the nurse.

iCare 6. **Drape the patient** (use a bath blanket if needed) to expose only the wound area.
   Draping provides privacy and emotional comfort.

7. **Place a waterproof pad** as needed.
   An underpad protects the linens from moisture and drainage.

8. **Prepare a sterile or clean field,** and add all supplies: gloves, scissors, irrigation supplies, gauze pad, selected wound dressings, tubing, and/or connectors.

9. **Don sterile or clean procedure gloves.** Use a gown and protective eyewear.
   Using sterile/aseptic versus clean technique is based on the wound type, physician preference, or facility protocol. A safe rule to follow is to use sterile gloves for a fresh noninfected wound and clean gloves for other wounds.

(continued on next page)

Procedure 35-6 ■ Applying a Negative Pressure Wound Therapy (NPWT) Device (continued)

10. **Irrigate the wound** with 10 to 30 mL of sterile saline or other prescribed solution before all dressing changes. Use a 35-mL syringe and a 19-gauge angiocatheter (needle removed) to direct the flow of the irrigation fluid from the clean end toward the dirty end of the wound.
Irrigation facilitates loosening of adherent tissue and removes debris and exudate while adhering to infection control principles of clean-to-dirty.

11. **Remove the excess solution** from the wound. Clean and dry the periwound skin with sterile gauze sponges, as needed. Consider a skin protectant around the wound edges.
Excess moisture predisposes skin to maceration and possible damage. Applying a skin protectant can assist the drape in sticking to the skin; it also protects the skin when the drape is removed (i.e., from stripping of skin by the adhesive).

12. **Remove soiled gloves** and don sterile ones for the procedure.
Change gloves during patient care if the hands will move from a contaminated body site (e.g., perineal area or wound) to a clean body site.

13. **To apply appropriate dressing** per preferred negative pressure wound therapy unit, follow Procedure 35-6A or 35-6B.

Procedure 35-6A ■ Open-Pore Reticulated Polyurethane Foam Therapy (i.e., Vacuum-Assisted Closure [VAC])

➤ When performing the procedure, always identify your patient according to agency policy, using two identifiers, and be attentive to standard precautions, hand hygiene, patient safety and privacy, body mechanics, and documentation.

Begin with Procedure Steps 1 through 13, at the beginning of Procedure 35-6. Then proceed as follows.

1. **Select the appropriate foam dressing:** black, white, or silver.
Black foam is sufficient for most wounds unless individual patient circumstances require white or silver. ***White foam*** *is denser and will limit granulation formation. It may be used for painful or superficial wounds, tunneling/sinus tracts/undermining, or where granulation tissue growth needs to be limited.* ***Silver dressings*** *may act as a barrier to bacterial penetration in the wound bed. Silver may eradicate biofilms of colonized bacteria.*

2. **Cut the foam dressing** to the appropriate size to fill the wound cavity. Do not cut the foam dressing over the wound. Rub the cut edges to remove any loose pieces.
If you cut the foam over the wound, particles may fall into the wound and create irritation ▼

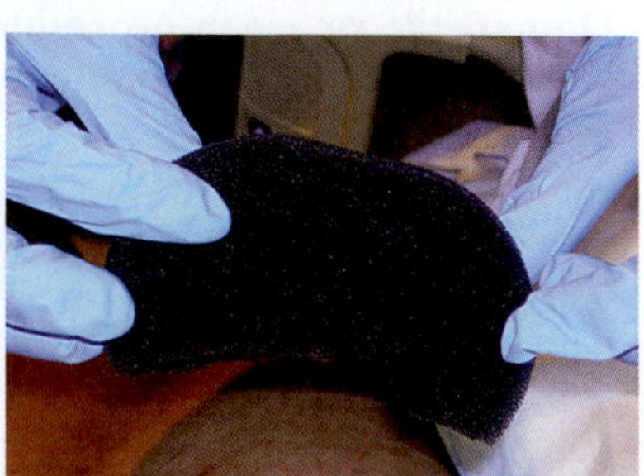

3. **Gently place the foam** dressing into the cavity without overlapping onto intact skin. Do not overfill the cavity or pack into deep crevices.
   a. Do not place foam into blind/unexplored tunnels.
   Forcing foam dressings into any area may damage tissue, alter the delivery of negative pressure, or hinder exudates or foam removal.
   b. Do not allow foam dressing to overlap onto healthy skin.
   Foam dressing becomes very wet during therapy and will macerate and damage intact skin.
   c. If you use more than one piece, note the total number of pieces that were placed into the wound, so you can document them on the transparent dressing and in the patient's health record.
   An accurate record of the number of foam pieces is necessary to prevent retained material within the wound.

4. **Apply a liquid skin preparation** product to periwound, if needed.
Skin preps can protect the periwound skin from excess fluid, adhesive stripping, or other damage.

5. **Apply transparent film/drape** 3 to 5 cm (1 to 2 in.) from wound margins without pulling, stretching, or wrinkling the drape. Do not push down or compress foam while placing drape.
The occlusive dressing creates a seal to help create negative pressure within the wound. Tension from pulling, stretching, or wrinkling the dressing may lead to tissue injury. More pressure will be placed on the wound bed than necessary if you have flattened the foam before turning on the suction unit.

6. **Avoid placing dressings that wrap** all the way around an extremity. If necessary, place several smaller pieces of drape rather than one continuous piece.
When pressure is applied, a circumferential dressing may interfere with circulation, if wrapped too tightly.

7. **Identify a site over the dressing** for the suction track tubing apparatus.

8. **Pinch up a piece of drape** and cut at least a 2-cm round hole. Do not make a slit or X because this may close off under pressure. ▼

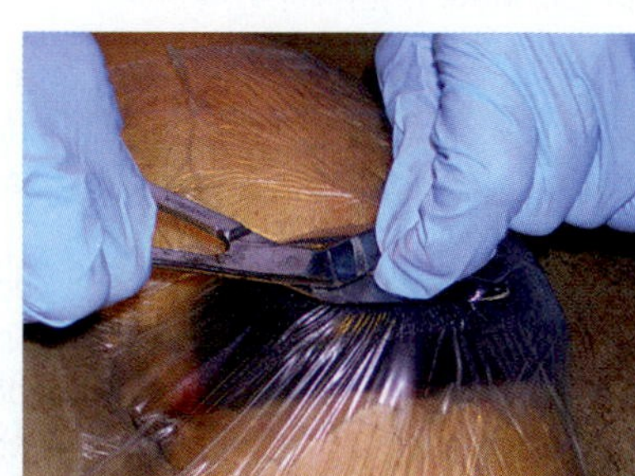

9. **Place the track adhesive** and suction device directly over the hole in the drape and apply gentle pressure to secure.
Negative pressure removes excess wound exudate from the wound bed.

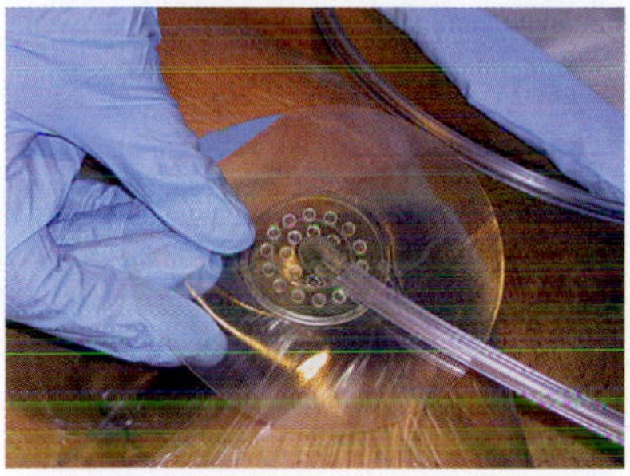

10. **Connect suction track tubing** to the canister tubing and open clamps. The canister is attached to a vacuum pump that provides either continuous or intermittent negative pressure, adjusted for the type of wound. Set suction to the prescribed pressure, which is typically in the range of –5 to –125 mm Hg (adjustable pressures, depending on the particular device used).
Suction draws excess exudate away from the wound and into an evacuation container.

11. **Connect tubing from the dressing** to the suction track tubing going to the collection canister.
Allows for collection and measurement of drainage.

12. **Position the tubing** and connector away from bony prominences and skin creases.
Prevents pressure injury to the skin.

13. **Ensure clamps are open** on all tubing.

14. **Turn on power to the pump** and set to the prescribed therapy settings to initiate therapy.
Therapy should be maintained for at least 22 out of 24 hours daily. Alternate wound care should be considered if the vacuum cannot be tolerated for this length of time.

15. **Listen for audible leaks** and observe dressing collapse or wrinkling as pressure is applied to the wound bed.
With an adequate seal, the dressing will collapse almost immediately. Any leak (e.g., between the dressing and drape, around tubing, at skin crevices, or at tubing connection sites) will prevent collapse.

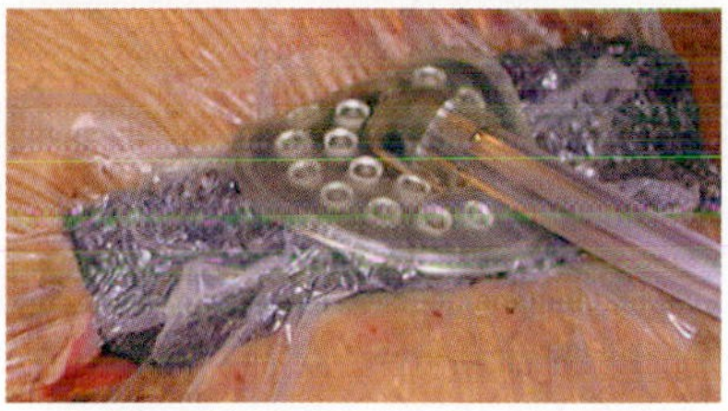

16. **Change the canister** at least once a week or when filled. Write the date on the canister.
This will help to know when it was changed last as well as how often it is being changed for fluid loss.

Procedure 35-6B ■ Gauze Dressing Application (i.e., Chariker–Jeter Method)

➤ When performing the procedure, always identify your patient according to agency policy and be attentive to standard precautions, hand hygiene, patient safety and privacy, body mechanics, and documentation.

Begin with Steps 1 through 13, at the beginning of Procedure 35-6. Then proceed as follows.

1. **Measure the length of drain** from wound margin, starting with the first hole perforation and pull back 1 cm.

2. **Moisten gauze** with normal saline.

3. **Wrap or "sandwich" the drain** in the moistened gauze and place in the wound base. Tuck gauze into any undermining areas to ensure contact with the wound bed.

4. **Apply a strip or small amount of ostomy paste** 1 cm from the wound edge and secure the drain as needed.
Paste is occlusive and will help maintain a seal between the drain and the transparent film dressing. Paste that is too close to the wound edge can get sucked into the drain and occlude pressure.

5. **Apply liquid skin preparation** product to periwound, if needed. Extra drape, hydrocolloid, or transparent dressing may be used to protect fragile skin.
Skin preps can protect the periwound skin from excess fluid, adhesive stripping, or other damage.

6. **Apply transparent film** approximately 1.0 to 2.5 cm ($^1/_2$ to 1 in.) beyond the wound margin to intact skin. Pinch the film around the drain tubing to ensure a tight seal.

7. **Avoid wrapping dressings** around an extremity. If necessary, place several smaller pieces of drape rather than one continuous piece.
When pressure is applied, a circumferential dressing may interfere with circulation.

8. **Attach filter tubing** to the canister spout.

9. **Connect tubing** from the dressing to the evacuation tubing going to the collection canister.
Allows for collection and measurement of drainage.

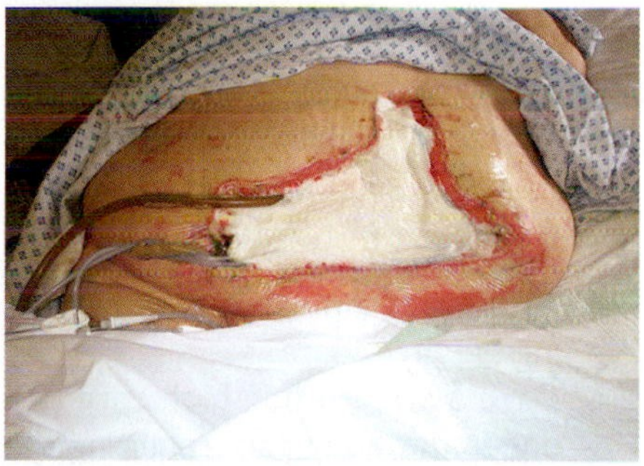

10. **Ensure clamps are open** on all tubing.

11. **Position the tubing** and connector away from bony prominences and skin creases.
Prevents pressure injury to the skin.

(continued on next page)

Procedure 35-6 ■ Applying a Negative Pressure Wound Therapy (NPWT) Device (continued)

12. Turn on power to pump and set to the prescribed therapy settings to initiate therapy.
Therapy should be maintained for at least 22 out of 24 hours daily. Alternate wound care should be considered if suction cannot be tolerated for this length of time.

13. Listen for audible leaks and observe dressing collapse as pressure is applied to the wound bed.
With an adequate seal, the dressing will collapse almost immediately. Any leak (i.e., between the dressing and drape, around tubing, at skin crevices, or at tubing connection sites) will prevent collapse.

14. Change the canister at least once a week or when filled. Document the date on the canister.
This will help to know when it was changed last as well as how often it is being changed for fluid loss.

? What if . . .

- **You are changing the dressing instead of applying it for the first time.**

Follow the procedure steps below.

NOTE: Dressings should be changed every 48 to 72 hours.

Dressings left in the wound longer than the recommended time frame can become difficult to remove if tissue grows into the foam. They can lead to infection or other adverse events.

a. Evaluate the need for analgesia.
b. Turn the suction pump unit off during the procedure.
c. Place a waterproof, biohazard pad under the body part requiring the dressing change.
d. Perform hand hygiene and don sterile or clean gloves as appropriate.
e. Remove the transparent dressing, using a push–pull method to gently pull up drape while pushing it slowly from the skin. Separating the drape from the skin in this manner will decrease the risk of tape stripping.
f. Gently remove gauze or foam dressing. If dressing is difficult to remove, instill normal saline onto the dressing for 15 to 30 minutes.
Dressing removal can damage new granulation tissue if tissue has grown into the dressing.
g. Count all pieces of gauze or foam dressing that were removed to ensure none remain in the wound bed. Ensure no dressing is left in tunneled or undermined areas.
Dressings are not bioabsorbable and can abscess if left in the wound.
h. Discard soiled dressings in a biohazardous waste receptacle.
i. Start at the beginning of Procedure 35-6 and perform Steps 1 through 13. Then, as instructed in Step 13, follow either Procedure 35-6A or 35-6B.

- **After 2 weeks, you see that the wound is not improving?**

Consult with the healthcare provider or a wound care specialist. Average length of therapy is usually 4 to 6 weeks. Therapy should be discontinued if the wound shows no improvement in 1 to 2 consecutive weeks, the patient is unwilling or unable to follow the medical plan, or the goal of therapy has been met.
The longer a wound is open, the longer it takes to heal, and places the patient at risk for complications. A steady decrease in wound size should be seen every week. If NPWT is not effective, alternate wound care should be evaluated.

- **You cannot find or remove a piece of foam?**

Notify the healthcare provider because this may necessitate surgery.
The material could be retained in the patient and create an inflammatory response.

- **There is a foul odor when the dressing is removed?**

Clean the wound with normal saline to ensure odor is not coming from the soiled dressing. If other signs of infection are present (i.e., fever, tenderness, redness, swelling, purulent drainage), notify the healthcare provider.

- **Suction cannot be maintained?**

Identify why the seal cannot be maintained. If the wound is very near the coccyx and gluteal fold, use a dollop of paste to help fill in the crack and maintain a seal. If the skin around the wound is moist, adhesive drape will not adhere to skin. Use a skin prep product or drape to protect the skin. If the tube is pulling away from the dressing or tension is being placed on the tube, anchor it with additional drape or tape several centimeters from the dressing or wound.

- **The canister is filling with blood?**

Immediately discontinue negative pressure therapy. The gauze or foam dressing will not stop the bleeding, so take measures to control bleeding (i.e., hold pressure on wound). Do not remove dressing until the treating healthcare provider is consulted.

- **Dressing does not collapse or the alarm sounds?**

a. Press firmly around the transparent dressing to seal.
b. Verify the machine is turned on, and all clamps are open, and tubing is not kinked.
c. Check tubing and drape for leaks. Listen for leaks with a stethoscope or by moving your hand around the wound margins while applying slight pressure.
d. Additional small pieces of transparent dressing may be used to seal around hardware, skinfold, or creases.
e. Do not place multiple layers of drape or adhesive dressing.
Several layers may decrease the dressing's moisture vapor transmission rate, increasing the risk of maceration.
f. Never leave foam in place without an adequate seal for more than 2 hours. If an adequate seal cannot be achieved in that time, remove the foam and apply a saline moistened gauze dressing.

Evaluation

- Note the patient's response to the procedure.
- Continue to monitor wound healing and changes in periwound tissues.
- Monitor dressing every 2 hours to ensure it is firm and collapsed in the wound bed while therapy is on.
- Monitor the seal of the dressing and pressure settings.
- Monitor for brisk or bright bleeding, evisceration or dehiscence, and symptoms of infection.
  These must be reported to the healthcare provider.

Home Care

- Refer the client to a home health agency for wound care.
- In limited circumstances, some patients or caregivers may be able to perform dressing changes. Determine their ability to perform dressing changes; teach and demonstrate as needed.
- Instruct the patient or family to visually check the dressing every 2 hours to ensure it is firm and collapsed in the wound bed.
- Review safety labeling, alarms, and pump instructions.
- Review conditions in which to seek medical care: bleeding, infection, unresolved alarms, or loss of suction.
- Review proper disposal of contaminated supplies.

Documentation

Document the following information:

- Date and time of dressing change
- Wound assessment: location of the wound, size (length, width, diameter), undermining or tunneling, amount and character of drainage, odor, wound bed including type and percentage of tissue seen, and periwound appearance
- Evaluation of therapy with evidence of healing
- Treatment selected: type of NPWT, type of gauze or foam, number of pieces placed in the wound
- Treatment settings: pressures, intermittent vs. continuous, or variable pressures
- Patient response to dressing change

Sample documentation for Procedure 35-6B: Chariker-Jeter Dressing Application

9/13/22. 1010 Patient reported pain rating 5 on a scale of 1 to 10. Administered hydrocodone 5.0 mg PO for pain at 0815 before initiation of negative wound pressure therapy. See MAR [medication administration record]. Stage 4 pressure injury to coccyx surgically débrided. Wound is 4 × 6 × 2 with no appreciable undermining. Wound bed is now clean of necrotic tissue with 100% pink tissue noted. Periwound has 2 cm of erythema to wound edges. Scant malodorous serosanguineous drainage. Using sterile technique, moistened saline gauze applied to wound bed with fenestrated drain. Ostomy paste applied at wound edge to assist in seal. Pump activated to 80 mm Hg continuous pressure. Patient rated pain in wound area as a 2 post-procedure. Plan: Begin dressing changes every 48 hours. ——— L. Opperta, RN

Practice Resources

Chariker, M. (2009); Gabriel, A., & Schraga, E. D. (2013, updated); McCulloch, J. M., & Kloth, L. C. (2010); Mattox, E. A. (2017); Moore, C., & Young, J., (2011); NCG (2006, revised 2011).

Thinking About the Procedure

The video **Open-Pore Reticulated Polyurethane Foam Therapy (i.e., Vacuum-Assisted Closure [VAC])**, along with questions and suggested responses, is available on the ***Davis's Nursing Skills Videos*** Web site on FADavis.com.

Procedure 35-7 ■ Applying and Removing a Transparent Film Dressing

➤ For steps to follow in *all* procedures, refer to the Universal Steps for All Procedures found on the page facing the inside back cover.

Equipment

- Clean nonsterile gloves
- Sterile gauze
- Normal saline solution or specified cleansing agent, warmed to body temperature when possible
  Cold solution lowers the temperature of the wound bed and slows the healing process.
- Scissors (if needed)
- Liquid skin preparation (if needed)
- Transparent film dressing

Delegation

Because assessment of the wound and knowledge of clean technique are important, you should not delegate this procedure to UAP.

Pre-Procedure Assessments

- Assess the area to determine whether a transparent film dressing is appropriate.
  Transparent film dressings are indicated as primary dressings (dressings that touch the wound or area to be treated) to protect

(continued on next page)

Procedure 35-7 ■ Applying and Removing a Transparent Film Dressing (continued)

high-risk intact skin; for superficial or partial-thickness wounds that have little to no drainage (i.e., stage 1 or 2 pressure injury); and to assist in débriding eschar by autolysis. Films may be used as a secondary dressing to protect other types of dressings from bodily fluids (i.e., wounds near the perineum).

- Assess the wound to determine if use of a transparent film is contraindicated.
  Films are contraindicated in third-degree burns, arterial ulcers, and infected wounds with moderate to heavy exudate. Films should not be used to fill dead space.
- Determine the size of the wound.
  Film dressings are available in many sizes. Select the appropriate size based on wound measurements, allowing for a 2.5 cm (1 in.) perimeter of intact skin around the wound for the adhesive to stick.
- Assess the periwound area.
  Film dressings should be attached to intact skin. The adhesive is not waterproof and will not adhere to wet or moist skin.

➤ When performing the procedure, always identify your patient according to agency policy, using two identifiers, and be attentive to standard precautions, hand hygiene, patient safety and privacy, body mechanics, and documentation.

Procedure Steps

1. **Place the patient in a** comfortable position that provides easy access to the wound.

Procedure Steps for Applying the Dressing

2. **If a dressing is present, wash your hands,** don clean, nonsterile gloves, and remove the old dressing.
3. **Dispose of the soiled dressing** and gloves in the biohazard waste receptacle.
   Observe universal precautions, preventing transfer of pathogens.
4. **Don clean nonsterile gloves,** and cleanse the skin surrounding the wound with normal saline or a mild cleansing agent. Be sure to rinse the skin well if you use a cleanser. Allow the skin to dry thoroughly.
   Cleansing prepares the skin for application of the dressing. Skin must be dry for the dressing to adhere.
5. **Cleanse the wound** as prescribed or according to agency procedure.
   Cleansing of wounds removes bacteria and necrotic debris from wound beds.
6. **Consider placing a skin barrier** around the wound before transparent film dressing application.
   Skin sealants may be applied to skin before tape to protect fragile skin from tears or epidermal stripping.
7. **Remove the center backing liner** from the transparent film dressing. ▼

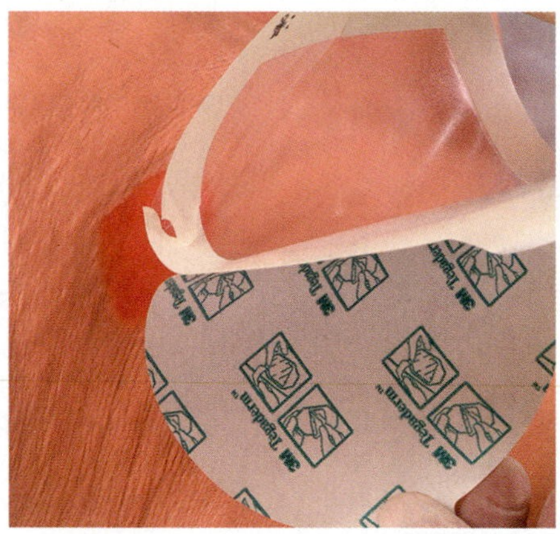

8. **Holding the dressing by the edges,** apply the transparent film to the wound without stretching or pulling the dressing or the skin.
   This reduces the risk of skin damage.
9. **Remove the edging liner** from the dressing.
10. **Gently smooth and secure** the dressing to skin from the center to outward.
    Allows the dressing to adhere fully to the patient's skin.
11. **Dispose of soiled equipment**; remove your gloves.

Procedure Steps for Removing the Dressing

Transparent film dressings are typically changed every 3 days. Change dressing sooner if drainage extends beyond the edges of the wound onto periwound skin. To remove the dressing, do the following:

12. **Grasp one edge** of the film dressing.
13. **Gently lift the edge.**
14. **Stabilize the skin** underneath the elevated edge with your finger.
    Stabilizing the skin as the adhesive is taken off will prevent epidermal stripping.
15. **With the other hand,** slowly peel the dressing back over itself, "low and slow," in the direction of hair growth. Use of an adhesive removal pad is recommended especially for sensitive skin.
    Removing the dressing at an angle will increase the risk of pulling on the epidermis and causing mechanical trauma.
16. **As dressing is removed,** keep moving your finger as necessary to avoid newly exposed skin.

? What if . . .

- **The adhesive will not adhere to the patient's skin because of excess hair?**
  Hair may be removed with clippers/scissors. Do not shave the site with a razor.
  Shaving can cause nicks or abrasions to the skin that could become a portal of entry for bacteria.

- **Your patient's skin is diaphoretic or excessively oily?**

Cleanse the skin with soap and water before the dressing change. Allow the skin to dry before continuing with the dressing. Also, polymer skin barriers may be used to place a seal over the skin and allow the tape adhesive to adhere.

- **Your patient has fragile skin (e.g., an elderly patient)?**

Skin sealant preparations may be used under adhesives.

The junction between the epidermis and dermis on the older adult is not as strong as with a younger person. Less pressure or tension is needed to break those bonds and cause skin damage.

- **The dressing sticks to itself before it can be applied?**

If a small portion of the dressing is stuck to itself, gently stretch or pull the edges in opposite directions. If a large portion is involved, throw the dressing away and start over.

Transparent dressings can be difficult to apply because they are polyurethane sheets coated on one side with an acrylic, hypoallergenic adhesive and are flimsy in nature, making them clumsy to work with at times.

- **Purulent-appearing fluid has collected underneath the film dressing?**

This does not necessarily mean the wound is infected. Remove the dressing and clean the wound per policy. Select an alternate dressing that will be more absorptive.

Because films do not have absorptive capabilities, any drainage produced by the wound will pool underneath.

Evaluation

- Verify the transparent film dressing is appropriate for the wound.
- Determine whether the dressing adheres comfortably to skin.
- Ensure that patient verbalizes understanding of treatment.

Patient Teaching

- Teach the patient about the expected healing process.
- Teach the patient about the use of transparent film dressings.
- Inform the patient and caregiver about signs and symptoms of infection and the need to report these findings.

Documentation

Document the following information (many agencies use a wound/skin flowsheet):

- Wound assessment: location of the wound, size (length × width × diameter) undermining or tunneling, amount and character of drainage, odor, wound bed including type and percentage of tissue seen, and periwound appearance
- Appearance and location of the wound, type and amount of exudate, and odor, if present, after cleansing
- The patient's pain level before the procedure. If the patient was medicated for pain, document the drug and dose used, time given, and the patient's response to analgesia.
- Method of cleansing the wound and surrounding skin
- Type of dressing applied to the wound
- Education provided to the patient

Sample documentation

2/22/22 2230 Transparent film dressing applied to stage I pressure injury on left lateral heel, 1 × 1 cm. Area is nonblanchable and painful to the touch. Cleaned with normal saline before dressing applied. Heel protectors placed bilaterally to keep heels suspended off the surface of the bed. Discussed pressure injury formation with patient, and the need to rotate positions and relieve heel pressure. Will continue to assist patient in turning every 2 hours. ——— M. K. Leonard, RN

Practice Resources

Association of periOperative Registered Nurses (AORN) (2018); Morgan, N. (2014).

Procedure 35-8 ■ Applying a Hydrating Dressing (Hydrocolloid or Hydrogel)

➤ For steps to follow in *all* procedures, refer to the Universal Steps for All Procedures found on the page facing the inside back cover.

Equipment

- Clean nonsterile gloves
- Hydrating dressing 3 to 4 cm (1.5 in.) larger than the wound
- Moisture-proof bag

Obtain the following items, only if needed:

- Normal saline solution warmed to body temperature when possible
  Cold solution lowers the temperature of wound bed and slows the healing process.
- Emesis basin
- Sterile gauze for cleansing
- Disposable clippers or scissors (to trim hair or dressing)
- Skin prep
- Measuring device
- Tape

Delegation

This procedure requires knowledge of wound healing, dressings, and infection control and prevention. You should not delegate this procedure to UAP.

Pre-Procedure Assessments

- Assess the area to determine whether a hydrating dressing is appropriate.
  Hydrating dressings are appropriate for wounds with minimal drainage. These dressings débride necrotic tissue from the wound bed. They may also be used to protect skin at risk for breakdown.
- Determine the size of the wound.
  Allows you to select a dressing of the appropriate size. Choosing a dressing size that extends beyond the injury ensures complete coverage.

➤ When performing the procedure, always identify your patient according to agency policy, using two identifiers, and be attentive to standard precautions, hand hygiene, patient safety and privacy, body mechanics, and documentation.

Procedure Steps

1. **Place the patient** in a comfortable position that provides easy access to the wound.
   Provides for patient comfort and proper nurse body mechanics during dressing change.

2. **If a dressing is present, perform hand hygiene**, don clean nonsterile gloves, and remove the old dressing.
   Prevents transfer of pathogens.

3. **Dispose of the soiled dressing** and gloves in the biohazard waste receptacle.
   Dressings may contain body fluids and other contaminants, so they must be disposed of in moisture-proof containers.

4. **Perform hand hygiene.** Don nonsterile gloves, and cleanse the skin surrounding the wound with normal saline or a mild cleansing agent. Be sure to rinse the skin well if you use a cleanser. Allow the skin to dry. Do not attempt to remove residue that is left on the skin from the old dressing.
   Cleansing and drying prepare the skin for application of the dressing. Removing residue irritates the surrounding skin.

5. **Cleanse the wound as directed.** Wound cleansing may be performed with clean or sterile technique, depending on the type of wound.
   Cleansing the wound removes microbes and necrotic debris from wound bed. Studies show using either saline or tap water is similarly effective for cleansing.

6. **Remove soiled gloves**; assess the condition of the wound. Note the size, location, type of tissue present, amount of exudate, and odor.
   Granulating tissue is beefy red with a velvety appearance. It appears with the growth of new blood vessels and connective tissue. Pale pink tissue may indicate compromised blood supply to the wound bed. Necrotic tissue, which is black, brown, or yellow in appearance, is nonviable and inhibits healing. A hydrocolloid dressing will interact with wound drainage to produce a thick, yellow gel that may have a foul odor. Clean the wound before assessing for exudate and odor.

7. **Apply skin prep** to the area covered by tape.
   Skin prep protects intact skin from breakdown from tape removal

8. **With the backing still intact,** cut the hydrating dressing, if necessary, to the desired shape and size. Size the hydrocolloid dressing so it will extend 3 to 4 cm (1.5 in.) beyond the wound margin on all sides and cover all areas of nonintact skin.
   Provides complete coverage of the wound.

9. **Don clean, nonsterile gloves**, and remove the backing of the hydrocolloid dressing, starting at one edge.
   - Place the exposed adhesive portion on the patient's skin.
   - Position the dressing to cover the wound. ▼

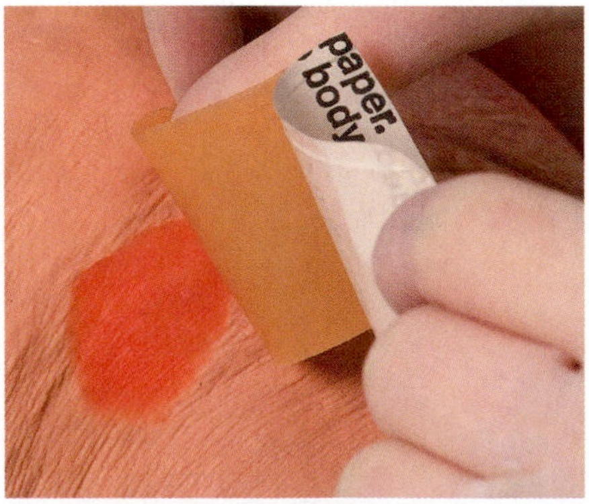

10. **Gradually peel away** the remaining liner; smooth the hydrocolloid dressing onto the skin by placing your hand on top of dressing and holding in place for 1 minute.
Warmth helps the dressing adhere to the skin.

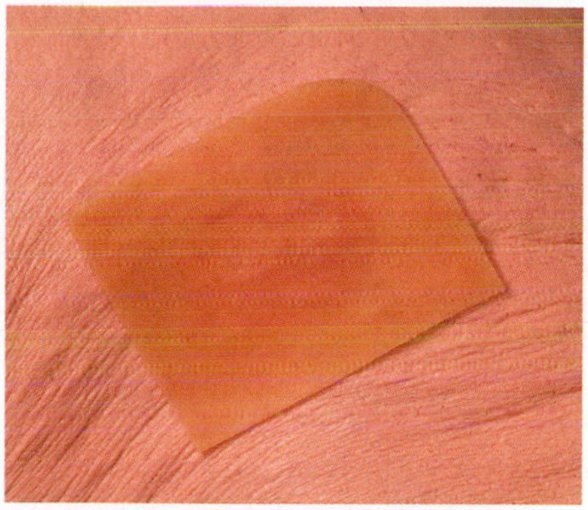

11. **Assist the patient to** a comfortable position; remove and discard your gloves. Wash your hands.

? What if . . .

- **Signs of infection are noted?**
Notify healthcare provider. Cultures may be prescribed. A different type of dressing may be prescribed as well.
- **The surrounding skin is not intact?**
Choose a larger size hydrocolloid dressing to cover the nonintact area. Document your observations and report new findings to the healthcare provider.

Evaluation

- Verify that a hydrocolloid dressing is still appropriate for the wound.
- Note whether the dressing adheres comfortably to the skin.
- Ensure the patient verbalizes understanding of treatment.
- Inspect the dressing daily. Change it if it becomes dislodged, leaks, or wrinkles or if it develops an odor.

Patient Teaching

- Teach the patient about the expected healing process.
- Inform the patient and caregiver about signs and symptoms of infection and the need to report these findings.

Home Care

- Hydrating dressings may be required in the home setting. Teach caregivers to use the appropriate size and change the dressing if it begins to leak, develops an odor, or begins to separate from the skin. Never reuse a dressing.

Documentation

Document the following information (many agencies use wound care flowsheets):

- Appearance, color, size, and location of the wound, type and amount of exudate, and odor, if present, after cleansing. Include wound measurements, if taken, and condition of surrounding skin.
- The patient's pain level before the procedure. If the patient was medicated for pain, document the drug and dose used, time given, and patient response.
- Method of cleansing the wound and surrounding skin
- Type of dressing applied to the wound
- Use of skin prep
- Education provided to the patient

Sample documentation

11/19/22 2230 Pt medicated with ibuprofen 600 mg by mouth for mild wound pain post-op. Pain rated as a 4 out of 10 prior to dressing change. Soiled hydrocolloid dressing removed from shear injury to left mid-scapular area. Wound cleansed with sterile saline and gauze. Shear is 3.5 × 4 cm and 100% covered with yellow slough. Moderate amount of nonodorous, serous drainage. Hydrocolloid reapplied as prescribed. Pain with no complaint of increase in pain. Educated pt. about autolytic action of hydrocolloid, plan of care, and expected outcomes for wound healing. ——— S. Terril, RN

Practice Resources

Dabri, G., & Phillips, T. (2016, January 12); Dumville, J. C., O'Meara, S., Deshpande, S., et al. (2013); Wound, Ostomy and Continence Nurses Society (WOCN), Doughty, D. B., & McNichol, L. L. (2016).

Thinking About the Procedure

The video **Applying a Hydrating Dressing (Hydrocolloid or Hydrogel),** along with questions and suggested responses, is available on the ***Davis's Nursing Skills Videos*** Web site on FADavis.com.

Procedure 35-9 ■ Placing Skin Closures

➤ For steps to follow in *all* procedures, refer to the Universal Steps for All Procedures found on the page facing the inside back cover.

Equipment

- Adhesive skin closures
- Tincture of benzoin or skin protectant pads
- Forceps
- Normal saline
- Gauze
- Gloves (sterile if indicated)

Delegation

This procedure may be delegated to UAP with the required training unless it is a new wound requiring sterile technique or has developed complications (e.g., dehiscence). Assessment of the incision line or wound is a licensed professional's responsibility and cannot be delegated.

Pre-Procedure Assessments

- Assess the type of wound to be closed.
  Adhesive closures are frequently used to keep surgical incisions well approximated. They may be used in conjunction with staples or sutures or following early staple/suture removal. Closures may be used to approximate the edges of lacerations or skin tears.
- Assess the wound for skin edge approximation.
  Wounds that are gaping or appear to have undermining should not be closed using adhesive closures.
- Assess the wound for drainage, amount, type, and odor.
  Adhesive skin closures might not be suitable for wounds that are draining heavily, because the adhesive would not stick to the skin.
- Assess the periwound area or surrounding skin. Assessment should include skin color, texture, temperature, and integrity of the surrounding skin. Look for maceration (caused by heavy drainage), excoriation (from caustic effluent), stripping (from inappropriate adhesive removal), pustules, papules, or lesions.
  Adhesive closures should be placed only on intact skin.
- Assess the length of the wound, the location (over a joint), or if edema may occur, to determine the size of the skin closure used. Consider elastic skin closures if distention or movement is anticipated.
  Closures come in several different lengths, widths, and flexibility capabilities to meet elasticity and conformability needs.

➤ When performing the procedure, always identify your patient according to agency policy, using two identifiers, and be attentive to standard precautions, hand hygiene, patient safety and privacy, body mechanics, and documentation.

Procedure Steps

1. **Don clean nonsterile** gloves.
   Gloving prevents cross-contamination.
2. **Cleanse the skin** at least 5 cm (2 in.) around the wound with saline-moistened gauze. Pat the skin dry, allowing it to dry thoroughly.
   The skin surrounding the wound must be clean and dry in order for the strips to adhere.
3. **Apply a skin preparation product**; allow it to dry (or follow agency procedures).
   Because the strips are prone to peeling off with moisture, benzoin enhances adhesion of the strips.
4. **Do not allow skin preparation** product to come into contact with the wound.
   It may impair healing.
5. **Peel back package tabs** to access the adhesive closures.
6. **Remove the card** from the package using modified sterile technique as necessary.
   Careful technique should be followed when applying to a surgical wound to minimize contamination and promote healing.
7. **Grasp end of the skin closure sheet** with forceps or gloved hand and peel strip from the card at a 90° angle.
   Closures lifted at a lesser angle or directly back on themselves may "curl," complicating handling.
8. **Starting at the middle** of the wound, apply strips perpendicular to the wound, drawing the wound edges together. Apply closures without tension; do not stretch or strap closures.
   a. Apply half of the closure to the wound margin and press firmly in place.
   b. Using fingers or forceps, ensure skin edges are approximated.
   c. Press free half firmly on the other side of the wound in a ladder fashion.
   d. Place the strips so that they extend at least 2 to 3 cm (¾ to 1 in.) on either side of the wound to ensure closure.
   e. Place the wound closure strips 3 mm (⅛ in.) apart along the wound. ▼

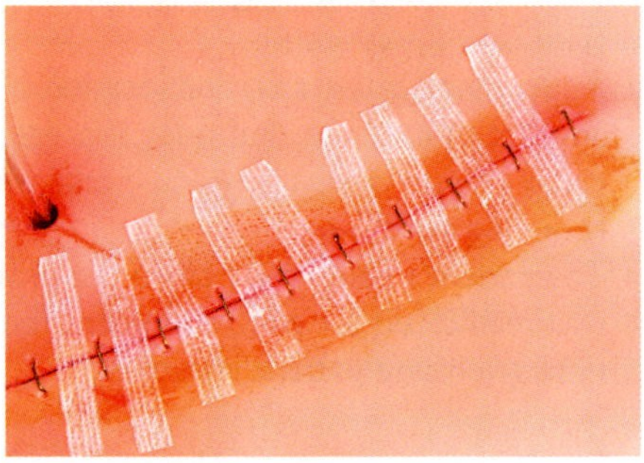

? What if . . .

- **A flap of skin rolls up on the edges?**

  Cleanse the wound with normal saline and reapproximate the edges of the skin flap with the intact epidermis. Apply skin closures across the flap.

- **The skin around the wound is swollen?**

  Apply skin closures without tension; reapply as swelling increases.

  This prevents pulling on the skin that can delay healing or disrupt the approximated borders of the wound, which is more likely to lead to scarring.

- **Edges are not accurately approximated or tension has been placed on the skin?**

  Remove the closure over the affected area, peeling each side toward the wound, and reapply.

  Use of adhesive products can cause superficial skin damage if the skin is stretched during application or with edema formation. Tension blisters are the most common problem associated with taping.

Evaluation

- Verify that skin closures are appropriate for the wound.
- Note whether the closures adhere comfortably to the skin.
- Ensure the patient verbalized understanding of the treatment.
- Inspect the wound daily. Lifted closure edges may be trimmed or closures replaced if less than half of the strip remains.

Patient Teaching

- Teach the patient about the expected healing process.
- Inform the patient or caregiver about signs and symptoms of infection and the need to report these findings.
- Instruct patients not to pull or tug on the strips.
  Improper removal may damage the underlying skin or the wound itself.
- Instruct patients that they do not need to keep the strips dry. They can bathe or shower as directed by the healthcare provider.
- Instruct the patient that adhesive strips are often kept in place until they begin to separate from the skin on their own.

Documentation

Document the following information (many agencies use specialized wound care flowsheets):

- Appearance and location of the wound, type and amount of exudates, and odor, if present, after cleansing
- The patient's level of pain before the procedure. If the patient was medicated for pain, document the drug and dose used, time given, and the patient response to analgesia.
- Method of cleansing the wound and surrounding skin
- Type of skin closures applied
- Education provided to the patient

Sample documentation

02/08/22 2040 Skin closures applied to surgical incision along right forearm. Wound edges are well approximated with slight erythema noted 4 mm from incisional site. Periwound skin is dry and intact with no drainage, induration, or odor noted. Wound cleansed with normal saline using sterile technique. Patient educated on the purpose of the closures and expected time and course of healing. Will continue to monitor. ——— S. Wong, RN

Practice Resources

Wound, Ostomy and Continence Nurses Society (WOCN); Doughty, D. B., & McNichol, L. L. (2016).

Thinking About the Procedure

The video **Placing Skin Closures,** along with questions and suggested responses, is available on the ***Davis's Nursing Skills Videos*** Web site on FADavis.com.

Procedure 35-10 ■ Applying Binders

➤ For steps to follow in *all* procedures, refer to the Universal Steps for All Procedures found on the page facing the inside back cover.

Equipment

- Abdominal binder, triangular arm binder, or T-binder
- Clean nonsterile gloves
- Measuring tape

Delegation

This procedure may be delegated to UAP. Assessment of the incision line or wound is a licensed professional's responsibility and cannot be delegated.

Pre-Procedure Assessments

- Assess the condition of the wound (if one is present). Note the amount and type of drainage. A wound must be dressed before it is bandaged; if there is a significant amount of exudate, you will need to apply a secondary dressing.
- Assess for pain; check the circulation of the underlying body parts before and after applying the binder. Look for cool, pale, or cyanotic skin, tingling, and numbness.
- Determine whether the patient or family has the skills to reapply the binder when necessary.

➤ When performing the procedure, always identify your patient according to agency policy, using two identifiers, and be attentive to standard precautions, hand hygiene, patient safety and privacy, body mechanics, and documentation.

➤ Observe Steps 1 through 7, regardless of the type of binder you use:

Procedure Steps

1. **Choose a binder** of the proper size, after measuring.
2. **Perform hand hygiene. Don nonsterile gloves.**
3. **Thoroughly clean and dry** the body part to be covered.
   Moisture contributes to skin breakdown.
4. **Place the body part** in its natural comfortable position (e.g., with the joint slightly flexed) whenever possible.
   Prevents strain on ligaments and muscles.
5. **Pad between skin surfaces** (e.g., under the axilla) and over bony prominences.
   Prevents pressure and abrasion of the skin.
6. **Fasten from the bottom up,** especially for abdominal binders.

   Make sure the binder is secured with enough pressure to provide the needed support and control bleeding, but not so tightly as to compromise circulation or impair breathing.

   Fastening from the bottom up gives upward support.
7. **Change binders** whenever they become soiled or wet.

Proceed to Step 8, 14, or 20, depending on the type of binder you are using.

Procedure Variation: Applying an Abdominal Binder

8. **Measure the patient** for the abdominal binder.
   a. Place the patient in supine position.
   b. With a measuring tape, encircle the abdomen at the level of the umbilicus. Note the measurement. This is the length of the binder.

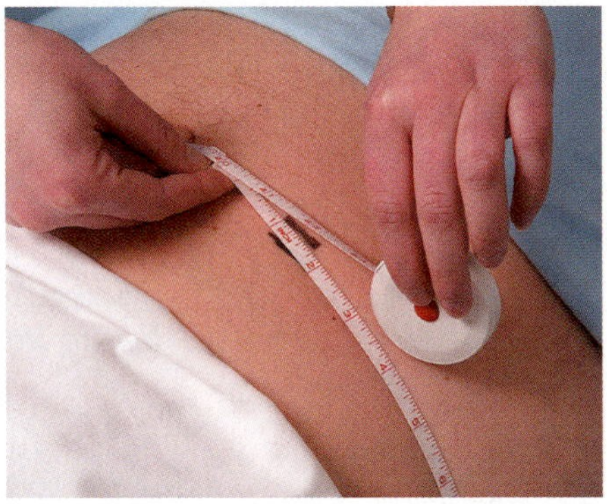

   c. Measure the distance from the costal margin to the top of the iliac crests. This is the width of the binder.
   d. Dispose of gloves and measuring tape; wash your hands.
   e. Based on the measurements, obtain an abdominal binder.
9. **Assist the patient to roll** to one side. Roll one end of the binder to the center mark. Place the rolled section of the abdominal binder underneath the patient. Position the binder appropriately between the costal margin and iliac crest.
10. **Make sure the binder** does not slip upward or downward.
    If the binder is positioned too high, it could impair lung expansion and gas exchange. If it is positioned too low, the binder will not provide adequate support.
11. **Assist the patient to turn** to the other side as you unroll the binder from underneath him. Pad any pressure areas or skin abrasions to avoid pressure injury.
12. **With your dominant hand, grasp the end of the binder** on the side farthest from you, and steadily pull toward the center of the patient's abdomen. With your nondominant hand, grasp the end of binder closest to you, and pull toward the center. Overlap the ends of the binder so that the hook and loop fasteners (e.g., Velcro) meet.

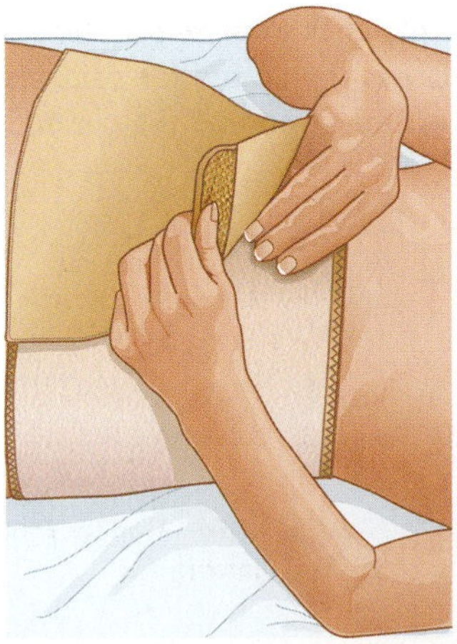

13. **Assess the abdominal binder** every 2 to 3 hours. Observe that the binder has not shifted up or down or compromised the patient's breathing. Remove it to assess the underlying skin and dressings. Change wound dressings if they are soiled, or as prescribed.

Procedure Variation: Applying a Triangular Arm Binder

A triangular arm binder or sling is used to support the upper extremities. Obtain a commercial sling (consisting of a sleeve for the arm and a strap to go around the neck) or a triangular piece of fabric. To form a splint from a triangular cloth, follow these steps:

14. **Ask the patient to place** the affected arm in a natural position across the chest, elbow flexed slightly.
    Slight flexion prevents swelling of the hand and relieves pressure on the shoulder.

15. **Place one end of the triangle** over the shoulder of the uninjured arm; allow the triangle to fall open so that the elbow of the injured arm is at the apex of the triangle.

16. **Move the sling** behind the injured arm.

17. **Pull up the lower corner** of the triangle over the injured arm to the shoulder of the injured arm.

18. **Tie the sling** with a square knot at the neck on the side of the arm requiring support.
    A square knot will not slip and is easy to untie.

19. **Adjust the injured arm** within the sling.
    To ensure patient comfort.

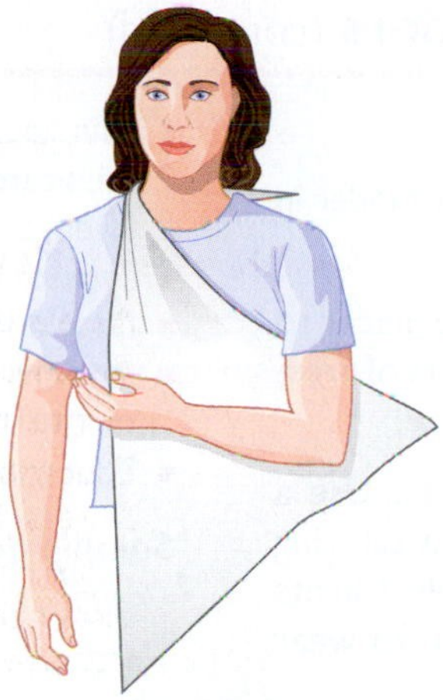

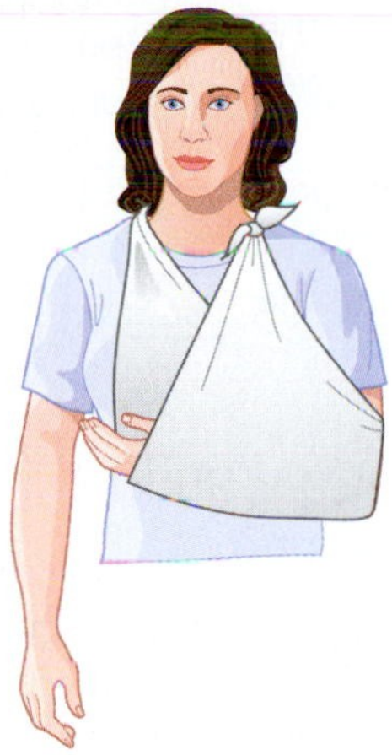

Procedure Variation: Applying a T-Binder

A T-binder is used to secure dressings or pads in the perineal area. A single T-binder is often used for women. A double T-binder is most commonly used for men. To apply a T-binder, follow these steps:

20. **Position the waist tails** under the patient at the natural waistline. Bring the right and left tails together; secure them at the waist with pins or clips.

21. **For a single T-binder,** bring the center tail up between the legs of the patient. Secure the tail at the waist with pins or clips.

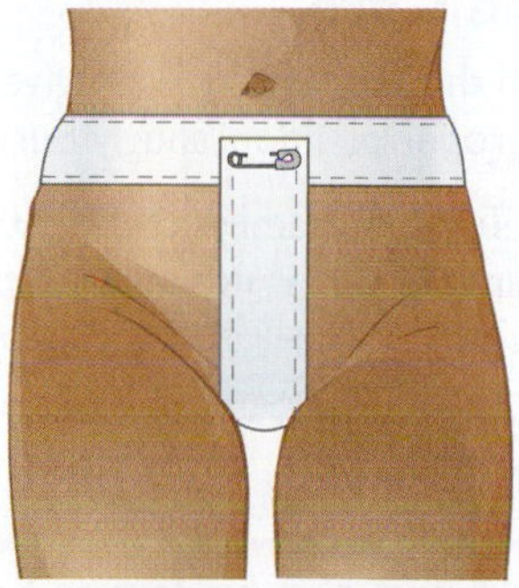

22. **For a double T-binder**, bring the tails up on either side of the penis. Secure the tail at the waist with pins or clips.

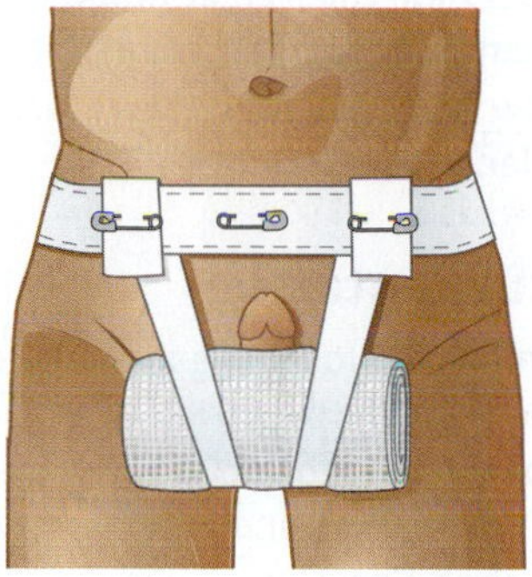

23. **Fasten the ties** at the waist using pins or clips.

? What if . . .

- **Your patient is obese?**

  Obtain the appropriate size binder before applying. Do not try to position a binder that is too small for the patient.
  A poorly fitting binder can constrict circulation, cause pressure points that can injure the skin, and restrict movement of the chest for adequate breathing. A binder that is too tight is uncomfortable, and it will not provide the proper support of an incision or wound needed for healing.

Evaluation

- Evaluate whether the patient's physical condition has changed since using the binder.
- Assess circulation to be sure the binder is not secured too tightly. Check color, warmth, tingling, sensation, and capillary refill.
- Assess the depth of breathing to be sure the binder is not restricting ventilation.
- Check the skin under the binder to be sure there are no areas of irritation, pressure, or skin abrasion.
- Assess incisions or wounds under the binder to be sure they are not bleeding and are healing properly.
- Monitor comfort regularly.
- Assess the client's ability to perform ADLs while wearing the binder.

(continued on next page)

Procedure 35-10 ■ Applying Binders (continued)

Home Care

- Teach the client and/or caregiver how to apply the binder in the proper position, snugly but not too tightly.
- Teach the family to inspect the site under the binder to be sure the skin is not pinched or with other points of pressure. This is especially crucial for older adults.
- Clean binders in warm, soapy water when soiled. Use a mesh laundry bag to keep the Velcro straps from catching other clothing in the washer. Air dry thoroughly. Clients should have two binders at home—a clean one to wear while the other is laundered.
- Apply and remove binder to promote comfort and ensure good circulation. This also allows the patient and caregiver to inspect any incision or wound underneath.
- Binders for children at home could be decorated with permanent marking pens.
- Allow children to help with applying and removing the binder.

Documentation

Document the following information (many agencies use specialized wound care flowsheets):

- Appearance and location of the wound or incision under the binder, type and amount of exudates, and odor, if present, after cleansing
- Pain level before and after the procedure. If the patient was medicated for pain, document the drug and dose used, time given, and patient response.
- Type of binder applied
- Date and time the binder was applied and removed
- Any change in the appearance of the wound or skin in contact with the binder
- Education provided to the patient

Sample documentation

01/23/22 1230 Abdominal binder applied. Vertical abdominal incision with dressing dry and intact. No sign of active bleeding or wound drainage noted. Oral pain medication given approximately 30 minutes before applying binder (see MAR). Pt reported pain at level 3 on a scale of 1 to 10 while applying binder but improved to a 1 afterward. No report of pressure points. Pt instructed to call if the binder feels too tight or too loose. — C. Marano, RN

Procedure 35-11 ■ Applying Bandages

➤ For steps to follow in *all* procedures, refer to the Universal Steps for All Procedures found on the page facing the inside back cover.

Equipment

- Appropriate bandage dressing
- Clean nonsterile gloves (2 pairs)
- Gauze sponges
- Normal saline
- Primary dressing (as prescribed)
- Scissors
- Tape or metal closures

Delegation

This procedure may be delegated to UAP who has the appropriate training. Assessment of the incision line or wound is a licensed professional's responsibility and cannot be delegated.

Pre-Procedure Assessments

- Determine the body part or area to be bandaged.
  This allows you to choose the correct width of gauze or elastic bandage to use.
- Assess the condition of the wound (if one is present).
  - Size (length, width, and depth in centimeters)
  - Location and depth of undermining or tunneling
  - Amount, character, and odor of drainage
  - Type and percentage of tissue present in wound bed (granulation, slough, fibrin, necrotic)
  - Periwound condition (intact, denuded, erythema, induration, or maceration)

  Wound dressings should be chosen based on the characteristics of the wound.
- Assess for pain
- Check the circulation of the underlying body parts before and after applying the bandage. Look for cool, pale, or cyanotic skin, tingling, and numbness.
  Circulation to an extremity can be compromised if the bandage is too tight or the extremity swells after application.
- Determine whether the client or family has the skills to reapply the bandage when necessary.
  Teaching might be needed for home care.

➤ When performing the procedure, always identify your patient according to agency policy, using two identifiers, and be attentive to standard precautions, hand hygiene, patient safety and privacy, body mechanics, and documentation.

Procedure Steps

Observe the following steps, regardless of the type of bandage you use:

1. **Choose a bandage** of the proper width. For example, use a 2.5-cm (1-in.) wide bandage for a finger, a 5-cm (2-in.) wide bandage for an arm, and a wider bandage for a leg.
   Prevents pressure and abrasion of the skin.
2. **Thoroughly clean and dry** the body part to be covered. Use a nontoxic cleansing solution, such as normal saline.
   Cleaning the wound removes debris, exudates, and bacteria. Drainage and moisture on the skin contribute to irritation.
3. **Remove excess moisture** by gently patting the wound and surrounding skin with gauze sponge.
   Drainage and moisture contribute to skin breakdown.
4. **Stand facing the patient.**
   In this position you can wrap the bandage evenly in the proper direction.
5. **Bandage the body part** in a comfortable position (e.g., with the joint slightly flexed), whenever possible.
   This prevents strain on ligaments and muscles. Movement of the extremity (extension) may cause skin damage if the bandage is too tight or the extremity is not properly positioned.
6. **Always work from distal** to proximal (or peripheral to central).
   This improves venous return and helps to prevent edema.
7. **If a wound is present,** apply a primary dressing, as prescribed, over the wound.
   A primary dressing is any dressing that is placed first in the wound bed. It provides exudates absorption, holds medications in place, provides antimicrobial coverage, or maintains a moist wound bed.
8. **Apply the bandage** with enough pressure to provide the needed support, but do not bandage too tightly. Make sure circulation to the area is not compromised.
9. **If possible, leave the fingers** (if you are bandaging an arm) or toes (if you are bandaging a leg or foot) exposed so that you can assess the circulation to the extremity. Begin the wrap along the pad of the foot or hand, just under the first bend of the toes or fingers (metatarsal or metacarpal joints).
10. **Begin the wrap** with the bandage against the skin. Unwind the bandage as if rolling it over the extremity.
    This helps to keep the bandage snug against the skin.
11. **Pad bony prominences** before bandaging if there are pressure concerns.
12. **Change bandages** whenever they become soiled or wet from external sources (stool, urine, etc.) and internal sources (drainage that has wicked on the outer surface of the bandage).
    Wound drainage contains chemicals, enzymes, and bacteria that can damage fragile healing tissues.
13. **After bandaging, assess** circulation and comfort.

Proceed to Step 14, 16, 19, 25, or 28, depending on the type of bandaging you are using.

Procedure Variation Circular Turns

Use this technique to wrap a finger or toe, or as an anchor at the beginning and end of another wrapping technique.

14. **With one hand, hold one end** of the bandage in place. With the other hand, encircle the body part two times with the bandage—the second wrap should partially cover the first wrap. At a 30° angle, continue to wrap the body part by overlapping two-thirds of the width of the bandage.
15. **Secure the bandage** with tape or fastener when you are finished, if circular turns are not being combined with another technique. ▼

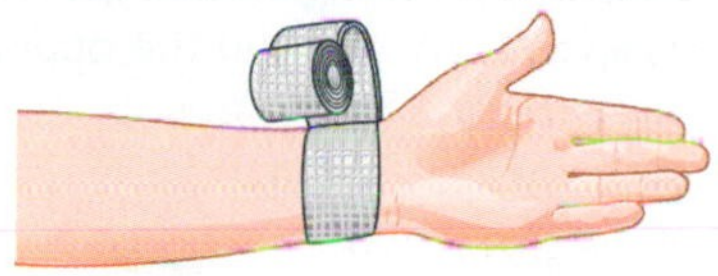

Procedure Variation Spiral Turns

Spiral turns are a variation of the circular turn technique. Spiral turns are most commonly used to wrap an extremity.

16. **Anchor the bandage** by making two circular turns—the second wrap completely covering the first one.
17. **Continue to wrap** the extremity by encircling the body part with each turn angled at approximately 30° so that you are overlapping the preceding wrap by two-thirds the width of the bandage.
18. **Complete the wrap** by making two circular turns and securing the bandage with tape or fastener. ▼

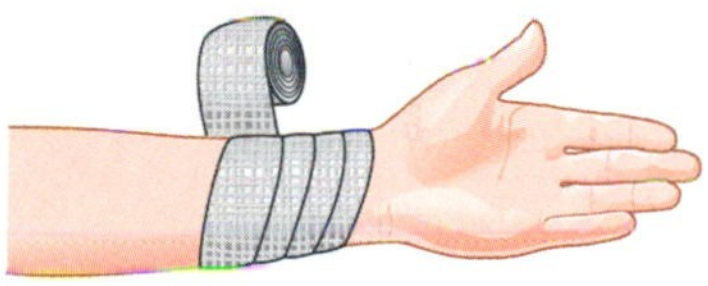

Procedure Variation Spiral Reverse Turns

Spiral reverse turns are used to bandage cylindrical body parts that are not uniform in size.

19. **Anchor the bandage** by making two circular turns.
20. **Bring the next wrap up** at a 30° angle, overlapping the wrap by two-thirds of the width of the bandage.
21. **Place the thumb** of your nondominant hand on the wrap to hold the bandage. ➤

(continued on next page)

Procedure 35-11 ■ Applying Bandages (continued)

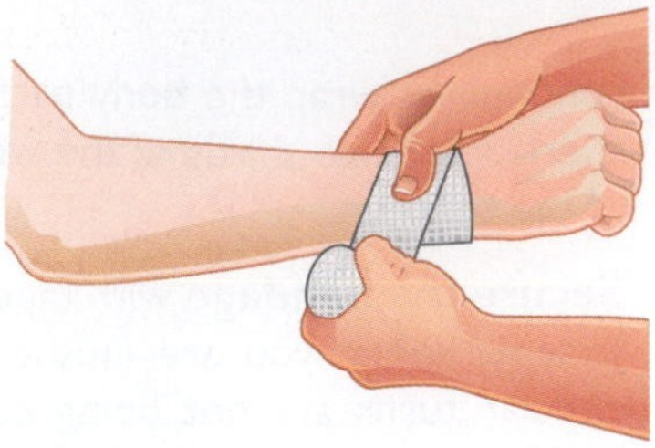

22. Fold the bandage back on itself; wrap at a 30° angle in the opposite direction.

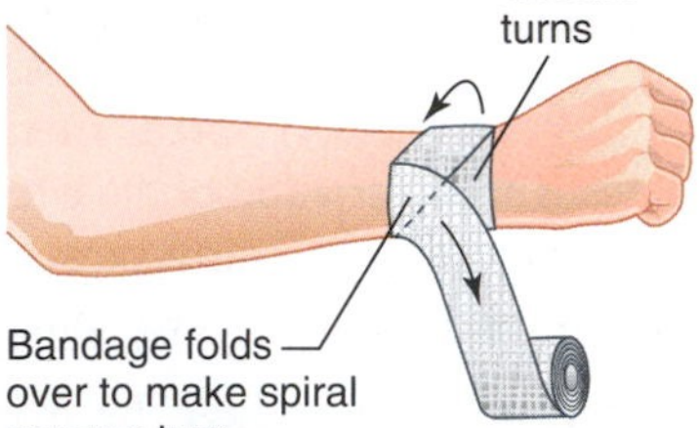

23. Continue to wrap the bandage, overlapping each turn by two-thirds. Align each bandage turn at the same position on the extremity.

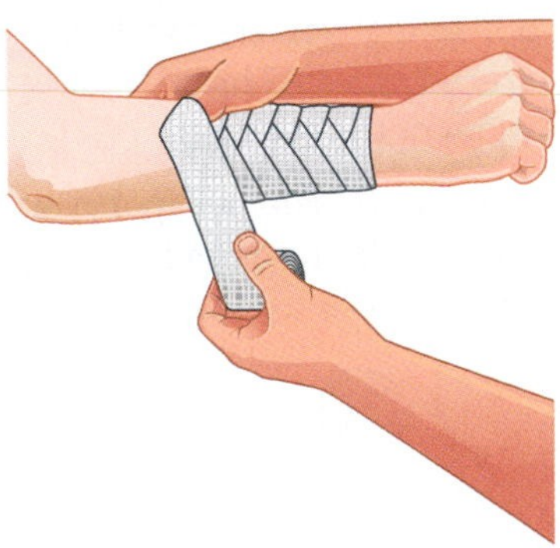

24. Complete the wrap by making two circular turns and securing the bandage with tape or fastener.

Procedure Variation Figure-8 Turns

The figure-8 wrap is used on joints (e.g., ankle, elbow).

25. Anchor the bandage by making two circular turns.

26. Wrap the bandage by ascending above the joint and descending below the joint to form a figure 8. Continue to wrap the bandage, overlapping each turn by two-thirds. Align each bandage turn at the same position on the extremity.

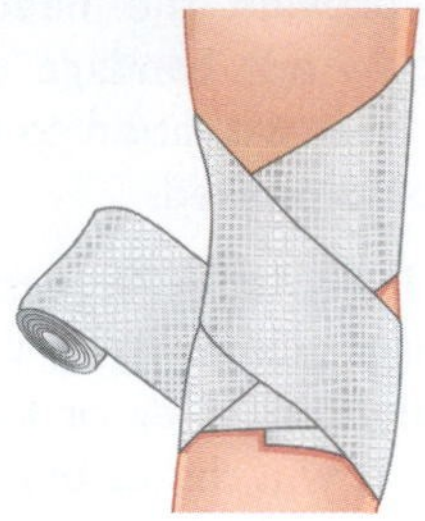

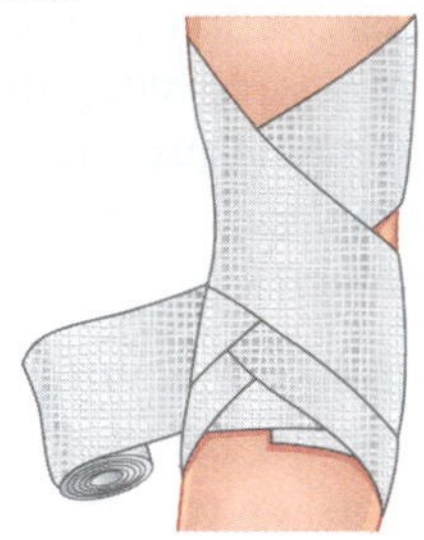

27. Complete the wrap by making two circular turns and securing the bandage with tape or fastener.

Procedure Variation Recurrent Turns

28. Anchor the bandage by making two circular turns.

29. Fold the bandage back on itself; hold it against the body part with one hand. With the other hand, make a half turn perpendicular to the circle turns and central to the distal end being bandaged.

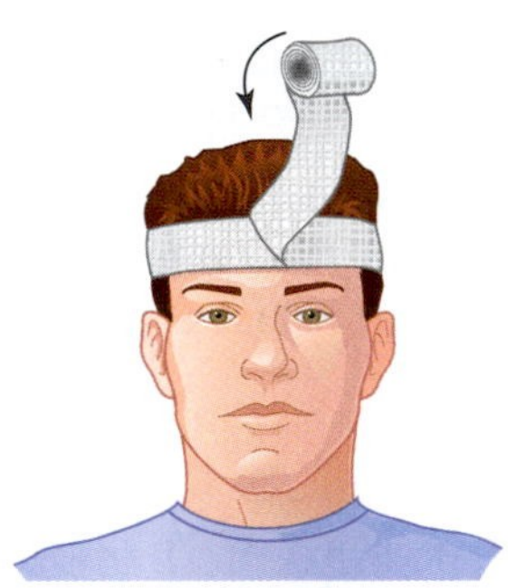

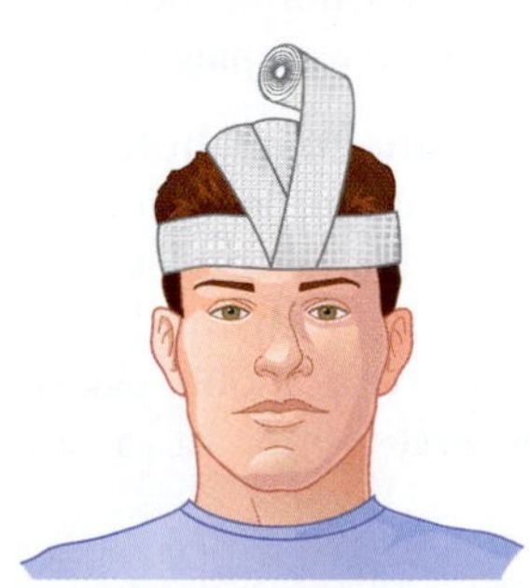

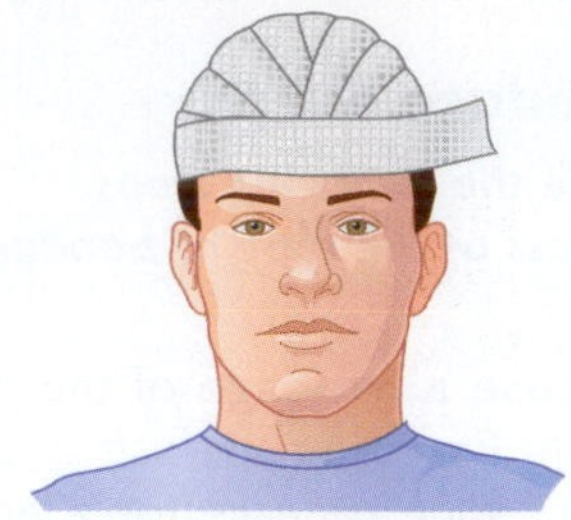

30. Hold the central turn with one hand; fold the bandage back on itself; bring it over the distal end of the body part to the right of the center, overlapping the center turn by two-thirds the width of the bandage.

31. Next, hold the bandage at the center with one hand as you bring the bandage back over the end to the left of center. Continue holding and folding the bandage back on itself, alternating right and left until the body part is covered. Overlap by two-thirds the bandage width with each turn.

32. Start and return each turn to the midline or center of the body part; angle it slightly more each time to continue covering the body part.

33. Complete the bandage by making two circular turns and securing the bandage with tape, clips, or fastener.

? What if . . .

- **Drainage breaks through the outer bandage more frequently than expected?**

  Determine the cause of the drainage if possible (i.e., is it blood or serum?). Increased drainage may be a sign of infection and should be evaluated. You might need to change the dressing more often or an alternate, more absorbent type of dressing may be needed.

  Wound exudates can harm healing tissues. Dressings that are saturated should be changed as soon as possible to prevent prolonged moisture exposure or maceration.

Evaluation

- Be sure the bandage is firmly wrapped without being too tight.
- Check the circulation is not compromised to the area distal of the bandage. Assess for color, temperature, sensation, movement, and capillary refill.
- Evaluate for numbness or pain around or distal to the bandaged area.

Patient Teaching

- Teach the patient about the expected healing process.
- Inform the patient and caregiver about signs and symptoms of infection and the need to report these findings.
- Instruct the patient and family about signs of circulation problems and how to remove the bandage if needed.

Home Care

- Refer the client to a home health agency for wound care.
- Some clients or caregivers may be able to perform dressing changes. Determine the client and/or caregiver's ability to perform dressing changes; teach and demonstrate as needed.

Documentation

Many agencies use wound care flowsheets.

- Appearance, size, color, and location of the wound, type and amount of exudates, and odor, if present, after cleansing.
- Level of pain before the procedure. If the patient was medicated for pain, document the drug and dose used, time given, and patient response.
- Method of cleansing the wound and surrounding skin, if performed
- Application of primary and secondary dressings
- Education provided to the patient
- Document neurovascular status distal to the bandage: color, temperature, sensation, movement, and capillary refill.

Sample EHR documentation

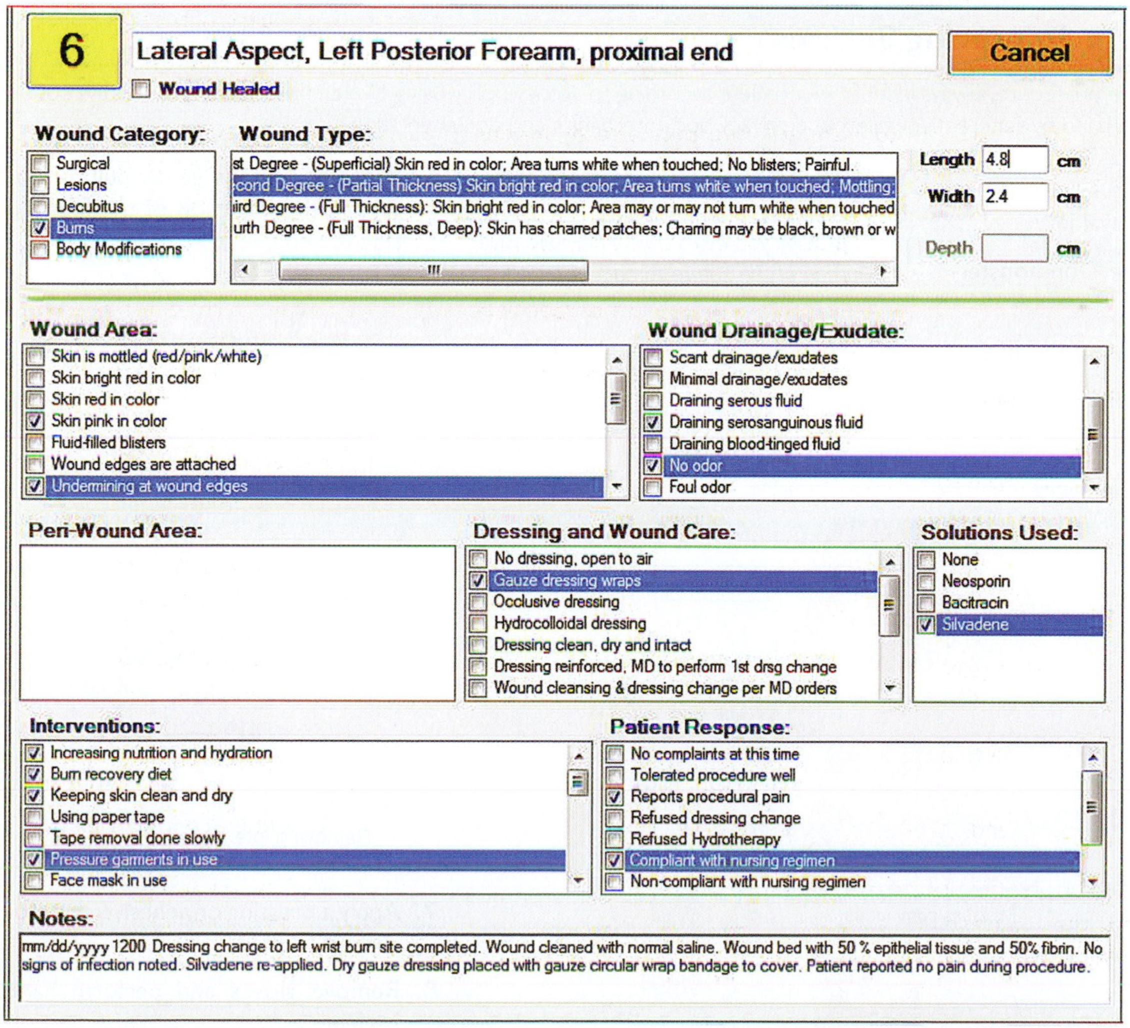

(continued on next page)

Procedure 35-11 ■ Applying Bandages (continued)

Practice Resources

Le Badour, G., Bergeron, J. D., Wesley, K. (2019).

Thinking About the Procedure

The video **Applying Bandages,** along with questions and suggested responses, is available on the ***Davis's Nursing Skills Videos*** Web site on FADavis.com.

Procedure 35-12 ■ Removing Sutures and Staples

➤ For steps to follow in all procedures, refer to the Universal Steps for All Procedures found on the page facing the inside back cover.

Equipment

- Nonsterile gloves
- Suture removal kit or sterile scissors and forceps (Procedure 35-12A)
- Staple remover (Procedure 35-12B)
- Gauze

Delegation

This procedure cannot be delegated to UAP. Assessment of the incision line or wound is a registered nurse's responsibility and cannot be delegated. The procedure requires assessment and judgment during removal and may require stopping the procedure if complications occur.

Pre-Procedure Assessment

- Assess staples to ensure none have rotated or turned instead of lying flat along the incision.

Procedure 35-12A ■ Removing Sutures

➤ When performing the procedure, always identify your patient according to agency policy, using two identifiers, and be attentive to standard precautions, hand hygiene, patient safety and privacy, body mechanics, and documentation.

Procedure Steps

1. Obtain a suture removal kit.
2. Perform hand hygiene. Don nonsterile gloves
3. Cleanse the wound or suture line.
4. Use the forceps to pick up one end of the suture.▼

Suture types

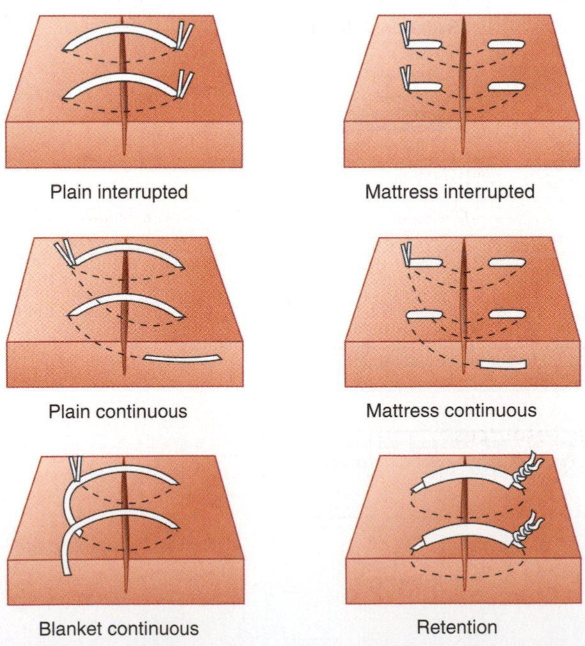

5. Slide the small scissors around the suture; cut near the skin.
   This helps you avoid pulling the exposed portion of the suture through the underlying tissue.
6. With the forceps, gently pull the suture in the direction of the knotted side to remove it.▼

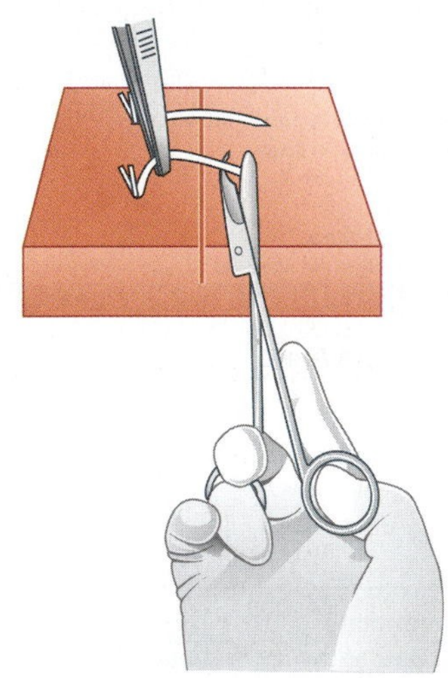

Removing interrupted sutures

7. Apply a dressing or adhesive skin closures if needed.
8. Remove gloves and perform hand hygiene.

Procedure 35-12B ■ Removing Staples

1. Perform hand hygiene. Don nonsterile gloves.
2. After cleansing the wound or incision, position the staple remover so that the lower jaw is on the bottom.
3. Place both tips of the lower jaw of the remover under the staple. ▼

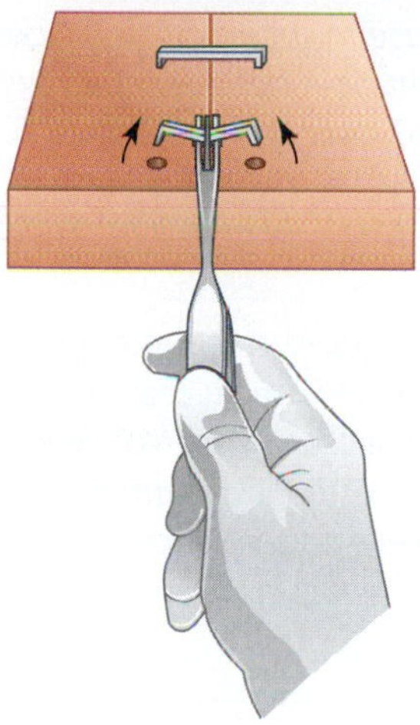

Removing staples

4. Ensure the staple is perpendicular to the plane of the skin. If not, reposition the staple with the tips of the lower jaw and apply gentle pressure, causing it to straighten the ends for easier removal.
5. Lift slightly on the staple ensuring that it stays perpendicular to the skin.
6. Continue to lift slightly as you gently squeeze the handles together to close.
   Spreads the ends of the staples apart, freeing them from the skin.
7. Lift the reshaped staple straight up from the skin.
8. Remove alternate staple; check the tension on the wound.
9. If there is no significant pull on the wound, remove the remaining staples.
   Where there are a large number of staples over an area of stress (abdomen, legs), the remaining staples are often removed a day or two later after ensuring the incision remains intact.
10. Place the removed staples on a piece of gauze.
    Staples are small and can be easily lost. Keeping them in one place prevents this.
11. Apply a dressing or adhesive closures, if needed.
12. Dispose of the removed staples in the sharps disposal container.
    Ends of the staples are sharp and should be handled with care.
13. Remove gloves and wash hands.

? What if . . .

- **A staple gets stuck?**
  Gently manipulate the staple with the remover until it is perpendicular to the skin.
  When the skin is stapled, the edges of the staple are crimped to hold the incision together. For the staple to be removed, those edges must be reshaped and straightened. If one edge of the staple is reshaped and the other is not, continuing to remove it can cause pain and tissue trauma.
- **The incision needs a dressing once the staples or sutures have been removed?**
  New surgical incisions should be covered with a sterile dressing the first 24 to 48 hours, but not necessarily after that time. Apply a dressing if you are concerned about soiling or per your institution's policy.
  In a healing incision, epithelial resurfacing is complete in 24 to 48 hours. Though only a few cells thick, this epithelium is enough to keep the wound closed and provide a bacterial barrier.

Evaluation

- Note whether the incision is well approximated after the procedure.
- Ensure that the patient verbalized understanding of the treatment.
- Inspect the wound daily.

Patient Teaching

- Teach the patient signs and symptoms of wound infections (e.g., redness, drainage) and the need to report these findings.
- Instruct the patient that he may be able to shower once sutures or staples are removed, if approved by the healthcare provider.

Documentation

Document the following information (many agencies use wound care flowsheets):

- Appearance and location of the wound, type and amount of exudates, and odor, if present, after cleansing
- The patient's level of pain before and after the procedure. If the patient was medicated for pain, document the drug and dose used, time given, and patient response.
- Method of cleansing the wound and surrounding skin, if performed
- Removal of staples or sutures. Note the number removed.
- Education provided to the patient

Sample documentation

02/23/22 1815 Staples removed from abdominal midline incision. Incision edges well approximated without erythema, drainage, or swelling. Dry dressing applied. Patient tolerated the procedure without discomfort. Discussed purpose of staple removal with patient. Will continue to monitor wound daily. ——————— M. Dali, RN

Practice Resources

Hin-Lun, L., & Hon-Ping, C. (2012).

Procedure 35-13 ■ Shortening a Wound Drain

➤ For steps to follow in *all* procedures, refer to the Universal Steps for All Procedures found on the page facing the inside back cover.

Equipment

- Nonsterile gloves
- Sterile gloves
- Sterile scissors
- Two safety pins or other clips (sterile)
- Sterile gauze

Delegation

Assessment of the incision line or wound and the drain is a registered nurse's responsibility and cannot be delegated. This procedure should not be delegated to UAP. The risking for accidentally losing the drain into the body or pulling it out of the wound is too high.

Pre-Procedure Assessments

- Inspect the site around the drain, noting skin excoriation, tenderness, erythema, warmth to the touch, and drainage seeping from the wound.
  Could indicate a wound infection or irritation of the drain at the skin site. Irritation can be the result of seeping drainage around the tube (e.g., if the tube diameter is not sufficient size to handle drainage output) or, more likely, an obstruction within the tubing.
- Assess the characteristics of the drainage, including color, volume of drainage, presence of blood, odor, pus, and any change in the type or amount of drainage through the tubing.
  A sudden decrease in drainage might indicate a blocked drain. Presence of fresh blood might be a sign of irritation within the wound. Pus and odor in the drainage could indicate wound infection.
- Check the suction apparatus to be sure it is functioning properly.
  A self-suction apparatus might need to be recompressed from time to time to maintain effective vacuum. Electric suction units can fail, delivering too much suction, which can lead to injury. Too little suction can contribute to insufficient drainage, which can lead to pressure on sutures if present, or cause the wound to become infected or heal more slowly.

➤ When performing the procedure, always identify your patient according to agency policy, using two identifiers, and be attentive to standard precautions, hand hygiene, patient safety and privacy, body mechanics, and documentation.

Procedure Steps

1. **Perform hand hygiene and don nonsterile gloves.** Remove wound dressings.
2. **Remove soiled gloves** and discard in a moisture-proof biohazard collection container.
3. **Open sterile supplies** (scissors, etc.).
4. **Don sterile gloves**; use sterile scissors to cut halfway through a sterile gauze dressing (for later use) or use a sterile precut drain dressing.
5. **If the drain is sutured in place**, use sterile scissors to cut the suture.
6. **Firmly grasp the full width** of the drain at the level of the skin and pull it out by the prescribed amount (e.g., 5 cm [2 in.]).
7. **Insert a sterile safety pin** through the drain at the level of the skin. Hold the drain tightly between your fingers, and insert another pin above your fingers.
   The pin keeps the drain from disappearing into the wound.

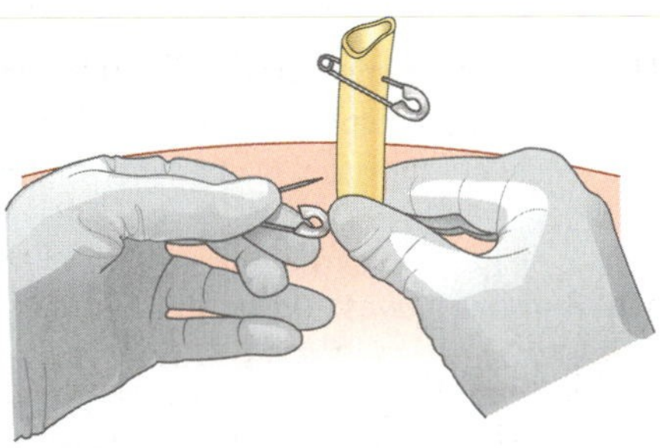

8. **Using sterile scissors, cut** the drain about 2.5 cm (1 in.) above the skin and pin. ▼

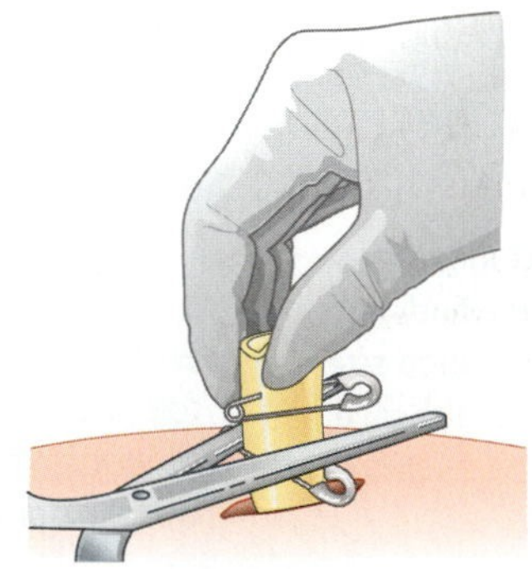

9. **Cleanse the wound,** using sterile gauze swabs and the prescribed cleaning solution. In some situations, you may use sterile forceps to manipulate the swabs.
10. **Apply precut sterile gauze** around the drain; then redress the wound. ▼

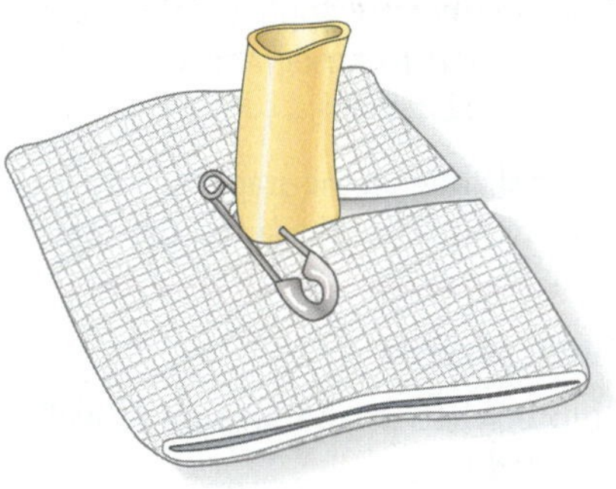

11. **Remove gloves** and discard in a biohazard container. Perform hand hygiene.
12. **Leave the patient** in a safe and comfortable position.

? What if . . .

- **You shorten the drain too much?**
  Immediately notify the surgeon who placed the drain.
  The drain will need to be evaluated to be sure it remains intact, which it mostly likely will. Drainage tubing is secured under the skin surface and will probably not be dislodged with shortening.

Evaluation

- Assess the local area of skin around the drain after manipulating it.
- Note the patency of the drain after shortening it.
- Be sure the drain is secure after shortening.
- Evaluate for complications occurring related to shortening procedure.

Patient Teaching

- Patients should not shorten their own drains. Consult a healthcare provider if concerned about the length of tubing or drains.

Documentation

- Record the intervention.
- Note the amount and characteristics of the drainage.
- Document the appearance of the wound.
- Note any complications that occur with shortening a drain (e.g., manipulation of tubing causes bleeding or drainage at the site).

Sample documentation

10/11/22 0930 Penrose shortened by 2.5 cm per post-op orders. Drain intact and not draining. Skin surrounding Penrose slightly erythematous but not warm to touch. Pt. denies tenderness. Pt tolerated procedure without complication. ——————— M. Garcia, RN

Thinking About the Procedure

The video **Shortening a Wound Drain**, along with questions and suggested responses, is available on the ***Davis's Nursing Skills Videos*** Web site on FADavis.com.

Procedure 35-14 ■ Emptying a Closed-Wound Drainage System

➤ For steps to follow in *all* procedures, refer to the Universal Steps for All Procedures found on the page facing the inside back cover.

Equipment

- Drainage container with graduated markings
- Nonsterile gloves
- Biomedical waste disposal sink
- Biohazard disposal receptacle

Delegation

This procedure may be delegated to UAP trained in the skill. Assessment of the wound and drainage characteristics is a licensed professional's responsibility and cannot be delegated.

Pre-Procedure Assessments

- Assess the appearance of the drainage tube site and sutures, if in place.
- Inspect for warmth, edema, redness, or pus where tubing penetrates the skin.
- Check to be sure the closed-wound drainage system is securely fastened at the connections and within the wound.
- Determine whether suction (electric, portable, or manual) is working properly.

➤ When performing the procedure, always identify your patient according to agency policy, using two identifiers, and be attentive to standard precautions, hand hygiene, patient safety and privacy, body mechanics, and documentation.

Procedure Steps

1. **Read the instructions** about the drainage device.
   Procedures vary among manufacturers and different systems.
2. **Don nonsterile gloves** and goggles or mask.
3. **Unfasten the drainage device** from the patient's gown.
   The drainage device is often pinned to the patient's gown to prevent it from dislodging.

(continued on next page)

Procedure 35-14 ■ Emptying a Closed-Wound Drainage System (continued)

4. **Open the drainage port**; empty the drainage into a small graduated container.

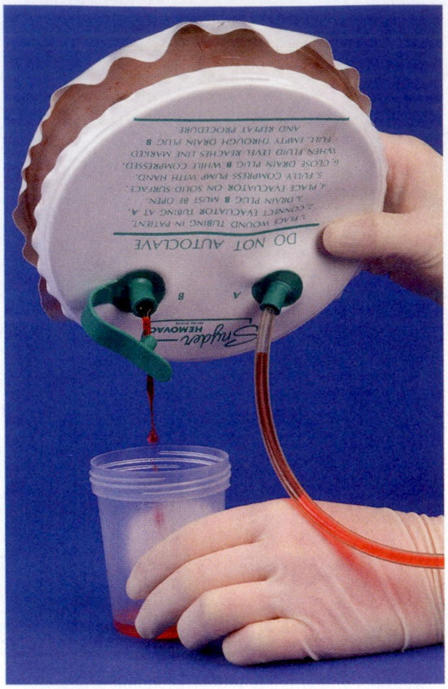

5. **With the port still open,** place the collection device on a firm, flat surface (e.g., the over bed table).

6. **Use the palm of one hand** to press down on the device and eject air from it. Do not stand directly over the air vent. Do not touch the drainage port.
   It can splash or bubble.

7. **Use your other hand to scrub** the port and plug with an alcohol-based antiseptic or povidone-iodine swab (Betadine), if the patient is not allergic to iodine.

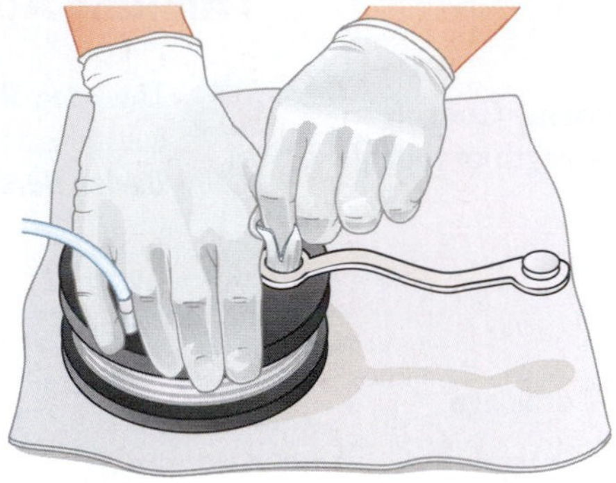

8. **Continuing to press down** on the device, replace the plug in the port. Do not touch the open port or the part of the plug that goes into the port.
   Creates a constant, negative pressure vacuum to facilitate suction.

9. **Attach the drainage device** to the patient's gown.
   Pinning keeps it secure and prevents it from accidentally dislodging.

10. **Measure the drainage** in the graduated container; discard drainage in the disposable container or sink for biohazardous material. Wash the graduated container. Do not stand in front of an air vent while doing so.
    Forced air in the room can cause the drainage to splash or bubble, introducing biohazardous material into the environmental air.

11. **Remove your gloves.** Perform hand hygiene.

12. **Document** in the patient's health record.

? What if . . .

- **The wound drainage spills?**

Don nonsterile gloves and protective clothing. Keep people away from the spill area. If sharps are present, remove with forceps. Contain the spill with absorbent pads and place all used materials in a red biohazard bag. Use an approved disinfectant. When finished place all materials including gloves and gowns in the bag and dispose of in the biohazard area.
Proper handling of contaminated biomedical materials is important to prevent transmission of infectious organisms.

Home Care

- Teach family members who are emptying drainage systems at home to wear gloves and avoid touching the drainage port.

Documentation

- Note the date and time the drainage system is emptied.
- Record the volume lost. Report excess fluid loss to the healthcare provider.
- Describe the appearance of drainage, including presence of blood or purulent material.

Sample documentation

03/12/2022 0750 Hemovac drained 18 mL serosanguineous fluid over 12 hours. No odor or purulent material noted at drainage site. ——— R. Ferretti, RN

Practice Resources

Memorial Sloan Cancer Center. (2016).

Thinking About the Procedure

The video **Emptying a Closed-Wound Drainage System,** along with questions and suggested responses, is available on the ***Davis's Nursing Skills Videos*** Web site on FADavis.com.

CLINICAL INSIGHTS

Clinical Insight 35-1 ➤ Applying Local Heat Therapy

Preparation

- Determine whether there are any contraindications to the treatment, such as impaired circulation, bleeding, wound complications, or inability to tolerate the treatment.
- Explain the application and rationale to the patient.

Moist Heat (Irrigations, Compresses, Hot Soaks)

If skin is intact:

- Soak a washcloth or towel in warm water (105°F to 115°F [40°C to 46°C]) and wring out the excess before applying to the skin. Reapply and change water frequently.
  To maintain a constant temperature.

For open areas, use a compress, a soak, or a bath:

- To make a compress, soak gauze in the heated solution (105°F to 115°F [40°C to 46°C]), and then apply it to the wound. Usually, you will use sterile gloves, gauze, and solution.
- Reapply compresses or towels; change the water frequently to maintain a constant temperature.
  Heat disperses quickly.
- **For a soak** you will need to immerse the affected area. Sterilized tubs are often used for this procedure.
- **A sitz bath** soaks the patient's perineal area. A special tub or chair may be used. Because of infection control concerns, disposable sitz baths are preferred. Check that the water temperature is from 105°F to 110°F (40°C to 43°C). Instruct the patient to soak for 15 minutes.

Dry Heat (Electric Heating Pads, Disposable Hot Packs, Hot Water Bags)

Aquathermia pads (also called K-pads) are plastic or vinyl pads that circulate water in the interior.

- Connect the pad via tubing to the electric heating unit, which constantly exchanges water that has been heated to the specified temperature.
- Fill the reservoir about two-thirds full of distilled water.
- Set the temperature control to 98°F to 105°F (37°C to 40.5°C).
- Cover the pad with a towel or fitted sleeve, and apply it to the body part.
  To prevent tissue injury.

Disposable Hot Packs and Hot Water Bags or Bottles

- Use water that is 115°F to 125°F (46°C to 52°C).
- Fill the bag about two-thirds full of warm tap water, expel the air from the bag, and close the top.
- Tip the bag upside down to test for leaking.
- Wrap the bag in a towel or fitted sleeve; place it on the patient.
- Never place a heat source directly on the patient's skin. Burns can occur.

Electric Heating Pads

- Be sure that the body part is dry or that the pad has a waterproof cover.
- Do not use pins (e.g., to hold a cover in place) or other sharp objects on the pad.
  The pin could go through a wire and cause an electric shock.
- Tell the patient to report any discomfort during the treatment.
- For home use, warn the patient about the danger of burns from high settings. Use pads with a switch that cannot be turned up.
- Avoid direct contact with the heating device. Cover the heat source with a washcloth, towel, or fitted sleeve.

General Safety Precautions for Applying Heat

- Never place a heat source (e.g., pad, bag) directly on the patient's skin. Burns can occur.
- Do not place the heating device (pad, bag) under the patient; place it over the body part.
  Helps prevent burns.
- Apply heat intermittently, leaving it on for no more than 15 minutes at a time in an area.
  This helps prevent tissue injury (e.g., burns, impaired circulation). It also makes the therapy more effective by preventing the rebound phenomenon: At the time the heat reaches maximum therapeutic effect, the opposite effect (vasoconstriction) begins.
- Check the skin frequently for extreme redness or blistering.
- When heat or cold is first applied, the thermal receptors react strongly, and the person feels the temperature intensely. Over about 15 minutes, the receptors adapt to the new temperature, and the person notices it less. Caution clients not to change the temperature when this occurs because doing so can cause tissue injury.
- Assess for hypotension and faintness. If they occur, discontinue the treatment. Have the patient lie down for several minutes, and check her BP. When the faint feeling passes, assist her to sit up slowly. Recheck the BP in the sitting position. If the BP remains low, encourage her to remain seated. If the patient is ambulatory, have her dangle her feet for several minutes before getting up.

Clinical Insight 35-2 ➤ Applying Local Cold Therapy

For patient safety, observe the following precautions when applying

- Check the skin frequently for extreme redness, blistering, cyanosis (blueness), or blanching. When heat or cold is first applied, the thermal receptors react strongly, and the person feels the temperature intensely. Over about 15 minutes, the receptors adapt to the new temperature, and the person notices it less. Caution clients not to change the temperature when this occurs because doing so can cause tissue injury.

Preparation

- Determine whether there are any contraindications to the treatment, such as impaired circulation, bleeding, wound complications, or inability to tolerate the treatment.
- Explain the application and rationale to the patient.
- Assess for indications for cold application (e.g., fever above 104°F [40°C]). Measure the patient's temperature.

Cooling Baths

A cooling bath is often used to treat a high fever (above 104°F [40°C]). It promotes heat loss through conduction and vaporization.

- Prepare a pan of water with a temperature from 65°F to 90°F (18°C to 32°C).
- You may add a fan to increase heat loss if the temperature is markedly elevated.
- Slowly sponge the face, arms, legs, back, and buttocks with the cool water. Do not dry the areas; cover with a damp towel.
- Take about 30 minutes to complete the bath.
  Cooling the body too rapidly will cause shivering, which will increase heat production.
- You may also place ice bags or cold packs on the forehead, in the axillae, and the groin.
- Assess the patient constantly during a cooling bath.
  If the patient begins to shiver, the temperature may actually begin to rise.

Cold Compresses

- Apply a cool, damp cloth or towel to the body part.
- Renew the compress or cloth frequently.
  The temperature of the compress or cloth will rapidly rise toward body temperature.

Ice Collars, Ice Bags, Commercially Prepared Cold Packs, Aquapads

- You can make an ice bag out of a nonsterile glove or small plastic bag by filling it with ice chips and tying a knot in the top.
- Fill the ice bag with ice chips or an alcohol-based solution.
- Cover ice bags or packs with a towel or soft cover to protect the skin.
- Apply to the skin for a maximum of 15 minutes, and then remove. You may reapply the cold pack in 1 hour.

Safety Precautions for Applying Cold

- Measure water temperature with a bath thermometer.
- Tell the patient to report any discomfort during the treatment.
- Avoid direct contact with the cooling device. Cover the cold pack with a washcloth, towel, or fitted sleeve.
- Apply cold intermittently, leaving it on for no more than 15 minutes at a time in an area.
  Helps to prevent tissue injury (e.g., impaired circulation). It also makes the therapy more effective by preventing the rebound phenomenon: At the time the cold reaches maximum therapeutic effect, the opposite effect (vasodilation) begins.
- Observe for tissue damage: bluish purple mottled appearance of the skin, numbness, and sometimes blisters and pain.
- Monitor for elevated blood pressure.

ASSESSMENT GUIDELINES AND TOOLS

Focused Assessment

History Questions for Skin and Wound Assessment

- ➤ What is your typical activity level?
- ➤ Do you ever use a wheelchair or mobile device to get around? Do you require assistance to get out of bed or a chair?
- ➤ Tell me about your usual diet.
- ➤ How much liquid do you drink each day?
- ➤ Do you have any areas of numbness and tingling?
- ➤ Have you had any recent changes in your skin?
- ➤ Do you have any sores or open areas? If so, how long have you had the wound?
- ➤ Have you ever had difficulty with wound healing?
- ➤ What kinds of healthcare problems have you been experiencing?
- ➤ What medications—prescribed, herbal, or over the counter—are you taking?
- ➤ What is your typical hygiene routine?
- ➤ Do you ever lose control of your bladder or bowels?
- ➤ Do you smoke?
- ➤ How much time do you spend outdoors?
- ➤ Do you have diabetes? If so, how often do you check your feet? How often do you see a podiatrist? What is your average blood sugar?

Focused Assessment

Physical Examination: Wound Assessment

All Wounds

Assess all wounds for the following:

Location

Describe the location of the wound in anatomical terms. For example, you would describe an incision from cardiac surgery as a midsternal incision extending from the manubrium to the xiphoid process.

Size

- Measure the length and width of the wound in centimeters.
- To measure wound depth, gently insert a sterile cotton-tipped applicator into the deepest part of the wound. Measure the applicator from the skin level to the tip.
- If possible, use photo documentation, indicating the dimensions on the photo. This is especially useful in the case of a wound with an irregular border.

Appearance

Your description of the appearance of the wound should be very detailed. You must describe the following:

- ***Type of wound*** *(open or closed)*
- ***If the wound is sutured,*** examine the closure. Are the wound edges approximated? Is there tension on any aspect of the wound? Are the stitches intact?
- ***The color of the wound.*** Redness and inflammation for the first 2 to 3 days is normal, but erythema or swelling beyond that time may indicate infection.
- ***Condition of the wound bed (in an open wound).*** A beefy red, moist appearance is evidence of healing. A pale color or dry texture indicates a delay in healing.
- ***Examine for necrosis, slough, and eschar.*** Examine for a tunnel or sinus tract in the wound bed; if there is one, inspect and probe it for depth and characteristics.
- ***The skin surrounding the wound.*** Observe for skin discoloration, hematoma, or additional injury to the surrounding tissue. Observe for maceration, tunneling, crepitus, blistering, or erythema. Examine the edges of the wound for epithelial tissue and contraction. Look for undermining beneath the wound margins.

Drainage

- ***Presence of drainage or exudate.*** Describe the color, consistency, amount, and odor.
- ***Assess the quantity of wound drainage*** by weighing dressings before they are applied and again when they have been removed. The change in weight reflects the amount of drainage that they have absorbed.
- ***If a drain is present,*** measure the amount of fluid in the collection container.
- ***Odor*** may indicate fistula formation or contamination with bacteria. If a new odor develops, assess carefully for presence of a fistula.

Patient Responses

Ask your patients about pain, discomfort, or itching related to the wound or wound care.

Assessing an Untreated Wound

Your assessment should determine what, if any, additional professional support is necessary. Assess the following same aspects as for treated wounds above: location, size, appearance, description of drainage, condition of wound margins, condition of surrounding skin, and effect of the wound on the patient. In addition, assess the following:

- ***Bleeding.*** If bleeding is profuse, apply direct pressure to the site. If bleeding continues after you apply pressure for 5 minutes or if blood is spurting from the wound, call the physician immediately.
- ***Severity of the wound.*** A gaping wound or a deep wound with fat, fascia, or muscle exposed will need additional care.
- ***Last tetanus immunization.*** Immunization should be given if (1) the last immunization was 10 years ago or longer, (2) the wound is contaminated with dirt or debris and the tetanus injection was given more than 5 years ago, or (3) it is uncertain when the patient last received an immunization.
- ***Whether the wound was caused by a bite.*** Determine whether the wound was caused by any type of bite, animal or human. A deep bite wound usually requires additional observation and/or antibiotics.
- ***Pain.*** Assess for pain. Any wound causing severe pain requires a comprehensive evaluation.
- ***Numbness or loss of movement.*** If any deficit is detected, the patient will need immediate evaluation.
- ***Presence of chronic medical conditions.*** Examples include diabetes, malnutrition, immunocompromise, a bleeding disorder. Patients with conditions that affect wound healing will need ongoing evaluation.

The Braden Scale for Predicting Pressure Sore Risk

BRADEN SCALE FOR PREDICTING PRESSURE SORE RISK

Patient's Name ____________ Evaluator's Name____________ Date of Assessment

SENSORY PERCEPTION ability to respond meaningfully to pressure-related discomfort	**1. Completely Limited** Unresponsive (does not moan, flinch, or grasp) to painful stimuli, due to diminished level of consciousness or sedation. OR limited ability to feel pain over most of body.	**2. Very Limited** Responds only to painful stimuli. Cannot communicate discomfort except by moaning or restlessness OR has a sensory impairment which limits the ability to feel pain or discomfort over $^1/_2$ of body.	**3. Slightly Limited** Responds to verbal commands, but cannot always communicate discomfort or the need to be turned. OR has some sensory impairment which limits ability to feel pain or discomfort in 1 or 2 extremities.	**4. No Impairment** Responds to verbal commands. Has no sensory deficit which would limit ability to feel or voice pain or discomfort.				
MOISTURE degree to which skin is exposed to moisture	**1. Constantly Moist** Skin is kept moist almost constantly by perspiration, urine, etc. Dampness is detected every time patient is moved or turned.	**2. Very Moist** Skin is often, but not always moist. Linen must be changed at least once a shift.	**3. Occasionally Moist:** Skin is occasionally moist, requiring an extra linen change approximately once a day.	**4. Rarely Moist** Skin is usually dry, linen only requires changing at routine intervals.				
ACTIVITY degree of physical activity	**1. Bedfast** Confined to bed.	**2. Chairfast** Ability to walk severely limited or non-existent. Cannot bear own weight and/or must be assisted into chair or wheelchair.	**3. Walks Occasionally** Walks occasionally during day, but for very short distances, with or without assistance. Spends majority of each shift in bed or chair.	**4. Walks Frequently** Walks outside room at least twice a day and inside room at least once every two hours during waking hours.				
MOBILITY ability to change and control body position	**1. Completely Immobile** Does not make even slight changes in body or extremity position without assistance.	**2. Very Limited** Makes occasional slight changes in body or extremity position but unable to make frequent or significant changes independently.	**3. Slightly Limited** Makes frequent though slight changes in body or extremity position independently.	**4. No Limitation** Makes major and frequent changes in position without assistance.				
NUTRITION usual food intake pattern	**1. Very Poor** Never eats a complete meal. Rarely eats more than $^1/_2$ of any food offered. Eats 2 servings or less of protein (meat or dairy products) per day. Takes fluids poorly. Does not take a liquid dietary supplement OR is NPO and/or maintained on clear liquids or IVs for more than 5 days.	**2. Probably Inadequate** Rarely eats a complete meal and generally eats only about $^1/_2$ of any food offered. Protein intake includes only 3 servings of meat or dairy products per day. Occasionally will take a dietary supplement. OR receives less than optimum amount of liquid diet or tube feeding.	**3. Adequate** Eats over half of most meals. Eats a total of 4 servings of protein (meat, dairy products per day. Occasionally will refuse a meal, but will usually take a supplement when offered OR is on a tube feeding or TPN regimen which probably meets most of nutritional needs.	**4. Excellent** Eats most of every meal. Never refuses a meal. Usually eats a total of 4 or more servings of meat and dairy products. Occasionally eats between meals. Does not require supplementation.				
FRICTION & SHEAR	**1. Problem** Requires moderate to maximum assistance in moving. Complete lifting without sliding against sheets is impossible. Frequently slides down in bed or chair, requiring frequent repositioning with maximum assistance. Spasticity, contractures or agitation leads to almost constant friction.	**2. Potential Problem** Moves feebly or requires minimum assistance. During a move skin probably slides to some extent against sheets, chair, restraints or other devices. Maintains relatively good position in chair or bed most of the time but occasionally slides down.	**3. No Apparent Problem** Moves in bed and in chair independently and has sufficient muscle strength to lift up completely during move. Maintains good position in bed or chair.					
				Total Score				

Source: U.S. Department of Health and Human Services. (1992). *Clinical practice guideline. Pressure ulcers in adults: Prediction and prevention* (pp. 16–17). PPPPUA Publication No. 92-0047. Rockville, MD: Public Health Service. Copyright © Barbara Braden and Nancy Bergstrom, 1988. Reprinted with permission.

The Norton Pressure Sore Risk Assessment Scale

Norton Scale for Assessing Risk of Pressure Ulcers

	Physical Condition		Mental Condition		Activity		Mobility		Incontinent		
	Good	4	Alert	4	Ambulant	4	Full	4	Not	4	Total Score
	Fair	3	Apathetic	3	Walk/help	3	Slightly limited	3	Occasional	3	
	Poor	2	Confused	2	Chair-bound	2	Very limited	2	Usually/urine	2	
	Very bad	1	Stupor	1	Bed	1	Immobile	1	Doubly	1	
Name/Date											

The Norton Scale uses five criteria to assess patients' risk for pressure ulcers. Scores of 14 or less indicate liability to ulcers; scores of <12 indicate very high risk.

Source: Norton, D., McLaren, R., & Exton-Smith, A. N. (1975). *An investigation of geriatric nursing problems in hospitals.* Edinburgh, Scotland: Churchill Livingstone. Used with permission.

The PUSH Tool for Evaluation of Pressure Ulcers

PUSH Tool - Version 3.0

Patient Name:____ Patient ID#:__________

Ulcer Location: _______________________________________ Date:__________

DIRECTIONS:

Observe and measure the pressure ulcer. Categorize the ulcer with respect to surface area, exudate, and type of wound tissue. Record a sub-score for each of these ulcer characteristics. Add the sub-scores to obtain the total score. A comparison of total scores measured over time provides an indication of the improvement or deterioration in pressure ulcer healing.

Length x Width	0 0 cm^2	1 <0.3 cm^2	2 0.3 - 0.6 cm^2	3 0.7 - 1.0 cm^2	4 1.1 - 2.0 cm^2	5 2.1 - 3.0 cm^2	**Subscore**
		6 3.1 - 4.0 cm^2	7 4.1 - 8.0 cm^2	8 8.1 - 12.0 cm^2	9 12.1 - 24.0 cm^2	10 > 24 cm^2	
Exudate Amount	0 None	1 Light	2 Moderate	3 Heavy			**Subscore**
Tissue Type	0 Closed	1 Epithelial Tissue	2 Granulation Tissue	3 Slough	4 Necrotic Tissue		**Subscore**
							Total Score

Length x Width: Measure the greatest length (head to toe) and the greatest width (side to side) using a centimeter ruler. Multiply these two measurements (length • width) to obtain an estimate of surface area in square centimeters (cm^2). **Caveat**: Do not guess! Always use a centimeter ruler and always use the same method each time the ulcer is measured.

Exudate Amount: Estimate the amount of exudate (drainage) present after removal of the dressing and before applying any topical agent to the ulcer. Estimate the exudate (drainage) as none, light, moderate, or heavy.

Tissue Type: This refers to the types of tissue that are present in the wound (ulcer) bed. Score as a "4" if there is any necrotic tissue present. Score as a "3" if there is any amount of slough present and necrotic tissue is absent. Score as a "2" if the wound is clean and contains granulation tissue. A superficial wound that is reepithelializing is scored as a "1". When the wound is closed, score as a "0".

4 - Necrotic Tissue (Eschar): black, brown, or tan tissue that adheres firmly to the wound bed or ulcer edges and may be either firmer or softer than surrounding skin.
3 - Slough: yellow or white tissue that adheres to the ulcer bed in strings or thick clumps, or is mucinous.
2 - Granulation Tissue: pink or beefy red tissue with a shiny, moist, granular appearance.
1 - Epithelial Tissue: for superficial ulcers, new pink or shiny tissue (skin) that grows in from the edges or as islands on the ulcer surface.
0 - Closed/Resurfaced: the wound is completely covered with epithelium (new skin).

Note: Refer to the NPUAP Website (www.npuap.org) for further information regarding development and use of the PUSH Tool.

Version 3.0: 9/15/98

PRESSURE ULCER HEALING CHART

(use a separate page for each pressure ulcer)

Patient Name:______________________________ Patient ID#:__________

Ulcer Location: ______________________________ Date:______________

Directions: Observe and measure pressure ulcers at regular intervals using the PUSH Tool. Date and record PUSH Sub-scale and Total Scores on the Pressure Ulcer Healing Record below.

	PRESSURE ULCER HEALING RECORD													
DATE														
Length × Width														
Exudate Amount														
Tissue Type														
Total Score														

Graph the PUSH Total Score on the Pressure Ulcer Healing Graph below.

PUSH Total Score	PRESSURE ULCER HEALING GRAPH													
17														
16														
15														
14														
13														
12														
11														
10														
9														
8														
7														
6														
5														
4														
3														
2														
1														
Healed 0														
DATE:														

Version 3.0: 9/15/98

Source: National Pressure Ulcer Advisory Panel (NPUAP). (1998). Pressure ulcer scale for healing (PUSH) Tool, version 3.0. Retrieved from http://www.npuap.org/wp-content/uploads/2012/03/push3.pdf

DIAGNOSTIC TESTING

Diagnostic Testing

Tests for Assessing Wounds

Test	Normal Range	Comments
Leukocyte (WBC) count	4,500–11,000/mm^3	Usually done as a part of a complete blood count (CBC) but may be ordered as an independent test. White blood cells (WBCs) may increase when a wound develops; continued elevation may signal infection. A low WBC count may delay wound healing. Leukocytes are responsible for an inflammatory reaction at the wound site, phagocytosis of bacteria and cellular debris, and the creation of antibodies.
Serum protein *Serum albumin* *Serum prealbumin*	6.0–8.0 g/dL 3.4–4.8 g/dL 12–42 mg/dL	Low serum levels indicate limited nutritional stores that delay wound healing or place the patient at high risk for pressure injuries. Serum protein may be monitored as an indicator of the ability to heal a wound or prevent a pressure injury. Serum protein and albumin levels are closely related. However, both fluctuate slowly. A more accurate measure of a patient's immediate protein stores is reflected in the prealbumin level.
Erythrocyte sedimentation rate (ESR)	<50 years old: 0–15 mm/hr >50 years old: 0–20 mm/hr	In the presence of an inflammatory and necrotic process, blood proteins are altered. This test indicates whether the red blood cells (RBCs) stick together, become heavier, and settle at the bottom of a tube when held vertically.
Coagulation studies: Partial thromboplastin time, activated (aPTT)	Varies with respect to equipment and reagents used. Critical values: >70 seconds or <53 seconds	Prolonged coagulation times may result in excessive blood loss or ongoing bleeding in the wound bed. Shortened coagulation times increase the risk for blood clot formation problems, such as deep vein thrombosis, pulmonary embolus, or stroke.
Prothrombin time (clotting time)	Critical values: >20 seconds (uncoagulated) or 3 times normal control (anticoagulated)	Altered coagulation may result from anticoagulant medications, a concurrent illness, trauma, or reaction to transfusions.
International normalized ratio (INR)	<2.0 for patients not receiving anticoagulation therapy; 2.0–3.0 for those receiving coagulation therapy	A standardized test to evaluate clotting times, considered the gold standard.
Wound cultures	Negative; no growth of pathogens	Wound cultures may be prescribed to determine the types of bacteria present in the wound. Cultures may be obtained by swab, aspiration, or tissue biopsy. A positive culture may not indicate an infection as chronic wounds are colonized with bacteria.
Tissue biopsy	Negative; no growth of pathogens	Wounds are not considered infected unless the bacteria count exceeds 100,000 organisms per gram of tissue. Exception: The presence of beta-hemolytic streptococci in any number indicates infection.

STANDARDIZED LANGUAGE

Standardized Language

Selected Standardized Outcomes and Interventions for Skin and Wound Diagnoses

Patient Situation (Data/Defining Characteristics)	NANDA-I Diagnosis	NOC Outcomes	Selected Indicators	Selected NIC Interventions and Specific Activities
Mrs. Whitefeather is 95 years old. She has cancer and has stopped eating and become very thin. Recently she has become too weak to move about in bed without help. However, her skin is intact with no redness, even over her bony prominences. She has a very low score on the Braden Pressure Ulcer Assessment Scale.	Risk for Impaired Skin Integrity	Tissue Integrity: Skin & Mucous Membranes *Other outcomes:* ➤ Immobility Consequences: Physiological ➤ Nutritional Status: Food & Fluid Intake ➤ Nutritional Status: Nutrient Intake	(5–Not compromised) Hydration Tissue perfusion Skin integrity (5–None) Erythema Blanching Skin lesions	***Bedrest Care*** ➤ Keep bed linen clean, dry, and wrinkle free. ➤ Facilitate small shifts of body weight. ***Pressure Injury Prevention*** ➤ Monitor any reddened areas closely. ➤ Turn every 1–2 hours, as appropriate. ➤ Turn with care (e.g., avoid shearing) to prevent injury to fragile skin. ➤ Post a turning schedule at the bedside, as appropriate. ➤ Avoid massaging over bony prominences. ➤ Utilize specialty beds and mattresses, as appropriate. ➤ Avoid use of "donut" types of devices in the sacral area. ***Other Interventions*** ➤ Nutrition Management ➤ Positioning ➤ Pressure Management ➤ Skin Surveillance
Mason Allen is 4 years old. He has a severe case of poison ivy, which has made blisters on his skin. He has been scratching and has bleeding, excoriated areas over his limbs, face, and trunk.	Impaired Skin Integrity	Tissue Integrity: Skin & Mucous Membranes *Other outcomes:* ➤ Infection ➤ Immune Hypersensitivity Response	(4–Mildly compromised) Skin integrity (4–Mild) Skin lesions Erythema (3–Moderate) Itching Localized inflammatory response	***Wound Care*** ➤ Monitor characteristics of the wound, including drainage, color, size, and odor. ➤ Cleanse with normal saline or a nontoxic cleanser, as appropriate. ➤ Apply an ointment to the skin/lesion, as appropriate or prescribed. ➤ Instruct the child and family member(s) about wound care procedures and signs of infection.

(Continued)

Standardized Language

Selected Standardized Outcomes and Interventions for Skin and Wound Diagnoses—cont'd

Patient Situation (Data/Defining Characteristics)	NANDA-I Diagnosis	NOC Outcomes	Selected Indicators	Selected NIC Interventions and Specific Activities
				Other Interventions ➤ Pruritus ➤ Management ➤ Skin Surveillance ➤ Wound Irrigation
Sabreen Hassen is an adolescent with paralysis to her lower extremities. She has a stage 2 pressure injury on her left heel.	Impaired Tissue Integrity	Wound Healing: Secondary Intention *Other outcomes:* Tissue Integrity: Skin & Mucous Membranes	(4–Substantial) Granulation Decreased wound size (4–Limited) Purulent drainage Surrounding skin erythema Wound inflammation Foul wound odor	*Pressure Injury Care* ➤ Débride the ulcer, as needed. ➤ Cleanse the ulcer with the appropriate nontoxic solution, working in a circular motion from the center. ➤ Cleanse the skin around the pressure injury with mild soap and water. ➤ Monitor for infection in the wound. ➤ Position every 1–2 hours to avoid prolonged pressure. *Other Interventions* ➤ Wound Care ➤ Pressure Management ➤ Infection Protection ➤ Medication ➤ Administration

Sources: Butcher, H. K., Bulechek, G. M., Dochterman, J. M., & Wagner, C. (2018). *Nursing intervention classification (NIC)* (7th ed.). St. Louis, MO: Elsevier. Used with permission; Johnson, M., Moorhead, S., Bulechek, G., et al. (2012). *NOC, and NIC linkages to NANDA-I and clinical conditions.* (3rd ed.). St. Louis, MO: Elsevier; Moorhead, S., Swanson, E., Johnson, M., & Maas, M. (Eds.). (2018). *Nursing outcomes classification (NOC)* (6th ed.). St. Louis, MO: Elsevier. and NANDA International. (2017). *Nursing diagnoses: Definitions and classification 2018-2020.* Philadelphia, PA: Author.

CLINICALJUDGMENT

Applying the Full-Spectrum Nursing Model

PATIENT SITUATION

Tio Santos is a 66-year-old obese man with diabetes and hypertension who is being seen for a wound on his right foot that doesn't seem to be healing. He injured his foot when repairing drywall at home. He is otherwise relatively sedentary at home. The wound is oozing, swollen, tender, and warm to the touch. Mr. Santos is now running a low-grade fever of 100.4°F at home. He tells you his foot is very painful, especially with any weight-bearing, and throbs when he is sitting or lying still. You measure the wound bed to be 6 cm × 4 cm and note purulent exudate at the distal edge. He is referred to an outpatient wound care center for treatment.

THINKING

1. *Theoretical Knowledge:*
   a. What is the Braden scale and why might it be used for Mr. Santos?
   b. What risk factors for delayed wound healing does Mr. Santos have?
2. *Critical Thinking (Considering Alternatives, Deciding What to Do):*
   a. To care for Mr. Santos's wound, should you use sterile gloves, clean nonsterile gloves, or no gloves? Explain your thinking.

DOING

3. *Practical Knowledge (Assessment):*
   a. What symptoms of infection does Mr. Santos have?
   b. To be certain the wound is infected, what would you need to know or do?

CARING

4. *Self-Knowledge:* Imagine you have had a wound on your foot for 6 weeks. It has not healed and you have all Mr. Santos's symptoms and, in fact, are in his situation. What would be the most troublesome symptom in your daily life? What would worry you the most?

Critical Thinking and Clinical Judgment

1. You are caring for a 22-year-old man who is paralyzed from the waist down secondary to an automobile accident. He has been admitted to the hospital with a urinary tract infection manifested by a fever of 102°F (39°C) and lethargy. His family reports he has been withdrawn and sits in his wheelchair watching TV all day long.
   a. What risk factors does this patient have for skin breakdown?
   b. What locations of his body should you be most concerned about in regard to pressure injury formation?
   c. What actions should you take to decrease the risk of pressure injury in this man? What further information do you need?
2. A 63-year-old man is admitted to your unit after an emergency appendectomy. His appendix was ruptured, and the surgeon has left the wound open to heal by secondary intention. A Jackson–Pratt drain is in place in the wound bed. A moderate amount of purosanguineous drainage is visible in the drain. The surgeon has ordered saline-moistened gauze packing every 4 hours.
   a. What actions should you take as you prepare to do the first dressing change?
   b. How will you secure the dressing?
3. For the following patients, write a nursing diagnosis related to skin integrity. Include problem, etiology, and defining characteristics. If you do not have enough data for one of those components, state what additional data you need.
   a. Mrs. Whitefeather is 95 years old. She has cancer, and she has stopped eating and has become very thin. Recently she has become too weak to move about in bed without help. However, her skin is intact with no redness, even over her bony prominences. She has a very low score on the Braden Scale for Predicting Pressure Sore Risk.
   b. Mason Allen is 4 years old. He has a severe case of poison ivy and has blisters on his skin. He has been scratching and has bleeding, excoriated areas over his limbs, face, and trunk.
   c. Sabreen Hassen has a stage 2 pressure injury on her left heel.

4. For each of the following concepts, use critical thinking to describe how or why it is important to nursing, patient care, or skin integrity and wound healing. Note that these are *not* to be merely definitions.

Shearing

Friction

Pressure

Wound healing process

Preventing pressure injury

Wound assessment

Dressing changes

What Are the Main Points in This Chapter?

- The layers of the skin are the epidermis (outermost), the dermis, and the subcutaneous layer (innermost).
- The major functions of the skin are protection of the internal organs, unique identification of an individual, thermoregulation, metabolism of nutrients and metabolic waste products, and sensation.
- Age, mobility, nutrition, hydration, moisture underlying conditions, medications, contamination or infection, diminished sensation, cognitive impairment, hygiene, and lifestyle are factors that influence the ability to maintain intact skin and heal wounds.
- If there are no breaks in the skin, a wound is described as **closed**. A wound is considered **open** if there is a break in the skin or mucous membranes.
- Acute wounds may be intentional (e.g., surgical incisions) or unintentional (e.g., from trauma) and are expected to be of short duration.
- Wounds that exceed the anticipated length of recovery are classified as chronic wounds. Chronic wounds include pressure, arterial, venous, and diabetic ulcers. A chronic wound may linger for months or years.
- **Clean wounds** are uninfected wounds with minimal inflammation. **Clean-contaminated wounds** are surgical incisions that enter the gastrointestinal, respiratory, or genitourinary tracts. **Contaminated wounds** include open, traumatic wounds or surgical incisions in which a major break in asepsis occurred. **Infected wounds** are wounds with evidence of infection, such as presence of microorganisms.
- A wound that involves minimal or no tissue loss and has wound edges that are approximated are said to heal by primary intention.
- A wound that involves extensive tissue loss and has margins that cannot be approximated, or is infected, heals by secondary intention.
- Tertiary intention healing, or delayed primary closure, occurs when two surfaces of granulation tissue are brought together. Initially the wound is allowed to heal by secondary intention.
- Healing occurs in three stages. The **inflammatory phase** lasts from 1 to 5 days and consists of two major processes: hemostasis and inflammation. The **proliferative phase** occurs from days 5 to 21. It is characterized by cell development aimed at filling the wound defect and resurfacing the skin. The **maturation phase** begins in the second or third week and continues until the wound is completely healed.
- Wound closure methods include adhesive strips (Steri-Strips), absorbent sutures, surgical staples, and surgical glue.
- Drainage is the flow of fluids from a wound or cavity. It is often referred to as exudate (fluid that oozes as a result of inflammation).
- Complications of wound healing include hemorrhage, infection, dehiscence, evisceration, and fistula formation.
- Pressure injury is caused by unrelieved pressure over time that compromises blood flow to tissue, resulting in ischemia in the underlying tissue.
- **A stage 1 pressure injury** is an area of persistent redness and does not blanch.
- **A stage 2 pressure injury** involves partial-thickness skin loss of the epidermis, dermis, or both.
- **A stage 3 pressure injury** is characterized by full-thickness skin loss involving damage or necrosis of subcutaneous tissue, which may extend down to, but not through, the underlying fascia. The ulcer appears as a deep crater.
- **A stage 4 pressure injury** involves full-thickness skin loss with extensive destruction; tissue necrosis; or damage to muscle, bone, or support structures. Undermining and sinus tracts (blind tracts underneath the epidermis) are common.
- Extrinsic factors leading to pressure injuries are those that alter the skin and tissue integrity and blood supply (e.g., aging, low blood pressure, neurological injury, poor nutrition, edema, and fever).

- Extrinsic factors include friction and shearing, and exposure to moisture and pressure.
- Not all lower extremity ulcers are related to pressure. Some are caused by poor perfusion, such as venous stasis ulcers, diabetic foot ulcers, and arterial ulcers.
- An eschar is a black leathery covering of necrotic tissue. An ulcer covered by an eschar cannot be classified because it is impossible to determine the depth.
- The Braden, Norton, and PUSH scales evaluate risk for problems with skin integrity.
- When assessing a wound, note the following: the type of wound, the color of the wound and surrounding skin, the condition of the wound bed, drainage and odor, and the level of pain associated with the wound or wound care.
- Prevention of pressure injury includes skin care, nutrition, turning and positioning, using therapeutic mattresses and cushions, and patient/family teaching.
- Five types of débridement are used: sharp, mechanical, enzymatic, autolytic, and biotherapy (maggot débridement).
- Wound care therapies to promote healing might include negative pressure wound therapy, electrical stimulation, tissue growth factors, ultrasound, bioengineered skin substitutes, and surgical options.
- Primary dressings are ones that are placed in the wound bed and have contact with the wound. A secondary dressing covers or holds a primary dressing in place. Many dressings can act as both.
- Types of wound dressings are absorption, alginate, antimicrobial, collagen, gauze, foam dressings, hydrocolloid, hydrogel, skin sealants, and moisture barriers.
- Ideal wound irrigation pressures range from 4 psi to 15 psi. Current recommendations are to use a 35-mL syringe attached to a 19-gauge angiocatheter. This will deliver the solution at approximately 8 psi.
- Heat application promotes vasodilatation, increases tissue metabolism, increases capillary permeability, reduces blood viscosity, and reduces muscle tension.
- The application of cold causes vasoconstriction, local anesthesia, reduced cell metabolism, increased blood viscosity, and decreased muscle tension.

Knowledge Map

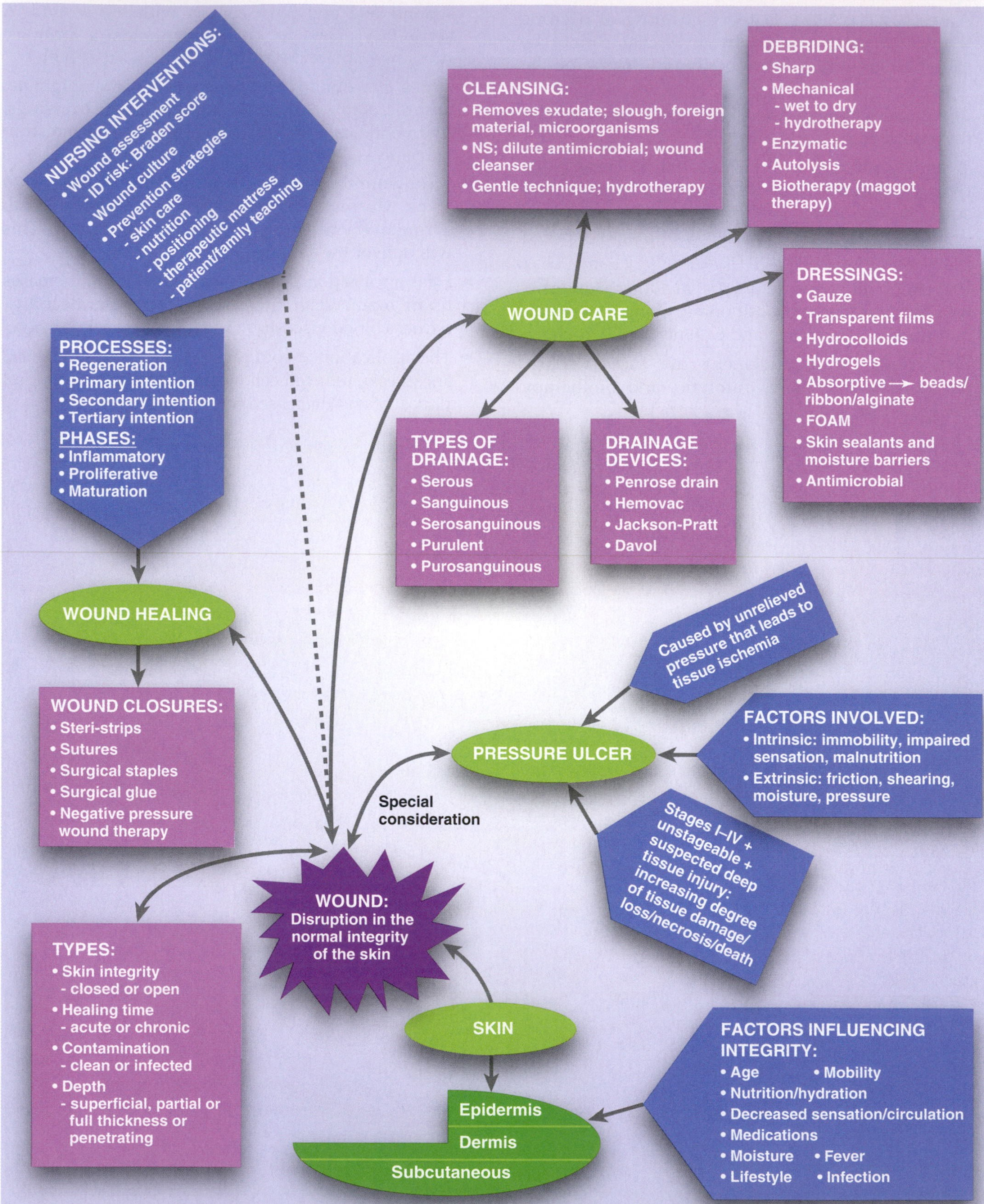

CHAPTER 36

Oxygenation

STUDENT RESOURCES

The questions and exercises in this book allow you to practice the kind of thinking you will use as a full-spectrum nurse. Critical-thinking questions usually have more than one right answer, so we do not provide "correct answers" for these features. Try to answer these questions yourself. It is more important to develop your nursing judgment than to just cover content. You will learn more by discussing the questions with your peers. If you are still unsure, see the Davis Advantage chapter resources for suggested responses.

To explore learning resources for this chapter,

Go to Davis Advantage and find:

Answers and Suggested Responses for all questions in this chapter

Concept Map

Knowledge Map

References and Bibliography

Lists of NOC Outcomes and NIC Interventions

Key Concepts

Oxygenation

Respiration

Ventilation

Related Concepts

See the Concept Map on Davis Advantage.

Example Problems

Pneumonia

URI and Influenza

Caring for the Nguyens

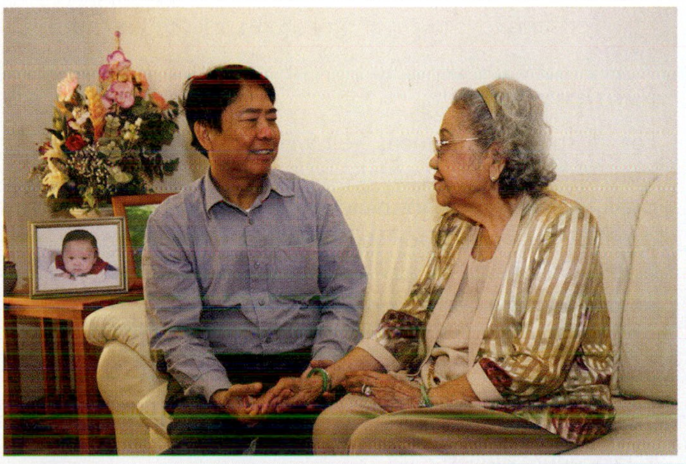

Mai Nguyen, Nam's 76-year-old mother, has been complaining of fatigue and a persistent cough for approximately 2 weeks. Nam has brought his mother to the family clinic where you are a nurse. Mrs. Nguyen appears disheveled. Her clothes are rumpled and her hair is tousled. Normally she is dressed neatly and wearing makeup. She has a hard time signing in at the desk and tells the receptionist she has a 1:00 p.m. appointment, but it is 9:00 a.m. Mrs. Nguyen's vital signs are as follows: BP, 142/90 mm Hg; pulse, 94 beats/min and regular; respirations 24 breaths/min and labored; temperature, 99.6°F (37.5°C) oral.

(Continued)

Caring for the Nguyens (continued)

A. What additional assessment data would be useful to gather at this time?

B. During her visit at the clinic, you notice that Mrs. Nguyen is very confused. Her weight has dropped 7 pounds since her visit last month, her mucous membranes are dry, and she is dyspneic with any activity. She is diagnosed with pneumonia. Because of her rapid decline, Mrs. Nguyen is admitted to the hospital to receive intravenous antibiotics. At the hospital, her initial pulse oximetry reading is 90%, and she is unable to cough up secretions. Write the most appropriate nursing diagnosis to focus interventions for Mrs. Nguyen.

C. What actions should you anticipate taking?

D. The hospitalist (hospital-based physician) writes prescriptions for IV fluids, antibiotics, suction prn, and continuous pulse oximetry. What additional prescriptions will you need to provide care for Mrs. Nguyen? What therapy would you suggest?

E. Mrs. Nguyen requires suctioning to help remove secretions. She has a weak cough and crackles and rhonchi throughout all lung fields. There are few secretions in her oropharynx, and she bites down on the catheter. What technique would you use to suction her? Explain your choice.

F. After 4 days in the hospital, Mrs. Nguyen is discharged to home. She asks the hospital nurse, "What can I do to make sure I never get that sick again?" How would you answer this question?

PracticalKnowledge clinical application

As you perform the procedures, apply the concepts and other theoretical knowledge you learned in Volume 1. This section will help you acquire the skills to safely provide for clients' oxygenation needs.

PROCEDURES

In this section you will find procedures necessary for supporting oxygenation. Some, but not all, of the procedures in this section can be delegated to qualified unlicensed assistive personnel (UAPs). Refer to the delegation notes in each procedure and to agency policies.

Procedure 36-1 ■ Collecting a Sputum Specimen

➤ For steps to follow in *all* procedures, refer to the Universal Steps for All Procedures found on the inside back cover.

Equipment

For all sputum specimens, you will need a patient identification label, a completed laboratory requisition form, and a small plastic bag with a biohazard label (or container designated by the agency) for delivering the specimen to the laboratory. Depending on how you obtain the specimen, you also need the following:

Procedure 36-1A: Collecting an Expectorated Sputum Specimen

- Sterile specimen container with lid
- Procedure gloves
- Glass of water
- Emesis basin
- Tissues
- Pillow (if abdominal or chest incision is present)

Procedure 36-1B: Collecting a Suctioned Sputum Specimen

- Sterile suction catheter or sterile suction kit
- Suction device (portable or wall)
- Sterile gloves
- Protective eyewear
- Inline sputum specimen container or trap
- Sterile saline solution
- Oxygen therapy equipment, if indicated
- Linen-saver pad or towel

Delegation

You can delegate collection of an expectorated sputum specimen to a UAP who has been adequately trained in performing the skill. Assess the patient's respiratory status first; if the patient's condition is unstable, do not delegate the procedure. Do not delegate obtaining a specimen by tracheal suctioning.

Pre-Procedure Assessments

- Assess the patient's comprehension of the procedure.
  Understanding allays anxiety and promotes cooperation.
- Assess breath sounds; respiratory rate, depth, and pattern; skin and nailbed color; and tissue perfusion.
  You may need to delay sputum collection if the patient is in respiratory distress.
- Assess ability to deep-breathe, cough, and expectorate.
  If the patient is unable to deep-breathe, cough, and expectorate, suctioning may be necessary to obtain an adequate sputum specimen.
- Determine when the patient last ate or had a tube feeding, especially for a specimen obtained by suction.
  Specimen collection should be delayed for 1 to 2 hours after eating because the procedure may cause vomiting, which creates a risk for aspiration of stomach contents.
- If suctioning is required to obtain the specimen, check for factors such as anticoagulant therapy, bleeding disorders, or low platelet count.
  These factors place the patient at risk for bleeding when the suction catheter is introduced.

➤ When performing the procedure, always identify your patient according to agency policy, using two identifiers, and be attentive to standard precautions, hand hygiene, patient safety and privacy, body mechanics, and documentation.

Procedure Steps

1. **Verify the medical prescription** for type of sputum analysis.
   The type of sputum specimen determines the number of specimens required and the time of day the specimen should be collected. For example, specimens to confirm tuberculosis typically require three consecutive morning samples.
2. **Position the patient** according to the required specimen collection technique.
   a. *For an expectorated specimen*, assist the patient to high or semi-Fowler's position or to a sitting position at the edge of the bed.
   b. *For a suctioned specimen*, position the patient in high or semi-Fowler's position.
   These positions facilitate insertion of the suction catheter and the ability to cough. They also promote lung expansion, and prevent aspiration should the patient vomit during the procedure.
3. **Drape a towel or linen-saver pad** over the patient's chest. Ask the patient to rinse his mouth and gargle with water.
   A towel or pad protects the patient's gown from soiling during specimen collection. Rinsing the mouth removes flora that may contaminate the specimen; however, evidence is not conclusive on this point.
4. **If the patient has an abdominal or chest incision, have the patient splint the incision with a pillow.**
   Splinting the incision decreases discomfort when the patient coughs.

Procedure 36-1A ■ Collecting an Expectorated Sputum Specimen

Procedure Steps

Follow Steps 1 through 4, above.

5. **Provide the patient with** the specimen container. Advise the patient to avoid touching the inside of the container. If you must hold the container for her, first don procedure gloves.
   The inside of the container should remain sterile. Wear gloves because you may come in contact with secretions or airborne bacteria when the patient coughs and expectorates. ▼

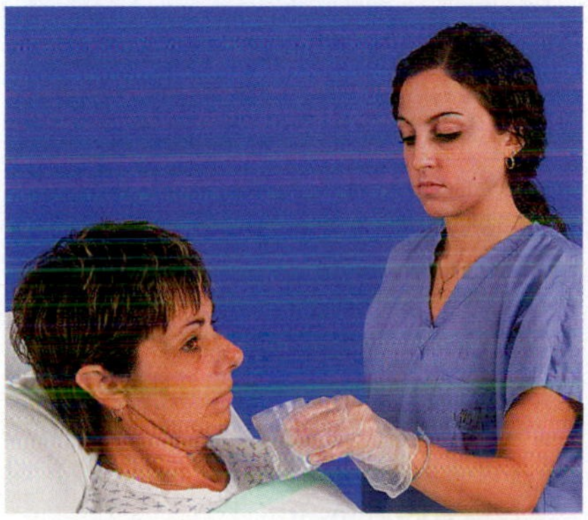

6. **Ask the patient to breathe** deeply for three or four breaths, and then ask him after a full inhalation to hold his breath and then cough.
   Deep breathing opens airways and stimulates the cough reflex. Coughing after a full inhalation creates enough force to mobilize secretions through the airways and into the pharynx.
7. **Instruct the patient to expectorate** the secretions directly into the specimen container.
   Prevents specimen contamination from outside organisms.

(continued on next page)

Procedure 36-1 ■ Collecting a Sputum Specimen (continued)

8. **Tell the patient to repeat deep breathing** and coughing until an adequate sample is obtained.
Typically 5 to 10 mL of sputum is required to ensure adequate sputum analysis.

9. **Don procedure gloves** if you are not already wearing them; cover the specimen container with the lid immediately after the specimen is collected.
Gloves protect you in the event the patient's coughing has contaminated the outside of the container. Covering the container immediately prevents spread of microorganisms.

10. **After the patient expectorates,** offer tissues and provide mouth care.
Promotes patient comfort.

11. **Label the specimen container** with patient identification label that contains the name of the test, and collection date and time.
Correctly identifying the specimen ensures accurate diagnosis and treatment.

12. **Place the specimen in** a plastic bag with a biohazard label. Attach a completed laboratory requisition form.
The plastic bag protects healthcare workers from exposure to microorganisms. The laboratory requisition form ensures proper processing of the specimen.

13. **Send the specimen** to the laboratory immediately, or refrigerate it if transport might be delayed.
If bacterial cultures are delayed, contaminating organisms may grow, producing false culture results and possibly inappropriate treatment.

Procedure 36-1B ■ Collecting a Suctioned Sputum Specimen

Procedure Steps

Follow Steps 1 through 4, above.

5. **Administer oxygen** to the patient, if indicated.
Suctioning may cause hypoxemia.

6. **Prepare the suction device**, and make sure it is functioning properly.

7. **Don protective eyewear.**
Protects your eyes from splattering of secretions during suctioning.

8. **Attach the suction tubing** to the male adapter of the inline sputum specimen container.

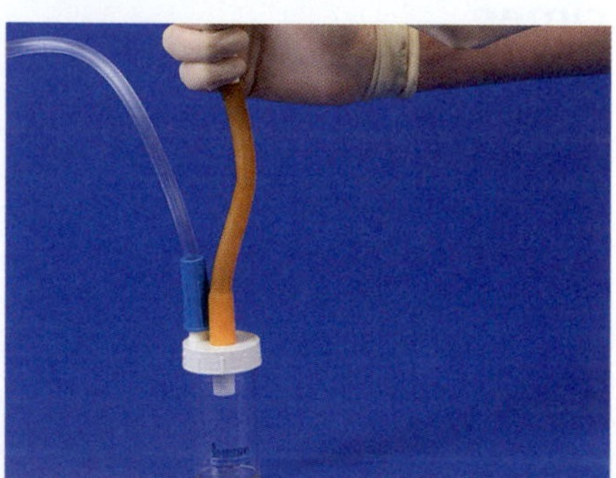

9. **Don sterile gloves.**
Protects the patient's sterile airways from contamination by outside organisms.

10. **Attach the sterile suction** to the flexible tubing on the sputum specimen container. The hand that touches the specimen container is no longer sterile.
Ensures that the sputum specimen goes directly into the specimen container instead of the suction tubing.

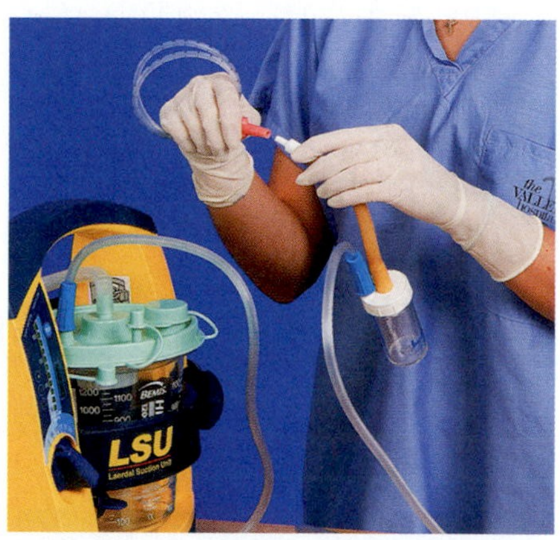

11. **Lubricate the suction catheter** with sterile saline solution.
Lubrication eases insertion and prevents trauma to mucosa.

12. **Insert the tip of the suction** catheter gently through the nasopharynx, endotracheal tube, or tracheostomy tube. Advance the tip into the trachea (see Procedure 36-6 or Procedure 36-8).
Gentle insertion prevents airway trauma.

13. **When the patient begins** coughing, apply suction by placing your finger over the suction control port for 5 to 10 seconds to collect the specimen.
Applying suction for longer than 10 seconds can cause hypoxia.

14. **If an adequate specimen** (5 to 10 mL) is not obtained, allow the patient to rest for 1 or 2 minutes, and then repeat the procedure. Administer oxygen to the patient at this time, if indicated.
Allowing the patient to rest and administering oxygen prevent hypoxia. You must assess your patient continually during this procedure to ensure patient safety and respiratory status.

15. **When you have collected** an adequate specimen, discontinue suction, then gently remove the suction catheter.
Applying suction during catheter removal can damage the airway mucosa.

16. **Remove the suction catheter** from the specimen container, and dispose of the catheter in the appropriate container.
Disposal of contaminated supplies prevents the spread of infection.

17. **Remove the suction tubing** from the specimen container, and connect the rubber tubing on the specimen container to the plastic adapter.

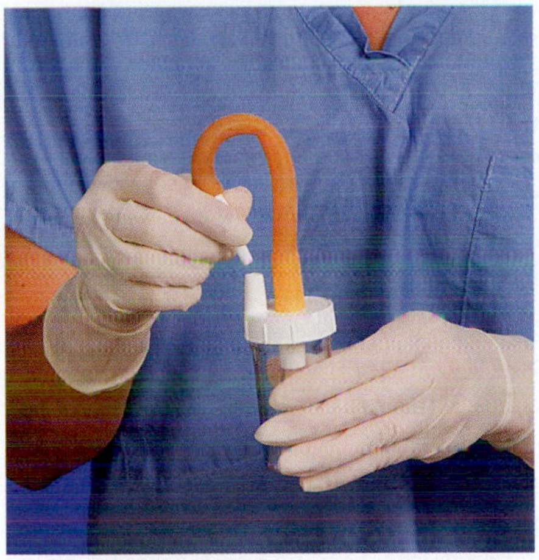

18. **If sputum comes in contact** with the outside of the specimen container, clean the outside with a disinfectant, according to agency policy.
Prevents spread of infection to staff members who must handle the specimen.

19. **Label the specimen container** with the patient identification, the name of the test, and collection date and time.
Correctly identifying the specimen ensures accurate diagnosis and treatment.

20. **Place the specimen** in a plastic bag with a biohazard label. Attach a completed laboratory requisition form.
Placing the specimen in a plastic bag protects healthcare workers from exposure to microorganisms. Completing the laboratory requisition form ensures proper processing of the specimen.

21. **Send the specimen to the laboratory** immediately, or refrigerate it if transport might be delayed.
If bacterial cultures are delayed, contaminating organisms may grow, producing false culture results and possibly inappropriate treatment.

Evaluation

- Evaluate the patient's respiratory status during and after the procedure, especially if suctioning was necessary.
- Examine the color, consistency, and odor of the sputum specimen.
- Promptly report laboratory results to the primary care provider.
- Evaluate the patient's understanding of the procedure and test results.

Patient Teaching

- Explain proper collection techniques to avoid specimen contamination.
- Show the patient proper coughing techniques to ensure an adequate specimen.
- Explain the importance of avoiding mouthwash before the procedure because it may alter laboratory results.
- If the patient has an incision, show him how to splint his incision to avoid discomfort during coughing and expectoration.

Home Care

Explain how to collect an expectorated sputum specimen and the importance of sending the specimen to the laboratory immediately after collection.

Documentation

- Record the date and time the specimen was collected, the method of collection, and the type of specimen ordered.
- Note the amount, color, consistency, and odor of the specimen.
- Document the patient's tolerance of the procedure.

Sample documentation:

06/05/20 0700 Patient suctioned via tracheostomy. Sputum specimen obtained and sent for acid-fast bacillus (AFB) analysis. Specimen contained 15 mL of yellow, tenacious, odorless sputum. Patient became short of breath with suctioning. 100% O_2 administered via tracheostomy hood for 10 minutes after suctioning. Shortness of breath abated with treatment. O_2 returned to 40% — S. Ryan, RN

Practice Resources

Centers for Disease Control and Prevention (CDC) (n.d.a); Texas Department of State Health Services, Laboratory Services Section Home (2009, updated May 2018).

Procedure 36-2 ■ Monitoring Pulse Oximetry (Arterial Oxygen Saturation)

➤ For steps to follow in *all* procedures, refer to the Universal Steps for All Procedures found on the inside back cover.

Equipment

- Nail polish remover, if necessary
- Oximeter and probe sensor appropriate for patient age, size and weight, and for the desired location.

Delegation

Because it is noninvasive and simple to perform, the registered nurse (RN) can delegate application of the pulse oximeter probe and measurement of arterial oxygen saturation (Sao_2) to a UAP or licensed practical nurse (LPN) who is adequately trained to perform the skill. Inform the UAP or LPN how often to take measurements, and instruct them to notify you immediately if Sao_2 falls below 95%. Although this procedure can be delegated, it is the responsibility of the RN to interpret the results, assess the patient, and notify the primary care provider.

Pre-Procedure Assessments

- Assess the need for Sao_2 monitoring: low hemoglobin level; confusion, decreased level of consciousness, or respiratory distress; or risk factors, such as heart or pulmonary disease, recovering from anesthesia, or ventilator-dependent.
  Sao_2 monitoring helps detect oxygenation problems early. Monitoring is especially important in patients with risk factors. Patients with underlying pulmonary disease may have adapted to low oxygen saturation levels, so you may need to adjust the lower limit alarm and, if you have delegated the procedure, the level for notification for these patients.
- Assess the patient's respiratory status, including breath sounds; respiratory rate, depth, and pattern; tissue perfusion; Sao_2; and skin and nailbed color.
  Assessment findings may suggest a decrease in oxygen saturation and validate oximetry readings.
- Determine the optimal location for the oximeter probe sensor, for example, the fingertip, earlobe, forehead, or bridge of the nose. Check the capillary refill and pulse at the pulse closest to the site.
  To ensure accurate monitoring, choose a site that has adequate circulation, is free of artificial nails, and contains no moisture. Clinical Insight 36-1 offers suggestions on site placement based on patient factors.
- Assess for factors that may interfere with pulse oximetry measurement, such as hypotension, hypothermia, and tremors.
  The sensor requires adequate circulation to recognize hemoglobin molecules that absorb the emitted light. Tremors may produce artifact that may be misinterpreted by the oximeter, causing false readings.
- Check patient history for allergy to adhesive.
  An allergic reaction may occur if an adhesive-backed disposable probe sensor is used in a patient with a history of allergy to adhesives.

➤ When performing the procedure, always identify your patient according to agency policy, using two identifiers, and be attentive to standard precautions, hand hygiene, patient safety and privacy, body mechanics, and documentation.

➤ *Note:* This procedure explains how to apply a pulse oximeter. Refer to Clinical Insight 36-1 for tips for obtaining accurate pulse oximetry readings.

Procedure Steps

1. **Choose a sensor appropriate** for the patient's age, size, and weight and for the desired location.
   - If the patient is allergic to adhesive, use a clip-on probe sensor.
   - If the patient's peripheral circulation is compromised, use a nasal sensor.
   An appropriate type of sensor is more comfortable for the patient and ensures accurate readings.
2. **Prepare the site by cleansing** and drying it. If the finger is the site, remove nail polish or an acrylic nail, if present.
   Dirt and skin oils on the site can interfere with passage of light waves. Nail polish or acrylic nails may interfere with signal transmission, causing inaccurate Sao_2 measurement. However, a recent study found that nail polish did not cause a clinically significant change in readings in healthy people (Chan, Chan, & Chan, 2013).
3. **Remove the protective backing** if you are using a disposable probe sensor that contains adhesive.
4. **Attach the probe sensor** to the chosen site. Make sure the photodetector and light-emitting diodes (LED) on the probe sensor face each other. Most probe sensors contain markings to facilitate correct placement.

When Using a Clip-on Probe Sensor

If you are using a clip-on probe sensor, warn the patient that he may feel a pinching sensation. Choose the site based on the status of circulation to the extremity and patient movement.
Inadequate circulation to the site and artifact caused by motion may alter Sao_2 results. The photodetector diodes and LED must be properly placed to ensure accurate readings.

5. **Connect the sensor probe** to the oximeter and turn it on. Check the pulse rate displayed on the oximeter to see whether it correlates with the patient's radial pulse. (Be sure the pulse oximeter is plugged in to an electrical socket.)

Correlation between the oximeter pulse display and the patient's radial pulse confirms accurate readings.

6. **Read the SaO_2 measurement** on the digital display when it reaches a constant value, usually in 10 to 30 seconds, but may take up to 2 minutes.
The oximeter requires time to detect the pulse, calculate oxygen saturation, and register an accurate reading.

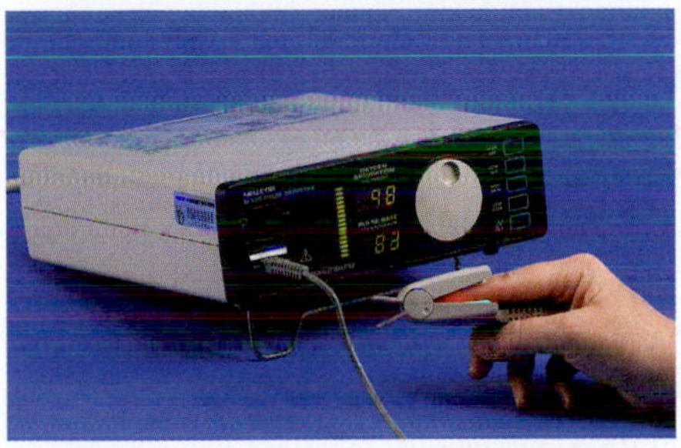

7. **Set and turn on the alarm** limits for SaO_2 and pulse rate, according to the manufacturer's instructions, patient condition, and agency policy if continuous monitoring is necessary.
Alarms must be set at appropriate levels to signify when SaO_2 or pulse rate falls below predetermined levels. Alarms help ensure prompt recognition and treatment of hypoxia.

8. **Obtain readings as prescribed** or indicated by the patient's respiratory status.
Some agencies require a prescription for pulse oximetry to ensure reimbursement.

9. **Rotate the site** if continuous monitoring is indicated.

For an Adhesive Probe Sensor

Rotate the site every 4 hours.

For a Clip-on Probe Sensor

Rotate the site every 2 hours.
Probe sensors and prolonged pressure may irritate the skin; rotating the site prevents skin breakdown.

10. **Remove the probe sensor,** and turn off the oximeter when monitoring is no longer necessary.
Some oximeters are battery powered; leaving them on after use depletes the battery.

Evaluation

- Evaluate the patient's understanding of the procedure and the obtained values.
- Compare pulse oximetry results with the patient's clinical presentation.
- Evaluate the effectiveness of therapy by comparing SaO_2 results before, during, and after treatment.
- Assess the site every 4 hours if you are using an adhesive probe sensor or every 2 hours if you are using a clip-on probe sensor.

Patient Teaching

- Demonstrate the procedure to the patient and caregiver, especially if the patient will be continuing pulse oximetry at home.
- Explain to the patient and caregiver the significance of SaO_2 results.
- Discuss the signs and symptoms of hypoxia (confusion, restlessness, shortness of breath, dyspnea, cyanosis, and somnolence) with the patient and caregiver.

Home Care

- Explain where to obtain a pulse oximeter.
- Tell the client and caregiver when to notify the primary provider of abnormal results or signs and symptoms of hypoxia.
- Help the client identify risk factors that decrease SaO_2 levels.

Documentation

- Record the date and time of each pulse oximetry reading obtained. Most agencies use a flowsheet if frequent monitoring is necessary.
- Document whether readings are intermittent or continuous.
- If readings are continuous, record alarm parameters.
- Chart the patient's vital signs and SaO_2 results, and indicate whether the patient is breathing room air or receiving oxygen therapy. For oxygen therapy, note the oxygen concentration and the mode of delivery.
- Document acute decreases in SaO_2, any precipitating factors, treatment interventions, and the patient's response.

Sample documentation

July 1, 2021 0300 Pt stated "short of breath." Crackles throughout lung fields. BP 140/92, apical pulse 110 beats/min, resp rate 32 breaths/min. Pulse oximetry applied to left index finger, and SaO_2 88% on room air. Places on O_2 at 4 L/min via nasal cannula. Dr. Jones notified. ——— Kate Jackson, RNC

Practice Resources

American Association of Critical-Care Nurses (AACN) (2016); Bunker, D. L. J., Kumar, R., Martin, A., et al. (2014); Chan, E. D., Chan, M. M., & Chan, M. M. (2013); Jones, M., Olorvida, E., Monger, K., et al. (2015).

Thinking About the Procedure

The video **Administering Oxygen,** along with questions and suggested responses, is available on the ***Davis's Nursing Skills Videos*** Web site on FADavis.com.

Procedure 36-3 ■ Performing Percussion, Vibration, and Postural Drainage

➤ For steps to follow in *all* procedures, refer to the Universal Steps for All Procedures found on the inside back cover.

Equipment

- Bed capable of being placed in the Trendelenburg position
- Pillows
- Patient gown
- Facial tissues
- Emesis basin
- Sputum specimen container, if needed
- Suction equipment, if needed
- Stethoscope

Delegation

You should assess the patient to determine the need for the procedure and to evaluate whether the patient can tolerate the procedure. You should perform the initial procedure, but you can delegate subsequent treatments to a respiratory therapist or UAP who is adequately trained. Instruct the respiratory therapist or UAP to report any changes in the patient's condition immediately. The RN is responsible for ongoing assessment and monitoring of airway clearance and respiratory status.

Pre-Procedure Assessments

- Check the patient's chest x-ray results.
  Identifies which lung fields require treatment.
- Assess the patient's respiratory status, including respiratory rate, depth, and rhythm; breath sounds; color; and pulse oximetry results.
  Determines the need for and effectiveness of percussion, vibration, and postural drainage.
- Determine when the patient last ate.
  Postural drainage should not be performed for at least 2 hours after meals to prevent nausea, vomiting, and aspiration.
- Assess the patient for dysrhythmias, coagulopathy (a defect in blood clotting), hypertension, and pain or tenderness in the chest area being treated.
  If any of these are present, the procedure should be avoided because it might worsen these conditions.

➤ When performing the procedure, always identify your patient according to agency policy, using two identifiers, and be attentive to standard precautions, hand hygiene, patient safety and privacy, body mechanics, and documentation.

Procedure Steps

1. **Help the patient assume the appropriate** position, based on the lung field that requires drainage.
   Helps mobilize secretions in the affected lung field by gravity.

   a. ***Apical areas of the upper lobes.*** Ask the patient to sit at the edge of the bed, if possible. If needed, place a pillow at the base of the spine for support. If the patient is not able to sit at the edge of the bed, place him in high-Fowler's position.

   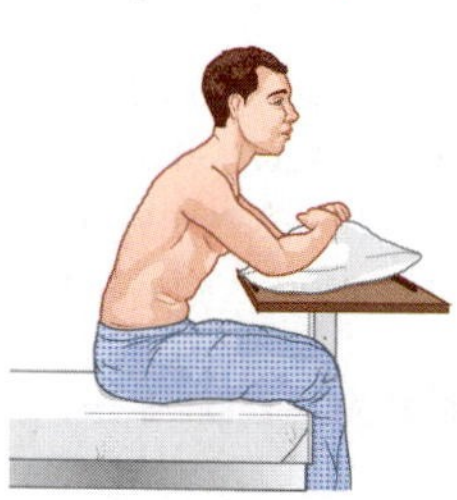

   b. ***Posterior section of the upper lobes.*** Position supine with a pillow under the hips and knees flexed. Have the patient rotate slightly away from the side that requires drainage.

   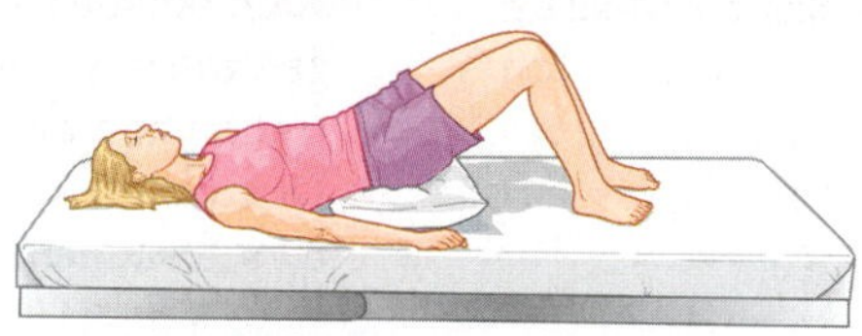

   c. ***Middle or lower lobes.*** Place the bed in the Trendelenburg position. Position the patient in Sims' position. To drain the left lung, position the patient on his right side. For the right lung, position the patient on his left side.

   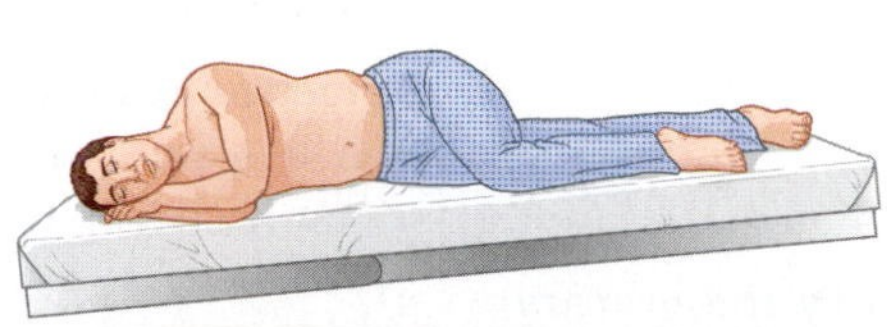

   d. ***Posterior lower lobes.*** Keeping the bed flat, position the patient prone with a pillow under her stomach.

   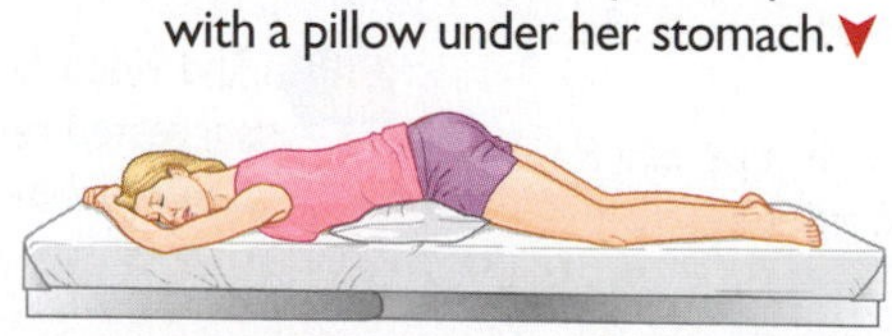

2. **Have the patient remain** in the desired position for 10 to 15 minutes, if tolerated.
   Allows adequate drainage of secretions by gravity from the desired lung field.

3. **Perform percussion** over the affected lung area while the patient is in the desired drainage position.
   Loosens and mobilizes secretions.

   a. Instruct the patient to breathe deeply and slowly.
   Relaxation helps the patient tolerate the procedure.

   b. Place a towel over the patient's skin or use the patient's gown to cover the area to be percussed.
   Protects the skin and promotes patient privacy and comfort.

   c. **Avoid clapping over bony prominences, female breasts, or tender areas of the chest.**
   Percussing over these areas may cause discomfort and compromise tissue integrity.

   d. Cup your hands, keeping your fingers flexed and your thumbs pressed against your index fingers.
   Cupping your hands promotes patient comfort during percussion.

   e. Place your cupped hands over the lung area that requires drainage.

f. Percuss the lung area for 1 to 3 minutes by alternately striking your cupped hands rhythmically against the patient.

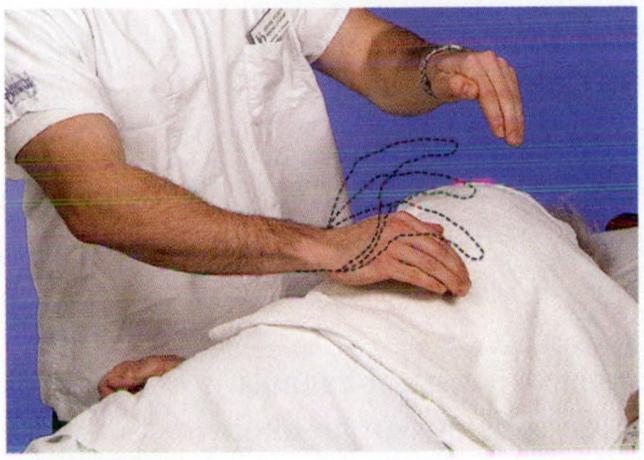

4. **Perform vibrations** while the patient remains in the desired drainage position.

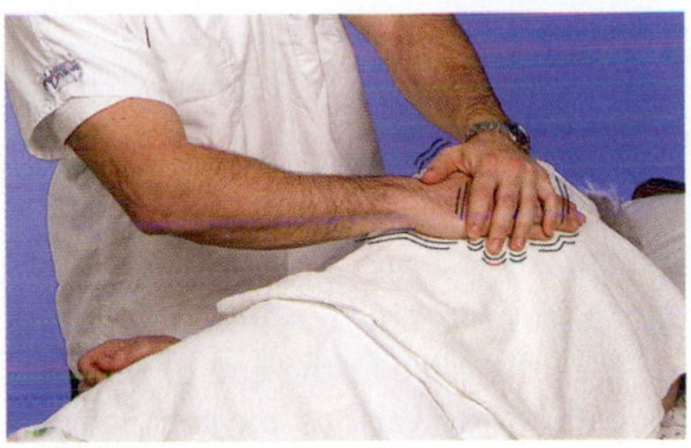

a. Place the flat surface of one hand over the lung area that requires vibration. Place your other hand on top of that hand at a right angle.
Using the flat surfaces of the hands provides a large surface area to transmit vibrations through the chest. Placing one hand on top of the other provides better leverage for vibrating.

b. Instruct the patient to inhale slowly and deeply.
Promotes relaxation and lung expansion.

c. Instruct the patient to make a "fff" or "sss" sound as she exhales.

d. As the patient exhales, press your fingers and palms firmly against her chest wall.
Vibrating during exhalation enhances the downward movement of the rib cage that occurs during exhalation.

e. Push down, and gently vibrate with your hands over the lung area.
Vibration helps mobilize secretions.

f. Continue performing vibrations for three exhalations.

5. **After performing postural** drainage, percussion, and vibration, allow the patient to sit up. Ask her to cough at the end of a deep inspiration. Suction the patient if she is unable to expectorate secretions. If a sputum specimen is needed, collect it in a specimen container.
Coughing helps clear the airway of secretions.

6. **Repeat Steps 1 through 5** for each lung field that requires treatment. The entire treatment should not exceed 60 minutes.
Treating for longer than 60 minutes fatigues the patient.

7. **Provide mouth care.**
Cleanses the mouth of secretions and promotes patient comfort.

Evaluation

- Evaluate the effectiveness of percussion, vibration, and postural drainage.
- Auscultate breath sounds every 2 to 4 hours, as indicated.
- Monitor pulse oximetry and arterial blood gas (ABG) results.
- Evaluate the need for further treatment.

Patient Teaching

- Demonstrate percussion, vibration, and postural drainage if the patient will be continuing it at home.
- Reinforce the importance of immediately reporting shortness of breath or any difficulty breathing.
- Explain the importance of drinking fluids to help thin and mobilize secretions.
- Teach coughing and deep-breathing exercises.

Home Care

- Be sure the client/family/caregiver knows how often the procedure should be done. There should be a prescription from the primary care provider.
- Most clients will not have a bed that can be placed in the Trendelenburg position.
- Demonstrate how to position the client with hips elevated on pillows, higher than the chest, or, if the client is able, to assume a knee–chest position.
- Provide the client and caregiver with contact information of healthcare personnel who can be reached for advice or emergencies.

Documentation

- Document the date and time you performed percussion, vibration, and postural drainage.
- Note the positions used and the length of time the patient maintained each position.
- Note the anatomical locations in which you performed percussion and vibration.
- Document the patient's tolerance of the procedure, as well as any complications and the nursing interventions you used to treat the complication.
- Document the amount, color, odor, and consistency of sputum obtained during the procedure and whether you sent a sputum specimen to the lab.

Sample documentation

June 15, 2020 Percussion and vibration done over Right lower lobe. Expectorated 10 mL thick, yellow, odorless mucus. Specimen to lab. BP 142/78, HR 98 beats/min, respirations 24 breaths/min. Few crackles auscultated over Right lung base, SaO_2 98% on 2 L/min nasal cannula. ——— Jeffrey Fine, RN

Practice Resources

Bilton, D. (2012); *Lippincott's Nursing Procedures* (2018).

Procedure 36-4 ■ Administering Oxygen

➤ For steps to follow in *all* procedures, refer to the Universal Steps for All Procedures found on the inside back cover.

Equipment

- Oxygen source
- Flow meter
- Oxygen tubing
- Nasal cannula, oxygen mask, or face tent
- Prefilled humidification device

Delegation

The RN is responsible for assessing respiratory function and initiating oxygen therapy. However, you may delegate reapplication and maintenance of oxygen therapy (e.g., adjusting the face mask) to appropriately trained assistive personnel when necessary.

Pre-Procedure Assessments

- Assess the patient's understanding of oxygen therapy.
- Assessment of the patient's respiratory status; includes respiratory rate, depth, and rhythm; breath sounds; color; capillary refill and pulse oximetry results.
  Determines the need for further treatment and effectiveness of oxygen therapy.
- Assess nares for patency (if a nasal cannula is being used) and behind the ears for signs of skin breakdown.

➤ When performing the procedure, always identify your patient according to agency policy, using two identifiers, and be attentive to standard precautions, hand hygiene, patient safety and privacy, body mechanics, and documentation.

➤ *Note:* Oxygen requires a medical prescription. In an emergency, administer oxygen to the patient to prevent respiratory distress, then notify the primary care provider for a prescription.

Procedure Steps

Also use Clinical Insight 36-3: Oxygen Therapy Safety Precautions.

1. **Attach the flow meter** to the wall oxygen source (in the photo the green meter on the wall). ▼

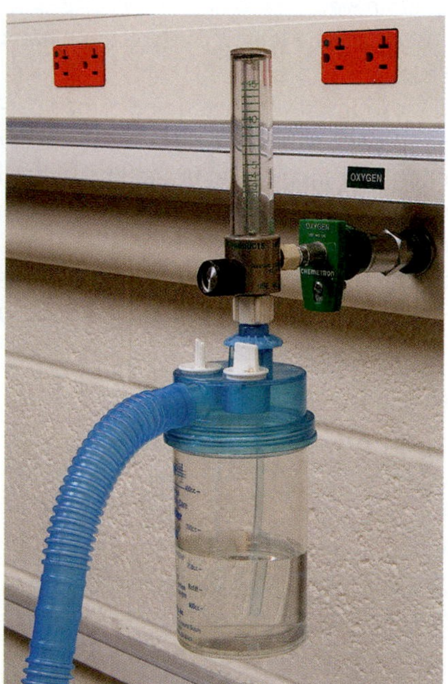

If Using a Portable Oxygen Tank

Attach the flow meter to the tank if it is not already connected. Once tubing is attached to the portable tank, check the amount of oxygen in the tank by looking at the meter.
The flow meter regulates the amount of oxygen delivered per minute. ▼

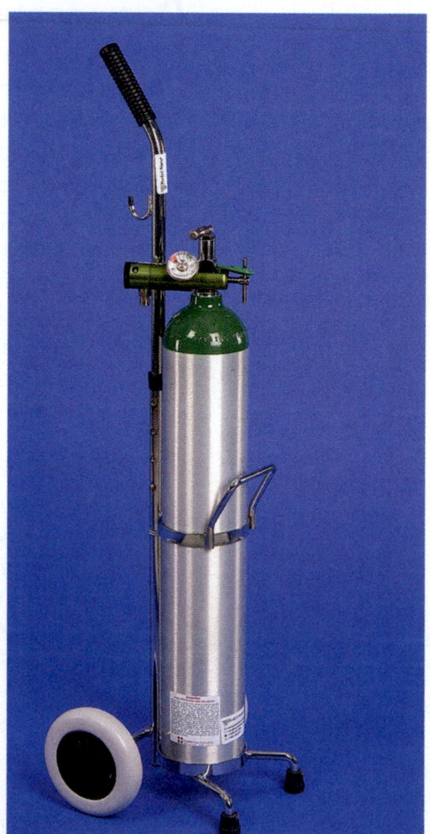

2. **Assemble the oxygen** equipment. (See the table at the end of this procedure for various oxygen delivery devices.)
3. **Attach the humidifier** to the flow meter. The humidifier is simply a small plastic container containing normal saline. If you are not using a humidifier, attach the adapter directly to the flow meter.
   The humidifier adds moisture in with the oxygen, which can dry the nasal or oral cavity.
4. **Turn on the oxygen** at the flow meter, and adjust the prescribed flow rate.

Then proceed to Step 5, 8, or 10.

Procedure Variation for Nasal Cannula

Follow Steps 1 through 4.

5. **Attach the nasal cannula tubing** to the humidifier or the adapter.
6. **Place the nasal prongs** in the patient's nares—prongs curved downward—and then place the tubing around each ear.
   Properly positions the device for optimal oxygen delivery.

7. Use the slide adjustment device to tighten the cannula in place under the patient's chin. It must fit securely, but not too tightly. **Then proceed to Step 12.**

The nasal cannula must fit securely to maximize the amount of oxygen inhaled by the patient. A good fit minimizes the amount of oxygen lost around the prongs. ▼

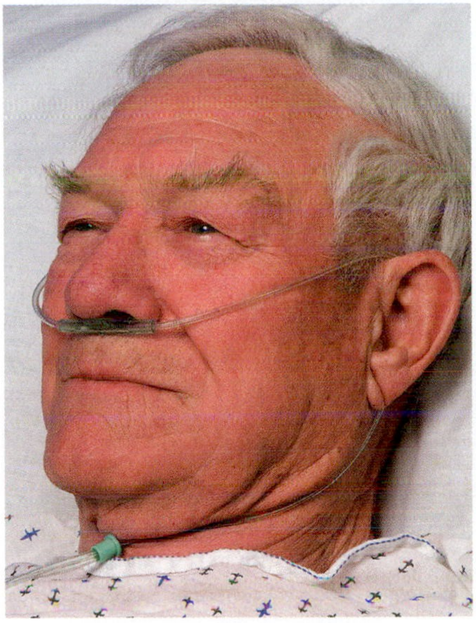

Procedure Variation for Face Mask

Follow Steps 1 through 4.

8. Gently place the mask on the patient's face, applying it from the bridge of the nose to under the chin.

9. Secure the elastic band around the back of the patient's head. Make sure the mask fits snugly but comfortably. **Then proceed to Step 12.**

The mask must fit snugly so that oxygen cannot escape around the edges of the mask. If the mask is too tight, it may cause skin breakdown. ▼

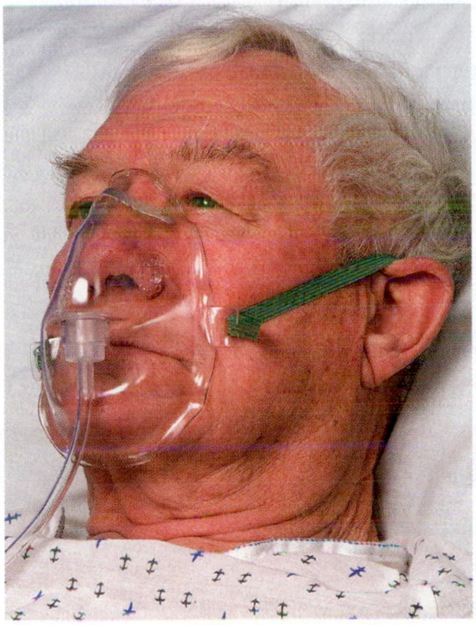

Procedure Variation for Face Tent

Follow Steps 1 through 4.

10. Gently place the face tent in front of the patient's face, making sure that it fits under the chin.

11. Secure the elastic band around the back of the patient's head.

To keep the face tent in place. ▼

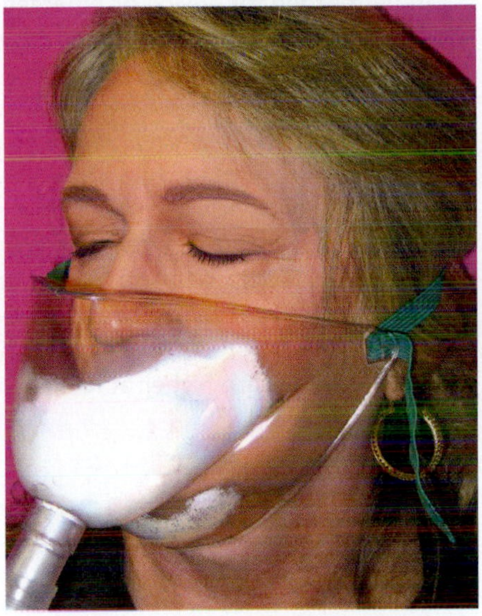

12. Double-check that the oxygen equipment is set up correctly and functioning properly.

Ensures that the oxygen is delivered at the prescribed rate. Oxygen delivered at an incorrect rate can cause patient injury.

13. Assess the patient's respiratory status before leaving the bedside.

To be certain it is safe to leave the patient.

Evaluation

- Assess respiratory rate, depth, and effort.
- Auscultate breath sounds before leaving the bedside, then monitor every 2 to 4 hours, and as indicated.
- Monitor pulse oximetry until respiratory status improves.
- Monitor ABG results if prescribed.
- Evaluate for skin breakdown, especially behind the ears, cheekbones, and under the chin—areas that are in contact with the oxygen delivery system.
- Notify the primary provider of respiratory status, oxygen, and response and any additional prescriptions needed.

Patient Teaching

- Demonstrate oxygen administration to the patient and caregiver if the patient will be continuing oxygen therapy at home. Allow for time to answer questions, and return demonstration of attaching and placing oxygen on.
- Explain the importance of immediately reporting shortness of breath or any difficulty breathing to the nursing staff before discharge. If the patient is at home, he will need to report the difficulty to the home health and/or primary care provider, and if needed, to call 911.

Home Care

- Explain to the client and caregivers where to obtain oxygen equipment and what services are available. Make sure they choose a supplier who has 24-hour emergency services.
- Instruct the client and caregiver about oxygen therapy and its use as well as safety measures that they must institute. Safety measures include keeping oxygen away from items that may cause ignition such as lighters, cigarettes, fireplaces, heaters, etc.
- To demonstrate the oxygen is on, client can hold nasal prongs on the side of the cheek to feel air flow or over a glass of water to see air moving water.
- Teach the client and caregiver to clean the nasal cannula or face mask with soap and warm water when it becomes soiled, and allow the mask to air-dry.

(continued on next page)

Procedure 36-4 ■ Administering Oxygen (continued)

- Provide contact information for healthcare personnel who can be reached for advice or emergencies.
- Explain the importance of immediately reporting shortness of breath or any difficulty breathing to the home health and/or primary care provider, and if needed, to call 911.
- In the home, liquid oxygen and oxygen concentrators are more commonly used than portable oxygen tanks. Liquid oxygen may be kept in small, portable containers; an oxygen concentrator removes nitrogen from room air and concentrates O_2. It requires a battery pack or electrical outlet for power. Oxygen concentrators can deliver flow up to 4 liters per minute (L/min) to create an FIO_2 of approximately 36%. Concentrations are higher at lower flow rates (e.g., an FIO_2 of 95% at 1 L/min).

Documentation

- Document the date, time, and reason oxygen therapy was initiated.
- Note the type of oxygen delivery system used, the amount of oxygen administered, and the patient's response to oxygen therapy.
- Document vital signs, pulse oximetry values, breath sounds, skin color, and respiratory effort.

Sample documentation

12/14/21 1005. Patient developed acute shortness of breath. RR 36/min & labored, P = 126 beats/min, and BP 212/110 mm Hg. Pulse ox 80% on room air. Crackles and expiratory wheezes auscultated throughout both lungs. Dr. Chow notified of patient's condition. Oxygen with partial rebreather mask @ 10 L/min and Lasix 40 mg IV prescribed and administered. Pulse ox using partial rebreather = 90%. —— S. Peters, RN

Practice Resources

Lippincott's Nursing Procedures (2018).

Oxygen Delivery Systems

DELIVERY METHOD	FIO_2	DISCUSSION	NURSING RESPONSIBILITIES
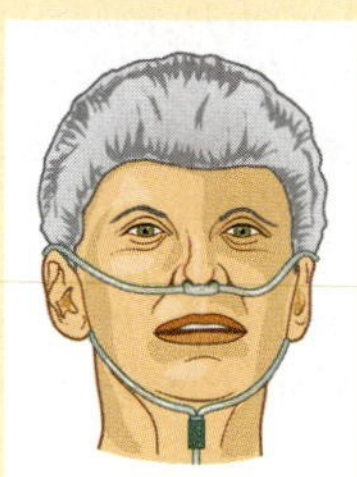 Nasal cannula	1 L/min = 24% 2 L/min = 28% 3 L/min = 32% 4 L/min = 36% 5 L/min = 40% 6 L/min = 44%	■ Relatively comfortable. ■ Patients can eat, talk, and cough with a nasal cannula in place. ■ Works best if the patient breathes through his nose.	■ Check frequently that the prongs are in the patient's nose. ■ Assess for dryness of the nasal mucosa. ■ Humidify flow at rates above 3 L/min (flow rates >3 L/min are drying). ■ Encourage the patient to take slow, deep breaths so he will inhale more oxygen and less room air.
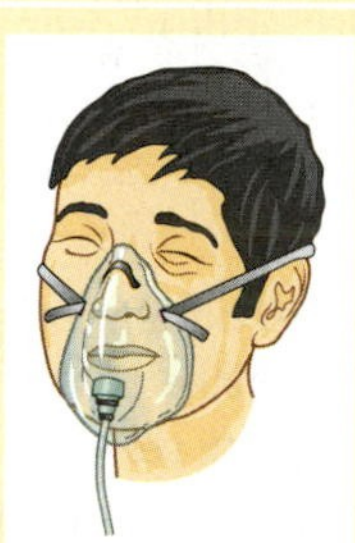 Simple face mask: A clear, flexible mask that covers the nose and mouth and delivers oxygen flow into the mask.	5–10 L/min = 40%–60% FIO_2	■ Requires flow rates greater than 5 L/min to prevent accumulation and rebreathing of exhaled CO_2 from within the mask. ■ Masks are not easily tolerated because they fit tightly and keep heat from radiating from the face, making patients feel hot. ■ Talking is muffled by the mask, and it must be removed for the patient to eat or drink.	■ Place face mask securely over the mouth and nose. ■ Elastic straps fit around the head to hold the mask in place. Place the straps well above the ears to prevent skin irritation and breakdown. ■ Place gauze or other soft material beneath the straps to prevent irritation. ■ Check the skin around the mask frequently. ■ Check the skin over the ears where the mask strap rubs. ■ Encourage the patient to take slow, deep breaths, so he will inhale more oxygen and less room air.

Oxygen Delivery Systems—cont'd

DELIVERY METHOD	FIO_2	DISCUSSION	NURSING RESPONSIBILITIES
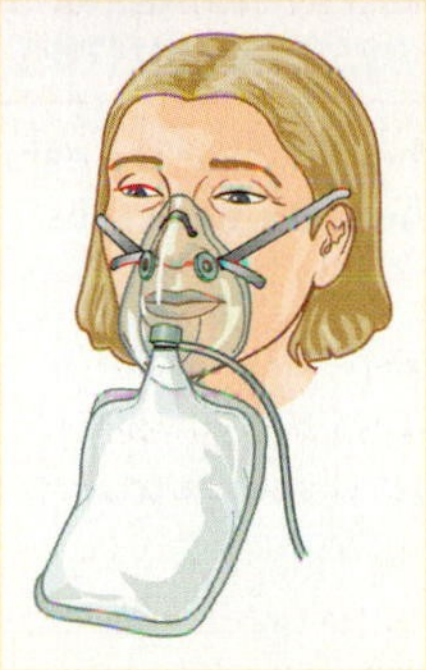 Partial rebreather mask: Uses the reservoir bag to capture some exhaled gas for rebreathing	6–15 L/min = 50%–90% FIO_2	▪ Allows higher FIO_2 levels to be delivered because O_2 is collected in the reservoir bag for inhalation. ▪ Exhalation ports allow most exhaled air to escape. ▪ Several types are available. ▪ Can deliver an FIO_2 above 50% at flow rates of 6–15 L/min. ▪ Patient rebreathes some exhaled air along with O_2.	▪ Maintain the flow at a high enough rate to prevent the reservoir bag from collapsing during inhalation. ▪ Encourage the patient to take slow, deep breaths, so he will inhale more oxygen and less room air.
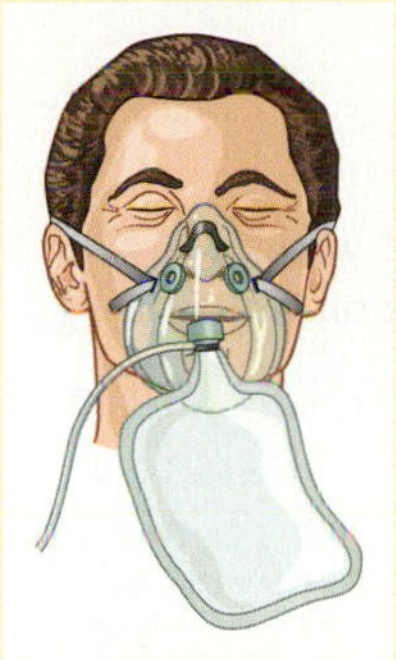 Nonrebreather mask: A type of reservoir bag mask; a valve keeps exhaled air from entering the reservoir bag.	6–15 L/min = 70%–100% FIO_2	▪ Contains only O_2, which allows higher FIO_2 delivery. An FIO_2 of 70%–100% can be delivered at flow rates of 6–15 L/min. ▪ This mask is the only external device capable of delivering an FIO_2 of 100% (in practice, it is rare to achieve a concentration above 75% because the mask does not seal perfectly with the face).	▪ Maintain the flow at a rate high enough to keep the reservoir at least one-third to one-half full during inhalation. ▪ Be sure the mask fits snugly so the patient will breathe in less room air.
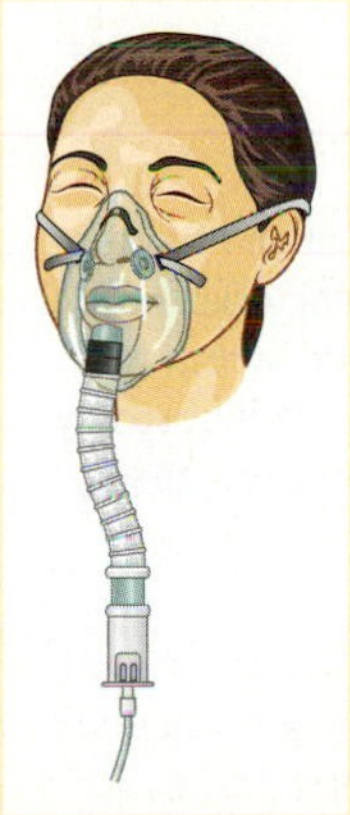 Venturi mask: A cone-shaped adapter that serves as a mixing valve to control the amount of O_2 and room air that flows through the mask.	24%–50% FIO_2	▪ The cone-shaped adapter at the base of the mask allows a precise FIO_2 to be delivered. This is very useful for patients with chronic lung disease. ▪ Exhalation ports keep CO_2 buildup to a minimum.	▪ The adapter indicates the required oxygen flow rate needed to deliver the desired FIO_2. Ensure that flow is set at the rate specified to deliver the FIO_2 desired.

(continued on next page)

Procedure 36-4 ■ Administering Oxygen (continued)

Oxygen Delivery Systems—cont'd

DELIVERY METHOD	FIO_2	DISCUSSION	NURSING RESPONSIBILITIES
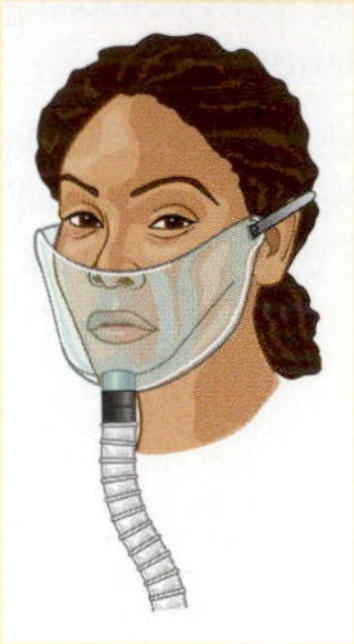 Face tent: A large, open plastic mask that fits under the chin. It is open at the top and is held in place with an elastic band around the head.	8–12 L/min = 30%–55% FIO_2	■ Less reliable than a face mask for delivering precise FIO_2 levels. ■ Allows moderate- to high-density aerosol delivery for humidification. ■ Patients who feel claustrophobic in a face mask often tolerate a face tent.	■ Check the skin over the ears where the mask strap rubs.
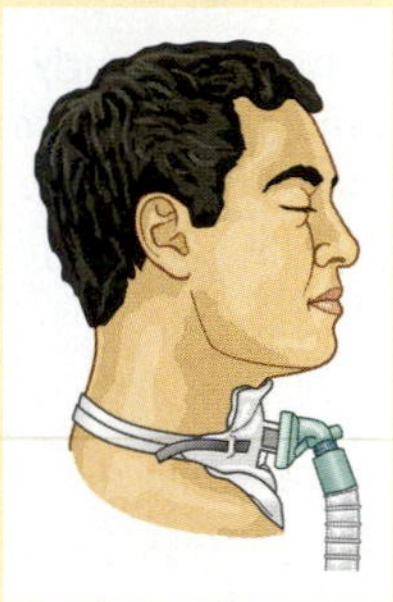 Tracheostomy collar: A small, cup-shaped device that fits over the tracheostomy opening and is held in place with elastic straps around the neck.	4–10 L/min = 24%–100% FIO_2	■ It is possible to deliver both high FIO_2 and high humidity with a tracheostomy collar. ■ Large-bore tubing is used to deliver humidification to the trachea; however, water frequently condenses inside the tubing and can be accidentally drained into the tracheostomy. Usually, a water trap of some sort is placed in the tubing to prevent this problem.	■ Watch for water accumulation in the tubing.
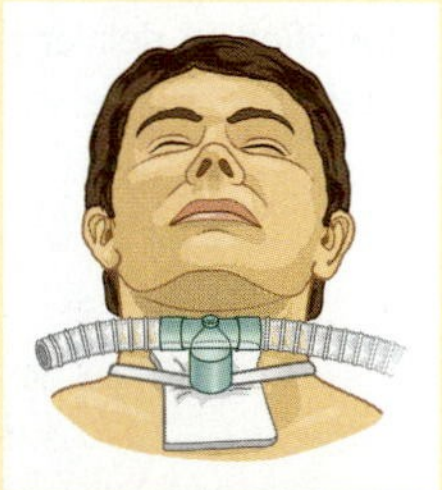 T-piece: A T-shaped plastic piece; the bottom of the T fits directly and tightly onto the tracheostomy tube.	4–10 L/min = 24%–100% FIO_2	■ Oxygen and humidity are delivered into one side of the T and exhaled through the other side.	■ Take care that the oxygen delivery tubing does not pull on the T-piece, which can dislodge the tracheostomy tube and create an airway emergency.

Thinking About the Procedure

The video **Administering Oxygen,** along with questions and suggested responses, is available on the ***Davis's Nursing Skills Videos*** Web site on FADavis.com.

Procedure 36-5 ■ Performing Tracheostomy Care

- For steps to follow in *all* procedures, refer to the Universal Steps for All Procedures found on the inside back cover.
- Also refer to Clinical Insight 36-4.
- Recall that the basic differences in sterile and modified sterile technique are that modified sterile technique uses a sterile catheter and supplies, but nonsterile procedure gloves.
- Using tap water for procedures exposes patients to waterborne pathogens; use distilled, filtered, or sterile solution if available. This differs among institutions, so follow agency requirements.

Equipment

- Tracheostomy suction equipment (see Procedure 36-6)
- Tracheostomy care kit or the following sterile supplies: several cotton-tipped applicators, two basins, a brush, sterile 4 in. × 4 in. gauze pads, sterile precut tracheostomy dressing
- Two pairs of sterile gloves (for modified sterile technique, use procedure gloves)
- Disposable inner cannula that is the same size as the tracheostomy, if available. Most tracheostomy tubes have disposable inner cannulas.
- Sterile normal saline solution (for modified sterile technique, you can use distilled or filtered water if agency policy allows)
- Hydrogen peroxide for cleaning of reusable inner cannula only
- Roll of twill tape or hook and loop fastener (Velcro) tracheostomy holder
- Bandage scissors
- Towel or linen-saver pad
- Overbed table
- Face shield and protective gown
- For modified sterile technique: disposable prepackaged wipes, or washcloth and distilled water and soap

Use only the sterile precut dressing, or open and refold a 4 in. × 4 in. gauze pad into a V-shape. Do not cut 4 in. × 4 in. gauze, and do not use cotton-filled gauze squares. The patient may aspirate the cotton or gauze fibers.

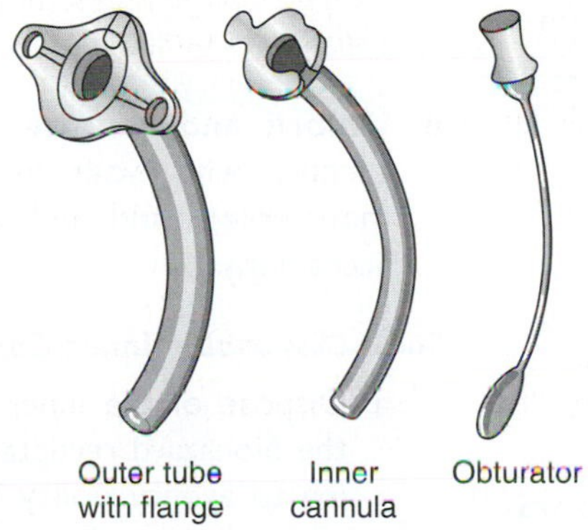

A, Nondisposable tracheostomy equipment

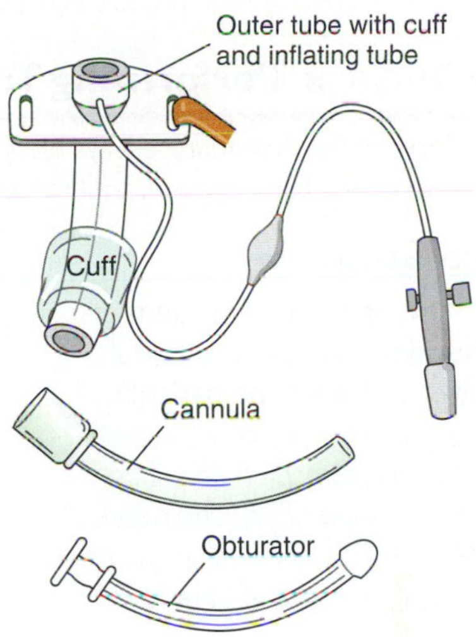

B, Disposable tracheostomy equipment

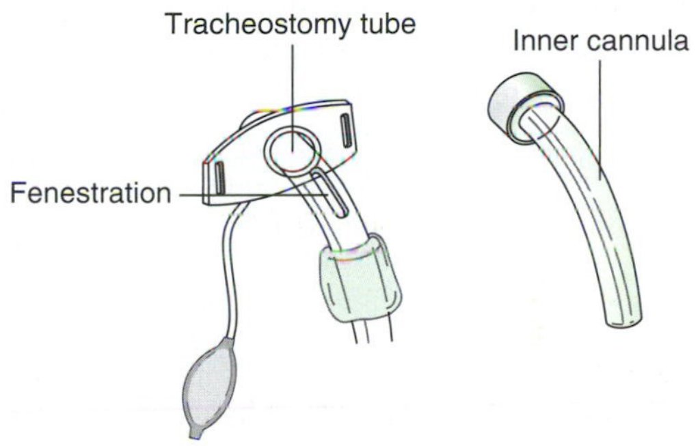

C, Fenestrated tracheostomy equipment

Delegation

In acute care settings and with new tracheostomies, you should not delegate this procedure to the UAP. For long-standing and well-healed tracheostomies, you can safely delegate care to the UAP or LPN who is adequately trained to perform the skill. This varies by state. In some states, only RNs can perform tracheostomy care. If you are not familiar with your state's nurse practice act, contact your state board of nursing.

(continued on next page)

Procedure 36-5 ■ Performing Tracheostomy Care (continued)

Pre-Procedure Assessments

- Assess respiratory rate, depth, and rhythm; breath sounds; color; and pulse oximetry results.
  Helps determine whether the patient can tolerate tracheostomy care.
- Assess the tracheostomy site for drainage, redness, or swelling.
  Drainage, redness, or swelling may indicate infection.
- Determine when the patient last ate.
  It is best to schedule this procedure at least 3 hours after a meal to decrease the risk of the patient vomiting and aspirating stomach contents.

Procedure 36-5A ■ Performing Tracheostomy Care Using Modified Sterile Technique

➤ When performing the procedure, always identify your patient according to agency policy, using two identifiers, and be attentive to standard precautions, hand hygiene, patient safety and privacy, body mechanics, and documentation.

Procedure Steps

1. **Position the patient** in semi-Fowler's position, and place a towel or linen-saver pad over the patient's chest.
   A semi-Fowler's position promotes lung expansion and prevents back strain for the nurse. A towel or linen-saver pad prevents soiling of the patient's gown.
2. **Don clean procedure gloves, gown, and face shield or mask.**
3. **Hyperoxygenate the patient as needed,** and suction the tracheostomy (see Procedure 36-6 or 36-7).
   Suctioning clears the tracheostomy of secretions that could occlude the outer cannula after the inner cannula is removed for care.

For a Passy–Muir Valve

Remove the Passy–Muir valve (PMV) before suctioning the patient to prepare for tracheostomy care. (A PMV is a device that is used to enable the patient with a tracheostomy to speak. It is attached to the end of the inner cannula at the tracheostomy site.)

4. **Remove and discard** the soiled tracheostomy dressing in the appropriate receptacle, and then remove and discard your gloves. Perform hand hygiene.
5. **Place the tracheostomy care** equipment on the overbed table, and prepare the equipment, keeping all supplies and equipment sterile.
   Ensures efficiency and helps maintain sterility during tracheostomy care.
   a. *Disposable inner cannula*—Pour filtered tap water or normal saline solution into the two sterile containers (per agency policy).
   b. *Reusable inner cannula*—Pour hydrogen peroxide into one of the sterile solution containers, and pour filtered tap water or normal saline solution into the other one. If the inner cannula is not disposable, use hydrogen peroxide to clean only the inner cannula. Use the filtered tap water to rinse the inner cannula and clean the faceplate and tracheostomy site.

   Steps c through g apply to both types of cannula.

   c. Obtain and open a package of disposable prepackaged wipes for cleaning the skin around the tracheostomy site.
   d. Open one cotton-tipped applicator package. Wet the applicators with normal saline solution. Wet the applicators with filtered tap water or normal saline solution.
   Prepares the applicators for cleaning the exposed surface of the outer cannula and the stoma site located under the faceplate of the tracheostomy tube, respectively.
   e. Open the package containing a new disposable inner cannula.
   Allows for quick replacement of the inner cannula.
   f. Open the package of Velcro tracheostomy ties, or cut a length of twill tape long enough to go around the patient's neck two times. Make sure to cut end of the tape on an angle.
   Allows for quick stabilization of the tracheostomy tube, preventing dislodgement. Cutting the twill tape on an angle allows for easy insertion through the faceplate eyelets.
   g. Position a biohazard receptacle within reach.
   Allows you to dispose of contaminated supplies safely as you use them without leaving the patient or interrupting the procedure.
6. **Don clean procedure gloves** Consider your dominant hand sterile and handle the sterile supplies with that hand only.
7. **For patients receiving oxygen:** With your nondominant hand, remove the oxygen or humidification source. Attach the oxygen source to the outer cannula, if possible. If not possible, have the respiratory therapist set up oxygen blow-by to use while you are cleaning the reusable inner cannula.
   Prevents oxygen desaturation in the patient during the procedure.
8. **Unlock and remove the inner** cannula with your nondominant (nonsterile) hand and care for it accordingly.

For a Disposable Inner Cannula

   a. Dispose of the inner cannula in the biohazard receptacle according to agency policy. You should never clean and reuse a disposable inner cannula.
   Prevents contamination by bacteria contained in the inner cannula.
   b. With your dominant hand, insert the new inner cannula into the patient's tracheostomy in the direction of the curvature. Following the

manufacturer's instructions, lock the inner cannula in place securely to prevent it from dislodging. Remember to keep your dominant hand sterile.

For a Reusable Inner Cannula

c. If a reusable inner cannula was used, place the inner cannula into the basin filled with hydrogen peroxide.
Hydrogen peroxide helps loosen tenacious (sticky) secretions.

d. Pick up the reusable inner cannula from the container of hydrogen peroxide with your nonsterile hand, and scrub it with the sterile nylon brush, using your dominant hand. ▼

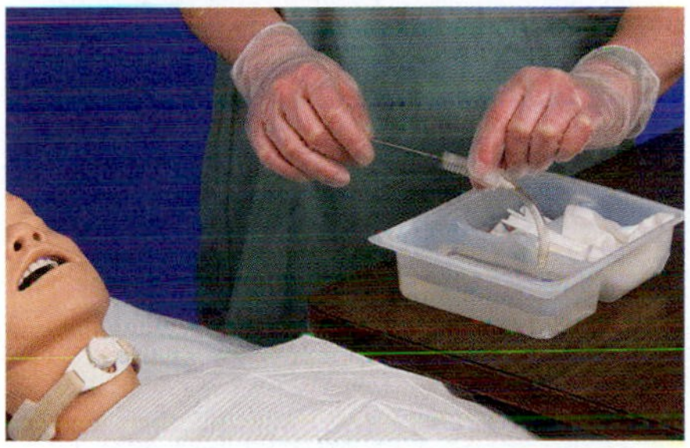

e. Immerse the inner cannula in the container of filtered tap water and agitate it until it is rinsed thoroughly.
Immersing the inner cannula in filtered tap water and agitating it removes the hydrogen peroxide and debris from the inner cannula minimizing tissue irritation.

f. Shake the cannula to remove water.
Removes excess fluid so the patient does not aspirate it when you reinsert the cannula.

g. With your dominant (clean) hand, reinsert the inner cannula into the patient's tracheostomy in the direction of the curvature. Following the manufacturer's instructions, lock the inner cannula in place securely to prevent it from dislodging. Remember to keep your dominant hand clean.

For a Passy–Muir Valve

h. Swish the PMV in warm filtered tap water with mild soap.

i. Rinse the PMV thoroughly in warm filtered tap water.

j. **Key Point:** ***DO NOT use hot water, peroxide, bleach, vinegar, alcohol, brushes, or cotton-tipped applicators to clean PMV, as this could damage the valve.***

k. Shake the PMV to remove excess fluid. If you are going to store the valve, be sure to air-dry the valve before placing it in a storage container.
Removes moisture, which can promote bacterial growth.

l. Set the PMV aside on clean surface to be replaced when the inner cannula is replaced.

For Patients Receiving Oxygen

m. Remove the humidification or oxygen source from the outer cannula, if indicated, using your nondominant hand.

n. Reinsert the inner cannula into the patient's tracheostomy in the direction of the curvature.

o. Following the manufacturer's instructions, lock the inner cannula in place securely. Remember to keep dominant hand clean.
Lock the inner cannula in place securely to prevent it from dislodging.

p. Reattach the humidification or oxygen source, if indicated.
Provides the patient with needed humidity or oxygen and prevents oxygen desaturation.

9. **Clean the stoma** under the faceplate with cotton-tipped applicators saturated with filtered tap water or normal saline solution, using a circular motion from the stoma site outward. Use each applicator only once, and then discard it.
Prevents contamination of the cleaned area. ▼

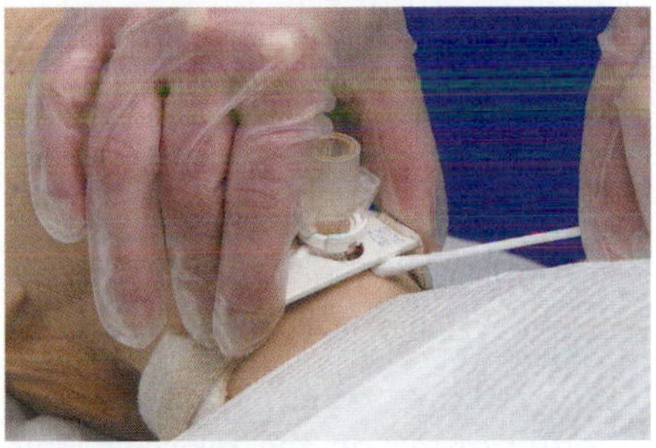

10. **Clean the top surface** of the faceplate and the skin around it with the gauze pads saturated with filtered tap water or normal saline solution. Use each gauze pad only once, and then discard it.
Removes secretions that provide a prime medium for microbial growth; prevents contamination of cleaned areas.

11. **Dry the skin and outer cannula** surfaces by patting them lightly with the remaining dry gauze pad.
Clean, dry skin is needed to avoid skin breakdown and removes moisture, which can promote bacterial growth around the stoma site.

To finish the procedure, skip to steps 12 through 17 of Procedure 36-5B.

Procedure 36-5B ■ Performing Tracheostomy Care Using Sterile Technique

➤ When performing the procedure, always identify your patient according to agency policy, using two identifiers, and be attentive to standard precautions, hand hygiene, patient safety and privacy, body mechanics, and documentation.

Procedure Steps

1. **Position the patient** in semi-Fowler's position and place a towel or linen-saver pad over the patient's chest.
A semi-Fowler's position promotes lung expansion and prevents back strain for the nurse. A towel or linen-saver pad prevents soiling of the patient's gown.

2. **Don clean procedure gloves.**

3. **Hyperoxygenate the patient,** as needed, and suction the tracheostomy (see Procedure 36-6 or 36-7).

(continued on next page)

Procedure 36-5 ■ Performing Tracheostomy Care (continued)

Suctioning clears the tracheostomy of secretions that could occlude the outer canula after the inner cannula is removed for care.

For a Passy–Muir Valve

Remove the Passy–Muir valve (PMV) before suctioning the patient to prepare for tracheostomy care. (A PMV is a device that is used to enable the patient with a tracheostomy to speak. It is attached to the end of the inner cannula at the tracheostomy site.)

4. **Remove and discard** the soiled tracheostomy dressing in the appropriate receptacle, and then remove and discard your gloves. Perform hand hygiene.

5. **Place the tracheostomy care equipment** on the overbed table and prepare the equipment, keeping all supplies and equipment sterile.
Ensures efficiency and helps prevent contamination during tracheostomy care.
   a. *Disposable inner cannula*—Pour sterile normal saline solution into the two sterile containers (per agency policy).
   b. *Reusable inner cannula*—Pour hydrogen peroxide into one of the sterile solution containers and pour sterile normal saline solution into the other one. If the inner cannula is not disposable, use hydrogen peroxide to clean only the inner cannula. Use sterile normal saline to rinse the inner cannula and clean the faceplate and tracheostomy site.

Steps c through g apply to both types of cannula.

   c. Obtain and open two 4 in. × 4 in. sterile gauze packages. Wet the gauze in one package with sterile normal saline solution, and keep the second package dry.
   You will use the second package of gauze to dry the skin around the tracheostomy site after cleaning.
   d. Open one cotton-tipped applicator package. Wet the applicators with sterile normal saline solution.
   Prepares the applicators for cleaning the exposed surface of the outer canula and the stoma site located under the faceplate of the tracheostomy tube, respectively.
   e. Open the package containing a new disposable inner cannula.
   Allows for quick replacement of the inner cannula.
   f. Open the package of Velcro tracheostomy ties, or cut a length of twill tape long enough to go around the patient's neck two times. Make sure to cut end of the tape on an angle.
   Allows for quick stabilization of the tracheostomy tube, preventing dislodgement. Cutting the twill tape on an angle allows for easy insertion through the faceplate eyelets.
   g. Position a biohazard bag within reach.
   Allows you to dispose of contaminated supplies safely as you use them without leaving the patient or interrupting the procedure.

6. **Don sterile gloves.** Consider your dominant hand sterile and your nondominant hand clean (nonsterile). Handle the sterile supplies with the dominant hand only.

7. **For patients receiving oxygen:** With your nondominant (nonsterile) hand, remove the oxygen or humidification source. Attach the oxygen source to the outer cannula, if possible. If not possible, have the respiratory therapist set up oxygen blow-by to use while you are cleaning the reusable inner cannula. (If not receiving oxygen, skip this step.)
Prevents oxygen desaturation in the patient during the procedure.

8. **Unlock and remove the inner cannula** with your nondominant (non-sterile) hand and care for it accordingly.

For a Disposable Inner Cannula

   a. Dispose of the inner cannula in the biohazard receptacle according to agency policy. You should never clean and reuse a disposable inner cannula.
   Prevents contamination by bacteria contained in the inner cannula.
   b. With your dominant hand (sterile), insert the new inner cannula into the patient's tracheostomy in the direction of the curvature. Following the manufacturer's instructions, lock the inner cannula in place securely to prevent it from dislodging. Remember to keep your dominant hand sterile.

For a Reusable Inner Cannula

   c. If a reusable inner cannula was used, place the inner cannula into the basin filled with hydrogen peroxide.
   Hydrogen peroxide helps loosen tenacious (sticky) secretions.
   d. Pick up the reusable inner cannula from the container of hydrogen peroxide with your nondominant hand and scrub it with the sterile nylon brush, using your dominant (sterile) hand.
   e. Immerse the inner cannula in the container of sterile normal saline solution and agitate it until it is rinsed thoroughly.
   Immersing the inner cannula in sterile saline solution and agitating it removes the hydrogen peroxide and debris from the inner cannula, minimizing tissue irritation.
   f. Tap the inner cannula against the side of the container to remove water.
   Removes excess fluid so the patient does not aspirate it when you reinsert the cannula.
   g. With your dominant (sterile) hand, reinsert the inner cannula into the patient's tracheostomy in the direction of the curvature. Following the manufacturer's instructions, lock the inner cannula

in place securely to prevent it from dislodging. Remember to keep your dominant hand clean.

For a Passy–Muir Valve

h. Swish the PMV in warm tap water with mild soap.

i. Rinse the PMV thoroughly in warm filtered tap water.

j. **Key Point:** ***DO NOT use hot water, peroxide, bleach, vinegar, alcohol, brushes, or cotton-tipped applicators to clean PMV, as this could damage the valve.***

k. Shake the PMV to remove excess fluid. If you are going to store the valve, be sure to air-dry the valve before placing it in a storage container.
Removes moisture, which can promote bacterial growth.

l. Set the PMV aside on clean surface to be replaced when the inner cannula is replaced.

For Patients Receiving Oxygen

m. Remove the humidification or oxygen source from the outer cannula, if indicated, using your nondominant hand.

n. Using your dominant (sterile) hand, reinsert the inner cannula into the patient's tracheostomy in the direction of the curvature.

o. Following the manufacturer's instructions, lock the inner cannula in place securely. Remember to keep dominant hand clean.
Lock the inner cannula in place securely to prevent it from dislodging.

p. Reattach the humidification or oxygen source, if indicated.
Provides the patient with needed humidity or oxygen and prevents oxygen desaturation.

9. Clean the stoma under the faceplate with cotton-tipped applicators saturated with sterile normal saline solution, using a circular motion from the stoma site outward. Use each applicator only once and then discard it.
Prevents contamination of the cleaned area.

10. Clean the top surface of the faceplate and the skin around it with the gauze pads saturated sterile normal saline solution. Use each wipe or gauze pad only once, and then discard it.
Removes secretions that provide a medium for microbial growth; prevents contamination of cleaned areas.

11. Dry the skin and outer cannula surfaces by patting them lightly with the remaining dry gauze pad.
Clean, dry skin is needed to avoid skin breakdown and removes moisture, which can promote bacterial growth around the stoma site.

The following steps apply to both modified sterile and sterile technique:

12. **Seek assistance from another** staff member to help with changing the tracheostomy stabilizers.
Prevents accidental dislodging should the patient begin coughing during the procedure.

13. Remove soiled tracheostomy stabilizers.

Removing a Soiled Velcro Tracheostomy Holder

a. With an assistant stabilizing the tracheostomy tube, disengage the Velcro on both sides of the soiled holder and remove it gently from the eyes of the faceplate. Discard the Velcro holder in the nearest biohazard receptacle.
Removing the soiled holder promotes hygiene and prevents the spread of infection.

Removing Soiled Twill Tape Tracheostomy Ties

b. With an assistant stabilizing the tracheostomy tube, cut the soiled tracheostomy ties using bandage scissors. *Do not* cut the tube of the tracheostomy balloon (if you do, the tracheostomy tube must be replaced). Remove the ties gently from the eyes of the faceplate and discard them in the nearest biohazard receptacle.
The tracheostomy balloon helps stabilize the tracheostomy in the trachea and prevents an air leak. Cutting the tube to the balloon prevents the balloon from holding air. Removing the soiled holder promotes hygiene and prevents the spread of infection.

14. Ask the patient to flex his neck, or, if he is unable, ask the assistant to hold the patient's head forward, and apply new tracheostomy ties.
Flexing the neck provides the same neck circumference as when the patient coughs and thus ensures you do not place and secure the tracheostomy stabilizers too tightly.

Using a Velcro Tracheostomy Holder

a. Unfasten the Velcro. Thread one end of the tracheostomy holder through the eyelet of the faceplate and fasten it.

b. Bring the holder around the back of the patient's neck.
The holder must be placed around the patient's neck to adequately secure the tracheostomy.

c. Thread the remaining end of the tracheostomy holder through the empty eyelet of the faceplate and fasten the Velcro, making sure that the holder fits securely.

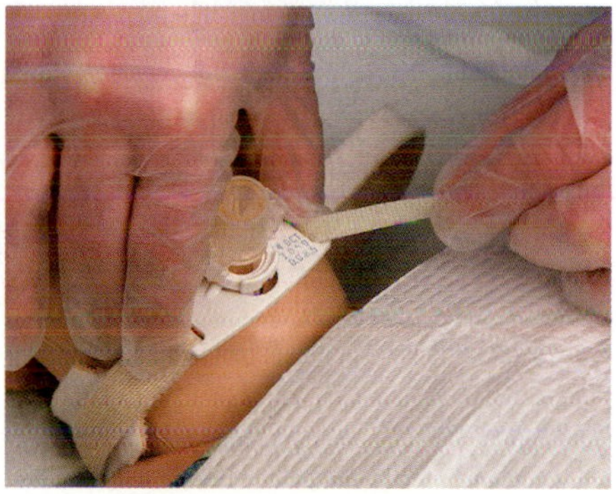

d. Place one finger under the holder to make sure that the holder is securing the tracheostomy effectively but isn't too tight.
Securing the tracheostomy too tightly might place pressure on the jugular veins, interfere with coughing, or cause necrosis at the tracheostomy insertion site.

(continued on next page)

Procedure 36-5 ■ Performing Tracheostomy Care (continued)

Using Twill Tape

e. Thread one end of the twill tape into one of the eyelets on the tracheostomy faceplate.

f. Continue to thread the twill tape through the eyelet, bringing both ends of the tape together.

g. Bring both ends of the twill tape around the back of the patient's neck.
To adequately secure the tracheostomy.

h. Thread the end of the twill tape that is closest to the patient's neck through the back of the eyelet on the faceplate.

i. Have your assistant place one finger under the twill tape while you tie the two ends together in a square knot.
Ensures you do not secure the tracheostomy too tightly.

j. Place one finger under the holder to make sure that the holder is securing the tracheostomy effectively but isn't too tight.
See step 14d.

15. Don a new pair of sterile gloves (after removing gloves and performing hand hygiene).

16. Insert a precut, sterile tracheostomy dressing under the faceplate and new tracheostomy stabilizers or fold a 4 in. × 4 in. gauze pad into a V shape (below). ▼

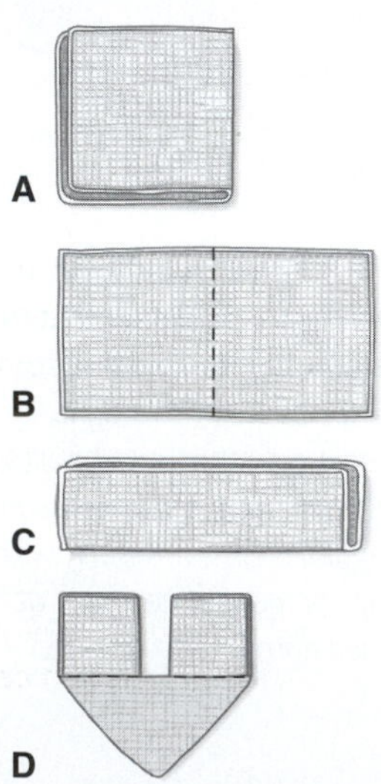

The new dressing absorbs secretions and prevents skin breakdown under the faceplate. Never cut the gauze to make a dressing because lint and fibers from the cut edge could enter the trachea and cause respiratory distress. ▼

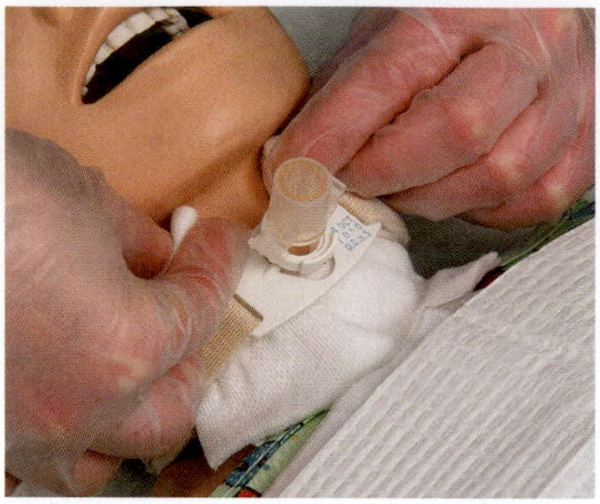

17. Dispose of the used equipment in the appropriate biohazard receptacle according to agency policy.
Helps prevent cross-contamination.

? What if . . .

■ **Your patient begins coughing?**

a. If the tracheostomy is still secured with ties or Velcro holder, wait to continue tracheostomy care until coughing has ended.

b. If tracheostomy is unsecured, stabilize the tube so that it does not become dislodged, being careful not to press too hard on the site. Continue with tracheostomy care when the patient finishes coughing.
Pressing too hard at the tracheostomy site will stimulate the coughing reflex.

c. If coughing continues, suspend tracheostomy care and suction the patient to remove any retained secretions.
Retained secretions may cause increased airway irritation and coughing. Removing secretions will reduce this irritation.

■ **You do not have an assistant to hold the cannula in place while you replace the soiled tracheostomy ties?**

Never cut the soiled tape before applying the clean tape. Always place the new tape/holders, be certain the tracheostomy is secured, and then cut off the soiled tape or holder.

■ **The tracheostomy tube becomes dislodged?**

a. To prevent this, plan ahead and always have another staff member with you to secure the tracheostomy tube while you change the tracheostomy ties or Velcro holder.

b. If the tracheostomy tube slips out slightly but is still in the trachea site, gently push it back into the stoma and secure it.
The pilot balloon will help to keep the tracheostomy tube from completely dislodging.

c. If the tracheostomy tube becomes completely dislodged, stay with the patient and ask your assistant to call for the respiratory therapist or trained person in your facility to insert a new tracheostomy tube.

■ **At step 9, there are crusts around the stoma when you are cleaning the stoma?**

Remove the crusts with a cotton-tipped swab soaked in hydrogen peroxide, then rinse with a swab soaked in filtered tap water or normal saline. Have the patient hold his breath while you remove crusts so he does not inhale them.

Evaluation

- Assess the area around the stoma site for signs of skin breakdown.
- Evaluate the patient's tolerance of the procedure. Note whether there were any signs of respiratory distress.

Patient Teaching

- Explain to the patient and his family that bloody secretions are normal for 2 to 3 days after tracheostomy tube insertion or for 24 hours after a tracheostomy tube change.
- Tell the patient and/or family to inform the nurse immediately if the tracheostomy tube becomes dislodged.
- Teach tracheostomy care to the patient and caregiver if the tracheostomy is expected to remain long term.

Home Care

- Clean, rather than sterile, technique can be used for tracheostomy care if the tracheostomy is more than 1 month old.
- Instruct the client and caregiver about home oxygen therapy and suctioning, if necessary.
- Demonstrate tracheostomy care to the caregiver and ask for a return demonstration.
- Provide the client and caregiver with information about where to obtain tracheostomy care supplies.
- Supply the client and caregiver with contact information of healthcare personnel who can be reached for advice or emergencies.
- Recommend ways of adding moisture to the air, with a goal of maintaining a relative humidity of 50% (e.g., a large humidifier, house plants, wearing damp gauze over the stoma, closing the bathroom door and turning on the hot water to fill the room with steam).
- The stoma should be cleaned using clean technique at least twice daily (or more often, depending on the amount of secretions).
- Stress good hand washing before and after doing any part of tracheostomy care.
- Remind client and caregiver not to use cotton or gauze. *These can leave fibers that may get into the airway and increase the incidence of infection.*

Documentation

- Document the date and time you performed tracheostomy care.
- Record the color, amount, consistency, and odor of secretions.
- Record the condition of the stoma and skin around the stoma site; note the presence of drainage, redness, or swelling.
- Document respiratory status, including respiratory rate, depth, and pattern; skin color; and breath sounds.
- Document the patient's tolerance of the procedure.
- If problems arose, document any interventions that were necessary.

Sample documentation

NOTE: Because this is only a partial computer screen, it may not show all the information you would need to record about the patient.

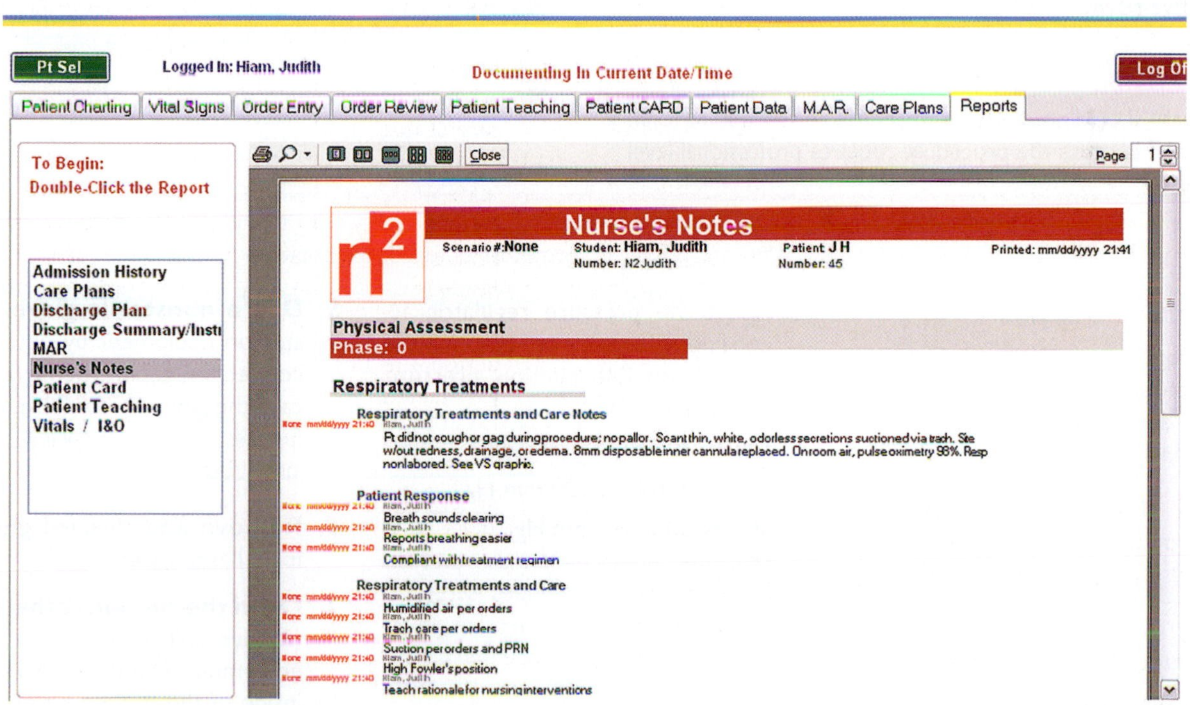

(continued on next page)

Procedure 36-5 ■ Performing Tracheostomy Care (continued)

Practice Resources

Barnett, M. (2012); Johnston, J., Davis, S., & Sherman, J. (n.d., updated 2016); Kozin, E., Straton, J., & Kapo, J. (2012); Mitchell, R. B., Hussey, H. M., Setzen, G., et al. (2013); Siddiqui, J., Sherren, P. B., & Birchall, M. A. (2013); Siegel, J., Rhinehart, E., Jackson, M., et al. (2007).

Thinking About the Procedure

The video **Performing Tracheostomy Care Using Sterile Technique,** along with questions and suggested responses, is available on the ***Davis's Nursing Skills Videos*** Web site on FADavis.com.

Procedure 36-6 ■ Performing Tracheostomy or Endotracheal Suctioning (Open System)

➤ For steps to follow in *all* procedures, refer to the Universal Steps for All Procedures found on the inside back cover.

Equipment

- Portable or wall suction device with tubing and a collection canister
- Linen-saver pad or towel
- Resuscitation bag connected to oxygen source
- Sterile suction catheter kit: adults: 12 to 18 Fr; children: 8 to 10 Fr; infants: 5 to 8 Fr
- If a kit isn't available, collect the following: sterile gloves, sterile suction catheter of the appropriate size, and a sterile container.
- Pour-bottle of sterile, normal saline solution
- Sterile basin or container for fluids
- Prefilled 10-mL containers of normal saline solution
- Face shield or goggles
- Sterile gloves (or procedure gloves; follow agency policy)
- Protective gown

Delegation

As a rule you should not delegate tracheostomy suctioning to an LPN or UAP because the procedure requires professional-level theoretical knowledge, assessment skills, and problem-solving ability. However, if the patient has a permanent tracheostomy tube in place and the patient will require long-term care, care can be delegated to trained personnel. Refer to individual state board of nursing for rules on delegating this procedure.

Pre-Procedure Assessments

- Assess the respiratory rate, depth, and rhythm; breath sounds; color; and pulse oximetry results.
- Assess for signs that indicate the need for suctioning: restlessness, cyanosis, labored respirations, decreased oxygen saturation, increased heart and respiratory rates, visible secretions in the airway, increased peak airway pressures on the ventilator, decreasing Sa_{O_2} or Pa_{O_2}, and adventitious breath sounds during auscultation.
  Suctioning should be performed only when necessary to prevent unnecessary oxygen desaturation and tissue trauma.

➤ When performing the procedure, always identify your patient according to agency policy, using two identifiers, and be attentive to standard precautions, hand hygiene, patient safety and privacy, body mechanics, and documentation.

Procedure Steps

1. **Position the patient** in semi-Fowler's position, unless contraindicated.
   Promotes lung expansion and oxygenation.
2. **Place the linen-saver pad** or towel on the patient's chest.
   Prevents soiling of the patient's gown during suctioning.
3. **Don face shield or goggles.**
4. **Turn on the wall suction** or portable suction machine, and adjust the pressure regulator according to agency policy, using the lowest possible suction pressure. Typically, this is:
   Adults: 100 to 150 mm Hg
   Children: 100 to 120 mm Hg
   Infants: 50 to 95 mm Hg
   Using the appropriate pressure prevents tissue trauma and ensures successful suctioning. Higher pressures are associated with hypoxemia, tissue trauma, and atelectasis, yet do not improve removal of secretions.
5. **Don a nonsterile glove.** Test the suction equipment by occluding the connection tubing. Remove and discard the glove. Perform hand hygiene.
   Ensures proper functioning before you insert suction catheter.
6. **Remove and discard glove.** Perform hand hygiene.
7. **Open the suction catheter kit** or (if a kit isn't available) the gathered equipment. Maintain sterility of the inside of the suction kit or the gathered equipment.

This prevents contaminating the upper airway when you introduce the suction catheter.

8. **Don gloves.** Follow agency policy, as some guidelines allow for clean non-sterile rather than sterile procedure gloves. Consider your dominant hand clean and your nondominant hand contaminated.

9. **Pour sterile saline** into the sterile container.
Sterile saline is used to clear the suction catheter of secretions after suctioning.

10. **Premeasure the catheter insertion distance** for 0.5 to 1 cm (¼ to ½ in.) past the distal end of the endotracheal tube (ETT); the ETT normally sits between 3 and 7 cm (1 to 2¾ in.) above the carina.

11. **Remove gloves and perform hand hygiene. Don sterile gloves.** Consider your dominant hand sterile and your nondominant hand unsterile.

12. **Pick up the suction catheter** with your dominant hand, and attach it to the connection tubing. Do not touch the connection tubing with your sterile (or clean) glove.
Prepares the suction catheter for use.

13. **Put the tip of the suction** catheter into the sterile container of normal saline solution, and suction a small amount through the suction catheter. Apply suction by placing a finger over the suction control port of the suction catheter.
Lubricates the catheter and helps ensure that the suction equipment is functioning properly. Sterile saline is necessary to clear the suction catheter of secretions after suctioning. The outside of the saline container is not sterile; it would contaminate your dominant hand.

14. **If the patient is receiving supplemental oxygen,** hyperoxygenate the patient according to agency policy. If the patient does not require oxygen, you do not need to hyperoxygenate.
Helps prevent hypoxia and related complications (cardiac arrhythmias, seizures, arrest) during suctioning. Suctioning clears secretions, but it also removes oxygen from airways.

If the Patient Requires Mechanical Ventilation

a. Press the 100% O_2 button on the ventilator. Some agencies require the nurse to manually hyperoxygenate the patient; follow agency policy.
Ventilators typically have a button that allows you to hyperoxygenate the patient for a total of 2 minutes. Once this time period elapses, the ventilator automatically resumes its previous settings.

If the Patient Does Not Require Mechanical Ventilation

b. Obtain the assistance of a second provider.

c. Have your partner attach the resuscitation bag to the tracheostomy tube or endotracheal tube, and hyperoxygenate the patient by compressing the resuscitation bag three to five times as the patient inhales. Remove the resuscitation bag, and place it next to the patient when finished.
You must perform hyperoxygenation manually if the patient does not require mechanical ventilation. ▼

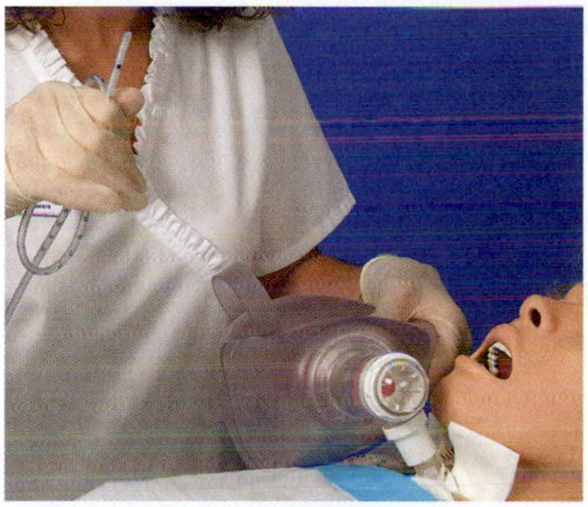

15. **Perform suctioning.**

a. Lubricate the suction catheter tip with the normal saline solution.
Lubrication eases passage of the suction catheter through the endotracheal or tracheostomy tube.

b. Using your dominant hand, gently but quickly insert the suction catheter into the endotracheal or tracheostomy tube. ▼

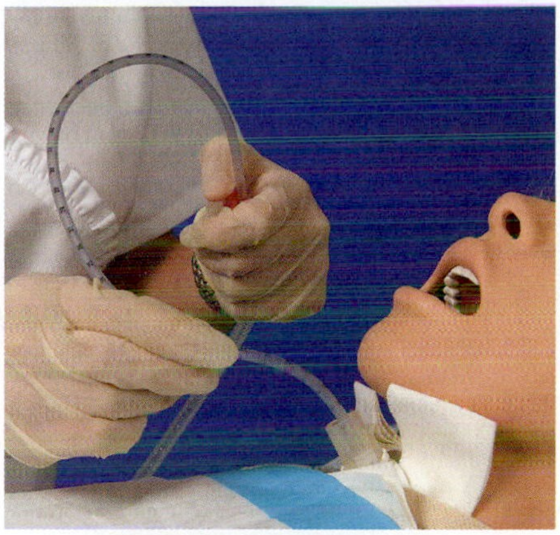

c. Advance the suction catheter, with suction off, gently aiming downward, and being careful not to force the catheter. Insert to the premeasured length: no farther than the **carina tracheae** (the ridge at the lower end of the trachea that separates the openings of the two mainstem bronchi); do not insert more than 6 in. (15 cm), and do not force against any resistance.
Forcing the catheter during insertion may cause tissue trauma.

d. Apply suction while you withdraw the catheter; rotate the catheter (roll it between your thumb and forefinger) as you remove it. Make sure to apply suction for no longer than 15 seconds.
Applying suction for longer than 15 seconds causes hypoxia and may cause tissue trauma.

16. **Repeat suctioning as needed.**
Several passes with the suction catheter may be needed to clear the airway of secretions.

a. Allow at least 30-second intervals between suctioning.

b. Hyperoxygenate the patient between each pass.

c. Limit total suctioning time to 5 minutes.

(continued on next page)

Procedure 36-6 ■ Performing Tracheostomy or Endotracheal Suctioning (Open System) (continued)

17. Coil the suction catheter in your dominant hand (alternatively, wrap it around your dominant hand). Pull the sterile (or clean) glove off over the coiled catheter. Discard the glove containing the catheter in a fluid-resistant receptacle designated by your agency.
Prevents contaminating the environment with secretions.

18. Replace the oxygen source if it was removed during suctioning.
To prevent hypoxia.

19. Using your nondominant hand, clear the connecting tubing of secretions by placing the tip into the container of sterile saline.
Prepares the tubing for later reuse.

20. Turn off the suction units (and the oxygen, if appropriate).

21. Remove gloves from nondominant hand, perform hand hygiene, and don clean procedure gloves.

22. Provide mouth care.

23. Reposition the patient.
Promotes comfort and prevents skin breakdown.

? What if . . .

- **Your patient has a cuffed tracheostomy tube?**
Check to see that it is properly inflated before suctioning. Usually this is 20 to 25 mm Hg or less, but follow the manufacturer's instructions and use a cuff manometer. See Clinical Insight 36-4 to learn how to check cuff inflation.

Evaluation

- Assess the color, amount, and consistency of secretions.
- Evaluate the patient's tolerance of the procedure (e.g., were there signs of respiratory distress during suctioning?)
- Evaluate the effectiveness of the procedure by comparing breath sounds, vital signs, and pulse oximetry before and after suctioning.

Patient Teaching

- Teach the patient and caregiver how to perform suctioning if the patient will be discharged with an artificial airway. Make sure they can successfully provide a return demonstration.
- Teach the caregiver strategies for managing the patient's airway at home.

Home Care

- Provide the family and caregiver information about where to obtain suction equipment, contact information for healthcare personnel who can be reached for advice or emergencies, and information about home oxygen therapy.
- Guidelines recommend clean technique for home care, and for repeated catheter use as long as the catheter is still clear.
- Teach the family and caregiver how to clean catheters for reuse (soak in hot, soapy water; rinse inside and out with clean water; air-dry; store in a dry container).

Documentation

Document the following:

- Date, time, and reason you performed suctioning
- The size of the suction catheter you used
- Amount, color, consistency, and odor of secretions
- Patient's respiratory status before and after the procedure
- Patient's tolerance of the procedure
- Any complications that occurred as a result of the procedure, and interventions you made in response

Sample documentation

Sept. 18, 2020 0900 Pulse ox 93%, VS elevated, upper airway rhonchi auscultated. Hyperoxygenated with 100% O_2; suctioned moderate amount thick, yellow mucus with #12 Fr suction catheter. After procedure lungs clear, pulse ox 98%, VS WNL. ——————— Jackie Estes, RN

Practice Resources

American Association for Respiratory Care (2010); Sole, M. L., Bennett, M., & Ashworth, S. (2015).

Thinking About the Procedure

The video **Performing Endotracheal Suctioning (Open System),** along with questions and suggested responses, is available on the ***Davis's Nursing Skills Videos*** Web site on FADavis.com.

Procedure 36-7 ■ Performing Tracheostomy or Endotracheal Suctioning (Inline Closed System)

➤ For steps to follow in *all* procedures, refer to the Universal Steps for All Procedures found on the inside back cover.

Equipment

For the once-a-day steps: Procedure gloves and inline suction catheter

When suctioning: Sterile normal saline and inline suction catheter

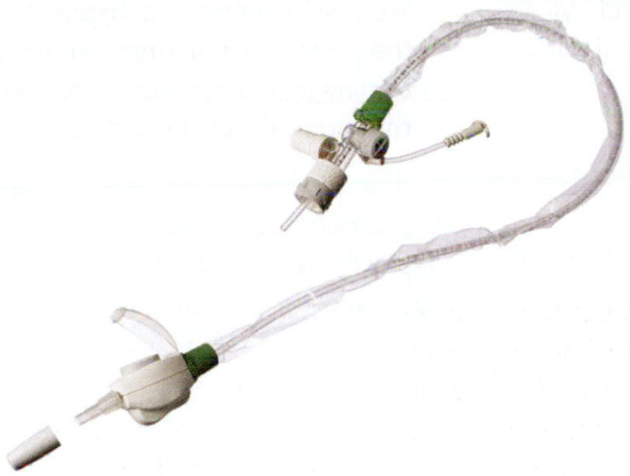

Inline suction catheter. (© Unomedical a/s, used with permission.)

Delegation

As a rule, you should not delegate tracheostomy or endotracheal suctioning to an LPN or UAP because both procedures require professional-level theoretical knowledge, assessment skills, and problem-solving ability. Refer to the individual state board of nursing for rules on delegating this procedure.

Pre-Procedure Assessments

- Assess respiratory status, including respiratory rate, depth, and rhythm; breath sounds; color; and pulse oximetry results.
- Assess for restlessness, cyanosis, labored respirations, decreased oxygen saturation, increased heart and respiratory rates, visible secretions in the airway, and the presence of adventitious breath sounds during auscultation.
  These assessments help determine whether the patient requires suctioning. Suctioning should be performed only when necessary to prevent unnecessary oxygen desaturation and tissue trauma.

➤ When performing the procedure, always identify your patient according to agency policy, using two identifiers, and be attentive to standard precautions, hand hygiene, patient safety and privacy, body mechanics, and documentation.

➤ *Note:* This procedure uses modified sterile technique.

Daily Procedure Steps

1. An inline suction unit is available only for patients on a mechanical ventilator. Most agencies require the respiratory therapy department to set up the inline suction equipment. If this is not the agency's policy, you may need to perform these steps once per day. Open the inline suction catheter package, using sterile technique.
2. Remove the adapter on the ventilator tubing.
3. Attach the inline suction catheter equipment to the ventilator tubing.
4. Reconnect the adapter on the ventilator tubing.
5. Attach the other end of the inline suction catheter to the connection tubing placed to suction.

Suctioning Procedure Steps

1. **Place the patient in semi-Fowler's position, unless contraindicated.**
   The suction catheter is contained within a sterile unit.
2. **Don clean procedure gloves.**
   You do not need to wear sterile gloves.
3. **Place a linen-saver pad** or towel on the patient's chest.
4. **If a lock is present** on the suction control port, unlock it.
5. **Turn on the wall suction** or portable suction machine, and adjust the pressure regulator according to agency policy or provider's prescription.
   Using the appropriate pressure prevents tissue trauma and ensures successful suctioning.
6. **Pick up the catheter** with your dominant hand and use your nondominant hand for the suction port.
   Using the dominant hand improves dexterity.
7. **Unlock the inline catheter** and gently insert the suction catheter into the airway by maneuvering the catheter within the sterile sleeve.

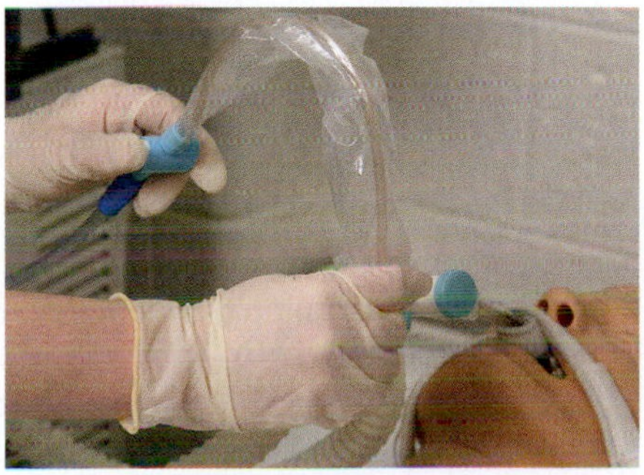

(continued on next page)

Procedure 36-7 ■ Performing Tracheostomy or Endotracheal Suctioning (Inline Closed System) (continued)

8. **Advance the suction catheter** into the airway, being careful not to force the catheter. Ask the patient to take slow, deep breaths if she can cooperate. Advance the catheter to the predetermined and premarked distance. Do not apply suction while advancing.
Forcing the catheter during insertion may cause airway trauma.

9. **Apply suction** by depressing the button over the suction control port as you withdraw the catheter. Apply suction for no longer than 15 seconds.
Applying suction for longer than 15 seconds causes hypoxia and may cause tissue trauma.

10. **Withdraw the inline suction** catheter completely into the sleeve. The indicator line on the catheter should appear through the sleeve.
The indicator line is a safety mechanism designed to make sure the suction catheter is withdrawn completely to prevent airway obstruction.

11. **Attach the prefilled 10-mL** container of normal saline solution to the saline port located on the inline equipment.
Provides a flush solution to clear the suction catheter of secretions.

12. **Squeeze the 10-mL container** while applying suction.
Clears the catheter of secretions, preparing the catheter for repeat use. If allowed to remain in the catheter or suction line, secretions may dry and harden, reducing line suction efficiency.

13. **Lock the suction regulator port.**
Prevents you from inadvertently applying suction.

? What if . . .

- **Your patient experiences a dysrhythmia?**

Stop suctioning and hyperoxygenate the patient. If a further attempt at suctioning promotes a dysrhythmia, notify the medical care provider.

For Evaluation, Patient Teaching, and Documentation, see Procedure 36-6. Typically, you would not be doing inline suctioning in the home.

Practice Resources

Letchford, E., & Bench, S. (2018); Restrepo, R. D., Brown, J. M., & Hughes, J. M. (2010).

Thinking About the Procedure

The video **Performing Tracheostomy Suctioning (Inline Closed System),** along with questions and suggested responses, is available on the ***Davis's Nursing Skills Videos*** Web site on FADavis.com.

Procedure 36-8 ■ Performing Orotracheal and Nasotracheal Suctioning (Open System)

➤ For steps to follow in *all* procedures, refer to the Universal Steps for All Procedures found on the inside back cover.

➤ *Note:* This procedure uses modified sterile technique. Although the oropharynx and nasopharynx are not sterile, you should keep the suction catheter free from other contaminants as much as possible. Some facilities do use sterile gloves for this procedure.

Equipment

- Portable or wall suction device with connection tubing and a collection canister
- Linen-saver pad or towel
- Sterile, flexible, multiple-eyed suction catheter kit (12 to 18 Fr for adults, 8 to 10 Fr for children, and 5 to 8 Fr for infants). If a kit isn't available, collect the following: sterile gloves, sterile suction catheter of the appropriate size, and a sterile container for fluids
- Pour-bottle of sterile water or sterile normal saline solution
- Face shield or goggles and gown
- Water-soluble lubricant for NT suctioning
- Sputum trap, if a specimen is needed
- Nasopharyngeal airway when frequent NT suctioning is required
- Resuscitation bag with mask

Delegation

You should not delegate orotracheal and nasotracheal suctioning to an LPN or UAP because these procedures require theoretical knowledge, assessment skills, and problem-solving ability.

Pre-Procedure Assessments

- Assess respiratory rate, depth, and rhythm; breath sounds; skin color; and pulse oximetry results.
- Assess for signs that indicate the need for suctioning: gurgling sounds during respiration, restlessness, labored respirations, decreased oxygen saturation, increased heart and respiratory rates, and the presence of adventitious breath sounds during auscultation.

  Suctioning removes oxygen from airways and can cause tissue trauma. It should be done only when essential (i.e., only when less invasive techniques have proved unsuccessful and when the secretions are causing physiological deterioration and/or distress).
- Assess the effectiveness of the cough.

➤ When performing the procedure, always identify your patient according to agency policy, using two identifiers, and be attentive to standard precautions, hand hygiene, patient safety and privacy, body mechanics, and documentation.

Procedure Steps

1. **Position the patient.**

Variation for Orotracheal Suctioning

a. Position the patient in semi-Fowler's position, with the head turned to face you.

Variation for Nasotracheal Suctioning

b. Position the patient in semi-Fowler's position, with his neck hyperextended, unless contraindicated.
Hyperextending the neck makes it easier to insert the suction catheter. Upright position helps to prevent back strain.

2. **Place the linen-saver pad** or towel on the patient's chest.
Prevents soiling of the patient's gown during suctioning.

3. **Put on a face shield or goggles and gown.**
Protects you from contamination with secretions that may splash during suctioning.

4. **Turn on the wall suction** or portable suction machine, and adjust the pressure regulator according to agency policy. Guidelines from American Association for Respiratory Care (AARC) specify:

   Adults: 100 to 150 mm Hg

   Children: 100 to 120 mm Hg

   Infants: 80 to 100 mm Hg

   Neonates: 60 to 80 mm Hg

   The suction regulator must be set appropriately to prevent tissue trauma and hypoxia and yet remove secretions effectively.

5. **Don a procedure glove** and test the suction equipment by occluding the connection tubing. Discard the glove and perform hand hygiene.
Testing the equipment ensures proper functioning before you insert the catheter in the patient's airway.

6. **Open the suction catheter kit** or, if a kit isn't available, the gathered equipment.
Nasal approach: If you are using the nasal approach, open the water-soluble lubricant and a nasopharyngeal airway.

7. **Don clean nonsterile gloves.** Consider your dominant hand clean and your nondominant hand contaminated.
Keeping the dominant hand sterile prevents contaminating the upper airways with a nonsterile suction catheter. This is a modified sterile suction technique because the catheter enters the trachea via nose or the mouth, which are not sterile. However, take care to keep the catheter free from other contamination.

If Using Sterile Technique

Don sterile gloves. Consider your dominant hand sterile and your nondominant hand unsterile. Alternatively, put a sterile glove on your dominant hand and a clean procedure glove on your nondominant hand.

NOTE: If you consider both hands sterile (i.e., for sterile technique), you must remove the cap from the sterile water before donning gloves.

8. **Pour sterile saline** into the sterile container using your nondominant hand.
Sterile saline will be used to clear the suction catheter of secretions after suctioning.

9. **Pick up the suction catheter** with your dominant hand, and attach it to the connection tubing, maintaining sterility of your hand and the catheter.
Prepares the suction catheter for use.

10. **Put the tip of the suction** catheter into the sterile container of normal saline solution, and suction a small amount of normal saline solution through the suction catheter. Apply suction by placing a finger over the suction control port of the suction catheter.
Lubricates the catheter and helps ensure that the suction equipment is functioning properly.

11. **Ask the patient to take several slow, deep breaths.** If patient's oxygen saturation is <94%, or if he is in any distress, you may need to give supplemental oxygen before, during, and after suctioning. See Procedure 36-4.
Promotes relaxation and helps hyperoxygenate the patient before suctioning.

12. **Using your nondominant hand,** remove the oxygen delivery device, if present (for nasal suctioning only).

For Oral Approach, Patient Receiving Nasal Oxygen

a. If the patient is receiving nasal oxygen and you are doing orotracheal suctioning, you do not need to remove the oxygen source.

(continued on next page)

Procedure 36-8 ■ Performing Orotracheal and Nasotracheal Suctioning (Open System) (continued)

For Nasal Approach, Patient Receiving Nasal Oxygen

b. Remove the nasal oxygen and place the nasal cannula in the patient's mouth. See Procedure 36-4.
Placing the cannula in the patient's mouth makes it easier to access the nares for suctioning while still delivering oxygen to the patient (orally).

13. Premeasure to approximate the depth you should insert the suction catheter. For adults, insert the catheter about 15 cm (6 in.) for an oral approach, and 20 cm (8 in.) for a nasal approach. Be careful not to contaminate the catheter while you measure.
Prevents trauma at the carina and ensures suctioning of the full length of the trachea.

For Oral Approach

a. Measure the distance between the edge of the patient's mouth to the tip of the earlobe and down to the bottom of the neck. ▼

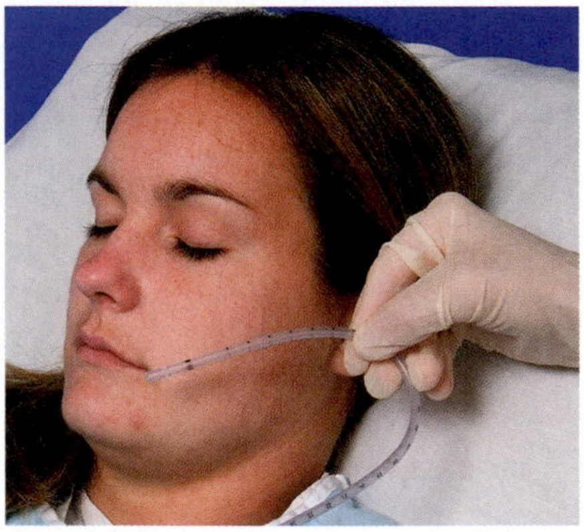

For Nasal Approach

b. Measure the distance from the tip of the nose to the tip of the earlobe and down to the bottom of the neck.
c. Insert nasopharyngeal airway gently into the nostril, with the bevel toward the septum (center of the nose), advance the airway straight in, following the floor of the nose. See Procedure 36-13.
Do not force nasopharyngeal airway into the nostril as this may cause unnecessary edema and trauma.

14. Lubricate and insert the suction catheter.
Lubrication makes it easier to pass a suction catheter through the nares.

For Orotracheal Suctioning

a. Lubricate the suction catheter tip with normal saline solution.
b. Using your dominant hand, gently but quickly insert the suction catheter along the side of the patient's mouth or through the endotracheal tube into the oropharynx.
Quick insertion along the side of the mouth prevents gagging.
c. When the patient inhales, advance the suction catheter to the predetermined distance, being careful not to force the catheter.
Advancing the suction catheter during inhalation ensures that the catheter enters the trachea rather than the esophagus. Forcing the catheter during insertion may cause tissue trauma.

For Nasotracheal Suctioning

d. Lubricate the catheter tip with the water-soluble lubricant.
Water-soluble lubricant is preferred because it will dissolve if it accidentally enters the lungs, whereas an oil-based lubricant (e.g., petroleum jelly) won't dissolve in the respiratory tract and causes complications if it enters the lungs.
e. Using your dominant hand, gently but quickly insert the suction catheter into the naris and down to the pharynx. When the patient inhales, advance the suction catheter, gently aiming downward to the predetermined distance, being careful not to force the catheter.
Ensures that the catheter enters the trachea. Forcing the catheter during insertion may cause tissue trauma.

15. Place a finger or thumb over the suction control port of the catheter. Apply suction while you withdraw the catheter, using a continuous rotating motion. Apply suction for no longer than 15 seconds.
Using a continuous rotating motion and suctioning while withdrawing the catheter prevents trauma to any one area of the airway. Limiting suctioning to less than 15 seconds prevents hypoxia. ▼

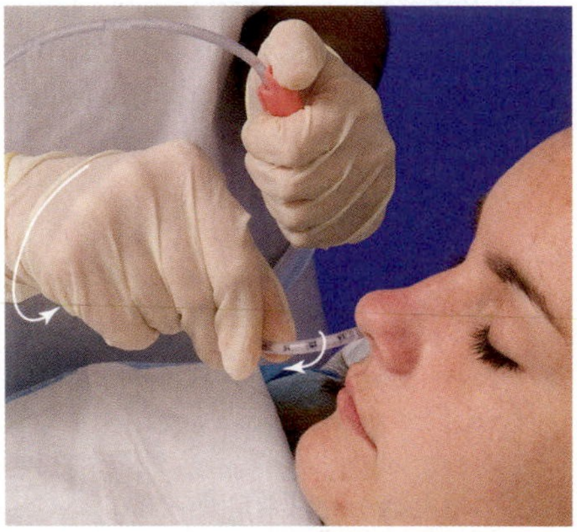

16. After you withdraw the catheter, clear it by placing the tip of the catheter into the container of sterile saline and applying suction. ▼

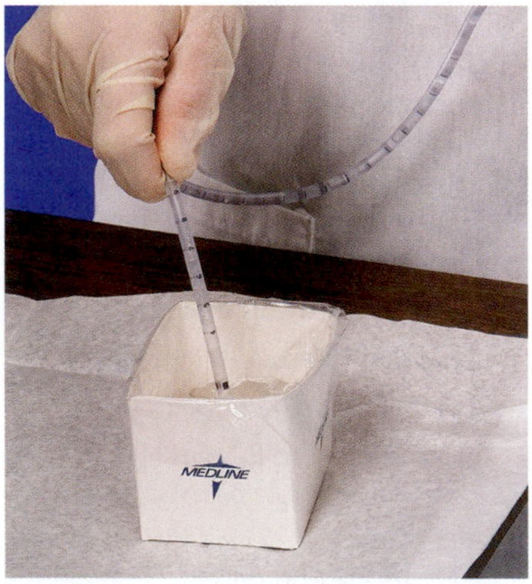

17. Lubricate the catheter, and repeat suctioning as needed, allowing intervals of at least 30 seconds between suctioning. Reapply oxygen between suctioning efforts, if required.
Several passes with the suction catheter may be needed to clear the airway of secretions. Total suctioning time should be limited to 5 minutes, however, to prevent trauma and hypoxia.

18. Replace the oxygen source.
Prevents hypoxia.

19. Coil the suction catheter in your dominant hand (alternatively, wrap it around your dominant hand). Hold the catheter while you pull the sterile glove off over it. Discard the glove containing the catheter in a biohazard receptacle (e.g., bag) designated by your agency.
These actions prevent contaminating the environment with secretions.

20. Using your nondominant hand, clear the connecting tubing of secretions by placing the tip into the container of sterile saline.

21. Dispose of equipment, and make sure new suction supplies are readily available for future suctioning.
The patient may require suctioning at any time, so equipment must be readily available.

22. Remove glove from nondominant hand and perform hand hygiene.

23. Don clean procedure gloves and provide mouth care.
Promotes patient comfort and clears the mouth of any secretions the patient may have expectorated.

24. Assist the patient to a comfortable position, and allow him to rest.
Comfort and rest help the patient recover from the stress of suctioning.

? What if . . .

- **Your patient's oxygen saturation is less than 94%, or if he is in any distress?**

  Administer supplemental oxygen before, during, and after suctioning. Notify the patient's primary provider if the patient does not respond to additional oxygen.

Evaluation

- Assess the color, consistency, and amount of secretions.
- Evaluate the patient's tolerance of the procedure. Note whether there were signs of respiratory distress during suctioning.
- Evaluate the effectiveness of the procedure by comparing breath sounds, vital signs, and pulse oximetry or blood gas data before and after the procedure.

Patient Teaching

- Explain the importance of administering supplemental oxygen or of taking several deep breaths before suctioning.
- Inform the patient that coughing typically increases with suctioning.
- Demonstrate orotracheal or nasotracheal suctioning to the caregiver, and ask for a return demonstration if suctioning will be required at home.

Home Care

- Instruct the family and caregiver about where to obtain suction equipment.
- Provide contact information of healthcare personnel who can be reached for advice or emergencies.
- Explain that the procedure can be performed using clean technique instead of sterile technique in the home.
- Instruct the caregiver that suction catheters can be cleaned for reuse by washing them with soapy water and then boiling them for 10 minutes. After they are cleaned, rinse the catheters with normal saline solution or tap water.
- Instruct to change the secretion collection container every 24 hours, or clean it according to home care agency guidelines every 24 hours.

Documentation

- Document the date, time, and reason you performed suctioning.
- Note the suction technique you used and the catheter size.
- Note the color, consistency, and odor of secretions.
- Document the patient's respiratory status before and after the procedure.
- Document the patient's tolerance of the procedure and any complications that occurred as a result of the procedure.
- Document any interventions you performed to address complications that occurred.

Sample documentation

July 31, 2020 0930 O_2 sat 89% on room air, bilateral rhonchi to bases auscultated, unproductive cough, heart rate 90, RR-18. Assistant nurse recruited for manual ventilation. Client placed in semi-Fowler's position, hyperventilated for 1 minute to 100% O_2 sat, oropharyngeal suctioning performed using sterile technique, resulting in moderate amounts of white, tenacious, yellow-tinged secretions. Improved breath sound with diminished rhonchi auscultated, O_2 sat at 97% on room air, heart rate 78, RR-14. Client smiles when asked how he feels. Bed in low position, call light and fluids in reach. ——— Kelton Jones, RN

Practice Resources

American Association for Respiratory Care (2010); American Red Cross (2011); Barnett, M. (2012); Restrepo, R. D. (2010).

Procedure 36-9 ■ Performing Upper Airway Suctioning

➤ For steps to follow in *all* procedures, refer to the Universal Steps for All Procedures found on the inside back cover.

➤ *Note:* Upper airway suctioning may be done via the oropharyngeal or nasopharyngeal route. However, nasal suction is usually required only to improve oxygenation in infants because most adult airway obstruction occurs in the mouth and oropharynx.

Vigorous nasal suction can induce epistaxis (nosebleed) and further complicate an already difficult airway.

Equipment

- Portable or wall suction device with connection tubing and a collection canister
- Linen-saver pad or towel
- Sterile suction catheter kit (12 to 18 Fr for adults, 8 to 10 Fr for children, and 5 to 8 Fr for infants). If a kit isn't available, collect the following: sterile suction catheter of the appropriate size, and a sterile container. If you plan to suction both the oropharynx and the nasopharynx, you need a separate sterile catheter for each.
- Yankauer device can be used for oropharyngeal suction.
- Pour-bottle of sterile normal saline solution
- Sterile basin or other container for fluids
- Face shield or goggles and gown
- Procedure gloves
- Water-soluble lubricant for nasopharyngeal suctioning
- Sputum trap, if a specimen is needed
- Biohazard bag

Delegation

Do not delegate oropharyngeal and nasopharyngeal suctioning to an LPN or UAP because these procedures require theoretical knowledge, assessment skills, and problem-solving ability. However, the UAP (and the client or family) can use a Yankauer tube to suction the oral cavity because there is less risk for trauma to mucosa than with oro- or nasopharyngeal suctioning.

Pre-Procedure Assessments

- Assess respiratory rate, depth, and rhythm; breath sounds; color; and pulse oximetry results. Note signs that indicate the need for suctioning: restlessness, cyanosis, labored respirations, decreased oxygen saturation, increased heart and respiratory rates, visible secretions in the airway, and the presence of adventitious breath sounds during auscultation.
  You must be certain the patient requires suctioning. Suctioning should be performed only when necessary to prevent unnecessary oxygen desaturation and tissue trauma.

➤ When performing the procedure, always identify your patient according to agency policy, using two identifiers, and be attentive to standard precautions, hand hygiene, patient safety and privacy, body mechanics, and documentation.

➤ *Note:* This procedure describes modified sterile technique: sterile supplies with clean procedure gloves. Although the oropharynx and nasopharynx are not sterile, you should keep the suction catheter free from other contaminants as much as possible. Some facilities do use sterile gloves for this procedure.

Procedure Steps

1. **Position the patient.** Explain that suctioning may stimulate coughing or gagging, but that coughing helps mobilize secretions.

Oropharyngeal Suctioning

Position the patient in a semi-Fowler's or high Fowler's position, with his head turned toward you.
Facilitates insertion of the suction catheter and prevents straining your back. It also promotes lung expansion and effective coughing.

For Nasopharyngeal Suctioning

Position the patient in semi-Fowler's or high Fowler's position with his neck hyperextended, unless contraindicated.

2. **Place the linen-saver pad** or towel on the patient's chest.
   Prevents soiling of the patient's gown during suctioning.

3. **Put on a face shield or goggles and gown.**
   Protects you from contamination with secretions that may splash during suctioning. Not all guidelines specify wearing a gown for this procedure.

4. **Turn on the wall suction** or portable suction machine, and adjust the pressure regulator according to agency policy, typically:
   Adults: 100 to 150 mm Hg
   Children: 100 to 120 mm Hg
   Infants: 50 to 95 mm Hg
   The suction regulator must be set appropriately to prevent tissue trauma and hypoxia and to function effectively to remove secretions. Higher pressures are associated with hypoxemia, tissue trauma, and atelectasis, yet do not improve removal of secretions.

5. **Test the suction equipment** by occluding the connection tubing.
   Ensures proper functioning before use.

6. **Open the suction catheter kit** or the gathered equipment. If you are using the nasal approach, open the water-soluble lubricant.

7. **Don procedure gloves**; consider (and keep) your dominant hand clean; consider your nondominant hand to be contaminated.
   This is not a sterile suction procedure, but care should be taken to keep the suction catheter free from other contaminants. Keeping the dominant hand clean prevents contaminating the upper airways with an unclean suction catheter.

8. **Pour sterile saline** into the sterile container, using your nondominant hand.
Sterile saline is necessary to clear the suction catheter of secretions after suctioning. The outside of the saline container is not sterile; it would contaminate your dominant hand.

9. **Pick up the suction catheter** with your dominant hand, and use your other hand to hold the connection tubing (to suction) while you attach it.

10. **Put the tip of the suction catheter** into the sterile container of normal saline solution, and suction a small amount of normal saline solution through the suction catheter. Apply suction by placing a finger over the suction control port. When using a Yankauer-type device, the suction is continuous and there is no port to occlude.
Ensures that the suction equipment is functioning properly. If you need to see a Yankauer device,

Go to **Figure 36-13C,** in Volume 1.

11. **Approximate the depth** to which you will insert the suction catheter.

For Oropharyngeal Suctioning

Measure the distance between the edge of the patient's mouth and the tip of the patient's earlobe.
Determines the proper distance you should insert the suction catheter for oropharyngeal suctioning.

For Nasopharyngeal Suctioning

Measure the distance between the tip of the patient's nose and the tip of the patient's earlobe.
Helps determine the correct distance you should insert the suction catheter for nasopharyngeal suctioning.

12. **Using your nondominant hand,** remove the oxygen delivery device, if present (for nasopharyngeal suctioning only). Have the patient take several slow, deep breaths.
Deep breathing helps to hyperoxygenate the patient and helps prevent hypoxia during suctioning.

13. **Lubricate and insert the suction catheter.**

For Oropharyngeal Suctioning

a. Lubricate the catheter tip with the normal saline solution.
b. Using your dominant hand, gently but quickly insert the suction catheter along the side of the patient's mouth into the oropharynx.
Inserting the suction catheter along the side of the mouth prevents gagging.

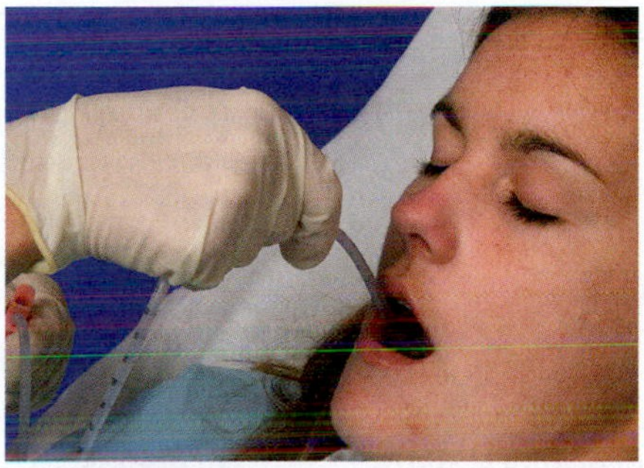

c. Advance the suction catheter quickly to the premeasured distance—usually 7.5 to 10 cm (3 to 4 in.) in the adult—being careful not to force the catheter.
Ensures that the suction catheter will reach the pharynx. Forcing the catheter during insertion may cause tissue trauma.

For Nasopharyngeal Suctioning

d. Lubricate the catheter tip with the water-soluble lubricant.
Eases passage of the suction catheter through the naris. Water-soluble lubricant is preferred because it will dissolve if it accidentally enters the lungs, whereas an oil-based lubricant (e.g., petroleum jelly or lotion) will not dissolve in the respiratory tract and causes complications if it enters the lungs.
e. Using your dominant hand, gently but quickly insert the suction catheter into the naris.
Prevents trauma to the naris.

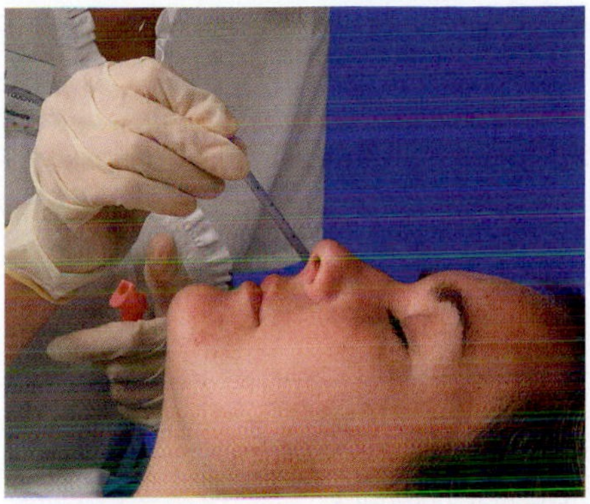

f. Advance the suction catheter, aiming downward to the premeasured distance—usually 13 to 15 cm (5 to 6 in.) in an adult—and being careful not to force the catheter. If you meet resistance, you may need to try the other naris.
Advancing the suction catheter the premeasured distance ensures that the suction catheter will reach the pharynx. Forcing the catheter during insertion may cause tissue trauma.

14. **Place a finger or thumb over** the suction control port of the suction catheter, and start suctioning the patient. Apply suction as you withdraw the catheter, using a continuous rotating motion.

> Limit suctioning to 10 to 15 seconds.
> *Using a continuous rotating motion while withdrawing the catheter prevents trauma to any one area of the airway. Limiting suctioning to less than 10 to 15 seconds prevents hypoxia.*

15. **After you withdraw** the catheter, clear it by placing the tip of the catheter into the container of sterile saline and applying suction.
Ensures patency of the catheter for repeat suctioning.

16. **Lubricate the catheter,** and repeat suctioning as needed, allowing at least 20-second intervals between suctioning. Limit total suctioning time to 5 minutes.

(continued on next page)

Procedure 36-9 ■ Performing Upper Airway Suctioning (continued)

Several passes with the suction catheter may be needed to clear the airway of secretions. The total suctioning time should be limited to 5 minutes, however, to prevent hypoxia and trauma to the mucosal membranes.

For Nasopharyngeal Suctioning

Each time you repeat suction, alternate nares.
Prevents trauma that would occur if you used only one naris.

17. **Coil the suction catheter** in your dominant hand. Pull the sterile glove off over the coiled catheter. (Alternatively, wrap the catheter around your dominant, gloved hand, and hold the catheter as you remove the glove over it.) Discard the glove containing the catheter in a biohazard receptacle designated by your agency.
Coiling the catheter inside the glove prevents contamination with secretions.

18. **Using your nondominant hand,** clear the connecting tubing of secretions by placing the tip of the tube into the container of sterile saline.
Ensures patency and prepares the equipment for future use.

19. **Dispose of equipment** in biohazard waste container/bag, and make sure new suction supplies are readily available for future suctioning needs.
The patient may require suctioning at any time, so equipment must be readily available.

20. **Provide mouth care.**
Promotes patient comfort and clears the mouth of any secretions the patient may have expectorated.

21. **Discard your other glove** and remaining supplies.

22. **Position the patient** in a comfortable position, and allow him to rest.
Promoting comfort and allowing for a period of rest helps the patient recover from suctioning, which may be very tiring.

? *What if . . .*

- **The patient's oxygen saturation is less than 94%, or if he is in any distress?**

  You may need to administer supplemental oxygen before, during, and after suctioning. See Procedure 36-4.

Evaluation

- Assess the color, consistency, and amount of secretions.
- Evaluate the patient's tolerance of the procedure. Note whether there were signs of respiratory distress during the procedure.
- Evaluate the effectiveness of the procedure by comparing breath sounds, vital signs, and pulse oximetry before and after the procedure.

Patient Teaching

- Explain the importance of administering supplemental oxygen to the patient before suctioning.
- Inform the patient that coughing typically increases with suctioning.
- Demonstrate oropharyngeal or nasopharyngeal suctioning to the caregiver, and ask for a return demonstration if suctioning will be required at home.

Home Care

- Instruct the family and caregiver where to obtain suction equipment.
- Provide contact information for healthcare personnel who can be reached for advice or emergencies.
- Explain that the procedure can be performed using clean technique instead of sterile technique in the home setting.
- Instruct the caregiver that suction catheters can be cleaned for reuse by washing them with soapy water and then boiling them for 10 minutes. After they are cleaned, rinse the catheters with normal saline solution or tap water.
- Teach to change the secretion collection container every 24 hours, or clean it according to home care agency guidelines every 24 hours.

Documentation

- Document the date, time, and reason you performed suctioning.
- Note the suction technique you used and the catheter size.
- Note color, consistency, and odor of secretions.
- Document the patient's respiratory status before and after the procedure.
- Document the patient's tolerance of the procedure and any complications that occurred as a result of the procedure, with resulting interventions.

Sample documentation

3/15/20 2200 Resp. labored, rate 28 breaths/min. Pulse oximetry on room air 92%. Breath sounds with rhonchi scattered throughout. Gurgling audible in upper airways. Patient unable to mobilize secretions with coughing. Suctioned by nasopharyngeal route using a 14-Fr. catheter. Approximately 30 mL thin, tan, odorless secretions obtained. After suctioning, resp. nonlabored, rate 20 breaths/min, and lungs clear on auscultation, with no gurgling audible. Pulse oximetry 96%. Patient tolerated procedure with no difficulty. ———————————— C.F. Hiam, RN

Practice Resources

McGrath, B. A., Bates, L., Atkinson, D., et al. (2012); Siegel, J., Rhinehart, E., Jackson, M., et al. (2007); Sole, M. L., Bennett, M., & Ashworth, S. (2015); Sole, M. L., Penoyer, D. A., Bennett, M. et al. (2011).

Thinking About the Procedure

The video **Performing Upper Airway Suctioning: Oropharyngeal,** along with questions and suggested responses, is available on the ***Davis's Nursing Skills Videos*** Web site on FADavis.com.

Procedure 36-10 ■ Caring for Patients Requiring Mechanical Ventilation

➤ For steps to follow in *all* procedures, refer to the Universal Steps for All Procedures found on the inside back cover.

TERM	EXPLANATION
FIO_2	Fraction of inspired oxygen.
Modes of Ventilation	Describes the setting on the ventilator that assists the patient to breathe. Can be controlled (CMV), intermittent mandatory (IMV), or synchronized intermittent mandatory (SIMV).
Tidal Volume	Amount of air delivered from the ventilator with each breath.
Assist-Control Mode—also known as Continuous Mechanical Ventilation (CMV)	The preset number of breaths per minute delivered by the machine. If the patient is able to initiate breaths, the machine will deliver a breath when the patient begins to inspire. If the patient is unable to breathe on his own, the machine will deliver the preset number of breaths in a rhythmic fashion.
Intermittent Mandatory Ventilation	A ventilator setting that delivers a minimum number of breaths per minute if the patient does not ventilate independently.
Synchronized Intermittent Mandatory Ventilation (SIMV)	A ventilator setting that delivers a minimum number of ventilations per minute if the patient does not ventilate independently. The ventilator breaths are synchronized with the patient's breaths. This mode is used for weaning patients from the ventilator.
Pressure Support	Provides positive pressure on inspiration to decrease the workload of breathing.
Continuous Positive Airway Pressure (CPAP)	Provides positive pressure during inspiration and expiration to keep alveoli open in a spontaneously breathing patient.
Positive End-Expiratory Pressure (PEEP)	Provides positive pressure on expiration to keep airways open for patients on CMV or SIMV mode ventilation.

Equipment

- Two oxygen sources
- Air source that provides 50 pounds per square inch (psi)
- Mechanical ventilator
- Humidification device
- Ventilator tubing, connectors, and adaptors
- Condensation collection device
- Inline thermometer
- Resuscitation bag with oxygen connection tubing
- Pulse oximetry device
- Procedure gloves, protective gown, and eye covering
- Sterile gloves, if you will perform suctioning
- Suction equipment (possibly)
- Sterile water for the humidifier. Some guidelines also recommend sterile water for rinsing the mouth.

Delegation

Care of a mechanically ventilated patient requires advanced knowledge of pulmonary anatomy and physiology and, therefore, should not be delegated to assistive personnel. In critical care settings, specially trained LPNs may provide care, but the RN is responsible for ensuring that procedures are implemented safely and effectively. RNs also provide ongoing assessment of the patient's ventilatory and oxygenation status. Patients requiring long-term ventilation are often cared for at home or in specialized long-term care units, where LPNs and family members may provide care.

Pre-Procedure Assessments

- Review the health record to make sure that mechanical ventilation is included in the options outlined in the patient's advance directive.
  The patient may not wish to pursue mechanical ventilation as a care option. If a patient who does not wish to be ventilated mechanically is currently on a ventilator, consult your hospital ethics committee.
- If the patient's condition allows, assess his understanding of mechanical ventilation therapy.
  Understanding helps allay anxiety and promotes cooperation.
- Assess respiratory rate, depth, and rhythm; breath sounds; color; and pulse oximetry results.
  Confirms the need for mechanical ventilation.
- Assess the oral cavity for bleeding, inflammation, odor, and presence of yeast or plaque.
  May indicate the need for more frequent oral care or for referral.
- Blood will probably be drawn for an ABG analysis
  To establish a baseline and, after that, to monitor response to therapy.

(continued on next page)

Procedure 36-10 ■ Caring for Patients Requiring Mechanical Ventilation (continued)

➤ When performing the procedure, always identify your patient according to agency policy, using two identifiers, and be attentive to standard precautions, hand hygiene, patient safety and privacy, body mechanics, and documentation.

Procedure Steps

Initial Ventilator Setup

1. **Prepare the resuscitation bag.**
The resuscitation bag should be readily available to provide ventilation in the event of an emergency.

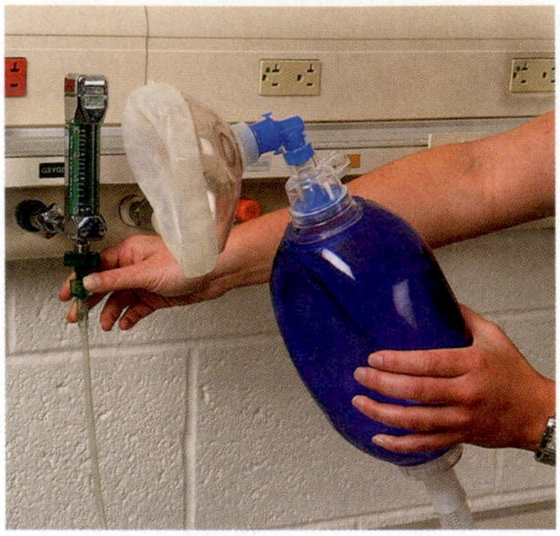

a. Attach a flow meter to one of the oxygen sources.
The flow meter helps regulate oxygen delivery.
b. Attach an adapter to the flow meter, and connect the oxygen tubing to the adapter.
c. Turn on the oxygen, and adjust the flow rate.

2. **Respiratory therapists** are responsible for setting up mechanical ventilation in most agencies. If you must assume the responsibility, refer to the manufacturer's instructions.

3. **Plug the ventilator into** a grounded electrical outlet and turn it on.

4. **Verify ventilator settings** and adjust as medically prescribed.
Ventilator settings must be individualized according to the patient's need for respiratory support. Incorrect settings may cause harm (e.g., hypoxia or barotrauma) to the patient.

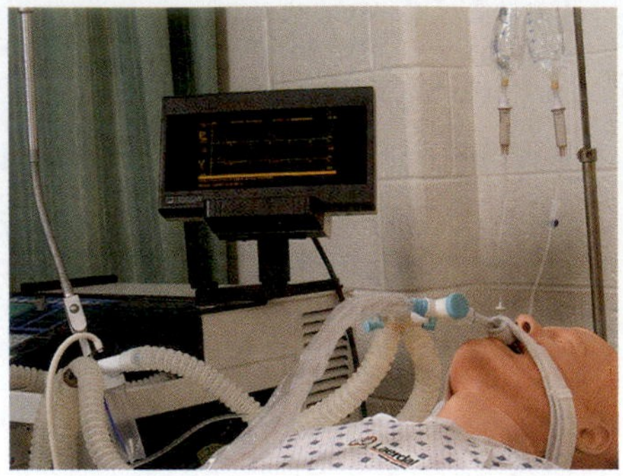

5. **Make sure that ventilator alarm** limits are set appropriately.
Inappropriately set alarm limits can result in harm to the patient.

6. **Make sure the humidifier** is filled with sterile distilled water.

7. **Don gloves, gown, and eye protection** if you have not already done so.

8. **Attach the ventilator tubing** to the endotracheal tube or tracheostomy tube.

9. **Place the ventilator tubing** in the securing device.
Prevents dislodging the endotracheal tube or tracheostomy when the patient moves.

10. **Attach a capnographic device,** if available.
To measure levels of carbon dioxide. These data are used to confirm placement of the endotracheal tube and disconnection from or malfunction of the ventilator. Oxygen levels alone are not sufficient for the ventilated patient.

11. **Prepare the inline (closed)** suction equipment (see Procedure 36-7).
Suctioning equipment should be readily available when the patient requires suctioning. Closed catheters are recommended to prevent ventilator-associated pneumonia.

After Initial Ventilator Setup

12. **Check respiratory status** and ABGs again about 30 minutes after setup. Also check whenever there are changes in the ventilator settings and as the patient's condition indicates.
To be certain the patient is being adequately ventilated and not experiencing oxygen toxicity.

13. **Check the ventilator tubing** frequently for condensation. Drain the fluid into a collection device, or briefly disconnect the patient from the ventilator and empty the tubing into a waste receptacle, according to agency policy.

Never drain the fluid into the humidifier.
Condensation in the ventilator tubing can cause resistance to airflow. Moreover, the patient can aspirate it. The fluid should not be drained into the humidifier because the patient's secretions may have contaminated it.

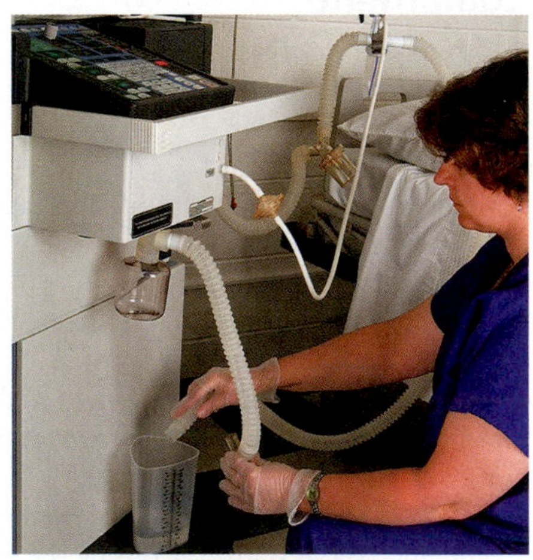

14. **Maintain the patient** in a semirecumbent position (head of bed elevated 30° to 45°). This is extremely important.
To promote lung expansion, reduce gastric reflux, and prevent ventilator-associated pneumonia.

15. **Check ventilator** and humidifier settings regularly.

16. **Check the inline thermometer.**
To ensure that the air being delivered to the patient is close to the body temperature to prevent scalding of the mucosal tissue or instead, cooling the patient (core temperature).

17. **Provide the patient with** an alternative form of communication, such as a letter board or white board.
A patient being mechanically ventilated is unable to speak, which can produce extreme anxiety. The patient must have a way to express her needs and concerns.

18. **Reposition the patient** regularly (every 1 to 2 hours), being careful not to pull on the ventilator tubing.
Repositioning protects skin integrity. However, pulling on the tubing creates pain. Patient comfort promotes relaxation, improving the effectiveness of the ventilator.

19. **Keep the patient's lips moistened** with a cool, damp cloth and water-based lubricant; and provide regular antiseptic oral care. A recommended regimen includes the following (American Association of Critical-Care Nurses, 2017):
    - Brush the teeth twice a day for 3 or 4 minutes.
    - Use a soft toothbrush.
    - Rinse the mouth with sterile water, according to agency policy.
    - Moisturize oral mucosa and lips every 2 to 4 hours.
    - Use a chlorhexidine gluconate (0.12%) rinse twice a day for intubated patients to reduce risk of VAP (adult patients).
    - Use mouthwash twice a day for adult patients (American Association of Critical Care Nurses, 2016).

    Mouth care provides comfort and preserves integrity of the mucous membranes. Patients being mechanically ventilated, even for a short period, are at high risk for developing ventilator-associated pneumonia (VAP). VAP is not uncommon, and it is associated with high mortality rates. This regimen is thought to help prevent VAP.

20. **Make sure the call device** is always within reach, and answer call device and ventilator alarms promptly.
Provides the patient with immediate access to help if a breathing problem occurs; reassures the patient and thus relieves anxiety.

21. **Monitor the tracheostomy** tube for proper cuff inflation (usually 20 to 25 mm Hg); see Clinical Insight 36-4.

22. **Check for gastric distention** and take measures to prevent aspiration.
Aspiration creates high risk for pneumonia.

23. **Clean, disinfect, or change** ventilator tubing and equipment according to agency policy.
There is no good evidence to indicate how often this should be done. Research so far indicates that tubing and equipment should not be routinely changed for infection control purposes (Liu, J., Ding, H., & Wang, Z. [2017]).

24. **Give sedatives or anti-anxiety drugs** as prescribed.

Evaluation

- After mechanical ventilation is instituted, assess for chest expansion and auscultate for bilateral breath sounds.
- Evaluate the patient's tolerance of mechanical ventilation. Verify that the patient is being adequately ventilated and that she is breathing in synchrony with the ventilator.
- Auscultate breath sounds every 2 to 4 hours, according to agency policy.
- When monitoring vital signs, count spontaneous breaths as well as those delivered by the ventilator.
- Monitor continuous pulse oximetry, capnography, and ABGs.

Patient Teaching

- Explain mechanical ventilation to the patient and family. Include information about the alarms they will hear.
- Demonstrate an alternative form of communication to the patient and family.
- When appropriate, explain the weaning process to the patient and family.
- If the patient requires mechanical ventilation after discharge, make arrangements for a home ventilator, and teach the patient and caregiver how to use it.

Home Care

- Consult with your facility discharge planning program and/or case management for discharge plans.
- Explain to the family and caregiver where to obtain a home ventilator, resuscitation bag, and oxygen equipment and what services are available. Make sure they choose a supplier who has 24-hour emergency services available.
- Help the client and caregiver devise a backup plan for ventilating the client in the event of a power failure.
- Tell the caregiver to notify the utility company and area emergency personnel that the client is being maintained on a ventilator at home.

(continued on next page)

Procedure 36-10 ■ Caring for Patients Requiring Mechanical Ventilation (continued)

- Instruct the client and caregiver about oxygen therapy and its use as well as safety measures that they must institute.
- Teach the client and caregiver to clean the ventilator tubing with soap and warm water when it becomes soiled.
- Provide the client and caregiver with contact information of healthcare personnel who can be reached for advice or emergencies.

Documentation

- Document the date and time mechanical ventilation was initiated.
- Note the type of ventilator used and the prescribed settings used.
- Document the client's response to mechanical ventilation, including vital signs, breath sounds, ease of breathing, pulse oximetry, intake and output, skin color, and ABG and chest x-ray results.

Sample documentation

02/26/20 0800 Patient found difficult to arouse. Dr. Henry made aware. ABG obtained; results included: pH 7.28; PCO_2 78 mm Hg; PO_2 48 mm Hg. Dr. Henry in to evaluate patient. Anesthesia called to intubate patient. Medicated with Versed 5 mg IV and intubated orally with a 7.5-Fr. ET tube. Placed on mechanical ventilator: TV 700 mL; FIO_2 80%, respiratory rate 14 breaths/min. Portable chest x-ray confirms ideal placement of ET tube as well as white-out of both lung fields. ABGs to be obtained in 30 min. Pulse oximetry 90% since being placed on ventilator. ———— L. Houck, RN

Practice Resources

American Association of Critical-Care Nurses (2016, 2017); Atay, S., & Karabacak, Ü. (2017); Boltey, E., Yakusheva, O., & Costa, D. K. (2017); El-Rabbany, M., Zaghlol, N., Bhandari, M., et al. (2015); Grap, M. J., Munro, C. L., & Gardner, M. (2016); Liu, J., Ding, H., & Wang, Z. (2017).

Procedure 36-11 ■ Setting Up Disposable Chest Drainage Systems

➤ For steps to follow in *all* procedures, refer to the Universal Steps for All Procedures found on the inside back cover.

Equipment

- Two disposable closed drainage systems
- Chest tube insertion kit (common tube size for adults is 36 Fr). Should contain povidone-iodine, local anesthetic, syringe, needles, drapes, scalpel, suture, sterile drapes, chest tube, connecting tubing, and necessary instruments.
- 5-in-1 or Y-connector for two chest tubes, if not contained in insertion kit
- Sterile water (for water-seal system)
- Two rubber-tipped hemostats
- Sterile gloves, masks, and sterile gowns
- Dressings: sterile 4 in. × 4 in. gauze dressings, precut drain dressings, petroleum (or other recommended) gauze dressings, and large drainage dressings
- Tape: 2-in. silk tape, 1-in. silk tape (or nylon banding system)

For disposable dry-seal systems:

- 50-mL syringe and 45 mL of sterile water or saline. Some dry-seal chest drainage units (CDUs) include these.

Delegation

Some agencies permit only registered nurses in the critical care units to perform dressing changes. The physician must perform dressing changes on other units. You should not delegate this procedure, because it requires advanced knowledge of pulmonary anatomy and physiology. As needed, teach the LPN and UAP how to safely provide care for the patient with chest tubes. Instruct them to notify an RN immediately if the chest drainage system becomes disconnected, the chest tube becomes dislodged, sudden bleeding occurs, or the patient develops respiratory distress.

Pre-Procedure Assessments

- Ensure that the patient has venous access.
- Assess vital signs.
- Assess the level of consciousness, orientation, responsiveness, anxiety, and restlessness.
  These can indicate hypoxemia.
- Assess the patient's knowledge of chest tube therapy.
  Understanding helps allay fears and anxiety.
- Assess cardiac status; respiratory rate, depth, and rhythm; breath sounds; skin color; pulse oximetry; and ABG results.
  Provides a baseline for comparison after chest tube insertion. Evaluates chest tube functioning afterward.

➤ When performing the procedure, always identify your patient according to agency policy, using two identifiers, and be attentive to standard precautions, hand hygiene, patient safety and privacy, body mechanics, and documentation.

Procedure Steps

Steps for Preparing the CDU

1. **Obtain and prepare** the prescribed chest drainage unit (CDU). ▼

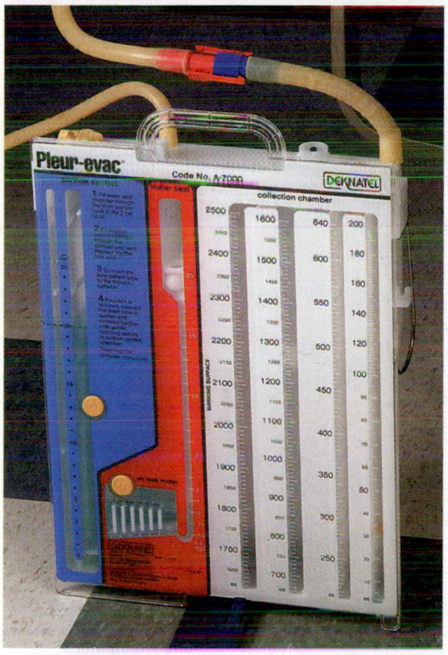

Disposable water-seal system.

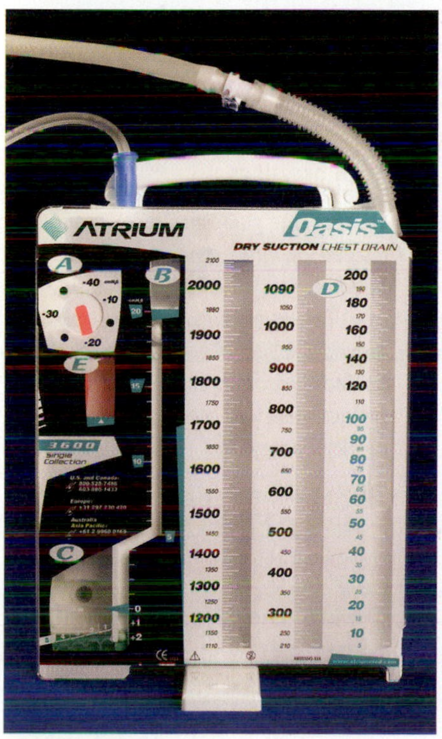

Disposable dry-seal system.

Procedure Variation for a Disposable Water-Seal CDU Without Suction

2. **Remove the cover** on the water-seal chamber, and, using the funnel provided, fill the second (water-seal) chamber with sterile water or normal saline. Fill the chamber to the 2-cm mark, or as indicated. (Note that some systems come prefilled.)
   The water-seal chamber allows air to exit from the pleural space during exhalation and prevents air from entering the pleural space during inspiration.

3. **Place the chest drainage unit (CDU)** upright, usually on the floor, and at least 30 cm (1 ft) below the patient's chest level.

4. **Replace the cover** on the water-seal chamber.
   Protects the chamber from contamination.

   ➤ **Go to Step 13.**

Procedure Variation for a Disposable Water-Seal CDU With Suction

5. **Remove the cover** on the water-seal chamber. If it is not a prefilled system, use a syringe or the funnel provided to fill the water-seal chamber (second chamber) with sterile water or normal saline to the 2-cm mark.
   The water-seal chamber allows air to exit from the pleural space during exhalation and prevents air from entering the pleural space during inspiration.

6. **Add sterile water or normal** saline solution to the suction control chamber. Add the amount prescribed by the clinician, typically 20 cm (7 in.). Place the CDU upright, usually on the floor, and at least 30 cm (1 ft) below the patient's chest level.
   Suction is regulated by the height of fluid in the suction control chamber.

7. **Attach the tubing** from the suction control chamber to the suction source tubing. Turn on the wall (or other) suction source. A wall suction of –80 cm H_2O is common.

   ➤ **Go to Step 13.**

Procedure Variation for a Disposable Dry-Seal CDU With Suction

8. **Remove the nonsterile** outer protective bag and the sterile inner wrapper following agency policy.

9. **Place the CDU upright,** usually on the floor, and at least 30 cm (1 ft) below the patient's chest level. Some CDUs have hangers for hanging at the bedside.

10. **If suction will be required,** attach the tubing from the suction control chamber to the connecting tubing attached to the suction source.

11. **Fill a syringe** with 45 mL of sterile water or saline (follow agency policy and the manufacturer's recommendation for type of fluid), or use the small bottle of sterile fluid in the CDU package. Fill the air leak monitor on the CDU by injecting the fluid via the needleless injection port on the back until it reaches the fill line.
    Once filled, the water may become colored for improved visibility of air leaks. Bubbles in this section of the CDU indicate an air leak.

    ➤ **Go to Step 13.**

Procedure Variation for a Heimlich Valve

12. **When a patient has little or no** drainage and does not require suction, the chest tube may be connected to a Heimlich valve instead of a CDU. These valves are attached to the end of the chest tube and allow one-way flow of air out of the chest tube. They contain "flutter" leaflets that allow air to exit but not reenter the pleural space. These valves can also be used for emergency transport until a chest drainage system is available.

    ➤ **Go to Step 13.**

(continued on next page)

Procedure 36-11 ■ Setting Up Disposable Chest Drainage Systems (continued)

Steps for Inserting and Connecting the Chest Tube

NOTE: The remaining steps apply to all variations.

13. Position the patient according to the indicated insertion site.
- For removing air: second intercostal space at the midclavicular line
- For fluid drainage: on the midaxillary line in the fifth or sixth intercostal space

14. Open the chest tube insertion tray and set up the sterile field. Using sterile technique, drop any necessary supplies on the field (e.g., 4 in. × 4 in. split gauze dressings, petroleum or other recommended gauze, syringes).

15. Don a mask, gown, and sterile gloves and organize the supplies you will need for dressing the chest tube insertion site.
Protective clothing prevents contamination of the surgical site and protects you from splashing.

16. Provide support to the patient while the physician or nurse practitioner prepares the sterile field, anesthetizes the patient, and inserts and sutures the chest tube.

17. As soon as the chest tube is inserted, attach it to the CDU tubing, using a connector.
Usually the nurse holds the nonsterile tubing that leads to the collection chamber and the physician attaches the sterile chest tube to it. Immediately attaching the chest tube to the drainage system prevents air from entering the pleural cavity.

18. If suction is prescribed, adjust the CDU suction to the level the clinician specifies, usually –20 cm H_2O. Also adjust the wall (or other) suction source, usually to –80 cm H_2O.

For a Water-Seal Drainage Unit

Adjust the suction source (e.g., wall suction) until gentle bubbling occurs in the suction control chamber. When the tube is functioning properly, the height of the fluid level in the drainage tube fluctuates with the respiratory cycle.

***NOTE: Increasing** suction at the suction source increases airflow through the system and creates more bubbling, but it does not increase the amount of suction placed on the chest cavity.*

For a Dry-Seal Drainage Unit

Adjust the CDU suction (e.g., to –20 cm H_2O) by turning the suction control dial on the CDU. Adjust the wall (or portable) suction pressure to –80 mm Hg or greater until the display on the suction-control chamber confirms adequate suction.

If Suction Is Not Prescribed

Leave the suction tubing on the drainage system open to maintain negative pressure. Follow the manufacturer's directions on the CDU as models will differ.

Steps for Dressing the Chest Tube

19. When the chest tube is functioning properly, the physician or nurse practitioner will suture it in place. Then don a new pair of sterile gloves. Using sterile technique, wrap petroleum, saline-soaked, or other recommended gauze around the chest tube at the insertion site.

***NOTE: Sometimes** the physician dresses the site.*

Theoretically, the moistened gauze creates a seal that prevents air from leaking around the site. However, continued use of petroleum gauze or ointments can macerate the skin, so use them with caution. Recent research suggests that saline-soaked, or even dry, gauze may be preferable to petroleum gauze; follow your agency's policy.

20. Place a precut, sterile split-drain dressing over the gauze around the chest tube.
Absorbs drainage from the insertion site, thereby reducing skin irritation and possible breakdown.

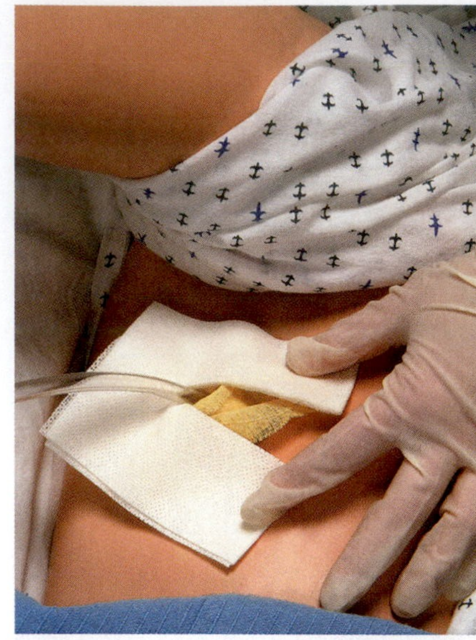

21. Place a second sterile, precut drain dressing over the first drain dressing with the opening facing in the opposite direction from the first.
The second drain dressing helps secure the first drain dressing and provides reinforcement against drainage.

22. Place a large drainage dressing (e.g., ABD) over the two precut drain dressings.

NOTE: Some guidelines recommend that instead of large amounts of tape and padding, a transparent dressing be used. This minimizes moisture collection around the site, allows nurses to inspect for leakage or infection, and does not restrict chest wall movement. Follow your agency's policy.

The large drainage dressing covers the insertion site, protecting it from outside sources of infection.

23. Secure the dressing in place, with wide tape, making sure to cover the dressing completely.
Creates an occlusive dressing that protects the chest tube from becoming dislodged and provides a seal over the insertion site, protecting it from outside sources of infection.

24. Date, time, and initial the dressing.
Informs other staff members when the dressing change was completed and by whom.

25. Using the spiral taping technique, wrap 1-in. cloth tape around the chest tube, starting above the connector and continuing below the connector. Reverse your wrapping by taping back up the tubing (using the spiral technique) until the wrapping is above the connector. The CDU may come with locking connections or bands; if so, use those.
Ensures a tight connection between the two tubings, thereby preventing an air leak at the connection site.

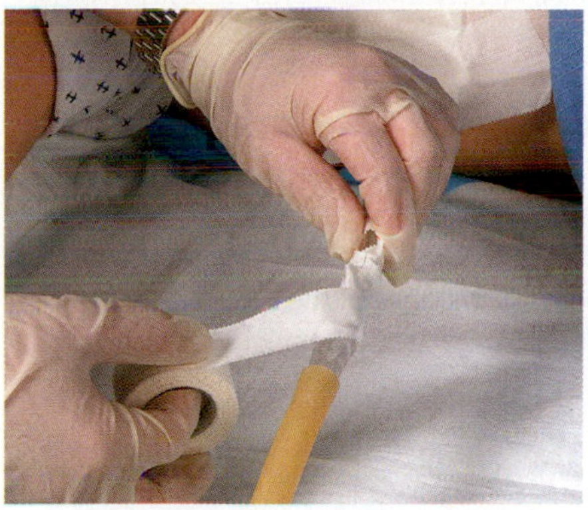

26. Cut an 8-in.-long piece of 2-in. tape. Loop one end around the top portion of the drainage tube, and secure the remaining end of the tape to the chest tube dressing.
Prevents pulling at the chest tube site when the patient moves.

27. Make sure the drainage tubing lies with no kinks from the chest tube to the drainage chamber.
Facilitates drainage and prevents fluid from accumulating in the pleural cavity.

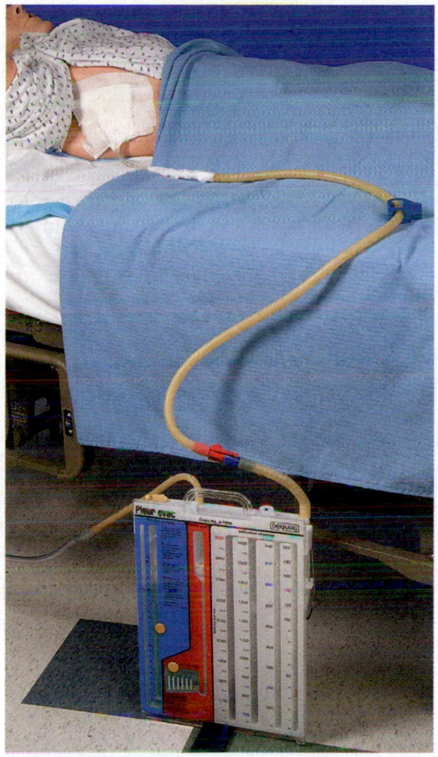

28. Prepare the patient for a portable chest x-ray exam.
A chest x-ray exam should be performed after the chest tube is inserted to ensure proper placement.

29. Institute safety measures:
a. Place two rubber-tipped clamps at the patient's bedside for special situations.
Rubber-tipped clamps are used to clamp the chest tube to check for an air leak, to change the drainage system, and to assess whether the chest tube can be safely removed.
b. Place a petroleum gauze dressing at the bedside.
In case the chest tube leaks or becomes dislodged, placing a petroleum gauze dressing over the insertion site helps keep air from entering the pleural cavity
c. Keep a spare disposable drainage system at the patient's bedside.
To use in case the drainage system in use is accidentally upended or the drainage collection chamber becomes filled.

30. Position the patient for comfort, as indicated, but with the head of the bed elevated to at least 30°.
- If the patient received a chest tube to relieve a pneumothorax, the preferred position is semi-Fowler's position.
- If the chest tube was inserted to promote fluid drainage, high-Fowler's position is recommended.

Evaluation

- Evaluate the patient's tolerance to the chest tube insertion. Determine whether the patient's respiratory status has changed.
- Auscultate breath sounds every 2 hours.
- Check chest drainage every 15 minutes for the first 2 hours, and then check as prescribed. Observe type, color, and amount.
- Monitor the chest tube insertion site for drainage and subcutaneous emphysema at least every 4 hours.
Crepitus is a sign that air is leaking into the subcutaneous tissues. Drainage is a sign that fluid is leaking around the insertion site. Both may indicate a compromise in tube patency.
- Confirm chest tube patency and determine whether bleeding is present.
- Monitor intake and output (I&O) every 8 hours.
- Check laboratory values to evaluate blood loss and oxygenation.
- Check the disposable chest drainage system for the presence of an air leak.
An air leak indicates that air is leaking from the chest and a tight seal has not yet formed over the site of injury.

Patient Teaching

- Teach the patient and family about chest tube insertion.
- Explain the importance of immediately reporting chest pain, shortness of breath, or tube dislodgement.

(continued on next page)

Procedure 36-11 ■ Setting Up Disposable Chest Drainage Systems (continued)

Home Care

- Explain to the client and caregiver how to care for the chest tube at home.
- Provide the client and caregiver with contact information should problems with the chest tube arise.

Documentation

- Assessment findings before, during, and after chest tube insertion (e.g., vital signs, breath sounds, cardiac status, pulse oximetry)
- Date and time of the chest tube insertion
- Name of the clinician who performed the procedure
- The location of the insertion site, the size of the chest tube, the type of drainage system, and the amount of suction applied, if any
- Any medications the patient received during the procedure
- Color and amount of drainage
- Chest tube output on the intake and output portion of the documentation record (often a flow sheet)
- Patient's tolerance to the procedure
- Presence of subcutaneous emphysema or air leak, if any
- Complications and any interventions performed as a result of the complications
- Chest x-ray findings

Sample documentation

8/25/20 0230 Patient presented with acute shortness of breath, pulse ox 84%, respirations 40 breaths/min and shallow, heart rate 132 beats/min. BP 188/100 mm Hg. Breath sounds absent on right side. Patient received morphine sulfate 4 mg IVP. #36 Fr chest tube placed by Dr. Phan under sterile conditions in right anterior chest, midclavicular line, above the 2nd ICS. Chest tube attached to 20 cm of water pressure. Small air leak present, no crepitus. Portable chest x-ray obtained after procedure, revealed chest tube in good placement and right lung re-expanded. Vital signs post-insertion: pulse ox 94%; BP 153/90 mm Hg, heart rate 100 beats/min, and respiratory rate 24 breaths/min. Breath sounds audible bilaterally. ——————— Pennie Bowen, RNC

Practice Resources

Kane, C. J., York, N. L., & Minton, L. A. (2013); Maliakal, M. (2013); Siegel, J., Rhinehart, E., Jackson, M., et al. (2007).

Thinking About the Procedure

The video **Disposable Chest Drainage Systems: Setting Up** and **Connecting & Dressing,** along with questions and suggested responses, is available on the ***Davis's Nursing Skills Videos*** Web site on FADavis.com.

Procedure 36-12 ■ Inserting an Oropharyngeal Airway

➤ For steps to follow in *all* procedures, refer to the Universal Steps for All Procedures found on the inside back cover.

The American Heart Association guidelines (2015) direct that you should insert an oropharyngeal airway only if you are trained in its use.

Equipment

- Oral airways in a variety of sizes
- Tongue blade
- Procedure gloves
- Suction equipment
- Resuscitation bag and oxygen source (depending on the patient's status)
- Padded tongue blade

Delegation

You should not delegate this procedure because it requires specialized knowledge, training, and assessment skills.

Pre-Procedure Assessments

- Determine the appropriate airway size by placing the airway on the outside of the patient's cheek. The length of the airway should extend from the front teeth to the end of the jawline.
- Assess respiratory status (breath sounds, respiratory rate and effort, skin color, and pulse oximetry findings).
  Findings confirm the need for the airway and provide a baseline for evaluating the effectiveness of the intervention.
- Assess for contraindications (e.g., patient is conscious or semiconscious; patient has loose teeth or recent oral surgery).
  An oropharyngeal airway may stimulate the gag reflex, causing vomiting or laryngospasm in a conscious patient.

➤ When performing the procedure, always identify your patient according to agency policy, using two identifiers, and be attentive to standard precautions, hand hygiene, patient safety and privacy, body mechanics, and documentation.

Procedure Steps

1. **Perform hand hygiene, and don** clean procedure gloves.
   Helps prevent transfer of microorganisms from the patient.

2. **Explain the procedure** to the patient, even if he appears to be unresponsive.
   Recall that hearing is the last sense lost, so the patient may be able to hear you. Information may help relieve the patient's anxiety, if present.

3. **Clear the mouth of any debris** or secretions. You may need to suction the mouth.

4. **Place the patient in supine** or semi-Fowler's position. Hyperextend the neck, unless contraindicated.
   Mild hyperextension allows the airway to slide naturally toward the pharynx.

5. **Gently open the mouth.** Remove dentures, if present.
   Dentures may cause further airway obstruction.

If Using Tongue Blade Technique

Open the patient's mouth and use the blade to depress the tongue.

If Using Crossed Fingers Technique

Place your thumb on the lower teeth. Cross your index finger over your thumb and place the finger on the upper teeth. Push the teeth apart.

6. **You may need to hold** the tongue down with a tongue blade as you insert the airway.

7. **Insert the airway** along the top of the tongue, in the upside-down position (the "C" faces upward toward the nose).
   Prevents pushing the tongue toward the pharynx.

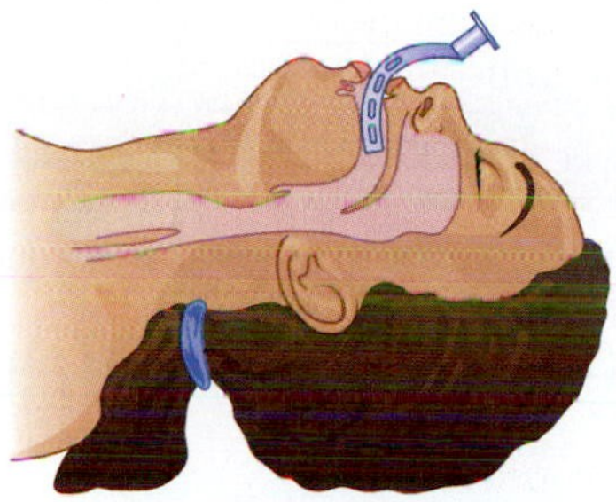

8. **As the airway approaches** the posterior wall of the pharynx, rotate the airway 180° so that the ends of the "C" turn downward over the back of the tongue. Continue to insert the airway until the front flange is flush with the lips.

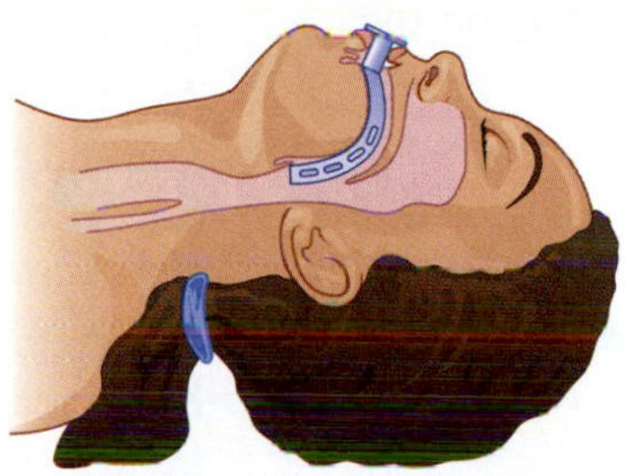

9. **Keep the patient's head tilted** slightly back and the chin elevated.
   This position helps the oropharyngeal airway to function optimally.

10. **Do not tape the airway** in place.
   You may need to remove the airway quickly for suctioning. Untaping would delay airway removal, increasing the risk of aspiration.

11. **Position the patient on her side.**
   To minimize the risk of aspiration.

12. **Provide oral hygiene** at least every 2 to 4 hours. Remove and cleanse the airway at that time; use hydrogen peroxide and then rinse with water.

? What if . . .

- **After inserting the airway, respirations are absent or inadequate?**

  Use a mouth-to-mask technique, a handheld resuscitation bag, or an oxygen-powered breathing device to ventilate the patient. Have someone call for help.

Evaluation

- After inserting the airway, verify patency by auscultating for bilateral breath sounds.
- Check for bleeding or tooth damage in the mouth.
  May be caused by airway insertion, especially if it must be done rapidly.
- Check to be certain the patient's lips and tongue are not caught between the teeth and the airway.
  Prevents trauma to the soft tissues.
- Monitor the airway position frequently.
  Ensures correct placement.
- Continually reassess the need for the airway. Remove it when the patient begins to cough or gag.
- Frequently assess oral mucous membranes when you remove the airway for care.
  Prolonged airway use can cause tissue irritation or ulceration.
- Keep suction available at the bedside. Suction the oropharynx as needed by inserting the suction catheter alongside the airway.

(continued on next page)

Procedure 36-12 ■ Inserting an Oropharyngeal Airway (continued)

Documentation

Document the following:

- Date and time of airway insertion
- Type and size of airway (oropharyngeal or nasopharyngeal)
- Assessments before and after the procedure, including breath sounds and focused respiratory assessment
- Any suctioning performed
- Patient's tolerance of the procedure
- Adverse reactions and interventions taken

Practice Resources

American Association of Critical-Care Nurses (2016); American Heart Association (2015); Brown, C. Sackles, J., Mick, N. (2017).

Procedure 36-13 ■ Inserting a Nasopharyngeal Airway

➤ For steps to follow in *all* procedures, refer to the Universal Steps for All Procedures found on the inside back cover.

The American Heart Association guidelines (2015) direct that you should insert a nasopharyngeal airway only if you are trained in its use.

Equipment

- Nasopharyngeal airway of the correct size
- Tongue blade
- Procedure gloves
- Water-soluble lubricant
- Penlight
- Suction equipment
- Resuscitation bag and oxygen source (depending on the patient's status)

Delegation

You should not delegate this procedure because it requires specialized knowledge, training, and assessment skills. Commonly, this procedure is performed by a respiratory therapist.

Pre-Procedure Assessments

- Determine the appropriate airway size: (1) Measure the diameter of the patient's nostril and use an airway that is slightly smaller than that; and (2) measure the distance from the tip of the patient's nose to the earlobe, and use an airway about 2.5 cm (1 in.) longer than that measurement. Airways are sized by their internal diameter. Generally, the larger the internal diameter, the longer the tube. Airways are available in a variety of pediatric and adult sizes.

  Small adult: 6 to 7 mm

  Medium adult: 7 to 8 mm

  Large adult: 8 to 9 mm
- Assess respiratory status (e.g., breath sounds, respiratory rate and effort, skin color, pulse oximetry findings).
  Findings confirm the need for the airway and provide a baseline for evaluating the effectiveness of the intervention.
- Assess for contraindications (e.g., anticoagulant therapy, hemorrhagic disorder, nasopharyngeal deformity, sepsis).
  Up to 30% of patients experience airway bleeding after insertion of a nasopharyngeal airway.

➤ When performing the procedure, always identify your patient according to agency policy, using two identifiers, and be attentive to standard precautions, hand hygiene, patient safety and privacy, body mechanics, and documentation.

Procedure Steps

1. **Perform hand hygiene** and don procedure gloves.
   Helps prevent transfer of microorganisms from the patient.
2. **Position the patient supine** or in semi-Fowler's position. Explain the procedure.
   A semi-Fowler's position facilitates airway insertions. Explaining may alleviate anxiety, enabling the patient to cooperate more with the procedure.
3. **Validate that the airway size** is correct. Hold the airway next to the patient's face. The length of the airway should measure from tip of nose to jawline below the ear.
4. **Lubricate the airway** with water-soluble lubricant.
   Prevents trauma to mucosa during insertion.
5. **Tilt the patient's head backward** to hyperextend the neck. Then push up the tip of the nose and gently insert the tip of the airway into the nose.
6. **Advance the airway** along the floor of the nostril into the posterior pharynx behind the tongue—until the outer flange rests on the nostril. If you meet resistance, rotate the tube slightly to enhance passage. Do not force against resistance.
   Forcing the tube can cause tissue trauma and airway kinking.

7. **Have the patient open her mouth.** Depress the tongue with a tongue blade and inspect the pharynx for proper placement of the tube tip. Use a penlight, if necessary, for better visualization.
When the tube is fully inserted, the outer flange of the tube should rest on the nostril, and only the tip of the tube should be visible at the top of the posterior pharynx. ▼

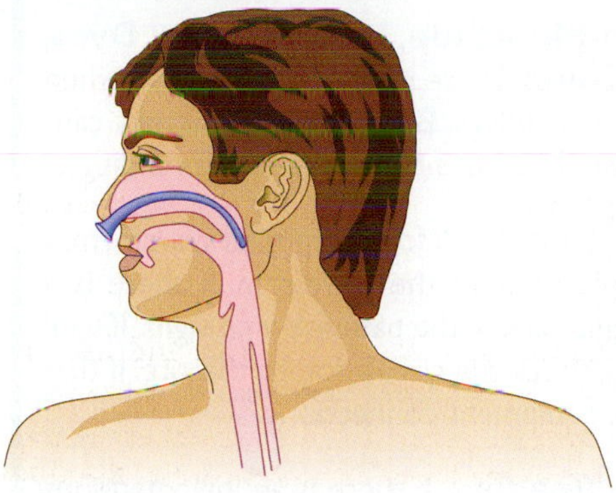

8. **Check for correct placement** and function: Close the patient's mouth, and place your finger close to the tube's opening to feel for air exchange.
9. **Auscultate the lungs** for the presence of bilateral breath sounds.
10. **Remove the airway** at least every 8 hours to check nasal mucous membranes for ulceration or irritation. Clean the airway at this time: Place in a basin, rinse with hydrogen peroxide, then rinse with water. Use a pipe cleaner to remove secretions, if necessary. Reinsert the airway in the other nostril.
To avoid skin and mucous membrane irritation and breakdown and to prevent infection

? What if . . .

- **After you insert the airway, the patient coughs, gags, vomits, or has laryngospasm?**

  The tube may be too long. If the tip extends beyond the top of the posterior pharynx, remove it and insert a shorter one.

Evaluation

- Assess respiratory rate and effort.
- Assess breath sounds.
- Observe for bleeding of nasal mucosa; suction as necessary.
- If the patient is receiving artificial ventilation, monitor for gastric distention and hypoventilation.
- Provide frequent oral and nares care; assess the skin around the nostril.

Documentation

Document the following:

- Date and time of airway insertion
- Type and size of airway (nasopharyngeal)
- Assessments before and after the procedure, including breath sounds, focused respiratory assessment, and condition of the mucous membranes
- Any suctioning performed
- Patient's tolerance of the procedure
- Adverse reactions and interventions taken
- Removal of the airway, cleaning, and replacement in the other nostril

Practice Resources

American Association of Critical Care Nurses (2017); American Heart Association (2015); American Red Cross (2011.); Brown, C. Sackles, J., Mick, N. (2017); Bullard, D., Brothers, K., Davis, C., et al. (2012).

CLINICAL INSIGHTS

Clinical Insight 36-1 ➤ Tips for Obtaining Accurate Pulse Oximetry Readings

Patient Movement. A nailbed is the most common site to place the probe. However, a tremor, twitch, shivering, or movement in bed can make pulse oximetry readings inaccurate. If the patient is unable to cooperate or control his movement, try using an ear probe or nasal sensor.

Acrylic Fingernails and Nail Polish. If the patient has acrylic nails, place the probe on a toe or earlobe. Many facilities stock individually packaged nail polish remover pads to remove nail polish before placing the probe.
Nail polish or acrylic nails may interfere with signal transmission, causing inaccurate Sao_2 measurement. However, a recent study found that nail polish did not cause a clinically significant change in readings in healthy people (Chan, Chan, & Chan, 2013).

Dirt and Skin Oils. Dirt and oils on the site can interfere with passage of light waves.

Poor Perfusion. A low reading may result from poor perfusion of the area where the probe is placed.

- A bent elbow, for example, may cause a slight decrease in circulation to the nailbed. If Sao_2 results are crucial to the patient's plan of care, use the earlobe to minimize the effect of movement on the reading.
- Keep the extremities warm to obtain a more accurate reading.
  Vasoconstriction due to cool extremities may also limit circulation.
- If poor perfusion is related to a disease process, use the earlobe or nose as the monitoring site.

Lighting. Bright fluorescent lighting may influence the accuracy of the reading. Dim the lights or cover the probe with bed covers or a towel to reduce error.

Anemia, Carbon Monoxide, Intravascular Dyes, and Dark Skin Color. These must be considered when interpreting oximetry readings. Because these factors cannot be controlled, watch for trend changes in the readings.

Equipment Function. Look for a displayed waveform; a reading is meaningless without the waveform. If there is a weak signal or no signal, check the patient's vital signs. If vital signs are satisfactory, check the circulation to the site. If that is satisfactory, check equipment connections.

Accuracy of the Reading. If there is an instantaneous change in saturation (e.g., from 99% to 82%), suspect an error. This is not physiologically possible. For any suspected inaccuracy, check the reading using the equipment on a healthy person. If it seems accurate, check the patient's medications and history of circulatory disorders; also check items listed above. When in doubt, rely on your clinical judgment more than the reading from the machine.

Clinical Insight 36-2 ➤ Guidelines for Preventing Aspiration

To prevent aspiration, use the following guidelines.

For At-Risk Patients

- Position the unconscious patient on his side to protect the airway.
- Request medications in elixir or liquid form.
- Break or crush pills, when appropriate.
- Keep a suction setup available for routine and emergency use.
- If the patient is intubated, keep the endotracheal or tracheostomy cuff inflated, and suction above the cuff before deflating the cuff.
- Do not offer food or fluids if the patient is heavily sedated or in the initial recovery phase of anesthesia.

Enteral Feedings

- Check the placement of the nasogastric tube before you administer enteral feedings.
- Check gastric residual volume before administering the next enteral feeding. Hold the feeding if the residual volume is high. (Note: The amount of acceptable residual volume depends on the amount and frequency of feedings.)
- If the patient is receiving continuous tube feedings, the head of the bed must remain elevated.
- Also see Procedure 27-3 for step-by-step instructions for administering feedings through gastric and enteric tubes.

Oral Feedings

- Position the patient upright or with the head of the bed elevated for feedings or meal.
- Be sure the head of bed remains elevated for at least 30 minutes after each feeding or meal.
- Offer small, frequent meals.
- Avoid thin liquids, or use thickening agents.
- Offer foods or liquids that can be formed into a bolus before they are swallowed.
- Cut food into small pieces.

Clinical Insight 36-3 ➤ Oxygen Therapy Safety Precautions

- Post signs indicating that oxygen is in use.
- Do not permit smoking near oxygen delivery systems.
- Ensure that three-pronged plugs are used for electrical devices (to prevent sparks).
- Allow no open flames (e.g., candles) near oxygen.
- Do not use electrical equipment with frayed wires or loose connections.
- Do not use petroleum products, aerosol products, and products containing acetone where oxygen is in use. (These are flammable substances that are easily ignited.)
- Secure oxygen tanks to rigid stands.
- Secure portable oxygen cylinders in holders or carriers provided.

Clinical Insight 36-4 ➤ Caring for Patients With Endotracheal Airways

Assisting With Endotracheal Airway Insertion

- **Gather equipment.** You will need an oxygen source and a bag (e.g., Ambu or nonrebreather bag) to inflate the lungs, a laryngoscope, endotracheal tubes of various sizes, water-soluble lubricant, a syringe to inflate the cuff, and tape to secure the tube in place.
- **Keep suction at the bedside** to clear the mouth and airway if secretions are obstructing your view of the cords.
- **You will need a surgical tray** if a tracheostomy is performed to create the direct opening into the trachea.
- **Remain calm, and explain** to the patient that the airway will enable him to breathe effectively.
- **Once the airway is in place, listen to breath sounds** to establish that both lungs are ventilated.
- **Reassess breath sounds periodically.** After the airway is inserted, record the type and size, as well as the patient's response to the procedure.
- **Expect that a portable chest x-ray will be prescribed** to confirm correct placement.

Managing and Monitoring Endotracheal and Airways

The following are activities associated with the care of all types of endotracheal airways.

- **Have emergency equipment,** including a duplicate tracheostomy kit, extra cannula, and suction setup, immediately available for reintubation if the tube should become dislodged.
- **Keep an extra cannula at the bedside** as patients may accidentally decannulate.
- **Secure the endotracheal tube** with ties, Velcro tapes, or a commercial holder to prevent accidental displacement.

- **Provide tracheostomy care every 4 to 8 hours** (Mitchell, Hussey, Setzen, et al., 2013).
- **Secure the orotracheal tube** to the opposite side of the mouth with each change of tape or ties to prevent skin erosion and breakdown.
- **Inspect skin around the tube** or tracheal stoma for redness, swelling, drainage, or irritation at least every 8 hours.
- **Provide skin care** around the tube and tape or holder at least daily.
- **Perform regular oral care.**
- **Inflate the cuff of the tube with a minimal occlusive volume and monitor cuff pressures** to prevent pressure necrosis inside the trachea. (This is a joint responsibility with the respiratory therapist.) Maximum acceptable tube cuff pressure is 25 mm Hg. The following is a method for checking for minimal occluding volume:
  1. Place stethoscope on patient's neck over the carotid pulse.
  2. Attach a 10-mL syringe to the pilot balloon of the inflated cuff.
  3. Remove air from the cuff—(1 mL at a time) until you hear a slight leak at the peak of inspiration.
  4. When you hear the leak, inject 1 mL of air back into the cuff.
- **Monitor and document cuff pressure** once per shift and when the tube is changed or repositioned.
- **Note the centimeter reference marking** on the endotracheal tube to monitor for possible displacement.
- **Minimize pulling and traction** on the artificial airway by supporting all tubing connected to the airway and using flexible catheter mounts and swivels.
- **Remind the conscious patient not to pull on the airway.**
- **Use a bite block between the teeth** to prevent the patient from occluding an orotracheal tube.
- **Provide 100% humidification** of inspired air. Check the oxygen setup regularly.
- **Routine saline instillation** to thin secretions is no longer recommended.
- **Ensure adequate hydration** with oral or IV fluids to keep the mucosa moist and thin secretions.
- **Suction the airway** when secretions collect. Remember, the patient probably can't cough effectively to clear secretions.

Clinical Insight 36-5 ➤ Managing Chest Tubes

Monitor Breathing, Gas Exchange, and Drainage

- **Frequently assess breathing patterns, breathing effort, and breath sounds.**
- **Assess mental status, heart rate and rhythm, and pulse oximetry readings.**
  These reflect adequacy of oxygenation.
- **Monitor character, color, and amount of chest drainage.** Immediately report sudden or large increases in drainage or new onset of bright red blood, along with an assessment of the patient's condition at that time.
  Drainage is usually greatest when the chest tube is initially inserted and decreases as the lung re-expands. You must replace the chest drainage unit (CDU) when the drainage compartment is almost full.

Prevent Complications or Intervene If They Occur

- **Observe the dressing at least every 4 hours.** Make sure that the dressing around the tube insertion site is occlusive (e.g., not wet or loose). Usually, petroleum gauze is wrapped around the insertion site to ensure occlusion.
- **Inspect for excessive, abnormal, or foul-smelling drainage.**
  This may indicate hemorrhage or infection.
- **Palpate around the dressing for subcutaneous emphysema** (air in the subcutaneous tissues).
  This may be caused by an incomplete seal at the chest tube insertion site.
- **Assess for pain**; medicate as needed.
- **Reposition the patient every 2 hours** and use pillows to keep the patient's weight off the chest tube.
  To prevent occlusion of the tube, promote drainage, and preserve skin integrity.
- **Encourage the patient to use the arm on the affected side.** Assist with range-of-motion exercises, if necessary.
  To maintain joint mobility.

- **Recollapse of the lung** can occur because of loss of negative pressure within the system. This is commonly caused by air leaks, disconnections, or breaks or cracks of the bottles or chambers. If any of these occur, immediately place the disconnected end nearest the patient into a bottle of sterile water or saline.

- **Do not clamp the chest tube.** Doing so can lead to a **tension pneumothorax.** Clamp chest tubes only for changing the drainage system. Limit the clamp time and monitor respiratory status constantly until the clamp is removed.

- **If the tube is accidentally pulled out,** immediately cover the wound with a dry, sterile dressing. Listen for air leaking out of the site. If you can hear air, tape the dressing loosely so that you do not occlude the site.
  If air cannot escape from the chest, a tension pneumothorax will occur, eventually compromising cardiovascular function.

Promote Lung Re-expansion

- **Encourage the patient to be as active as his condition permits.**
  Chest drainage systems are bulky, but with disposable systems, patients can still get out of bed and ambulate, but will need assistance to protect and monitor the system and the patient.
- **Instruct the patient to perform deep breathing and coughing every 2 hours,** unless contraindicated. Assist the patient to sit upright and splint the chest with a pillow or the hands, and provide analgesia as needed.
  These interventions help to minimize discomfort.

Key Points for Managing a One-Bottle System

- **Keep the intake tube below the fluid level in the drainage bottle.**
  To prevent drawing air into the pleural space with inhalation.
- **Maintain the tubing about 2 cm below the water level.** As tubing length below the water increases, more effort is required to exhale.
- **Take precautions to see that the bottle is not accidentally tipped over,** uncovering the long vent tube and allowing air to enter the pleural space.

Maintain the Drainage System

For All Types of CDUs:

- **Make sure the drainage system is located below the insertion site.**
  If the drainage system is higher than the insertion site, fluid may flow back into the pleural cavity, compromising the patient's respiratory status.
- **Regularly inspect tubing** to ensure that connections are airtight and tubing is not kinked or occluded.
  Kinks in the drainage tubing increase pressure in the pleural cavity and prevent fluid drainage.
- **Monitor drainage.**
  Blood or purulent matter can occlude the tubing.
- **Inspect the air vent in the drainage system** to make sure it is patent.
  If air builds up in the pleural cavity, pneumothorax may occur.
- **Monitor to ensure the system is maintaining consistent negative pressure levels.**

- **Do not "milk" or strip the tubing.**
  Doing so can create excess negative pressure and damage lung tissue. Always be sure to verify operation through the users' manual or with the product's vendor. Most systems will have some type of check system to ensure that the system is operating correctly.

- **To transport or ambulate a patient**: (1) Keep the CDU upright below chest level; (2) disconnect the CDU from suction source and make sure the air vent is open.

Water-Seal Drainage Systems:

- **Take precautions that the CDU is not tipped over** (e.g., tape it to the floor).

Clinical Insight 36-5 ➤ Managing Chest Tubes—cont'd

- **Observe for tidaling** (fluctuations in the water-seal chamber's fluid level that correspond with respiration). The level will increase on inspiration and decrease on exhalation. This will be opposite for a patient on a mechanical ventilator.
- **Bubbling in the bottom of the water-seal chamber indicates an air leak.** When this occurs, check for poor tubing connections. A small amount of bubbling right after insertion or with exhalation or cough is normal.
- **Check the water in the suction control chamber**; replace as needed.
  The water can evaporate.
- **If the chest tube disconnects from the drainage unit,** establish a temporary water seal by immersing the open end of the chest tube in a bottle of sterile water to a depth of 2 cm until a new system can be connected. Cleanse the end of the patient connector on the drain system with alcohol and reconnect it if it has not been contaminated. If the patient connector on the drain system is contaminated, you must initiate a new CDU.

Dry-Seal Drainage Systems:

- **Inspect the air vent in the drainage system** to make sure it is patent.
  The air vent must remain patent to allow air to escape. If air builds up in the pleural cavity, pneumothorax may occur.
- **Check the indicators on the CDU to be certain that suction is operating properly.**
  A dry chest drainage system doesn't use water in the suction chamber. A valve inside the regulator continuously balances the forces of suction and the atmosphere. The valve automatically responds and adjusts to changes in patient air leaks and fluctuations in suction source vacuum to deliver accurate suction to the patient. Pressure can be set from –10 cm H_2O to –40 cm H_2O by adjusting the rotary dry suction dial.
- **Observe for bubbling.**
  If the water in a dry-seal CDU is bubbling, it means there is an air leak.

ASSESSMENT GUIDELINES AND TOOLS

Focused Assessment

Oxygenation

Part I. Questions to Assess Risk for Impaired Oxygenation

Demographic Data

- ➤ What is your age?
- ➤ Where do you live?
- ➤ What is your occupation?

Health History

- ➤ What healthcare problems are you currently being treated for?
- ➤ Have you ever been hospitalized or had surgery? If so, when and for what reason?
- ➤ Do you have a history of allergies or asthma?
- ➤ What medications do you currently take?
- ➤ What over-the-counter medications or alternative treatments do you use? What do you use them for?

Respiratory History

- ➤ Have you ever been diagnosed with a respiratory problem? If so, what was the diagnosis? When was the diagnosis made?
- ➤ Have you noticed any changes in your breathing?
- ➤ How often do you cough?
- ➤ When you do cough, is it productive?
- ➤ What do the secretions you cough up look like and smell like?
- ➤ How much sputum do you produce?
- ➤ How do you treat your cough? What effect did it have?
- ➤ Do you ever wheeze or feel short of breath?
- ➤ What causes you to wheeze or feel short of breath?
- ➤ Do body positions affect your breathing pattern?
- ➤ What position do you lie in when you sleep? Do you use more than one pillow?
- ➤ Do you ever wake up short of breath?

Environmental History

- ➤ Are there pets in the house?
- ➤ What response, if any, do you have to pets, dust, pollen, or plants?
- ➤ Are you exposed to smoke or fumes in the home and workplace?
- ➤ Are you exposed to respiratory irritants such as asbestos, chemicals, coal dust, fungus, molds, or soot in the home or workplace?
- ➤ What type of heating, air-conditioning, or air-filtering system do you have in the home or workplace?

(Continued)

Focused Assessment

Oxygenation—cont'd

Lifestyle

- What is your current stress level? What are your major sources of stress?
- What is your usual diet? Is your current diet typical, or have you recently changed your eating habits?
- What is your usual activity level?
- What level of activity makes you feel short of breath?
- Do you smoke now, or have you ever smoked?
- If you smoke, how many packs per day and for how many years have you smoked?
- Do you smoke marijuana or use other substances?

Part II. Focused Physical Examination

Pulmonary System

- ***Inspect*** to observe respiratory patterns, signs of respiratory distress, chest structures and movement, skin and mucous membrane color, presence or absence of edema, sputum characteristics, and overall general appearance.
- ***Palpate*** skin temperature and areas of tenderness.
- ***Percuss*** over the lung fields (for consolidation or excess air pockets).
- ***Auscultate*** breath sounds and vascular sounds.
- ***Assess breathing patterns:*** eupnea, tachypnea, bradypnea, apnea, Kussmaul's breathing, Biot's breathing, and Cheyne-Stokes respirations.
- ***Assess cough and related symptoms:***

  Nasal congestion, sneezing, watery eyes, and nasal discharge suggest allergies.

  Fever, chest congestion, noisy breath sounds, sputum production suggest a URI.

  Dyspnea, chest tightness, and wheezing suggest airway obstruction (e.g., asthma).
- ***Assess sputum:*** appearance, color, odor, amount, and timing.
- ***Obtain sputum samples*** as needed.
- ***Assess respiratory effort:*** Breathing should be effortless. Observe for shortness of breath, dyspnea, nasal flaring, head bobbing, retractions, use of accessory muscles during inspiration, grunting, needing to sit upright to breathe, paroxysmal nocturnal dyspnea, conversational dyspnea, stridor, and wheezing.

DIAGNOSTIC TESTING

Diagnostic Testing

Tests Related to Oxygenation

Test	Purpose
Angiogram	A contrast dye is injected into a vein, and serial films are taken to assess patency of the vessels.
Arterial blood gases (ABG)	An analysis of arterial blood that evaluates the effectiveness of gas exchange
Bronchoscopy	Insertion of a flexible endoscope to examine the larynx, trachea, and bronchial tree
Cardiac catheterization	A catheter is passed into the heart to assess pressures, blood flow, and the size and patency of chambers.
Chest x-ray study (CXR)	Provides an anterior–posterior or lateral view of the heart and lungs, shows tissue density (e.g., to evaluate size, masses, fluid)
Hemoglobin (Hgb)	A serum measurement that affects the oxygen-carrying capacity of the blood. May be measured separately or as part of a complete blood count.
Pulmonary function studies	A series of tests to detect lung volume and capacity
Sputum culture	A microscopic evaluation of the sputum
Thoracentesis	Insertion of a large-bore needle through the chest wall into the pleural space to obtain fluid specimens, to instill medication, or to drain accumulations of fluid
Throat culture	A swab of the pharynx or tonsils is performed to assess pathogens present in the pharynx.
Ventilation–perfusion scan	Used to assess for pulmonary embolus, this scan entails injection of a radioactive substance that allows blood flow to the lungs to be evaluated. A second substance is inhaled that maps out oxygen distribution in the lungs.
White blood cell (WBC) count	A serum measure to assess for the presence of infection

Diagnostic Testing

Lung Volumes and Capacities

The norms presented in this table are based on averages for a young adult man. The following are measured by spirometry.

Title	Definition	Significance
Tidal volume (V_T)	The amount of air moved into and out of the lungs with each normal breath. Normally around 500 mL.	In a healthy state, V_T increases when oxygen demand increases. Diseases that restrict lung inflation, create muscular weakness, or paralyze the diaphragm limit the ability of the body to increase tidal volume. When such disorders become severe, V_T will fall too low to support even resting oxygen demands.
Inspiratory reserve volume (IRV)	The maximum amount of air that can be inhaled above and beyond the normal tidal volume. Ranges from 2,000 to 3,000 mL.	IRV determines how much the tidal volume can increase when oxygen demands increase.
Expiratory reserve volume (ERV)	The maximum extra amount of air that can be forcefully exhaled after the end of a normal tidal expiration. Ranges from 1,000 to 1,500 mL.	Some diseases (e.g., emphysema) cause collapse of alveoli and airways, which traps extra air in the lungs. This "trapped" air cannot be exhaled and lowers ERV.
Residual volume (RV)	The amount of air remaining in the lungs after the most forceful exhalation. Ranges from 1,000 to 1,500 mL.	Diseases that reduce ERV lead to an increase in RV. As more air is trapped in the lungs and cannot be exhaled even with forceful attempts (ERV), it becomes part of the residual volume that is never completely exhaled.
Inspiratory capacity (IC)	The combination of the tidal volume and inspiratory reserve volume (V_T + IRV). Ranges from 2,500 to 3,500 mL.	This is the amount of air that can be inhaled with maximum effort. It reflects the capacity one has to inhale deeply.
Functional residual capacity (FRC)	The combination of expiratory reserve volume and residual volume (ERV + RV). Ranges from 2,000 to 3,000 mL. Exhalation of additional air requires effort to force more air out.	This is the amount of air that stays in the lungs at the end of a normal, passive quiet exhalation. Disorders that cause air trapping increase the FRC.
Vital capacity (VC)	The combination of inspiratory reserve volume and expiratory reserve volume (IRV + ERV). Ranges from 3,000 to 4,500 mL.	This is the maximum amount of air that can be forcefully exhaled after filling the lungs to their maximum level with the deepest possible inspiratory effort.

Diagnostic Testing

Reading a Tuberculin Skin Test Result

Size of Induration	Considered Positive For
>5 mm	People who have had recent close contact with someone with active TB
	People who have HIV or risk factors for HIV
	People with previous history of TB
	IV drug users known to be HIV-negative
>10 mm	People with medical conditions that increase the risk of progressing from latent TB to active TB (e.g., diabetes mellitus, use of steroids, chronic renal failure, some malignancies)
	Residents and employees of high-risk congregate settings: prisons, skilled nursing facilities (SNFs) and other long-term facilities, healthcare facilities, and homeless shelters
	Foreign-born persons recently arrived (i.e., within the past 5 yr) from countries having a high incidence of TB
	Low-income groups
	Children younger than 4 years of age or exposed to adults in high-risk categories
>15 mm	People who do not meet any of the above criteria

CLINICALJUDGMENT

Applying the Full-Spectrum Nursing Model

PATIENT SITUATION

Haley, a 15-year-old female high school student, was admitted to the hospital with shortness of breath and right-sided chest pain when breathing. She states that she has had "the flu" for 3 days. She has a history of asthma since age 6 and smokes half a pack of cigarettes a day. Both her parents are heavy smokers. An IV was initiated, and she is receiving 800 mg of vancomycin (an antibiotic) intravenously every 12 hours. She is not on oxygen therapy, but receives 10 incentive spirometer treatments per hour while awake. Her heart rate is 80 beats/min, respiratory rate, 24 breaths/min, and blood pressure, 110/70 mm Hg. Her skin is pale but warm, and capillary refill time is 2 seconds. She has no clubbing of the fingers. She is urinating approximately 400 mL of clear yellow urine every 8 hours and maintaining a normal bowel elimination pattern. Laboratory results are:

Red blood cell count (RBCs): 3.56×10^6 (3.56 million/mm^3)
White blood cell count (WBCs): 11,800/mm^3
Hemoglobin: 11.2 g/dL
Hematocrit: 32.7%
Haley says, "I feel really tired, and too weak to even pick up a glass of water." Her cough produces white, thick sputum. Sputum culture on admission confirms a diagnosis of streptococcal pneumonia.

THINKING

1. *Theoretical Knowledge:*

   a. According to the Centers for Disease Control and Prevention, should Haley have received a pneumonia immunization? Why or why not?

   b. What is clubbing of the fingers? You may wish to refer to Chapter 22 for review, or to a medical-surgical nursing text.

2. *Critical Thinking (Analyzing Assumptions):*
   Why is it a positive finding for Haley that she does not have clubbed fingers?

DOING

3. *Practical Knowledge:*
Twenty-four hours after the antibiotics were started, Haley's respiratory status becomes worse. She says, "It's so hard to breathe." It is decided to begin administering oxygen. Another sputum culture is prescribed. You are to collect a sputum specimen from the patient.

   a. What position should Haley assume for this procedure?

   b. What kind of protective clothing do you need for this procedure?

   c. You remove the lid from the specimen container. When you hand it to Haley, she touches the inside of the container with her fingers. What should you do?

   d. What would you tell Haley to do in order to expectorate the sputum specimen?

4. *Nursing Process (Assessment):*
In the admission data, what important information is missing with regard to her respiratory status?

CARING

5. *Self-Knowledge:*
Describe one or two patient care experiences you might draw upon to help you in caring for Haley. In what ways were those patients similar to Haley, and how might that help you?

6. *Ethical Knowledge:*
After you finish collecting the sputum specimen, what do you think Haley's biggest concern is right now?

Critical Thinking and Clinical Judgment

1. Recall the three patients discussed in the Meet Your Patients scenario in your textbook in Volume 1:

   - Mary is a 4-year-old girl with a history of asthma. Her mother, Ms. Green, has brought her in because of an "asthma attack." Mary is sitting on her mother's lap and breathing rapidly through an open mouth. Her cough sounds congested and wheezy. The nurse practitioner has ordered a nebulized treatment containing albuterol (Proventil) and ipratropium bromide (Atrovent).

   - Mr. Chu is a 78-year-old man complaining of cough, sore throat, fatigue, and weakness. His temperature is 100.4°F (38°C), pulse is 90 beats/min, respirations are 26/min, and blood pressure (BP) is 166/82 mm Hg.

   - William is a 19-year-old male who has had a sudden onset of right-sided chest pain and shortness of breath. His chest x-ray revealed a right pneumothorax, and he is currently receiving 35% oxygen by face mask while waiting for an ambulance to transport him to the hospital for further evaluation.

   a. Which patients are experiencing problems with ventilation? Explain your answer.

   b. Which patient appears to be experiencing problems with hypoxia? Does the problem appear to be related to oxygenation or perfusion? Explain your answers.

   c. Mr. Chu has smoked two packs of cigarettes per day for 50 years. ABGs reveal a low Po_2 and a high Pco_2 consistent with chronic lung disease. He is diagnosed with an acute exacerbation of chronic bronchitis. He is placed on oral antibiotics and long-acting bronchodilators by metered-dose inhaler (MDI). What teaching could you offer to help Mr. Chu mobilize and expectorate secretions?

   d. Mary receives her nebulizer treatment and markedly improves. The physician has prescribed a variety of take-home medications that you must teach her mother about. The treatment plan includes a protocol based on peak expiratory flow monitoring. Discuss how you might involve Mary in her own care.

   e. William's chest x-ray film reveals a spontaneous pneumothorax. There is no apparent fluid in the pleural space. What chest tube systems can be used to treat his pneumothorax? Explain your thinking.

2. You are caring for a 68-year-old woman during the night shift. Earlier today she had an abdominal hysterectomy under general anesthesia. You note that her respiratory rate has steadily risen from 16 to 26 and that she has developed a mild, nonproductive cough. When you listen to her chest, you hear crackles throughout. She has a 40-pack-per-year cigarette smoking history. Identify an appropriate nursing diagnosis for this patient. Explain the reasons for your choice.

3. For each of the following concepts, use critical thinking to describe how or why it is important to nursing, patient care, or oxygenation. Note that these are not to be merely definitions.

Ventilation	Hypoventilation
Gas exchange	Hyperventilation
Artificial airways	Supplemental oxygen
Suctioning	Pulse oximetry
Negative pressure in the chest	

What Are the Main Points in This Chapter?

- The structures of the airways, lungs, chest cavity, heart, and blood vessels function together to supply oxygen to the tissues; thus, abnormalities in any of these structures can interfere with tissue oxygenation.
- Developmental stage, environment, individual characteristics, lifestyle, medications, and pathological factors can interfere with ventilation, circulation, or gas exchange, leading to problems with tissue oxygenation.
- A health assessment related to oxygenation includes assessment of ventilation (breathing), circulation (blood flow), and gas exchange (exchange of oxygen and carbon dioxide). The length and focus of the assessment varies with the purpose and urgency of the clinical situation.
- A physical examination related to adequacy of oxygenation includes observations of adequacy of breathing, circulation, and gas exchange.
- Pulse oximetry and arterial blood gases are used to monitor oxygen saturation.
- Small changes in oxygen saturation are associated with large shifts in the amount of oxygen available to the tissues and organs.
- Interventions to promote optimal respiratory function include deep regular breathing, flu and pneumonia immunizations for at-risk individuals, frequent position changes, incentive spirometry, and preventing aspiration.
- Deep breathing, coughing exercises, and hydration promote deep inhalation and forceful expulsion of secretions.
- Supplemental oxygen is used to prevent hypoxemia. It may be delivered by a variety of methods.
- Artificial airways provide an open airway for patients who cannot maintain their own airway. The most common artificial airways are oropharyngeal, nasopharyngeal, and endotracheal.
- Airways can be suctioned to remove secretions and maintain patency. Signs that indicate the need for suctioning include gurgling sounds during respiration, restlessness, labored respirations, decreased oxygen saturation, increased heart and respiratory rates, and the presence of adventitious breath sounds during auscultation.
- Mechanical ventilation with a positive pressure ventilator requires the patient to have an artificial airway.
- Chest tubes remove air or fluid from the pleural space so that the lungs can fully expand. Chest tubes should be clamped only for changing the drainage system; clamping can lead to tension pneumothorax.
- Respiratory medications promote ventilation and oxygenation by their effects on the respiratory system. The major types of respiratory medicines include bronchodilators, corticosteroids, cough preparations, decongestants, antihistamines, and mucolytics.

Knowledge Map

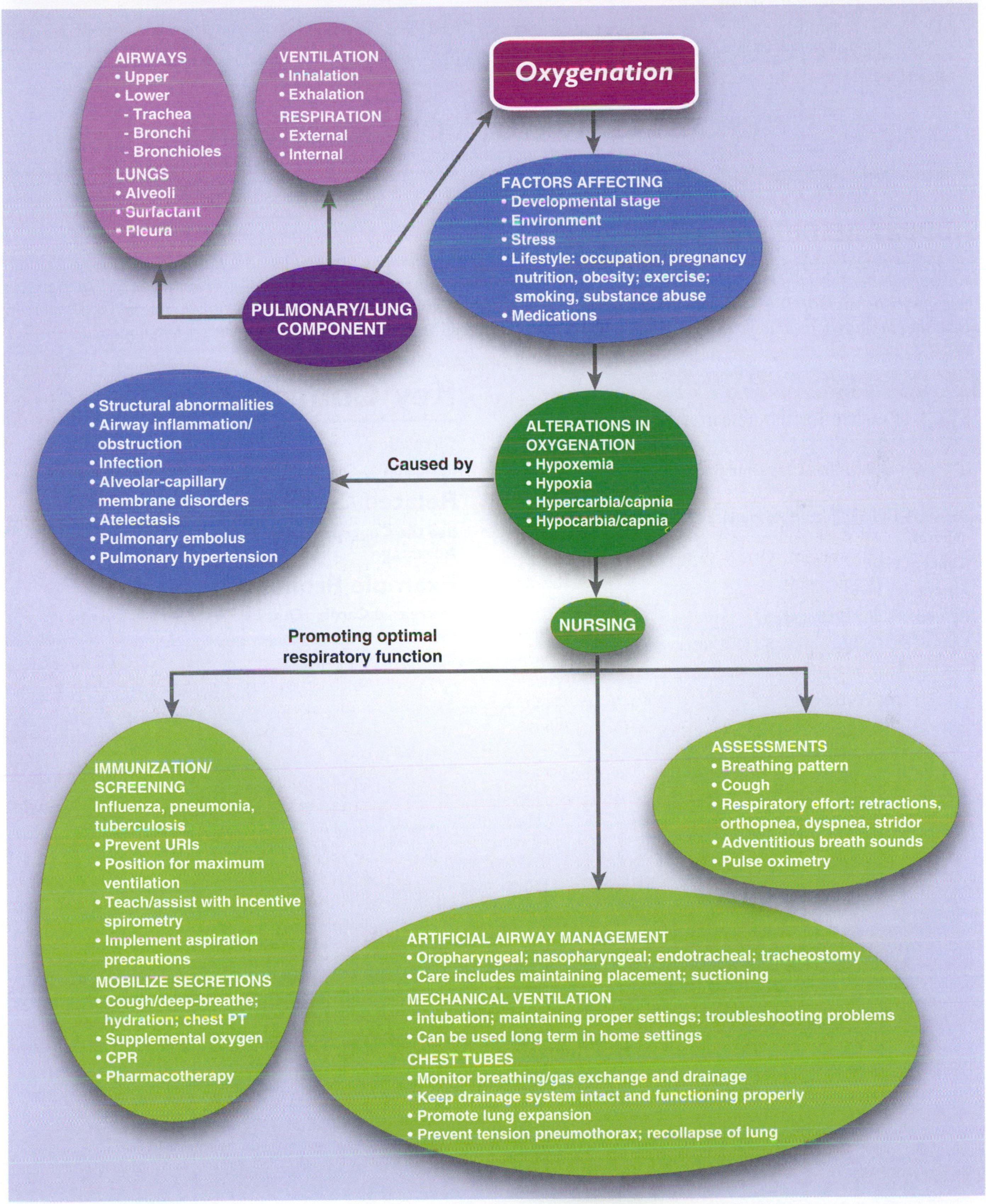

CHAPTER 37

Circulation & Perfusion

STUDENT RESOURCES

The questions and exercises in this book allow you to practice the kind of thinking you will use as a full-spectrum nurse. Critical-thinking questions usually have more than one right answer, so we do not provide "correct answers" for these features. Try to answer these questions yourself. It is more important to develop your nursing judgment than to just cover content. You will learn more by discussing the questions with your peers. If you are still unsure, see the Davis Advantage chapter resources for suggested responses.

To explore learning resources for this chapter,

Go to Davis Advantage and find:

Answers and Suggested Responses for all questions in this chapter

Concept Map

Knowledge Map

References and Bibliography

Lists of NOC Outcomes and NIC Interventions

Key Concepts

Circulation

Perfusion

Related Concepts

See the Concept Map on Davis Advantage

Example Problem

Decreased Cardiac Output

Caring for the Nguyens

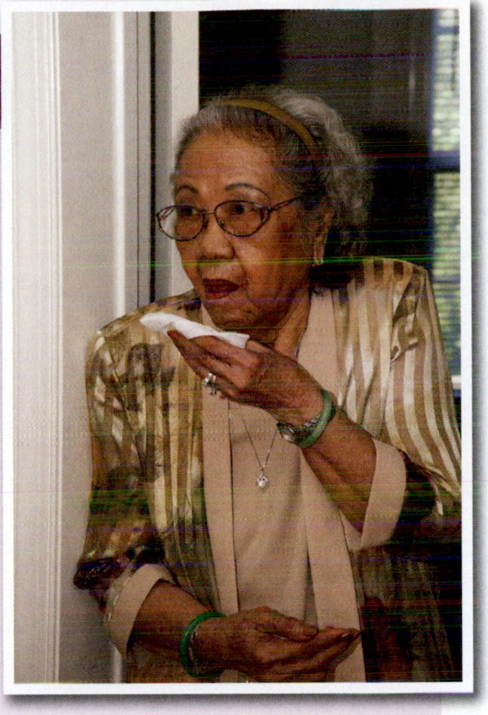

Mai Nguyen, Nam's 76-year-old mother, has been complaining she feels tired all the time; she just can't do what she normally does. She describes having a hard time catching her breath as she walks up stairs and goes about her day. Nam has noticed that his mother's ankles are more swollen than he has ever seen them. He schedules an appointment for his mother at the family clinic where you are the nurse. Mrs. Nguyen appears pale and not her usual energetic self. Nam tells you that his mom is "not right" and seems to be confused about things at home, which is not like her. She has a history of chronic congestive heart failure.

A. What additional health history data would be useful to gather at this time?

B. During her visit at the clinic, you observe that Mai has a cough. She spits a small amount of pink, frothy mucus into a tissue. Mrs. Nguyen's vital signs are as follows: BP, 142/90 mm Hg; pulse, 96 beats/min and with some irregular beats; respirations, 38 breaths/min and shallow; temperature, 97.8°F (36.5°C) oral.
- Which of these symptoms and vital signs is/are not within normal limits?
- For each abnormal finding, explain why you think it is occurring.

C. You decide to include a nursing diagnosis of Acute Confusion in Mrs. Nguyen's plan of care.
- What symptoms does she have that support this nursing diagnosis?
- What physiological changes are causing these symptoms?

D. In addition to angiotensin-converting enzyme (ACE) inhibitor, beta blocker, diuretic, and digoxin, what additional therapies do you anticipate the physician will prescribe?

E. Mrs. Nguyen asks you, "What can I do to make sure I never get this sick again?" How would you answer this question?

PracticalKnowledge clinical **application**

PROCEDURES

In this section you will find the procedures necessary for supporting circulation and perfusion. As you perform the procedures, apply the theoretical knowledge and concepts you obtained in Volume 1. The registered nurse is responsible for assessing patients' circulation and perfusion and their responses to procedures.

Procedure 37-1 ■ Performing Cardiac Monitoring

➤ For steps to follow in *all* procedures, refer to the Universal Steps for All Procedures found on the inside back cover.

Equipment

- Alcohol pads
- Gauze dressing
- Washcloth
- Shaving supplies or scissors, if necessary
- Disposable electrodes

For hardwire monitoring, add:

- Cardiac monitor
- Cable with lead wires
- Safety pin
- 1-in. tape

For telemetry, add:

- Transmitter with lead wires (with a new battery inserted before each use)
- Pouch to carry transmitter

Delegation

You should not delegate this procedure to the licensed practical nurse or unlicensed assistive personnel because it requires knowledge of anatomy, physiology, and advanced assessment techniques.

Pre-Procedure Assessment

- Assess cardiovascular status, including heart sounds, pulse rate, and blood pressure, and check for the presence of pain.
- Assess skin integrity of the chest before applying electrodes.
  Skin lesions contraindicate the application of leads to the affected area.
- Assess for history of dysrhythmias.
  Early recognition of dysrhythmias allows for prompt treatment, which improves patient outcomes.

➤ When performing the procedure, always identify your patient according to agency policy, using two identifiers, and be attentive to standard precautions, hand hygiene, patient safety and privacy, body mechanics, and documentation.

Procedure Steps

1. **Prepare the monitoring equipment.**

For Hardwire Monitoring

a. Plug the cardiac monitor into an electrical outlet, and turn it on.
Allows the monitor to warm up while you prepare the patient for monitoring.

b. Connect the cable with lead wires into the monitor.
The cable and lead wires must be properly connected to the monitor to obtain an accurate electrocardiogram (ECG) tracing. Most are color coded.

For Telemetry Monitoring

c. Insert a new battery into the transmitter.
A new battery should be inserted with each use to ensure transmitter function.

d. Turn on the transmitter.
Tests the unit to make sure that the battery is functional.

e. Connect the lead wires to the transmitter, if they are not permanently attached. Be sure to attach each one to its correct outlet.
The lead wires must be properly connected to the transmitter to obtain an accurate ECG tracing.

2. **Expose the patient's chest** and identify electrode sites based on the monitoring system being used and the patient's anatomy. Gently rub the placement sites with a washcloth or gauze pad until the skin reddens slightly.
The monitoring system will dictate lead placement. Sites over soft tissues or close to bone provide accurate waveforms; sites over bony prominences, thick muscles, and skinfolds can produce artifact.

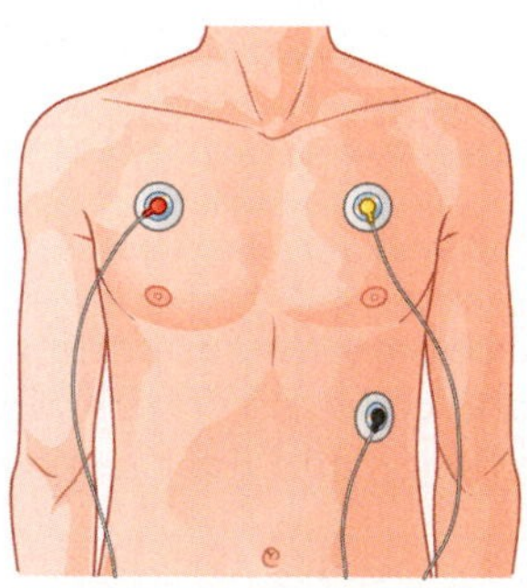

3. **If the patient's chest has dense hair,** shave or clip the hair with scissors at each electrode site.
Hair may interfere with electrical contact, preventing accurate ECG waveform transmission.

4. **With an alcohol pad** clean the areas chosen for electrode placement, and allow them to dry.
Alcohol removes oil on the skin that may prevent the electrodes from adhering.

5. **Remove the electrode backing** and make sure the gel is moist. Discard the electrode if the gel is dry. The number of electrodes needed will depend on the monitoring system being used. It will be three to five electrodes.
A dry electrode will not conduct electrical activity.

6. **Attach the lead wires** to the electrodes by snapping or clipping them in place.

7. **Apply the electrode** to the site by pressing it firmly. Repeat with the remaining electrodes.
Pressing the electrode firmly creates a tight seal, which ensures electrical contact.

8. **Secure the monitoring equipment.**

For Hardwire Monitoring

a. Wrap a piece of 1-in. tape around the cable, and secure it to the patient's gown with a safety pin.
Secures the cable so leads are not disconnected with patient movement.

For Telemetry Monitoring

b. Place the transmitter in the pouch, and tie it around the patient's neck. Place the transmitter into the patient's robe or gown pocket if a pouch is not available.
Allows the patient independence with ambulation.

9. **Check the patient's ECG** tracing on the monitor. If necessary, adjust the gain to increase the waveform size.
The ECG tracing should be large enough to accurately assess all of the waveform components.

For Telemetry Monitoring

You may need to call a monitoring room to verify ECG tracing and rhythm.

10. **Set the upper and lower** heart rate alarm limits according to agency policy or patient condition, and turn them on.

11. **Obtain a rhythm strip** by pressing the "record" button.
You must obtain a rhythm strip to document the patient's cardiac rhythm.

For Hardwire Monitoring

a. Press the "record" button on the bedside monitor.
The "record" button, located on the monitor at the bedside, allows you to print a rhythm strip immediately when cardiac symptoms occur.

For Telemetry Monitoring

b. Press the "record" button on the transmitter of the telemetry unit, or call the monitoring room to have the ECG trip printed.
The "record" button on the telemetry transmitter allows you or the patient to print a rhythm strip immediately when cardiac symptoms occur.

12. **Interpret the rhythm strip**, and then mount it appropriately (e.g., with transparent tape) in the patient's chart.
Provides a permanent record of the patient's heart activity; identifies rhythm abnormalities in the patient's rhythm.

? What if . . .

- **Your patient is diaphoretic?**
Remove electrodes, clean the area with alcohol, allow the area to dry, and then reapply electrodes.
To obtain an accurate ECG tracing.
- **Your patient is receiving a cardiac medication?**
Print a strip before giving medication and after giving medication. You may also need to call the telemetry station to have the ECG monitored.
To assess and monitor effects of medication.
- **You are not getting a good reading on the monitor?**
Recheck the leads; replace leads or move leads if necessary.

Evaluation

- Evaluate changes in the patient's cardiac rhythm.
- Check skin integrity, and replace the electrodes at least every 24 hours.
Avoids skin irritation at the electrode sites. In addition, the gel begins to dry, so replacement ensures an adequate waveform.

Patient Teaching

- Explain the rationale for cardiac monitoring.
- Teach the patient that if he experiences symptoms (e.g., shortness of breath, chest pain, dizziness, palpitations) he should notify the nurse immediately so a rhythm strip can be recorded.
- Tell the patient being monitored by telemetry to remove the transmitter before showering. Ask the patient to inform you before removing it.
- Discuss home telemetry monitoring with the patient and caregiver if the patient requires telemetry monitoring after discharge.

Home Care

- Evaluate the client's and caregiver's ability to continue telemetry monitoring at home with help from an outside agency.
- Help the client and caregiver contact the monitoring agency and arrange for home telemetry monitoring.
- Explain to the caregiver and patient that the emergency medical service will be notified by the monitoring agency if a dysrhythmia develops.
- Instruct the caregiver and patient about proper lead placement and the need to rotate electrode sites to prevent skin breakdown.

Documentation

- Document the date and time that monitoring was instituted.
- Note the monitoring lead selected.
- Document a rhythm strip every 8 hours and with changes in the patient's condition according to agency policy. Label the rhythm strip (if the monitor does not label it for you) with the date, time, patient's name, and room number. Indicate on the strip when symptoms and treatment interventions occurred.
- Document the patient's response to treatment.

Practice Resources

Hancock, E. W., Deal, B. J., Mirvis, D. M., et al. (2009); Ladha, E., House-Kokan, M., & Parker, L. (2018); Morrison, L. J., Neumar, R. W., Zimmerman, J. L., et al. (2013).

ASSESSMENT GUIDELINES & TOOLS

Focused Assessment

Assessing Circulation

Part I. Questions to Assess Risk for Impaired Circulation

Demographic Data

- What is your age?
- Where do you live?
- What is your occupation?

Health History

- Do you have current health problems? Describe.
- Do you have past health problems? Describe.
- Have you ever been hospitalized or had surgery, If so, when and for what reason?
- Do you take medication for your heart, blood pressure, cholesterol, or erectile dysfunction, diabetes, breathing difficulty, or other conditions?
- Do you have chronic fatigue, heartburn, anxiety, swelling of the ankles, difficulty breathing, chest discomfort, palpitations, dizziness or fainting spells, dental problems, pain in the calf when walking that stops with rest, chronic cough or wheezing, shortness of breath, or unexplained weight loss?
- Do you take over-the-counter products, such as vitamins, supplements, or aspirin?
- What else do you want to tell me about your physical or mental health history?

Family History

- Did your father or a brother develop coronary artery disease or have a heart attack before the age of 55?
- Did your mother or sister develop coronary artery disease or have a heart attack before the age of 65?

Cardiovascular History

- Have you ever had or been diagnosed with a heart attack, angina, coronary artery disease, peripheral artery disease, stroke, aortic aneurysm?
- Do you have high or low blood pressure? Do you feel dizzy if you stand up quickly?
- Have you ever had chest pain? If so, describe the circumstances? What was done to relieve the symptoms? What measures do you take to prevent the pain?
- Do you become easily fatigued or feel your heart rate is rapid? Do you ever feel heart palpitations?
- Do you have pain in your legs when you are walking uphill or walking for a long time?
- Do you experience cold hands and feet? If so, how often?
- Do you have pain or tingling in your feet or toes with exercise? Do they feel numb when you are at rest? Does the pain worsen when your leg is elevated and/or improve when you dangle your legs over the side of the bed?
- Do you have pain in your leg, foot, or toes that is so severe that shoes or the weight of a sheet at night is painful?
- If you are male, do you experience impotence?
- Do you have ulcers that do not heal?

Nutrition History

- In a typical day, how many servings of whole grains, fruits, vegetables, dairy products, eggs, nuts, and red meat or fish do you eat or drink per day?
- How many meals per week do you eat fast food or other high-fat food?
- How many sugar-sweetened soft drinks and sodas do you drink per day?
- How many meals per week do you eat out? Where?
- How many times per day do you add salt or eat salty foods?
- How many times per week do you skip a meal?
- Do you have diabetes or prediabetes? Are you a normal weight?

Lifestyle and Health Promotion Activities

- What is your current stress level? What are your major sources of stress? How do you relieve stress?
- What is your usual diet? Is your current diet typical, or have you recently changed your eating habits?
- What is your usual activity level? Do you exercise regularly? If so, how many minutes per week of moderate to vigorous physical activity do you get?
- Do you check your lipid profile (cholesterol and triglycerides) and blood sugar (fasting blood sugar and hemoglobin A_{1C}) on a regular basis?
- Do you smoke now, or have you ever smoked? If you smoke, how many packs per day and for how many years have you smoked?
- Do you use crack cocaine or other illicit substances?

Part II. Focused Physical Examination

Cardiovascular System

- Review Procedure 22-13: Assessing the Heart and Vascular System.
- ***Inspect the neck*** for carotid and jugular pulsations. Palpate each carotid separately. Auscultate the carotid arteries and jugular veins for bruits and hums.
- ***Inspect the precordium*** for pulsations. Palpate for pulsations, lifts, heaves, and thrills. Auscultate for heart sounds.
- ***Assess peripheral circulation:*** Palpate peripheral pulses, assess skin color and temperature, note hair distribution on extremities. Inspect for skin ulcers and edema of the feet and ankles.
- ***Inspect*** for venous valve competence.
- ***Perform the capillary refill test*** anywhere you note signs of diminished blood flow.

DIAGNOSTIC TESTING

Diagnostic Testing

Tests Related to Circulation

Test	Purpose
Angiogram	A contrast dye is injected into a vein, and serial films are taken to assess patency of the vessels.
Arterial blood gases (ABG)	An analysis of arterial blood evaluates the effectiveness of gas exchange and perfusion.
Cardiac catheterization	A catheter is passed into the heart to assess pressures, blood flow, and the size and patency of chambers.
Chest x-ray study (CXR)	Provides an anterior–posterior or lateral view of the heart and lungs, shows tissue density (e.g., to evaluate size, masses, fluid).
Cholesterol, lipid profile	Indicates risk for cardiovascular disease long term.
Creatine kinase-MB (CK-MB)	The MB isoenzyme is present only in the heart muscle. A serum measurement of the MB band is used to detect a myocardial infarction (MI). Levels rise with an acute MI.
Echocardiogram	An ultrasound evaluation of the heart that examines heart function and blood flow.
Electrocardiogram (ECG)	Electrodes placed on the extremities and chest wall conduct electrical activity from the heart. ECG illustrates heart rate, rhythm, and size and helps evaluate heart damage.
Hemoglobin (Hgb)	A serum measurement that affects the oxygen-carrying capacity of the blood. May be measured separately or as part of a complete blood count.
Holter monitor	A continuous ECG tracing used to correlate symptoms and cardiac activity. Typically the tracing lasts 48 hours to 7 days.
Magnetic Resonance Angiography	This is an MRI exam of the blood vessels. Unlike a traditional **angiography (MRA)**, there is no angiography tube (catheter) placed into the body. MRA is noninvasive.
Technetium scan	Technetium-99m sestamibi is injected intravenously. Approximately 90 to 120 minutes later, the heart is scanned. Areas of myocardial damage appear as "hot spots" on the scan.
Treadmill test	Evaluates the effect of exercise on the heart and circulation via continuous ECG and vital sign monitoring during exercise.
Troponin	A serum evaluation of a complex of proteins is used to detect MI. Levels of these contractile proteins remain elevated for up to 7 days after MI.
Ultrasound (Doppler)	A transducer, which directs high frequency sound waves to the artery of vein, is used to examine blood flow. A normal result shows no areas of narrowing or closure in the blood vessel.
Venography	Using dye and x-ray technology, a narrow tube (catheter) is inserted into a large vein to identify any blood clots or unusual narrowing or blockage of venous blood flow.
VQ Scan	Used to detect a blood clot in the lungs.

STANDARDIZED LANGUAGE

Standardized Language

Examples of NOC Outcomes and NIC Interventions Linked to Circulation Diagnoses

Nursing Diagnosis	NOC Outcomes	NIC Interventions
Activity Intolerance (could also be related to pulmonary functioning)	Energy Conservation Self-Care: Activities of Daily Living (ADL)	Energy Management Exercise Promotion: Strength Training Self-Care Assistance
Decreased Cardiac Output	Blood Loss Severity Cardiac Pump Effectiveness Circulation Status Tissue Perfusion: Cardiac Tissue Perfusion: Abdominal Tissue Perfusion: Cerebral Tissue Perfusion: Peripheral Tissue Perfusion: Pulmonary Vital Signs	Bleeding Reduction Cardiac Care Cerebral Perfusion Promotion Circulatory Care: Arterial Circulatory Care: Venous Insufficiency Hemodynamic Regulation Intravenous (IV) Therapy Shock Management
Impaired Peripheral Tissue Perfusion Alteration	Circulation Status Fluid Overload Severity Tissue Integrity: Skin & Mucous Membranes	Circulatory Care: Arterial Insufficiency Circulatory Care: Venous Insufficiency Fluid Management Peripheral Sensation Management Skin Surveillance
Risk for Impaired Cerebral, Gastrointestinal, or Renal Perfusion	Circulation Status Cognition Electrolyte & Acid/Base Balance Fluid Balance Neurological Status: Consciousness Kidney Function Tissue Perfusion: Abdominal Organs	Cerebral Perfusion Promotion Neurologic Monitoring Hypovolemia Management Fluid/Electrolyte Management Circulatory Care: Arterial Insufficiency Circulatory Care: Venous Insufficiency Circulatory Precautions Hemodialysis Therapy

Source: Johnson, M., Moorhead, S., Bulechek, G., et al. (2012). *NOC and NIC linkages to NANDA-I and clinical conditions.* St. Louis, MO: Elsevier; Butcher, H., Bulechek, G., Dochterman, J., et al. (Eds.). (2018). *Nursing interventions classification (NIC)* (7th ed.). St. Louis, MO: Elsevier; Moorhead, S., Swanson, E., Johnson, M., et al. (Eds.). (2018). *Nursing outcomes classification (NOC)* (6th ed.). St. Louis, MO: Elsevier. Used with permission.

CLINICALJUDGMENT

Applying the Full-Spectrum Nursing Model

PATIENT SITUATION

Margarita, a 62-year-old director of management technology for a large company, was admitted to the hospital with shortness of breath, sudden and intense fatigue, and intense chest pressure that she describes as feeling like a steel band tightening around her rib cage. She reports the pain moved up to her jaw. The pain began suddenly but lasted approximately 5 to 7 minutes. During the episode, her husband tells you that Margarita acted as though she had a feeling of doom.

Margarita also has a history of sudden onset neck pain that seems to be triggered by heightened stress at work. Margarita is pale and clammy. She states she feels nauseated and has burning in her epigastric area. Her heart rate is 80 beats/minute, respiratory rate, 12 breaths/min, and blood pressure, 168/92 mm Hg. Skin is pale but warm, and capillary refill time is 4 seconds. Height is 5 ft 4 in. Weight is 156 lb. Body mass index (BMI) is 29.2. Waist circumference is 36 in.

The health history includes type 2 diabetes mellitus, high blood pressure, and tobacco use (half a pack of cigarettes a day). Margarita's mother had a heart attack in her 50s.

Lab work prior to admission:

Fasting lipids: total cholesterol, 288 mg/dL; LDL, 148 mg/dL; HDH, 44 mg/dL; triglycerides, 222 mg/dL
Serum glucose: 244 mg/dL
Hs-CRP: 3.1 mg/dL

THINKING

1 *Theoretical Knowledge:*

a. What predisposing factors increase Margarita's risk for myocardial infarction?

b. What does it mean to have infarcted myocardial tissue?

2 *Critical Thinking (Analyzing Assumptions):*
Based on your knowledge of vascular causes of myocardial infarction, what are the most likely causes in this patient?

DOING

3. *Practical Knowledge:*
After your patient's vital signs are stable and her pain is controlled, the emergency physician prescribes further diagnostic testing to determine the extent of damage to her heart.

a. What tests would you expect your patient to have?

b. You attempt to adhere electrodes for cardiac monitoring to Margarita's chest. The ECG tracing shows a great deal of artifact rather than a clear ECG tracing. What should you do to obtain an accurate tracing?

c. You notice your patient is experience multiple "runs" of aberrant heartbeats. What should you do in response to the abnormal ECG tracing?

4. *Nursing Process (Assessment):*
In the admission data, what important information is missing with regard to her cardiac status?

CARING

5. *Self-Knowledge:*
Describe a personal experience involving someone in your own family or a friend who experienced a life-threatening event. How did you feel when your loved one was faced with a potentially life-altering heart condition? How might you draw upon this experience to help you in caring for Margarita?

6. *Ethical Knowledge:*
   a. After Margarita is finished with the last diagnostic test, what do you think her biggest concern is likely to be?
   b. Margarita tells you that she does not want anyone to know she has a heart problem. Yet her husband wants to tell other family members. How do you best respond to her concerns for privacy?

Critical Thinking and Clinical Judgment

1. Recall the patient discussed in the Meet Your Patient scenario in Volume 1 of your textbook: Ms. Saunders is a 55-year-old accountant. She says she has been extremely tired, easily becomes short of breath, and is unable to complete her chores without frequent rest breaks. She is pale and seems tired. Her vital signs are as follows: temperature, 98.4°F (36.7°C); pulse, 86 beats/min; respirations, 24 breaths/min and unlabored; BP, 136/78 mm Hg; and pulse oximetry, 98% on room air. She is now waiting for her lab results, which include a complete blood count (CBC).

   Which of the following nursing diagnoses can you make, based on the patient data given here? Use a nursing diagnosis handbook and the standardized language table in this chapter.

   Decreased Cardiac Output

   Risk for Impaired Cardiac Tissue Perfusion

   Impaired Peripheral Tissue Perfusion

   Activity Intolerance

2. Ms. Saunders is diagnosed with severe anemia. She is hospitalized because her hemoglobin is 8.9 g/dL. How will this affect her oxygenation? What interventions would improve her fatigue?

3. For the following concept, use critical thinking to describe how or why it is important to nursing, patient care, or oxygenation. Note that this is *not* to be merely a definition.

   Perfusion

What Are the Main Points in This Chapter?

- The structures of the airways, lungs, chest cavity, heart, and blood vessels function together to supply oxygen to the tissues; thus, abnormalities in any of these structures can interfere with tissue oxygenation.
- Developmental stage, environment, individual characteristics, lifestyle, medications, and pathological factors can interfere with circulation and perfusion, leading to problems with tissue oxygenation.
- A health assessment related to circulation includes assessment of ventilation (breathing), circulation (blood flow), perfusion, and gas exchange (exchange of oxygen and carbon dioxide). The length and focus of the assessment varies with the purpose and urgency of the clinical situation.
- A physical examination related to adequacy of circulation includes observations of adequacy of circulation, and perfusion.
- Cardiovascular function is influenced by developmental stage, environment, lifestyle, substance abuse, medications, and pathophysiological conditions such as heart failure, coronary artery disease, and peripheral vascular disorders.
- The purposes of cardiac monitoring are to identify the patient's baseline rhythm and rate, recognize significant changes in the baseline rhythm and rate, and recognize life-threatening dysrhythmias that require immediate intervention.
- Promoting circulation ensures that oxygenated blood reaches tissues and organs and venous blood returns to the heart. Activities that promote venous return and peripheral arterial circulation and prevent clot formation assist with circulation.
- Cardiovascular drugs are used to enhance cardiac output, thus providing increased blood flow and oxygenation to organs and tissues. They include vasodilators, beta-adrenergic blocking agents, diuretics, and positive inotropes.

Knowledge Map

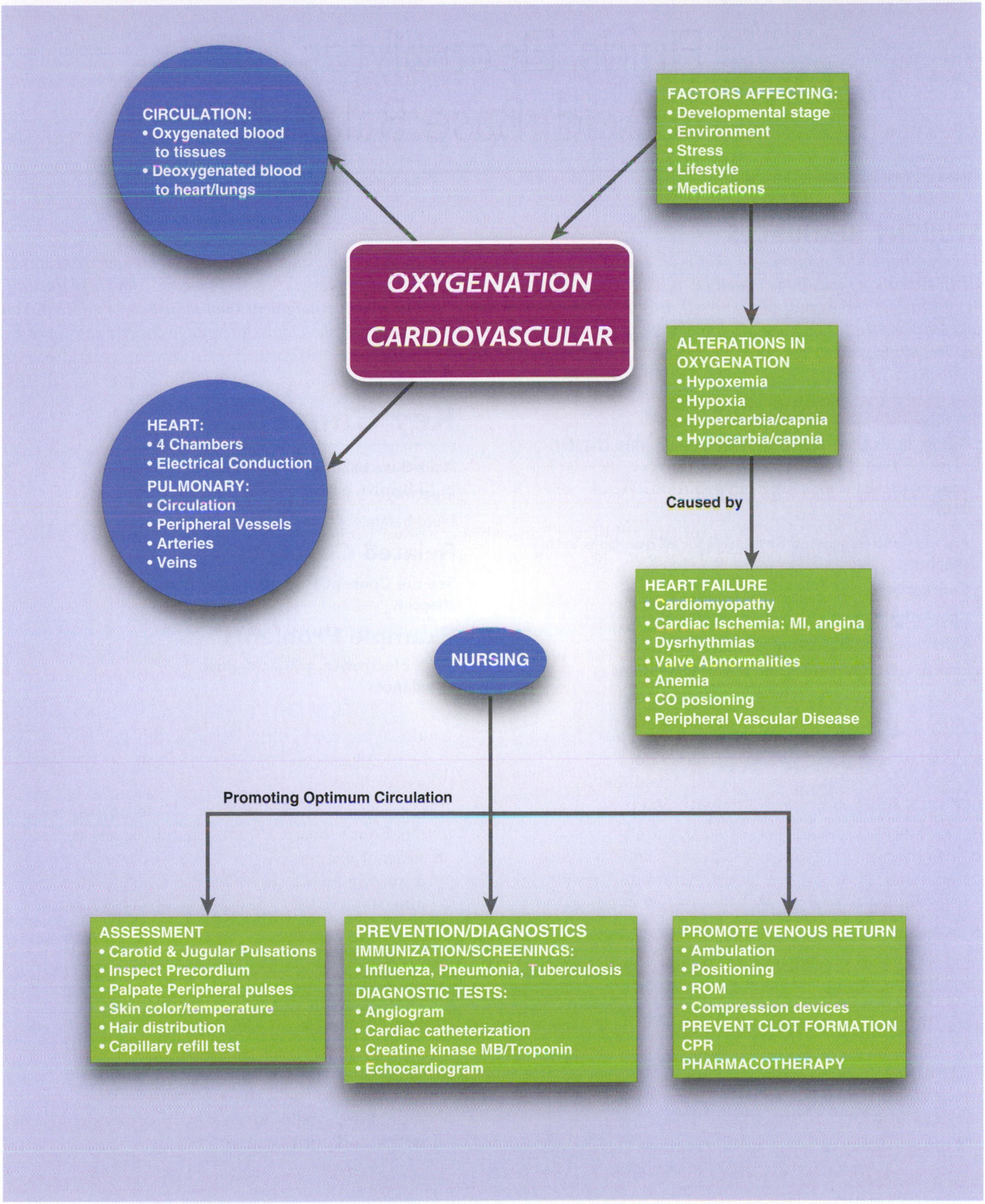

CHAPTER 38

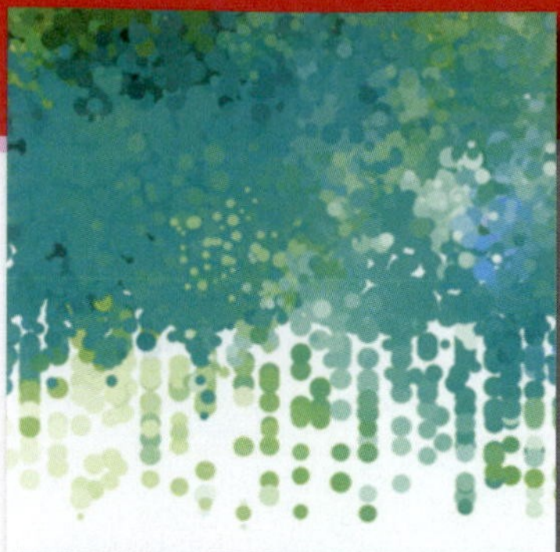

Fluids, Electrolytes, & Acid–Base Balance

STUDENT RESOURCES

The questions and exercises in this book allows you to practice the kind of thinking you will use as a full-spectrum nurse. Critical-thinking questions usually have more than one right answer, so we do not provide "correct answers" for these features. Try to answer these questions yourself. It is more important to develop your nursing judgment than to just cover content. You will learn by discussing the questions with your peers. If you are still unsure, see the Davis Advantage chapter resources for suggested responses.

To explore learning resources for this chapter,

Go to **Davis Advantage** and find:

- Answers and Suggested Responses for all questions in this chapter
- Concept Map
- Knowledge Map
- References and Bibliography
- Lists of NOC Outcomes and NIC Interventions

Key Concepts

Acid–Base balance
Electrolyte balance
Fluid balance

Related Concepts

See the Concept Map at the end of this chapter.

Example Problems

Fluid, Electrolyte, and Acid–Base Imbalances

Caring for the Nguyens

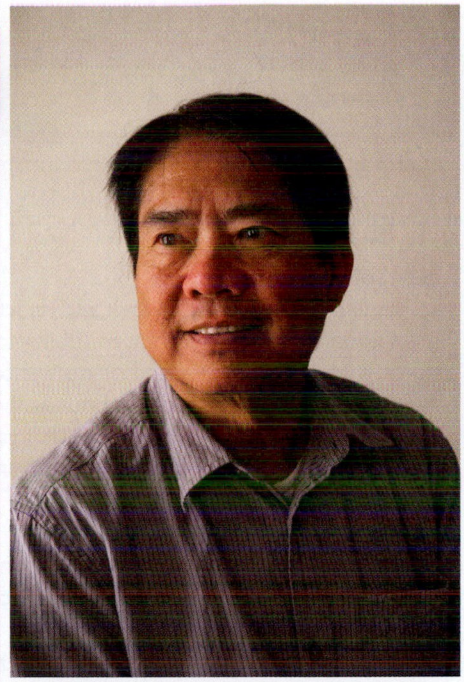

Nam Nguyen has been prescribed the following medicines:

lisinopril 20 mg PO daily
hydrochlorothiazide 25 mg PO daily in the a.m.
metformin 500 mg PO before breakfast and lunch

Today he had blood drawn for analysis. Following are the electrolyte panel results.

Sodium	136 mEq/L
Potassium	3.0 mEq/L
Chloride	96 mEq/L
Bicarbonate	24 mEq/L
BUN	18 mg/dL
Creatinine	0.8 mg/dL

A. Review the lab results. Compare Nam's lab work with the established norms for these values. Based on the lab results, what kind of assessment questions would be appropriate to ask Nam?

B. Use your pharmacology text to review Nam's medications. Which, if any, of these medicines might be contributing to Nam's lab results?

C. What teaching would be appropriate for Nam?

Practical Knowledge clinical application

To prevent, identify, and treat fluid, electrolyte, and acid–base problems, you will need to be skilled at initiating and managing intravenous infusions of fluids and blood, performing focused history and physical assessments, and interpreting arterial blood gas (ABG) values. When performing the procedures, apply the concepts and other theoretical knowledge you have learned.

PROCEDURES

Procedure 38-1 ■ Initiating a Peripheral Intravenous Infusion

➤ For steps to follow in *all* procedures, refer to the Universal Steps for All Procedures found on the inside back cover.

Equipment

- IV solution
- Administration set or IV lock and injection caps. (For a glass solution container, use vented tubing; for a plastic container you may use either vented or nonvented tubing.)
- Extension tubing with or without saline lock.
- Appropriately sized intravenous (IV) catheter
- Prefilled syringe to prime extension tubing.
- Clean, unsterile gloves
- Scissors
- Antiseptic swabs that contain solutions such as chlorhexidine (preferred INS, 2016) or 70% alcohol wipes.
- Tourniquet (non-latex, if available)
- Sterile manufactured catheter stabilization device or ½-in. tape.
- Transparent semipermeable occlusive dressing (preferred) and/or 2 in. × 2 in. sterile gauze,
- 1-in. nonallergenic tape, preferably clear
- Labels, time tape
- Linen-saver pad
- Arm board, if necessary

Delegation

In some states and agencies, you can delegate peripheral IV catheter insertion to a licensed practical nurse (LPN) who is adequately trained in the procedure.

Pre-Procedure Assessments

- Assess the patient's need for IV therapy by checking vital signs, laboratory values, urine output, skin turgor, breath sounds, and the condition of mucous membranes.
- Check for any situations that may contraindicate administering the prescribed fluids to the patient.
- Assess for allergy to tape.
- Assess the veins on the arms and hands for a potential insertion site.
  The upper extremities are preferred because of better blood flow, easier access, and less potential for complications than in other locations.
- Check the medical record for factors such as anticoagulant therapy, bleeding disorders, or low platelet count.
  These factors place the patient at risk of bleeding during IV catheter insertion.

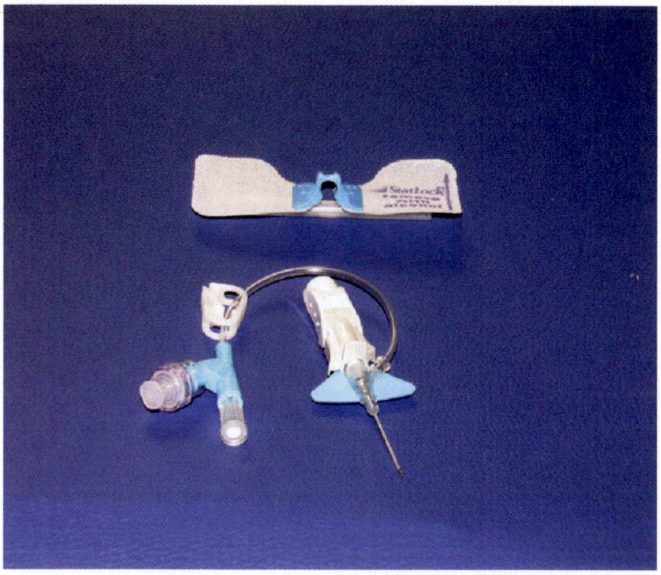

Catheter stabilization device

➤ *When performing the procedure, always identify your patient according to agency policy, using two identifiers, and be attentive to standard precautions, hand hygiene, patient safety and privacy, body mechanics, and documentation.*

Procedure Steps

NOTE: Maintain scrupulous aseptic technique throughout this procedure.
Any microorganisms introduced can cause infection at the site, which could quickly migrate into the bloodstream and cause sepsis.

1. **Place the patient in** a comfortable position, the bed at a comfortable working height, and supplies within reach. Explain the procedure to the patient.
   Makes the procedure safer, easier, and decreases the risk for the nurse to develop back problems from improper body mechanics.

2. **Prepare the IV solution** and administration set or IV lock.
   a. Following the "rights" of medication administration, check the IV solution to make sure that you have the proper solution with the prescribed additives.
   IV solution is considered medication, and you should check it carefully to avoid administration and compatibility errors.
   b. Check the expiration date on the IV solution. Do not use IV solution after the expiration date.
   c. Check the IV solution for discoloration or particulate matter.
   Indicates contamination and should not be used.
   d. Label the IV solution container with the patient's name, date, and your initials. Place a time tape on the solution container with the prescribed infusion rate, time the infusion begins, and the time it is to be completed.
   Policies govern when solution containers, administration sets, dressings, and IV catheters need to be changed to avoid complications such as infection. Although not all agencies require a time tape, labeling infusion rates on the solution containers in this manner will alert others and makes it easy to see at a glance whether the solution is infusing on time.

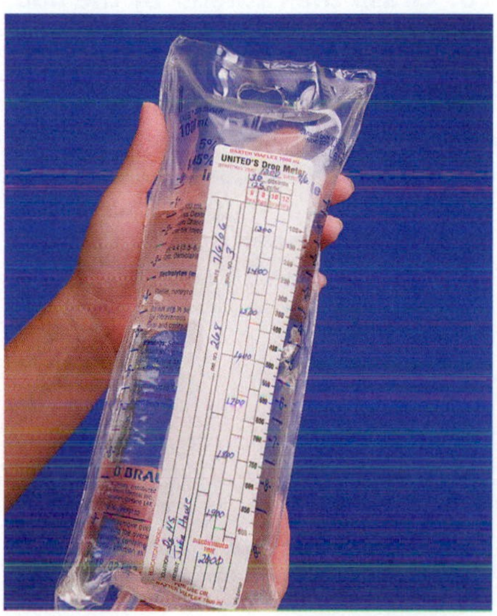

   e. Take the administration set from the package and close the roller clamp by rolling it downward. Label the tubing with the date and time.
   Ensures that fluid does not flow through inadvertently after the bag is spiked.
   f. Remove the protective cover from the solution container port.
   g. Remove the protective cover from the spike on the IV administration set, keeping the spike sterile. Insert the spike into the port of the solution container.

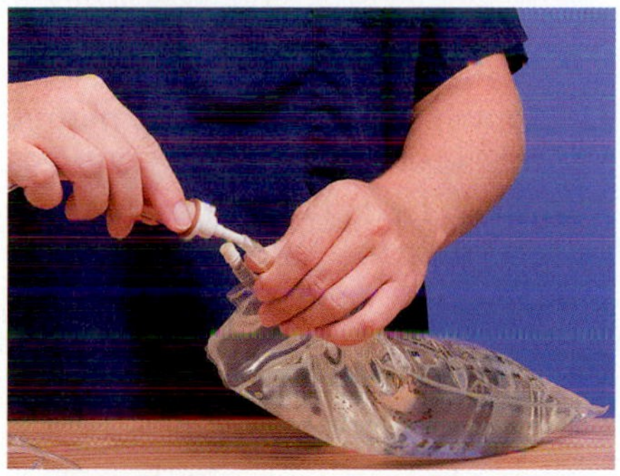

When Using a Glass Bottle

Clean the rubber stopper on the top of the bottle with an alcohol pad. Then insert the spike of the administration set through the stopper.

   h. Be certain the tubing is clamped. Hang the IV solution container on an IV pole.
   Clamping prevents leakage of fluid.
   i. Lightly compress the drip chamber, and allow it to fill up halfway.
   Overfilling the drip chamber will impair your ability to see the drips and adequately regulate the IV flow rate.

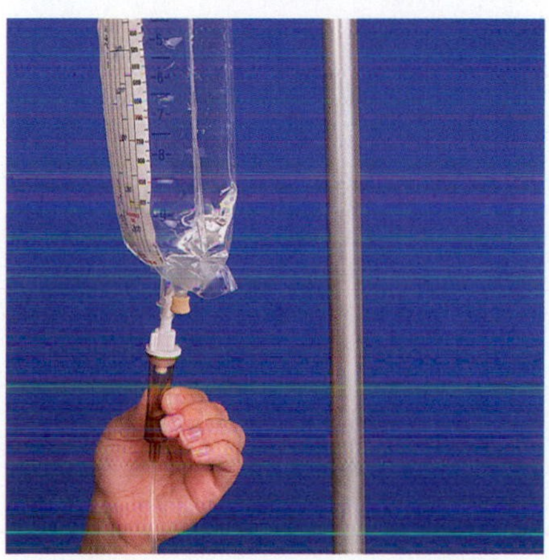

When Not Using Extension Tubing

Prime the tubing by opening the roller clamp and allowing the fluid to slowly fill the tubing. When tubing is filled, close the clamp.

When Using Extension Tubing

Either attach it to the end of the administration set now and prime it with the rest of the IV line, or prime it separately, as follows:

   j. Scrub the injection port of the extension tubing with an antiseptic pad and let it dry.
   k. Attach a flush syringe filled with normal saline to the injection port or to the non–luer-lock end and slowly push the fluid through the tubing until completely primed. (Consult packaging instructions for the amount of saline needed to flush the tubing.)
   l. Leave flush syringe attached to the extension tubing.
   IV extension tubing makes it easier to convert an IV to a saline lock without disturbing the IV dressing and catheter. Manipulation of the IV catheter increases the risk of complications such as phlebitis, inflammation, infection, and infiltration.
   m. Inspect the tubing for air. If air bubbles remain in the tubing, flick the tubing with a fingertip to mobilize them into the drip chamber. Recap the end of the tubing firmly.
   Air in the tubing creates the potential for air embolism.

3. **Place a linen-saver pad** under the patient's arm.
Protects the bed from soiling during venipuncture.

4. **Place the patient's arm** in a dependent position.
Gravity helps fill and dilate the vein, making venipuncture easier.

5. **Apply a tourniquet** 10 to 20 cm (4 to 8 in.) above the selected site. Palpate the radial pulse. If no pulse is present, loosen the tourniquet, and reapply it with less tension.
Occluding the arterial flow diminishes venous filling, making venipuncture difficult.

(continued on next page)

Procedure 38-1 ■ Initiating a Peripheral Intravenous Infusion (continued)

6. **Locate a vein for inserting the IV catheter.** Select the best most distal vein on the hand or arm. Check with the medical provider before using an arm or hand that contains a dialysis graft or fistula, or the affected arm of a patient who has undergone a mastectomy. See Clinical Insight 38-3 for more guidelines.
Choose the most distal veins on the hand or arm so that you can perform subsequent venipunctures proximal to the previous site. This preserves veins for long-term therapy and prevents extravasation of fluid and medicines.

7. **Palpate the vein and press it** downward, making sure that it rebounds quickly. If the vein is not adequately dilated, ask the patient to open and close his fist; apply heat (e.g., a warm towel, a warming mitt); lightly tap the vein site; or stroke the extremity from distal to proximal, beginning below the selected venipuncture site. If available in your agency, use an infrared or other visualization device to assist in locating a vein.
These actions bring blood to the local area to dilate the vein, making it easier to locate and making venipuncture easier.

8. **Loosen the tourniquet.** If excessive hair is present at the venipuncture site, clip it with a scissor.
Loosening the tourniquet restores blood flow and allows for patient comfort while preparing for venipuncture. Clipping the hair helps the dressings to adhere after catheter insertion. Shaving is not recommended because it may abrade the skin, providing a portal of entry for pathogens.

9. **Don clean nonsterile gloves.**
Provides protection from inadvertent exposure to blood. Note that some nurses don gloves routinely, even when preparing supplies and equipment. However, there is no risk for coming in contact with body fluids before this step, so strictly speaking, CDC standard precautions require gloves only from this step forward.

10. **Select an IV catheter** appropriate for the size of the vein, the solution to be infused, and the expected duration of therapy. Using aseptic technique, open the package touching only the outside of it.
Reduces the risk of extravasation and phlebitis. Always use the smallest diameter and shortest catheter that will deliver the desired solution flow. For most adults this will be a 20- to 24-gauge to minimize venous irritation and promote blood flow around the catheter. Aseptic handling reduces the risk of infection.

11. **Gently reapply the tourniquet** and scrub the site, using an antiseptic swab that contains >0.5% chlorhexidine gluconate (preferred, INS, 2016); if this is not available, use 70% alcohol wipes. Cleanse using a back and forth motion for 30 seconds (INS, 2016). If povidone iodine must be used, apply with an applicator and allow to remain on the skin for 1.5 to 2 minutes until completely dry. Remove with sterile normal saline or sterile water for patients with compromised skin integrity.
Removes microorganisms from the skin so that they do not enter the venous system during venipuncture. ▼

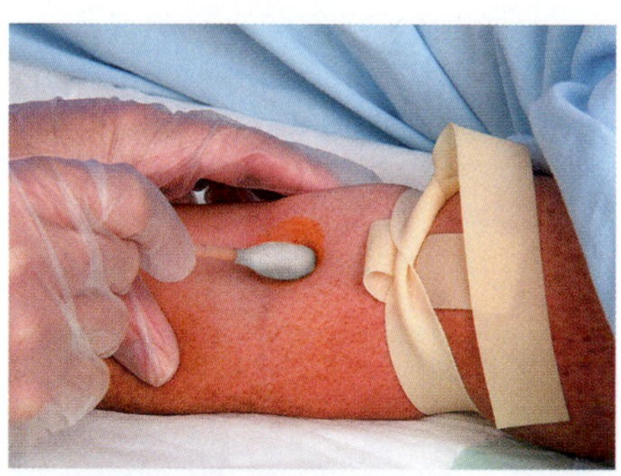

12. **Allow the antiseptic to air-dry.** Do not fan.
The antiseptic promotes adherence of the dressing. Fanning can cause contamination of the skin.

13. **Pick up the catheter and inspect the tip.**
There should be no burrs (rough spots, ridges) on the needle or peeling of the catheter material.

14. **Inform the patient** that you are about to insert the catheter and that it may be uncomfortable.
Keeping the patient informed promotes cooperation and lessens anxiety.

Procedure Variation If Using a Wing-Tipped Catheter (Butterfly)

15. **Grasp the catheter by the wings, using the thumb and forefinger of your dominant hand, making sure that the bevel is up. Remove the protective cap from the needle.**
Stabilizes the catheter for insertion. Inserting the needle bevel up makes it less likely that you will pierce both vein walls (go "through" the vein) as well as making piercing the skin less painful for the patient. ▼

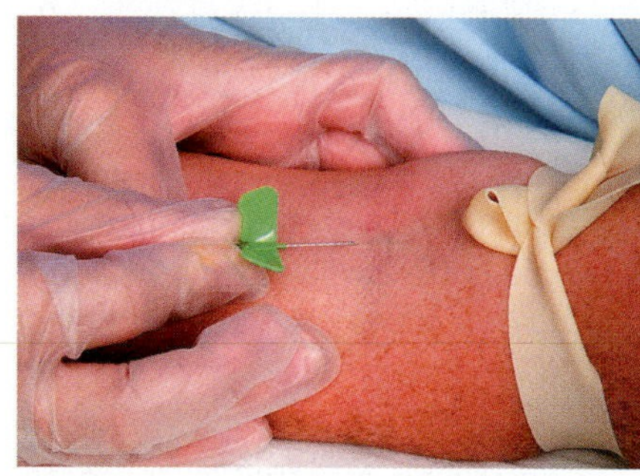

Procedure Variation If Using an Over-the-Needle Catheter

16. **Grasp the catheter by the hub,** using the thumb and forefinger of your dominant hand, making sure that the bevel is up.
See Wing-Tipped Catheter rationale, preceding. ▼

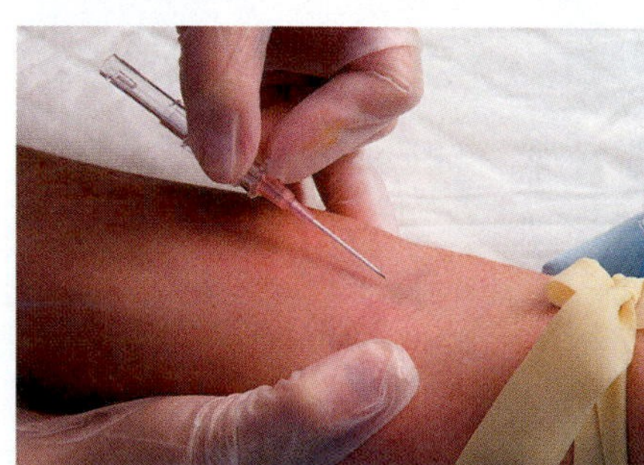

17. **Using your nondominant hand,** stabilize the vein by continuously pulling the skin taut below the puncture area (pull downward toward the hand or fingers). Do not press too hard, and make sure not to contaminate the insertion site.
Stabilizing the vein eases insertion and prevents damage to the underside of the vein as well as preventing the vein from rolling. Pressing too hard compresses blood flow in the vein and causes it to collapse.

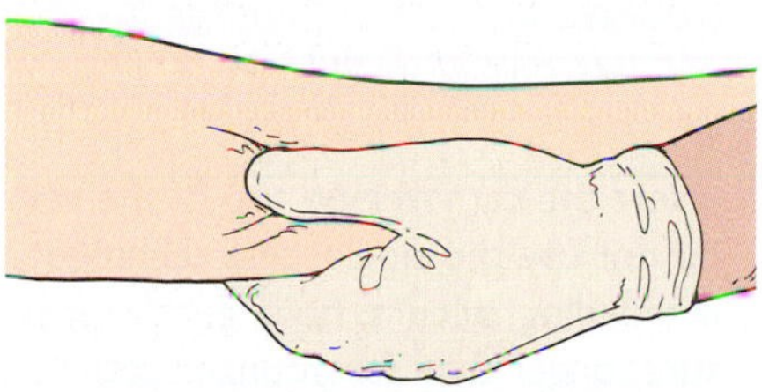

18. **Holding the catheter at** a 30° to 45° angle, pierce the skin directly over the vein. Penetrate all layers of the vein with one quick, smooth motion.
A 30° to 45° angle allows you to pierce the skin without inadvertently passing through the vein and allows backflow of blood into the catheter.

19. **Look for a flashback of blood** into the chamber of the catheter or the tubing of the winged catheter.
The flashback of blood indicates that the vein has been entered, but only by the needle when using an over-the-needle catheter.

20. **Lower the angle of the catheter** and needle to skin level and advance them into the vein.

For a Wing-Tipped Catheter

Fully advance the catheter.

For an Over-the-Needle Catheter

Still maintaining traction on the skin with your nondominant hand, hold the catheter hub with your thumb and middle finger, and use your index finger to advance the catheter to at least half of its length before you begin withdrawing the needle. When a steady backflow of blood occurs, partially withdraw the needle while advancing the catheter fully into the vein.

Withdrawing the needle too early will result in the catheter not fully entering the vein, only the needle. There will be no bleeding from the catheter and infiltration will occur when starting the IV solution. The patient will also experience pain.

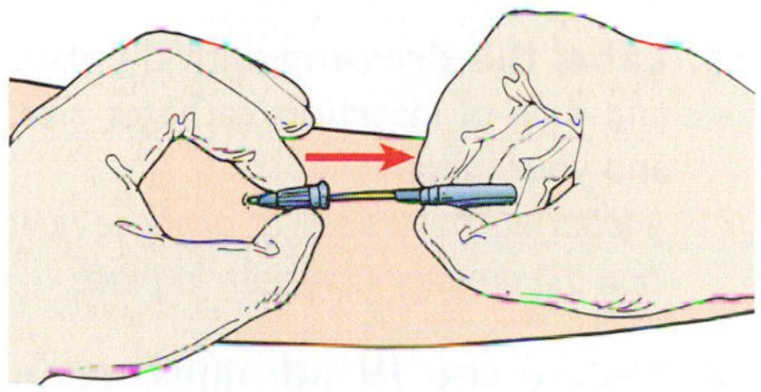

21. **While holding the catheter** in place with one hand, release the tourniquet and remove or retract the needle.

For an Over-the-Needle Catheter

Hold the catheter in place by placing light pressure on the catheter, away from the hub and venipuncture site.

> Never attempt to reinsert the needle after it is withdrawn. This can damage the catheter and even cause bits of it to break off within the vein.

For a Winged Needle

Place a finger lightly on the same area plus a finger farther along the vein away from the needle so the needle does not go through the vein.

Releasing the tourniquet restores full circulation to the patient's extremity and prevents injury. Placing light pressure on the catheter or vein minimizes bleeding from the catheter or needle while you complete the procedure.

22. **Quickly connect** the administration set to the IV catheter, using aseptic technique.
To minimize bleeding and prevent infection.

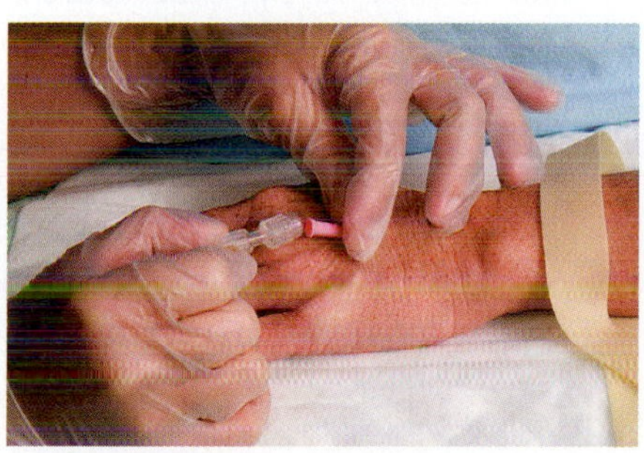

If Using a Peripheral IV Lock

Once the lock is connected, flush with normal saline and then disconnect the flush. A common amount is 1 to 2 mL, but tubing varies, so check package instructions for the exact amount needed.
Flushing the catheter both clears it and keeps it sterile.

23. **While still stabilizing the catheter** in place, slowly open the roller clamp. Observe that flow is achieved. Adjust the drip to the prescribed flow rate.

24. **Secure the connection** between the tubing and the catheter. Many sets have luer-lock connections, so no further securing is needed. If not using luer-lock tubing, clasping devices and threaded devices can be used. Do not use tape.
Secure the connection to prevent separation of tubing from the hub.

> Taping is not recommended because the junction is not visible under tape; therefore, the tubing could separate from the catheter without being discovered, possibly leading to air embolism, bleeding, or infection.

25. **Stabilize the catheter** to directly hold it in place on the skin. Use an agency-approved device. Catheter stabilization devices include manufactured devices (such as StatLok), or tape.

When Stabilizing With Tape

Place a narrow (¼-in.) strip of tape under the catheter hub and crisscross the ends over the hub to form a chevron. Apply tape only to the catheter hub, not to the catheter itself, and do not apply tape directly to the site where the catheter enters the skin.
Luer-locks are designed to prevent accidental disengagement of tubing and catheter; they do not stabilize the catheter. Catheter stabilization (or primary securement) is important to minimize catheter movement and help prevent complications such as phlebitis, inflammation, infiltration, and infection.

(continued on next page)

Procedure 38-1 ■ Initiating a Peripheral Intravenous Infusion (continued)

26. Dress the site, following agency policy. If needed, clean the site with an antiseptic swab and allow it to dry before applying the dressing.

If Using a Transparent Dressing (Preferred)

a. Open the package containing the dressing. Remove the protective backing from the dressing, making sure not to touch the sterile surface.

b. Cover the insertion site and the hub or winged portion of the catheter with the dressing. Do not cover the junction with the administration tubing.

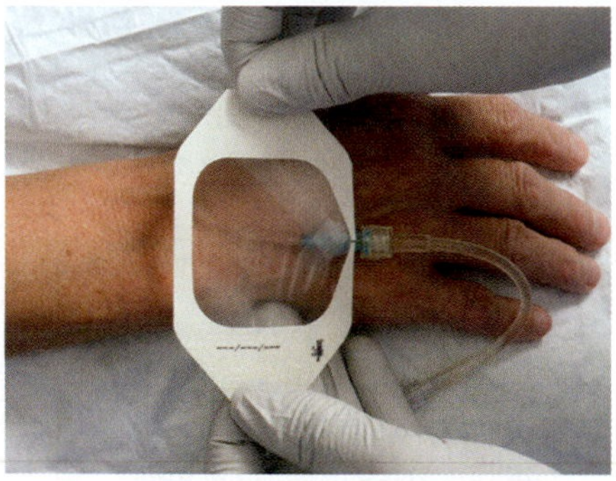

c. Gently pinch the transparent dressing around the catheter hub to secure the hub further (primary securement). Smooth the remainder of the dressing so that it adheres to the skin.

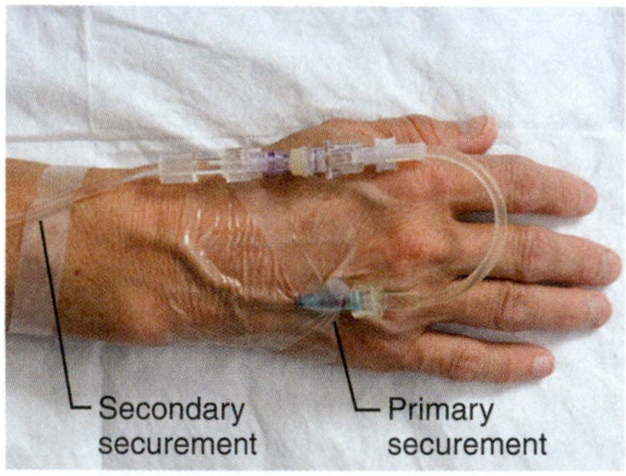

The INS (2016) recommends that butterfly catheter is used for venipunctures or an intermittent infusion. It should not be used for regular infusions.

If You Must Use a Gauze Dressing

d. Fold a 2 in. × 2 in. sterile gauze dressing in half, cover it with 1-in. tape (about 3 in. long).

e. Place under the tubing/hub junction and press down on the tape.
Raises hub off the skin and prevents pressure on the skin.

f. Place a sterile gauze pad over the insertion site and catheter hub—but not over the catheter–hub junction.

g. Secure all edges with tape.

27. Label the dressing with the date and time of insertion, catheter size, and your initials.
A label lets nurses see at a glance how long the dressing has been in place.

28. Secure the IV administration tubing by looping and taping the tubing to the skin (secondary securement). See Step 26c, preceding.
Helps prevent the IV catheter from becoming dislodged and decreases movement of the catheter, thereby decreasing the risk of phlebitis, inflammation and infiltration.

29. Place an arm board under the joint and secure it with tape if the insertion site is located near a joint.
An arm board stabilizes the joint and helps prevent the catheter from becoming dislodged. However, avoid inserting an IV near a joint when possible because there is increased potential for movement of the IV catheter, leading to an increased risk of complications. IVs placed in the antecubital fossa are difficult to assess for infiltration. Arm boards are not widely used because of the high acuity of inpatients, many of whom have central lines instead of peripheral IVs.

30. Dispose of all supplies, including sharps, into appropriate receptacles; raise the siderail; lower the bed; and be sure the patient call system is within reach. Wash your hands.
Prevents infection and ensure patient and staff safety.

? What if . . .

■ **The patient is an older adult?**

Do not scrub skin too vigorously.
This can damage fragile surface tissue, creating a portal for pathogens.

Use a softer tourniquet and do not apply tightly; for well-dilated veins, do not use one at all.
This decreases the risk of rupture of fragile veins.

Use the smallest catheter possible to meet the infusion needs.

Insert the needle at an almost flat angle (10° to 20°).
In most older adults, veins are close to the skin surface.

Before penetrating the skin, apply traction to the vein below the insertion site.
Stabilizes the vein and makes it easier and less painful for the needle to enter the skin.

Insert the catheter on top of the vein; do not use the side access technique.

If bleeding occurs, hold gentle pressure longer than for younger patients.
A clot may take longer to form.

■ **The patient is an infant younger than 2 months old?**

Allow the antiseptic to air-dry on the skin. Do not fan.
Increases the antiseptic's effectiveness; promotes patient comfort on puncture of the skin; promotes adherence of dressing. Fanning increases exposure to airborne microbes.

■ **The patient is allergic to iodine or shellfish?**

Use 70% alcohol or chlorhexidine for 30 seconds to cleanse the site (not povidone-iodine or iodine).

■ **You are not successful with the first venipuncture attempt?**

Use a new cannula and make a second attempt on the other arm; or if unsuccessful, higher up on the same arm. Do not make more than two attempts without seeking assistance.

■ **When you insert the needle and catheter and connect the tubing, you see bright red blood quickly appear and start to advance up the tubing?**

You may have inadvertently entered an artery. If this occurs, remove the catheter and apply direct pressure for at least 5 minutes. Notify the primary care provider. Monitor the extremity distal to the insertion site for pulses, color, and temperature.

Evaluation

- Monitor the IV site and flow rate regularly (many agency standards require hourly) while IV fluid is infusing. Check for signs of infiltration, inflammation, and phlebitis.
- Monitor the patient's tolerance of IV therapy by auscultating breath sounds and monitoring vital signs, urine output, laboratory values, and neck vein distention. Report to the primary provider any signs of fluid overload, such as crackles, edema, shortness of breath, diminished urine output, increased blood pressure, increased heart rate with bounding pulse, and distended neck veins. Fluid overload can lead to pulmonary edema and heart failure.

Patient Teaching

- Instruct the patient about IV therapy.
- Teach the patient the importance of notifying staff immediately if the catheter or administration set becomes dislodged; the insertion site becomes tender, red, or swollen; or the patient notices moisture or fluid leakage.
- Explain the desired and adverse effects of IV therapy, and tell the patient to notify staff if he develops discomfort or breathing difficulty.
- Teach the patient measures to avoid dislodging the catheter.

Home Care

- Explain home IV therapy to the client and caregiver, and teach them how to identify complications.
- Provide the client with the name and phone numbers of people to contact in case problems arise with the catheter site or if there is a change in level of comfort (e.g., increased pain, swelling).

Documentation

- Date and time of insertion, gauge and type of catheter, number of attempts, and location of the insertion site
- Tourniquet use (or nonuse)
- Blood return in catheter; whether the IV flushes, type and amount of flush solution used
- Dressing and tape type used
- Method of securing or stabilizing the IV line
- Type and rate of the IV fluid infusing
- Patient's tolerance of the procedure, any adverse reactions to the insertion or IV therapy, and the interventions required
- Patient teaching
- Often, IV care is documented on a flowsheet. Fluids infused are documented on the intake and output (I&O) record as well.

Sample documentation

06/07/22 0200. 20-gauge, winged catheter inserted in cephalic vein, with tourniquet, without difficulty on first attempt. Obtained blood return. Catheter flushed easily. Dressed site with a transparent, semipermeable dressing and clear tape. Catheter stabilized with fixation device. 1 L of D_5/NS hung at 125 mL/hr. Patient tolerated venipuncture with no difficulty. Instructed to notify nursing staff immediately if pain or swelling occurs at the site. Also taught precautions to take to avoid dislodging IV catheter and importance of notifying staff immediately should it become dislodged. ——— S. Jiminez, RN

Practice Resources

Czajka, C., Frey, A., & Scbears, G. (2018); Grange, K. (2015); Infusion Nurses Society (INS) (2016); Shlamovitz, G. (updated 2017a).

Thinking About the Procedure

The video **Initiating a Peripheral Intravenous Infusion,** along with questions and suggested responses, is available on the ***Davis's Nursing Skills Videos*** Web site on FADavis.com.

Procedure 38-2 ■ Regulating the IV Flow Rate

➤ For steps to follow in *all* procedures, refer to the Universal Steps for All Procedures found on the inside back cover.

Equipment

- IV solution hanging on an IV pole and attached to an administration set
- Watch with a second hand or digital seconds
- Time tape

Delegation

Refer to your state nurse practice act and agency policy regarding delegation of this task to an LPN.

Pre-Procedure Assessments

- Assess the IV catheter for patency and date of insertion before starting the infusion and then regularly (many agencies specify hourly) while the IV fluid infuses.
  Decreases risk of complications related to incorrect infusion rate, expired infusion solution, tubing, or catheter dwell time.
- Assess the IV site for signs of phlebitis, infiltration, infection, or inflammation.
  You must change the IV catheter before regulating the flow rate if any of these complications occur.

(continued on next page)

Procedure 38-2 ■ Regulating the IV Flow Rate (continued)

- Confirm the patient's need for IV therapy by verifying the prescription and checking laboratory values, urine output, vital signs, and breath sounds.
  Ensures that the patient still needs IV fluids and that the solution is correct. Laboratory values and assessment findings verify the need for the IV treatment plan. IV therapy creates a risk for fluid overload.

➤ When performing the procedure, always identify your patient according to agency policy, using two identifiers, and be attentive to standard precautions, hand hygiene, patient safety and privacy, body mechanics, and documentation.

Procedure Steps

1. **Follow all the "checks" and "rights"** of medication administration, including verifying the prescription. Check the solution to make sure that you have the proper IV fluid hanging with the prescribed additives, and that there is no discoloration of or particles or crystallization in the fluid. Also verify the infusion rate.
   IV solution is considered medication, and you should check it carefully to avoid administration and compatibility errors. Do not simply pull a bag of fluid from a shelf assuming that the shelf is labeled properly. Bags are often misplaced, and this is a potential source of error.

2. **Calculate the hourly rate** if it is not specified in the prescription. Divide the volume to be infused by the number of hours it is to be infused. For example, if the physician prescribes 1,000 mL to run over the course of 4 hours, the infusion rate is 250 mL/hr.
   You must carefully calculate the infusion rate to ensure that the patient receives the correct volume of fluid.

   NOTE: If you are using a volume-control pump, you can omit Steps 3 and 4.

3. **Calculate the drip rate** by multiplying the number of milliliters to be infused in 60 minutes by the drop factor in drops [gtts]/per milliliter; then divide by 60 minutes:

$$\frac{\text{Hourly rate in mL} \times (\text{gtts/mL})}{60 \text{ minutes}} = \text{drip rate}$$

   For example, an hourly rate of 100 mL multiplied by 15 gtts/mL and divided by 60 minutes equals 25. Therefore, the drip rate equals 25 gtts/minute. Each administration set has a drip factor that is determined by the manufacturer. The drip factor is the number of drops necessary to deliver 1 mL of solution. Microdrip tubing has a drip factor of 60 gtts/mL; blood administration tubing typically has a drip factor of 10 gtts/mL; macrodrip tubing has a drip factor of 15 gtts/mL.

4. **Verify your calculations.**
   To prevent dosage errors, either have a second person verify your calculations or check them a second time yourself.

5. **Apply a time tape** when hanging a new bag to the IV solution container next to the volume markings. Mark the time tape with the time that the infusion was started. Continue to mark 1-hour intervals on the time tape until you reach the bottom of the container.
   The time tape allows all nurses to accurately monitor the rate of administration.

6. **Open the roller clamp** so that IV fluid begins to flow (when hanging a new bag).
   The roller clamp must be opened to allow the flow of fluid.

7. **Set the rate.**

For Gravity Drip

Using a watch placed next to the drip chamber, count the number of drops entering the drip chamber in 1 minute. Adjust the roller clamp by increasing or decreasing the flow until you achieve the prescribed drip rate.
Timing the drip rate for 1 minute helps to accurately achieve the correct drip rate and having the watch next to what you are counting will ensure that you do not miss seeing any drops. ▼

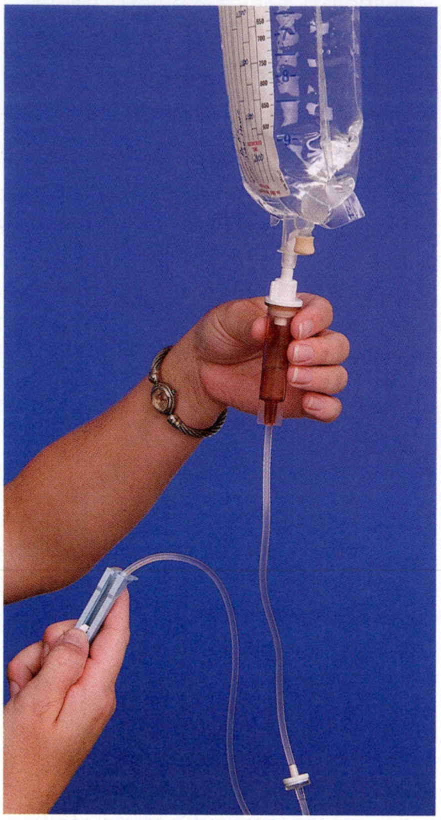

For a Volume-Control Pump

Program the prescribed rate into the pump.
IV solution is considered a medication and must infuse at the prescribed rate.

8. **Monitor manually regulated** infusion rates closely for the first 15 minutes after you begin an infusion; then monitor at least hourly by counting drops per minute or reading the numbers on the pumps.
   Changes in the patient's position may speed up or slow down the infusion rate; frequent monitoring of the infusion rate ensures that the correct volume of fluid infuses over the correct length of time.

? What if . . .

- **The prescription for the IV flow rate changes?**
  Recalculate the new flow rate and adjust the drops/minute to obtain the desired new flow rate. Also, remove the old time tape and place a new time tape with the new rate of infusion.
- **When you check the rate, you discover that the IV has been running too slowly for the past hour?**
  Adjust to the correct rate, but do not attempt to catch up by adjusting the flow to a rate higher than prescribed. *Too rapid IV infusion can lead to fluid overload for patients with congestive heart failure or other cardiopulmonary problems.*
- **When you check the rate, you discover that the IV has been running too fast for the past hour?**
  Slow the rate and assess the patient for signs of fluid volume excess.

Evaluation

- Evaluate the patient's response to IV therapy by checking for signs of excessive or deficient fluid volume.
- Evaluate the IV site for signs of infiltration, inflammation, infection, and phlebitis.
- Check laboratory studies to help evaluate the effectiveness of IV therapy.
- Monitor for correct IV rate at least hourly.
- Evaluate the tubing for kinks, or patient lying on the tubing. *Kinked tubing will interfere with the flow rate.*

Patient Teaching

- Explain the desired and adverse effects of IV therapy.
- Discuss the importance of notifying staff immediately if the catheter or administration set becomes dislodged; if the insertion site becomes tender, red, or swollen; if the patient notices moisture or fluid leakage; or if he has difficulty breathing.
- Teach safety measures if the patient is permitted to ambulate while the IV is infusing.

Home Care

- Explain home IV therapy to the client and caregiver, and teach them how to identify complications.
- Provide the client and caregiver with the name and phone numbers of people to contact in case problems arise with the catheter, insertion site, or level of comfort.

Documentation

Often IV care is documented on a flowsheet, and includes the following.

- Date and time the infusion was started
- Type of IV fluid, rate of infusion, and IV catheter site
- Whether rate is manual or pump controlled
- Patient's tolerance of IV therapy, any complications, and the interventions taken
- Document the volume infused on the intake and output (I&O) record.

Practice Resources

INS (2016); Shlamovitz, G. (updated 2017).

Procedure 38-3 ■ Setting Up and Using Volume-Control Pumps

➤ For steps to follow in *all* procedures, refer to the Universal Steps for All Procedures found on the inside back cover.

Equipment

- Nonsterile gloves
- Alcohol wipes or chlorhexidine/alcohol antiseptic product
- Volume-control pump and IV pole
- Administration set appropriate for the pump
- IV fluid or medicated solution
- Tape for IV fluid solution time tape

Delegation

You can delegate the task of setting up a volume-control pump to an LPN who is specially trained in IV therapy, if covered by the agency's policy. Do not delegate this task to unlicensed assistive personnel (UAP). Do, however, instruct the UAP to notify you of any pump alarms that sound.

Pre-Procedure Assessments

- Confirm the patient's need for IV therapy by checking vital signs, laboratory values, urine output, skin turgor, breath sounds, and the moisture of mucous membranes.
  IV therapy creates a risk for fluid overload and electrolyte imbalance, which may be revealed by assessment data.
- Assess the existing IV catheter for patency.
  Occlusion of the IV catheter prevents the infusion of IV fluid. If not patent, you will need to change the IV.
- Assess the IV site hourly for signs of phlebitis, infiltration, infection, and inflammation.
  Complications of IV therapy interfere with the therapeutic benefit of the fluids, as well as increase medical concerns and treatment cost for the patient. You must change the IV catheter and site if any of these complications occur.

(continued on next page)

Procedure 38-3 ■ Setting Up and Using Volume-Control Pumps (continued)

➤ When performing the procedure, always identify your patient according to agency policy, using two identifiers, and be attentive to standard precautions, hand hygiene, patient safety and privacy, body mechanics, and documentation.

Procedure Steps

1. **Calculate the infusion rate** by dividing the volume to be infused by the number of hours it is to be infused. For example, if the prescription states 1,000 mL to run over 8 hours, divide 1,000 mL by 8 hours to determine the infusion rate of 125 mL/hr.
This ensures that the patient receives the correct dose. Pumps are usually programmed in milliliters per hour instead of drops per minute.

2. **Verify your calculations.**
To prevent dosage errors, either ask a second person to verify your calculations or check them a second time yourself.

3. **Attach the pump to the IV pole,** and plug it into the nearest electrical outlet.

Check to be sure that the infusion pump has a safety sticker on it and that the cord and plug are intact.

Volume-control pumps need regular maintenance checks. Using an electrical outlet saves battery power if needed for transport or electrical outage. As with gravity flow, the IV solution container needs to remain above the pump to prevent occlusion and for proper drainage of the container.

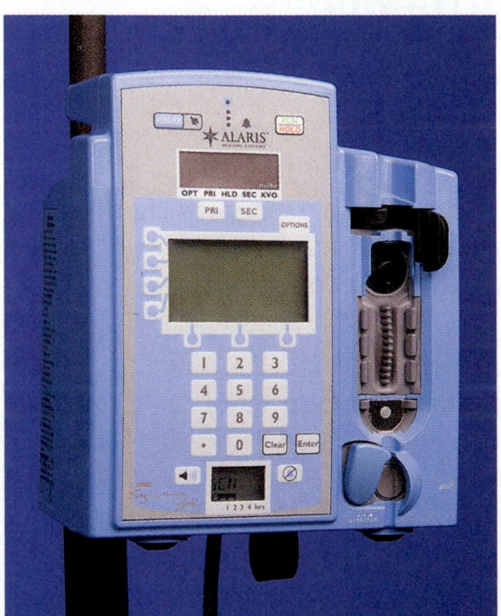

4. **Take the administration set** from the package, and close the clamp on it.
To prevent inadvertent loss of fluid.

5. **Attach a filter to the end** of the administration set, if required.
Filters are sometimes used to filter minute particles from the solution.

6. **Remove the protective covers,** and spike the port of the solution container with the administration set, maintaining sterility. Label the IV tubing and solution container with the date and time, and place a time tape on the solution container. Hang the container on the IV pole.
Labeling the administration set with the date and time informs the nursing staff when the administration set should be changed. The time tape allows you, and other nurses, to see at a glance whether the correct volume is infusing.

7. **Compress the drip chamber** of the administration set, and allow it to fill halfway. Consult the manufacturer's instructions for setup as pumps differ. (On older gravity pumps, place the electronic eye on the drip chamber between the fluid level and the origin of the drop.)
Prepares the administration set for priming and prevents air from entering the tubing with the solution. Infusion pumps compress the tubing to move fluid; they measure the amount internally. On older gravity-type pumps, an electronic eye counts the number of drops to ensure the proper rate.

8. **Prime the administration set** with fluid by opening the roller clamp and allowing the fluid to flow slowly through the tubing. Close the clamp.
Priming removes air from the tubing to prevent air embolus.

9. **Inspect the tubing** for air. If air bubbles remain in the tubing, flick the tubing with a fingertip to mobilize the bubbles into the drip chamber.
Air bubbles in the administration tubing interrupt flow and they can cause air emboli, which can be dangerous to the patient if they accumulate in the circulation.

10. **Turn on the pump, and load** the administration tubing into the pump according to the manufacturer's instructions.
NOTE: This process differs among manufacturers; thus, consult their instructions.

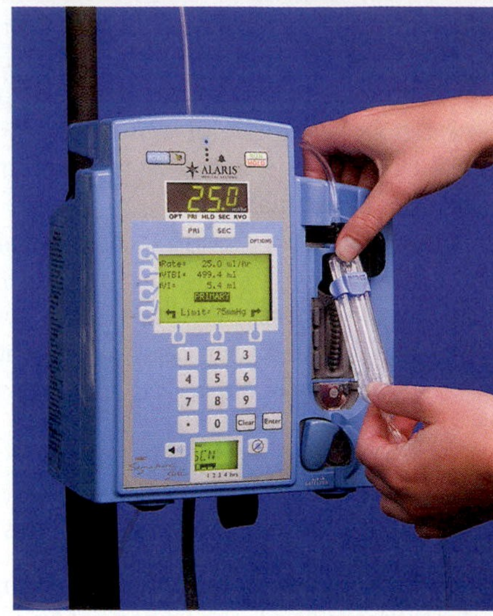

11. **Program the pump** with the prescribed information: total hours, infusion rate (hourly rate), and the volume to be infused (usually the total amount in the IV bag). *NOTE: Some pumps have only total hours and volume to infuse and do not have a feature that allows you to program in the infusion rate.*

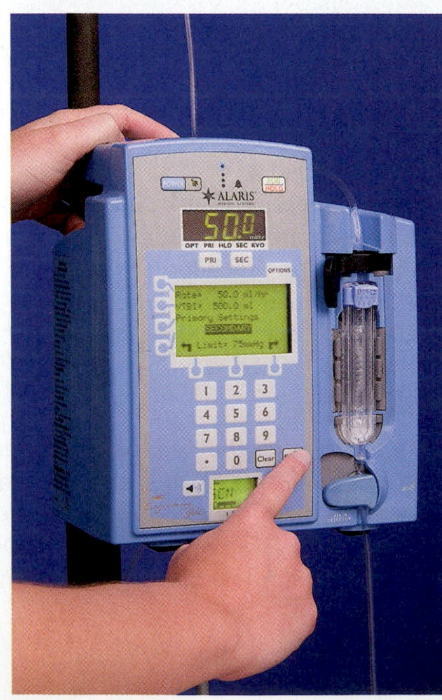

12. **Don clean nonsterile gloves,** check the IV site for patency, and scrub all surfaces of the primary line injection port or needleless connector, including the threads, with an antiseptic pad for at least 15 seconds. Allow it to dry.
Clean nonsterile gloves protect from exposure to body fluids when you connect the tubing to the IV catheter or port. Scrubbing the port helps prevent infection.

13. **Connect the administration set** adapter to the injection port, keeping the connecting ends sterile.
Aseptic technique decreases the risk for contamination.

14. **Unclamp the administration set** tubing (open the roller clamp all the way), and press the start button on the pump.
Allows the IV fluid to flow through the administration set.

15. **Make sure the alarms** are turned on and audible.
The alarms must be functioning so that the pump can alert you of problems, such as kinks, air in the tubing, or catheter occlusion.
Key Point: ***Do not depend completely on the pump alarms to indicate IV patency. Pumps can infuse fluid, even if the line is clogged or infiltrated into the surrounding tissue.***

16. **Check the pump regularly** to make sure the correct volume is infusing. Checks are commonly done hourly.
Infusion pumps sometimes malfunction, so frequent monitoring is essential.

17. **At the end of your shift** (or at the time specified by your healthcare facility), clear the pump of the volume infused and record the volume on the patient's I&O form.
This helps the oncoming shift accurately monitor the fluid infused during their shift.

? What if . . .

- **You later find the IV free flowing and not running via the pump setting?**

Immediately slow the IV fluid down. At the same time, begin assessing the patient: vital signs, mental awareness, lung sounds, pulse oximetry. Depending on the type of fluid running, you may need to make other assessments. Calculate the amount of IV fluid actually infused compared with the prescribed amount. Notify the provider and write out an occurrence report. If the pump is malfunctioning, set it aside, label it as "not working," and notify biomedical engineering so they can repair it.
Labeling the pump will prevent others from using it, until it can be repaired.

Evaluation

- Monitor the correct functioning of the pump regularly, perhaps hourly.
- Assess the IV site hourly for signs of phlebitis, infiltration, infection, and inflammation.
Complications of IV therapy interfere with the therapeutic benefit of the fluids and increase medical concerns, and treatment costs for the patient. You must change the IV catheter and document if any of these complications occur.

Patient Teaching

- Explain use of the IV infusion pump to the patient.
- Teach the patient the importance of notifying staff immediately if the infusion pump alarm sounds; the catheter or administration set becomes dislodged; the insertion site becomes tender, red, or swollen; or the dressing becomes wet.
- Teach the patient safety measures if he is able to ambulate while the infusion pump is in use.

Home Care

- Explain home IV infusion pump use to the client and caregiver, and teach them how to identify complications. Most home infusion pumps are smaller than institutional pumps.
- Provide the client with the name and phone numbers of people to contact in case problems arise with the catheter, insertion site, IV infusion pump, or other equipment.

Documentation

- Type and volume of IV fluid infusing, along with the infusion rate
- Use of the infusion pump, and patient's tolerance of IV therapy
- Any complications of IV therapy and the interventions taken
- Document volume infused on the patient's I&O record and/or an IV flowsheet.

Sample documentation

01/26/21 0600 Patient admitted from the ED with dehydration. NSS infusing at 250 mL/hr via infusion pump through an 18-gauge catheter. No signs of infiltration. No tenderness, redness, or swelling at the insertion site. Temp 102.6°F orally. HR 118 beats/min, RR 24 breaths/min, and BP 90/46 ——— R. Brill, RN

Practice Resources

Cummings, K., & McGowan, R. (2011); Franklin, B. (2017); Phillips, L. & Gorski, L. (2018).

Thinking About the Procedure

The video **Setting Up and Using Volume-Control Pumps,** along with questions and suggested responses, is available on the ***Davis's Nursing Skills Videos*** Web site on FADavis.com.

Procedure 38-4 ■ Changing IV Solutions and Tubing

➤ For steps to follow in *all* procedures, refer to the Universal Steps for All Procedures found on the inside back cover.

Equipment

- Nonsterile gloves
- Administration set
- IV solution
- IV pole
- Antiseptic swabs that contain solutions such as 70% alcohol or 2% chlorhexidine (chlorhexidine is not recommended in infants younger than age 2 months). You may use iodine-based products if alcohol or chlorhexidine are contraindicated and the patient is not allergic to iodine.
- 1-in. nonallergenic tape
- Time tape
- Watch with a second hand or digital seconds

Delegation

You can delegate the tasks of changing IV solutions and tubing to an LPN who is specially trained in IV therapy. The task should not be delegated to a UAP. However, do instruct the UAP to notify you of any problems that occur with IV therapy, such as the disconnecting of the administration set; catheter dislodging; or complaints of pain, swelling, or redness at the insertion site.

Pre-Procedure Assessments

- Assess the IV catheter for patency before changing the solution container or administration set.
- Assess the IV site for signs of phlebitis, infiltration, infection, or inflammation.
  If any of these complications occur, discontinue the IV and start a new IV at a different site.
- Check IV catheter insertion date.
  IV catheters are replaced per agency guidelines, which are based on the CDC recommendations of changing a peripheral IV site when clinically indicated (e.g., signs of phlebitis, infiltration, irritation).

Procedure 38-4A ■ Changing the IV Solution

➤ When performing the procedure, always identify your patient according to agency policy, using two identifiers, and be attentive to standard precautions, hand hygiene, patient safety and privacy, body mechanics, and documentation.

Procedure Steps

1. **Following the rights** of medication administration, prepare and label your next container of IV solution at least 1 hour before the present infusion is scheduled to finish.
   Preparing the next IV solution container reduces the risk of the present container running dry, thereby causing clots to form that would occlude the catheter.
2. **Close the roller clamp** on the infusing administration set.
   Prevents air from entering the tubing while changing the IV solution container.
3. **Wearing clean nonsterile gloves,** remove the old IV solution container from the IV pole. Remove the spike from the bag, keeping the spike sterile.
   The spike must remain sterile to prevent contamination of the new IV fluid. Clean nonsterile gloves protect you from exposure to body fluids.
4. **Remove the protective cover** from the new IV solution container port.
5. **Place the spike into the port** of the new solution container.

For a Glass Bottle

First scrub the rubber stopper on the top of the bottle with an antiseptic pad; then, insert the spike of the administration set through the rubber stopper.
Cleansing the stopper removes particulate matter and microbes.

6. **Hang the IV solution** container on the IV pole.
   Allows the fluid to infuse by gravity.
7. **Inspect the tubing** to be sure that it is free of air bubbles and the drip chamber remains half-filled. Flick the tubing with a finger to mobilize the bubbles into the drip chamber.
   Prevents air from entering the system as the new solution is hung. If the drip chamber becomes too full, it will be difficult to impossible to count the drip rate properly and regulate the IV.
8. **Open the roller clamp** and adjust the drip rate, as prescribed.
   IV solution is considered a medication and must infuse at the prescribed rate for therapeutic effect and to prevent fluid overload.
9. **Affix the time tape** to the new IV solution container, if practiced within your agency. Mark the tape with the time the infusion was started, and mark 1-hour intervals on the tape until you reach the bottom of the container.
   The time tape allows you and other nurses to monitor the rate of administration easily.
10. **Dispose of used supplies** into appropriate receptacles, according to agency policy in line with CDC guidelines.

Procedure 38-4B ■ Changing the IV Administration Tubing and Solution

➤ When performing the procedure, always identify your patient according to agency policy, using two identifiers, and be attentive to standard precautions, hand hygiene, patient safety and privacy, body mechanics, and documentation.

Procedure Steps

1. **Prepare the IV solution** and tubing as you would when initiating a new IV. (See Procedure 38-1, Step 2.)
2. **Hang the new administration** set on the IV pole.
3. **Close the roller clamp** on the old administration set.
   Stops the flow of fluid from the old container.
4. **Disconnect the old tubing**
   a. Wearing clean nonsterile gloves, place a sterile swab under the catheter hub.
   The swab absorbs any leakage from the catheter hub when you disconnect the tubing.
   b. Apply pressure to the vein about 3 inches above the insertion site, using the fourth or fifth finger of your nondominant hand. Hold the catheter hub firmly with the thumb and index finger of that hand, but do not apply downward pressure.
   Prevents blood from leaking out of the catheter during the tubing change. Holding the hub firmly keeps the catheter from moving about and traumatizing the vein.
   c. Then carefully remove the device securing the connection between the catheter and tubing. This may be as simple as unscrewing a luer-lock. The connection should not be covered by tape, but if it is, remove it so you can access the connection.
5. **Remove the protective cover** from the distal end of the new administration set.
   Cover keeps the distal end sterile until you are ready to connect it to the IV catheter.
6. **Continue to stabilize the IV** catheter with your nondominant hand while applying pressure over the vein.▼

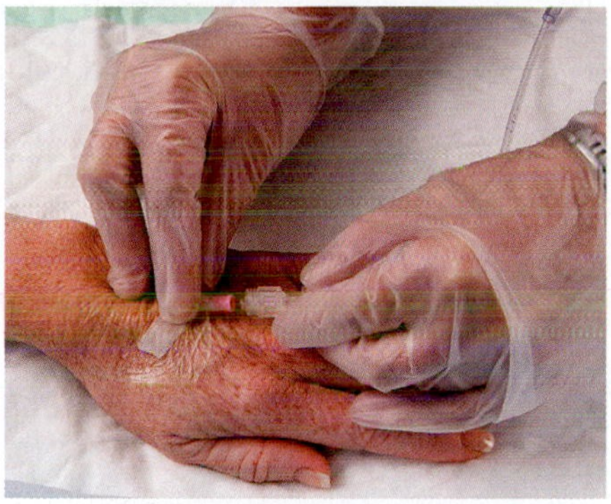

7. **Gently disengage the used** tubing from the IV catheter, and place it in a basin or other receptacle. Quickly insert the new tubing into the catheter hub.
   The CDC recommends IV tubing should be changed no less frequently than at 96-hour intervals, but at least every 7 days, depending on agency policy and solution. Certain solutions (e.g., blood, blood products, fat emulsions) require more tubing changes within 24 hours of initiating the infusion (CDC, updated 2017). Change it quickly to prevent microorganisms from entering the IV catheter.
8. **Open the roller clamp** on the new administration set, and allow the IV solution to infuse.
   Clears the IV catheter of blood, preventing catheter occlusion.
9. **Program and turn on** the volume-control pump. Or, for a gravity drip, use the roller clamp to adjust the flow to the prescribed rate.
   IV solution is considered a medication and must infuse at the prescribed rate.
10. **Cleanse the IV site** and secure the IV catheter and tubing connection.
   Removes microorganisms and media for growth; helps preserve the integrity of the intact line; and prevents air and microorganisms from entering the line.
11. **Loop and tape tubing** to patient's skin.
   Helps minimize catheter movement, which contributes to phlebitis.
12. **Label tubing and solution** with date, initials, rate, and time tape.
   Alerts staff to when tubing and solution was changed and to when they will need to be changed again to decrease the incidence of infection.
13. **Dispose of used supplies** into appropriate receptacles according to agency policy in line with CDC guidelines.

? What if . . .

- **The drip chamber becomes too full (over half) so that drops cannot be adequately counted?**
  Close the roller clamp, invert the bag or bottle, and squeeze the excess fluid back into the bag/bottle.
- **The tubing will not separate from the catheter connection when you attempt to disconnect it?**
  If the lock does not twist off, gently try using a hemostat ("mosquito" clamp) to twist the lock. Do not lock the hemostat; merely use it lightly as a grip. After the lock is off, if the tubing will not separate, use the hemostat to gently twist the tubing back and forth. If the catheter needs to be stabilized, wear a sterile glove or use a sterile hemostat.

(continued on next page)

Procedure 38-4 ■ Changing IV Solutions and Tubing (continued)

Evaluation

- Assess the IV insertion site for signs of infiltration, inflammation, infection, and phlebitis.
- Evaluate the effectiveness of IV therapy by assessing the patient's hydration status or expected effect of the intravenous medication/solution.
- Monitor the IV rate regularly (usually hourly).

Patient Teaching

- Discuss the importance of notifying staff immediately if the catheter or administration set becomes dislodged; if the insertion site becomes tender, red, or swollen; or if the IV dressing becomes wet.

Home Care

- Explain home IV therapy to the client and caregiver and teach them how to identify complications.
- Obtain a return demonstration to ensure the caregiver is able to perform fluid and tubing changes, when necessary.

Documentation

- Fluid and tubing changes are usually documented on a flowsheet.
- Document the date and time the IV fluid and tubing were changed; type of IV fluid and rate of infusion; and the location and condition of the IV catheter insertion site.
- Any complications of IV therapy and the interventions taken.

Sample documentation

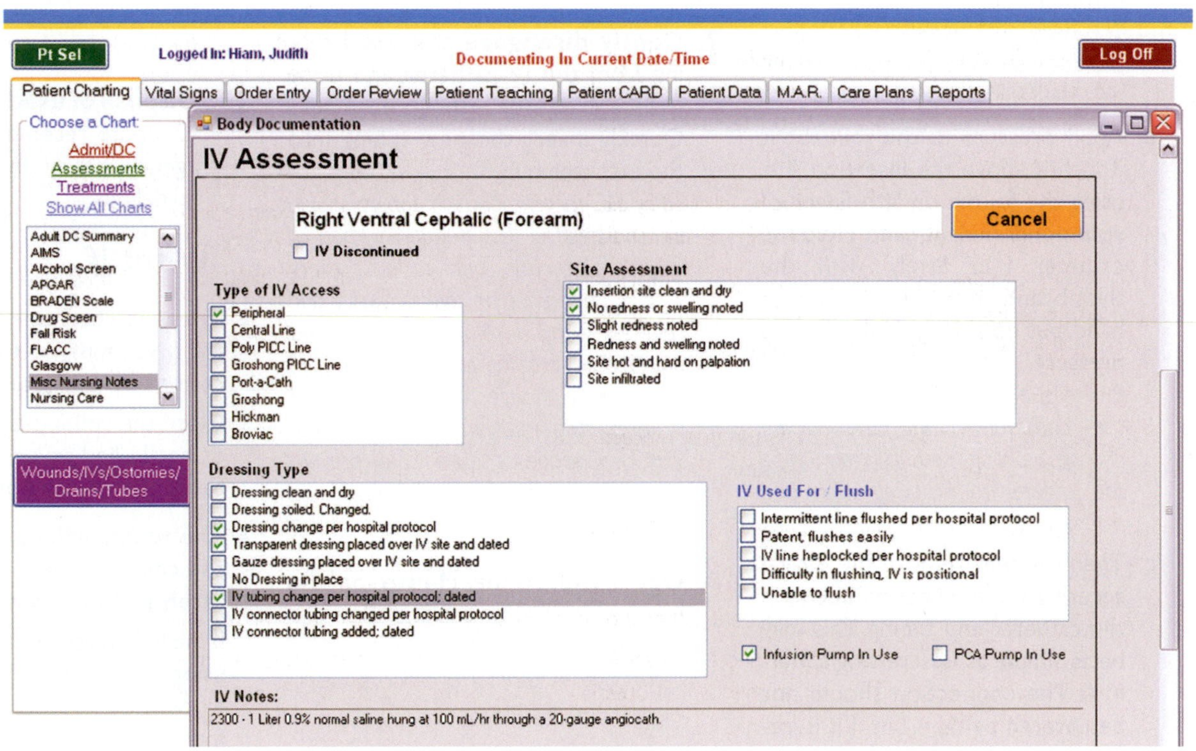

Practice Resources

CDC (2016); CDC (updated 2017); INS (2016); Philips, L. & Gorski, L. (2018).

Procedure 38-5 ■ Changing IV Dressings

➤ For steps to follow in *all* procedures, refer to the Universal Steps for All Procedures found on the inside back cover. For this procedure, also refer to Clinical Insights 23-1 through 23-4 and Procedures 23-7 and 23-8 if you need to review information about medical and surgical asepsis.

Equipment

Peripheral IV Dressings

- Clean nonsterile gloves
- Sterile transparent semipermeable dressing or dressing specified by institution
- Antiseptic swabs: alcohol or chlorhexidine

NOTE: Use iodine-based products only if the preferred antiseptics cannot be used. Chlorhexidine is not recommended in infants younger than age 2 months.

- 1-inch nonallergenic tape or manufactured stabilization device

Central Line Dressings

- Clean nonsterile gloves
- Central line dressing kit. It should include sterile gloves, a mask, a sterile transparent semipermeable dressing, sterile tape, an antimicrobial agent, and a sterile catheter stabilization device. If it does not, obtain them.

NOTE: It is acceptable to use povidone-iodine followed by alcohol as the antimicrobial if the preferred chlorhexidine is contraindicated.

- A sponge containing the antimicrobial agent chlorhexidine gluconate may be used as a part of the dressing, as well.
  To reduce the risk for catheter-related infection
- Mask for patient (possibly)

NOTE: Some institutions do not include this in their procedure and a few patients cannot tolerate wearing a mask.

Delegation

You can delegate the tasks of changing dressings to an LPN who is specially trained in IV therapy. The task should not be delegated to a UAP. Do, however, instruct the UAP to notify you of any problems that occur with dressing such as soiling, blood, leakage, or loosening.

Pre-Procedure Assessments

- Assess the IV catheter for patency before changing the dressing.
  Ensure that the IV is still working properly.
- Assess the IV site for signs of phlebitis, infiltration, infection, or inflammation.
  If any of these complications exist, the current IV will need to be discontinued and a new IV started.
- Assess for allergy to tape.
- Assess IV catheter start date.
  IV catheters are replaced per agency guidelines, which are based on the CDC recommendations of changing a peripheral IV site no more frequently than every 72 to 96 hours in adults. Changing more often than recommended actually increases the risk of infection.

Procedure 38-5A ■ Peripheral IV Dressings

➤ When performing the procedure, always identify your patient according to agency policy, using two identifiers, and be attentive to standard precautions, hand hygiene, patient safety and privacy, body mechanics, and documentation.

➤ *Note:* This procedure is usually performed at the same time the IV tubing is changed because the old dressing may need to be removed to do that. The CDC recommends that dressing be changed when damp, loosened, or visibly soiled. You should follow your agency's policy.

Procedure Steps

1. **Wearing clean nonsterile gloves,** stabilize the catheter with your nondominant hand, avoiding direct pressure on the catheter/hub junction, and carefully remove and discard the dressing and the catheter stabilization device.
   Remove the dressing gently to avoid dislodging the catheter.
2. **Inspect the insertion site.** Look for erythema and drainage, and note any tenderness. Remove procedure gloves and perform hand hygiene.
   If signs of infection, phlebitis, or infiltration are present, you must remove the IV catheter.
3. **Don a clean pair of nonsterile gloves.**
4. **Cleanse the insertion site,** and then allow the antiseptic to dry on the skin. Do not fan.

If Using Chlorhexidine

Apply using a back-and-forth motion and friction for at least 30 seconds. (Avoid using chlorhexidine in infants younger than age 2 months.)

If Using Alcohol or 2% Tincture of Iodine

Using a circular motion, start at the insertion site and work outward 2 to 3 inches. Do not go back over any cleansed area.
Removes microorganisms from the skin to minimize the risk of their entering the venipuncture site. Allowing the antiseptic to dry increases its effectiveness.

5. **Perform hand hygiene** and change procedure gloves. Apply a new sterile catheter stabilization device and dressing. For illustrations, see Procedure 38-1.

(continued on next page)

Procedure 38-5 ■ Changing IV Dressings (continued)

If Using a Transparent Dressing

a. Open the package containing the sterile, semipermeable, transparent dressing. Remove the protective backing from the dressing, making sure not to touch the sterile surface.

b. Cover the insertion site and the hub with the dressing. Do not cover the junction with the tubing of the administration set.

c. Gently pinch the transparent dressing around the catheter hub to secure the hub. Smooth the remainder of the dressing so that it adheres to the skin.
Pinching the dressing around the hub prevents pressure of the hub on the underlying skin.

If Using a Gauze Dressing

d. Fold a 2 in. × 2 in. sterile gauze dressing in half, cover it with 1-inch tape (about 3 inches long).

e. Place under the tubing/hub junction and press down on the tape.
Raises the hub to prevent pressure on the skin.

f. Place a sterile gauze pad over the insertion site and catheter hub—but not over the catheter/hub junction

g. Secure all edges with tape.

6. **Secure the connection between** the catheter and the tubing, but do not cover the catheter-tubing junction with tape.
Securing the connection helps maintain a closed system and prevents entry of microorganisms. You should not cover the junction with tape because removing the tape may interfere with your ability to disconnect the tubing from the hub quickly, should you need to do so. Removing tape requires much manipulation; the more the catheter is manipulated, the higher the risk for infection and dislodging.

7. **Secure the IV administration** tubing by looping and taping the tubing to the skin (referred to as *secondary securement*). See Procedure 38-1, Step 26C.
Looping the tubing provides slack to prevent the IV catheter from becoming dislodged.

8. **Label the dressing with the date** and time of insertion, catheter size, and the date the dressing was changed and your initials.
Peripheral IV catheters should be replaced as clinically indicated (e.g., phlebitis, infiltration, irritation) to prevent complications. Labeling the dressing with the date and time of insertion helps communicate to other nurses the date of the IV insertion and dressing change.

9. **Discard all supplies** in the appropriate containers according to agency policy in line with CDC guidelines.

? What if . . .

■ **The patient is immunocompromised? Or the peripheral midline catheter must be in the same site for an extended time?**

Use sterile gloves and a mask when changing the dressing and giving site care.

Thinking About the Procedure

The video **Peripheral IV Dressings,** along with questions and suggested responses, is available on the ***Davis's Nursing Skills Videos*** Web site on FADavis.com.

Procedure 38-5B ■ Central Line Dressings

➤ When performing the procedure, always identify your patient according to agency policy, using two identifiers, and be attentive to standard precautions, hand hygiene, patient safety and privacy, body mechanics, and documentation.

➤ *Note:* This procedure focuses on dressing change. Refer to Clinical Insight 38-4 for assessments and maintenance of CVCs.

Procedure Steps

1. **Obtain a sterile central line** dressing kit (or equivalent supplies if there is no kit) and mask for the patient, if one is needed.
Because central lines have direct access to the central circulation, the risk of systemic infection is greater. Therefore, the procedure uses aseptic technique. All supplies must be sterile.

2. **Place the patient** in a semi-Fowler's position, if tolerated. Lower the siderail and adjust the bed to working height.
Semi-Fowler's position and bed adjustments facilitate site cleansing and dressing application and reduce strain on the nurse's back.

3. **Explain the procedure** and ask the patient to turn his head to the opposite side from the insertion site. If he cannot cooperate, place a mask on the patient.
Explanation may reduce anxiety and enhance cooperation; turning helps prevent contamination of the insertion site.

4. **Put on your mask** and clean nonsterile gloves. Carefully remove the old dressing and catheter stabilization device, if present.

5. **Inspect the site** for signs and symptoms of infection and other complications.
If a complication is suspected, notify the person who placed the central line.

6. **Remove and discard your gloves,** along with the soiled dressing. Perform hand hygiene.

7. **Set up a sterile field** and open the dressing kit.
To prevent contamination of the insertion site and the sterile supplies.

8. **Don the sterile gloves** contained in the kit and arrange sterile supplies as needed.

9. **Scrub the insertion site** and surrounding skin with an antiseptic swab.

If Using Chlorhexidine

Use a back-and-forth motion with friction and scrub for at least 30 seconds.

If Using Povidone-Iodine and Alcohol

The kit should contain three swabs of each. Beginning with a povidone-iodine swab, start at the insertion site and work outward several inches ("dirty to clean"). Repeat with the other two povidone-iodine swabs. Then, using the same method, clean with the three alcohol swabs. With each swab, do not "go back over" an area you have just cleaned with that swab.
To rid the site of any potential infectious microorganisms, work "from clean to contaminated."

10. **Scrub the sutures (if any),** and the catheter from insertion site to the hub or bifurcation, for at least 15 seconds with an alcohol swab or chlorhexidine/alcohol antiseptic product.

11. **Allow the site to dry**—do not fan.
Allows the antiseptic time to work completely and allows the dressing to stick properly. Povidone-iodine requires 1 minute to air-dry completely; chlorhexidine requires 30 seconds.

12. **Apply the transparent dressing** that comes in the kit.

If You Place Gauze Under the Catheter Hub

You may first place a small piece of folded sterile gauze under the catheter hub.
To reduce pressure on the skin under the hub.

If Chlorhexidine Gluconate Sponge Is Part of the Dressing

Apply the sponge directly over the catheter insertion site, ensuring that the sponge is in full contact with the skin. Then apply the transparent dressing over the sponge.
Reduces the risk for catheter-related infection, especially in units with high infection rates or in high-risk patients (CDC, 2016; Marschall, Mermel, Fakih, et al., 2014)

13. **Apply a new catheter** stabilization device, if one is used.

14. **Remove the drape,** if you used one.

15. **Loop the catheter gently** and secure it with tape to the skin. Avoid securing it to the dressing. Or, depending on type of CVC, place a piece of clear tape across the ends of the catheter lumens, near but not on the hubs.
Ensures that accidental tugging on the catheter does not dislodge the catheter. Do not cover the hubs because you may need to access them.

16. **Label the dressing** with the date changed, time, and your initials.
Alerts staff to when the next dressing change will be due.

17. **Dispose of supplies** into the appropriate receptacles according to agency policy in line with CDC guidelines.

18. **Place the patient in** a comfortable position, raise the siderail, and be sure the call device is accessible.

19. **Remove your mask and gloves** and the patient's mask.

Thinking About the Procedure

The video **Central Line Dressings,** along with questions and suggested responses, is available on the ***Davis's Nursing Skills Videos*** Web site on FADavis.com.

Procedure 38-5C ■ PICC Line Dressings

➤ When performing the procedure, always identify your patient according to agency policy, using two identifiers, and be attentive to standard precautions, hand hygiene, patient safety and privacy, body mechanics, and documentation.

Procedure Steps

1. **Obtain a sterile PICC** (central) line dressing kit (or equivalent supplies if there is no kit) and mask for the patient, if one is needed.
Because central lines have direct access to the central circulation, the risk of systemic infection is greater. Therefore, this procedure uses aseptic technique, even though the insertion site is peripheral. All supplies must be sterile.

2. **Place the patient in a semi-Fowler's position,** if tolerated. Lower the siderail and adjust the bed to working height.
Semi-Fowler's position and bed adjustments facilitate site cleansing and dressing application and reduce strain on the nurse's back.

3. **Explain the procedure** and ask the patient to turn his head to the opposite side from the insertion site. If the patient cannot cooperate, place a mask on him, if consistent with agency policy.

(continued on next page)

Procedure 38-5 ■ Changing IV Dressings (continued)

Explanation may reduce anxiety and enhance cooperation; turning helps prevent contamination of the insertion site from nasal and oral airborne secretions.

4. **Inspect the site** for signs and symptoms of infection and catheter migration.
5. **Put on your mask and** clean nonsterile gloves and carefully remove the old dressing by pulling toward the insertion site and catheter stabilization device, if present. Discard your gloves with the dressing.
   The mask helps prevent contamination of the insertion site from the nurse's nasal and oral airborne secretions. Pulling toward the insertion site minimizes the possibility of dislodging the catheter.
6. **Perform hand hygiene,** open the kit, and remove and don the sterile gloves.
7. **Unfold drape and establish your sterile field.** Transfer items from kit to your sterile field.
   Ensures that strict sterile technique is maintained.
8. **Use a sterile tape measure** to compare the external length of the PICC with the baseline insertion length (if consistent with agency's policy).
   Detects catheter migration, which may indicate that the PICC line is not in the correct location.
9. **Scrub the insertion site** and surrounding skin with an antiseptic solution. Ensure that blood or encrustations are removed from the site and catheter. (Refer to Procedure 38-5B: Central Line Dressings, Steps 9 and 10.)
10. **If you are using a chlorhexidine gluconate sponge** as part of the dressing, apply it directly over the catheter insertion site, ensuring that it is in direct contact with the skin.
    Minimizes the proliferation of microorganisms.
11. **Allow the site to air dry.**
12. **Apply a commercial stabilization device, if applicable.**
13. **Apply a transparent dressing** over catheter site.

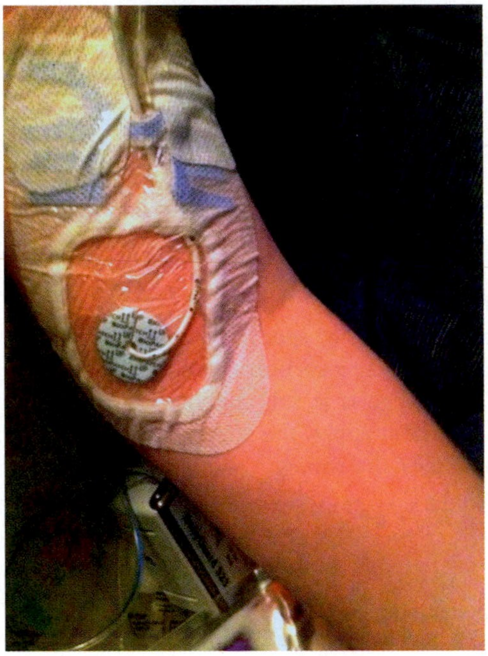

14. **Label the dressing** with the date, time, and your initials.
    Used to identify the next scheduled dressing change.
15. **Loop and anchor the catheter tubing, as needed;** secure it with tape.
    Reduces the risk of accidental dislodgement.
16. **Place the patient** in a comfortable position, raise the siderails, and place the call light so it is accessible to patient.
17. **Dispose of used supplies** into the appropriate receptacles according to agency policy and consistent with CDC guidelines.

Evaluation

- Evaluate the IV insertion site and surrounding tissue for signs of infiltration, inflammation, infection, and phlebitis.
- Monitor the dressing for dampness, blood, soiling, or loosening.
  If these occur, the dressing must be changed.

Patient Teaching

- Explain the importance of notifying staff if the IV dressing becomes soiled, dampened, or loosened.
- Remind the patient to notify staff immediately for bleeding, pain, or swelling around the catheter or dressing area or discomfort in the hand, arm, or shoulder on the same side as the catheter.

Home Care

- Explain home IV therapy to the client and caregiver and teach them how to identify complications.
- Obtain a return demonstration by the client or caregiver to ensure competent performance of fluid, tubing, and dressing changes when necessary.

Documentation

- Chart the date and time the dressing was changed. Document the location and condition of the IV catheter insertion site.
- Document any complications of IV therapy and the interventions taken.
- Document the dressing change on your IV record. Often, IV care is documented on a flowsheet.

Sample documentation

mm/dd/yyyy 2300 New transparent semipermeable dressing applied over PICC insertion site in left forearm. No redness, tenderness, swelling, or exudate at the site. ——————— Mary Ramirez, RNC

Practice Resources

CDC (2016); INS (2016); Marschall, J., Mermel, L., Fakih, M., et al. (2014); Moureau, N., & Chopra, V. (2016).

Thinking About the Procedure

The video **PICC Line Dressings,** along with questions and suggested responses, is available on the ***Davis's Nursing Skills Videos*** Web site on FADavis.com.

Procedure 38-6 ■ Converting a Primary Line to a Peripheral IV Lock

➤ For steps to follow in *all* procedures, refer to the Universal Steps for All Procedures found on the inside back cover.

Equipment

- Clean nonsterile gloves
- Peripheral intermittent IV lock adapter
- Two syringes containing saline solution (one syringe with dilute heparin solution, if required by agency policy)
- Linen-saver pad
- Transparent semipermeable dressing
- Alcohol or chlorhexidine/alcohol or other antiseptic swab

Delegation

You can delegate the task of converting a primary IV line to an intermittent lock device to an LPN who is specially trained in IV therapy. The task should not be delegated to UAP. However, you should instruct the UAP to notify you of any problems with the intermittent lock device, such as dislodging of the catheter or client complaints of pain, swelling, or redness at the insertion site.

Pre-Procedure Assessments

- Assess the patient's readiness to have the IV fluid discontinued (e.g., tolerating oral fluids, adequate urine output, and laboratory values within normal limits).
  If the patient's condition indicates that he still requires IV fluids, notify the primary care provider and do not discontinue the IV line.
- Assess for allergy to tape.
- Assess the IV site for signs of phlebitis, infiltration, extravasation, or infection.
  If complications are present or the IV has been in place longer than 96 hours, remove the IV catheter instead of converting it to an intermittent lock.

➤ When performing the procedure, always identify your patient according to agency policy, using two identifiers, and be attentive to standard precautions, hand hygiene, patient safety and privacy, body mechanics, and documentation.

➤ Maintain sterility of supplies and equipment (e.g., do not touch catheter opening or ends of the IV lock; keep flush syringe connector sterile).

Procedure Steps

1. **Help the client assume** a comfortable position that provides access to the IV site.
   Promotes cooperation and facilitates your ability to perform the procedure.

2. **Lower siderails, raise the bed** to working height, and place linen-saver pad under extremity with the IV.
   Protects linens from blood and fluid that might leak from the vessel during catheter removal and ensures good body mechanics.

3. **Don clean nonsterile gloves.** Remove the IV lock from the package and flush the adapter with the syringe of saline or dilute heparin, according to agency policy. Leave the syringe of saline attached to the adapter. The saline will be used again for flushing the catheter once the adapter is attached to the IV catheter. **Continue with Step 4.**
   Removes air from the lock. ➤

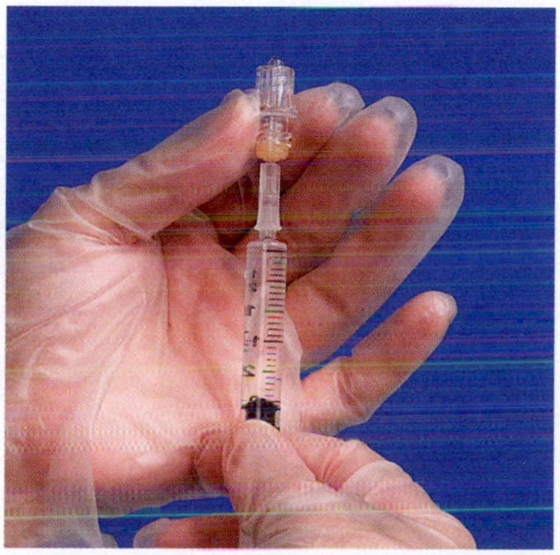

(continued on next page)

Procedure 38-6 ■ Converting a Primary Line to a Peripheral IV Lock (continued)

Variation for Primary Tubing Set-Up With Extension Tubing With a Lock

Discontinue the IV solution and disconnect the primary tubing from the extension tubing with lock. Then flush extension tubing per agency policy and **skip to Step 12.**

4. **Carefully remove the IV dressing** and the tape that is securing the tubing.
   Provides access to the IV catheter.

5. **Close the roller clamp** on the administration set.
   Prevents loss of IV fluid during the procedure.

6. **With the side of your** nondominant hand, apply pressure over the vein just above the insertion site but not directly on the catheter/hub junction. At the same time, stabilize the catheter hub with your thumb and forefinger.
   Applying pressure over the vein stops blood from flowing from the catheter as you change the administration tubing.

7. **Gently disengage the used** tubing from the IV catheter. If the tubing does not separate from the catheter, see the What If ... section at the end of Step 13.

8. **Quickly insert the lock adapter** into the IV catheter and turn it to lock it in place.
   Insert the adapter quickly to prevent bleeding from the IV catheter.

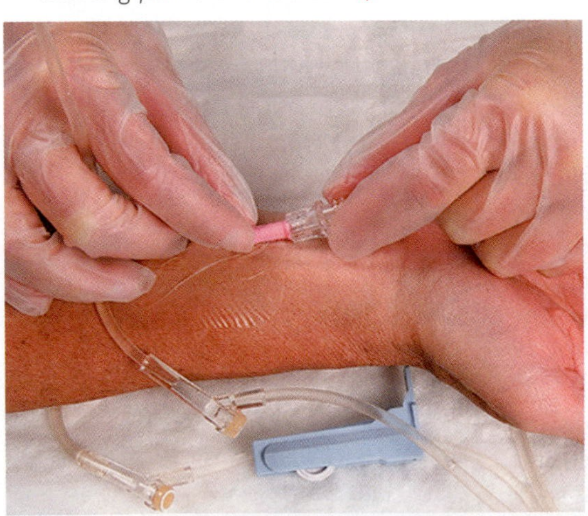

9. **With the attached syringe** of saline or dilute heparin, flush the catheter using the method recommended according to agency policy (e.g., push-stop-push or a slow, steady push).
   Some experts recommend a turbulence (push-stop-push method) on the theory that turbulence ensures patency of the IV catheter by clearing the catheter and helping prevent reflux of blood back into the catheter. Others believe this method has undesired effects and recommend, instead, a steady, slow push. There is no evidence to support the turbulence theory (INS, 2016). In the meantime, follow agency policy regarding the flushing technique.

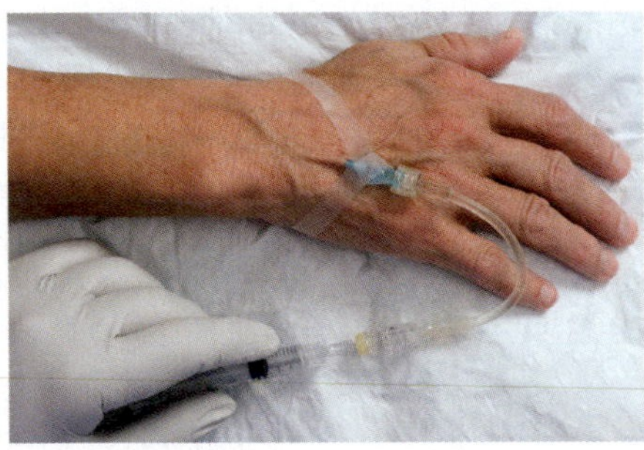

10. **Using aseptic technique,** cover the insertion site and catheter hub with a sterile transparent semipermeable dressing. Do not cover the junction of the catheter hub and the IV lock. See Procedure 38-5A for review of dressings.
    Secures the IV catheter and prevents contamination of the site.

11. **Label the dressing** with the date changed and your initials.

12. **Discard used supplies** into appropriate receptacles according to agency policy in line with CDC guidelines.
    Discarding used equipment properly keeps the healthcare environment safe.

? What if . . .

- **At Step 7, the tubing will not separate from the catheter?**

  First, if it is a luer-lock connection, be sure you have twisted the luer-lock "open." If so, place a hemostat ("mosquito" clamp) on the IV tubing and gently twist back and forth to loosen the connection. Then if the IV tubing still does not come loose, use the hemostat to gently twist the lock back and forth to loosen the connection. Do not lock the hemostat; merely use it lightly as a grip.
  Use of hemostat may help loosen tubing from the catheter, but placement is critical so that the IV catheter and connector are not damaged.

- **At Step 7, the IV catheter becomes dislodged while trying to disconnect the tubing?**

  If you can see as much as three-fourths of the catheter emerging from the site, you must remove it and start a new IV at a different site.
  Trying to re-advance the catheter might cause it to pierce through the vein as well as increase the risk of infection from reinserting a catheter that is no longer sterile. It also causes tissue trauma and increases the risk of phlebitis from catheter manipulation.

Evaluation

- Assess the patency of the catheter before each use according to institutional policy. Patency check and flushing are usually done every 8 to 24 hours.
- Evaluate the patient's tolerance to intermittent IV therapy.
- Inspect the insertion site for signs of complications.

Patient Teaching

Explain the importance of notifying staff if the IV site becomes red, painful, or swollen; or if the dressing becomes soiled, damp, or loosened (indicating that the catheter has become dislodged or the connection is loose). Include the family in the teaching because the patient may not be able to assess his own IV therapy.

Home Care

- Explain home use of the intermittent lock to the patient and caregiver. Teach them how to flush the catheter before and after administering prescribed medications.
- Provide the patient and caregiver with the name and phone numbers of people to contact in case problems arise with the catheter or insertion site.

Documentation

- Document the date and time the IV line was converted to an intermittent lock device.
- Note the size and location of the catheter, as well as the type and amount of flush solution used.
- Record on the I&O record the amount of IV fluid infused.
- Document the condition of the IV site and any complications noted.
- Often, IV care is documented on a flowsheet or the electronic patient record.

Practice Resources

Goossens, G. (2015); INS (2016).

Thinking About the Procedure

The video **Converting a Primary Line to a Peripheral IV Lock,** along with questions and suggested responses, is available on the ***Davis's Nursing Skills Videos*** Web site on FADavis.com.

Procedure 38-7 ■ Discontinuing a Peripheral IV

➤ For steps to follow in *all* procedures, refer to the Universal Steps for All Procedures found on the inside back cover.

Equipment

- Clean nonsterile gloves
- Sterile 2 in. × 2 in. gauze dressings
- 1-in. tape or transparent semipermeable dressing
- Linen-saver pad

Delegation

You can delegate the task of discontinuing an IV to an LPN who is specially trained in IV therapy. The task should not be delegated to UAP. However, you should instruct the UAP to notify you of any bleeding from the insertion site.

Pre-Procedure Assessments

- Assess the patient's readiness to have the IV fluid discontinued and verify the prescription. For example, determine whether he is tolerating oral fluids and has adequate urine output and whether laboratory values are within normal limits.
  If the patient's condition indicates that he still requires IV fluids, notify the provider and do not discontinue the IV line.

➤ When performing the procedure, always identify your patient according to agency policy, using two identifiers, and be attentive to standard precautions, hand hygiene, patient safety and privacy, body mechanics, and documentation.

Procedure Steps

1. **Assist the client to a comfortable** position and raise the bed to working height.
   Helps ensure patient cooperation with the procedure; supports good body mechanics for the nurse.

2. **Place a linen-saver pad** under the extremity with the IV.
   Protects linens from blood and fluid that might leak from the vein during catheter removal

3. **Don clean nonsterile gloves,** and close the roller clamp on the administration set.
   Closing the roller prevents IV fluid from spilling onto the bed or client during catheter removal. Procedure gloves protect you from body fluid exposure.

4. **Carefully remove the IV dressing,** catheter stabilization device, and the tape that is securing the tubing.
   Removing tape and dressings can be painful especially if over hair or sensitive or thin skin.

If the IV Is Running Through an Extension Tubing or a Saline Lock

Disconnect the administration set tubing and close the slide clamp on the extension tubing.

(continued on next page)

Procedure 38-7 ■ Discontinuing a Peripheral IV (continued)

5. **Scrub the catheter–skin junction** with an alcohol prep pad or chlorhexidine/alcohol antiseptic product for at least 15 seconds.
Removes microorganisms from the skin entry site.

6. **Apply a sterile 2 in. × 2 in. gauze** pad above the IV insertion site and gently remove the catheter, directing it straight along the vein. Do not press down on the gauze pad while removing the catheter.
Directing the catheter along the vein prevents vein injury while you are removing the catheter.

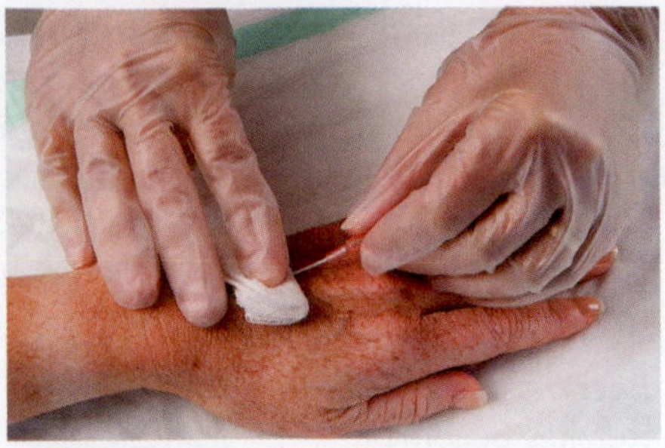

7. **Immediately apply firm pressure** with the gauze pad over the insertion site. Hold pressure for 1 to 3 minutes; hold longer if bleeding persists.
This typically stops bleeding by hastening clot formation.

8. **Remove the soiled 2 in. × 2 in.** gauze pad, and replace it with a sterile 2 in. × 2 in. gauze pad folded over to form a pressure dressing. Secure it with 1-inch tape or a transparent semipermeable dressing.
Protects the site from contamination.

9. **Return the bed to a low position.** Discard all supplies in the appropriate receptacles according to agency policy in line with CDC guidelines.

Evaluation

- Assess the integrity of the removed catheter; compare the length with the original insertion length to ensure the entire catheter is removed. If a catheter defect is noted, report to the manufacturer and regulatory agencies and complete an incident report according to agency policy.
- Evaluate the patient's response to oral fluids after IV therapy is discontinued.
- Monitor for changes in the patient's condition to assess whether IV therapy should be re-established.

Patient Teaching

- Instruct the client and family to notify staff if bleeding or discomfort occurs at the insertion site.
- Teach the importance of drinking adequate amounts of fluid, within the prescribed treatment plan, to prevent dehydration. (Some patients have fluid restrictions.)

Documentation

- Document the date and time that IV therapy was discontinued.
- Note the condition of the site, including the presence of any complications. If complications are present, document your interventions, including provider notification.
- Often you will record this procedure on a flow sheet or in the electronic patient record.

Sample documentation

mm/dd/yyyy 2100 Discontinued RA#2, 22-gauge catheter. Site without redness, swelling, tenderness, or exudates. Pressure applied to site for 3 minutes. Bleeding stopped and sterile 2 in. × 2 in. gauze dressing applied. Informed patient to notify staff if bleeding or discomfort occurs. ——— S. Horowitz, RN

Practice Resources

CDC (2017); INS (2016).

Thinking About the Procedure

The video **Discontinuing a Peripheral IV,** along with questions and suggested responses, is available on the ***Davis's Nursing Skills Videos*** Web site on FADavis.com.

Procedure 38-8 ■ Administering a Blood Transfusion

➤ For steps to follow in *all* procedures, refer to the Universal Steps for All Procedures found on the inside back cover.

Equipment

- Clean nonsterile gloves
- Blood product
- Normal saline IV solution, 250 mL

Key Point: *Normal saline solution is the only solution that is compatible with blood products; other IV solutions cause hemolysis of blood cells.*

- Blood administration set (with a 200-micrometer filter and luer-lock connection). If there is no filter on the tubing, you must attach one.
- IV pole
- Watch with a second hand or digital seconds
- Thermometer
- Blood pressure cuff with sphygmomanometer
- Stethoscope

Delegation

Do not delegate this procedure to the LPN or UAP because blood product administration requires advanced assessment and critical-thinking skills. The LPN and UAP can assist by monitoring vital signs. Instruct both about the complications associated with blood product administration, and instruct them to inform you if any occur.

Pre-Procedure Assessments

- Confirm the patient's need for blood products by assessing vital signs, urine output, and laboratory studies.
  Blood products may cause life-threatening complications; therefore, they should be administered only when needed.
- Check the patient's history for previous blood transfusions and reactions and verify her blood type.
  If the patient has a history of a blood transfusion reaction, precautions must be taken before she receives additional transfusions. For example, she may need premedication with acetaminophen, a corticosteroid, and diphenhydramine; specially treated blood products; and the use of a specialized administration set with greater filtering capabilities.
- Assess patency of the existing IV catheter, and make sure that it is the proper size for blood product administration.
  Nurses often use a 20-gauge catheter for blood administration. However, for routine transfusion, a 22-gauge or even a 24-gauge catheter can be used. You would need an 18- or 20-gauge catheter when large amounts of blood must be transfused rapidly. The primary consideration should be the size of the patient's veins and not an arbitrary catheter size.
- Assess for allergy to tape.

Procedure 38-8A ■ Administering Blood and Blood Products

➤ When performing the procedure, always identify your patient according to agency policy, using two identifiers, and be attentive to standard precautions, hand hygiene, patient safety and privacy, body mechanics, and documentation.

Procedure Steps

1. **Verify that informed consent** has been obtained.
   Informed consent is required for blood product administration, as for any invasive or risk-bearing procedure.
2. **Verify the medical prescription,** noting the indication, rate of infusion, and any medications. If there are any pretransfusion medications, administer them as prescribed.
   Helps prevent administration errors.
3. **Obtain a blood administration set** and 250 mL of IV normal saline solution or as prescribed. Some agencies may require a flush with normal saline between infusions.
4. **Obtain infusion pump,** if possible, and blood warmer, if necessary
   Having all supplies and equipment on hand minimizes delays in starting the transfusion.
5. **Obtain the blood product** from the blood bank, according to your institution's policy. Wear clean nonsterile gloves whenever handling blood products.
   Some blood banks require a pickup slip that verifies the presence of a functioning IV catheter, signed informed consent, and a prescription because blood must be discarded after it has been out of refrigeration for 30 minutes.
6. **Verify that the blood product** matches the prescription. Inspect the blood. If you note any of the following abnormalities, return the blood to the blood bank and obtain a new bag:
   a. Pink plasma indicates hemolysis.
   b. The red cells should be red, not purple or black.
   c. There should be no large clots visible.
   d. There should be no leakage.
7. **Verify the patient and blood** product identification with another qualified staff member (as deemed by your institution).
   Only one of the staff members is required by The Joint Commission to be qualified to administer blood products; however, agency policies may specify those requirements.
   a. Use two patient coidentifiers (e.g., ask the patient to tell you her full name and date of birth) and compare it with the name and date of birth located on the blood bank form and patient ID band.
   Allowing the patient to confirm her identity and comparing the information against the blood bank form is a safety measure to ensure that the correct patient is receiving the correct blood product.
   b. Compare the patient name and hospital identification number on the patient's identification bracelet with the patient name and hospital identification number on the blood bank form attached to the blood product.
   Verifies that the correct patient is receiving the correct blood product.
   c. Compare the unit identification number located on the blood bank form with the identification number printed on the blood product container.
   Verifies that the blood bank has dispensed the correct blood product. ▼

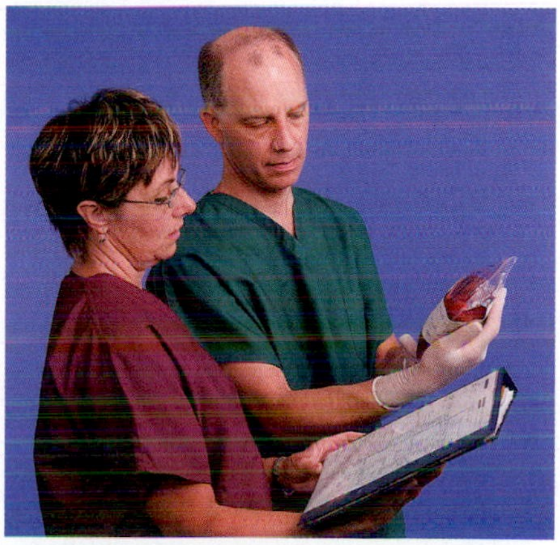

   d. Compare the patient's blood type listed on the blood bank form with the blood type listed on the blood product container.

(continued on next page)

Procedure 38-8 ■ Administering a Blood Transfusion (continued)

Verifies that the blood type of the product matches the patient's blood type.

e. If all verifications are in agreement, both staff members should sign the blood bank form attached to the blood product container.

> Contact the blood bank immediately if any discrepancies occur during the identification process. If there are any discrepancies, do not administer the blood product.
> *Signing the blood bank form confirms that the blood product was identified and verified by two qualified staff members.*

f. Document on the blood bank form the date and time that the transfusion was started.
Blood cannot be infused past the expiration time; documenting the start time alerts the nurse of the expiration time.

g. Make sure that the blood bank form remains attached to the blood product container until administration is complete.
Ensures product identity should a transfusion reaction occur.

8. **Remove the blood** administration set from the package, and label the tubing with the date and time. Then, close all clamps on the administration set.
Labeling the administration set with the date and time informs the nursing staff when the administration set should be changed.

9. **Remove the protective covers** from the normal saline solution container port and from one of the spikes located on the "Y" of the blood product administration set. Place the spike into the port of the solution container.

10. **Hang the normal saline solution** container on the IV pole. Refer to the photo in Step 16.

11. **Compress the drip chamber** of the saline administration set and allow it to fill halfway.
Prevents air from entering the tubing with the solution.

12. **Open the roller clamp** and prime the administration set tubing with normal saline.
Removes air from the tubing.

13. **Close the roller clamp.** Inspect the tubing for air. If air bubbles are in the tubing, flick the tubing with a fingertip to mobilize the bubbles up into the drip chamber.
Air bubbles in the administration tubing can cause an air embolus.

14. **Gently invert the blood** product container several times, but do not shake the bag.
Mixes the blood product with the preservatives that are added to the container without causing trauma (lysis) to the cells.

15. **Hang the blood product bag** on the IV pole and thread the line through the infusion pump.
Enables the blood to flow by gravity.

16. **Remove the protective covers** from the blood spike on the blood tubing and the blood product port. Carefully spike the blood product container through the port.
Prevents inadvertent puncturing of the container.

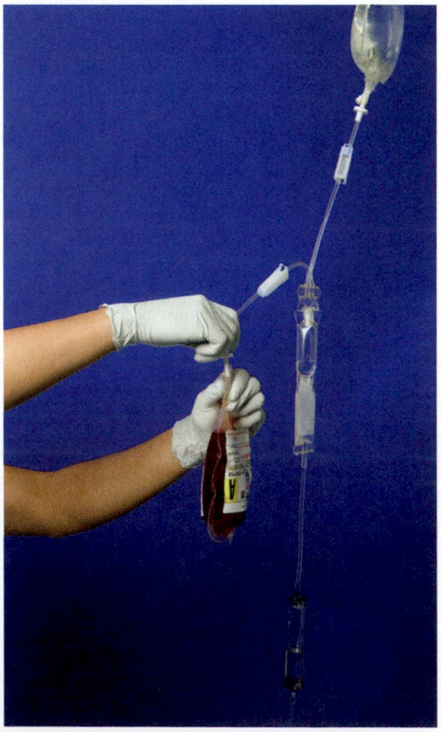

17. **Obtain and record** the patient's vital signs, including temperature, pulse, and blood pressure, before beginning the transfusion.
Establishes a baseline to help monitor for transfusion reactions.

18. **Using aseptic technique**, attach the distal end of the administration set to the IV catheter.
Prevents contamination of the IV catheter and administration set.

19. **Slowly open the roller clamp** closest to the blood product.
Allows the blood product to slowly fill that side of the "Y" of the administration set tubing.

20. **Set the infusion rate.** Start the infusion rate slowly (2 mL/min) for the first 15 minutes (INS, 2016). If no reaction occurs after 50 mL has infused, set it to the prescribed rate.
A unit of blood cannot hang for more than 4 hours; otherwise, bacterial growth may occur.

For a Volume-Control Infusion Pump

Program the rate. Push "Start." Start the rate slowly at 2 mL/min until 50 mL have infused. If no reaction occurs, set it to the prescribed rate.

For Gravity Flow

Using the roller clamp, adjust the drip rate. Keep in mind that blood administration sets have a drip factor of 10 gtts/mL.

NOTE: When using a 24-gauge needle, you will usually (but not always) use gravity infusion instead of a pump.

Forcing red blood cells through a smaller size catheter could result in some cell damage. Allowing the blood to flow by gravity allows time for the cells to change shape as they naturally do when flowing through small capillaries. However, only pumps that have been approved for blood transfusions should be used, because they prevent hemolysis.

21. **Remain with the patient** for the first 5 minutes and obtain vital signs within 5 to 15 minutes after initiating the infusion (INS, 2016).

Although the literature indicates that most severe blood transfusion reactions occur during the transfusion of the initial 50 mL of blood, recent research found that the average time to react was over 1.5 hours into the infusion (Cortez-Gann, Gilmore, Foley, et al., 2017). However, the first 10 to 15 minutes are the most critical (AABB, 2012).

22. **Ensure that the patient's** call device is readily available and have her alert you immediately of any signs or symptoms of a transfusion reaction, such as back pain, chills, itching, or shortness of breath.
If the patient alerts you immediately, you should be able to stop the transfusion in time to prevent serious complications.

23. **Obtain vital signs** again in 15 minutes (follow agency procedures), then again in 30 minutes, and then hourly while the transfusion infuses. Blood and blood product infusions must be completed within 4 hours (AABB, 2012; INS, 2016).
Frequent monitoring alerts you to detect early signs of transfusion reaction or fluid overload.

24. **After the unit has infused,** close the roller clamp to the blood product container and open the roller clamp to the normal saline solution to flush the administration set with normal saline solution.
Flushing the tubing with normal saline solution clears the tubing of any blood and avoids wasting any of the blood product.

25. **Close the roller clamp** to the normal saline and then disconnect the blood administration set from the IV catheter, if an additional unit of blood has not been prescribed.

26. **If another unit of blood** is required, change the transfusion administration set and filter after the completion of each unit; or, if more than 1 unit can be infused within the 4-hour time frame, change the transfusion set and filter every 4 hours (INS, 2016).
The same administration set can be used for two units of blood or per agency policy.

27. **Discard the empty blood** container and administration set in a biohazard receptacle, according to your institution's policy.
Promotes a safer healthcare environment.

? What if . . .

- **Two individuals are not available to verify that the blood and the patient are a match, and the blood must be hung now?**

In this instance, if it is available, an automated identification technology (e.g., bar coding) may be used.

Procedure 38-8B Managing a Transfusion Reaction

➤ When performing the procedure, always identify your patient according to agency policy, using two identifiers, and be attentive to standard precautions, hand hygiene, patient safety and privacy, body mechanics, and documentation.

Procedure Steps

1. **If signs or symptoms of a transfusion reaction occur, stop the transfusion immediately. Do not flush the tubing.**
Flushing the tubing causes the patient to receive the blood that remains in the tubing.

2. **Disconnect the administration** set from the IV catheter. Call for help. Obtain vital signs, and auscultate heart and breath sounds.
Severe transfusion reactions may cause respiratory distress and shock; early recognition and treatment improve patient outcomes.

3. **Maintain patency of the IV** catheter by hanging a new infusion of normal saline solution, using new tubing.
Maintaining a patent IV catheter with normal saline solution provides IV access in which emergency medication can be administered if necessary.

4. **Notify the primary provider** as soon as you have stopped the blood, assessed the patient, and hung the new normal saline solution.

5. **Place the administration set** and blood product container, with the blood bank form attached, inside a biohazard bag. Send the bag to the blood bank immediately.
The remainder of the blood must be sent to the blood bank, where it can be analyzed to help determine the cause of the reaction.

6. **Obtain blood** (from the extremity opposite the transfusion site) and urine specimens according to your institution's policy.
Blood banks typically require (a) a specimen for a type and crossmatch to compare with the pretransfusion type and crossmatch, (b) a specimen for free hemoglobin, and (c) a specimen for serum bilirubin level. A urine sample should also be sent to check for hemoglobinuria, a sign of acute hemolytic reactions.

7. **Continue to monitor vital signs** frequently, at least every 15 minutes.
To quickly detect worsening of the patient's condition.

8. **Administer medications,** as prescribed.
Medications will vary depending on the type of transfusion reaction.

? What if . . .

- **At Step 3, you do not have a new bag of normal saline to hang?**

Clamp the normal saline line until you can obtain a new bag of normal saline, then disconnect the old normal saline. Do this as quickly as possible.
Preserves the patency of the IV catheter.

(continued on next page)

Procedure 38-8 ■ Administering a Blood Transfusion (continued)

Evaluation

- Evaluate the patient's response to the blood transfusion by checking for changes in blood pressure and oxygenation, improvement in color, or for signs of fluid overload.
- Monitor for signs and symptoms of transfusion reaction.
- Assess the IV insertion site for signs of infiltration, phlebitis, infection, or inflammation.
- Monitor laboratory studies, such as complete blood count, to help evaluate the effectiveness of therapy and/or transfusion reaction.

Patient Teaching

- Explain the signs and symptoms of transfusion reactions and tell the client and family to notify staff immediately should they occur.
- Warn the client or family to notify staff immediately if tenderness, redness, or swelling occurs at the IV catheter insertion site.
- Explain the importance of notifying staff immediately if the administration set becomes disconnected from the IV catheter or the IV catheter becomes dislodged.

Documentation

- Document the date, time, and reason the transfusion was started.
- Document transfusion vital signs according to institution policy (many institutions have a special form for transfusion vital signs).
- Record the amount of blood transfused on the I&O record.
- Document any complications and the interventions taken.

Sample documentation

mm/dd/yyyy 0600, 1 unit (250 mL) PRBCs hung at 0300 and infused through 20-gauge catheter in LA, for Hgb of 8.3 mg/dL. Pretransfusion vital signs: T 98.9°F, BP 100/68 mm Hg, HR 114 beats/min, and RR 22 breaths/min. See frequent vital sign sheet for other transfusion vital signs. Breath sounds remained clear throughout the transfusion. No evidence of reaction. Post-transfusion lab due at 1200. ———— L. Gilmore, RN

Practice Resources

Cortez-Gann, J., Gilmore, K., Foley, K., et al. (2017); American Association of Blood Banks (AABB) (2012); INS (2016);

Thinking About the Procedure

The video **Administering Blood and Blood Products,** along with questions and suggested responses, is available on the ***Davis's Nursing Skills Videos*** Web site on FADavis.com.

Procedure 38-9 ■ Assisting With Percutaneous Central Venous Catheter Placement

➤ For steps to follow in *all* procedures, refer to the Universal Steps for All Procedures found on the inside back cover.

Equipment

- Sterile gloves (two or three pairs)
- Masks, hats, barrier gowns
- 10-mL vials of normal saline (three or four)
- Syringes with 1-in. needle (two or three)
- 25-gauge ⅝-in. and 18-gauge 1½-in. needles (two or three of each)
- Central venous catheter (CVC) kit containing an introducer, antiseptic solution/swabs, sterile drapes, 10-mL syringe, 1% or 2% Xylocaine without epinephrine, suture, sterile scissors and needle holder, CVC catheter (single- or multilumen)
- Injection caps
- Alcohol wipes

Delegation

Do not delegate this procedure because complex assessment and support skills are needed. The nurse must be alert to changes in the patient's condition and signs of developing complications. CVC placement at the bedside is associated with pneumothorax, hemothorax, cardiac tamponade, and air emboli.

Pre-Procedure Assessments

- Obtain baseline vital signs.
- Verify that informed consent has been given.
- Assess for allergy to tape.

➤ When performing the procedure, always identify your patient according to agency policy, using two identifiers, and be attentive to standard precautions, hand hygiene, patient safety and privacy, body mechanics, and documentation.

Procedure Steps

1. **Explain the procedure** to the patient.
To relieve anxiety and increase the patient's ability to cooperate with the procedure.

2. **Verify informed consent** and obtain vital signs.

3. **Gather supplies and perform** meticulous hand hygiene.
Promotes efficiency; removes contaminants to help prevent infection.

4. **Set up the sterile field** and add supplies. Position the table so it is easily accessible by the physician or advanced practice nurse (APN) during the procedure.
Promotes efficiency and makes the procedure faster and therefore less burdensome for the patient.

5. **Position the patient** to facilitate the procedure, usually in the Trendelenburg position with a rolled towel between the shoulders.
To prevent air embolism and dilate neck veins.

6. **Offer mask, gown, and sterile gloves** (and possibly hat, depending on agency policy) to the physician or APN after she performs hand hygiene.
Maximum barrier precautions are required for central line placement.

7. **Don mask and then sterile gloves.**
To prevent contamination of sterile areas and of the insertion site as you cleanse it. Don mask first to keep gloves sterile.

8. **Prep the marked site** with >0.5% chlorhexidine preparation in alcohol (CDC, updated 2017). A 2% chlorhexidine gluconate in 70% alcohol applicators, using a friction scrub, is commonly used.
   a. Use a back-and-forth motion to scrub an area at least 20 to 25 cm (8 to 10 in.) in diameter. Do not go back over an area with the same applicator.
   b. Repeat with three applicators. Total scrub should take at least 30 seconds (2 minutes for a moist site such as the femoral vein).
   c. Allow site to air-dry completely (about 2 minutes). Never wipe or blot dry.
   Insertion kits and agency policies may vary. Follow agency policy. If it does not conform to evidence-based guidelines, work for policy change.

9. **Drape the insertion site** with a large sterile drape, exposing only the prepared skin area. Use other large drapes to cover the patient from head to toe. If your agency does not have a policy that the patient wear a mask, have the patient turn his head in the opposite direction of insertion site.
Creates a sterile field and decreases the chance of contamination by the patient's exhalations. Turning the head to the opposite side also helps to make it easier to advance the catheter when it passes through the subclavian site.

10. **Observe while the physician** or APN performs the following steps:
   a. Anesthetizes the area with lidocaine.
   b. Primes the central venous catheter with saline.
   c. Performs venipuncture with the insertion needle (in the internal jugular or subclavian site). The femoral site may be used in emergencies, but it is associated with a higher rate of complications than other sites.
   d. Attaches a syringe to the needle and aspirates for blood.
   To ensure the needle is in the vein.
   e. After obtaining blood return, removes syringe from the needle and inserts a guidewire through the needle.
   The guidewire guides the flexible catheter into the vein.
   f. Aspirates all air out of the catheter lumens and then flushes them with normal saline.
   To reduce the risk of air embolism.
   g. Places injection caps on each lumen.
   To prevent blood loss and maintain sterility of the lumens
   h. Sutures the catheter in place.
   To minimize movement and prevent catheter migration (in or out).

11. **Apply sterile transparent dressing** over the site after the physician or APN is finished.
Minimizes contamination of the site. The most common route of infection is via migration of skin organisms at the insertion site into the cutaneous catheter tract with colonization of the catheter tip. Transparent dressing allows for observation of the site without removing the dressing and manipulating the catheter.

12. **If there are clamps** on the lumens, close them.

13. **Place tape over the lumens** near the ends, but not on the injection caps.
To minimize movement of the catheter that increases the risk of dislodgement.

14. **Remove sterile drape** and assist the patient to a comfortable position. Monitor for complications, especially respiratory distress.

15. **Dispose of used supplies** and equipment in the appropriate receptacles according to agency policy in line with CDC guidelines.

16. **Remove and dispose of mask** and gloves. Perform hand hygiene.
Observes standard precaution guidelines.

17. **Follow provider's prescriptions** (e.g., obtain chest x-ray)

(continued on next page)

Procedure 38-9 ■ Assisting With Percutaneous Central Venous Catheter Placement (continued)

Guidelines

- The patient and all staff in the room should wear a mask.
- A health professional who has received appropriate education (e.g., a nurse) should observe the CVC insertion to ensure that aseptic technique is maintained.
- This person should stop the procedure if aseptic technique errors are made.
- A central line checklist should be used during the procedure. You may be responsible for auditing the procedure and completing the checklist.

? What if . . .

- **In Step 9, a large sterile drape is not available?**

  Use two small drapes to cover the patient from head to toe.

  Evidence-based guidelines advise maximal barrier precautions for insertion of CVCs.

Evaluation

- Obtain vital signs.
- Auscultate the lungs and assess for respiratory distress, sharp chest pain, and coughing. Monitor for 24 hours for these signs.

  To detect pneumothorax or cardiac tamponade.
- Obtain a chest x-ray.

  To verify correct location of catheter tip in the distal third of the superior vena cava, as well as absence of thorax and cardiac puncture.
- Assess the patient daily to determine continuing need for the CVC.

  Risk of infection is closely related to the length of time the CVC is in place.
- For further evaluation and follow-up, refer to Clinical Insight 38-4: Caring for Patients With a Central Venous Access Device (CVAD): CVC and PICC; and Procedure 38-5B: Central Line Dressings.

Documentation

- Date and time of catheter insertion
- Catheter type and size
- Site location
- Assessments and interventions performed at insertion and immediately after
- Patient's tolerance of procedure (subjective and objective data)
- X-ray verification of catheter placement

Practice Resources

CDC (updated 2017); INS (2016); Moureau, N. & Chopra, V. (2016)/

CLINICAL INSIGHTS

Clinical Insight 38-1 ➤ Assessing for Trousseau's and Chvostek's Signs

Positive Trousseau's and Chvostek's signs are signs of hypocalcemia. To check for these signs, follow these instructions.

Trousseau's Sign

Inflate a blood pressure cuff above systolic pressure. Flexion of the wrist and hand constitutes a positive sign.

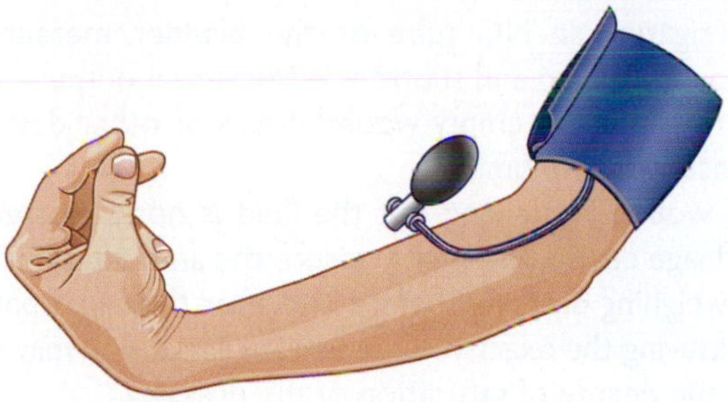

Chvostek's Sign

Tap the face in front of the ear and below the zygomatic bone (cheek bone). Facial twitching constitutes a positive sign.

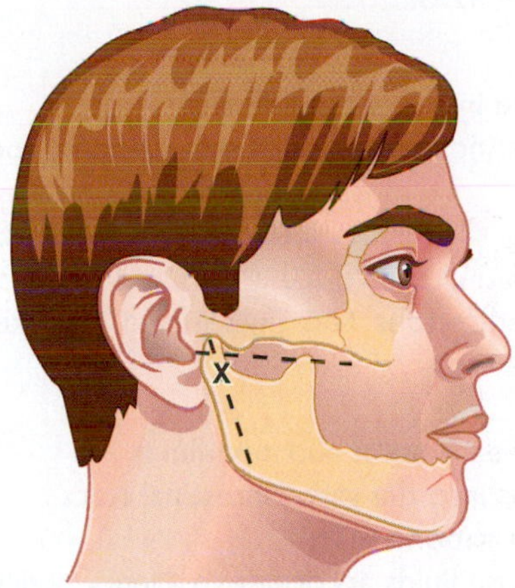

Clinical Insight 38-2 ➤ Guidelines for Measuring Intake and Output (I&O)

General Guidelines

Assessing

- Identify factors that can affect the patient's fluid intake or output (e.g., surgery, medical condition, or medications such as diuretics).
- Measure all fluids the patient consumes or excretes.
- Enlist the patient's help in keeping track of I&O if she is able.
- If you delegate the task of recording intake and output:
  - Be sure the assistive person understands its importance and knows how to perform the procedure correctly.
  - Be certain to evaluate the totals and the fluid sources. A patient or UAP can collect the data, but an RN must make the assessments.
- For accuracy, use a graduated container and hold it at eye level when measuring fluids.

Recording

- You will usually record measurements on a bedside I&O form and transfer the 8-hr total to a graphic sheet or the 24-hr I&O on the patient's record. You may sometimes need hourly measurements. See Chapter 18, "Intake and Output Records," and Figure 18-2.
- Document your findings in milliliters (mL). Describe any fluid restrictions and the patient's compliance with them.

Measuring Intake

It is most accurate to premeasure fluids before they are consumed. However, if that is not possible, you can use the following estimates:

Equivalents

1 oz = 30 mL
1 teaspoon = 5 mL
1 tablespoon = 15 mL
1 home measuring cup of fluid = 8 oz (240 mL)
1 pint of fluid = 16 oz (480 mL)
1 quart of fluid = 32 oz (960 mL)

Various Containers

Record ice chips as fluid at half their volume (1 cup ice = ½ cup fluid)
Bowl (soup) = 180 mL
Creamer (small) = 30 mL
Custard cup = 100 mL
Drinking cup = 180 mL
Coffee mug = 240 mL
Gelatin cup = 100 mL
Ice cream serving = 120 mL
Juice glass = 120 mL
Paper cup, large = 200 mL

(Continued)

Clinical Insight 38-2 ➤ Guidelines for Measuring Intake and Output (I&O)—cont'd

Paper cup, small = 120 mL
Water glass = 200 mL
Water pitcher = 1,000 mL

Examples of Fast-Food Drinks
Child-size drink = 12 oz
Small drink = 16 oz
Medium drink = 21 oz
Large drink = 32 oz

Assessing

- Fluid intake includes the following:
  - Oral fluids, including the liquid in prepared foods
  - Soups
  - Everything that melts into liquid at room temperature (e.g., gelatin, custard, ice cream, and ice)
  - Liquid medications and fluids used to take tablets or capsules
  - IV fluids
  - Enteral or parenteral nutrition fluids
  - Instillations into the gastrointestinal tract
  - Bladder irrigations
- Measure oral fluids according to agency policy.
- For increased accuracy, use a graduated cup to measure and record fluid amounts before the patient consumes them. Subtract from the total any fluid that the patient throws away or saves for future consumption.
- Wash the measuring cup after each use, except after measuring water.
- Measure and teach the patient to measure and record the amount of fluid he drinks with each meal, with medicine, and between meals.
- In the home, cups come in many different sizes, so do the following:
  - Use a measuring cup to measure how much the drinking cups and glasses hold.
  - Always use the same drinking cup or glass.
  - Explain that the labels on cans and bottles will help to determine precise fluid amounts.

Recording

- At least every 8 hours, record the type and amount of all fluids the patient has received and indicate the route (oral, parenteral, rectal, or enteric tube).
- Record all forms of intake except blood and blood products

Measuring Output

Assessing

Refer to Procedure 30-1: Measuring Urine, to review how to measure urine.

Fluid output includes everything that leaves the body in fluid form: urine, watery stool, vomitus, wound drainage, surgical drains, NG tubes, chest tubes, and any fluid aspirated from a body cavity.

- Use a calibrated container to measure fluids. Observe it at eye level and take the reading at the bottom of the fluid meniscus.
- Use a different graduated container for each patient; clean after use.
- Teach the patient to keep toilet paper out of the urine for accurate measurement.
- If irrigating an NG tube or the bladder, measure the amount instilled and subtract it from total output.
- You will need to empty wound drains or other devices to measure this volume.
- If a wound is draining, but the fluid is not collected in a drainage device, you may measure the amount of fluid lost by weighing dressings before and after they are applied. If measuring the exact volume is not crucial, you may evaluate the degree of saturation of the dressing.

Recording

- Record the type, route, and amount of all fluids the patient loses.
- Insensible fluid losses can't be easily quantified. However, unusual losses (e.g., saturated dressing, excessive perspiration, rapid breathing patterns, and large burn areas) should be objectively described in narrative charting.

Tips for Analyzing I&O

- Measure and record all intake and output.
- Determine if output is more or less than intake.
- Evaluate trends over for a period of 24 to 48 hours.
- To identify problems, when evaluating total urine output, ask how many times the patient voided. For example, was a total of 300 mL obtained from 2 voids or from 10 voids of 30 mL each?
- Evaluate patterns and values outside the normal range (e.g., frequent voiding, infrequent voiding), keeping in mind the normal range for 24-hour intake and output.
- The amount of output is important, but consider color, color changes, and odor.
- Analyze intake and output holistically. Take into account the patient's usual pattern and amounts, age, medical problem, and type of surgical procedure.
- You must correlate I&O with daily weights to accurately determine overall fluid status (Collins & Claros, 2011; Davies, H., Leslie, G., Morgan, D., et al., 2018; Shells, R. & Morrell-Scott, M., 2018)

Clinical Insight 38-3 ➤ Guidelines for Selecting a Peripheral Venipuncture Site

- As a general rule, select the most distal vein on an upper extremity.
- If available, use visualization technologies such as portable ultrasound or imaging devices.
  This minimizes the number of needlesticks the patient must undergo.
- For adults, you will usually use veins in the hand or arm; for infants, veins in the scalp or dorsum of the foot can also be used.
- If possible, select a vein on the patient's nondominant hand or arm.
  Helps to preserve functional ability.

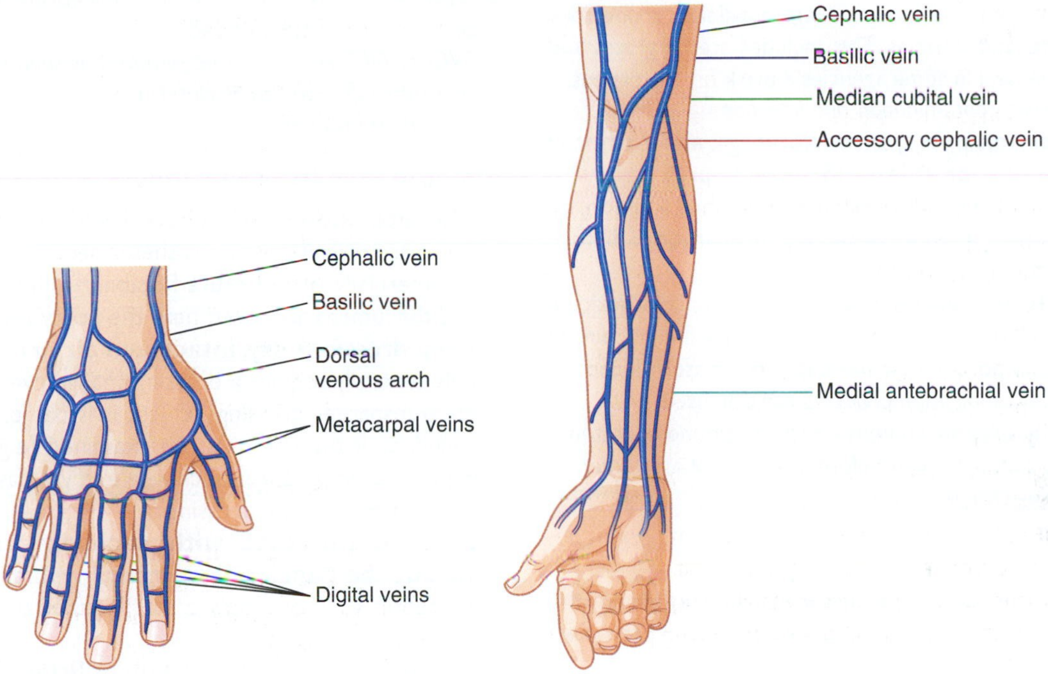

A Superficial veins of the hand **B Superficial veins of the forearm**

- Look for a vein that has a firm, round appearance with a relatively straight pathway. Do not use a red, hot, or hard vein.
- Avoid veins that are highly visible; they tend to roll.
- The cephalic vein of the arm is one of the best veins to use because it is relatively large, and the forearm provides a natural splint
- The dorsal veins of the hand are easy to access and are splinted by the metacarpals, but these veins are often quite small and fragile.
- Avoid the antecubital veins if possible. If the patient flexes her arm, the IV catheter may become displaced, so you would probably need to splint her elbow to prevent that. Furthermore, if a PICC line is needed at a later time, you will still have the antecubital veins available for it.
- For the following situations, you need to use the largest vein available, keeping other selection criteria in mind:
  - Hypertonic solutions, viscous solutions, or irritating medications
  - Rapid rates (also require a larger IV catheter)
- If the infusion is to be ongoing, begin the infusion with the best lowest vein and move proximal to the previous site (toward the heart) for subsequent insertions. Peripheral IV catheters are routinely changed no more frequently than every 72 to 96 hours (CDC, updated 2017).
  If you start the next IV below an already used site (i.e., to change the site or after a failed attempt at insertion), fluid may leak from the old site.
- Avoid areas at which the vein crosses over joints. If you must use such an area, splint the joint to limit movement.
  Splinting the joint helps preserve the vein for use, but it limits functional ability.
- Avoid areas with scarring, or with impaired circulation or neurological status (e.g., the affected arm following a mastectomy; an area with signs of infection, previous infiltration, or thrombosis; an arm with an arteriovenous fistula [shunt for dialysis]; or the affected side after cerebrovascular accident [stroke, brain attack]). **Key Point.** ***If you must use such an area, first obtain a medical prescription.***
- Do not use veins in the legs and feet unless there is no other option.
  Peripheral circulation may not be adequate in the lower limbs, so there is increased danger of thrombus formation. In adults, this location also interferes with mobility. Foot veins may be used for infants if the IV is taped securely.

Clinical Insight 38-4 ➤ Caring for Patients With a Central Venous Access Device (CVAD): CVC and PICC

Asepsis

- **Use good hand hygiene and follow agency protocols** for site care.
  To protect yourself and the patient.
- **Use strict aseptic technique** when manipulating injection ports, catheter hub and extension legs, needleless connectors, insertion site, and dressing. This includes sterile gloves and supplies, mask, and in some agencies a mask for the patient.
  To minimize line contamination and infection.
- **Scrub injection ports, extension legs, and catheter hubs** vigorously for at least 15 seconds, preferably with 70% alcohol, >0.5% chlorhexidine in alcohol solution, or iodophors (i.e., povidone-iodine) preparation, before accessing them (INS, 2016).
- **Appropriate antiseptics** include alcohol and chlorhexidine gluconate (CHG). Do not use povidone-iodine and tincture of iodine to scrub ports unless there is some reason alcohol or CHG-alcohol combination products can't be used.
- **Do not apply organic solvents,** such as acetone or acetone-based products, to the skin before insertion of a catheter or during dressing changes.

Assessments

- **Check the patient record for radiographic confirmation** of correct tip location before beginning prescribed therapies.
- **Inspect catheter–skin junction sites** through the transparent dressing and palpate for tenderness daily.
- **Do not remove transparent dressing except** when dressing change is required. If site is dressed with gauze, remove it to inspect the site.
  A high-risk route of infection is via migration of skin organisms at the insertion site into the cutaneous catheter tract, with colonization of the catheter tip.
- **Observe for excessive bleeding** at the insertion site.
  You may need to obtain a prescription for a topical hemostatic agent and use with a pressure dressing.
- **If symptoms of infection occur** (e.g., fever without obvious cause; redness, edema, induration, exudates, or tenderness at the site), remove the dressing and inspect the site directly. Anticipate that blood cultures will be needed from both the peripheral site and the central catheter.
- **Be aware that risk of infection is higher** with femoral catheters and with multilumen catheters.
  Multilumen catheters require more manipulation, which encourages more colonization and bacterial growth within the catheter lumen.
- **Assess for compromised catheter integrity** (wet dressing; kinked, cracked, or leaking external catheter).
- **Inspect catheter connections** and pump function, including flow rate.
- **Observe for symptoms of catheter migration** to the right atrium or ventricle (i.e., mid- to lower sternal pain, dysrhythmias).
- **If there are signs of complications,** notify the medical provider.
- **Assess the patient daily** for indications that the CVC or PICC line is still needed.
  CVCs or PICC line should be removed as soon as possible because the infection rate is closely related to the length of time the catheter is in place.

Maintenance Interventions

- **The site should be covered** with a semipermeable transparent dressing, the catheter secured with a sterile commercially manufactured stabilizer (instead of tape), and the lumens anchored near the ports with clear tape.
- **Keep dressings dry, intact, and air occlusive.** Protocols generally require a dressing change every 5 to 7 days for transparent dressings, unless it is damp, loosened, or soiled, or if the site must be examined (e.g., because of pain or odor). A dressing change every 2 days is required for a gauze and tape dressing.
- **Perform site care with each dressing change.** Cleanse the catheter–skin junction with an appropriate antiseptic solution, apply a sterile stabilizer, and apply a new sterile dressing.
- **Manipulate the catheter hub as little as possible.**
  To minimize catheter movement, phlebitis, and contamination of the line. Less catheter manipulation is associated with fewer bloodstream infections.
- **Flush catheters before and after any infusions** or per agency protocol. This may be every 12 to 24 hours when not in use.
  - **Flush volume** should be twice the volume of the catheter and add-on devices (consult package label).
  - **Use a syringe size recommended** by the catheter manufacturer (10 mL is the smallest size recommended because of the pressure generated).
  - **Type of flush solution depends on agency policy** (saline versus heparin).
  - **Use single-use, labeled syringes of flush solution** to prevent cross-contamination.
  - **If you have trouble flushing,** the catheter may be kinked or malpositioned, the inline filter may be clogged, or a clamp may need to be released. You can correct these problems.
  - **Never flush against resistance.**
    The catheter might be clogged, and you would risk dislodging a small clot. This could also rupture the catheter.
  - **If the patient has a PICC line,** take blood pressures on the alternate arm.

Clinical Insight 38-4 ➤ Caring for Patients With a Central Venous Access Device (CVAD): CVC and PICC—cont'd

Using the arm with the PICC can cause bleeding at the site, thrombus formation, retrograde blood flow, and increased risk of catheter occlusion.

- **If the patient is receiving parenteral nutrition,** reserve and label one lumen just for that purpose.

Documentation

- **Document routine assessments and the condition of the catheter–skin junction site.** When site care is given, also document the patient's response and any actions taken to correct or prevent adverse reactions.

Related Information

- **For information about dressing changes,** refer to Procedure 38-5B: Central Line Dressings.
- **For information about administering medications** through a CVAD, see Procedure 26-18: Administering Medication Through a Central Venous Access Device.

Practice Resources

CDC (2016); Infusion Nurses Society (2016); Marschall, J., Mermel, L., Fakih, M., et al. (2014).

Clinical Insight 38-5 ➤ Managing Infiltration and Extravasation

- At the first sign or symptom of infiltration or extravasation, stop the IV. Symptoms include slowed or stopped flow, swelling, tenderness, pallor, hardness, and coolness at the site. The patient may complain of pain or a burning sensation in the area.

For a Central Venous Access Device: CVC or PICC

- Clamp and cap the catheter hub.
- Do not remove the catheter.
- Follow agency policy when you suspect infiltration or extravasation.
- If the patient has an implanted port, aspirate, remove the port access needle, and apply a dressing.
- Notify the provider who inserted the catheter, who may order an x-ray to help determine the cause of the problem.

For a Short Peripheral Catheter

- Assess capillary refill, sensation, and motion distal to the infiltrated site.
- Disconnect the tubing from the catheter hub; attach a 3- to 5-mL syringe and try to aspirate fluid from the catheter lumen. Use aseptic technique.
- Photograph the site to create a record of its condition, if agency policy allows.
- Wearing gloves, remove the catheter and hold a dry gauze pad over the site to stop the bleeding. Apply a dry dressing.
- Do not apply excessive pressure to the site.
- Use a skin marker to outline the areas of infiltration/extravasation to monitor changes.
- If you need to start a new IV, use the other arm, if possible. If it is not possible, start it in a more proximal location on the same arm.
- Measure the circumference of the arm and compare it with the opposite arm.
- Apply cold or warm compresses, depending on which fluid has escaped into the tissues.
  - For alkaloids (e.g., vincristine) and epipodophyllotoxins (e.g., etoposide), use heat.
  - For nonirritant hypertonic fluids or medications, use dry, cold compresses.
  - For isotonic or hypotonic fluids or medications, choose either heat or cold, or alternate them, based on patient comfort.
- Apply compresses for 15 to 30 minutes every 4 to 6 hours; continue for 24 to 48 hours.
- Estimate the volume of fluid that escaped into the tissues; notify the prescriber.
- Some medications leaked into the surrounding tissue can cause damage and even necrosis. For instance, when dopamine extravasates, you might need to give a prescribed amount of antidote (e.g., phentolamine [Regitine] injected subcutaneously), as well as hydrocortisone and an anti-inflammatory to minimize tissue damage. Be sure to check the protocol at your facility.
- Elevate the extremity and advise the patient to rest.
- Document all fluids and medications involved, equipment being used (e.g., pump), size and type of the catheter, description of the site (including location, size, and color), methods used to assess the site before administering the fluids (e.g., aspiration), patient's signs and symptoms, interventions, notifications, and patient teaching.
- Complete an occurrence (or incident) report, as required by your facility.

Practice Resources

Gahart, B. & Nazareno, A. (2019). INS (2016)

ASSESSMENT GUIDELINES AND TOOLS

The following questions and guidelines will help you obtain subjective and objective data about patients' fluid, electrolyte, and acid–base balance.

Focused Assessment

Assessing Fluids, Electrolytes, and Acid–Base Balance

Nursing History

Demographic Data

Age, gender, height, weight, body mass index

Past Medical History

- Have you ever been hospitalized or had surgery? If so, when and for what reason?
- For what healthcare problems are you currently being treated?
- Have you ever been diagnosed with kidney disease, high blood pressure, diabetes, or thyroid or parathyroid problems?

Current Health Concerns

- What symptoms are you currently experiencing?
- Have you recently experienced any of the following symptoms?

Excessive thirst
Fever
Excessive perspiration
Nausea, vomiting, or diarrhea
Dry skin or mucous membranes
Dark, concentrated urine
Limited amounts of urine
Difficulty breathing
Swelling of your hands, feet, or ankles
Dizziness or feeling faint
Muscle weakness
Excessive fatigue
Numbness, tingling, or cramping sensations

- Is your weight stable? Have you had any recent changes in your weight?
- Do you believe you have any problems with fluid loss?

Food and Fluid Intake

- How much fluid do you usually drink in a 24-hour period?
- Do you believe you drink adequate amounts of fluid?
- Describe your usual diet.
- Have you recently changed your diet or fluid intake?
- Are you following a special diet?
- Have you ever been placed on a restricted diet?
- Have you experienced any recent changes in your appetite or thirst?
- Do you salt your food?
- Do you ever use a salt substitute?

Fluid Elimination

- How often do you urinate in a 24-hour period? Has that changed recently?
- How often do you get up during the night to urinate?
- Have you noticed any recent changes in the amount or appearance of your urine?
- How often do you experience vomiting, diarrhea, or constipation? Describe your experience.
- Do you have any wounds? If so, where are they and how did they happen? What is the color of drainage and how much drainage are you experiencing?
- Do you have any breaks in your skin? If so, describe the problem and show me the area.

Medications

- What prescribed medications do you currently take?
- What over-the-counter medications or alternative treatments do you use? Why do you use them?
- How often do you take laxatives or antacids?
- What vitamins, herbals, or supplements do you take?

Lifestyle

- What is your usual activity level?
- What type of exercise do you engage in? How often?
- How much fluid do you consume before, during, and after exercise?
- Do you drink alcohol? If so, how much do you consume in a day, a week?
- Do you smoke? If so, how much? For how long?
- Do you use any illegal medications or drugs?

Physical Assessments

Skin

Assess the skin for the following:

- Color and temperature may be cues to the presence of fever and circulation status.
- Moisture content offers some indication of fluid status. A diaphoretic client is losing fluid at a faster rate than a client with dry skin. Dry, scaling skin may indicate a fluid deficit. Any breaks in the skin are potential areas for fluid loss.
- Turgor varies with age, weight, and skin condition but does offer information on fluid status. Pinch the skin over the sternum. Normally skin immediately returns to its usual position. In fluid volume deficit or malnutrition the skin may remain "tented" for a period of time before returning to its original position. You must, however, correlate skin turgor with context and other clinical signs. For example, the skin loses elasticity with aging, so clients older than age 65 often have decreased turgor, which is normal for them.
- Edema in dependent areas is a cue for fluid volume excess. In an ambulatory client, assess the lower extremities and

Focused Assessment

Assessing Fluids, Electrolytes, and Acid–Base Balance—cont'd

hands. In a bedridden client, edema will shift as the client is turned.

- To grade edema (on a scale +1 to +4, +1 represents minimal edema and +4 represents the most severe edema),

Mucous Membranes

- Inspect the tongue and buccal mucosa. Mouth breathing alone usually does not change these areas.
- Assess tongue turgor in all age groups because it is not affected by age.
- Assess the color, moisture, and continuity of the mucous membranes
- Dry, cracked, or dull mucous membranes are signs of fluid volume deficit.

Cardiovascular System

- Assess vital signs (see later section).
- Pulse and blood pressure are affected by fluid and electrolyte status.
- If you suspect fluid volume deficit, assess for orthostatic hypotension:
  - Assess blood pressure while client is lying or sitting.
  - Have the client rise to a seated or standing position, and reassess the blood pressure (BP).
  - A drop in systolic BP of >15 mm Hg is a sign of orthostatic hypotension.
- Check capillary refill. Delayed capillary refill is a sign of fluid volume deficit; rapid capillary refill indicates adequate circulation and volume. If capillary refill is delayed, evaluate feet and hands bilaterally. Delays in just one area indicate impaired circulation to the extremity rather than volume changes.
- Assess venous filling by observing the jugular and hand veins. Flat jugular or hand veins indicate low fluid volume. Distended vessels are a sign of overload.
- Assess peripheral edema (discussed earlier).

Respiratory System

- Assess respiratory rate, depth, and pattern. The respiratory system rapidly responds to changes in pH. Similarly, alterations in gas exchange at the alveolar–capillary membrane may trigger pH changes.
- Assess breath sounds. Crackles or moist rales may indicate fluid overload. Areas of consolidation indicate impaired gas exchange.

Neurological System

- Assess level of consciousness and orientation.
- Assess neuromuscular irritability.
- Assess energy level and fatigue.
- Assess reflexes

For specific neurological cues to alterations in fluid, electrolyte, or acid–base balance,

Go to Chapter 38, **Table 38-5: Electrolyte Imbalances** and **Table 38-7: Acid-Base Imbalances,** in Volume 1.

Vital Signs

- Temperature. An elevated body temperature increases the loss of body fluids.

  In hypernatremia, body temperature elevates because less fluid is available for sweating.

  In uncomplicated fluid volume deficit, body temperature decreases.
- Pulse:
  - Tachycardia is an early sign of fluid volume deficit.
  - Pulse rate is affected by fluid status and some electrolytes (primarily sodium, potassium, calcium, and magnesium).
  - Dysrhythmias are seen with potassium and magnesium imbalances.

  The pulse volume is directly affected by fluid status. As fluid volume increases, the pulse volume also increases. Similarly, a drop in fluid volume leads to a drop in pulse volume.
- Respiratory rate. Alterations in respiratory rate may cause acid–base imbalances or be associated with compensation for a metabolic disorder.
- Blood pressure:
  - Assess for orthostatic hypotension (a drop in the systolic BP from lying or sitting to standing positions greater or equal to 20 mm Hg).
  - Blood pressure rises and falls with fluid volume.
  - Blood pressure is elevated by hypernatremia and fluid volume excess.
  - Respiratory acidosis causes increased heart rate, resulting in BP elevation.
  - High potassium intake may lower blood pressure.

Daily Weights

Daily weights are an accurate method of assessing fluid status.

- Use the same balanced scale each day to monitor fluid status accurately.
- Weigh the client at the same time of day, making sure that the client is wearing the same amount of clothing.
- Each kilogram (2.2 lb) of weight is equivalent to 1 liter (1,000 mL) of fluid.
- For clients undergoing hemodialysis (blood cleansing through an artificial kidney), weigh the client before and after dialysis treatments. Many lose 3 to 4 kg (6.6 to 8.8 lb) after several hours of dialysis.
- You may institute weight monitoring as an independent nursing prescription, which can be delegated to an assistive personnel.
- Important when it is impractical or impossible to measure I&O accurately (breastfeeding intake, incontinence, draining wounds).

Fluid Intake and Output

See Clinical Insight 38-2.

DIAGNOSTIC TESTING

Diagnostic Testing

Assessing Fluid, Electrolyte, and Acid–Base Balances

Venous Blood Sample	Normal Ranges
Sodium	135–145 mEq/L
Potassium	3.5–5 mEq/L
Chloride	97–107 mEq/L
Bicarbonate	22–26 mEq/L
BUN	10–31 mg/dL
Creatinine	0.5–1.2 mg/dL
Serum osmolality	275–295 mOsm/kg
Urine osmolality	250–900 mOsm/kg
Hematocrit	43%–49% in men
	38%–44% in menstruating women
Freshly Voided Urine Sample	
pH	5.0–9.0
Specific gravity	1.001–1.029
Arterial Blood Sample	
pH	7.35–7.45
P_{CO_2}	35–45 mm Hg
HCO_3^-	22–26 mEq/L

CLINICALJUDGMENT

Applying the Full-Spectrum Nursing Model

PATIENT SITUATION

Darlene Malone, age 42, has been admitted to the emergency department with complaints of fatigue, extreme weakness, and heart palpitations. She says she has not seen a healthcare provider in nearly 10 years. Suddenly, she slumps and falls over. She is not breathing, has no pulse, and does not respond to verbal stimuli. She is resuscitated with CPR and IV epinephrine, and an endotracheal tube is placed. STAT lab results show a potassium level of 7.7 mEq/L, BUN of 102 mg/dL, and creatinine of 5 mg/dL. A physician diagnoses acute renal failure. Among other interventions, an IV is started to administer 10% calcium chloride solution, 1,000 mg, by slow IV push to counteract the toxic effects of hyperkalemia on the cell membranes. The nurse used a 20-gauge over-the-needle catheter in Ms. Malone's right cephalic vein, about 5 cm (2 in.) above her wrist.

THINKING

1. *Theoretical Knowledge:*
   a. Which lab results are abnormal? Are they high or low?
   b. Which lab results directly reflect her renal failure?
   c. What term correctly describes serum potassium of 7.7 mEq/L?

2. *Critical Thinking (Considering Alternatives):*

   a. What do you think is causing Ms. Malone to have hyperkalemia? You should be able to think this through and make a reasonable guess even if you have not studied pathophysiology.

   b. Ms. Malone is to be given 50 mEq of sodium bicarbonate by slow IV push for an acid–base imbalance that is often associated with hyperkalemia. Which imbalance do you think would be treated with sodium bicarbonate: metabolic acidosis or metabolic alkalosis?

DOING

3. *Practical Knowledge:*

   a. When you prepare to administer the sodium bicarbonate (in question 2b), you notice that the IV infusion is barely flowing and that the insertion site is swollen and pale. What is the first thing you should do?

   b. You aspirate the catheter and do not obtain a blood return. Ms. Malone absolutely must have this medication. Describe what you would do in the order you would do it.

4. *Nursing Process (Planning Goals):* NOC outcome best suited to evaluating Ms. Malone's hyperkalemia is Electrolyte & Acid–Base Imbalance. Based on the function of this electrolyte, what is the primary indicator that you could use to evaluate her goal achievement for this problem?

CARING

5. *Self-Knowledge:* Ms. Malone will need dialysis to replace her inadequate renal function and control her serum potassium level. It is likely that her renal failure was brought on by years of illegal drug abuse. She has never held a full-time job and has not worked at all for the past 7 years. Her dialysis treatments will need to be paid for by Medicaid, which is funded by tax dollars. How do you feel about this—specifically, how do you feel about the issues of (a) a person's responsibility for her own health and (b) compassion for people who cannot afford to pay for healthcare? Focus on your own feelings, not on issues of what "should" be done.

Critical Thinking and Clinical Judgment

1. Recall the Meet Your Patients scenario in Volume 1. When you review Jackson LaGuardia's medical records to prepare for the clinical day, you find that he is in the emergency department (ED) with four other members of the LaGuardia family. All of them have come to the ED complaining of nausea, vomiting, and diarrhea related to severe gastroenteritis, a viral intestinal disorder. The family members include the following:

   8-month-old Jason, grandson of Jackson

   26-year-old Susanna, Jackson's daughter and Jason's mother

   60-year-old Jackson

   58-year-old Gemma, Jackson's wife

   82-year-old Martha, Jackson's mother

   Jason, Jackson, and Martha are being admitted to the hospital. However, Susanna and Gemma have been asked to follow up tomorrow in the urgent care clinic. The following questions pertain to this scenario.

   a. Martha LaGuardia's prescriptions call for lactated Ringer's solution with 20 mEq KCl per liter to infuse at 150 mL/hr. After 4 hours of infusion, Martha begins to complain of shortness of breath and develops a cough. What do you suspect may be happening? What actions should you take?

b. What theoretical knowledge will you use in caring for Ms. LaGuardia's immediate problem?

c. Jason LaGuardia has been prescribed 250 mL of 0.9% saline solution over 8 hours. What type of equipment should you consider using?

d. Calculate the drip rate for Jason's infusion if a gravity flow device is used. What further information do you need to perform this calculation?

e. As you may recall, Jackson LaGuardia has end-stage renal disease. His lab work reveals a hemoglobin of 7.6 mg/dL and a hematocrit of 21%. He has been prescribed two units of packed red blood cells over 8 hours. Given his condition, for what fluid balance problem is he at risk? What additional parameters should you assess while he is receiving the transfusion?

2. You are asked to administer an antibiotic intravenously via piggyback. You are not familiar with the equipment that this facility uses. As a student, what approach should you take to solve this problem?

3. Identify techniques that you have observed that may contribute to contamination of an IV site.

4. Interpret the following ABG results. Explain your thinking.

a. pH 7.47	Pco_2 45 mm Hg	HCO_3^- 32 mEq/L
b. pH 7.32	Pco_2 50 mm Hg	HCO_3^- 25 mEq/L
c. pH 7.30	Pco_2 41 mm Hg	HCO_3^- 18 mEq/L
d. pH 7.45	Pco_2 30 mm Hg	HCO_3^- 22 mEq/L

5. For each of the following concepts, use critical thinking to describe how or why it is important to nursing; patient care; or fluids, electrolytes, and acid–base balance. Note that these are *not* to be merely definitions.

Homeostasis

Selectively permeable membranes

Fluid imbalance

Electrolyte imbalances

Acid–base imbalances

Parenteral fluid and electrolyte replacement

What Are the Main Points in This Chapter?

- Water is the largest single constituent of the body. Total body water content varies with age, gender, and the number of fat cells.
- Intracellular fluid (ICF) is contained within the cells. It is essential for cell function and metabolism and accounts for approximately 40% of body weight.
- Extracellular fluid (ECF) consists of three types of fluid: interstitial, intravascular, and transcellular fluid. ECF carries water, electrolytes, nutrients, and oxygen to the cells and removes the waste products of cell metabolism. ECF accounts for 20% of body weight.
- Electrolytes that carry a positive charge are called cations. These include sodium (Na^+), potassium (K^+), calcium (Ca^{2+}), and magnesium (Mg^{2+}). Electrolytes that carry a negative charge are called anions.
- Potassium and magnesium are the major cations in the ICF. Phosphate and sulfate are the major anions.
- The major electrolytes of ECF are sodium, chloride, and bicarbonate. Albumin is also present in the ECF.

- The functions of the major electrolytes include the following:
  - Sodium is essential to regulate fluid volume.
  - Chloride works with sodium to regulate osmotic pressure, and with the bicarbonate buffer system to regulate acid–base balance.
  - Potassium is essential for cellular metabolism.
  - Calcium is responsible for bone health and neuromuscular and cardiac function, and is an essential factor in blood clotting.
  - Magnesium is a mineral used in more than 300 biochemical reactions in the body.
  - Phosphorus is important in the formation of bones and teeth and has an inverse relationship with calcium.
- Osmosis, diffusion, filtration, and active transport are mechanisms used to maintain a balance between fluids and solutes in the body.
- General recommendations for total fluid intake are 2,700 mL per day for women and 3,700 mL per day for men.
- When the body is in a healthy state, fluid losses through urine, skin, insensible losses, and feces are equivalent to fluid intake.
- Fluid volume deficit occurs when there is a proportional loss of water and electrolytes from the ECF.
- Fluid volume excess involves excessive retention of sodium and water in the ECF.
- Bicarbonate is important in acid–base regulation and is regulated by the kidneys to maintain pH.
- The amount of acid or base present in a solution is measured as pH. The pH is reported on a scale of 1 to 14, with 1 to 6.9 being acidic, 7 neutral, and 7.1 to 14 basic, or alkaline. Normal blood pH is slightly alkalotic, between 7.35 and 7.45.
- A buffer system consists of a weak acid and a weak base. These molecules react with strong acids or bases to keep them from altering the pH by either absorbing free hydrogen ions or releasing free hydrogen ions. The principal buffer system in the ECF is the carbonic acid (H_2CO_3) and sodium bicarbonate ($NaHCO_3^-$) system.
- When the serum pH falls below 7.35, the patient is acidotic. When the serum pH increases above 7.45, the patient is alkalotic. ABGs are used to monitor acid–base balance.
- When the serum pH is too acidic (pH is low), the lungs remove carbon dioxide through rapid, deep breathing. If the serum pH is too alkaline (pH is high), the lungs try to conserve carbon dioxide through shallow respirations.
- The kidneys affect pH by regulating the amount of bicarbonate (base) that is kept in the body.
- Assessment of a client's fluid, electrolyte, and acid–base balance includes history; laboratory data; physical examination of the skin, mucous membranes, and neurological status; and assessment of cardiovascular and respiratory systems.
- I&O are monitored to assess fluid status. To monitor, measure all fluids consumed and excreted in a 24-hour period.
- Tests used to monitor fluid, electrolyte, and acid–base balance include serum electrolytes and osmolality, complete blood count, urinalysis, and measurement of arterial blood gases.
- Nursing interventions for patients experiencing alterations in fluid, electrolyte, or acid-base balance include preventing imbalances modifying oral intake, providing parenteral replacement, and transfusing blood products.
- Intravenous fluids are classified as isotonic, hypotonic, and hypertonic solutions, based on their comparison to the osmolality of blood serum.
- Vascular access devices may provide access to peripheral or central veins.
- Intravenous equipment consists of the IV catheter, an administration set, extension tubing, and the IV solution.
- Nurses are responsible for using established formulas to calculate and maintain the correct rate of flow and for monitoring the client's response to the infusion.
- Assess for local IV site complications (e.g., infiltration, extravasation, infection, thrombus, and thrombophlebitis) and systemic complications (e.g. fluid volume excess, sepsis, and embolus).
- Meticulous aseptic technique is required for initiation and care of intravenous infusions to prevent bloodstream infection.
- Blood products are infused when the client has experienced significant blood loss, diminished oxygen-carrying capacity, or a deficiency in one of the blood components.
- Nurses must administer the correct blood type to patients to prevent a hemolytic reaction.

Knowledge Map

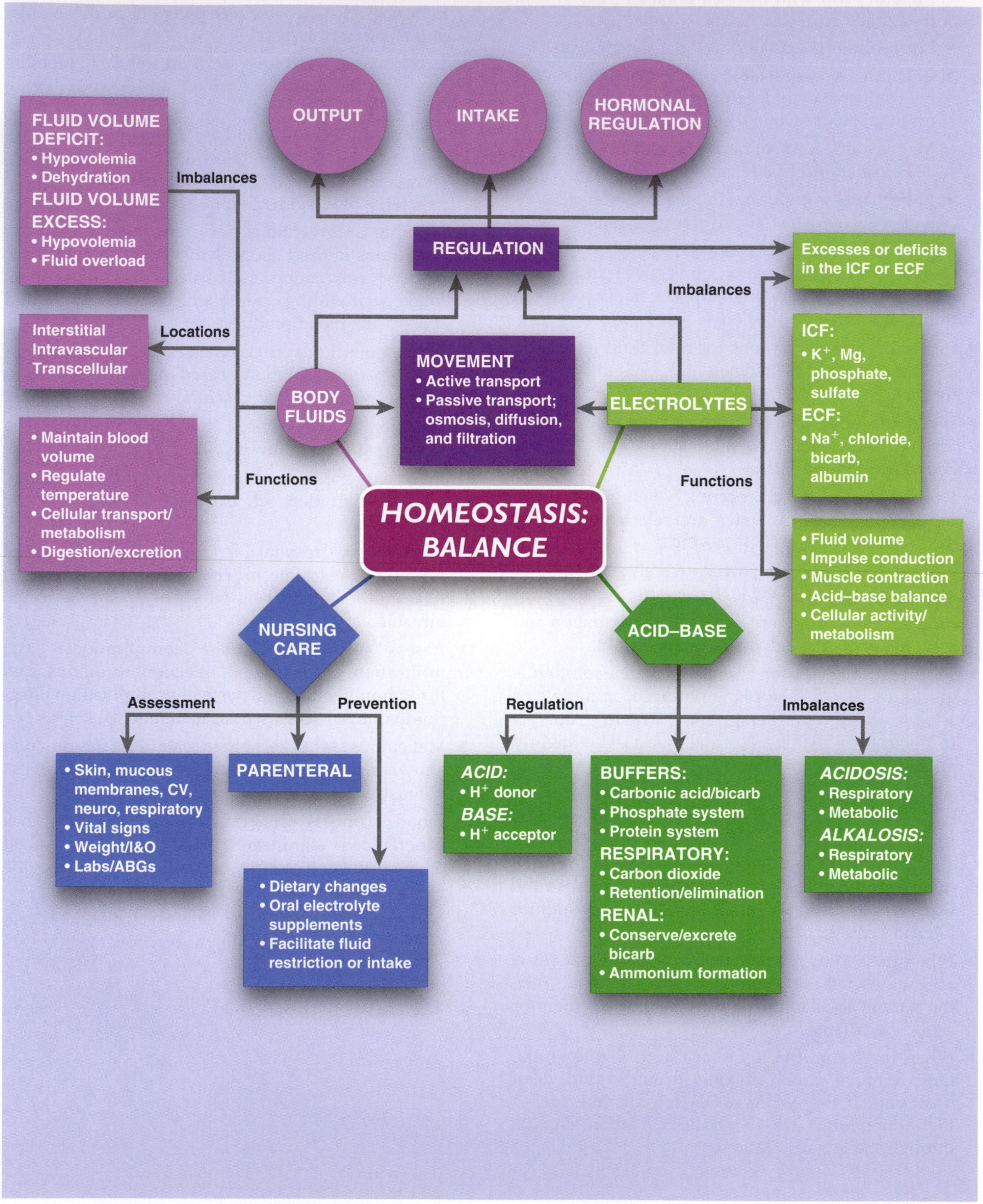

UNIT 5

Nursing Functions

CHAPTER 39

Perioperative Care

STUDENT RESOURCES

The questions and exercises in this book allow you to practice the kind of thinking you will use as a full-spectrum nurse. Critical-thinking questions usually have more than one right answer, so we do not provide "correct answers" for these features. Try to answer these questions yourself. It is more important to develop your nursing judgment than to just cover content. You will learn more by discussing the questions with your peers. If you are still unsure, see the Davis Advantage chapter resources for suggested responses.

To explore learning resources for this chapter,

Go to Davis Advantage and find:

Answers and Suggested Responses for all questions in this chapter

Concept Map

Knowledge Map

References and Bibliography

Lists of NOC Outcomes and NIC Interventions

Key Concepts

Intraoperative care

Perioperative nursing

Preoperative care

Postoperative care

Related Concepts

See the Concept Map on Davis Advantage.

Caring for the Nguyens

Mai Nguyen, the 76-year-old mother of Nam Nguyen, has been experiencing blurred vision and decreased visual acuity. A local ophthalmologist diagnosed bilateral cataracts. The ophthalmologist has recommended cataract removal in the left eye, with insertion of an intraocular lens. He told Mrs. Nguyen to schedule the surgery "at your convenience" and explained that the surgery would be performed on an outpatient basis. The ophthalmologist gave Mrs. Nguyen the following list of activities to prepare for the surgery:

- Schedule a date for your surgery. My receptionist will set up a time for your surgery. All surgeries are performed

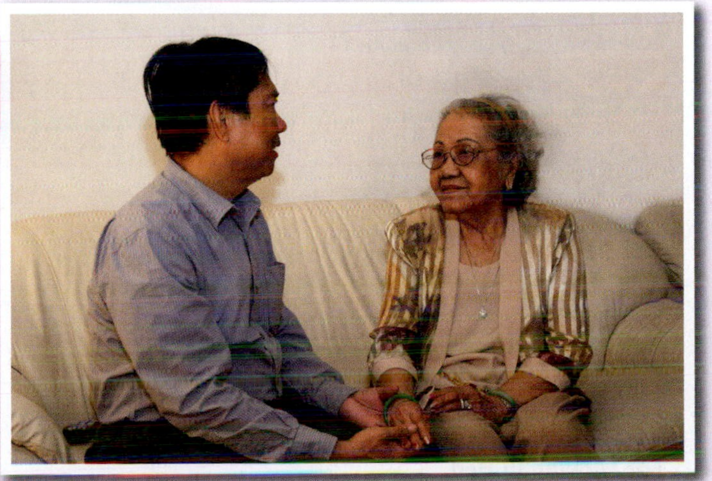

(Continued)

Caring for the Nguyens (continued)

at Western Medical Center Same-Day Surgery Department.

- Please arrange to be seen by your primary care provider 1 to 2 weeks prior to the surgery to receive clearance for surgery.
- Make an appointment with the Preoperative Center at Western Medical Center Same-Day Surgery Department 1 to 2 days before surgery.
- Arrange to have a ride to and from the surgery.

A. What preoperative testing is Mrs. Nguyen likely to undergo? Explain your rationale.

B. The preoperative list states that the client must be seen by the primary care provider to receive clearance for surgery. Why is this an essential part of the preoperative period?

C. What theoretical knowledge do you need to perform preoperative teaching for Mrs. Nguyen? How could you obtain that information? Be specific about your sources.

D. What content would you include in Mrs. Nguyen's preoperative teaching?

E. The ophthalmologist has planned anesthesia via conscious sedation. What factors, if any, might keep Mrs. Nguyen from receiving this form of anesthesia? What additional information do you need to answer this question?

PracticalKnowledge clinical application

Perioperative nursing care includes procedures and techniques designed for prevention and early detection of complications. Recall that full-spectrum nursing involves thinking, doing, and caring—all are equally important, in perioperative as well as other settings.

PROCEDURES

The procedures in this section will help you to prevent postoperative complications. Preoperative teaching of coughing, deep breathing, moving in bed, and leg exercises help to prevent thrombophlebitis, atelectasis, and pneumonia. Antiembolism stockings and sequential compression devices are designed to promote peripheral circulation and prevent thrombus formation. Gastrointestinal suction is used to relieve or prevent abdominal distention.

Procedure 39-1 ■ Teaching a Patient to Deep-Breathe, Cough, Move in Bed, and Perform Leg Exercises

➤ For steps to follow in *all* procedures, refer to the Universal Steps for All Procedures found on the inside back cover.

Equipment

For Teaching Deep Breathing and Coughing

- Folded blanket or a pillow (if teaching will include splinting of a surgical incision site)
- Tissues

For Moving in Bed

- Small pillow or folded blanket
- Pillows

Delegation

You or another registered nurse (RN) should perform the initial teaching. You may delegate reinforcement of the teaching to a licensed vocational nurse/licensed practical nurse (LVN/LPN) or unlicensed assistive personnel (UAP).

Pre-Procedure Assessments

- Assess the patient's cognitive level and level of consciousness.
  Helps assess the patient's ability to understand and follow directions and select the appropriate teaching method.

- Assess the patient's pain level.
  Even preoperatively, pain must be well controlled to ensure full patient participation.
- Determine whether the surgical procedure and/or a physical disability will limit the patient's participation.
  For example, a fractured arm that has not yet been repaired will impair the patient's ability to hold a pillow for splinting.
- Determine whether the surgical procedure may entail special exercises or equipment. In addition, assess for any special equipment, such as braces, slings, or abductor wedges that may be needed when turning a patient in bed.

Knee and hip surgeries often involve special exercises or equipment postoperatively. Consult the surgeon before teaching the patient any leg exercises. Spinal and neurological surgeries often limit movement in the postoperative period. For example, some spinal surgeries require the patient to logroll (move from head to toe as one unit). Some neurological procedures require limiting the amount of time the patient's head of bed is above 30°. Identify these restrictions preoperatively, and inform the patient and family about them during your teaching session.

- Assess the patient's belief about the ability of the surgical incision to remain intact.
  If the patient believes that the incision will not stay together if he coughs or moves, he is less likely to comply.

Procedure 39-1A ■ Teaching a Patient to Deep-Breathe and Cough

➤ When performing the procedure, always identify your patient according to agency policy, using two identifiers, and be attentive to standard precautions, hand hygiene, patient safety and privacy, body mechanics, and documentation.

Deep breathing and coughing expand the lungs, improve ventilation, promote gas exchange, and help prevent atelectasis and pneumonia. Coughing after deep breathing mobilizes secretions, which keeps airways and alveoli open and provides greater surface area for gas exchange.

Procedure Steps

1. **Assist the patient to a Fowler's or semi-Fowler's position,** with the shoulders relaxed.
   Allows for best chest and lung expansion.
2. **Assist the patient who will have a chest or abdominal incision** to practice splinting the site with a folded blanket or pillow (see the photo in column 2).
   Counterpressure supports the incision and decreases pain. ➤

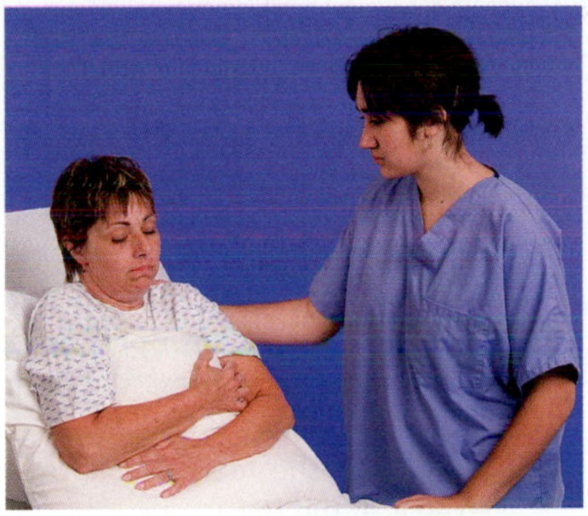

3. **Teach the patient diaphragmatic/deep breathing.** Tell the patient to:
   a. Place her hands anteriorly, along the lower end of the rib cage. The tips of the third fingers should touch at the midline.
   b. Slowly take a deep breath in through the nose. Tell the patient that she should feel her chest expanding as the diaphragm moves down.
   c. Hold her breath for 2 to 5 seconds.
   Stimulates surfactant production and helps prevent alveolar collapse.
   d. Slowly and completely exhale the breath through her mouth.
4. **Teach the patient to cough** in conjunction with diaphragmatic breathing. Instruct her to:
   a. Complete two or three cycles of diaphragmatic breathing.
   b. On the next breath in, have the patient lean forward and cough rapidly, through an open mouth, using the muscles of the abdomen, thighs, and buttocks. Cough several times on that breath.
   This information helps the patient to distinguish coughing from merely clearing her throat.

For a Patient Experiencing Weakness

If the patient is too weak to perform this maneuver, have the patient inhale deeply, bend forward slightly, and perform three or four "huffs" against an open glottis to move secretions forward.

Procedure 39-1B ■ Teaching a Patient to Move in Bed

➤ When performing the procedure, always identify your patient according to agency policy, using two identifiers, and be attentive to standard precautions, hand hygiene, patient safety and privacy, body mechanics, and documentation.

Moving in bed promotes blood circulation, stimulates respiratory function, and helps mobilize gas in the intestines.

Procedure Steps

1. **Start with the patient in** supine position, bedrails up. Then instruct the patient as follows.
2. **To turn to the left side:** Bend the right leg, sliding the foot flat along the bed and flexing the knee.
   Enables the patient to push herself over to the opposite side.

(continued on next page)

Procedure 39-1 ■ Teaching a Patient to Deep-Breathe, Cough, Move in Bed, and Perform Leg Exercises (continued)

3. **Reach the right arm across the chest,** and grasp the opposite bedrail.
   Helps the patient to turn, reduces the need to use the abdominal muscles for turning, and minimizes incision pain.

4. **Breathe deeply, and practice splinting** any potential abdominal or chest incisions. Assist the patient to practice as needed.
   Facilitates comfort during movement.

5. **Pull on the bedrail** while pushing off with the right foot.
   Assists patient to turn to the left.

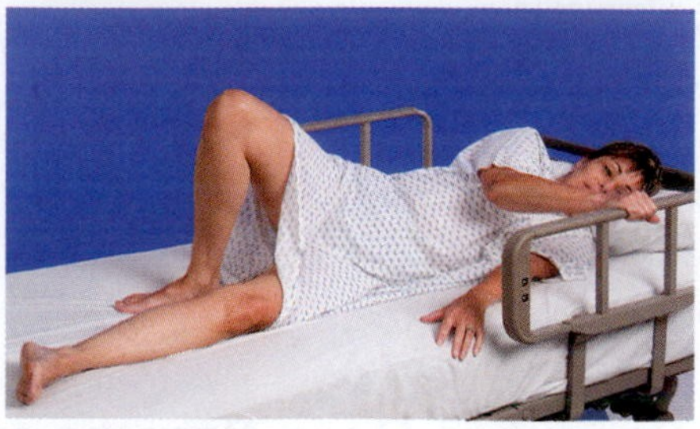

6. **If the patient cannot maintain** this position independently, place a folded pillow or blanket along her back for support.

7. **Teach the patient to change** positions every 2 hours, repeating the turning process with the opposite arm and leg. For patients who need pillows placed for support, you will need to assist with turning.

Procedure 39-1C ■ Teaching Leg Exercises

➤ When performing the procedure, always identify your patient according to agency policy, using two identifiers, and be attentive to standard precautions, hand hygiene, patient safety and privacy, body mechanics, and documentation.

Leg exercises flex and extend the leg muscles to increase peripheral circulation and help prevent thrombus formation. Thrombus formation is a common postoperative complication.

Procedure Steps

1. **Instruct the patient to lie supine** in the bed.

   NOTE: Although these exercises can be done when the patient is up in a chair, the effect will be diminished by the effects of gravity.

2. **Perform ankle circles.** Instruct the patient to:
   a. Start with one foot in the dorsiflexed position.
   b. Slowly rotate the ankle clockwise.
   c. After three rotations, repeat the procedure in a counterclockwise direction.
   d. Repeat this exercise at least three times in each direction, then switch and exercise the other ankle.

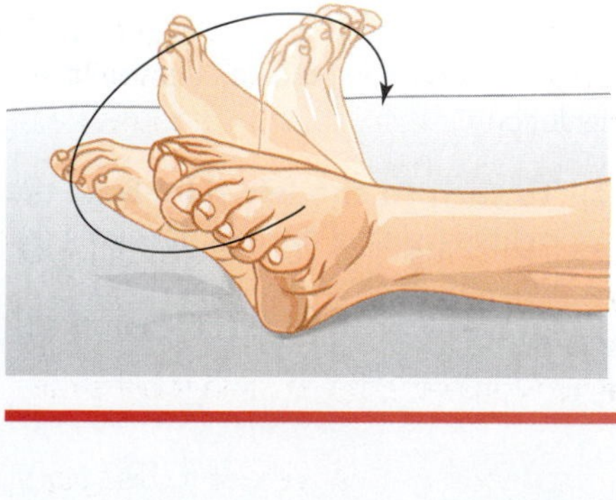

3. **Perform ankle pumps.** Instruct the patient to do the following:
   a. Start with one foot, leg extended.
   b. Point the toe until her foot is plantar flexed.
   c. Pull the toes back toward her head until the foot is dorsiflexed; at the same time, press the back of the knee into the bed.
   d. Make sure she feels a pull, or a stretch, in the calf.
   e. Repeat the alternation between plantar and dorsiflexion several times.
   f. Repeat the cycle with the other foot.

4. **Perform leg exercises.** Instruct the patient to:
   a. Lie supine in the bed.
   b. Slowly begin bending one knee, sliding the sole of the foot along the bed until the knee is in a flexed position.

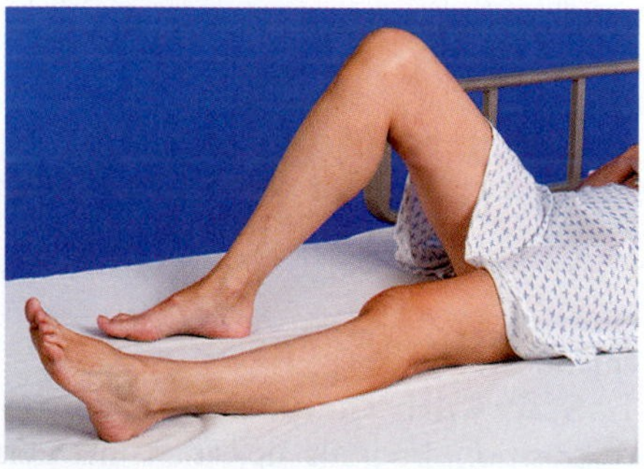

   c. Reverse the motion, extending the knee until the leg is once again flat on the bed.

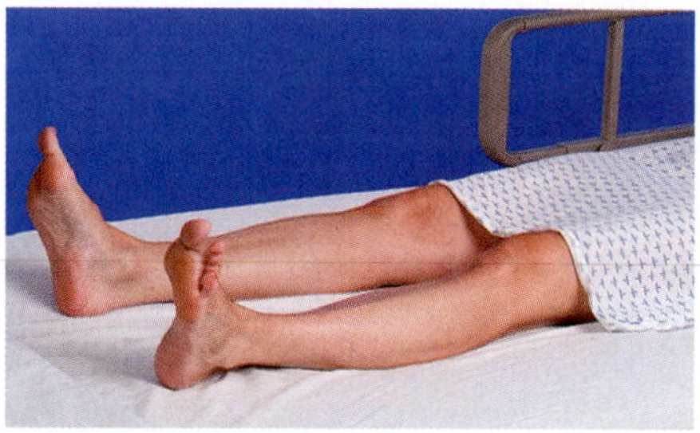

   d. Repeat several times.
   e. Repeat using the opposite leg.

? What if . . .

- **The patient has had knee, hip, or back surgery?**
  Leg exercises may be contraindicated in patients having knee, hip, or back surgery. Check the surgeon's prescriptions and/or collaborate with the physical therapist.

- **The patient has had nasal, ophthalmic, or neurological surgery?**
  Coughing and deep-breathing exercises are contraindicated.
  To avoid increasing intracranial pressure.

Evaluation

Make sure that the patient performs correctly a return demonstration of the procedures taught.

Documentation

In many healthcare facilities, checklists and charts have special areas in which to document patient teaching. Documentation should identify the person who completed the teaching, the person to whom the procedures were taught, what procedures were taught, and whether the patient understood the teaching. Also include the name and type of any printed materials given.

Sample electronic documentation

Note that because this is just one screen of a documentation system, not all of the information is visible. For example, you cannot see the date or the name of the nurse.

Practice Resources

Cao & Zhang (2015); Vancouver Coastal Health (2014).

Thinking About the Procedure

The videos **Teaching a Patient to Deep-Breathe and Cough, Teaching a Patient to Move in Bed,** and **Teaching Leg Exercises,** along with questions and suggested responses, is available on the ***Davis's Nursing Skills Videos*** Web site on FADavis.com.

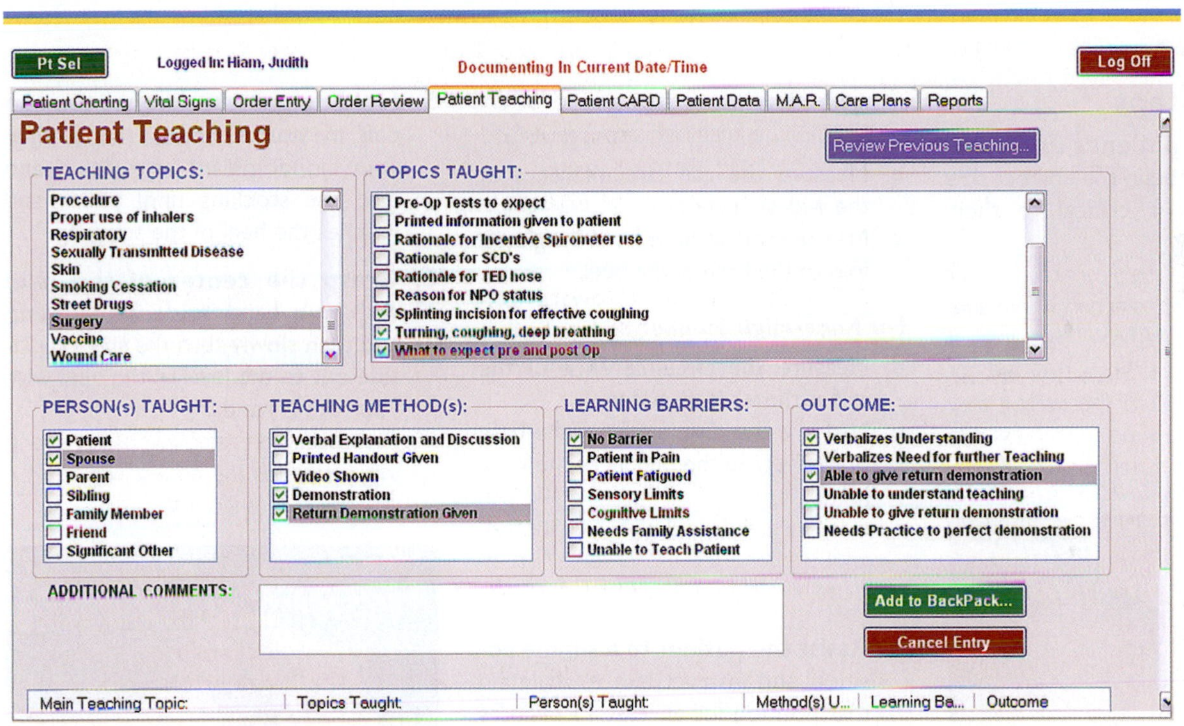

Pt Sel | Logged In: Hiam, Judith | Documenting In Current Date/Time | Log Off

Patient Charting | Vital Signs | Order Entry | Order Review | Patient Teaching | Patient CARD | Patient Data | M.A.R. | Care Plans | Reports

Patient Teaching

Review Previous Teaching...

TEACHING TOPICS:
- Procedure
- Proper use of inhalers
- Respiratory
- Sexually Transmitted Disease
- Skin
- Smoking Cessation
- Street Drugs
- Surgery
- Vaccine
- Wound Care

TOPICS TAUGHT:
- ☐ Pre-Op Tests to expect
- ☐ Printed information given to patient
- ☐ Rationale for Incentive Spirometer use
- ☐ Rationale for SCD's
- ☐ Rationale for TED hose
- ☐ Reason for NPO status
- ☑ Splinting incision for effective coughing
- ☑ Turning, coughing, deep breathing
- ☑ What to expect pre and post Op

PERSON(s) TAUGHT:
- ☑ Patient
- ☑ Spouse
- ☐ Parent
- ☐ Sibling
- ☐ Family Member
- ☐ Friend
- ☐ Significant Other

TEACHING METHOD(s):
- ☑ Verbal Explanation and Discussion
- ☐ Printed Handout Given
- ☐ Video Shown
- ☑ Demonstration
- ☑ Return Demonstration Given

LEARNING BARRIERS:
- ☑ No Barrier
- ☐ Patient in Pain
- ☐ Patient Fatigued
- ☐ Sensory Limits
- ☐ Cognitive Limits
- ☐ Needs Family Assistance
- ☐ Unable to Teach Patient

OUTCOME:
- ☑ Verbalizes Understanding
- ☐ Verbalizes Need for further Teaching
- ☑ Able to give return demonstration
- ☐ Unable to understand teaching
- ☐ Unable to give return demonstration
- ☐ Needs Practice to perfect demonstration

ADDITIONAL COMMENTS:

Add to BackPack...

Cancel Entry

Main Teaching Topic: | Topics Taught: | Person(s) Taught: | Method(s) U... | Learning Ba... | Outcome

Procedure 39-2 ■ Applying Antiembolism Stockings

➤ For steps to follow in *all* procedures, refer to the Universal Steps for All Procedures found on the inside back cover.

Equipment

- Measuring tape
- Antiembolism stockings
- Disposable wipes or washcloth and towel (if needed to cleanse legs)
- Talcum powder (optional: check manufacturer's recommendations)

Delegation

You can delegate application of antiembolism stockings to UAP who have been trained in the task. Instruct the UAP as follows:

- Report the presence of any abnormalities on the lower extremities, such as lesions, sores, or redness, before applying the stockings.
- Instruct the patient to maintain a recumbent position for at least 15 minutes before applying the stockings.
- Do not massage the legs.
- Make sure there are no wrinkles in the stockings once they have been applied.

(continued on next page)

Procedure 39-2 ■ Applying Antiembolism Stockings (continued)

Pre-Procedure Assessments

- **Assess the level of consciousness and cognitive ability.**
  If the patient is unconscious or confused, you will need to call for assistance to hold and stabilize the lower extremities as you apply the stockings.
- **Assess for signs and symptoms of severe peripheral arterial disease, such as weak or absent pulses, discoloration or cyanosis, or gangrene.**
  Antiembolism stockings should not be used in patients with any of these findings because stockings compress the vessels and, therefore, further impede the already compromised arterial flow.
- **Assess skin condition. Note lesions, dermatitis, or major edema, as evidenced by shiny, taut skin.**
  If skin is overstretched by edema, antiembolism stockings may irritate or worsen skin conditions and cause skin breakdown.
- **Note the patient's position and length of time she has been in that position.**
  Place the patient supine for at least 15 minutes before stocking application. This prevents trapping of pooled venous blood.

➤ When performing the procedure, always identify your patient according to agency policy, using two identifiers, and be attentive to standard precautions, hand hygiene, patient safety and privacy, body mechanics, and documentation.

➤ If possible, apply stockings in the morning, before the patient gets out of bed. This prevents venous distention and edema that occur when the patient is sitting or standing.

Procedure Steps

1. **Measure the patient's lower extremities** to obtain the correct size stockings. This is critical to their effectiveness.
   Stockings must be sized correctly in order to apply the correct amounts of pressure at the ankle, mid-calf, and upper thigh. If they are not tight enough, they will not improve venous return effectively. If they are too tight, they may compress the veins and impair circulation to the skin.▼

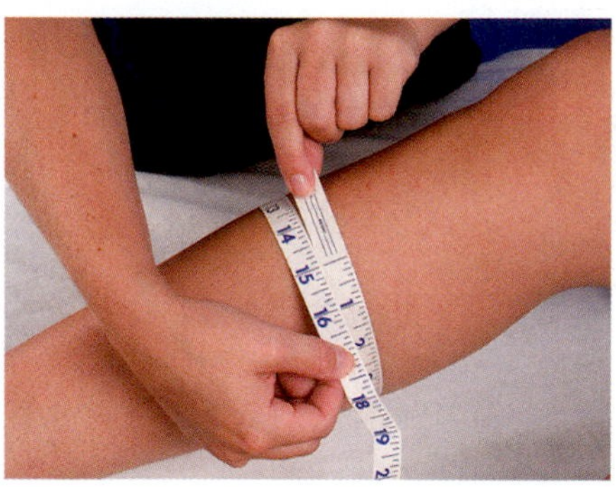

For Thigh-High Stockings

NOTE: *Thigh-high elastic stockings have not been proved to be more effective in preventing thromboembolism than knee-high ones, and should probably be avoided because of the tendency to roll and have a tourniquet effect (Gerhard-Herman, Gornik, Barrett, et al., 2017).*

   a. Measure the circumference of the upper thigh at the gluteal fold.
   The manufacturer of thromboembolic deterrent (TED) stockings recommends that thigh-high stockings not be applied if the thigh circumference exceeds 82 cm (32 in.). Use knee-high stockings instead.

   b. Measure the calf circumference at the widest section.

   c. Measure the distance from the gluteal fold to the base of the heel.

For Knee-High Stockings

   d. Measure the circumference of the calf at the widest section.

   e. Measure the distance from the base of the heel to the middle of the knee joint.
   Evidence is not conclusive, but it increasingly supports the use of knee-high instead of thigh-high hose.

2. **Assist the patient to a supine** position, and instruct him to maintain that position for at least 15 minutes before you apply the stockings.
   Prevents trapping of pooled venous blood by the antiembolism stockings.

3. **Cleanse the patient's legs and** feet if necessary. Dry well.
   Removing surface dirt and bacteria will decrease the likelihood of infection and odor.

4. **Lightly dust the legs and feet** with talcum powder to ease the application of the stockings, if recommended by the manufacturer. **Key Point:** ***Do not use powder if the patient is or is likely to become diaphoretic. Powder eases the application of the stockings, but perspiration will cause the powder to clump.***

5. **Holding one stocking at the top** cuff in your dominant hand, slide your nondominant arm down and into the stocking until your hand reaches the heel of the stocking.

6. **Grasp the center of the heel** with your hand inside the stocking, and then slowly turn the stocking inside out to the level of the heel with your other hand.
   The elastic in the stockings is very strong; this method is the easiest way to fit it over the foot and calf.▼

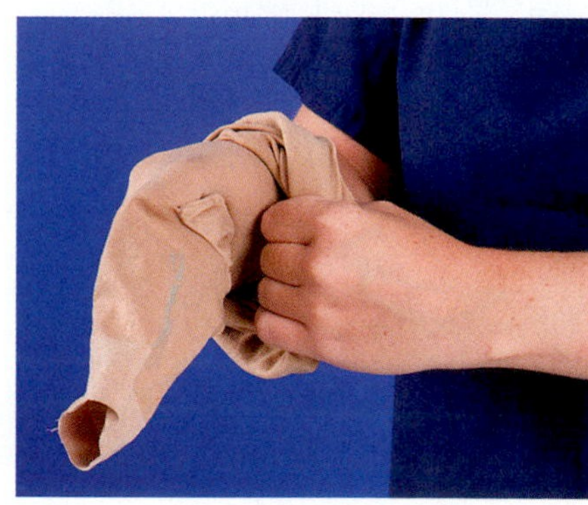

7. **Ask the patient to point his toes** as you grasp the turned foot of the stocking and ease it onto his foot and heel (like putting on a sock). Center the patient's heel in the heel of the stocking.
   Ensures that the pressure of the stocking is over the correct anatomical areas.

8. **Gradually pull the remainder** of the stocking up and over the leg, turning it right side out as you

proceed. Be certain the stocking is straight.

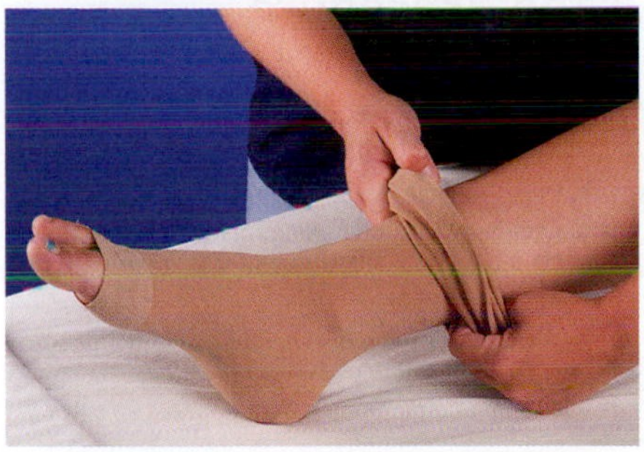

For Knee-High Stockings

a. Pull up to 2.5 to 5 cm (1 to 2 in.) below the knee

For Thigh-High Stockings

b. Pull up to the gluteal fold of the thigh, rotating inward so the gusset is centered over the femoral artery, slightly toward the inside of the leg.
Stockings apply varying amounts of compression between ankle, calf, and thigh areas. Keeping the stocking straight ensures that the pressure occurs over the correct areas.

9. **Smooth out any excess** material; keep stockings free of wrinkles and bunching.
Decreases the risk of skin breakdown and areas of inappropriate and potentially dangerous constriction.

10. **When using stockings with closed** toes, tug gently on the stocking toe to create a small space between the end of the toes and the stocking.
Prevents compression of small vessels in the toes, which may impede circulation.

11. **Repeat the procedure** on the other leg.

12. **Remove the stockings** and bathe and dry the legs daily.

13. **Launder the stockings** at least every 3 days; dry them on a flat surface.
Soiled stockings can irritate the skin; dry flat to prevent stretching.

? What if . . .

- **Both legs do not measure the same?**
Order two different sizes of stockings and use one from each package to make two pairs.

Evaluation

- Evaluate patient comfort.
Severe, continuous discomfort may indicate that the stockings are the wrong size.
- Check the stockings for wrinkles and/or rolling down at the top, especially when sitting.
Wrinkles and rolling down can cause skin breakdown and areas of constriction.
- Evaluate and monitor skin condition.
Elastic stockings should be removed for 20 to 30 minutes every 8 to 12 hours to allow you to inspect the patient's skin and evaluate the adequacy of his circulation.
- Evaluate the patient's ability to ambulate.
It is important to reduce the time the patient is immobile due to pain, sedation, mechanical ventilation, and so on.
- Re-measure the legs regularly.
To prevent complications related to swelling and weight gain.

Home Care

- Teach the client and/or caregiver to apply the stockings.
- Encourage the client to have two pairs of stockings on hand so that one pair can be used while the other is being laundered.
- Instruct the client to follow the manufacturer's directions for washing the stockings.
- Teach the client not to roll down the tops of the stockings.

Documentation

- Document leg measurements and size of the stockings used, to provide a baseline.
- Document the time and date applied.
- Note the condition of the skin, including any abnormalities.

Sample electronic documentation

Note that because this is just one screen of a documentation system, not all of the information is visible. For example, you cannot see the date or the name of the nurse.

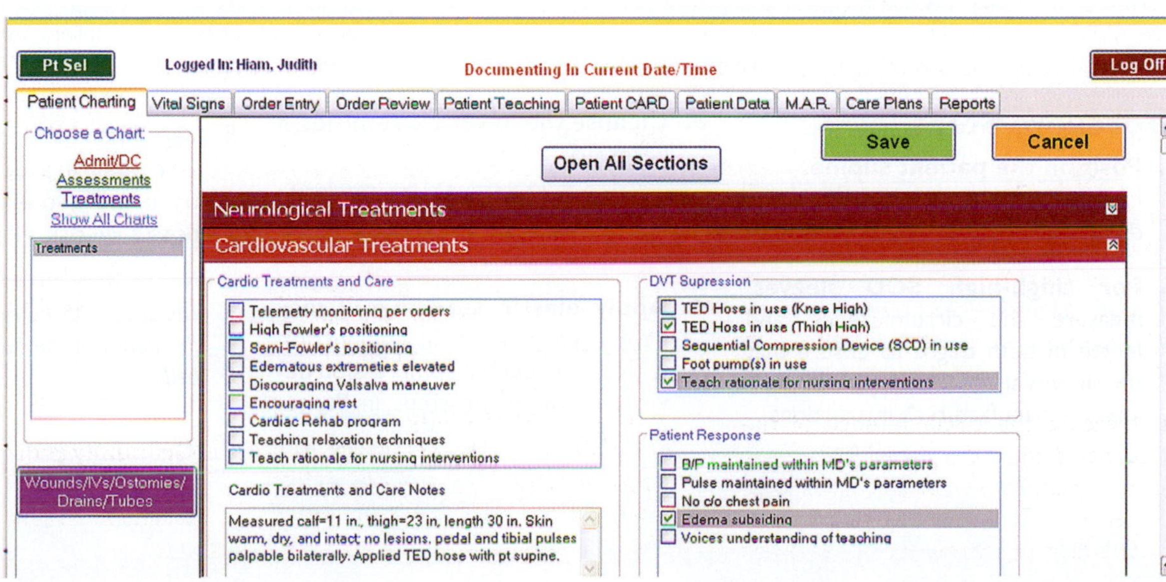

(continued on next page)

Procedure 39-2 ■ Applying Antiembolism Stockings (continued)

Practice Resources

American Association of Critical-Care Nurses (2016); Wade, R., Sideris, E., Paton, R., et al. (2015).

Thinking About the Procedure

The video, **Applying Antiembolism Stockings**, along with questions and suggested responses, is available on the ***Davis's Nursing Skills Videos*** Web site on FADavis.com.

Procedure 39-3 ■ Applying Sequential Compression Devices

➤ For steps to follow in *all* procedures, refer to the Universal Steps for All Procedures found on the inside back cover.

Equipment

NOTE: Sequential compression devices may be referred to by several different brand names, including SCDS (sequential compression decompression stockings), Flowtrons, and PAS (pneumatic air stockings).

- Compression pump, motor, or machine
- Connecting tubing, if applicable (In some devices, the tubing is preconnected to the sleeves.)
- Compression sleeve (knee-high or thigh-high, depending on the order and the type of device)
- Elastic stockings (if also prescribed)
- Disposable wipes or washcloth and towel as needed to cleanse the lower extremities
- Measuring tape

Delegation

You may delegate the application of the sequential compression device to UAP who has had training in that task. Instruct the UAP to report any redness, irritation, or open areas on the lower extremities. SCDs should not be removed for long periods because they are needed to support the patient's peripheral circulation. Instruct the UAP to ensure that all cords and connecting tubing are in a place that will not create a fall risk for the patient or visitors.

Pre-Procedure Assessments

- Assess cognitive level and level of consciousness.
  Patients with altered cognition may be at higher risk for falls related to the presence of the connecting tubing and attachment to the compression pump. Patients who are unconscious will not be able to report a device that is creating too much pressure.
- Assess signs and symptoms of severe peripheral arterial disease, such as weak or absent pulses, discoloration or cyanosis, or gangrene.
  Increased compression of vessels by the sequential device may further impede arterial flow.
- Assess skin condition. Note lesions, dermatitis, or major edema, as evidenced by shiny, taut skin.
  If skin is overstretched by edema, the sequential compression sleeve may irritate or worsen skin conditions and cause skin breakdown.

➤ When performing the procedure, always identify your patient according to agency policy, using two identifiers, and be attentive to standard precautions, hand hygiene, patient safety and privacy, body mechanics, and documentation.

Procedure Steps

1. **Position the patient supine.**
   Prevents venous pooling. Allows for easier application of the compression sleeve.
2. **For thigh-high SCD sleeves,** measure the circumference and length of both thighs to ensure that the sleeves are of the proper size. Follow the manufacturer's instructions.
3. **Cleanse the lower extremities,** if necessary.
   Removes surface dirt and bacteria to decrease the likelihood of infection and odor.
4. **Apply elastic stockings** if they have been ordered in conjunction with the sequential compression device, following the steps in Procedure 39-2.
5. **Place the compression device** pump in a location near an electrical outlet so that the cord will not pose a fall risk. Plug in the pump.
   NOTE: Many compression pumps come equipped with hangers so you can hang the device at the bottom of the patient's bed.

6. Apply the compression sleeve.

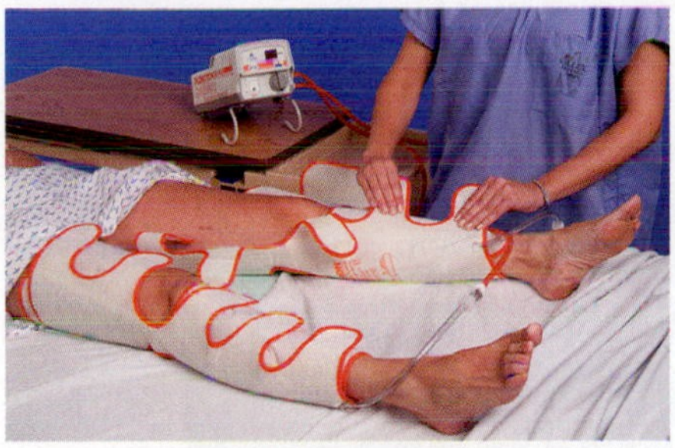

For Flowtron Brand (available in knee-length only)

a. Open the Velcro fasteners on the sleeve.

b. Place the sleeve under the lower leg below the knee, with the "air bladder" side down on the bed.

c. Bring the ends of the sleeve up, and wrap them around the lower leg, leaving one to two fingerbreadths of space between the leg and the sleeve.
Prevents excess pressure and overcompression.

For SCDS/PAS Brands

d. Open the Velcro fasteners on the sleeve.

e. For thigh-high sleeves, place the opened sleeve under the leg, ensuring that the knee opening is at the level of the knee joint and that the fastener will close on the anterior surface.
Ensures that compression occurs over the correct structures. Prevents restricted range of motion (ROM) of the knee joint.

f. Bring the ends of the sleeve up, and wrap them around the leg, leaving one to two fingerbreadths of space between the leg and the sleeve.
Prevents excess pressure and overcompression.

7. Connect the sleeve to the compression pump.

8. Turn the pump on and, if applicable, set the compression pressure on the pump device to the manufacturer's recommended setting.

NOTE: In some facilities, the compression pressure amount is preset and can be changed only by the central supply/equipment department.

Evaluation

After applying the device, make the following ongoing assessments:

- Inflation and deflation of the sleeve
Ensures that the device is actually working.
- Kinking or pinching of the connecting tubing
Interferes with inflation of sleeves and may cause overheating or malfunction of the unit.
- Circulation, sensation, and motion of the foot, including skin color, pulses, temperature, capillary refill, motion, and sensation
- Patient comfort
Increasing discomfort may indicate excess or incorrect pressure.
- Skin condition. Remove the compression sleeves at intervals so that you can inspect skin and evaluate the adequacy of circulation.
NOTE: If elastic stockings are being used in conjunction with the sequential compression device, follow the recommendations in Procedure 39-2.
- Signs and symptoms of deep vein thrombosis
Even with sequential compression device therapy, a patient can still develop thrombi.

Patient Teaching

Teach the patient to call for assistance when disconnecting the tubing from the compression pump to ambulate.

Prevents patient falls. The SCD tubing is a tripping hazard, and injuries from falls involving SCDs are likely to be more severe than injuries associated with general patient falls (Edwards & Holthaus, 2017).

Documentation

- Document the date and time you applied the device.
- Note the type and size (if applicable) of the compression sleeve used.
- Document the skin condition, including any abnormalities.

Sample documentation

11/11/21 1100. Knee-high SCD applied per prescription. Skin warm, dry, and intact at time of application. Peripheral pulses palpable. Pt's wife instructed on use of SCD. Pt unresponsive. No evidence of discomfort, no grimace or movement with application. ——— S. Bee, RN

Practice Resources

Edwards & Holthaus (2017); Sadaghianloo, N., & Dardik, A. (2016)

Thinking About the Procedure

The video **Applying Sequential Compression Devices,** along with questions and suggested responses, is available on the ***Davis's Nursing Skills Videos*** Web site on FADavis.com.

Procedure 39-4 ■ Managing Gastric Suction

➤ For steps to follow in *all* procedures, refer to the Universal Steps for All Procedures found on the inside back cover.

Equipment

Procedure 39-4A Initial Equipment Setup

- Nonsterile procedure gloves
- Suction source (either a portable machine or piped-in wall source)
- Suction container and tubing
- Stopcock (to connect the nasogastric [NG] tube to suction tubing)

Procedure 39-4B Emptying the Suction Container

- Clean nonsterile procedure gloves
- Graduated container
  To measure gastric output when emptying the suction container. Not needed if suction canister is marked for measuring.
- Alcohol wipes or chlorhexidine/alcohol antiseptic product

Procedure 39-4C Irrigating the Nasogastric Tubing

- Nonsterile procedure gloves
- Irrigating set (basin and bulb syringe or catheter-tipped syringe)
- Normal saline irrigant (unless another irrigant is prescribed)
- Linen-saver pads

Procedure 39-4D Providing Comfort Measures

- Nonsterile procedure gloves
- Emesis basin, cup, and water for mouth care
- Water-soluble lubricant
- Cotton-tipped applicators
- Tissues or damp washcloth

NOTE: This procedure assumes an NG or other enteric tube is already in place and that its correct placement has already been verified. If you need to insert an NG tube or check placement, refer to Chapter 27. Tubes for gastric decompression are typically large-lumen tubes such as a Salem sump or Levin tube. See the table at the end of this procedure for more information about tubes.

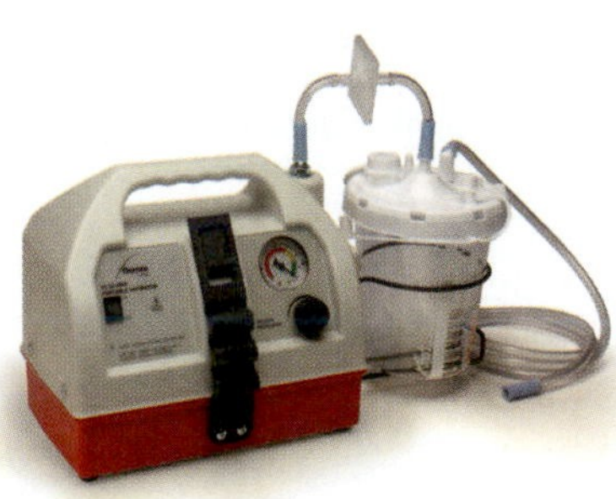

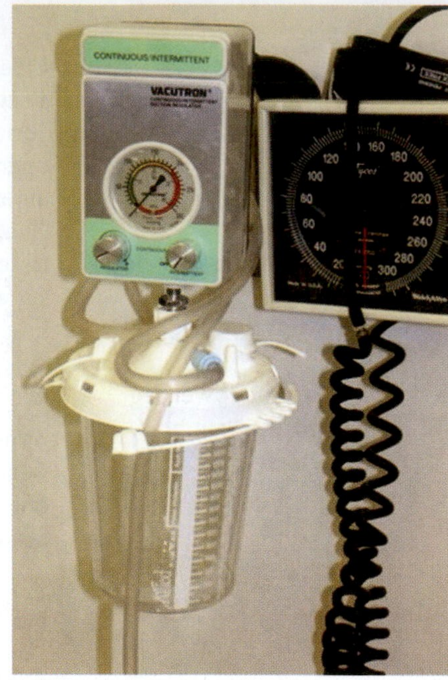

Delegation

A registered nurse should do the initial setup and any subsequent irrigation. You may delegate UAP to empty and measure drainage and perform comfort measures. You must monitor equipment functioning and the patient's responses to the decompression. Instruct the UAP about observations that should be reported to you.

Pre-Procedure Assessments

- Determine that the NG tube has been inserted and placement has been verified.
- Verify the prescriber's order for type of tube and whether it is to be placed to suction or a drainage bag; also verify the type of suction to be used (low, high, continuous, intermittent).
- Auscultate for bowel sounds.
- Assess the patient's ability to cooperate with the procedure and understand explanations.
- Refer to the Evaluation section of this procedure. This procedure assumes an NG tube is already in place, so assessments are ongoing.

Procedure 39-4A ■ Initial Equipment Setup

➤ When performing the procedure, always identify your patient according to agency policy, using two identifiers, and be attentive to standard precautions, hand hygiene, patient safety and privacy, body mechanics, and documentation.

Procedure Steps

1. **Place the collection container** in the holder (either on the portable suction machine or on the wall). Plug the power cord into a grounded outlet if using a portable suction machine.
2. **Connect the short tubing** between the container and the suction source. In some systems, the port will be marked "vacuum."
3. **Connect the long suction tubing** to the container (it may be marked "patient"); if one is available, connect a stopcock to the open end nearest the patient.
4. **Don nonsterile procedure gloves.**
   Helps prevent transfer of microorganisms.
5. **After the NG tube has been** inserted and placement verified, attach the end of the NG tube to the suction tubing.
   See Chapter 27 to review importance of tube placement. You must be certain the NG tube is in the stomach, not in the esophagus or airways.
6. **If the patient has a double-lumen** tube (e.g., Salem sump), instill 10 to 20 mL of air into the vent lumen to make sure it is patent. This should create a soft hissing sound.
7. **Check that the NG tube is secured** to the client's nose and gown, or secure if needed (see Chapter 27 to review).
   Minimizes movement of the tube, helping to prevent irritation of the nares or other insertion site, as well as helping to keep the tube from migrating up out of the stomach.
8. **Turn on the suction source** to the prescribed amount. In an emergency when there is no order, always use low suction. Open the stopcock; note the direction of the arrows.
9. **Observe that drainage appears** in the collection container.
   It may take up to 5 minutes for air to be removed from the canister before the stomach contents will drain.▼

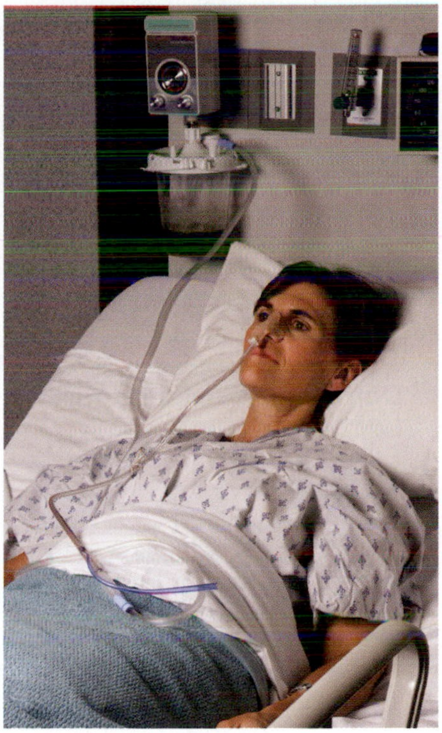

Procedure 39-4B ■ Emptying the Suction Container

➤ When performing the procedure, always identify your patient according to agency policy, using two identifiers, and be attentive to standard precautions, hand hygiene, patient safety and privacy, body mechanics, and documentation.

1. **Don clean nonsterile gloves.**
   Limits the transfer of microorganisms; protects your hands from contact with body secretions.
2. **Turn off the suction source** and close the stopcock on the tubing (or clamp the tubing, if there is no stopcock).
   Prevents suction flow during emptying of the container.
3. **Empty the suction canister.**

For a Suction Container Marked With Measurements

Note the amount, color, and odor of the contents. Empty and rinse the container.

For a Suction Container Not Marked Incrementally

Remove the cap from the lid of the suction container and pour the drainage into a graduated measuring container. Note color, odor, and amount. Empty and rinse the container.
A container with graduated markings enables you to monitor intake and output (I&O) accurately. Rinsing removes organic material that could be a reservoir for microorganisms.

4. **Wipe the port of the suction** container with an alcohol wipe. Place the suction container back in its holder and close the stopper on the lid.
5. **Turn on the suction source** to the prescribed amount. Note the direction of the arrows and turn the stopcock to the "On" position. If there is no stopcock, unclamp the tubing.
6. **Observe for proper functioning** of the suction and patency of the tubing.
   Prevents complications that would result from malfunction.
7. **Remove and discard your gloves.** Perform hand hygiene.

(continued on next page)

Procedure 39-4 ■ Managing Gastric Suction (continued)

Procedure 39-4C ■ Irrigating the Nasogastric Tubing

➤ When performing the procedure, always identify your patient according to agency policy, using two identifiers, and be attentive to standard precautions, hand hygiene, patient safety and privacy, body mechanics, and documentation.

1. **Place a linen-saver pad** on the bed under the NG tube.
2. **Open the irrigation set** and pour saline into the basin.
   Water is not used because it may cause electrolyte imbalances.
3. **Place patient at a 30° to 45°** elevation (unless contraindicated or not tolerated).
   This position helps avoid gastric reflux of irrigant.
4. **Don clean procedure gloves.**
   Limits the transfer of microorganisms; protects your hands from contact with body secretions.
5. **Check for correct placement** of the NG tube using at least two bedside methods (see Chapter 27 as needed).
   Prevents accidental instillation of irrigant into the airways.
6. **Fill the syringe with 10 to 30 mL** of saline and place it on the linen-saver pad.
7. **Clamp the NG tube** or turn off the stopcock connecting to the suction tubing. Then disconnect the NG tube from the suction tubing.
   Prevents backflow of drainage and soiling of linens and clothing.
8. **Hold the drainage tubing up** until suction clears it. Then place it on the linen-saver pad or hook it over the suction machine.
   Keeps secretions from soiling the bed linens or clothing.
9. **Turn off the suction machine.**
10. **Unclamp the NG tube** or turn on the stopcock.
11. **Unpin the NG tube** (or remove tape) from the patient's clothing.
12. **Attach the syringe and instill** the irrigant slowly into the NG tube. Do not force the solution. Be careful not to instill fluid into the air vent.
    Clears the NG tube of gastric contents to keep it patent and helps keep the tube from adhering to the gastric mucosa. Partially digested food, clotted blood, or tissue debris may clog the tube and prevent effective drainage.
13. **Lower the end of the NG tube** and then release the syringe bulb (or, depending on the type of syringe, pull back the plunger) to withdraw fluid. Instill and withdraw until fluid flows in and out freely.
    Uses the force of gravity with negative pressure to withdraw instilled fluid and gastric contents.

For a Double-Lumen NG Tube

Draw 30 mL of air into the syringe and inject it into the "pigtail" (the smaller-bore tube). Follow agency policy for this.
This clears the air-vent tube of any secretions. It must be patent in order to equalize pressure and prevent gastric tissue trauma at the drainage ports. The air also keeps the tube from draining fluid out of the stomach by capillary action.

14. **Reclamp the NG tube** or turn off the stopcock.
    Prevents backflow of drainage.
15. **Reconnect the NG tube** to the suction tube. Then release the clamp or turn on the stopcock.
16. **Reattach the NG tube** to the patient's clothing (with a pin or tape—see Chapter 27 as needed).
    Prevents pulling on and irritating the patient's nostril.
17. **Provide comfort measures** (e.g., mouth care).
18. **Remove and discard gloves.** Perform hand hygiene.

Procedure 39-4D ■ Providing Comfort Measures

➤ When performing the procedure, always identify your patient according to agency policy, using two identifiers, and be attentive to standard precautions, hand hygiene, patient safety and privacy, body mechanics, and documentation.

1. **Don clean nonsterile procedure gloves.**
2. **Provide mouth care** (see Procedures 25-6, 25-7, and 25-8 if you need to review). Use mouthwash as desired. Avoid using lemon-glycerin swabs. Apply water-soluble lubricant to the lips if they become dry and crusty.
   The patient most likely has a dry mouth from not receiving oral intake and from mouth breathing. Lemon-glycerin swabs cause even more drying of tissues.
3. **Remove nasal secretions** with a tissue or a damp washcloth. Moisten a cotton-tipped applicator and wipe the inside of each nostril. If secretions are encrusted, moisten the applicator with hydrogen peroxide, then follow with an applicator moistened with water.
   To soften, dissolve, and remove secretions and prevent tissue irritation.
4. **Apply a small amount of** water-soluble lubricant to the inside of each nostril.
   Soothes and softens dried skin. Avoid petroleum-based lubricants, as complications may occur if they are inhaled.

5. **Check that the tape or tube** fixation device is secure. If it is not, replace it (see Procedure 27-2 as needed).
Prevents irritation of the nasal skin and mucosa. Helps prevent migration of the NG tube from the stomach.

? What if . . .

- **Resistance is met when you irrigate the NG tube?**

Check the tubing for kinks or evidence of obstruction. Have the patient turn to the left side.
Turning to one side changes the position of the distal tip of the NG tube.

- **The patient complains that the NG tube is pulling against her nostril?**

The tube may not be properly anchored to her clothing. Reattach the safety pin (or tape) closer to the nose so that there is more slack in the tube.

- **The NG tube causes excoriation of the nares?**

Remove the tape or fixation device from the nose. Remove the residual adhesive from the skin. Apply skin sealant and anchor the tube so that the adhesive touches in a different place on the skin. Keep the excoriated areas clean and dry.

- **The NG tube does not drain?**

Check tubing for kinks or blockage. Check the suction apparatus. If the collection container is higher than the patient's abdomen, lower it. If these aspects are working properly, irrigate the tube (see Procedure 39-4C, preceding). If the tube still is not draining and the patient is uncomfortable, document and notify the primary care provider. Encourage the patient to relax and breathe slowly through her nose. If the patient has abdominal distention, pain, or vomiting, notify the provider immediately.

If the container is too high, the negative pressure of low suction may not be enough to overcome the force of gravity. Abdominal distention, pain, or vomiting may mean the system is not working. Continued distention creates undue strain on the suture line. You should notify the care provider of these symptoms even when the mechanical aspects of the suction seem in working order.

Gastric Decompression Tubes

TYPE	LUMEN(S)	USE	MANAGEMENT	DISCUSSION
Levin	1, unvented	Decompression, feedings, or irrigation	Use low intermittent suction; may require irrigation.	If the tube opening(s) rest(s) against the gastric mucosa, the suction may irritate or injure the tissue.
Salem Sump	2	Decompression, suction, gastric lavage	Vented. May use high continuous suction.	The air vent helps keep the tube away from the gastric mucosa during suction.
Sengsten–Blakemore	3	Decompression; treatment of active bleeding from esophageal or gastric varices	Use low intermittent suction.	Gastric or esophageal balloons hold the tube in place.
Cantor	1, unvented	Decompression	Use intermittent suction.	Distal end is weighted with a balloon. Used in bowel obstruction. Rarely used because of the hazard posed by the mercury in the weighted balloon.
Miller–Abbott	2	Decompression	Use intermittent suction.	Distal end weighted with a balloon. Used in bowel obstruction. Rarely used because it contains mercury in the weighted balloon.
Ewald or other very large-bore tube	May be passed orally for emergency evacuation of stomach contents to prevent absorption of ingested medications, poisons, or products. A piston-tipped syringe is placed on the end of the tube for manual suction. Typically, the stomach is washed repeatedly with saline and all contents are withdrawn. Because of its large diameter, this type of tube is not tolerated by patients who are alert and is not left in place after lavage is completed.			
Weighted Small-Bore Tubes (e.g., Keofeed)	For feedings only. Suction collapses the tube.			

(continued on next page)

Procedure 39-4 ■ Managing Gastric Suction (continued)

Evaluation and Maintenance

- Periodically assess placement of the tube by a combination of methods (i.e., checking pH of aspirate, by listening over the stomach with a stethoscope while injecting air into the tube, and by reviewing radiographic reports). See Chapter 26 for review, as needed.
- Monitor patency of the tube and the effectiveness of the suction. Check tube connections.
- Monitor patient comfort (e.g., sore throat).
  The continuing presence of a tube in the nose and throat is bothersome to patients. The major nuisance is the pressure of the tube against the internal mucous membranes, irritating the nostril, pharynx, and esophagus.
- Auscultate for bowel sounds; turn off suction while auscultating.
  Bowel sounds indicate the return of peristalsis and the success of gastric decompression. You may hear the sound of the suction apparatus and misinterpret it as bowel sounds.
- Monitor for gastric distention, vomiting, and abdominal pain.
  These symptoms probably indicate the suction is not working effectively. See the What If . . . section, preceding.
- Examine skin and mucous membranes around the insertion site (e.g., nares, abdomen).
- Follow agency policy or the primary care provider's prescription for irrigation of the gastric tube. It is common to irrigate with 10 to 30 mL of normal saline every 3 to 4 hours.
- Monitor the color of the drainage (should be green to gold). If there is blood in the drainage, notify the primary care provider.
- For clients undergoing prolonged gastrointestinal (GI) suction, observe for signs and symptoms of hyponatremia and hypokalemia (i.e., fatigue, lethargy, confusion, seizures, muscle weakness, paresthesia, and cardiac dysrhythmias). Review lab results and report any symptoms to the primary care provider.
- Assess the patient's ability to move about in bed while attached to the suction source.

Patient Teaching

- Instruct the patient to notify you of any discomfort, and to not tug on or try to reposition the NG tube if it becomes uncomfortable.
- Instruct the patient to notify you if feeling nauseated.
  This could mean the tube is blocked and not draining effectively.

Home Care

Usually, gastric suction is performed in a hospital. If the client is to go home with gastric suction (e.g., a terminally ill person who has a bowel obstruction and wants to be in his or her own home), teach the family how to use the device before the person is discharged. Also arrange for home healthcare.

Documentation

- Record all drainage as output on the I&O record.
- Record the time, type, and volume of irrigations and the drainage returned.
- Be sure to include irrigation fluids as input on the I&O record.
- Note color, odor, and consistency of drainage.
- Document patient's emotional and physical responses to NG intubation.
- Document any evidence of tube or equipment malfunction.
- Document epigastric pain, discomfort, distention, or vomiting.

Practice Resources

Allied Healthcare Products, Inc. (n.d.); Best Practices: Evidence-Based Nursing Procedures (2nd ed.). (2007).

Thinking About the Procedure

The videos **Managing Gastric Suction: Initial Equipment Setup, Emptying the Suction Container** and **Irrigating the Nasogastric Tubing,** along with questions and suggested responses, are available on the ***Davis's Nursing Skills Videos*** Web site on FADavis.com.

CLINICAL INSIGHTS

Clinical Insight 39-1 ➤ Preoperative Teaching

Explain What to Expect Before Surgery

- Explain the planned preoperative testing—lab tests, x-ray studies, ECG, and so on.
- Discuss skin preparation, including preoperative wash with an antibacterial product if this is included in the treatment plan.
- Discuss prescribed preoperative medications.
- Outline activities that will occur before surgery, such as insertion of an IV, placement of a urinary catheter, or cardiac monitoring.
- Review the preoperative restriction of fluid and food.
- Tell the patient that a member of the anesthesia team will speak with him about the proposed anesthesia before surgery.
- If the patient is having surgery on the GI tract, an additional bowel prep may be ordered (e.g., a low-residue diet beginning 1 week before surgery, and a liquid diet for the 48 hours preceding surgery). Patients having GI surgery also may have enemas before surgery.
- Explain the need to remove jewelry, makeup, hearing aids, glasses, contact lenses, and any removable dental prostheses before being transported to the operating suite. It is best to have a family member take valuable belongings home for safekeeping.
- Give the patient and family a tentative schedule for the operative day, including the time to arrive at the hospital or surgery center.

Explain What to Expect in the Operative Suite

- Inform the patient and family where they can go to wait during surgery.
- Describe the operating room and the activities that the patient may anticipate before the surgery.
- Describe the types of people who may be present in the operative suite. This is particularly important if the patient is not receiving a general anesthetic.
- Explain that the anesthesiologist or nurse anesthetist will monitor the patient and is responsible for keeping him comfortable with medications throughout the entire procedure.
- Describe the activities that may occur in the preoperative holding area.

Explain What to Expect After Surgery

- Explain that the patient will initially be cared for in the postanesthesia care unit. After a period of observation, he will be transferred to the surgical unit. Note that some patients may be transferred directly to a critical care unit after surgery. If this is expected, tell the patient and family about this preoperatively.
- Family may visit after the patient has been admitted and assessed on the surgical unit.
- Tell the patient what to expect in terms of dressings, equipment, and monitoring devices.
- Describe the types of assessments that will be performed.
- Explain that pain medication will be given to keep the patient comfortable. If he experiences pain, he should tell the nursing staff.
- Discuss the usual progression of recovery, including activity level, deep breathing, coughing, leg exercises, and dietary intake.
- Discuss the usual progression of recovery, including activity level, deep breathing and coughing, leg exercises, and dietary intake.
- Discuss the anticipated length of stay.
- Teach the patient how to move into and out of bed after surgery.
- Teach the importance of deep breathing and coughing, especially after general anesthesia. Demonstrate how to splint the incision to facilitate deep breathing and coughing. Refer to Procedure 39-1.
- Teach and emphasize the importance of leg exercises to minimize the risk of thrombus formation. Refer to Procedure 39-1.
- If decreased activity or prolonged bedrest is anticipated, explain the use of antiembolism stockings or sequential compression devices. Refer to Procedures 39-2 and 39-3.

NOTE: If the patient is to be discharged the day of surgery, inform him in advance about what to wear to the facility, and explain that he must arrange for a responsible adult to drive him home.

Clinical Insight 39-2 ➤ Preparing a Room for a Patient's Return From Surgery

In many institutions, the patient is transported to surgery using the bed that is in his hospital room, so these steps may vary.

- Put clean linens on the bed, including pads to protect the linen from drainage.
- Fold the linens back to the end of the bed.
- Raise the bed to stretcher height, and lock the wheels.
- Move furniture and equipment so that the stretcher can be placed directly against the bed.
- If needed, set up suction, oxygen, or other special equipment.
- Place the following equipment in the room:
  Stethoscope, manometer, thermometer (to measure vital signs)
  IV pole
  Emesis basin
  Tissues
  A clean gown, washcloth, and towel
  Extra pillows for positioning the patient

Clinical Insight 39-3 ➤ Creating an Operative Field

- A nonsterile team member (usually the circulating nurse) performs a surgical prep, using a scrub agent and "paint," to cleanse the operative site. Antiseptic agents must be approved by the U.S. Food and Drug Administration and by the agency's infection control professional. Chlorhexidine and povidone-iodine solutions are most commonly used.
- The **operative field** encompasses the patient and the immediate surrounding area.
- Creation of the sterile field proceeds as follows:
  - Don head covering and shoe covers before entering the surgical suite.
  - Perform a surgical scrub.
  - Don sterile gown, gloves, and other surgical attire (e.g., mask).
  - Cover the area surrounding the operative site with sterile drapes so that only the patient's operative area is exposed.
  - Place sterile draping over the remainder of the patient's body.
  - In most cases suspend a vertical drape at neck level so the client's head and airway are accessible to the anesthesiologist or nurse anesthetist (who is not sterile). For neurosurgery, even the head is draped, and the anesthesiologist or nurse anesthetist sits to the side of the head.

ASSESSMENT GUIDELINES AND TOOLS

Focused Assessment

Example of a Preoperative Checklist (AORN)

AORN *SAMPLE* Preoperative Assessment Form
(Facility Name and Address)

NOTE: *This record is a sample only. Clinical records should be customized to incorporate data fields that represent the setting, facility, procedure, and patient.* Reproductions and variations are encouraged, provided credit is given to AORN.

Addressograph

(Patient Information:
name, age, gender, medical record number, date)

Date:____________

Structural Data:

Admitted via:
☐ Ambulatory ☐ Wheelchair ☐ Stretcher
☐ Other assistive devices:____________
Admitted from:
☐ Home ☐ Transferring hospital
☐ Acute rehab facility ☐ Extended/skilled care facility

Identity confirmed (I26): ☐ Yes ☐ No
Advance directive signed: ☐ Yes ☐ No
Location:____________

Date of preoperative assessment:____________
Planned procedure:____________
Language(s) spoken: ☐ English ☐ Spanish ☐ Other:____________

Operative procedure, surgical site, and laterality verified (I143): ☐ Yes ☐ No
Consent for planned procedures verified (I124): ☐ Yes ☐ No
NPO status verified (I138): ☐ Yes ☐ No
Since: (date/time)____________

☐ Patient's records, belongings, valuables secured (I115)
Belonging inventory: ☐ Watch ☐ Jewelry
☐ Contacts/glasses ☐ Dentures/partial(s) ☐ Hearing aid

Preadmission testing
☐ CBC____________ ☐ Urinalysis____________
☐ Potassium level____________ ☐ EKG____________
☐ CXR____________ ☐ Pregnancy test:____________
☐ Type and cross # of units:____________

Nursing Data Elements:

General health status: (check when present)
☐ Diabetes ☐ Cancer ☐ Obesity ☐ Pregnancy
☐ Hematologic disorders (anemia, sickle cell disease or conditions)

☐ Vital signs:
Temperature:________ Pulse:________ BP:________
Respirations:________ Height:________ Weight:________

☐ Allergies verified (note type of reaction) (I123)
Latex allergy: ☐ Yes ☐ No
Medications: ☐ Yes:____________ ☐ No
Food: ☐ Yes:____________ ☐ No

☐ Daily medications (prescription, OTC, vitamins, alternative medication, herbal remedies, chemotherapy):
____
Medications taken day of surgery:____________

☐ Alcohol/Drug social use:____________

☐ **Neurologic assessment:** ☐ Alert and oriented
☐ Speech intact ☐ Follows simple commands
☐ Risk of falls ☐ History of seizures
LOC: ☐ Alert/oriented ☐ Drowsy ☐ Sedated
☐ Asleep ☐ Unresponsive ☐ Disoriented
☐ Other:____________

☐ **Sensory assessment:**
☐ No limitations ☐ Hearing impairment ☐ Visual impairment

☐ **Cardiovascular assessment:**
☐ Pacemaker ☐ Implanted defibrillator
☐ Chest pain
☐ Peripheral edema: Location:____________
☐ DVT/PE risk:
☐ None ☐ Low ☐ Med ☐ High
____

☐ **Respiratory assessment:**
☐ Tracheotomy
☐ Intubated
☐ Chest tube
Respirations: ☐ Regular ☐ Labored
Smoking history ☐ Yes ☐ No
Packs/day:____ Years smoked:________
Quit date:____________
☐ Cough ☐ Cold symptoms
☐ Current or recent respiratory infection
☐ Preexisting respiratory problems (specify):
____

☐ **Musculoskeletal assessment:**
☐ No limitations
☐ Paralysis
☐ Traction
☐ Limited ROM
☐ Amputation:____________
☐ Prosthesis:____________

(Continued)

Example of a Preoperative Checklist (AORN)—cont'd

Nursing Data Elements (continued):

☐ **Skin assessment:**
- ☐ Cool ☐ Warm ☐ Intact
- ☐ Dry ☐ Moist
- ☐ Body jewelry removed
- ☐ Makeup removed
- ☐ Tattoos: ____________
- ☐ Rash: ____________
- ☐ Bruises: ____________
- ☐ Wounds: ____________
- ☐ Ostomy: ____________
- ☐ Catheter/Drain: ____________
- ☐ Venous access device: ____________

☐ **Gastrointestinal assessment:**

Last bowel movement (date/time): ____________

Usual diet: ____________

____

Recent unexplained weight loss
- ☐ Yes: Amount: ______ Time frame: ______
- ☐ No

Problems chewing or swallowing
- ☐ Yes ☐ No

Special needs:
- ☐ Chewing ☐ Swallowing
- ☐ Appetite ☐ Diet preferences

☐ **Genitourinary/Gynecology assessment:**
- ☐ Voided on call to OR
  Time: ______ Amount: ______
- ☐ Urinary catheter: Amount in bag: ______
- ☐ Urinary incontinence

☐ **Psychosocial assessment:**
- ☐ Calm/relaxed ☐ Anxious ☐ Talkative
- ☐ Crying ☐ Restless ☐ Withdrawn
- ☐ Other: ____________
- ☐ Concerns regarding surgery or hospitalization:
  ____
- ☐ Religious/cultural concerns/requests:
  ____
- ☐ Receives help from:
  - ☐ Children ☐ Support person
  - ☐ Other (specify):
  ____
- ☐ Patient cares for:
  - ☐ Children: Ages: ______
  - ☐ Self ☐ Spouse
  - ☐ Other (specify):
  ____

☐ Determine level of knowledge (I135):
- ☐ Barriers to learning: ____________
- ☐ Motivation to learn
  - ☐ excellent ☐ average ☐ limited

☐ Abuse screening

Have you ever felt threatened verbally, emotionally, or physically in any of your relationships?
- ☐ Yes ☐ No

Have you been hit, slapped, kicked, or otherwise physically hurt by an intimate partner?
- ☐ Yes ☐ No

Are you afraid of your partner or anyone you live with?
- ☐ Yes ☐ No

If yes, describe and make appropriate referral

☐ **Pain assessment**
- ☐ Instructed on use of pain scale
- ☐ Pain assessment (0-10): ____________
  Location: ____________

☐ **Discharge planning**

Will require assistance after discharge
- ☐ Yes ☐ No

Discharge plan:
- ☐ Home
- ☐ Home nursing service
- ☐ Short-term care facility
- ☐ Extended care facility
- ☐ Other: ____________

Individual who will escort patient home:

Name: ____________

Phone number: ____________

Relationship: ____________

Comments:

____

____

____

____

____

Preoperative nursing diagnoses
- ☐ Anxiety/fear (X4)
- ☐ Therapeutic regimen management ineffective (X33)
- ☐ Deficient knowledge (X30)
- ☐ Risk for injury (X29)
- ☐ Pain (X38)
- ☐ Other: ____________

Comments:

RN Signature:
X

Source: Reprinted with permission from Association of periOperative Registered Nurses (AORN) Perioperative Patient-Focused Model.

Focused Assessment

Intraoperative Care Questionnaire

Common nursing interview questions include the following:

- What is your name?
- What type of surgery are you going to have today?
- Is someone here with you?
- Are you allergic to any medications, latex, or tape?
- When is the last time that you had anything to eat or drink?
- Do you have false teeth, contact lenses, or any other prostheses that need to be removed?
- Have you taken any medications today?
- Do you have any implants, such as metal plates or a pacemaker?
- Do you have any scratches, bruises, or other wounds on your body at this time?
- Are there any parts of your body that are painful, such as a stiff shoulder or leg?

Also see the World Health Organization (WHO) Surgical Safety Checklist, following.

Focused Assessment

Example of a Surgical Safety Checklist

Surgical Safety Checklist

World Health Organization | Patient Safety
A World Alliance for Safer Health Care

Before induction of anaesthesia

(with at least nurse and anaesthetist)

Has the patient confirmed his/her identity, site, procedure, and consent?
- ☐ Yes

Is the site marked?
- ☐ Yes
- ☐ Not applicable

Is the anaesthesia machine and medication check complete?
- ☐ Yes

Is the pulse oximeter on the patient and functioning?
- ☐ Yes

Does the patient have a:

Known allergy?
- ☐ No
- ☐ Yes

Difficult airway or aspiration risk?
- ☐ No
- ☐ Yes, and equipment/assistance available

Risk of >500ml blood loss (7ml/kg in children)?
- ☐ No
- ☐ Yes, and two IVs/central access and fluids planned

Before skin incision

(with nurse, anaesthetist and surgeon)

- ☐ **Confirm all team members have introduced themselves by name and role.**
- ☐ **Confirm the patient's name, procedure, and where the incision will be made.**

Has antibiotic prophylaxis been given within the last 60 minutes?
- ☐ Yes
- ☐ Not applicable

Anticipated Critical Events

To Surgeon:
- ☐ What are the critical or non-routine steps?
- ☐ How long will the case take?
- ☐ What is the anticipated blood loss?

To Anaesthetist:
- ☐ Are there any patient-specific concerns?

To Nursing Team:
- ☐ Has sterility (including indicator results) been confirmed?
- ☐ Are there equipment issues or any concerns?

Is essential imaging displayed?
- ☐ Yes
- ☐ Not applicable

Before patient leaves operating room

(with nurse, anaesthetist and surgeon)

Nurse Verbally Confirms:
- ☐ The name of the procedure
- ☐ Completion of instrument, sponge and needle counts
- ☐ Specimen labelling (read specimen labels aloud, including patient name)
- ☐ Whether there are any equipment problems to be addressed

To Surgeon, Anaesthetist and Nurse:
- ☐ What are the key concerns for recovery and management of this patient?

This checklist is not intended to be comprehensive. Additions and modifications to fit local practice are encouraged.

Revised 1 / 2009

Source: Reprinted with permission from the World Health Organization. Retrieved from http://apps.who.int/iris/bitstream/10665/44186/2/9789241598590_eng_Checklist.pdf

Focused Assessment

Postanesthesia Assessment: Essential Elements

AORN (2009, updated 2014) has identified the essential elements of assessment in the PACU.

- **Vital signs**
  - Blood pressure, cuff or arterial
  - Respiratory rate, respiratory competence, and breath sounds
  - Respiratory adequacy, including skin color and condition
  - Temperature (record type of measurement used, for example, skin, tympanic, oral)
  - Pulse (apical and peripheral)
  - Oxygen saturation (e.g., pulse oximeter reading)
- **Peripheral circulation** (postoperative tissue perfusion), for example, peripheral pulses and sensation at extremities
- **Neurological status,** including pupil response and intracranial pressure (if indicated)
- **Mental status,** including level of consciousness, alertness, lucidity, orientation
- **Intravenous therapy**, including patency, location of sites, rates of solution(s), and/or blood products infusing
- **Allergies and sensitivities**
- **Pain**
- **Motor abilities,** including return of sensory and motor control in areas affected by local or regional anesthetics
- **Skin integrity**
- **Temperature regulation**
- **Positioning**
- **Surgical incision site,** including condition of suture line(s) if visible
- **Nausea and vomiting**
- **Fluid and electrolyte balance**
- **Safety needs** (e.g., siderails raised)
- **Central venous pressure (CVP), pulmonary wedge pressure**
- **Airway:** patency, presence of artificial airway, mechanical ventilator settings
- **Condition of dressing(s)**
- **Drainage,** including type; patency; and amount and type of drainage from dressings, tubes, and catheters

DIAGNOSTIC TESTING

Diagnostic Testing

Common Preoperative Screening Tests

Test	Uses
Urinalysis	To detect urinary tract infections (UTIs) and the presence of glucose or protein in the urine, which may indicate poorly controlled diabetes or renal disease
Complete blood count (CBC)	To detect irregularities in hemoglobin (Hgb) and count (CBC) hematocrit (Hct)
	A low Hgb level is an indication of anemia, which may place the client at risk if significant blood loss occurs
	Measures white blood cell (WBC) count as an indicator of immune function
	Measures platelet count, which affects clotting ability
ECG	To detect cardiac dysrhythmias (electrocardiogram) and other cardiac pathology
Chest x-ray	To detect for or evaluate underlying pulmonary disease; also to reveal heart size, as an indicator of heart function.
Blood type and crossmatch	To identify blood type in the event that blood transfusion becomes necessary
Serum electrolytes	To detect sodium, potassium, chloride, magnesium, calcium, and pH imbalances, which affect cardiac and other organ function and fluid balance
Fasting blood sugar	To detect diabetes or poorly controlled diabetes
Comprehensive metabolic panel	Includes electrolytes, blood glucose, liver function tests (ALT, AST), serum albumin and protein, and renal function tests (BUN and creatinine); used to detect underlying health problems that may affect surgical risk or outcome

STANDARDIZED LANGUAGE

Standardized Language

Preoperative Patients: Selected Standardized Nursing Diagnoses, Outcomes, and Interventions

Selected NOC Outcomes and Goals Using NOC Indicators	Selected NIC Interventions and Nursing Activities (*Note:* Interventions and activities marked with an asterisk (*) are routinely performed for ALL surgery patients.)
Nursing Diagnosis: Anxiety related to change in health status	
NOC Outcomes: Anxiety Level Anxiety Self-Control ***NOC Goals:*** Patient will exhibit: ➤ (5) No restlessness ➤ (4) Only mild muscle and facial tension ➤ (4) Only mild difficulty concentrating ➤ (5) No increased blood pressure, pulse rate, or respiratory rate ➤ (5) No physical signs of anxiety such as: dilated pupils, sweating, and dizziness ➤ (3) Moderate verbalized anxiety	***Anxiety Reduction*** ➤ Use a calm, reassuring approach.* ➤ Explain all procedures, including sensations likely to be experienced during the surgical procedure.* ➤ Seek to understand the patient's perspective of the situation. ➤ Provide accurate factual information about the surgery.* ➤ Discuss common feelings and concerns that patients have about surgery. This helps the patient feel supported and less anxious.*
Individualized Goals: ➤ Identifies symptoms that are indicators of her anxiety. ➤ Communicates need for assistance.	***Calming Technique*** ➤ Maintain eye contact with patient.* ➤ Maintain calm, deliberate manner.* ➤ Encourage slow, purposeful deep breathing. ***Presence*** ➤ Stay with the patient and provide assurance of safety and security during periods of anxiety. ➤ Listen to the patient's concerns.* ➤ Administer medications as appropriate to reduce anxiety.
Nursing Diagnosis: Fear related to unknown outcome of surgery and fear of pain that may result	
NOC Outcomes: Fear Level Fear Self-Control ***NOC Goals:*** ➤ (5) Exhibits no restlessness or irritability. ➤ (5) Reports no difficulty concentrating. ➤ (5) No physical signs of fear: increased BP, radial pulse rate, respiratory rate, sweating, dilated pupils, pale skin ➤ (5) No verbalized fear ➤ (5) No crying ***Individualized Goals:*** ➤ Does not exhibit physical signs of fear (e.g., pupil dilation; dry mouth; increased BP, pulse and respiratory rate). ➤ Reports understanding of pain control measures to be used during and after surgery.	***Anxiety Reduction*** See Anxiety diagnosis. ***Coping Enhancement*** ➤ Assist the patient in developing an objective appraisal of the event ➤ Evaluate the patient's decision-making ability.* ➤ Encourage the use of spiritual resources, if desired. ***Preparatory Sensory Information*** ➤ Identify the typical sensations (what will be seen, felt, smelled, tasted, heard) the majority of patients describe as associated with each aspect of the procedure/treatment.* ➤ Personalize the information by using personal pronouns.* ***Security Enhancement*** ➤ Explain all tests and procedures to the patient/family.* ➤ Assist the patient to use coping responses that have been successful in the past.

(Continued)

Standardized Language

Preoperative Patients: Selected Standardized Nursing Diagnoses, Outcomes, and Interventions—cont'd

Selected NOC Outcomes and Goals Using NOC Indicators	Selected NIC Interventions and Nursing Activities (*Note:* Interventions and activities marked with an asterisk (*) are routinely performed for ALL surgery patients.)
Nursing Diagnosis: Knowledge Deficit of preoperative procedures and postoperative expectations *Knowledge-Related Diagnoses* (e.g., Health Maintenance Alteration, Infection Risk)	
NOC Outcomes: Knowledge: Disease Process Knowledge: Treatment Regimen ***NOC Goals:*** Provides: ➤ (3) Moderate description of specific disease process ➤ (4) Substantial description of strategies to minimize disease progression ➤ (4) Substantial description of signs and symptoms of disease complications ***Individualized Goals:*** ➤ Verbalizes rationale for pre- and postoperative interventions. ➤ Describes or demonstrates postoperative expectations (i.e., deep breathing, turning/position changes).	***Teaching: Preoperative*** ➤ Inform the patient/significant others how long surgery is expected to last.* ➤ Determine the patient's previous surgical experiences and level of knowledge related to surgery.* ➤ Provide time for the patient to ask questions and discuss concerns.* ➤ Instruct the patient or caregiver how to participate in the care.* ➤ Describe preoperative routines (e.g., anesthesia, diet, bowel preparation, tests/labs, voiding, skin preparation, IV therapy, clothing, family waiting area, transportation to operating room).* ➤ Describe any preoperative medications, the effects these will have on the patient, and the rationale for using them.* ➤ Inform significant others of the place to wait for the results of the surgery.* ➤ Introduce the patient to perioperative staff as appropriate.* ➤ Discuss possible pain control measures.* ➤ Describe postoperative routines/equipment (e.g., medications, respiratory treatments, tubes, machines, support hose, surgical dressings, ambulation, diet, family visitation) and explain their purpose.* ➤ Instruct the patient in postoperative deep-breathing exercises, splinting incision, coughing.* ➤ Reinforce information provided by other healthcare team members, as appropriate.* ➤ Include the family/significant others [in the teaching-learning process] as appropriate.*
Nursing Diagnosis: Sleep Pattern Disturbance related to anxiety about the upcoming surgery	
NOC Outcome: Sleep ***NOC Goals:*** ➤ (4) Mild interrupted sleep ➤ (5) Hours of sleep (at least 5 hr/24 hr), not compromised ➤ (4) Sleeps through the night consistently, mildly compromised. ***Individualized Goals:*** ➤ Reports minimal compromise in hours of sleep and sleep pattern. ➤ No difficulty falling and staying asleep reported or observed.	***Sleep Enhancement*** ➤ Determine the patient's usual sleep-activity pattern.* ➤ Determine effects of patient's current medications on sleep pattern.* ➤ Adjust environment (lighting, noise, temperature, etc.) to promote sleep.* ➤ Demonstrate and explain the procedure for progressive muscle relaxation. ➤ Administer medication to promote sleep, as appropriate.

Sources: Butcher, H. K., Bulechek, G. M., Dochterman, J. M., et al. (Eds.). (2018). *Nursing interventions classification (NIC)* (7th ed.). St. Louis, MO: Elsevier; Moorhead, S., Swanson, E., Johnson, M., et al. (Eds.). (2018). *Nursing outcomes classification (NOC)* (6th ed.). St. Louis, MO: Elsevier; Saba, V. K. (2017). *Clinical Care Classification (CCC) System, Version 2.5.* Retrieved October 26, 2018, from www.sabacare.com.

Standardized Language

Intraoperative Patients: Selected Standardized Nursing Diagnoses, Outcomes, and Interventions

NOC Outcomes and Indicators	NIC Interventions and Activities (*Note:* Interventions and activities marked with an asterisk (*) are routinely performed for ALL surgery patients.)
Nursing Diagnosis: Aspiration Risk related to depressed respirations and reflexes secondary to anesthesia *Collaborative Problem:* Potential Complication of anesthesia: Aspiration ***Comments:*** This is especially relevant for patients who have weak muscles for coughing or a poor gag reflex.	
NOC Outcome: Respiratory Status: Airway Patency ***NOC Goal:*** ➤ (5) No choking or adventitious breath sounds	***Artificial Airway Management**** ➤ Institute endotracheal suctioning, as appropriate.* ***Aspiration Precautions**** ➤ Monitor pulmonary status.* ➤ Keep suction setup available.* ➤ Maintain an airway.* ***Sedation Management**** ➤ Ensure that emergency resuscitation equipment is readily available, specifically source to deliver 100% O_2, emergency medications, and a defibrillator.* ➤ Initiate an IV line. ➤ Ensure availability of and administer antagonists as appropriate, per physician's order or protocol. ***Vomiting Management**** ➤ Position to prevent aspiration.
Nursing Diagnosis: Perioperative Hypothermia Risk related to exposure in cool environment and administration of cool IV fluids *Collaborative Problem:* Potential complication of surgery and anesthesia: hyperthermia, hypothermia, malignant hyperthermia ***Comments:*** Applies especially to very young, very old, and very thin patients	
NOC Outcome: Thermoregulation ***NOC Goals:*** ➤ (5) No hyperthermia ➤ (5) No hypothermia ➤ (4) Mild increased (or decreased) skin temperature	***Temperature Regulation: Intraoperative**** ➤ Begin warming preoperatively and continue during intraoperative phase.* ➤ Adjust operating room temperature for therapeutic effect.* ➤ Apply head covering.* ➤ Cover exposed body parts.* ➤ Warm or cool all irrigating, IV, and skin preparation solutions, as appropriate.* ➤ Continuously monitor the patient's temperature.* ➤ Cover patient with heated blanket for transport to postanesthesia care unit.* ***Malignant Hyperthermia Precautions**** ➤ Maintain emergency equipment for malignant hyperthermia, per protocol, in operative areas.* ➤ Notify anesthesiologist and surgeon of patient history.* ➤ Provide a cooling blanket.* ***Vital Signs Monitoring**** ➤ Monitor blood pressure, pulse, temperature, and respiratory status, as appropriate.* ➤ Monitor skin color, temperature, and moistness.*

(Continued)

Standardized Language

Intraoperative Patients: Selected Standardized Nursing Diagnoses, Outcomes, and Interventions—cont'd

NOC Outcomes and Indicators	NIC Interventions and Activities (*Note:* Interventions and activities marked with an asterisk (*) are routinely performed for ALL surgery patients.)

Nursing Diagnosis: Fluid Volume Alteration Risk related to NPO status and blood loss from surgery.

Collaborative Problem: Potential complication of surgery: Fluid and electrolyte imbalance

Comments: Clients undergoing surgery are at risk for vascular, cellular, and/or intracellular dehydration. Patients with renal or cardiac problems are at higher than normal risk for fluid and electrolyte imbalance.

NOC Outcomes:

Blood Loss Severity

Fluid Balance

Urinary Elimination

Vital Signs

NOC Goals:

- (4) Systolic and diastolic blood pressures, mild deviation from normal range
- (5) Mean arterial pressure not compromised
- (5) Central venous pressure not compromised
- (5) Pulmonary wedge pressure not compromised
- (4) Peripheral pulses mildly compromised
- (4) 24-hr intake and output balance mildly compromised
- (5) Adventitious breath sounds not present
- (5) Neck vein distension not present
- (5) Peripheral edema not present

Fluid Management*

- Maintain accurate intake and output record.*
- Insert urinary catheter, if appropriate.*
- Administer IV therapy, as prescribed.*
- Monitor hemodynamic status, including CVP, MAP, PAP, and PCWP, if available.*
- Prepare for administration of blood products (e.g., check blood with patient identification and prepare infusion setup), as appropriate.*

Fluid Monitoring*

- Determine possible risk factors for fluid imbalance (e.g., renal pathologies, liver dysfunction).*
- Monitor color, quantity, and specific gravity of urine.*
- Monitor for distended neck veins, crackles in the lungs, peripheral edema, and weight gain.*
- Monitor blood pressure, heart rate, and respiratory status.*
- Monitor serum and urine electrolyte values.*

Intravenous (IV) Therapy*

- Monitor IV flow rate and IV site during infusion.*
- Monitor for IV patency before administration of IV medication.*

Nursing Diagnosis: Latex Allergic Response Risk; or Latex Allergic Response related to multiple previous exposures to latex

Comments: Use these diagnoses only if the patient has the necessary defining characteristics or risk factors. Do not use them routinely for all patients.

NOC Outcomes:

Immune Hypersensitivity Response

Symptom Severity

NOC Goals:

- (5) No localized inflammatory responses
- (5) Respiratory, cardiac, renal, and neurological functions not compromised

Latex Precautions (Intraoperative)

- Place allergy band on patient [if not already done preoperatively].
- Record allergy or risk in patient's medical record [or check to see that it was done].*
- Post sign indicating latex precautions.
- Survey environment and remove latex products.
- Monitor latex-free environment.
- Report information to physician, pharmacist, and other care providers, as indicated.

Latex Precautions (Preoperative)*

- Question patient or appropriate other about history of neural tube defect (e.g., myelomeningocele) or congenital urological condition (e.g., extrophy of the bladder).*

Standardized Language

Intraoperative Patients: Selected Standardized Nursing Diagnoses, Outcomes, and Interventions—cont'd

NOC Outcomes and Indicators	NIC Interventions and Activities (*Note:* Interventions and activities marked with an asterisk (*) are routinely performed for ALL surgery patients.)
	➤ Question patient or appropriate other about systemic reactions to natural rubber latex (e.g., facial or scleral edema, tearing eyes, urticaria, rhinitis, and wheezing).* ➤ Question patient or appropriate other about allergies to foods such as bananas, kiwi, avocado, mango, and chestnuts.*

Nursing Diagnosis: Risk for Perioperative Positioning Injury related to patient factors such as edema, emaciation, obesity, and sensory perceptual disturbances secondary to anesthesia

Collaborative Problem: Potential complication of surgery: Neuromuscular, skeletal, or skin injury

NOC Outcomes and Indicators	NIC Interventions and Activities
NOC Outcomes: Circulation Status Mobility Neurological Status Physical Injury Severity Tissue Perfusion: Peripheral ***NOC Goals:*** ➤ (4) Pa_{O_2} mild deviation from normal range ➤ (4) Pa_{CO_2} mild deviation from normal range ➤ (4) Pallor and dependent rubor mild ➤ (5) Joint movement not compromised ➤ (5) Spinal sensory/motor function not compromised ➤ (5) Central motor control not compromised ➤ (5) No burns, bruises, extremity or back sprains, impaired mobility ➤ (4) Capillary refill (fingers and toes) mild deviation from normal range ➤ (5) No numbness ➤ (5) All pulses no deviation from normal range ➤ (5) Skin integrity not compromised	***Circulatory Precautions**** ➤ Perform a comprehensive appraisal of peripheral circulation (e.g., check peripheral pulses, edema, capillary refill, color, and temperature of extremity).* ***Positioning: Intraoperative**** ➤ Use assistive devices for immobilization.* ➤ Lock wheels of stretcher and operating room bed.* ➤ Use an adequate number of personnel to transfer patient.* ➤ Support the head and neck during transfer.* ➤ Immobilize or support any body part, as appropriate.* ➤ Maintain patient's proper body alignment.* ➤ Apply padding to bony prominences.* ➤ Apply safety strap and arm restraint, as needed.* ➤ Record position and devices used.* ***Surgical Precautions***** ➤ Verify surgical site.* ➤ Verify client's blood type.* ➤ Verify that there is blood on reserve.* ➤ Verify client's identity.* ➤ Verify patient's allergies.* ➤ Check ground isolation monitor.* ➤ Verify the correct functioning of equipment.* ➤ Check suction for adequate pressure and complete assembly of canisters, tubing, and catheters.* ➤ Count sponges, sharps, and instruments before, during, and after surgery, per agency policy; record results of counts.* ➤ Provide an electrosurgical unit, grounding pad, and active electrode, as appropriate.* ➤ Verify the integrity of electrical cords.* ➤ Verify the proper functioning of electrosurgical unit.* ➤ Verify that the client is not in contact with metal.* ➤ Check for the presence of implants, pacemakers, and metal prostheses pacemakers contraindicating use of electrosurgical cautery.*

(Continued)

Standardized Language

Intraoperative Patients: Selected Standardized Nursing Diagnoses, Outcomes, and Interventions—cont'd

NOC Outcomes and Indicators	NIC Interventions and Activities (*Note:* Interventions and activities marked with an asterisk (*) are routinely performed for ALL surgery patients.)
	➤ Verify the patient's skin integrity at site of [electrocautery] grounding pad.* ➤ Verify that skin prep solutions are nonflammable.* ➤ Adjust coagulation and cutting currents, as instructed by physician or per agency policy.* ➤ Inspect the patient's skin for injury [at conclusion of procedure].* ➤ (non-NIC) Monitor sterile technique throughout procedure.*

Sources: Butcher, H. K., Bulechek, G. M., Dochterman, J. M., et al. (Eds.). (2018). *Nursing interventions classification (NIC)* (7th ed.). St. Louis, MO: Elsevier; Moorhead, S., Swanson, E., Johnson, M., et al. (Eds.). (2018). *Nursing outcomes classification (NOC)* (6th ed.). St. Louis, MO: Elsevier; Saba, V. K. (2017). *Clinical Care Classification (CCC) System, Version 2.5.* Retrieved October 26, 2018, from www.sabacare.com.

Standardized Language

Postoperative Patients: Selected Standardized Nursing Diagnoses, Outcomes, and Interventions

Outcomes and Goals	Nursing Interventions and Activities
Nursing Diagnosis: Activity Intolerance r/t pain and the surgical procedure and stressors of surgery	
NOC Outcomes: Activity Tolerance Endurance Energy Conservation Psychomotor Energy ***Goals Using NOC Indicators:*** ➤ O_2 saturation, heart rate, respiratory rate, systolic and diastolic blood pressure not compromised with activity ➤ Ease of breathing with activity not compromised ➤ Walking pace and distance not compromised ➤ Ease of performing activities of daily living (ADLs) not compromised ➤ Ability to speak with physical activity not compromised ➤ Energy restored after rest, not compromised ➤ Uses naps to restore energy, often demonstrated. ➤ Exhibits concentration, consistently demonstrated.	***NIC Interventions:*** Activity Therapy Energy Management Exercise Promotion: Strength Training ***Nursing Activities:*** ➤ Collaborate with other disciplines to plan and monitor activity program as appropriate. ➤ Assist to choose appropriate activities. ➤ Assist to focus on strengths rather than weaknesses. ➤ Assist to identify activity preferences. ➤ Instruct the client and family how to perform desired activities. ➤ Refer to community centers, programs as appropriate. ➤ Arrange physical activities to reduce competition for oxygen supply to vital body functions (e.g., avoid activity immediately after meals). ➤ Avoid care activities during scheduled rest periods. ➤ Assist to sit on side of bed ("dangle"), if unable to transfer or walk. ➤ Monitor location and nature of pain during activity. ➤ Teach activity organization and time management techniques to prevent fatigue.

Standardized Language

Postoperative Patients: Selected Standardized Nursing Diagnoses, Outcomes, and Interventions—cont'd

Outcomes and Goals	Nursing Interventions and Activities
Nursing Diagnosis: Acute Pain r/t (1) inflammation or injury in the surgical area, (2) abdominal distention secondary to decreased peristalsis, (3) muscle pain secondary to positioning and tension	
NOC Outcomes: Pain Level Pain Control ***Goals Using NOC Indicators:*** ➤ Consistently rates pain as controlled. ➤ No moaning or crying ➤ No facial expressions of pain ➤ Describes causal factors. ➤ Uses preventive measures. ➤ Uses nonanalgesic relief measures. ➤ Uses analgesics as recommended. ➤ Reports changes in symptoms to a health professional. ***Other Goals:*** ➤ No guarding of incision	***NIC Interventions:*** Analgesic Administration Pain Management: Acute Patient-Controlled Analgesia (PCA) Assistance ***Nursing Activities:*** ➤ Assess location, characteristics, onset, duration, frequency, quality, and intensity of pain and predisposing factors. ➤ Observe for nonverbal discomfort cues. ➤ Assure the client of analgesic availability. ➤ Consider cultural influences of responses to pain. ➤ Utilize developmentally appropriate assessment method. ➤ Determine necessary frequency of pain assessment and formulate pain assessment plan. ➤ Control environmental factors that may contribute to the client's response. ➤ Provide information about the pain, such as causes of the pain, how long it will last, and anticipated discomforts from procedures (e.g., teach the client to splint incision when ambulating). ➤ Provide optimal pain relief with analgesics as appropriate. ➤ Implement PCA as appropriate. ➤ Intervene before pain becomes severe. ➤ Medicate before activity to increase participation. ➤ Teach nonpharmacological pain relief measures (e.g., visualization, progressive muscle relaxation). ➤ Utilize multidisciplinary approach to pain management.
Nursing Diagnosis: Anxiety r/t change in health status, hospital environment	
NOC Outcomes: Anxiety Level Anxiety Self-Control ***Goals Using NOC Indicators:*** ➤ Consistently uses effective coping strategies. ➤ Often seeks information to reduce anxiety. ➤ Consistently uses relaxation techniques to reduce anxiety. ➤ Often maintains concentration. ➤ Verbalizes that anxiety is mild. ➤ Minimal restlessness, hand wringing, muscle tension, facial tension, difficulty concentrating. Minimal changes in vital signs; no dilated pupils, sweating, or dizziness ➤ Controls anxiety response consistently.	***NIC Interventions:*** Anxiety Reduction ***Nursing Activities:*** ➤ Use calm, reassuring approach. ➤ Observe for verbal and nonverbal signs of anxiety. ➤ Explain all procedures and activities. ➤ Provide information concerning diagnosis, treatment, prognosis. ➤ Administer back rub or neck rub as appropriate. ➤ Listen attentively. ➤ Create trusting atmosphere. ➤ Assist the client to identify stressful situations. ➤ Assist the client to recognize that she is anxious. ➤ Assess the client's ability to make decisions.

(Continued)

Standardized Language

Postoperative Patients: Selected Standardized Nursing Diagnoses, Outcomes, and Interventions—cont'd

Outcomes and Goals	Nursing Interventions and Activities
	➤ Encourage verbalization of feelings, perceptions, and fears related to the surgical procedure. ➤ Encourage family visits if these ease the client's stress. ➤ Support use of appropriate defense mechanisms. ➤ Instruct the client in use of relaxation techniques.

Nursing Diagnosis: Nausea r/t manipulation of gastrointestinal tract, decreased peristalsis secondary to anesthesia

Outcomes and Goals	Nursing Interventions and Activities
NOC Outcomes: Nausea & Vomiting Control Nausea & Vomiting: Disruptive Effects Nausea & Vomiting Severity Nutritional Status: Food & Fluid Intake ***Goals Using NOC Indicators:*** ➤ No nausea, or intensity only mild ➤ Reports nausea, retching, and vomiting controlled. ➤ Mild or no intolerance of odors ➤ Mild or no intolerance of movement ➤ Recognizes onset of nausea. ➤ Recognizes precipitating stimuli. ➤ Frequency, intensity, and distress of nausea are mild. ➤ Uses preventive measures often. ➤ Only mild decrease in food and fluid intake ➤ No weight loss ➤ Reports bothersome side effects from antiemetics. ➤ Reports failure of antiemetic treatment.	***NIC Interventions:*** Nausea Management Medication Management ***Nursing Activities:*** ➤ Provide information about the cause of nausea and vomiting and the expected duration. ➤ Provide information about the goals, effects, and possible side effects of treatment with antiemetics. ➤ Describe the limited role of administering parenteral fluids to prevent dehydration and to administer supplemental electrolytes (e.g., potassium). ➤ Encourage the client to monitor own nausea experience, including use of a symptom diary. ➤ Encourage the client to learn strategies for managing own nausea. ➤ Perform complete assessment including frequency, duration, severity, and precipitating factors. ➤ Observe for nonverbal cues of discomfort. ➤ Evaluate past experiences with nausea. ➤ Identify strategies that have been successful in relieving nausea. ➤ Discuss relaxation and distraction techniques if anxiety is suspected of playing a role (e.g., guided imagery, self-hypnosis, biofeedback, music therapy). ➤ Encourage frequent oral hygiene unless it stimulates nausea. Keep tissues and water to rinse the mouth nearby. ➤ Give cold, clear, odorless foods, as appropriate. ➤ Encourage the client to eat high-carbohydrate and low-fat foods and to eat small, frequent meals. ➤ Drink cola, but not too cold; suck on an ice cube, sorbet, or a piece of frozen fruit. ➤ Have the client sit in an upright position for 30 to 45 min after eating. ➤ Control odors and unpleasant visual stimuli in the room. ➤ Administer antiemetic medications. ➤ Refer to a dietitian as needed.

Postoperative Patients: Selected Standardized Nursing Diagnoses, Outcomes, and Interventions—cont'd

Outcomes and Goals | **Nursing Interventions and Activities**

Nursing Diagnosis: Constipation r/t decreased activity, decreased food or fluid intake, decreased peristalsis secondary to anesthesia, pain medication

Outcomes and Goals

NOC Outcome:
Bowel Elimination

Goals Using NOC Indicators:
- Elimination pattern not compromised
- Reports ease of stool passage not compromised.
- Bowel sounds not compromised
- Muscle tone to evacuate stool not compromised
- Passes soft, formed stool in amount appropriate for diet.
- No pain with passage of stool

Other:
- Bloating not present

Nursing Interventions and Activities

NIC interventions:
Bowel Management

Constipation/Impaction Management

Nursing activities:
- Monitor for signs and symptoms of constipation.
- Note date of last bowel movement.
- Monitor bowel sounds.
- Monitor frequency, consistency, shape, volume, and color of bowel movements.
- Teach the client about specific foods that assist promotion of bowel regularity.
- Insert a rectal suppository, enema, or irrigation, as needed.
- Evaluate medication profile for GI side effects (e.g., narcotic analgesics).
- Give warm liquids after meals.
- Instruct the client in foods high in fiber.

Nursing Diagnosis: Urinary Retention r/t anesthesia, preoperative medications (anticholinergics), pain, fear, unfamiliar surroundings, client's position

Outcomes and Goals

NOC Outcome:
Urinary Elimination

Goals Based on NOC Indicators:
- Empties bladder completely.
- Fluid intake not compromised
- No hesitancy with urination

Other:
- Bladder not palpable
- Reports subjective feeling of empty bladder.
- 24-hr intake and output balanced

Nursing Interventions and Activities

NIC Interventions:
Urinary Retention Care

Urinary Catheterization

Nursing Activities:
- Perform comprehensive urinary assessment (fluid intake, urinary output, voiding pattern, cognitive function, preexisting urinary problems).
- Provide privacy for elimination.
- Use power of suggestion (run water, flush toilet).
- Provide ample time (at least 10 minutes) for client to empty bladder.
- Use spirits of wintergreen in bedpan or urinal.
- Insert urinary catheter as appropriate.
- Use percussion and palpation to estimate degree of bladder distention.
- Catheterize for post-voiding residual as appropriate.

Nursing Diagnosis: Surgical Recovery Delay (etiologies will vary with pathology)
- ***Note:*** This diagnosis is broad and encompasses some of the other diagnoses. If the client has Delayed Surgical Recovery, you will not, for example, need a diagnosis of Nausea on the plan of care.
- This diagnosis is appropriate when the patient requires more days to recover than the anticipated length of stay for the surgery.

Outcomes and Goals

NOC Outcomes:
Post-Procedure Recovery

Wound Healing: Primary Intention

Ambulation

Nursing Interventions and Activities

NIC Interventions:
Embolus Precautions

Exercise Therapy: Ambulation

Incision Site Care

(Continued)

Standardized Language

Postoperative Patients: Selected Standardized Nursing Diagnoses, Outcomes, and Interventions—cont'd

Outcomes and Goals	Nursing Interventions and Activities
Blood Loss Severity Endurance Hydration Infection Severity Nausea & Vomiting Severity Pain Level ***Goals Using NOC Indicators:*** ➤ Systolic BP within 20 mm Hg of baseline ➤ Ambulation tolerance in normal range ➤ No nausea, vomiting, shivering ➤ Only mild pain ***Other:*** ➤ Ready for discharge within prescribed length of stay for surgery performed ➤ No postoperative complications (e.g., bleeding, infection, delayed wound healing, pneumonia)	Nutrition Management Pain Management: Chronic Self-Care Assistance ***Nursing Activities:*** ➤ Monitor for postoperative complications. ➤ Monitor the healing process in the incision site. ➤ Provide incision care as needed. ➤ Teach the client and family how to care for the incision. ➤ Facilitate early ambulation postoperatively. ➤ Encourage increased intake of protein, iron, and vitamin C, as appropriate. ➤ Determine, in collaboration with the dietician as appropriate, number of calories and type of nutrients needed to meet nutrition requirements. ➤ Select and implement a variety of measures (e.g., pharmacological, nonpharmacological, interpersonal) to facilitate pain relief, as appropriate. ➤ Teach principles of pain management. ➤ Encourage independence, but intervene when the client is unable to perform.

Sources: Butcher, H. K., Bulechek, G. M., Dochterman, J. M., et al. (Eds.). (2018). *Nursing interventions classification (NIC)* (7th ed.). St. Louis, MO: Elsevier; Moorhead, S., Swanson, E., Johnson, M., et al. (Eds.). (2018). *Nursing outcomes classification (NOC)* (6th ed.). St. Louis, MO: Elsevier; Saba, V. K. (2017). *Clinical Care Classification (CCC) System, Version 2.5.* Retrieved October 26, 2018, from www.sabacare.com.

CLINICALJUDGMENT

Applying the Full-Spectrum Nursing Model

PATIENT SITUATION

Recall Nishad Singh (Meet Your Patient, in Volume 1). He is a 68-year-old man who came to the emergency department (ED) with sudden onset of rectal bleeding. He had been "tired and dragging for several months." The ED nurse identified nursing diagnoses of Mild Anxiety, Pain, and Risk for Bleeding. Preoperatively, his vital signs were as follows:

BP: 138/88 mm Hg
Pulse: 104 beats/min and regular; 120 beats/min; 134 beats/min
Respiratory rate: 20 breaths/min
Temperature: 36.7°C (98.0°F)
Oxygen saturation: 98%

Mr. Singh was admitted to the hospital where he received an IV of 1,000 mL of lactated Ringer's solution and a unit of packed red blood cells. He was to undergo emergency colon resection surgery; however, a left hemicolectomy including the sigmoid colon and the anus was required. He spent 4 hours in the PACU, until his vital signs stabilized. Mr. Singh now has a colostomy high in his descending colon, with a stoma on his left abdomen slightly superior to the level of his umbilicus. He also has an abdominal incision that was made for exploration. On the next day after the surgery, the surgeon informed Mr. Singh that he has widespread adenocarcinoma (cancer) of the colon with metastasis to the liver. The nurse has identified these four nursing diagnoses (among others):

Knowledge Deficit (colostomy care) r/t lack of prior experience and no preparation prior to surgery
Fear r/t diagnosis of colon cancer, liver metastasis, and possible terminal illness
Pain secondary to surgical incision and manipulation of abdominal organs during the surgical procedure
Risk for Impaired Skin Integrity r/t irritation from fecal drainage and ostomy pouch

THINKING

1. *Theoretical Knowledge:*
   a. What is a left hemicolectomy? If you do not know the answer, consult an appropriate reference.
   b. What does "metastasis to the liver" mean? If you do not know the answer, consult an appropriate reference.
2. *Critical Thinking (Inquiry):*
   a. Why might Mr. Singh have needed a colostomy instead of having his transverse colon reconnected to the remaining lower colon or rectum? State the reference you used to answer this question.
   b. Why do you think Mr. Singh has a colostomy above the level of the umbilicus and not lower down in his abdomen? State the reference you used to answer this question.

DOING

3. *Practical Knowledge:* Mr. Singh returned from surgery with knee-high antiembolism stockings.
   a. You notice that the stockings have slid down and become wrinkled between his knees and ankles. After you straighten them and pull them up, the tops reach to about 7.6 cm (3 in.) below Mr. Singh's knees. What does this probably mean, and what should you do?
   b. Which of the following instructions should you give when delegating care of Mr. Singh's antiembolism stockings to the nursing assistant? (Mr. Singh's stockings have closed toes.)
      - Remove the stockings and bathe and dry the legs every 8 to 12 hours.
      - Massage the legs after removing Mr. Singh's stockings.
      - Before reapplying stockings, report the presence of any lesions, sores, or redness of the lower extremities.
      - Instruct the patient to remain supine for at least 15 minutes after removing the stockings.
      - Make sure there are no wrinkles in the stockings once they have been applied.
      - Tug gently on the end of the stocking to create a small space between the end of the toes and the stocking.
4. *Nursing Process (Nursing Diagnosis):* List Mr. Singh's four nursing diagnoses in order of priority. List the highest priority first. Explain how you decided the priorities.

CARING

5. *Self-Knowledge:*
   a. If you were assigned to care for Mr. Singh today, what aspect of care would you feel best prepared to give? Explain your thinking.
   b. What aspect of Mr. Singh's care would you be most uncomfortable providing? Explain your thinking.
6. *Ethical Knowledge:* You want to provide culturally competent care. What is the first thing you will need to do in order to address Mr. Singh's cultural needs? Review Chapter 15 if you need to.

Critical Thinking and Clinical Judgment

1. You are speaking with several classmates about an upcoming surgical rotation. During the rotation, you will have an opportunity to work with a circulating nurse and a scrub nurse. One of your classmates says that she is very nervous. "I don't know whether I will be able to handle this rotation. I'm afraid I might not be able to watch the surgery. I've never really seen anything gross like that before." Another classmate confides that she is worried that she will contaminate everything and put the client at risk. What advice can you give them, and what actions can you take to prepare yourself for your experience in the OR?

2. You are working on a busy surgical unit on the evening shift. There is one UAP on the unit this evening. You are caring for the following clients:
   - Mr. Singh (Meet Your Patient, in Volume 1), who underwent a colon resection and colostomy for colon cancer. He is now in postoperative day 2. Mr. Singh is complaining of chest pain and shortness of breath.
   - Ms. Yasmin, a 52-year-old woman admitted to the unit from PACU 1 hour ago after total abdominal hysterectomy and bilateral salpingo-oophrectomy (TAH-BSO—removal of the uterus, ovaries, and fallopian tubes).
   - Steven Stellanski, a 16-year-old with trisomy 21 who underwent an emergency appendectomy early this morning.

   The PACU calls to inform you that they are ready to transport Mrs. Bauer back to the unit. She is an 87-year-old woman from the local skilled nursing facility who underwent an extensive debridement of a stage IV pressure ulcer on the coccyx. The PACU nurse tells you Mrs. Bauer is confused and agitated and will need close monitoring.

   a. What problem(s) does admission of this new patient present for you? To answer this question, identify the priority nursing activity for each of the three patients you already have, as well as for Mrs. Bauer.

   b. How will you handle this situation? Identify three options, and explain their advantages and disadvantages.

3. You will be caring for a 23-year-old client who underwent emergency surgery after an automobile accident. He has had no preoperative teaching. What concerns does this raise for you? How will you address these concerns?

4. For each of the following concepts, use critical thinking to describe how or why it is important to nursing, patient care, or perioperative nursing. Note that these are *not* to be merely definitions.

   Preoperative teaching

   Preoperative physical preparation

   Intraoperative safety measures

   Anesthesia

   Postoperative complications

What Are the Main Points in This Chapter?

- Perioperative nursing includes care of patients during the preoperative, intraoperative, and postoperative phases.
- Perioperative nursing requires the systematic integration and synthesis of the nursing process with established standards of practice.
- The Association of periOperative Registered Nurses (AORN) is the organization that developed the standards of care that inform perioperative nursing and the standardized language, the Perioperative Nursing Data Set (PNDS).
- "Never events" are serious and costly errors resulting in severe consequences for the patient and are mostly preventable. Medicare will not reimburse institutions for care related to complications caused by never events.

- Surgical risk is associated with the type of surgery and the condition of the patient (e.g., age, general health, personal habits).
- During the preoperative period, it is essential to determine whether the client is physiologically, cognitively, and psychologically prepared for the intraoperative and postoperative phases of surgery.
- Preoperative care includes assessment, preoperative teaching, confirming that surgical consent has been obtained; preventing wrong patient, wrong site, wrong surgery; communicating with the surgical team; preparing the patient physically for surgery; transferring the patient to the operative suite; and preparing the postoperative room on the surgical unit.
- The surgical consent form is a witnessed legal document that ensures that the surgical patient has given informed consent for the surgical procedure. The physician is legally responsible for obtaining informed consent; however, the nurse sometimes obtains the patient's signature on the form after verifying that the patient has been informed.
- A great deal of perioperative nursing care is standardized, aimed at preventing potential complications, and applicable to all patients having surgery.
- General anesthesia produces rapid unconsciousness and loss of sensation. Regional anesthesia produces loss of pain sensation without loss of consciousness.
- Intraoperative care includes skin preparation, positioning the patient for surgery, and protective measures to ensure patient safety during surgery.
- The PACU RN integrates knowledge of common complications of surgery, well-established nursing diagnoses for the postoperative client, and data from an individualized comprehensive postoperative assessment to plan and implement appropriate outcomes and interventions for the client during the postoperative stage.
- Assessments during postoperative recovery are the same as those performed in the PACU, but they can be performed less frequently.
- Antiembolism stockings and sequential compression devices may be used to help prevent thrombophlebitis.
- Incentive spirometry may be used to help prevent atelectasis and pneumonia.
- Gastrointestinal suction may be used for gastric decompression after certain surgeries to prevent gastric distention, which can increase respiratory complications, place a strain on suture lines, and interfere with wound closure.

Knowledge Map

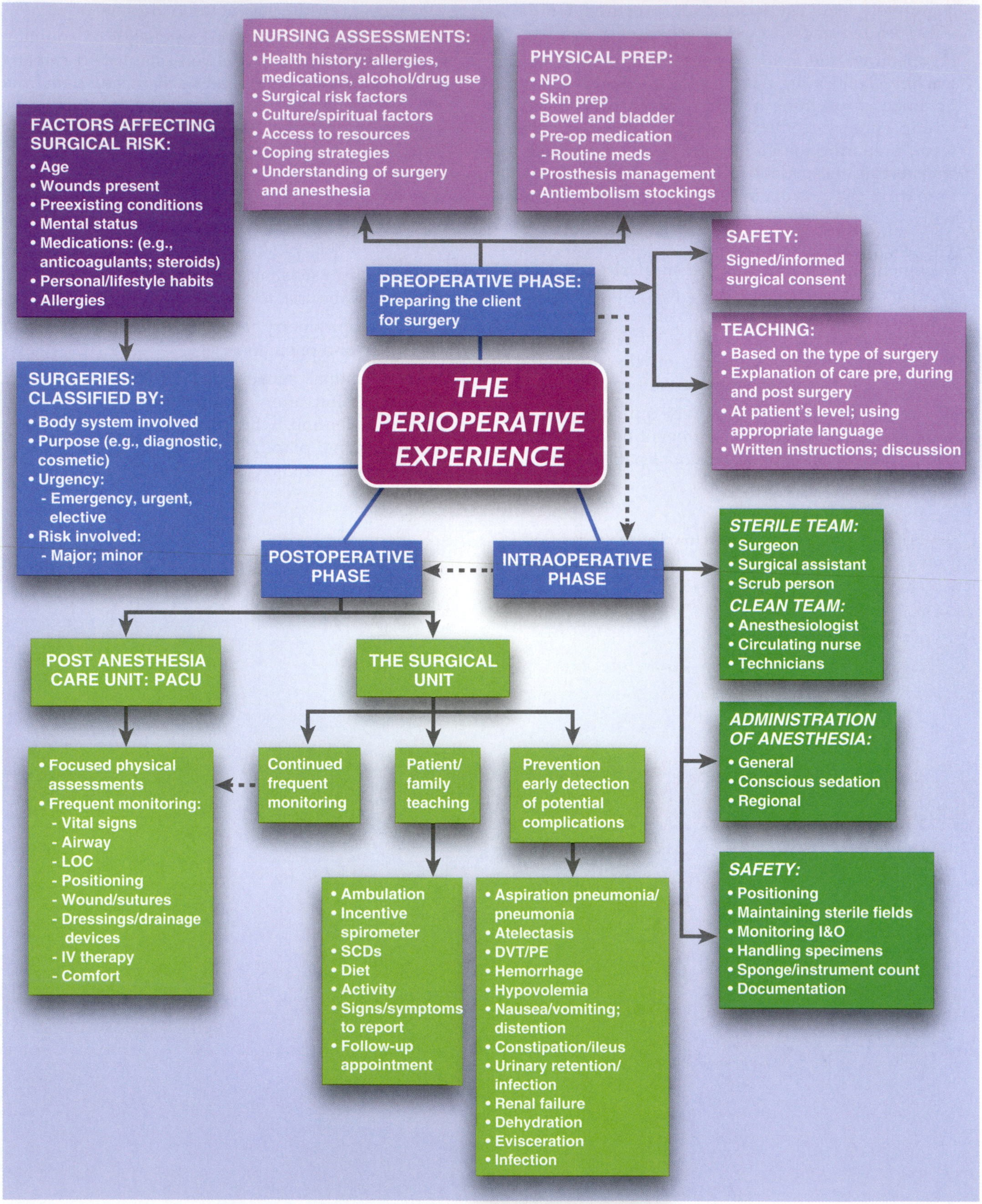

CHAPTER 40

Leading & Managing

STUDENT RESOURCES

The questions and exercises in this book allow you to practice the kind of thinking you will use as a full-spectrum nurse. Critical-thinking questions usually have more than one right answer, so we do not provide "correct answers" for these features. Try to answer these questions yourself. It is more important to develop your nursing judgment than to just cover content. You will learn more by discussing the questions with your peers. If you are still unsure, see the Davis Advantage chapter resources for suggested responses.

To explore learning resources for this chapter,

Go to Davis Advantage and find:

Answers and Suggested Responses for all questions in this chapter
Concept Map
Knowledge Map
References and Bibliography
Lists of NOC Outcomes and NIC Interventions

Key Concepts

Change
Followership
Leadership
Management

Related Concepts

See the Concept Map on Davis Advantage

Caring for the Nguyens

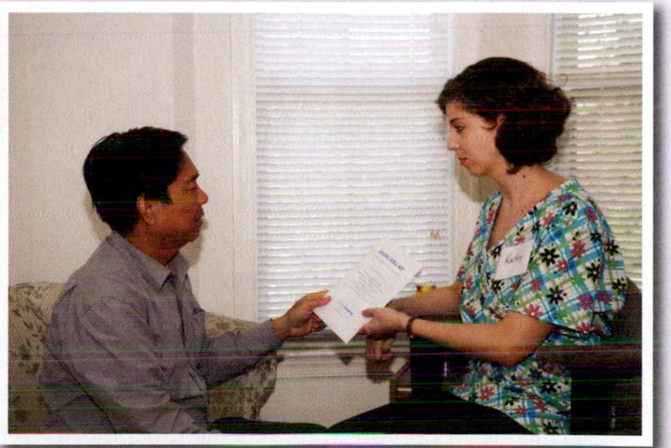

Anh Chu, Nam's aunt, is scheduled for outpatient cataract surgery later this week at the local hospital. Nam reports to the clinic wishing to discuss the plan for his aunt's surgery "with whoever is the boss." Nam is concerned that his aunt will not be staying at the hospital. "She's having surgery. I don't understand this! She's 78 years old. She's going to need help. This doesn't make sense. You have to change things. It won't be safe to do this as planned."

Nam tells you that he has discussed his concerns with the ophthalmologist. He tells you that the ophthalmologist

(Continued)

Caring for the Nguyens (continued)

told him he was "overreacting. We always do it this way. You just don't understand." Nam is visibly upset. He believes that his aunt is receiving inadequate care. He appeals to you to help him take care of his aunt. "This is where Aunt Chu gets her care. You know her. You have to change this."

Anh Chu has been seen at the family clinic several times over the past few years. She takes a medication for osteoporosis and has been counseled about the need for exercise and weight loss. She has also begun to experience problems with "accidents"—that is, urine leakage. She has never had surgery before, and her only hospitalizations have been for childbirth. Ms. Chu's husband recently passed away, and she has been living alone since then.

A. Devise a plan to resolve this conflict with Nam.

PracticalKnowledge clinical **application**

CLINICALJUDGMENT

Applying the Full-Spectrum Nursing Model

ORGANIZATIONAL SITUATION

A small, not-for-profit hospice center in a small community has received a generous memorial gift from the family of a client who recently died. The family asked only that the money be "put to the best possible use." Everyone in the facility has an opinion about the best use for the money.

The administrator wants to renovate their old, run-down headquarters. The financial officer wants to put the money in the bank "for a rainy day." The chaplain wants to add a small chapel to the building. The nurses want to create a food bank to help the poorest of their clients. The social workers want to buy a van to transport clients to healthcare providers. The staff has agreed that all the ideas have merit and all the needs are important. Unfortunately, there is enough money to fund only one of them.

The more the staff members discuss how to use this gift, the more insistent each group becomes about defending its own idea. At the last meeting, it is clear that some are becoming angry and frustrated. A shouting match even occurs between the administrator and the financial officer.

THINKING

1. *Theoretical Knowledge:*
   Which is appropriate at this point, a problem-solving approach or informal negotiation? Explain your answer.

DOING

2. *Practical Knowledge:*
   If you were to conduct the informal negotiation, list the steps of the plan you would follow.

CARING

3. *Self-Knowledge:*
   Which idea do you think has the most merit? Why did you select the one you did?

4. *Ethical Knowledge:*
   Which groups or individuals seem to demonstrate the value of caring for clients? Explain your thinking.

Critical Thinking and Clinical Judgment

1. Identify a personal or professional change that you would like to see take place, and outline the steps needed to implement the change.

2. Eleanor, a LPN returning to school to obtain her associate's degree in nursing, is faced with a multitude of responsibilities. A wife, a mother of two toddlers, and a full-time staff member at a local hospital, Eleanor suddenly finds herself in a situation in which there just are not enough hours in a day. She is convinced that becoming a registered nurse is an impossible goal. You are Eleanor's mentor. When you ask where she wants to be in 5 years, she answers, "At this moment, I think, on an island in Tahiti!"

   a. Help Eleanor develop a personal time inventory. To help her determine specifically what to include, make your own personal time inventory to share with her as an example.

   b. Once Eleanor has finished her time plan, how would you advise her to use it to make better use of her time? Make specific suggestions.

3. What strategies could you use to better manage your time?

4. Why is it important to learn good time management habits while you are a student?

5. This is your first semester in the nursing program. Although you have attended college to complete the prerequisite courses, this seems to be so different. All of a sudden, you have to attend clinical rotations in addition to classes. And you have to prepare ahead of time for the clinical experience, often even going to the hospital the night before to obtain information related to your patients. You feel like you are drowning! What can you do?

Go to Chapter 40, **Table 40-4: Components of Time Management,** in Volume 1.

Work through the table, asking yourself questions such as the following. Be very specific in your answers; give examples.

   a. *Prioritizing:*
      - What tasks do you have to complete on a daily basis? Weekly? During the semester?
      - List the tasks in order of importance.
      - Which of the tasks do you have control over (e.g., scheduling a haircut or setting aside time to read the next assignment versus taking a test that is scheduled)?

   b. *Assigning priorities:* Assign priorities to the tasks you have identified.

   c. *Questioning effectiveness, efficiency:* Ask yourself, "How can I accomplish these tasks in the least amount of time but to the best of my ability?"

   d. *Rechecking:* Review your plan. Mentally and physically recheck the plan. Revise the plan as needed.

   e. *Self-reliance:* Carry out your plan. Use critical-thinking skills, and adapt the plan as needed so that you "go with the flow."

   f. *Treating:* Be good to yourself, but commit yourself to time management and excellence. How can you do that? What treats will you give yourself?

6. For each of the following concepts, use critical thinking to describe how or why it is important to nursing, patient care, or managing or leading. Note that these are *not* to be merely definitions.

Leadership skills

Management skills

Becoming a mentor

Being a mentee

Time management

Resolving conflicts

Delegating appropriately

Understanding the change process

What Are the Main Points in This Chapter?

- Leadership is the ability to influence other people.
- Transformational leaders communicate their vision in a way that reduces negativity and inspires commitment in people.
- Three common behavioral leadership styles are authoritarian, democratic, and laissez-faire.
- A manager is an employee of an organization who has power, authority, and responsibility for planning and directing the work of others.
- Effective managers possess a combination of qualities: leadership skills, clinical expertise, and business sense.
- A manager's activities are generally organizational, interpersonal, and informational.
- Not all leaders should be managers; but all managers should be leaders.
- It is never too early in your career to develop a SWOT (strengths, weaknesses, opportunities, threats) or SOAR (strengths, opportunities, aspirations, results) analysis. Throughout your nursing program, revisit the analysis, and update it as you gain new knowledge and skills.
- A mentor is a role model who develops the novice nurse to be a professional by coaching, encouraging, supporting, and guiding him or her.
- Be mindful of nurses who demonstrate strong mentor qualities. Do not be afraid to ask for their support and guidance. Develop mentor qualities of your own, so you can also mentor a new student.
- At times throughout our nursing careers, we will all assume the role of follower.
- Followers need to be self-directing, actively participating experts who work on behalf of the organization.
- Sources of power include authority, reward, expertise, and coercion.
- Nurses have expertise, power, and authority over other healthcare workers. It is important that you understand your sources of power and use them wisely.
- Empowerment is the feeling of self-determination, competence, and recognition that your expertise and power within the healthcare system have meaning and positive impact.
- Evaluative feedback is a leadership responsibility that reinforces constructive and discourages undesirable behavior, provides recognition, and develops employee skills.
- Delegation of patient care tasks to other healthcare workers is one of the most important responsibilities of the registered nurse.
- Nurses must understand change and act as change agents within today's healthcare setting.
- Managing change involves recognizing and decreasing resistance.
- Conflict is inevitable, but it does not need to be destructive.
- One of a manager's responsibilities is to facilitate conflict resolution and, if necessary, function as an informal negotiator.
- Effective time management is essential to planning safe, effective patient care and demonstrating management skills.
- Time management includes goal setting and organizing and streamlining your work.
- Do not forget to get rest and "time off" when managing time.

Knowledge Map

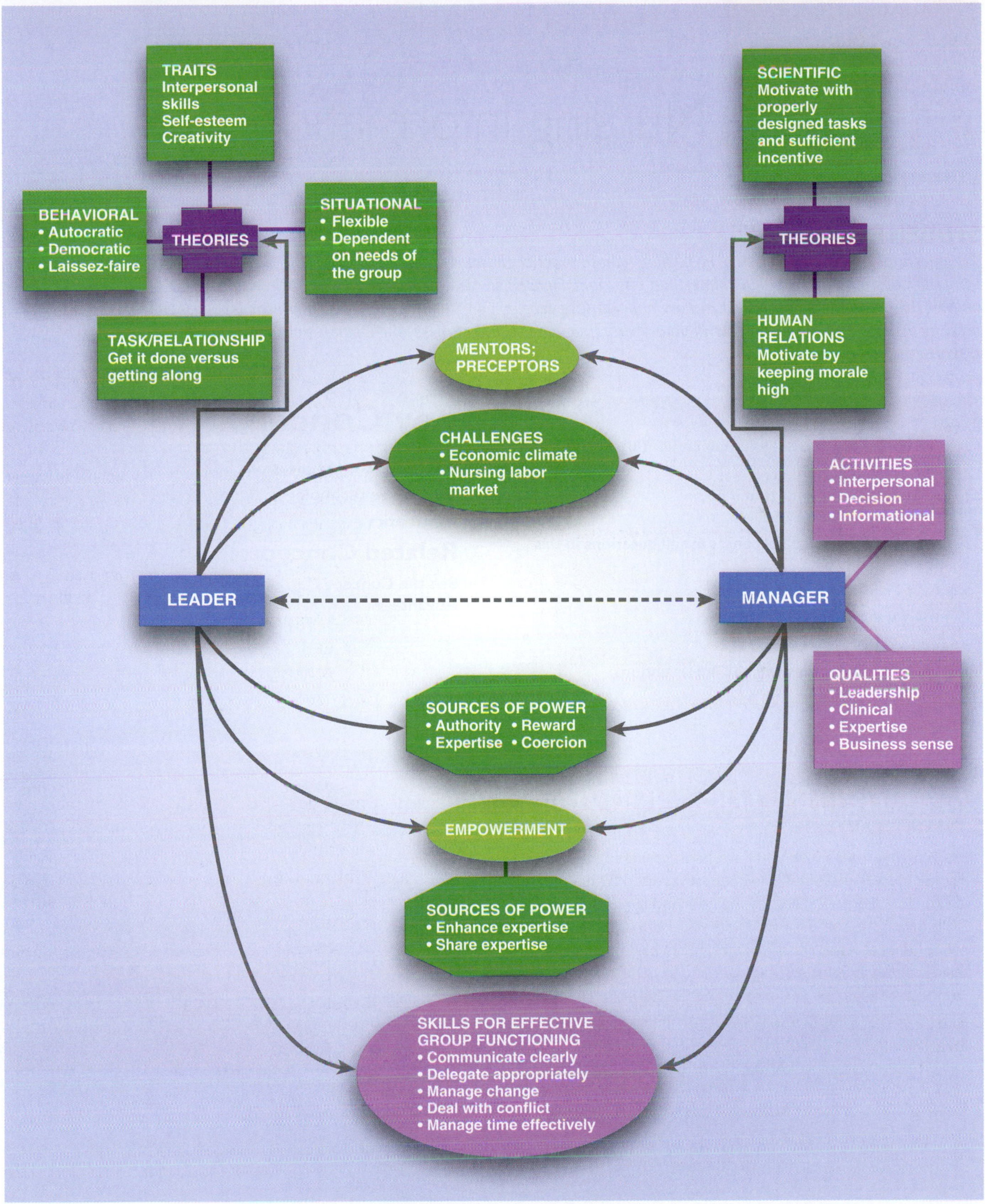

CHAPTER 41

Nursing Informatics

STUDENT RESOURCES

The questions and exercises in this book allow you to practice the kind of thinking you will use as a full-spectrum nurse. Critical-thinking questions usually have more than one right answer, so we do not provide "correct answers" for these features. Try to answer these questions yourself. It is more important to develop your nursing judgment than to just cover content. You will learn more by discussing the questions with your peers. If you are still unsure, see the Davis Advantage chapter resources for suggested responses.

To explore learning resources for this chapter,

Go to Davis Advantage and find:

Answers and Suggested Responses for all questions in this chapter
Concept Map
Knowledge Map
References and Bibliography
Lists of NOC Outcomes and NIC Interventions

Key Concepts

Electronic communication
Healthcare technology
Informatics

Related Concepts

See the Concept Map on Davis Advantage

Caring for the Nguyens

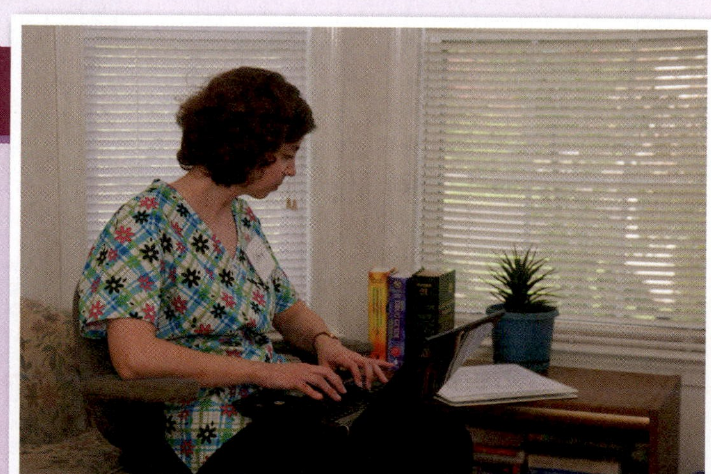

Nam Nguyen, a patient you have been caring for at the Family Medicine Center, has been devastated by his recent diagnoses of type 2 diabetes mellitus and hypertension. "Oh my, this is bad. This stuff kills you. I don't understand what I did to cause this," he sighs. He is having difficulty following his medication regimen and says he doesn't understand what he is supposed to do. You have supplied him with information at each of his clinic visits as well as handouts, medication information, and a reminder sheet for his medicines. Nam asks you whether there is any information available on the Internet.

A. What advice would you give him about looking up medical information on the Internet?

B. What sources would you recommend to Nam?

Practical Knowledge clinical application

STANDARDIZED LANGUAGE

Standardized Language

American Nurses Association Recognized Languages for Nursing

Language	Description	Recognition Date
Diagnosis Related Group (DRG)	DRG is a classification system for most health conditions to establish a standardized reimbursement system for Medicare.	1983
NANDA International	The NANDA-I taxonomy provides a way to classify and categorize areas of actual or potential concern for patient care. The taxonomy includes 13 Domains (areas of interest) with diagnostic labels that contain definitions, defining characteristics, related factors, at-risk population, and associated conditions. Nursing diagnoses can be problem-focused, potential risk, or health promotion.	1992
Clinical Care Classification (CCC)	Developed by Virginia Saba, CCC is used primarily by home health agencies and community settings. The taxonomy contains nursing diagnoses and interventions developed to code, index, classify, document, track, and analyze clinical care processes.	1992
Omaha System	The Omaha System is standardized healthcare terminology used to document care in community and home care agencies. This system consists of the following: ➤ Problem Classification Scheme for client assessment ➤ Intervention Scheme for planning care and client services ➤ Problem Rating Scale for Outcomes for evaluating client changes The Omaha System provides a framework for collection, aggregation, analysis, and sharing of clinical data.	1992
Nursing Outcomes Classification (NOC)	NOC presents standardized terminology for nursing-sensitive patient outcomes. Each outcome represents the measurable state of the client, caregiver, family, or community before and after a nursing intervention to evaluate the effectiveness of care.	1997
Nursing Interventions Classification (NIC)	NIC is a system for identifying, organizing, documenting, and communicating the care that nurses provide to clients, families, and other healthcare professionals. Each intervention includes a concept label, definition, and activities.	1992
Nursing Management Minimum Data Set (NMMDS)	This data set describes the healthcare and nursing environment associated with the diagnosis, intervention, and outcome segments from the administrative, management, and resource management perspectives. It is composed of data elements in three categories: environment, nurse resources, and financial resources.	1998
Perioperative Nursing Data Set (PNDS)	The PNDS language supports evidence-based, perioperative nursing practice and provides support for structured documentation of nursing activities. It provides a common language for clinical research and assists with the measurement and evaluation of patient outcomes. This was the first nursing language developed by a nursing specialty.	1999
Statistical Nomenclature of Medicine Clinical Terminology (SNOMED CT)	SNOMED CT is a reference terminology that includes clinical concepts used to describe assessment, diagnosis, intervention, and outcome. Although it includes nursing concepts, it was not developed specifically for nursing, but rather for a broad spectrum of healthcare domains.	2002
Nursing Minimum Data Sets (NMDS)	This data collection establishes comparability of nursing data across population settings, geographic areas, and times. It describes the nursing care of patients or clients and their families in a variety of settings, both institutional and noninstitutional.	1999
International Classification for Nursing Practice (ICNP)	ICNP describes nursing practice in various clinical settings worldwide using common language. It includes nursing phenomena or diagnoses, outcomes, and actions.	2000

CLINICALJUDGMENT

Applying the Full-Spectrum Nursing Model

PATIENT SITUATION

Sarita, a nurse working in the surgical intensive care unit (ICU), is ordering patient lab work and recording patient information in the electronic health record (EHR). While at the computer terminal, a physician walks over to her and requests an update on a postoperative patient's condition. They go to the bedside to assess the patient's color and perfusion. Another nurse, Janelle, needs to order a STAT x-ray exam using the central computer in the unit. When Sarita goes back to the computer screen to order lab work and finish her documentation, Janelle has stepped in and is now accessing another patient's record.

THINKING

1. *Theoretical Knowledge:*
   a. Name five benefits of using an electronic health record for storing and retrieving patient data in a busy critical care unit.

   b. List five potential areas of difficulty in using this same electronic health record.

2. *Critical Thinking (Considering Alternatives):*
   a. Brainstorm about possible solutions for dealing with bottlenecks among staff using a centralized computer.

DOING

3. *Practical Knowledge:*
   a. Where would you look to find out who has accessed the patient record?

CARING

4. *Ethical Knowledge:*
   a. What violation has Sarita committed in this situation? What should she have done instead?

   b. What is the nurse's responsibility in protecting patient information in the electronic record? What kinds of things should the nurse do?

5. *Self-Knowledge:*
   a. Have you ever been so busy that you felt as though you just needed to take a "necessary" shortcut to save time? Describe your experience.

Critical Thinking and Clinical Judgment

1. Refer to the following table. For each of the uses listed, what kind of information do you think the database should provide? That is, what kind of data would you need? For example, look at the first item under In Nursing Practice. For "Literature access and retrieval," you would use a database that contains information about journals, books, reports, and their content, perhaps CINAHL. For all of the following (Use in Nursing Practice), what kind of database would you use? What kind of information would you need? The first one is done for you.

Work with your classmates. Share your knowledge and experience to answer these questions. Consult your instructor as needed.

USE	TYPE OF INFORMATION NEEDED
In Nursing Practice Literature access and retrieval (e.g., for evidence-based practice)	***Suggested response:*** CINAHL; information about books, journals, and their content; possibly the Internet
Care planning	***Clues:*** What information would you need for care planning? Where would you find it?
Client records (e.g., documenting, order entry, retrieving lab results) Telenursing (e.g., in home health) Case management	
In Nursing Education Literature access and retrieval Computer-assisted instruction (CAI) programs Classroom technology Distance learning Testing and grading Student records	
In Nursing Administration Quality assurance/improvement and utilization review Employee records (e.g., to track licenses, immunizations) Staffing patterns, hiring Buildings and facilities management Finance and budgets Accreditation reviews (e.g., monitoring quality control)	***Clues:*** What information would you need to evaluate the quality of care in your institution? Where would you find it?
In Nursing Research Literature review Data collection Data analysis (both qualitative and quantitative) Research dissemination Applying for grants	

2. Search for "online nursing journals" on the Internet. Make a list of nursing journals that provide full-text articles that are available on the Web, and at no charge.

3. For each of the following concepts, use critical thinking to describe how or why it is important to nursing, patients, or to nursing informatics. Note these are *not* to be merely definitions.

Nursing informatics

Data

Knowledge

Wisdom

Evidence-based practice

Computers

Hardware

Storage media

Connectivity

Group messaging by text or application

Telehealth

Electronic health records

Standardized nursing language

Literature databases

The World Wide Web

Evaluating Web sites

What Are the Main Points in This Chapter?

- Whatever their roles—staff nurse, administrator, educator, researcher, primary care provider—nurses use data, information, and knowledge in their daily work.
- Informatics is the processing and management of data, information, and knowledge necessary for making practice decisions.
- The nursing informatics specialist uses nursing science, computer science, and information science to manage and communicate data, information, knowledge, and wisdom in nursing practice.
- A computer has four main functions: input, processing, output, and storage. Together they are known as information processing (or data processing).
- *Connectivity* is a term referring to the ways in which computers and other hardware communicate and share information.
- Some forms of electronic communication include electronic mail and text and application-based messaging, Web conferencing and webinars, online forums, social networking, and telehealth applications.
- Electronic health records are a platform for communication among the interdisciplinary healthcare team regarding patient healthcare needs, patient data, and plan for care.
- EHRs allow clinicians to create, store, edit, and retrieve patient charts via the Internet or local intranet software.
- An important benefit of EHRs is reduced errors resulting from illegible handwriting.
- EHRs equip providers with clinical support tools to conveniently access information to assist with clinical decision making.
- Computer- and application-based tools for providing and managing care (including tracking patients and equipment, managing workflow) reduce errors with automation and aid patients in self-care.
- Standardized languages within the EHR facilitate research to improve healthcare. They also aid in billing, recordkeeping, and scheduling follow-up care.
- It is important to use and protect passwords to guard the privacy of patient records.
- Computer illiteracy and discomfort with technology is a common reason for resisting use of an EHR. Many claim documentation in the system is time consuming, especially when less familiar with the system.
- Evidence-based practice requires the ability to organize and manage information to identify a clinical problem, search the literature, evaluate the evidence, and plan an intervention.
- An information literate person seeks authoritative, current, and reliable sources of information from trusted Internet sources.
- CINAHL and MEDLINE are two important databases to search for nursing literature.

Knowledge Map

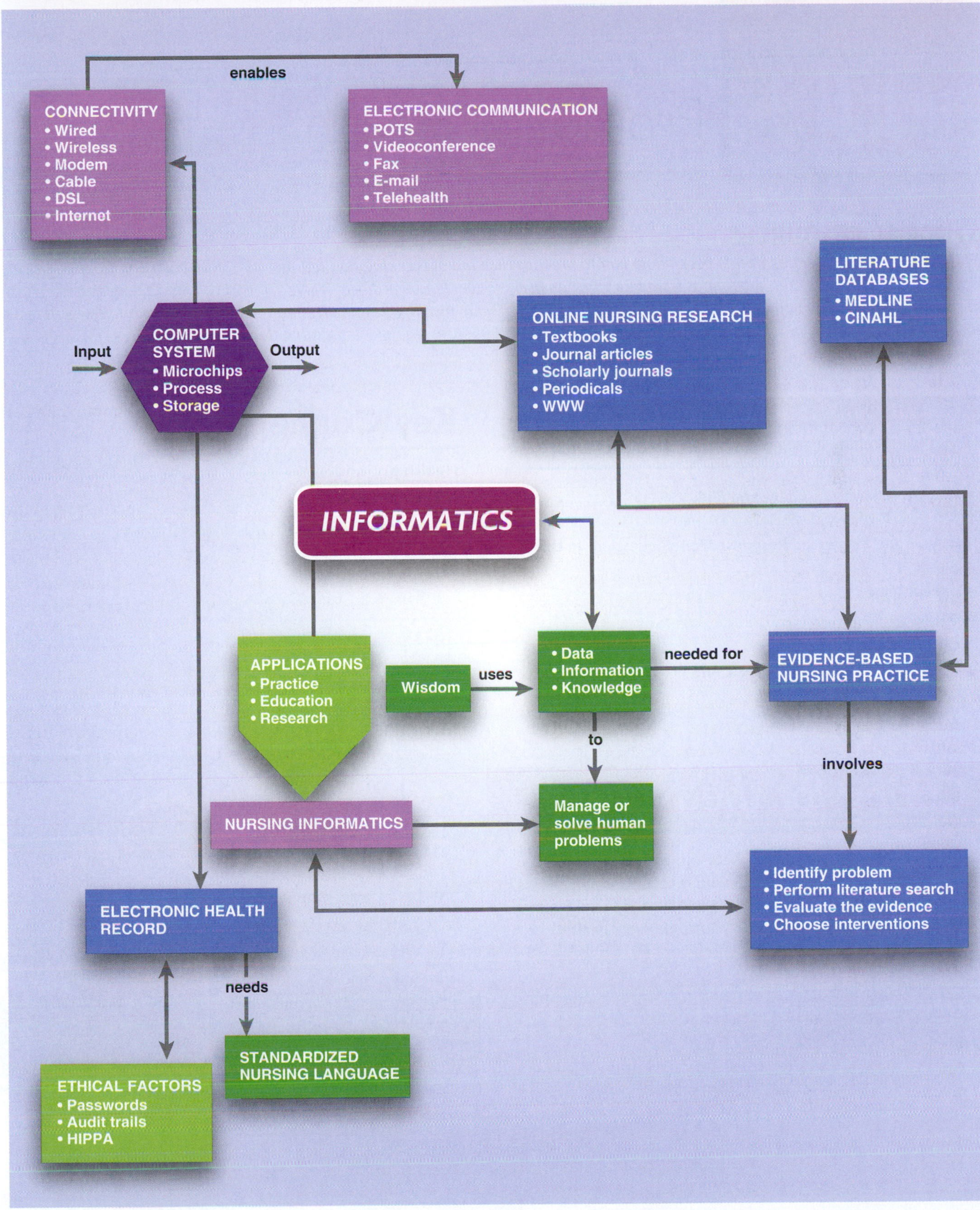

CHAPTER 42

Promoting Health

STUDENT RESOURCES

The questions and exercises in this book allow you to practice the kind of thinking you will use as a full-spectrum nurse. Critical-thinking questions usually have more than one right answer, so we do not provide "correct answers" for these features. Try to answer these questions yourself. It is more important to develop your nursing judgment than to just cover content. You will learn more by discussing the questions with your peers. If you are still unsure, see the Davis Advantage chapter resources for suggested responses.

To explore learning resources for this chapter,

Go to Davis Advantage and find:

Answers and Suggested Responses for all questions in this chapter
Concept Map
Knowledge Map
References and Bibliography
Lists of NOC Outcomes and NIC Interventions

Key Concepts

Health promotion
Health protection
Illness prevention
Wellness

Caring for the Nguyens

Nam and Yen Nguyen; their 3-year-old grandson, Kim Phan; and Mai Nguyen, Nam's 76-year-old mother, are all patients at the Family Medicine Center. Zach Miller, the family nurse practitioner at the center, asks you to devise a health promotion program for each member of the family.

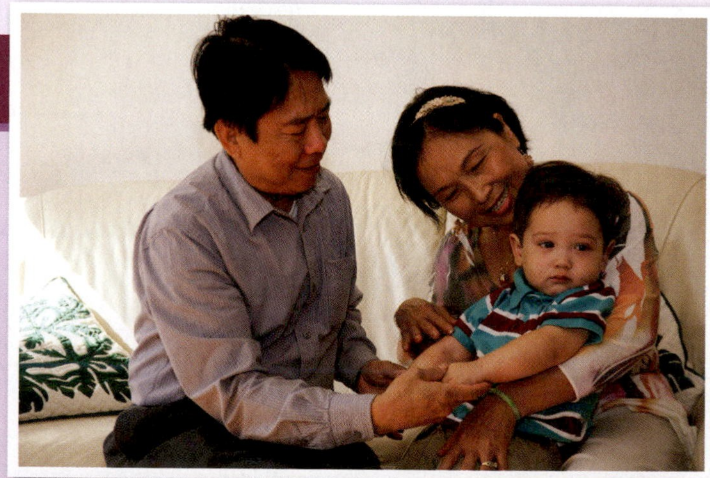

Caring for the Nguyens (continued)

A. What information should you gather before you begin?

B. How might you obtain this information?

C. How will the plans differ for each?

D. Review Meet the Nguyens in the front of this textbook; also review Nam's physical exam findings in Chapter 22. What health promotion strategies and health screenings should you recommend to Nam?

E. How would you begin to organize and prioritize a health promotion program for Nam?

F. Using therapeutic communication, give examples of appropriate questions to ask Nam about his health beliefs.

ASSESSMENT GUIDELINES AND TOOLS

Focused Assessment

Health Promotion: Physical Fitness Assessment

Cardiorespiratory Fitness

There are many different modes of testing, such as field tests (walking or running), motor-driven treadmills, stationary bicycles, and step testing.

- **Field tests** for running are good for children. A 9-year-old child should be able to complete a 1-mile run in approximately 10 minutes, and a 17-year-old boy should be able to complete a 1-mile run in approximately 7½ minutes (Presidential Youth Fitness Program, n. d.).
- **The step test** is appropriate for most adults. Using a 12-inch bench, instruct the participant to step up and down at a rate of 24 steps per minute for 3 minutes. At the end of 3 minutes, he should check his heart rate. Stop testing immediately if the participant experiences any chest pain, shortness of breath, or light-headedness. Results depend on age and gender and are available below.

Step Test Evaluation Charts

3-Minute Step Heart Rate Test (Men)

Physical Condition	18–25 yr	26–35 yr	36–45 yr	46–55 yr	56–65 yr	65+ yrs
Excellent	<79	<81	<83	<87	<86	<88
Good	79–89	81–89	83–96	87–97	86–97	88–96
Above average	90–99	90–99	97–103	98–105	98–103	97–103
Average	100–105	100–107	104–112	106–116	104–112	104–113
Below average	106–116	108–117	113–119	117–122	113–120	114–120
Poor	117–128	118–128	120–130	123–132	121–129	121–130
Very poor	>128	>128	>130	>132	>129	>130

3-Minute Step Test (Women)

Physical Condition	18–25 yr	26–35 yr	36–45 yr	46–55 yr	56–65 yr	65+ yr
Excellent	<85	<88	<90	<94	<95	<90
Good	85–98	88–99	90–102	94–104	95–104	90–102
Above average	99–108	100–111	103–110	105–115	105–112	103–115
Average	109–117	112–119	111–118	116–120	113–118	116–122
Below average	118–126	120–126	119–128	121–129	119–128	123–128
Poor	127–140	127–138	129–140	130–135	129–139	129–134
Very poor	>140	>138	>140	>135	>139	>134

(Continued)

Focused Assessment

Health Promotion: Physical Fitness Assessment—cont'd

Muscular Fitness

- **Muscle strength** is recorded as a ratio of weight pushed (or lifted) divided by body weight. For example, a woman weighing 150 pounds who is able to lift 86 pounds will have a ratio of 86 divided by 150, or 0.57.
  - Instruct the participant warm up and stretch before the test. Weight benches are ideal sites for testing upper body and leg strength.
  - Compare the ratio obtained with normative standards or with previous personal scores to evaluate improvement.
- **Muscle endurance** is evaluated by the push-up or curl-up (crunch) test. Ask the participant to perform as many push-ups or curl-ups as possible without pausing.
- The number of repetitions is the score. Once again, compare scores with norms or previous performance.

Flexibility

The sit-and-reach test evaluates low back and hip (trunk) flexion.

- Ask the participant to sit on a floor mat with legs fully extended and feet flat against a box. Have her extend her arms and hands forward as far as possible and hold for a count of 3.
- Using a ruler, measure the distance in inches that the client can reach beyond the proximal edge of the box. If the client cannot reach the edge, measure the distance of the fingertips from the edge, and report it as a negative number.
- Norms for trunk flexion vary among men and women. The desired range for men is +1 to +5 inches, and for women it is +2 to +6 inches (Murdaugh, Pender, & Parsons, 2019).

Focused Assessment

Lifestyle and Risk Assessment

The following is an example of a health risk assessment (HRA).

Name ______________ Age __________ Gender _______

Health View

In general, would you say your present health is?

□ Excellent

□ Very good

□ Good

□ Fair

□ Poor

General Practices

1. **Physical activity.** How many days each week do you get at least 30 minutes of physical activity, such as brisk walking, cycling, active gardening, active dance, swimming, jogging, or active sports? __________
2. **Strength exercises.** How many days each week do you do strength-building exercises, such as weight lifting or isometric exercises? __________
3. **Smoking status.** Indicate your present smoking status.

   □ Current smoker □ Ex-smoker

   □ Nonsmoker, never smoked regularly.

   Environmental smoke. Do you live with or work with smokers and breathe secondhand smoke regularly?

   □ Yes □ No
4. **Alcohol.** How many drinks do you typically have on a day you drink? *One drink is a bottle or can of beer (12 oz), a glass of wine or wine cooler (3.5 oz), or a shot glass of liquor (1.5 oz).*

   □ Never drink.

   □ Have no more than one drink in a day.

   □ Have no more than two drinks in a day.

   □ Sometimes have three or four drinks in a day.

   □ Sometimes have five or more drinks in a day.
5. **Sleep.** How many hours of sleep do you usually get each night? ________

Eating Practices

6. **Breakfast.** How many days each week do you usually eat breakfast (more than just coffee and a roll)? ________
7. **Bread/grains.** How many servings of whole-grain breads and cereals do you eat daily? *One serving = 1 slice bread, ½ cup dry cereal, ½ cup cooked oatmeal or other whole-grain cereal or brown rice.* __________
8. **Fruits and vegetables.** How many servings of fruits and vegetables do you eat daily? *One serving = 1 medium fruit, 6 oz fruit or vegetable juice, 1 cup raw fruit or vegetables, ½ cup cooked fruit or vegetables.* __________
9. **High-fat and high-cholesterol foods.** How often do you eat foods high in saturated fat and cholesterol (e.g., steak, hamburger, hot dog, sausage, bacon, cheese, fried chicken, French fries, ice cream, cheesecake, or other desserts)?

   □ Daily

   □ Eat these foods three or more times a week.

   □ Seldom or never eat these foods.
10. **Nuts/seeds.** How many servings of nuts do you usually eat each week? *One serving = 1 oz or a small handful, or 2 tablespoons of natural nut butter.* __________

Focused Assessment

Lifestyle and Risk Assessment—cont'd

11. **Legumes.** How many times a week do you eat legumes (peas, beans, lentils, garbanzos)? *One serving = ½ cup cooked.* ________

12. **Refined foods.** How often do you eat highly refined foods (soda pop, snack foods, chips, refined cereals, pastry, candy)?
    - ☐ Daily
    - ☐ Eat these foods three or more times a week.
    - ☐ Seldom or never eat refined foods.

13. **Weight.** How many pounds have you gained since you were 21 to 24 (enter 0 if you weigh the same, weigh less, or are younger than 21 years). ________

14. **Water Intake.** How many glasses (8 oz) of water do you typically drink each day? ______

Mental/Social Health

15. **Happiness.** How happy have you been during the past month?
    - ☐ Very happy
    - ☐ Pretty happy
    - ☐ Not too happy
    - ☐ Very unhappy

16. **Mood/Feelings**
    - (a) During the past month, have you often been bothered by feeling down, depressed, or hopeless?
      ☐ Yes ☐ No
    - (b) During the past month, have you often been bothered by having little interest or pleasure in doing things?
      ☐ Yes ☐ No
    - (c) Have your feelings in the past month caused you significant distress or impaired your ability to function socially or at work (or school)?
      ☐ Yes ☐ No

17. **Stress and coping.** How much of the time do you feel stressed out and unable to cope with life?
    - ☐ Seldom or never
    - ☐ Occasionally
    - ☐ Much of the time
    - ☐ Most of the time

Social Support

18. **Support.** Do you have family or friends you can get help from if needed?
    ☐ Yes ☐ No

19. **Social Interaction.** Do you have frequent social contact with family or friends?
    ☐ Yes ☐ No

Community

20. **Community Support.** Do you meet regularly with a faith community or other group that gives you support, comfort, meaning, and direction in your life?
    ☐ Yes ☐ No

Safety

21. **Seat belts.** What percentage of the time do you wear seat belts when riding in a car? ________

22. **Smoke alarm.** Do you have a working smoke alarm on each floor of your home, including the area in which you sleep?
    ☐ Yes ☐ No ☐ Don't know for sure.

23. **Helmet.** When biking or rollerblading, do you always wear a helmet and protective gear?
    ☐ Yes ☐ No

24. **Substance use and driving.** Do you ever drive soon after drinking alcohol or taking drugs or ride with someone who has been using illicit substances, including alcohol?
    ☐ Yes ☐ No

Safer Sex

25. **Practice safer sex.**
    - (a) Are you in a monogamous relationship?
      ☐ Yes ☐ No
    - (b) Do you always use condoms, or abstain from sexual relations?
      ☐ Always ☐ Don't always practice safer sex

Preventive Exams

26. Do you keep current on recommended preventive exams (see list below) and immunizations?
    ☐ Yes ☐ No ☐ Don't know for sure.

Recommended Preventive Exams

- Periodic checkup, including blood pressure, height and weight, and cholesterol check as recommended by your doctor.
- Pap tests within the last year, for women 21 or older
- Mammogram within last year, for women 45 or older
- Colorectal cancer screening, for all persons 45 or older
- Flu immunization, for everyone 6 months and older
- Pneumonia immunizations, for everyone 65 or older

Height ________

Weight ________

Blood pressure ________

Blood cholesterol ________ (mg/dL)

(Continued)

Focused Assessment

Lifestyle and Risk Assessment—cont'd

Scoring

Your score is the number of good health indicators you meet out of the 17 possible listed (below) in this assessment. The higher your score, the healthier your lifestyle. The Average Health Style Score is 9.4

Health Indicator	Guidelines for Good Health
1. Physical activity	Get 30 or more minutes of physical activity most days of the week.
2. Strength training	Do strength-building exercises at least twice per week.
3. Not smoking	Avoid all tobacco use and frequent exposure to secondhand smoke.
4. Alcohol use	Alcohol is not recommended, but if you drink alcohol, limit to one to two drinks in a day.
5. Adequate rest	Get adequate rest, at least 7 to 8 hours of sleep daily for best health.
6. Breakfast daily	Eat a nutritious breakfast daily for optimal physical and mental performance.
7. Whole grains	Choose whole-grain breads and cereals, at least three or more servings/per day.
8. Fruits and vegetables	Eat at least five servings of fruits and vegetables daily.
9. Fats, cholesterol	Limit high-fat meats, whole milk, and butter. Vegetable oils are healthier than oils from animals.
10. Nuts and Legumes	Nuts, such as almonds, contain healthy fats and protect against heart disease. Legumes prevent carbohydrate cravings, prevent metabolic syndrome, provide protein and energy, protect against cancer, and are a source of calcium and other vitamins and minerals.
11. Healthy weight	Maintain a healthy weight by eating well and participating in regular, moderate-intensity physical activity.
12. Mental health	Develop effective coping skills, and maintain a happy, hopeful outlook.
13. Social support	Maintain good social support and frequent contact with family and friends.
14. Community	Participate regularly in a faith community or other group that provides meaning, direction, and support in your life.
15. Safety	Be safety conscious; wear safety belts in the car and helmets when biking.
16. Safer sex	Remain in a monogamous relationship, or always use condoms, or abstain.
17. Regular exams	Get regular exams, including age/gender recommended preventive exams.

Source: Hall, D. R. (2004). Lifestyle check assessment. Vanderbilt University Health and Wellness.

STANDARDIZED LANGUAGE

Standardized Language

Health Promotion Diagnoses

Nursing Diagnosis	Selected NOC Outcomes and Goals Using NOC Indicators	Selected NIC Interventions and Nursing Activities
Sedentary Lifestyle	***NOC Outcomes*** Exercise Participation Physical Fitness ***Goals*** Meets mutually defined goals of increased mobility. Verbalizes feeling of increased strength and ability to move.	***NIC Interventions*** Exercise Promotion Self-Modification Assistance ***Nursing Activities*** Screen for mobility skills: ➤ bed mobility ➤ supported and unsupported sitting ➤ transition movements standing and walking Prior to activity, treat pain. Obtain any assistive devices needed. Encourage independence in ADLs. Develop mutually agreed on goals of increased activity.
Risk for Frail Elderly Syndrome	***NOC Outcomes*** Self-Care Status Nutritional Status: Food and Fluid Intake ***Goals*** Maintains ability to perform basic tasks and personal care independently with or without assistive device.	***NIC Interventions*** Hope Inspiration Health Education Self-Care Assistance ***Nursing Activities*** Assess home environment for safety. Evaluate depression or cognitive impairment. Provide suggestions for managing energy use. Encourage participation in low-intensity aerobic chair exercise. Provide opportunities for socialization and sensory stimulation.
Deficient Community Health	***NOC Outcomes*** Community Health Status Community Immune Status Community Risk Control: Communicable Disease ***Goals*** Community actions reduce the spread of infectious agents that threaten public health.	***NIC Interventions*** Communicable Disease Management Health Screening Program Development Surveillance: Community ***Nursing Activities*** Monitor immunization status of community. Facilitate access to immunizations. Provide immunizations to prevent communicable disease. Provide health education. Teach handwashing. Participate in community surveillance.

(Continued)

Standardized Language

Health Promotion Diagnoses—cont'd

Nursing Diagnosis	Selected NOC Outcomes and Goals Using NOC Indicators	Selected NIC Interventions and Nursing Activities
Readiness for Enhanced Health Management	***NOC Outcomes*** Compliance Behavior Health Promoting Behavior Participation in Healthcare Decisions ***Goals*** Participates in activities to enhance management of therapeutic regimen.	***NIC Interventions*** Decision-Making Support Health Education Health System Guidance Mutual Goal Setting Risk Identification Self-Modification Assistance Teaching: Individual ***Nursing Activities*** Create an accepting, nonjudgmental atmosphere. Encourage consideration of values underlying choices and consequences of the choice. Determine ability and motivation of patient and partner to correctly participate in therapeutic regimen. Include family/support person in instruction. Provide financial resource assistance if needed.

Sources: Butcher, H. K., Bulechek, G. M., Dochterman, J. M., Wagner, C.M. (Eds.). (2018). *Nursing interventions classification (NIC)* (7th ed.). St. Louis, MO: Elsevier. Used with permission; Moorhead, S., Swanson, E., Johnson, M., Maas, M., et al. (2018). *Nursing outcomes classification (NOC)* (6th ed.). St. Louis, MO: Elsevier. Used with permission; NANDA International. (2017). *Nursing diagnosis: Definitions and classifications 2018–2020*. Thieme. Used with permission.

CLINICALJUDGMENT

Applying the Full-Spectrum Nursing Model

PATIENT SITUATION

Shandra Shane is a single 37-year-old woman with three children, ages 12, 15, and 17. She is raising the children on her own, although her sister occasionally helps with transportation or advice about disciplining her teenage daughters. Ms. Shane is a night-shift worker at the hospital. Her typical schedule is 3 to 4 hours of sleep in the morning soon after she gets home and then a short nap in the early evening before going back to work. She smokes 1 to 1½ packs of cigarettes per day but tells you she has been trying to smoke less around her children. Her job stress is high, as the hospital is cutting back on the number of staff. Ms. Shane also takes care of her aging mother, who has Alzheimer's and lives with her. Ms. Shane's outlet for stress is going out with friends and drinking beer on the weekend. She is seeking your professional guidance to lose some weight (about 60 pounds) and to feel more energetic.

THINKING

1. *Theoretical Knowledge:*
   List health behaviors that negatively influence health status.

2. *Critical Thinking (Contextual Awareness):*
   What factors in this situation would you consider threatening to Ms. Shane's health and could lead to disease later in life?

DOING

3. *Nursing Process (Planning/Intervention):*
   What suggestions might you make about Ms. Shane's diet that could help her to lose weight? Why might these actions be effective for weight loss?

4. *Practical Knowledge:*
   What areas of her daily living other than her diet might you explore further and offer recommendations for improving to promote better health and prevent illness?

CARING

5. *Self-Knowledge:*
   Have you ever been in a situation in which you felt stressed, tired, and wanting gratification offered by food, nicotine, or alcohol? Describe your experience.

6. *Ethical Knowledge:*
   In what ways could you demonstrate genuine caring for Shandra?

Critical Thinking and Clinical Judgment

1. While working in a physician's office, a 70-year-old woman is referred to you for counseling regarding health protection activities. She is hypertensive and obese.
   a. How does her age affect your assessments and communication?
   b. What type of learning aids might be needed?
   c. What health screenings are appropriate for this client?

2. Below is a group of clients who wish to enroll in a health promotion program.
   - Jennifer Kaska is 23 years old and was diagnosed with diabetes mellitus at the age of 12 years. She checks her blood sugar and administers insulin as needed. She runs 3 miles, 3 days per week.
   - Maurice Rosenthal is 47 years old with no known illness. He is 6 feet tall and weighs 240 pounds. His body mass index (BMI) is 33 kg/m^2, indicating obesity. He takes no routine medication, only acetaminophen for occasional headaches.
   - Clara Fenton is 83 years old and has been diagnosed with hypertension, emphysema, and osteoporosis. She takes 10 prescription medications daily in addition to a multivitamin and an occasional laxative.

   Discuss the pros and cons of providing a group program that includes all three of these clients.

3. L. F. is a 50-year-old man with heart disease. He had coronary artery bypass surgery 1 month ago. He has stopped going to his prescribed cardiac rehabilitation program because of the distance he must travel to the rehabilitation center. Discuss at least two approaches for working with this client.

4. Cecelia Kent is 32 years old. She takes no medications and has annual physical exams. She walks 4 to 5 miles, 5 days per week, and lifts light weights two to three times per week. She eats a low-fat, low-salt, low-sugar diet. She has never smoked, and drinks only limited alcohol.
   a. She asks you to recommend further health promotion activities. How would you respond?
   b. How could you incorporate Cecelia into a health promotion class that includes Jennifer Kaska, Maurice Rosenthal, and Clara Fenton (from question 2)?

(continued)

5. For each of the following concepts, use critical thinking to describe how or why it is important to nursing, patient care, or health promotion. Note that these are *not* to be merely definitions.

Health promotion	Hardiness
Illness prevention	Health screenings
Lifestyle	Health education

What Are the Main Points in This Chapter?

- *Health promotion* refers to helping clients develop an optimal state of health.
- Intention is the difference between health promotion and health protection (illness prevention).
- There are three levels of activities for health protection: primary, secondary, and tertiary prevention. *Primary interventions* are designed to prevent or slow the onset of disease. *Secondary interventions* are designed to detect illnesses in early stages. *Tertiary interventions* focus on stopping the disease from progressing and on rehabilitation.
- The *Healthy People 2020* initiative is designed to achieve four overarching goals:
  - Attain high-quality, longer lives free of preventable disease, disability, injury, and premature death.
  - Achieve health equity, eliminate disparities, and improve the health of all groups.
  - Create social and physical environments that promote good health for all.
  - Promote quality of life, healthy development, and healthy behaviors in all life stages.
- Pender's Health Promotion Model (HPM) identifies three groups of variables that affect health behavior: (1) individual characteristics and experiences; (2) behavior-specific cognitions and affect; and (3) behavioral outcome.
- A Wellness Wheel identifies six dimensions of health: emotional, intellectual, physical, spiritual, social/family, and occupational.
- The Transtheoretical Model of Change identifies four stages of change: contemplation, determination, action, and maintenance.
- Health promotion activities for all age groups include nutrition, exercise, safety concerns, changing unhealthy lifestyles, immunizations, and screenings.
- Health promotion activities may be conducted in acute care facilities, the workplace, local communities, or schools.
- A health promotion assessment involves obtaining a health history, physical examination, fitness assessment, lifestyle and risk appraisal, life stress review, assessment of healthcare beliefs, nutritional assessment, and screening activities.
- Health screening activities are designed to detect disease at an early stage so that treatment can begin before there is an opportunity for disease to spread or reduce the quality of life.
- Health screening activities vary based on developmental stage and identified risk factors.
- Nurses promote health through role models, counseling, health education, and providing and facilitating support.

Knowledge Map

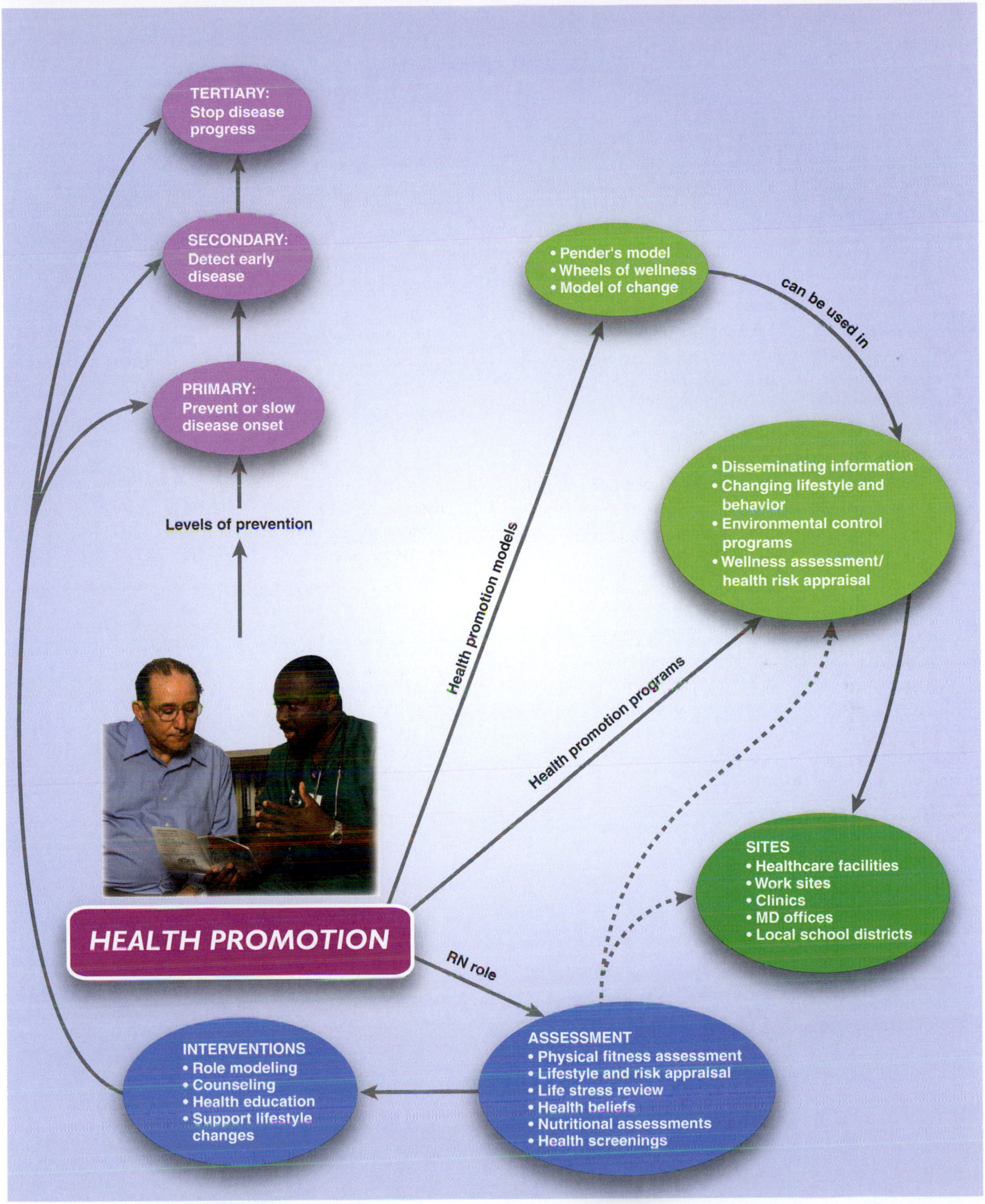

UNIT 6

The Context for Nurses' Work

CHAPTER 43

Community & Home Health Nursing

STUDENT RESOURCES

The questions and exercises in this book allow you to practice the kind of thinking you will use as a full-spectrum nurse. Critical-thinking questions usually have more than one right answer, so we do not provide "correct answers" for these features. Try to answer these questions yourself. It is more important to develop your nursing judgment than to just cover content. You will learn more by discussing the questions with your peers. If you are still unsure, see the Davis Advantage chapter resources for suggested responses.

To explore learning resources for this chapter,

Go to Davis Advantage and find:

Answers and Suggested Responses for all questions in this chapter
Concept Map
Knowledge Map
References and Bibliography
Lists of NOC Outcomes and NIC Interventions

Key Concepts

Community nursing
Home healthcare
Population

Related Concepts

See the Concept Map on Davis Advantage.

Caring for the Nguyens

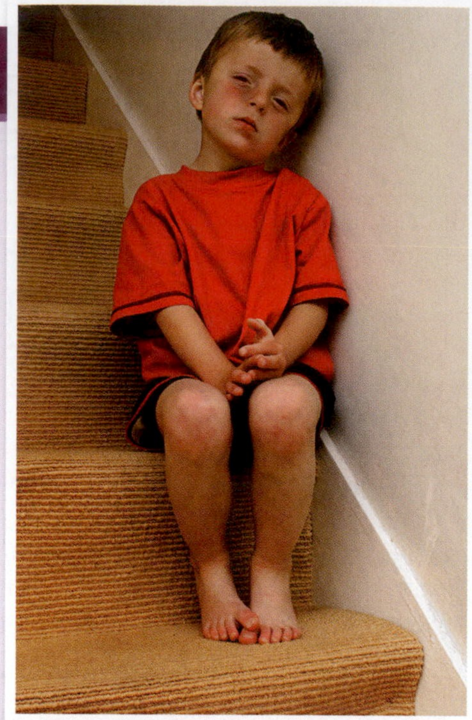

Yen Nguyen works as preschool teacher in her community. Andre is a 4-year-old boy in her class. Over the past few months, she has noticed that Andre has many bruises in various stages of healing. He seems withdrawn and does not interact much with the other children. She is concerned that Andre might be a victim of child abuse, but she is reluctant to make that accusation, especially because her assistant doesn't seem to have noticed anything amiss.

Yen talks to her husband, Nam, about her concerns: "I'm worried about a child at school, but I'm afraid to say anything. What if I'm wrong? I'd probably lose my job. But if I'm right and I don't say anything, I could still lose my job, and this boy could be hurt even worse." Nam suggests that she contact the clinic nurse at the Family Medicine Center for confidential advice on how to proceed.

A. Imagine that you are the clinic nurse. Use the full-spectrum nursing model to identify at least 10 questions that you would need to answer to investigate Yen's concerns further.

B. *Self-knowledge:* What personal values do you have that would affect the manner in which you handle this situation? Explain.

C. *Ethical knowledge:* What is the most important ethical issue in this situation? That is, what is the most important goal? Note that there may be several moral and legal issues, but you are being asked to identify the *most* important one. Note also that we are not asking you what the nurse *can* do, but rather what the nurse ideally *should* do.

D. You share the questions you have with Yen. She believes that there is a real need to investigate child abuse. You advise her to call the local child protective services (CPS) agency. Based on your knowledge of community and public health nursing, what aspects of the community health role will the nurse from CPS use as she investigates this situation?

PracticalKnowledge clinical **application**

Practical knowledge in community and home-care nursing requires you to apply the nursing process to both individuals and groups.

CLINICAL INSIGHTS

Clinical Insight 43-1 ➤ Safety Considerations in Home Care

Before the Visit

- **Plan ahead.** Know where you are headed. Use a map or global positioning system (GPS). Contact the client or family for directions if it is unclear where you are headed. File a visit plan with your office each day.
- **Dress in appropriate clothing** as dictated by your agency. Wear a nametag clearly identifying you and the agency. Wear comfortable, non-skid shoes that will enable you to move quickly if necessary.
- **Carry a cell phone.** Be sure it is fully charged. Know how to quickly access 911 in case of emergency.
- **Do not carry a purse,** multiple credit cards, or excess cash. Instead, use a waist or fanny pack and conceal it under clothing. Carry enough money or other payment method for emergency transportation, telephone numbers for clients and home health agency, and emergency contact information.
- **Keep your car in good repair** and always have enough gasoline in the tank. Be prepared for inclement weather, and always carry an emergency car safety pack.
- **Do not get out of your car for any reason if driving in an area that might not be safe.** Carjacking involves minor car impact ("fender bender") as a strategy to get a person to exit the vehicle, leaving her vulnerable for attack, assault, or theft.
- **Observe your surroundings** as you drive to the visit. Notice the location of emergency services, local gas stations, and public places if help is required.
- **Carry mace or other items to aid in self-defense** in situations in which you feel threatened.
- **Park as close to your destination as possible.** If possible, park your car facing the direction you plan to go when you leave. Never enter dead-end streets or alleys.
- **Check your surroundings before you leave your car.** If you feel unsafe, leave the area immediately and call your office.
- **Lock the car. Leave no valuables in sight.**
- **Prepare your bag while you are still in the car.**
- **Carry your bag on one arm. In the opposite hand, carry your keys.** Always have them ready. You may need them if you decide to exit quickly. Also, you can use keys to defend yourself by placing the pointed ends of the keys between your fingers.
- **Walk directly to the client's house.** Walk in the middle of the sidewalk. Use common walkways. Avoid isolated and poorly lighted areas. Do not take shortcuts.
- **Knock or ring the doorbell before entering.** Never enter without being invited. If there is no answer at the door, call or text the patient.
- **If for any reason you feel that the neighborhood is unsafe, do not get out of the car.** Instead, leave the neighborhood immediately and phone your agency.

During the Visit

- **Introduce yourself** and clearly identify your agency. Show your name badge.
- **Sit where you have access to an exit.** When you enter the home, observe all exits.
- **Notice who is present in the home. Request introductions.** This information is useful for planning care as well as for ensuring safety.
- **Leave immediately if you suspect substance use** or drunken behavior.
- **Leave immediately if there is a violent domestic argument.** Do not attempt to intervene. When you return to your car, drive to a safe location and call 911 to report the event.
- **Request that animals be kept in another room** while you make your visit.
- **If weapons are visible, request that they be put away** immediately. Leave the home if this request is not met.
- **If household members interfere with the visit,** discuss the problem with the client. You may need to arrange a time to visit when they are not present.

After the Visit

- **Continue to observe the safety precautions** you used when getting to the visit. Do not let down your guard as you return to your car.
- **If you are in an unsafe neighborhood or poorly lighted area, leave immediately and do not consult the map** for directions to your next visit. Drive to a secure public location, and then consult the map.
- **Inform your agency** if you believe the home or neighborhood is potentially hazardous.
- **Request a security escort service** if future visits are required.
- **Document your assessments** and the care delivered.
- **Report abuse** if you suspect it in the home.

Other

You also need to protect yourself from infection and accidental injury, as you would in a hospital (see Clinical Insight 43-2).

- Use safe lifting techniques, especially because you might have to improvise more than in the hospital. There will probably be no one to assist with patient transfer, ambulation, or lifting. Mechanical lifts are not often available in the home.
- Do not dispose of loose sharps in household trash containers, toilets, or recycling bins. Place them immediately in a sharps disposal container. If a sharps container is not available, use a puncture- and leak-resistant plastic household container (e.g., a plastic milk jug).

Clinical Insight 43-2 ➤ Infection Control in the Home

The following suggestions can help you maintain infection control during a home visit.

Hand Hygiene

- Keep antibacterial cleanser and protective equipment approved by the Occupational Safety and Health Administration in your nursing bag.
- Perform hand hygiene using soap and warm water or an antibacterial handrub at the beginning and end of each visit and before and after any treatment.
- Always perform hand hygiene before handling your nursing bag.
- If the home conditions are dirty or your hands become soiled, wash your hands with soap and warm water as soon as possible.

Supplies

- In homes that you know are not clean, limit the supplies you bring into the home. For example, leave your nursing bag in the car, and bring only the supplies you need for the visit.
- If necessary, use a 1:10 dilution of chlorine bleach in water to disinfect surfaces or equipment in the home. Some equipment may need to be disinfected by boiling in a covered pan of water for 15 to 20 minutes. Do not boil plastic or rubber items.
- You can disinfect hard plastic items by wrapping them with a wet paper towel and placing them in a zippered plastic bag. Microwave the entire bag on high for 10 minutes.

Nursing Bag Hygiene

- Do not bring the bag into the home in any of the following circumstances. The home is:
  - Known to be colonized with a multidrug-resistant organism (e.g., vancomycin-resistant *Enterococcus* [VRE], methicillin-resistant *Staphylococcus aureus* [MRSA], *Clostridium difficile*)
  - Infested with bedbugs, pests
  - Grossly contaminated with human or pet urine or feces (McGoldrick, 2017)
- **Non-wheeled bag—** Place on an impermeable surface barrier with antimicrobial additives to protect the bag from contact with microorganisms. In the car, you should place it on a visibly clean, dry surface. Avoid using paper towels, newspaper, or other products that may wick moisture from the environmental surface.
- **Wheeled bag—**If the bag is brought into the home, keep it on the floor and do not allow the front flap to have contact with the surface of the floor.
- If you use items from your nursing bag during the visit, always clean them with an approved antibacterial wipe or solution before placing them back into your bag.
- Clean the interior and exterior surfaces of the bag monthly when a surface barrier is used, or weekly if it is not, and anytime it is visibly soiled.

Biohazard and Sharps Disposal

- Flush wound irrigation or potentially contaminated liquids down the toilet while wearing gloves and any other appropriate protective equipment.
- Double-bag dressings, equipment, or disposable supplies that have been contaminated with body secretions to prevent leakage. The bags should be labeled *Biohazard.*
- Carry small biohazard sharps containers. Place syringes and sharps in the container without recapping them. If clients or family must use syringes or sharps, you may wish to leave a sharps container in the home. An alternative solution is to have them use a metal coffee can with lid, for example.

Client Teaching

- Provide instruction on home cleanliness, hygiene, hand hygiene, food preparation, and instructions to avoid contact with persons who are ill, as needed.
- If the client is immunocompromised, teach the signs and symptoms of infection. Advise the client to immediately notify the primary care provider of any changes.

Special Situations

- If the patient has a multidrug-resistant infection or pulmonary tuberculosis, use appropriate barrier precautions, including an N95 respirator. Leave reusable equipment in the home; and if possible, schedule these clients as the last appointment of the day.

STANDARDIZED LANGUAGE

This section provides guidelines for using NANDA International (NANDA-I), Nursing Outcomes Classification (NOC), Nursing Interventions Classification (NIC), the Clinical Care Classification System (CCC), and the Omaha System to develop problem statements, goals, and nursing orders to use in planning care for aggregates and communities. If you need to review these five standardized languages,

Go to **Chapters 4, 5, and 6,** in Volume 1.

The Omaha System

The Omaha System is a problem-solving model for community health practice, education, and research. The taxonomy consists of *diagnostic labels* organized into four *domains* (categories), along with two sets of *modifiers*. Within those domains, the system classifies 42 client problems or areas of concern (see Omaha System: Domains, Problem Modifiers, and Examples of Problem Labels, following). As you can see, the problem labels in the environment domain are especially useful in community nursing. For the complete problem classification scheme,

Go to the **Omaha System Web site,** at http://www.omahasystem.org

Omaha Problem Classification Scheme

To create a diagnostic statement, choose an appropriate problem label, and add a modifier to it from each of the two sets in the accompanying Standardized Language box, Omaha System: Domains and Examples of Problem Labels. For a community-based diagnosis, you would add "group" as the modifier.

For example, a group Environment diagnosis for workers in a meatpacking plant with lax safety standards might read ***Deficit in Group*** Workplace Safety. If only one worker were at risk (perhaps because of her inattention to safety rules), you could write *Potential Deficit in Individual* Workplace Safety.

Domain: Environment
Modifiers: (1) Health Promotion, Potential Deficit, or Deficit (2) Family, Individual, or Group
Diagnostic Statements:
Deficit in Group Workplace Safety
Potential Deficit in Individual Workplace Safety

Standardized Language

Omaha System: Domains, Problem Modifiers, and Examples of Problem Labels

Domains

Environmental Domain—The material resources, physical surroundings, and substances both internal and external to the client, home, neighborhood, and broader community

Problem (Diagnosis) Labels: Income, Sanitation, Residence, Neighborhood/Workplace Safety

Psychosocial Domain—Patterns of behavior, communication, relationships, and development

Problem (Diagnosis) Labels: Social Contact, Role Change, Interpersonal Relationships, Spirituality, Grief, Mental Health, Sexuality, Caretaking/Parenting, Neglect, Abuse

Physiological Domain—Functional status of processes that maintain life

Problem (Diagnosis) Labels: Hearing, Vision, Oral Health, Speech and Language, Pain, Respiration, Digestion-Hydration, Communicable/Infectious Condition

Health Related Behaviors Domain—Activities that maintain or promote wellness, promote recovery, or maximize rehabilitation potential

Problem (Diagnosis) Labels: Nutrition, Personal Hygiene, Prescribed Medication Regimen, Sleep and Rest Patterns, Family Planning, Physical Activity

Problem Modifiers

Set 1—Health Promotion, Potential Deficit, Deficit

Set 2—Family, Individual, Group*

*Martin and Scheet (1992, p. 67) suggest that *Group* be added to these modifiers.

Source: Martin, K. S., & Scheet, N. J. (1992). *The Omaha System: Applications for community health nursing*. Philadelphia: W. B. Saunders, pp. 67–74. Used with permission; Omaha System (2009). *Solving clinical data-information: Problem rating scale for outcomes*. Retrieved from http://www.omahasystem.org

Using the NOC and Omaha Systems to Write Aggregate Goals

NOC Outcomes

NOC standardized outcomes in the Community Health domain include the following (Moorhead, S., Swanson, E., Johnson, M., et al., 2018):

- Community Competence
- Community Disaster Readiness
- Community Disaster Response
- Community Health Status
- Community Immune Status
- Community Risk Control: Chronic Disease
- Community Risk Control: Communicable Disease
- Community Risk Control: Lead Exposure
- Community Risk Control: Obesity
- Community Violence Level

You can use these NOC labels to write goals by adding the appropriate NOC indicators and scales (see NOC Measurement Scales, in the Standardized Language section of Chapter 5, in this volume).

Omaha System Outcomes

Using the Omaha System, you will develop goals/outcomes from the words in the nursing diagnosis. Recall that all nursing diagnoses are identified as *individual, family,* or *group,* so a group nursing diagnosis will automatically indicate a group goal. For example, for the diagnosis Deficit in Group Workplace Safety, you would build the outcomes around the words "Group Workplace Safety." The Omaha System includes a five-point Problem Rating Scale for Outcomes (see the accompanying table) that describes what you expect to achieve in terms of the client's knowledge, behavior, and status.

Standardized Language

Omaha Problem Rating Scale for Outcomes

Concept	1	2	3	4	5
Knowledge The ability of the client to remember and interpret information	No knowledge	Minimal knowledge	Basic knowledge	Adequate knowledge	Superior knowledge
Behavior The client's observable responses, actions, or activities fitting the occasion or purpose	Never appropriate	Rarely appropriate	Inconsistently appropriate	Usually appropriate	Consistently appropriate
Status The condition of the client in relation to objective and subjective defining characteristics	Extreme signs/ symptoms	Severe signs/ symptoms	Moderate signs/ symptoms	Minimal signs/ symptoms	No signs/ symptoms

Source: The Omaha System. (2009, May 11, updated). *Solving clinical data-information: Problem rating scale for outcomes.* Retrieved on February 1, 2019 from http://www.omahasystem.org/problemratingscaleforoutcomes.html

Using the above table, you would create expected outcomes by applying this scale to Group Workplace Safety, as follows.

Standardized Language

Creating Outcomes for the Diagnosis Group Workplace Safety

***Nursing Diagnosis*: Deficit in Group Workplace Safety**

Rating Scale Concept	Present Status, Before Interventions	Expected Outcome, After Interventions
Knowledge	(2) Minimal knowledge of workplace safety	(4) Adequate knowledge of workplace safety
Behavior	(2) Rarely appropriate safety behaviors	(4) Usually appropriate group safety behaviors
Status	(2) Severe signs/symptoms (e.g., frequent accidents or injuries)	(4) Minimal signs/symptoms (e.g., few accidents or injuries)

The outcomes in this table mean that after your interventions, you expect the group to have adequate knowledge of workplace safety, demonstrate usually appropriate behaviors (e.g., usually follow the safety rules), and demonstrate minimal accidents or injuries. To evaluate the client's progress, you would assign a scale number to the group's actual knowledge, behavior, and status *after interventions*.

Using the NIC and Omaha Interventions Labels for Community Healthcare

The NIC Interventions Taxonomy

The NIC taxonomy includes 16 interventions specifically designed for community health grouped into two Classes: Community Health Promotion, and Community Risk Management. (See the following box.)

Standardized Language

NIC Community Health Classes and Interventions

Class: Community Health Promotion—Interventions promote the health of the whole community

Interventions:

Case Management
Community Health Advocacy
Community Health Development
Fiscal Resource Management
Health Education
Health Policy Monitoring
Immunization/Vaccination Management
Program Development
Social Marketing

Class: Community Risk Management—Interventions that assist in detecting or preventing health risks to the whole community

Interventions:

Bioterrorism Preparedness
Communicable Disease Management
Community Disaster Preparedness
Environmental Management: Community
Environmental Management: Worker Safety
Environmental Risk Protection
Health Screening
Risk Identification
Surveillance: Community
Vehicle Safety Promotion

Source: Butcher, H., Bulechek, G., Dochterman, J., et al. (Eds.). (2018). *Nursing interventions classification (NIC)* (7th ed.). St. Louis, MO: Elsevier.

The Omaha Interventions Taxonomy

The Omaha System taxonomy provides four "intervention categories" you can use in community-oriented nursing practice:

- **Health Teaching, Guidance, and Counseling.** These primary prevention activities include giving information; anticipating client problems; encouraging client action and responsibility for self-care; and assisting with coping, decision making, and problem-solving. As a community-oriented nurse, you should spend most of your time offering this level of intervention.
- **Treatments and Procedures.** These are secondary interventions directed toward preventing disease, identifying risk factors and early signs and symptoms, and decreasing or alleviating signs and symptoms.
- **Case Management.** Case management is a tertiary intervention that includes coordination, advocacy, and referral. These activities involve facilitating service delivery on behalf of the client, communicating with health and human service providers, promoting assertive client communication, and guiding the client toward appropriate community resources.
- **Surveillance.** These nursing activities include detection, measurement, critical analysis, and monitoring to indicate client status in relation to a given condition or phenomenon.

To write an intervention statement, you must combine one of those four "categories" of interventions with one of the "targets" (objects of the nursing interventions), such as bowel care and nutrition. Then you must add patient-specific information to individualize the nursing order. See the accompanying box for intervention categories, examples of targets, and intervention statements (nursing orders). To see the entire set of intervention targets,

Go to the **Omaha System Web site,** at http://www.omahasystem.org/interventionscheme.html

You will notice that the targets can be used for individuals as well as groups. It is the designation of the nursing diagnosis as *individual, family,* or *group* that determines this.

Standardized Language

Omaha Intervention Categories and Examples of Targets

Categories

I. Teaching, Guidance, and Counseling
II. Treatments and Proceduress
III. Case Management
IV. Surveillance

Examples of Targets

Anatomy/physiology
Behavior modification
Communication
Discipline
Feeding procedures
Homemaking/housekeeping
Substance use cessation
Wellness

Examples of Aggregate Targets

Caretaking/parenting skills
Day care/respite
Durable medical equipment
Education
Employment
Environment
Finances
Legal system
Transportation
Other community resource

Examples of Nursing Intervention Statements

Treatments and Procedures (II): Feeding procedures (Demonstrate to Mrs. Adams how to feed Mr. Adams at the next visit.)

Surveillance (IV): Feeding procedures (After teaching, observe a feeding. Monitor for choking.)

Source: The Omaha System. (2009, May 11, updated). Solving the clinical data-information scheme: Intervention scheme. Retrieved February 1, 2019 from http://www.omahasystem.org/interventionscheme.html

Clinical Care Classification System for Home Healthcare

Standardized Language

Clinical Care Classification: 21 Care Components (Version 2.5) Coded by Alphabetic Classes*

Code	Component	Code	Component
A	Activity	L	Respiratory
B	Bowel/Gastric	M	Role Relationship
C	Cardiac	N	Safety
D	Cognitive/Neuro	O	Self-Care
E	Coping	P	Self-Concept
F	Fluid Volume	Q	Sensory
G	Health Behavioral	R	Skin Integrity
H	Medication	S	Tissue Perfusion
I	Metabolic	T	Urinary Elimination
J	Nutritional	U	Life Cycle
K	Physical Regulation		

*The Clinical Care Classification system is copyrighted, placed in public domain, and cannot be sold, but is available with written permission (Saba, V. K. [1994, 2004, 2012, 2017]. Clinical Care Classification System [Version 2.5] [2nd ed.]. New York, NY: Springer. Retrieved from https://www.sabacare.com).

Standardized Language

An Example of Clinical Care Classification (CCC) Nursing Diagnoses and Interventions

A—ACTIVITY COMPONENT *(1 of 21 Care Components)*—
A cluster of elements that involve the use of energy in carrying out musculoskeletal and bodily actions.

01 Activity Alteration *(Major Nursing Diagnosis)*—Change in or modification of energy used by the body.

Subcategories that provide greater definition of the problem (of "01 Activity Alteration")

01.0	Activity Alteration
01.1	Activity Intolerance
01.2	Activity Intolerance Risk
01.3	Diversional Activity Deficit
01.4	Fatigue
01.5	Physical Mobility Impairment
01.6	Sleep Pattern Disturbance
01.7	Sleep Deprivation

Actions performed to carry out physiological or psychological daily activities:

Example: Teach Passive Range of Motion

Adapted: Saba, V. K. (2017). About. Clinical Care Classification System (Version 2.5) (2nd ed.). New York, NY: Springer. Retrieved February 1, 2019, from https://sabacare.com/Custom/Tables/Components.php

CLINICALJUDGMENT
Applying the Full-Spectrum Nursing Model

PATIENT SITUATION

While honeymooning in the Caribbean, Lorenzo and Elvia learn that the area has infected *Aedes aegypti* mosquitos, which can spread the Zika virus. Later she learns that she conceived when traveling to this area and seeks healthcare for her first trimester pregnancy in south Florida. The couple is concerned about the possibility of contracting Zika virus.

THINKING

1. *Theoretical Knowledge:*
   a. How is Zika virus spread?
   b. What symptoms would Elvia show if she has the Zika infection?
2. *Critical Thinking (Contextual Awareness):*
   Why is it important to detect and treat Zika infection in women of childbearing age?

DOING

3. *Nursing Process (Assessment):*
   How might you assess the extent of the problem of Zika virus infection within the southern Florida community (Dade County)?
4. *Practical Knowledge:*
   a. As the Community Health nurse, you design a *primary* intervention program to prevent women of childbearing age to acquire Zika virus infection during pregnancy. What might you do for this program?
   b. What *secondary* interventions would you include in your patient education?

CARING

5. *Self-Knowledge:*
   a. When showing compassion for your client, what information about her pregnancy might you offer?
   b. How would you feel if you were exposed to the Zika virus during your first trimester of pregnancy?

Critical Thinking and Clinical Judgment

1. You are nearing completion of your fundamentals course. One night while you are preparing for your next clinical, the telephone rings. It is your neighbor, Tanya. Her 5-year-old daughter, Tiffany, attends kindergarten at the local public school. Tiffany came home with a letter from the school nurse stating that another child in the class was ill with H1N1 and that all the students in the class had been exposed to this flu virus.

   Tanya is concerned about the risks to Tiffany and the rest of the family. Tiffany was vaccinated against H1N1. Tanya is 8 months pregnant, and the family has no health insurance. She states that because you are a nursing student, she thought you might know what she should do or where she might go for assistance.

   What are the key pieces of information (both theoretical knowledge and patient data) you need to solve your neighbor's situation?

2. You are a nurse in a public health clinic providing routine childhood immunizations. A 16-year-old mother comes into the clinic requesting "shots" for her newborn baby as well as a birth control "shot." She indicates that she has no money to pay for the shots because her 20-year-old boyfriend gave her only enough to get to the clinic.

   Which of the following is your nursing priority for this situation?

   What will you do next?

   Explain *how* you have chosen your priority diagnosis.

   On what did you base your choice?

   - Give the newborn the immunizations; and arrange for the client to meet with the social worker regarding securing healthcare coverage.
   - Educate the mother about birth control.
   - Take the client and child to a private room and discuss the general health of the newborn and the plans for a healthcare provider to see the child. Also ask about the health needs of the mother.
   - Ask the mother whether she is being abused and report the incident if so.

3. Your assignment is to conduct a community assessment of your own neighborhood.

   How will your membership in the community affect your assessment? What activities could you delete from the assessment?

4. You are driving home from nursing school clinical day and happen upon a car overturned along a deserted country road. You recall what you learned about the Good Samaritan laws.

   Under these circumstances, are you liable for the care you provide? What is your best course of intervention?

5. As a beginning home health nurse, you have been assigned to visit the following clients today:

   - Roland Escobar (Meet Your Patients, Volume 1), a 78-year-old man recovering from a cerebrovascular accident (stroke)
   - Sally Littlemoon, a 48-year-old woman with diabetes mellitus, blindness, and lower extremity cellulitis (a skin infection)
   - Beatrice Wayne, a 67-year-old woman who has undergone elective coronary artery bypass graft surgery (open-heart surgery)
   - Kent Churchill, an 80-year-old man with a recent hip fracture and surgical repair

- Chana Padir, a 50-year-old woman with severe pain secondary to breast cancer with extensive metastases. She is receiving hospice care.

a. Explore some alternatives for your schedule. How would you prepare to make these five visits in one day? How would you determine how to arrange your schedule?

b. The report you receive from the home health supervisor includes the following information:
   - Ms. Littlemoon and Mr. Churchill require dressing changes.
   - Mr. Escobar and Ms. Wayne require teaching about their medications.
   - Mr. Escobar, Ms. Littlemoon, and Mr. Churchill require venipuncture for lab work.
   - Ms. Padir is having increasing pain.

   Based on this information, what else do you need to know and/or do before you begin your visits?

   What practical knowledge will you need to provide care for these clients?

c. How might the care you deliver to Ms. Wayne differ from the care you give to Ms. Padir? To answer the question, consider the context for each woman. How are their situations different?

d. When visiting Ms. Padir, you realize that her husband and children are very fearful of her impending death. They seem overwhelmed by the care she requires.

   What values and beliefs do you have about death and dying that might influence your care of the Padir family? (Review Chapters 15, 16, and 17 if necessary.)

   What must you consider when planning your interventions? How might you intervene?

e. When you arrive at the home of Ms. Wayne, she is dressed and out of bed. She tells you she is able to walk around her house independently with very little pain. She can identify the medications she is receiving, their purpose, and their schedule for administration. Her chest wound is healing nicely, and her breath sounds are clear. She informs you that she is planning on going to her cabin in the mountains this upcoming weekend with her husband and children.

   What actions must you take with regard to continuing her home visits? Why?

   What rules/guidelines will influence your choice of action?

6. For each of the following concepts, use critical thinking and summarize how or why it is important to nursing, patient care, or community nursing. Note that these are *not* to be merely definitions.

Community

Aggregates

Census tracts

Vulnerable populations

Healthy People 2020

Windshield survey

Primary intervention

Secondary intervention

Tertiary intervention

Disaster preparedness

Omaha System

7. For each of the following concepts, use critical thinking to describe how or why it is important to nurses, patient care, or nursing in the home. Note that these are *not* to be merely definitions.

Delivering healthcare in the home setting	Developing rapport at the home visit
Skilled services	Assessment of the home environment
Caregiver role strain	Documentation of home healthcare services
Preparing for the home visit	Clinical Care Classification System

What Are the Main Points in This Chapter?

- A community can be defined as a place with defined boundaries, a group of people with a common language, rituals, or customs.
- Each community determines the meaning of health and nursing activities to promote health.
- A vulnerable population is defined as an aggregate that is at increased risk of adverse health outcomes. Members of vulnerable groups have a higher probability of developing illness.
- The community nurse assesses three general dimensions of a community: structure, status, and process.
- Common practice areas for community-based nurses include schools, churches, prison systems, disaster relief services, occupational and public health clinics, and international relief organizations.
- Community health nursing focuses on the health of individuals, families, and groups and how their individual health affects the community as a whole.
- Public health nursing focuses on the community at large and the eventual effect of the community's health status on the health of individuals, families, and groups.
- Community-oriented nursing combines components of community and public health. Nurses practicing community-oriented nursing are fluid in their approach. Their focus is a comprehensive look at the individual, family, group, and community at large. Community-based nurses serve as advocates, educators, collaborators, counselors, and effective communicators.
- Community-based nurses may provide care at three levels: primary (preventive), secondary (early detection and early treatment), and tertiary (halt disease progression). The focus is on primary prevention.
- The Omaha classification system is a commonly used documentation system for generating a care plan for a community or an individual within the community setting.
- A community health nurse might practice as a school nurse, public health nurse, parish or prison nurse, international health nurse, or disaster service.
- Home healthcare is delivered in the community setting.
- Home health nursing fosters client and family independence and promotes self-care.
- In the home setting, many factors, such as cleanliness and noise level, are not within the nurse's control. In addition, the home health nurse works without immediate on-site access to other healthcare professionals.
- Home health agencies may be public, voluntary, proprietary, or hospital-based agencies. They may provide direct or indirect care and may specialize in certain types of clients.
- As a full-spectrum nurse working in home healthcare, you will function in the following roles: communicator, direct care provider, client/family educator, client advocate, and care coordinator (case manager).
- Hospice nurses work in hospitals, special hospice facilities, or the homes of patients who are dying. The goal of their care is to provide comfort and manage symptoms.
- Home healthcare is reimbursed by Medicare, by Medicaid, and by private insurance, or paid for through direct payment from the client. Medicare and Medicaid are the largest payors.
- To be eligible for continuing care under most government healthcare programs and private insurers, a client must be homebound and require skilled nursing care.
- Preparation for a home visit includes obtaining information from the referral, identifying the purpose of the visit, gathering required supplies, contacting the client to arrange the visit, and providing for your own safety.
- During a home visit, you will establish a rapport with the client and family, assess the needs of the client and caregivers, develop and discuss the plan of care and needed services with the client and caregivers, provide skilled care, and evaluate the need for continued services.
- Medicare requires specific client assessments using a form called the Outcome and Assessment Information

Set (OASIS). It must be completed at the start of care, with each recertification (every 60 days), and at the termination of care.

- The Clinical Care Classification (CCC) system is a system of care and documentation used by most home-care agencies.
- Interventions to reduce caregiver strain include providing emotional support and arranging additional home and community services to support the client and caregiver.
- As a nurse delivering home care, you will need to follow standard precautions but recognize how infection control techniques may be modified to the home environment.
- In addition to infection control, nursing interventions usually include assisting with medication management, assessing and supporting home safety, and providing caregiver support.
- After a home visit you must document care, coordinate services for the client, and prepare for future visits.

Knowledge Map

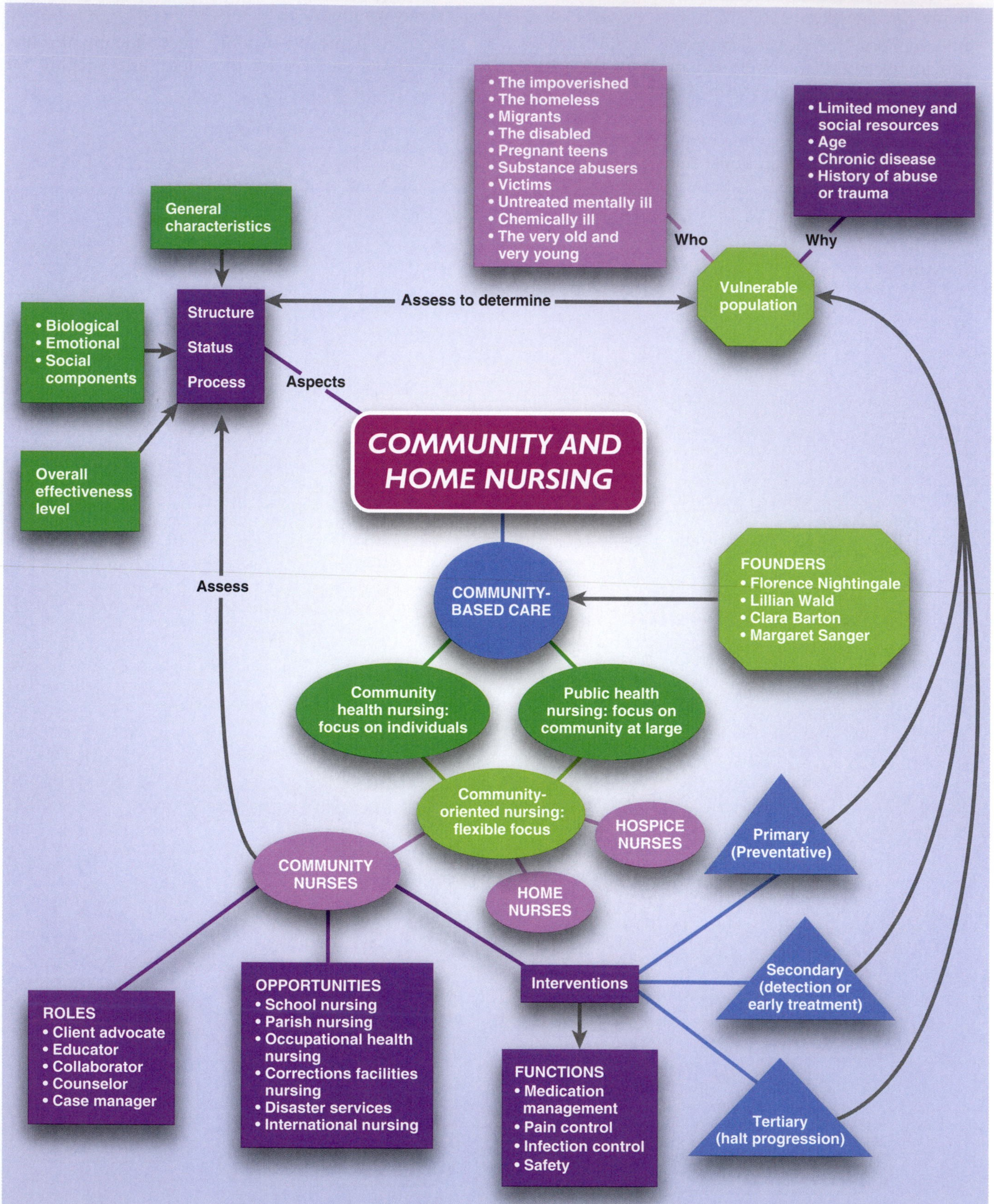

CHAPTER 44

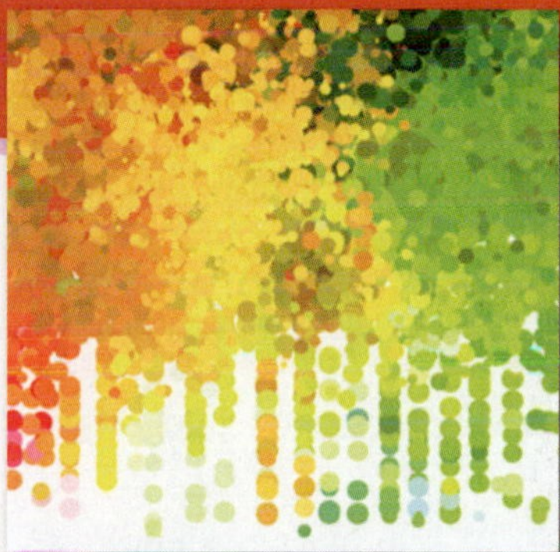

Ethics & Values

STUDENT RESOURCES

The questions and exercises in this book allow you to practice the kind of thinking you will use as a full-spectrum nurse. Critical-thinking questions usually have more than one right answer, so we do not provide "correct answers" for these features. Try to answer these questions yourself. It is more important to develop your nursing judgment than to just cover content. You will learn more by discussing the questions with your peers. If you are still unsure, see the Davis Advantage chapter resources for suggested responses.

To explore learning resources for this chapter,

Go to Davis Advantage and find:

Answers and Suggested Responses for all questions in this chapter

Concept Map

Knowledge Map

References and Bibliography

Lists of NOC Outcomes and NIC Interventions

Key Concepts

Morals

Nursing ethics

Values

Related Concepts

See the Concept Map on Davis Advantage

Example Problems

Moral distress

Whistleblowing

Caring for the Nguyens

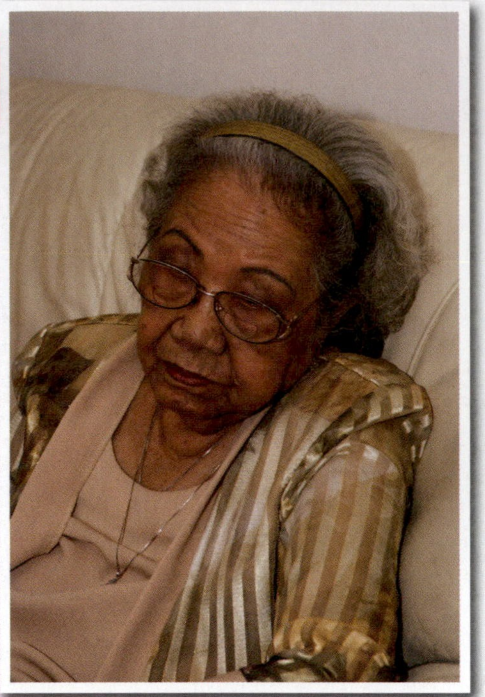

Mai Nguyen, Nam Nguyen's mother, has hypertension. She is forgetful about taking her medicines. Since her husband died, she has experienced periods of depression. When asked about her medicines she often replies, "It doesn't really matter since my husband died. If I die, what difference will it make?"

Mai Nguyen was scheduled to have lunch with friends but did not arrive. When her friends called the house, they got no answer. At the end of lunch, one of Mai's friends decided to call Nam to inform him of her concerns about his mother. Nam found his mother unresponsive on the kitchen floor. He called 911, and she was brought to the hospital by ambulance. At the hospital, the emergency department (ED) physician tells Nam that his mother has had a massive stroke (brain attack) brought on by uncontrolled hypertension. He asks Nam whether Mrs. Nguyen has an advance directive. She does not. The physician asks Nam to consider what level of care to offer his mother. He tells Nam that comprehensive treatment would include intubation, mechanical ventilation, and tube feeding support. The physician feels it is unlikely that she will experience significant recovery from this stroke.

Nam tells you, "I want everything done for my mother. I lost my father this year, and I'm not going to lose her, too." Yen, Nam's wife, reminds you that Mai has been depressed since her husband died and has expressed a desire to die. Because Nam and Yen are not in agreement about the course of action, no decision is communicated. Mai Nguyen's condition continues to deteriorate, and the ED physician feels he must intubate her, place her on a ventilator, and admit her to the ICU according to hospital protocol.

A. You are aware of Mai's statements and her poor compliance with treatment. What, if any, concerns do you have about this course of action?

B. Mai continues to decline. Nam is informed that the "only thing keeping your mother alive is the ventilator and IV medicines." Do you consider this heroic treatment?

C. How would you approach Mr. Nguyen to speak with him about how he is feeling?

D. Nam and Yen have asked to meet with the team providing care to Mai. They announce that they would like all the "heroic measures to end." They request that Mai be allowed to die. Could you participate in this care? With what actions would you be comfortable? With what actions would you be uncomfortable?

PracticalKnowledge clinical **application**

Practical knowledge in nursing ethics primarily involves communication and problem-solving skills. We have included one model of ethical decision making as well as guidelines for patient advocacy for your quick reference in clinical situations.

CLINICAL INSIGHTS

Clinical Insight 44-1 ➤ Using the MORAL Model for Ethical Decision Making

- **M-Massage the dilemma.** Identify and define the issues in the dilemma. Consider the options of all the major players in the dilemma and their value systems. This includes patients, family members, nurses, physicians, religious representatives, and other interdisciplinary healthcare members. Identify the information gaps.
- **O-Outline the options.** Examine all the options, including those that are less realistic and conflicting. This stage is designed only for considering options and not for making final decisions.
- **R-Resolve the dilemma.** Review issues and options, applying basic principles of ethics to each option. Decide the best option based on the views of all those concerned in the dilemma.
- **A-Act by applying the chosen option.** This step is usually the most difficult because it requires actual implementation, whereas the previous steps allow only for dialogue and discussion.
- **L-Look back and evaluate.** Reflect on the entire process and evaluate all steps, including the implementation. No process is complete without thorough evaluation. Ensure that those involved are able to follow through on the final option. If not, a second decision may be required, and the process must begin again at the first step.

Practice Resources

Badruddin, S. (2016); Yoder-Wise, P. (2019).

Clinical Insight 44-2 ➤ Guidelines for Advocacy

The following principles will help you to function effectively as an advocate.

- **Keep the ethical principle of patient autonomy always in mind.**
- **Know and document the facts** of the case.
- **Know the arguments** of those who oppose the patient. Use role playing to develop a strategy for responding to the arguments.
- **Have a sound base of support for your actions.** Be familiar with any policies or laws that apply.
- **Form a coalition of allies,** if you can. Get consultation. Communicate, inform, and clarify their collaborative roles.
- **Intervene high enough in the hierarchy** to get the job done. If the difficulty is with a provider or an organizational policy, merely going to the charge nurse will not be enough. You will need to communicate with nurse administrators or other agency administrators.
- **Demonstrate to the system** how it is defeating its own goals (e.g., for patient care).
- **Avoid getting into a power struggle** if possible (use the preceding steps first). If you must, decide how far you need to go and whether you are willing to go that far. You will need to enlist people with more power in the system than you have (e.g., family members, providers, administrators).
- **Be aware of client vulnerability.** When possible, avoid confrontation. If there is risk for the client (as in a power contest), be sure the client is aware of his risks and possible gains; then let him choose how far to take the situation.
- **Have alternative actions.** Assess risks realistically. Weigh them against potential gains.

CLINICALJUDGMENT

Applying the Full-Spectrum Nursing Model

PATIENT SITUATION

Read the following summary of the Kithari and Kirschner article:

Kothari, S., & Kirschner, K. (2006). Abandoning the Golden Rule: The problem with "putting ourselves in the patient's place." ***Topics in Stroke Rehabilitation, 13*****(4), 68–73.**

A large body of evidence documents the difficulties healthcare professionals have in predicting what their patient believes or wishes. These difficulties extend from the predictions of:

- Very specific patient wishes, such as for life-sustaining therapies
- More global assessments of patients' lives as a whole (e.g., their quality of life)

One explanation for this phenomenon is that healthcare professionals, either consciously or unconsciously, adopt "Golden Rule thinking." This refers to our attempts to understand another person's situation by imagining what we would believe or want under similar circumstances, in other words, "putting ourselves in the patient's place."

Although Golden Rule thinking would seem to be a promising strategy, studies show that it actually results in inaccurate presumptions of a patient's wishes or beliefs. These presumptions, in turn, have significant clinical and ethical implications. That is, they cause healthcare professionals and families to make decisions for the patient that are, in reality, *not* what the patient would want. The thinking goes:

I should put myself in the patient's place.
If I were the patient, I would want X.
Therefore, the patient probably wants X.
Because the patient probably wants X, we will do X.

This thinking process can have different results: (1) The patient really does want X, so you have met his needs. (2) The patient really wanted Y, so you did not meet his needs.

THINKING

1. *Theoretical Knowledge:* What is the Golden Rule, or what does it say?

2. *Critical Thinking (Inquiry):* What is one thing that could be done ahead of time to prevent the need for Golden Rule thinking? Explain why that would work.

DOING

3. *Nursing Process (Assessment):* If you do not know what the patient would want, instead of thinking what *you* would want, how might you get an idea of what the patient might want?

CARING

4. *Self-Knowledge:* What is your earliest memory of being taught the Golden Rule?

5. *Ethical Knowledge:* Which ethical principle does the Golden Rule seem to try to follow: autonomy, nonmaleficence/beneficence, fidelity, veracity, or justice?

Critical Thinking and Clinical Judgment

1. Some examples of ethical issues you may encounter are end-of-life issues, abortion or other reproductive issues, breaches of patient confidentiality, and incompetent or illegal practices of colleagues. Stop for a moment and think about a time when you have witnessed an ethical challenge in the clinical area.
   a. Describe the situation.
   b. How well equipped did you feel to handle the situation?
   c. What guided your thoughts and actions?

2. At the beginning of this chapter in Volume 1, Alan (Meet Your Patients), a teenager, had been injured in a soccer game. Without a blood transfusion, he may die, but because his family is of the Jehovah's Witnesses faith, Alan's parents have refused to sign permission for his transfusion. Taking each of the abilities required for ethical agency, state whether or not you think these people have the abilities listed below: Alan, Alan's parents, the physician, the nurse. Explain your thinking. An ethical agent must be able to:

   a. Perceive the difference between good and evil, right and wrong.

      Alan

      Parents

      Physician/surgeon

      Nurse

   b. Understand abstract ethical principles.

      Alan

      Parents

      Physician/surgeon

      Nurse

   c. Reason and apply ethical principles to make decisions, weigh alternatives, and plan ways to achieve goals.

      Alan

      Parents

      Physician/surgeon

      Nurse

   d. Decide and choose freely.

      Alan

      Parents

      Physician/surgeon

      Nurse

   e. Act according to his choice; this assumes both the power and the capability to act.

      Alan

      Parents

      Physician/surgeon

      Nurse

(continued)

3. Consider Alan's situation again. Analyze the situation (a) using a deontological framework and ethical principles and then (b) using a utilitarian framework. Focus on this question: Is it ethical to try hard to influence the parents to consent to allow a blood transfusion?
   a. Deontology
   b. Utilitarianism
   c. Did you reach a different conclusion depending on the framework you selected?

4. You are a busy nurse caring for a caseload of eight patients. One patient, Lily, is the mother of the hospital administrator. She had surgery 3 days ago and is progressing nicely, but she is very demanding and requires a great deal of assistance to be repositioned in bed and to move from bed to chair. She has frequent visitors, including children and young grandchildren. In the next room is a young Haitian woman whose bill is paid by Medicaid. She has a history of drug abuse and had surgery this morning. She speaks little English and seems very anxious. She is experiencing nausea and pain and needs a transfusion of a unit of packed red blood cells this evening. Her boyfriend is at the desk requesting to bring her 3-year-old daughter to the unit so that she may see her mother. The visiting policy says that children must be at least 12 years old to visit the unit. Consider what aspects of justice apply to this situation and how it might be most equitably handled. Focus on the principle of justice.

5. An example of the feminist ethical approach arises in deciding whether to allocate federal healthcare resources to younger people (e.g., education, day care, free immunizations) or to older adults (e.g., prescription drug insurance, long-term care). Feminist reasoning would be as follows:
   - In the United States, older women outnumber older men.
   - Older women tend to be poorer and are more likely to be alone than are men.
   - Therefore, if healthcare for older adults were to be rationed, it would negatively affect women more than it would men.
   - Thus, more healthcare resources should be allocated to older adults, especially women.

   a. Analyze this decision using a deontological framework. Explain your reasoning, as was done above.
   b. Analyze this decision using a consequentialist framework. Explain your reasoning.

6. Deception can take different forms, from intentional lying to nondisclosure of information or partial disclosure of information. Think about your duty to tell the truth. Is there ever a time when being completely honest is not the best nursing intervention? Do you consider withholding information the same as lying?

7. Review the following scenario. Examine your self-knowledge, and work through the steps of the values clarification process (choosing, prizing, and acting). A 40-year-old couple with no other children learn that their unborn child has Down syndrome. The couple needs to make a difficult decision because the mother is 18 weeks pregnant.
   a. How would you feel about this couple if they chose to have this child and insisted on doing everything possible to keep the baby alive even if it is born with severe handicaps?
   b. Do you think that your professional relationship with this couple would change if they chose to terminate the pregnancy?

c. How can you help the couple clarify their values?

(1) List alternatives.

(2) Examine the possible consequences of the alternative choices.

(3) Choose freely.

(4) Feel good about the choice that has been made.

(5) Affirm the choice to others.

(6) Act on the choice.

(7) Act with a consistent pattern.

What Are the Main Points in This Chapter?

- Ethics is a formal process for deciding right and wrong conduct in situations where issues of values and morals arise.
- *Nursing ethics* refers to ethical questions that arise out of nursing practice.
- Morals are learned and internalized throughout the life span. Carol Gilligan proposed that moral development and reasoning are different among men and women.
- Ethical agency is the ability to make ethical choices and to be responsible for one's ethical actions. In practice, nurses sometimes make moral decisions that they are not able to carry out.
- Moral distress is the inability to carry out moral decisions.
- Whistleblowing occurs when a person identifies in the workplace an incompetent, unethical, or illegal situation or actions of others, and then appeals to someone who may have the power to stop it.
- Nursing ethics problems arise from technological advances, the needs of a multicultural population, cost containment efforts in healthcare, the nature of nursing work, and the nature of the nursing profession.
- Nurses have complex obligations and multiple complex relationships within healthcare organizations (e.g., with employers, providers, patients, families, and other nurses).
- Ethical decisions are affected by a person's developmental stage, values, moral frameworks and principles, and professional guidelines.
- Attitudes are mental dispositions or feelings toward a person, object, or idea.
- A belief is something that one accepts as true.
- A value is a belief that you have about the worth of something; a value is highly prized and expressed through behaviors, feelings, and decisions.
- Values are transmitted through social interaction.
- Value neutrality means that we attempt to understand our own values regarding an issue and to know when to put them aside, if necessary, to become nonjudgmental.
- Six important ethical principles are autonomy, nonmaleficence, beneficence, fidelity, veracity, and justice.
- Consequentialist theories are ethical theories in which the rightness or wrongness of an action depends on the consequences of the act, rather than on the nature of the act itself.
- The principle of utility states that a "good" act is one that produces the greatest good for the greatest number of people.
- Deontological theories consider an action to be right or wrong independent of its consequences.
- Feminist ethics asserts that focusing on deontological principles distracts one from dealing with larger social issues and that objectivity is impossible.
- An ethics of care directs attention to a patient's specific situation viewed within the context of his or her life narrative. It emphasizes feelings, but not at the expense of some conventional ethical principles, such as autonomy, nonmaleficence, or beneficence.
- Nurses can obtain ethical guidance from professional codes of ethics, standards of practice, and the American Hospital Association's *Patient Care Partnership.*

(continued)

- The principle of autonomy underlies informed consent—clients' right to decide for themselves whether or not they will agree to a proposed procedure or treatment.
- Specific ethical issues the nurse is likely to encounter may involve AIDS, abortion, allocation of resources, issues of confidentiality, end-of-life issues (e.g., advance directives, DNAR/AND prescriptions, life-sustaining treatments, informed consent, organ transplantation), and reproductive technologies.
- A value is a belief you have about the worth of something; it serves as a principle or a standard that influences your decision making.
- Values clarification is the process of becoming conscious of and naming one's values. Nurses can assist clients with values clarification.
- Not all moral problems are dilemmas. A dilemma is a particular kind of moral problem: It is a painful situation in which a choice must be made between two equally undesirable actions. There is no clearly right or wrong option.
- One method of working through an ethical problem is to perform assessment and diagnosis, as in the nursing process; then use the mnemonic MORAL: **M**assage the dilemma, **O**utline the options, **R**esolve the dilemma, **A**ct by applying the chosen option, and **L**ook back and evaluate.
- A good compromise preserves the integrity of all parties when there is disagreement among them in a moral situation.
- Nurses should be patient advocates because (1) their professional role requires it, (2) they have special knowledge that the patient does not have, (3) they have a special relationship with patients, and (4) one aspect of the nursing role is to defend patient's autonomous decisions.
- The nurse's role as an advocate is to inform, support, and communicate.

Knowledge Map

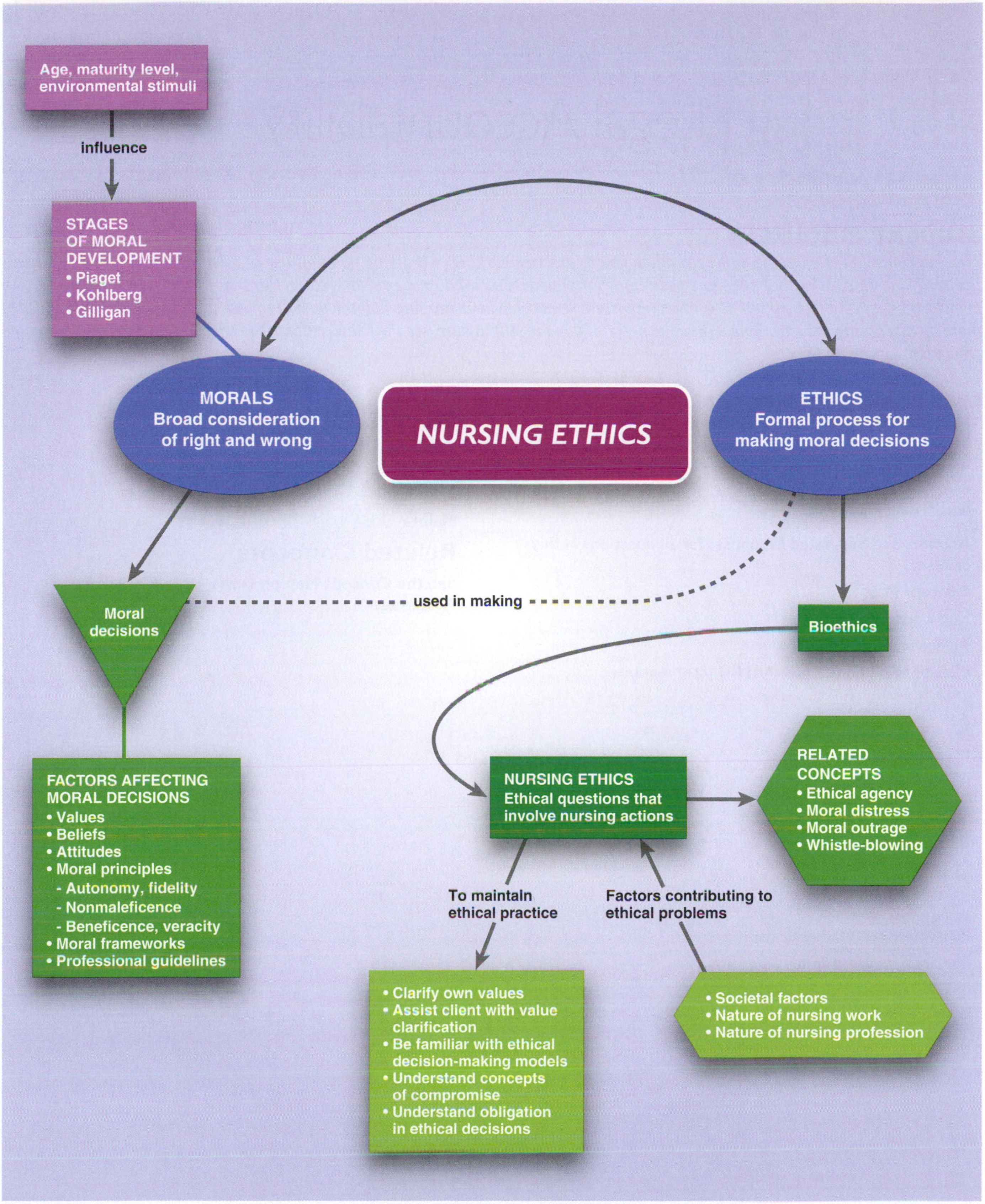

CHAPTER 45

Legal Accountability

STUDENT RESOURCES

The questions and exercises in this book allow you to practice the kind of thinking you will use as a full-spectrum nurse. Critical-thinking questions usually have more than one right answer, so we do not provide "correct answers" for these features. Try to answer these questions yourself. It is more important to develop your nursing judgment than to just cover content. You will learn more by discussing the questions with your peers. If you are still unsure, see the Davis Advantage chapter resources for suggested responses.

To explore learning resources for this chapter,

Go to Davis Advantage and find:

Answers and Suggested Responses for all questions in this chapter

Concept Map

Knowledge Map

References and Bibliography

Lists of NOC Outcomes and NIC Interventions

Key Concepts

Law

Liability

Malpractice

Related Concepts

See the Concept Map on Davis Advantage

Caring for the Nguyens

Nam and Yen Nguyen have requested an appointment with you, the nurse at the Family Medicine Clinic, to discuss advance directives. Their experience with Nam's mother, Mai, has created concerns about end-of-life care.

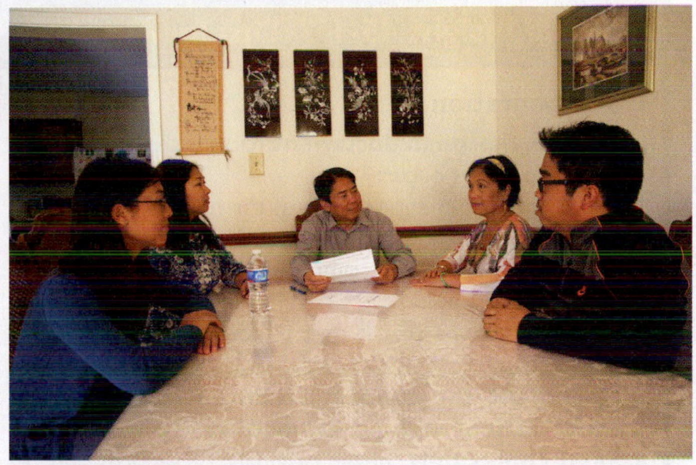

A. Nam asks you, "Do you think it's appropriate to create an advance directive at my age?" How would you respond?

B. Nam tells you that he believes in "natural death." He states, "I don't want extraordinary measures, and I never want to be resuscitated." Yen responds that she is extremely uncomfortable with blanket statements about treatment. "If he got hit by a car or had some accident, I would want you to do everything in your power to treat him. I couldn't carry out his wishes," she states. What actions should you take to help Nam and Yen resolve this discrepancy?

PracticalKnowledge clinical application

CLINICAL INSIGHTS

Clinical Insight 45-1 ➤ Tips for Avoiding Malpractice

Client Relationships

- **Develop open, honest, respectful, and caring relationships** with patients and families. Patients are less likely to sue if they feel that you were caring and professional.
- **Maintain client privacy and confidentiality.**
- **Recognize "problem" clients.** Try to identify the basic problem or complaint and intervene to resolve it. Angry clients who feel mistreated are more likely to bring a malpractice lawsuit.

Professional Interactions

- **Don't blame or criticize other healthcare providers** in the presence of clients (e.g., "Sorry you didn't get your pain medication. The night shift was a little short-staffed last night").
- **Don't make statements that may appear to be an admission of guilt** (e.g., "Oh my gosh, I forgot to shut off that IV!"). Errors should not be included on the client's health record, but instead recorded in an incident report.

Client Assessments

- **Perform timely assessments and recognize significant assessment cues;** notify primary care providers of changes in the client's condition or client complaints.
- **Recognize significant assessment cues** and notify primary care providers of changes in the client's condition or client complaints.
- **Use the proper chain of command** to ensure appropriate and timely care when the primary healthcare provider is not available.
- **Perform falls risk assessments,** document, and take measures to ensure client safety. Falls are a common cause of client injury.

(Continued)

Clinical Insight 45-1 ➤ Tips for Avoiding Malpractice—cont'd

Documentation

- **Careful, thorough documentation** is the best defense if a lawsuit does occur:
  - Use and document all steps of the nursing process.
  - Be especially thorough when documenting care for patients who will not comply with treatments or who complain a lot.
  - Courts assume that if care is not documented, it was not given.
- **Document the time and content of telephone conversations with other healthcare providers.**
- **Send copies only,** never originals, of records and reports requested by other professionals.

Competent Practice

- **Know and follow applicable laws:** (1) federal and state laws, (2) your state's nurse practice act (perform only the activities within your scope of practice and competence).
- **Know and follow agency policies and procedures.**
- **Know and follow standards of care** set forth in the state nurse practice act, by professional organizations, in professional literature, by agency policy, and so on.
- **Stay competent in your area of practice;** for example, attend continuing education, webinars, and in-service programs to improve your knowledge and skills.
- **Don't accept a clinical assignment that you think you are not competent to perform.** Evaluate your assignment with your supervisor if there is a question.

Medication Administration

- **Follow the "rights" of medication administration** (see Chapter 26).
- **Follow medical prescriptions,** but clarify them as needed. Do not implement a questionable prescription or one you do not understand.

Practice Resources

Brown, G. (2016); Fall Documentation and Injury Prevention. (2018); Singh, T. & Singh, N. (2016).

Clinical Insight 45-2 ➤ Using Equipment Safely

The following will help you to ensure proper and safe use of equipment:

1. Obtain appropriate training on equipment use.
2. Follow the healthcare agency's protocols, policies, and procedures on the use of the equipment.
3. Follow the manufacturer's operating instructions.
4. Be sure medical equipment has been properly inspected.
5. Perform safety checks regularly and before each use.
6. Position and use equipment properly during treatment.
7. Know how the equipment functions; be alert to signs that it is not working properly.
8. Make sure rooms are not cluttered with equipment.
9. Follow agency policies regarding equipment brought from the client's home (e.g., hair dryers, electric shavers, radios); usually these should be inspected for proper grounding and safe cords.
10. Remove and label equipment that is malfunctioning to prevent others from using it until it can be repaired or replaced.

Practice Resources

Mattox, E. (2012); Watson, E. (2014).

Clinical Insight 45-3 ➤ Guidelines for Documenting Care

To be accurate and complete, your reporting and documentation of client care must address the following:

1. Client status (e.g., symptoms and responses to treatments)
2. The nursing care given
3. Providers' prescriptions
4. Medications and treatments
5. Client responses
6. Consultations with other members of the healthcare team regarding client status

You might find the 5 Cs mnemonic helpful for documenting care. Documentation should be:

Complete
Clear
Correct
Comprehensive
Chronological

Practice Resources

Brown, G. (2016); Malpractice outcome could hinge on what ED nurses documented. (2017); Watson, E. (2014).

CLINICALJUDGMENT

Applying the Full-Spectrum Nursing Model

PATIENT SITUATION

A nurse employed by a temporary agency is assigned to a neurology unit for a 12-hour shift. On arrival, she discovers that the registered nurse (RN) assigned for the shift called in sick, leaving her with two unlicensed assistive personnel (UAPs) to provide client care and administer medication, including controlled substances. The nursing supervisor informs her that she will be responsible for the unit with 22 clients, 12 of whom are acutely ill and require close observation and frequent care. The nursing supervisor is not available to work on the unit and has no additional RNs to provide client care. The nurse decides not to accept the assignment, to report the decision and reasons to her agency supervisor, and to leave the neurology unit immediately before starting the shift.

THINKING

1. *Theoretical Knowledge:*
   a. In addition to protecting her nursing license, what other factors should the nurse have considered in deciding whether to stay on or leave the unit?
   b. Because the nurse decided not to accept the assignment, would this have been considered abandonment?
   c. What standards, guidelines, and laws would apply to determine whether the nurse's behavior was in accordance with standards of practice?
2. *Critical Thinking (Contextual Awareness):*
   a. Which statements in the ANA Nurses' Bill of Rights should the nurse have considered before deciding whether to accept the assignment?
   b. What factors in this situation could create legal problems for the nurse?

DOING

3. *Nursing Process (Planning/Intervention):* The nurse's action (leaving the unit) might be viewed, under some laws in some situations, as abandonment of clients. What are some alternative actions the nurse might have taken to avoid that risk?

CARING

4. *Self-Knowledge:* Have you ever been in a situation in which you felt a moral obligation to help, yet knew you would be in over your head? Describe your experience.
5. *Ethical Knowledge:* In your opinion, did the nurse do the right thing when she decided not to accept the assignment and to leave the nursing unit immediately? Explain your thinking.

Critical Thinking and Clinical Judgment

1. Think about the Meet Your Nurse Role Model scenario you read at the beginning of the chapter in Volume 1. A nurse with 3 years of experience on a medical-surgical unit arrives to work and discovers that two of her colleagues called in sick, including the charge nurse. The nursing supervisor informs her that she will need to assume the charge nurse role, in addition to assuming care for three clients. Feeling frustrated, the nurse ponders whether she should just quit and find another job, but then decides to accept the assignment. Two hours into the shift, one of her clients begins to experience complications, requiring blood glucose checks every 2 hours and frequent monitoring. In addition, one of the nurses becomes ill and is replaced by a float nurse from the labor and delivery unit, who spends her time continuously texting on her cell phone. The nurse contacts the nursing supervisor and requests additional assistance but is told no other nurse is available and that the supervisor is involved with an emergency situation on another unit. The nurse begins to analyze this situation from a legal perspective to determine the best course of action.

Use the critical-thinking model to identify questions to ask yourself in reflecting and deciding what to do.

Go to Chapter 2, **Box 2-2: Critical-Thinking Model,** in Volume I.

a. What questions do you need to ask about context?

b. What knowledge do you need to make an informed and credible decision?

c. What questions do you need to ask when considering alternatives?

d. What questions do you need to ask about analyzing your assumptions?

e. What questions do you need to ask about reflecting and deciding?

2. Analyze this passage:
Nursys is the national database for verification of nurse licensure and contains information on disciplinary information for RNs and LVN/LPNs. The e-Notify feature of Nursys provides free real-time information to employers about their nurse employees (https://www.nursys.com/)
   - Do you think there is a need for Nursys?
   - What rights does it help protect?

3. Imagine that you are working in a large medical center in an area where there have been several robberies and assaults in the past 6 months, mostly late at night. Although the parking lot is nearly a block from the employees' exit and is not well lit, there is only one security guard on duty outside the hospital after 2200. Despite repeated requests from employees all the way up the chain of command, no efforts are being made to improve lighting or to hire more security guards. What standards and laws might be helpful to the employees?

4. George Agnew, 75 years old, is admitted to the emergency department after being involved in a serious car accident. His wife is with him, and she is very upset—to the point of being hysterical. It is likely that Mr. Agnew will die, but providers are considering whether he will need a ventilator in the next hour or so. You need to know Mr. Agnew's wishes on this issue, but he is not conscious. The charge nurse tells you not to ask Mrs. Agnew because it will just upset her more.

   a. What is happening in the situation that may influence the outcome?

   b. What factors may influence your behavior and the behavior of others in this situation?

   c. What values or biases do you have that influence your behavior in this situation?

   d. Where might you get the information you need instead of asking Mrs. Agnew?

   e. What would you do? What legal support, if any, do you have?

5. Compare and contrast the following definitions of practical nursing and professional nursing taken from the Nurse Practice Act in Missouri and then discuss the differences in the scope of practice for the LPN/LVN and the RN. Identify two tasks/responsibilities that only the RN can perform.
   DEFINITION 1. Practical nursing is the performance for compensation of selected acts for the promotion of health and in the care of persons who are ill, injured, or experiencing alterations in normal health processes. Such performance requires substantial specialized skill, judgment, and knowledge. All such nursing care shall be given under the direction of a person licensed by a state regulatory board to prescribe medications and treatments or under the direction of a registered professional nurse. For the purposes of this chapter, the term "direction" shall mean guidance or supervision provided by a person licensed by a state regulatory board to prescribe medications and treatments or a registered professional nurse, including, but not limited to, oral, written, or otherwise communicated orders or directives for patient care. When

practical nursing care is delivered pursuant to the direction of a person licensed by a state regulatory board to prescribe medications and treatments or under the direction of a registered professional nurse, such care may be delivered by a licensed practical nurse without direct physical oversight.

DEFINITION 2. Professional nursing is the performance for compensation of any act which requires substantial specialized education, judgment, and skill based on knowledge and application of principles derived from the biological, physical, social and nursing sciences, including, but not limited to:

a. Responsibility for the teaching of health care and the prevention of illness to the patient and his or her family;

b. Assessment, nursing diagnosis, nursing care, and counsel of persons who are ill, injured, or experiencing alterations in normal health processes;

c. The administration of medications and treatments as prescribed by a person licensed by a state regulatory board to prescribe medications and treatments;

d. The coordination and assistance in the delivery of a plan of health care with all members of a health team;

e. The teaching and supervision of other persons in the performance of any of the foregoing. (Missouri Revised Statutes, 2013)

6. The patient was an older adult with various medical conditions and receiving multiple medications. The nurse determined the patient was a high fall risk, 8 on a scale of 0 to 10. The nurse decided to initiate the hospital's fall prevention plan, which meant raising the siderails and placing restraints on the patient without a provider's prescription. Hospital policy, however, did require a nurse who initiated restraints on a patient for fall prevention to notify a provider within 1 hour after doing so.

   The next day another nurse, seeing that no prescriptions for restraints had been received, removed the restraints. The patient was getting up out of bed on his own. His nursing neurological assessment showed signs of dementia and confusion. His oxygen saturation was low, and his heartbeat was irregular. The provider was notified by phone but declined to prescribe restraints. Later that evening the patient was found on the floor with a closed-head injury. He was transferred to a university hospital, where he died a few weeks later. The case was dismissed against the hospital (Sturgill v. Ashe Memorial Hosp., 2008).

   a. In this case, the nurse was caring for a patient at high risk for fall but did not have a prescription to use restraints. Why do you think the court dismissed the case against the hospital?

   b. What other action might the nurse have taken to prevent this patient's fall?

7. For each of the following concepts, use critical thinking to describe how or why it is important to nurses, patients, or legal issues. Note that these are *not* to be merely definitions.

   Civil law

   The U.S. Constitution Bill of Rights and the Patient Care Partnership

   The ANA Code of Ethics; the ANA Standards of Practice; and the ANA Nurses' Bill of Rights

   Patient advocacy

   Battery

   Vicarious liability

What Are the Main Points in This Chapter?

- The law is a binding practice, rule, or code of conduct that guides a community or society and is enforced by a controlling authority.
- Laws are primarily derived from four sources: (1) the Constitution, (2) statutes, (3) administrative bodies, and (4) the courts.
- The right of privacy comes from the Bill of Rights.
- A living will gives directions to others about a person's wishes regarding life-prolonging treatments if the person becomes unable to make those decisions; it must be prepared when the person is alert and oriented (competent).
- A durable power of attorney for healthcare identifies a person who will make healthcare decisions in the event the client is unable to do so.
- State laws affecting nursing practice include mandatory reporting laws, Good Samaritan laws, safe harbor laws, and nurse practice acts.
- The ANA Code of Ethics describes the standards of professional responsibility for nurses and provides insight into ethical and acceptable behavior.
- The ANA Nurses' Bill of Rights identifies the rights nurses should expect from their workplace and work environment that are necessary for sound professional practice.
- A primary function of the medical malpractice system is to encourage healthcare providers to adhere to standards of practice and perform their responsibilities in a competent manner.
- Standards of practice look to what a reasonable and prudent nurse would do in the same or similar situation.
- Nurse practice acts are established by state boards of nursing to govern the practice of nursing.
- In most states, nurses are obligated legally to report suspected or actual client abuse, impaired health professionals, and communicable diseases.
- State boards of nursing are empowered under the nurse practice act to approve prelicensure nursing education programs, determine the criteria for licensure, define the practice of nursing, and establish grounds for disciplinary actions against nurses.
- Criminal law deals with wrongs or offenses against society. Civil law deals with wrongs to individuals.
- Intentional torts include assault, battery, false imprisonment, fraud, and invasion of privacy.
- Quasi-intentional torts involve those actions that injure a person's reputation.
- Unintentional torts that involve healthcare professionals are negligence and malpractice.
- Negligence is a wrong committed against an individual by one who has failed to use ordinary care.
- Malpractice is negligence committed against an individual by a licensed professional involving a duty, breach of that duty, an injury, and damages.
- Litigation is the formal process whereby the legal issues, rights, and duties between the parties are heard and decided. The stages include (1) pleading and pretrial motions, (2) discovery, (3) alternative dispute resolution, (4) trial, and (5) appeal.
- Malpractice claims, in general, result from failure to maintain the standard of practice, including failure to assess, diagnose, plan, implement, and evaluate client responses to care.
- Nurses can help reduce their legal risks by developing open, honest, respectful, caring relationships with clients and families; observing standards of care; and accurate documentation.
- You may witness a client's signature on a consent form, but you are not legally responsible for explaining the treatments and options, nor are you responsible for evaluating whether the provider has adequately explained them.

Knowledge Map

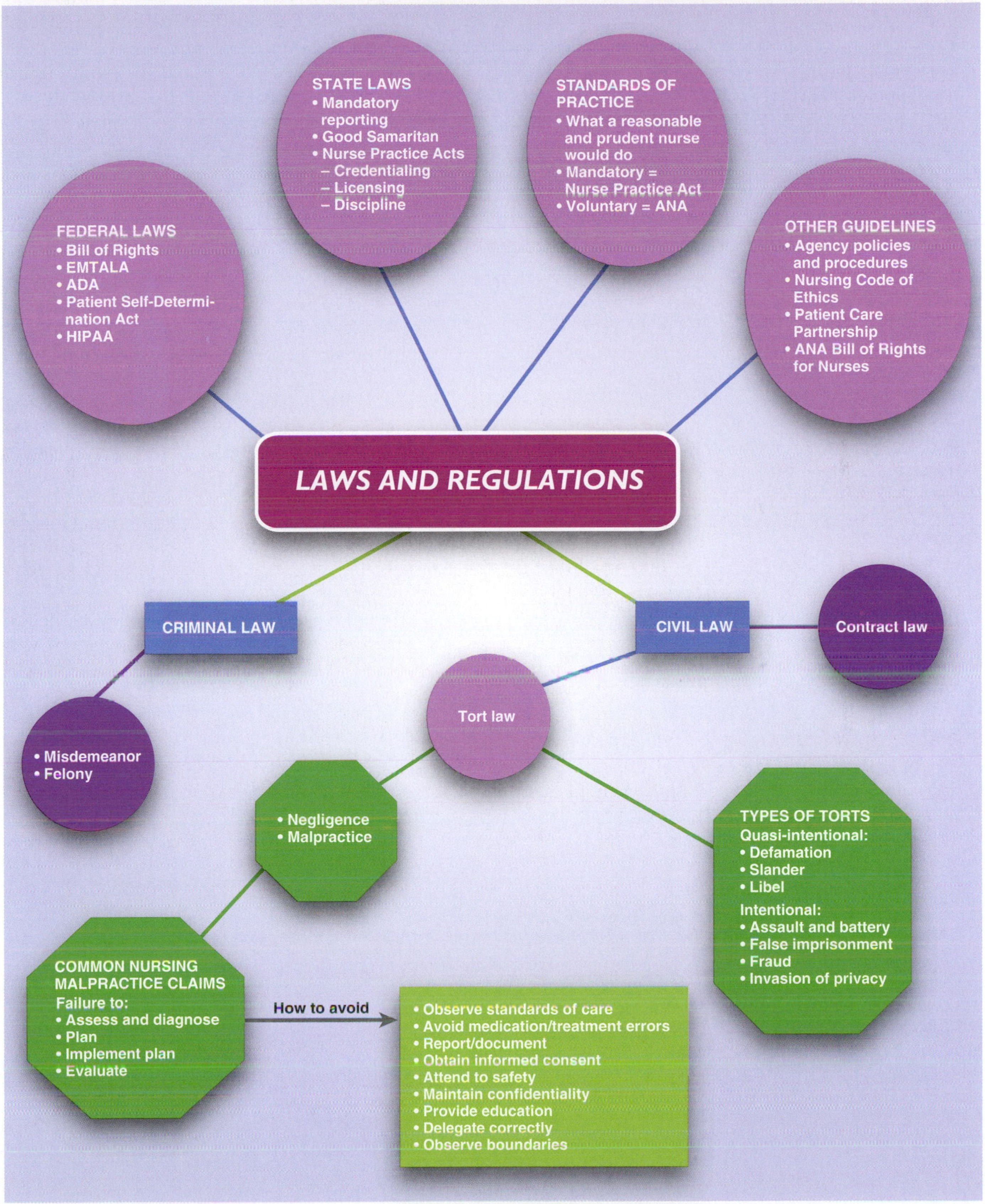
STATE LAWS
• Mandatory reporting
• Good Samaritan
• Nurse Practice Acts
– Credentialing
– Licensing
– Discipline
STANDARDS OF PRACTICE
• What a reasonable and prudent nurse would do
• Mandatory = Nurse Practice Act
• Voluntary = ANA
FEDERAL LAWS
• Bill of Rights
• EMTALA
• ADA
• Patient Self-Determination Act
• HIPAA
OTHER GUIDELINES
• Agency policies and procedures
• Nursing Code of Ethics
• Patient Care Partnership
• ANA Bill of Rights for Nurses
LAWS AND REGULATIONS
CRIMINAL LAW
CIVIL LAW
Contract law
Tort law
• Misdemeanor
• Felony
• Negligence
• Malpractice
TYPES OF TORTS
Quasi-intentional:
• Defamation
• Slander
• Libel
Intentional:
• Assault and battery
• False imprisonment
• Fraud
• Invasion of privacy
COMMON NURSING MALPRACTICE CLAIMS
Failure to:
• Assess and diagnose
• Plan
• Implement plan
• Evaluate
How to avoid
• Observe standards of care
• Avoid medication/treatment errors
• Report/document
• Obtain informed consent
• Attend to safety
• Maintain confidentiality
• Provide education
• Delegate correctly
• Observe boundaries

Credits

Note: Unless cited below, text credits appear within the text.

CHAPTER 11

Discharge Assessment/Instructions, Patient Education Form: Fisherman's Hospital, Marathon, FL. Used with permission.

CHAPTER 22

Procedure 22-2, Step 1, Skin Color Changes, Jaundice: From Chapman, L. (2009). *Core components of maternal nursing*. Philadelphia: F.A. Davis.

Procedure 22-2, Step 1a and b, Step 1, Skin Color Changes: Cyanosis and Vitiligo, Step 7, Step 7d, Herpes, Venous Star, Petechiae, and Ringworm; Procedure 22-3, Step 1, Alopecia Areata; Procedure 22-4, Step 3, Fungal Infection and Half-and-Half Nails; Procedure 22-5, Steps 2 and 4; Procedure 22-6, Steps 4a and b, 5a through f, Step 6e (2), Step 6j, Step 7, Step 8d [1 and 2], Step 8e [1 and 2]; Procedure 22-7, Step 1a [i through iii], Steps 1b, 3e, 5, 6 [a and c]; Procedure 22-8, Steps 5a and b; Procedure 22-10, Steps 2 and 3a; Procedure 22-12, Step 5c, Steps 6 [a through c], 7b, and 9; Procedure 22-13, Steps 1 [b and c], 2, 8, and8b; Procedure 22-14, Steps 5, 6, and 7 [c and d]; Procedure 22-14, Deep Palpitation (one-hand technique) and Bimanual Deep Palpation; Procedure 22-15, Steps 1 [c1 through d], 1c, Lordosis, Scoliosis, Kyphosis, 2b [1 through 7], Step 2b, Abnormal Gaits: Propulsive gait, Scissors gait, Spastic gait, Steppage gait, Waddling gait, 3 [a through b 2], 4a, 6c [1 and 2], 9; Procedure 22-15: Using a goniometer (image); Procedure 22-16, Steps 11c, 13a, 18a, 20, 21 22, 23, 24a through e, and 25; Procedure 22-17, Step 5 [a and c], 6, and 7 [1 and 2]; Procedure 22-18, Step 3 [a and d] and 4: From Dillon, P. M. (2016). *Nursing health assessment: The foundation of clinical practice* (3rd ed.). Philadelphia: F. A. Davis.

Procedure 22-2, Step 1, Skin Color Changes, Port-Wine Stain; Procedure 22-2, Step 7d, Capillary Hemangioma and Vesicles; Procedure 22-4, Step 3, Paronychia: From L. A. Goldsmith. (1997). *Adult and pediatric dermatology: A color guide to diagnosis and treatment*. Philadelphia: F. A. Davis.

Clinical Insight 22-1 [a and b]; Clinical Insight 22-3 [1 through 3b]; Procedure 22-1, Various types of thermometers; Procedure 22-8, Step 4d; Procedure 22-2, Describing Skin Lesions; Procedure 22-9, Step 2b [1 and 2]; Procedure 22-11, Step 4a through c; Procedure 22-15, Step 8 [1 through 13]: From Dillon, P. M. (2003). *Nursing health assessment: A critical thinking case studies approach*. Philadelphia: F.A. Davis.

Procedure 22-3, Step 1, Pediculosis; Procedure 22-5, Step 2, Bell's Palsy; Procedure 22-6, Steps 6b, Hordeolum, Step 6e, Pterygium and Subconjunctival Hemorrhage, and Step 8e(2): Courtesy of Wills Eye Hospital, Philadelphia.

Procedure 22-5, Step 2, Cushing's Syndrome; Procedure 22-9, Step 4, Black Hairy Tongue; Procedure 22-15, Step 7, Degenerative Joint Disease and Rheumatoid Arthritis; Procedure 22-17, Step 3d, Abnormalities: Male Genitourinary System, Syphilitic Chancre and Genital Warts: Courtesy MCP-Hahnemann University Department of Dermatology, Philadelphia.

Procedure 22-6, Step 3b, Procedure 22-12, Step 2b: From Scanlon, V. C. (2019). *Essentials of anatomy and physiology* (8th. ed.). Philadelphia, PA: F. A. Davis.

Procedure 22-7, Step 3e, Otitis Media and Perforated TM: Courtesy of Welch Allyn, Skaneateles Falls, NY.

Procedure 22-7, Step 3e, Normal TM, left ear: Courtesy of Ann Marie Ramsey, RN, MSN, CPNP.

Procedure 22-9, Step 3: Courtesy Robert A. Levine, DDS, and Sheryl Radin, DDS.

Procedure 22-9, Step 4, Red beefy tongue: From Custom Medical Stock Photo, Inc. Chicago, IL.

Procedure 22-9, Step 4, Geographic tongue, Leukoplakia, and Cancer of the tongue: Courtesy of Tina S. Liang, DMD.

CHAPTER 23

Procedure 23-1B, Step 3: © iStockphoto

Procedure 23-2, Step 1e: Courtesy of Moldex-Metric, Inc., Culver City, CA, www.moldex.com

CHAPTER 24

Procedure 24-1, Step 1: Infrared-Beam Detector, Cord-Activated Sensor: Courtesy of Smart Caregiver Corporation.

CHAPTER 25

Procedure 25-9, Step 10: Courtesy of EZ Access, Auburn, WA.

CHAPTER 26

Procedure 26-10, Equipment 1: Courtesy of Edward Lin, MD, Ingenious Technologies Corporation. Training video link: http://ingenious.com/NS/ns.htm

Procedure 26-17A, Step 7: Dr. Brian Oxhorn, Roseman University, Henderson, NV. Used with permission.

CHAPTER 27

Clinical Insight 27-1 a and b: From Lutz, C., Mazur, E., & Litch, N. (2019). *Nutrition and diet therapy* (7th ed.). Philadelphia, PA: F. A. Davis.

Procedure 27-2, Step 11: From Scanlon, V. C. (2019). *Essentials of anatomy and physiology* (8th ed.). Philadelphia, PA: F. A. Davis.

Procedure 27-2, Step 20g: Courtesy Dale Medical Products, Plainville, MA.

Procedure 27-3A, Step 5h: Nestle Healthcare Nutrition Inc.

Procedure 27-5, Equipment: Permission for use granted by Cook Medical Incorporated, Bloomington, IN.

CHAPTER 28

Guidelines for Physical Assessment for Urinary Elimination: From Dillon, P. M. (2016). *Nursing health assessment: The foundation of clinical practice* (3rd ed.). Philadelphia: F. A. Davis.

CHAPTER 29

Procedure 29-6, Equipment: From Williams, L., & Hopper, P. (2019). *Understanding medical surgical nursing* (6th ed.). Philadelphia: F. A. Davis.

Procedure 29-8, Equipment, and Procedure 29-8B, Steps 8 and 11: Courtesy of Hollister Incorporated, Libertyville, IL.

CHAPTER 35

Procedure 35-6A, Steps 2, 8, 9, and 15, and Procedure 35-6B, Step 9: From Rhoads, J., & Meeker, B. J. (2008). *Davis's guide to clinical nursing skills.* Philadelphia: F. A. Davis.

Braden Scale for Predicting Pressure Ulcer Score Risk: Copyright © Barbara Braden and Nancy Bergstrom, 1988. Reprinted with permission.

Norton Scale for Assessing Risk of Pressure Ulcers: Copyright © D. Norton, R. McLaren, & A. N. Exton-Smith. 1975. Reprinted with permission.

The PUSH Tool for Evaluation of Pressure Ulcers: Copyright © D. National Pressure Ulcer Advisory Panel (NPUAP) 1998 Reprinted with permission.

CHAPTER 38

Procedure 38-1, Steps 17 and 20: From J. Rhoads & B. J. Meeker. (2008). *Davis's guide to clinical nursing skills.* Philadelphia: F.A. Davis.

CHAPTER 39

Procedure 39-4, Equipment 1: Courtesy of Allied Healthcare Products, St. Louis, MO.

INDEX

Note: References are to volume and page number(s). Page numbers followed by *f* refer to figures; page numbers followed by *t* refer to tables; page numbers followed by *b* refer to boxes; page numbers followed by *p* refer to procedures; page numbers followed by "e" refer to bonus chapter content available in eBook on Davis Advantage.

A

C

D

E

G

I

J

K

L

N

P

Q

R

U

V

W

X

Y

Z

MODEL OF FULL-SPECTRUM NURSING

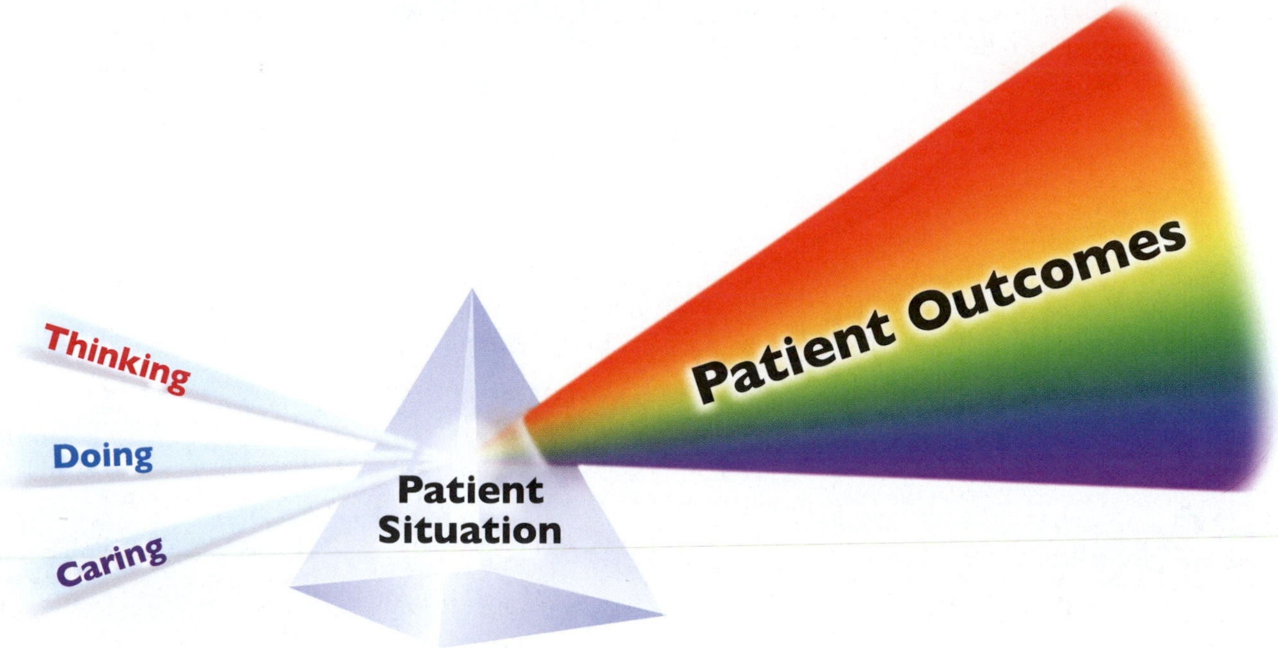

This illustration depicts the full-spectrum model of nursing used throughout this learning package. A full-spectrum nurse uses critical thinking and the nursing process to apply various types of knowledge (theoretical, practical, ethical, and self-knowledge) to the patient situation to bring about desired health outcomes. Truly, thinking and doing.